Whitcup and Nussenblatt's

UVEITIS

Fifth Edition

Whitcup and Nussenblatt's

UVEITIS

Fundamentals and Clinical Practice

SCOTT M. WHITCUP, MD
Department of Ophthalmology
David Geffen School of Medicine at UCLA
UCLA Stein Eye Institute
Los Angeles, CA, USA
Founder and CEO
Akrivista and Whitecap Biosciences
Irvine, CA, USA

H. NIDA SEN, MD, MHSc
Lasker Clinical Research Scholar
Director, Uveitis Clinic and Fellowship Program
Head, Clinical and Translational Immunology Unit
National Eye Institute
Bethesda, MD, USA;
Professor
George Washington University School of Medicine
Washington, DC, USA

Contributor

ALAN PALESTINE, MD
Professor, School of Medicine
Chief, Uveitis and Ocular Immunology Section
Director of Resident Research
University of Colorado School of Medicine
Denver, CO, USA

ELSEVIER London New York Oxford Philadelphia St Louis Sydney 2022

First edition 1989
Second edition 1996
Third edition 2004
Fourth edition 2010

Library of Congress Control Number: 2020952350

ISBN: 9780323480147

Content Strategist: Kayla Wolfe
Content Development Specialist: Louise Cook
Project Manager: Julie Taylor
Design: Patrick Ferguson
Illustration Manager: Narayanan Ramakrishnan
Marketing Manager: Kate Bresnahan

Printed in India

Last digit is the print number: 9 8 7 6 5 4 3 2 1

CONTENTS

FOREWORD

Our knowledge of basic immunology, the human immune response, and how to either augment or inhibit this response has exploded over the last decade. These advances have led to changes in the way we assess and treat patients with uveitis. In addition to furthering our understanding of the pathogenesis of a large number of uveitis conditions, we have been challenged with new infectious causes of uveitis diseases caused by viruses including the Zika virus, Ebola virus, and West Nile virus. Finally, advances in diagnostic testing and imaging have changed the way we diagnose uveitis and monitor our patients' response to therapy. It is the perfect time for a new edition of *Whitcup and Nussenblatt's Uveitis: Fundamentals and Clinical Practice.* I was very happy to see Dr. Whitcup take on the leadership role for the new 5th edition, and for ensuring that this important book continues to be available to clinicians around the world.

This textbook remains the go-to guide for diagnosing and managing patients with uveitis. It is both comprehensive, covering all the key topics related to uveitis, but also practical, readable, and useful to both ophthalmologists and other clinicians managing patients with inflammatory eye diseases. I have known and worked closely with both Dr. Whitcup and Dr. Nussenblatt for over 40 years, and spent time seeing patients with both of them for many years. Their organized and thoughtful approach to diagnosing, treating, and managing patients with uveitis is clearly elucidated in this book. Although Dr. Nussenblatt was not involved with this edition of the book, having passed away suddenly in 2016, his imprint on the book continues.

Part 1 of the book provides an overview of the basic science of ocular immunology with specifics on the role of the immune response on disease pathogenesis. It also discusses advances in our understanding of ocular inflammation and how these advances have led to novel therapies for autoimmune and inflammatory disease.

Part 2 of the book concentrates on the diagnosis of uveitis. As expected, the section discusses advances in testing such as the use of polymerase chain reaction (PCR) in diagnosing infectious causes of uveitis. However, an important part of this section is a practical approach to diagnosis by detailing tips on obtaining the medical history, examining the uveitis patient, and developing a differential diagnosis. We as clinicians tend to overlook the benefits and pitfalls of diagnostic testing, and this is beautifully discussed in the chapter on diagnostic testing. Finally, a new chapter on the use of optical coherence tomography (OCT) in uveitis has been added in this edition.

Part 3 of the book concentrates on the treatment of uveitis: both medical and surgical. What is useful in this section is that in addition to the multitude of new immunotherapies, the book also supplies a philosophy and approach to treatment decisions in patients with uveitis.

Part 4 focuses on infectious causes of uveitis. It covers the usual suspects in uveitis like syphilis and tuberculosis (TB), with up to date information on diagnostic tests and antimicrobial therapy. It also covers new infectious causes of uveitis like Ebola and Zika.

The last section of the book, Part 5, covers noninfectious causes of uveitis, more specifically, those not caused by an active acute infection. In addition, the section includes chapters on anterior uveitis, scleritis, and the masquerade syndromes.

I met Bob Nussenblatt at the ARVO meeting in 1976 and for over four decades was able to follow his academic and scientific career as he flourished at the National Eye Institute and developed an international reputation as a model for the clinician-scientist. One of his many qualities was his ability to identify and nurture colleagues both nationally and internationally, forming other great leaders in the field of uveitis. This book is part of Bob's legacy. Bob and Scott Whitcup had similar backgrounds, both completing residencies in internal medicine in addition to ophthalmology. This solid knowledge of medicine, ophthalmology, and basic science contribute to the strong foundation of the book. Importantly, their high ethical standards, always placing the patient first, gives the book a unique tone and perspective. Two giants working together under a friendship and professional partnership for decades also comes through in reading the book. In spite of working at one of the most advanced technological medical centers in the world, Bob never lost his special and humble way of interacting with patients and colleagues in a friendly way. That was Bob. I am sure he would continue to be proud of Scott, Nida, and Alan and the latest edition of the book. This edition under the leadership of Scott will continue to help ophthalmologists practice their best medicine, exactly as Bob did his whole life.

I was happy to hear that Dr. Nida Sen had become involved with this edition of the book. Nida is an outstanding clinician-scientist and heads the uveitis program at the National Eye Institute. I was also pleased to see that Alan Palestine has contributed several chapters to the book. As with Dr. Whitcup, Dr. Palestine spent time at the National Eye Institute and has been a major contributor to the uveitis literature for several decades. In summary, *Whitcup and Nussenblatt's Uveitis* is both an authoritative review of the subject with a practical approach that clinicians will find useful. It is a book that I and others frequently pull off the shelf and that improves the care of our patients.

Rubens Belfort Jr, MD, PhD, MBA
Vision Institute, Federal University of Sao Paulo, Brazil
President, National Academy of Medicine, Brazil
2020

PREFACE TO THE FIFTH EDITION

Over the past decade there has been a scientific explosion in both interest and research in immunology and the role it plays in disease. Not only have we learned more about how the immune system leads to disease pathogenesis, but we have also advanced our understanding on how modulating the immune response can lead to meaningful improvements in therapeutic outcomes. This research on downregulating the immune response has led to the development of new immunomodulatory agents that block the immune system at different sites of action including T cells, B cells, and cytokines. These new therapies provide clinicians with a number of additional therapeutic options for treating a host of immune-mediated inflammatory diseases including uveitis.

However, from an immunologic perspective, the last 10 years of research are likely to be remembered as the decade of cancer immunotherapy. Data now show that augmenting the existing antitumor immune responses results in the most significant clinical responses and the best opportunities for long-term disease remission and cure. These immunotherapies include the checkpoint inhibitors and chimeric antigen receptor T-cell therapy (CAR-T). But how do these new immunotherapies relate to uveitis? First, uveitis has occurred as an adverse effect of some immunotherapies. For example, both anterior and posterior uveitis have been reported in patients treated with checkpoint inhibitors. These observations provide further insight into the immune mechanisms of ocular inflammatory disease and identify novel potential therapeutic targets for uveitis. Second, it is interesting that this new-found success in cancer therapy is based on enhancing the body's own anticancer immune response. This is analogous to advances in treating autoimmune and inflammatory diseases. Despite development of new immunosuppressive drugs like methotrexate and cyclosporine for inflammatory diseases, corticosteroids remain the mainstay of treatment for most forms of uveitis today. Hench and colleagues described the antirheumatic effects of the hormones released by the adrenal gland including adrenocorticotropic hormone (ACTH) in 1949 and corticosteroids were used to treat uveitis shortly thereafter. Similarly, recent advances in the treatment of autoimmune diseases have resulted not from the synthesis of new anti-inflammatory compounds, but by specifically modulating the patient's immune response, for example, with monoclonal antibodies against key proinflammatory cytokines like tumor necrosis factor (TNF)-alpha, IL-17, and IL-23.

It is clear that studies on the pathogenesis of uveitis have furthered our understanding of ocular immunology and provided novel targets for therapeutic interventions, but this science has been the foundation for examining the role of inflammation in other nonuveitis conditions including age-related macular degeneration (AMD) and diabetic retinopathy. AMD is the leading cause of central vision loss in developed countries and is a great example of how our understanding of ocular immunology has augmented our knowledge about diseases other than uveitis. Genetic data from genome wide association studies and rare variant analyses pointed to involvement of the complement system in AMD. Other studies have supported the role of inflammation in the development or severity of AMD including inflammasome activation and dysregulated para-inflammation. Para-inflammation was defined by Medzhitov as a low level of inflammation that can exist between basal homeostasis and a progressive and more active inflammatory response. These data have supported the development of immune strategies for the treatment of atrophic AMD, including drugs to block the complement system.

In addition to progress in our understanding of the immune response, there have been a number of other advances that have improved the treatment of uveitis. Prompt and accurate diagnosis of uveitis remain crucial to patient outcomes. There have been a couple of key technical advances that aid clinicians in the diagnosis of uveitis. Greater availability and accuracy of polymerase chain reaction (PCR) related tests for a number of infectious agents have improved our diagnosis of infectious uveitis, and these are discussed in the chapters that discuss viral, bacterial, and fungal causes of disease. Improvements in optical coherence tomography (OCT) have increased the utility of the instrument in characterizing inflammatory disease in the eye and in assessing the response to therapy.

There have also been changes in how we deliver drugs locally to the eye. The treatment of uveitis has always utilized local therapy of drugs to the eye. This started with topical corticosteroids for anterior uveitis in the 1950s followed by periocular corticosteroid injections for intermediate and posterior uveitis. Starting with the use of intravitreal injections of ganciclovir and foscarnet, uveitis specialists became aware of both the safety and efficacy of delivering drugs into the vitreous for treating CMV retinitis. Clinical trials of intravitreal injections of the anti-VEGF agents added to the safety and efficacy of this approach. Today, intravitreal injections of triamcinolone or sustained-release corticosteroid implants is increasing, while the use of periocular injections of corticosteroids is decreasing.

As with previous editions of *Uveitis: Fundamentals and Clinical Practice,* our goal remains the same: to provide a comprehensive text that provides both a practical and coherent approach to the diagnosis and treatment of the various forms of the disease. The book reviews the basic immunology of uveitis but focuses on the clinical aspects of the underlying science. We also hope that our book will be of value to clinicians and scientists outside of eye care, including internists, rheumatologists, and researchers in the field of inflammation.

The book is divided into five parts. The first part reviews the fundamentals of immunology and pathogenesis of ocular inflammatory disease. The second part focuses on diagnosis, including medical history, clinical examination, and diagnostic testing. A chapter on evidence-based medicine in uveitis is also included in this section. Part 3 reviews the principles of medical therapy for uveitis and details the commonly used drugs. A discussion of the role of surgery in the management of uveitis is also included in this part. The infectious causes of uveitis are included in the chapters in Part 4. These include bacterial, viral, fungal, and parasitic diseases. This section also includes a chapter on postsurgical causes of uveitis, because many of these are due to infection. Finally, the last section includes chapters on uveitis conditions that are predominantly caused by noninfectious etiologies: often autoimmune diseases or masquerade syndromes like cancer or toxicity. However, it is important to note that some of these conditions, like white dot syndromes, may have infectious causes.

There have been a number of important additions and updates to this edition of the book. Because of the increase in use of OCT in both the evaluation and management of the uveitis patient, a new chapter on OCT has been added (Chapter 6). With advances in our understanding of immunology and the development of a number of new medications for the treatment of uveitis, the chapters on fundamentals (Chapter 1) and medical therapy (Chapter 8) have been extensively updated. Chapters in the section on infectious causes of uveitis have also been extensively revised, incorporating information on new diagnostic testing such as PCR. Furthermore, there have been a number of new infectious causes of uveitis, like Ebola virus, and most recently severe acute respiratory syndrome coronavirus 2 (SARS-CoV-2), that have been added to this section. Importantly, we have added many new figures to better illustrate clinical features of uveitis and added new case histories where useful.

This edition of *Whitcup and Nussenblatt's Uveitis: Fundamentals and Clinical Practice* is the first I have written without my colleague and friend Bob Nussenblatt. Bob passed away in 2016. To those of us who know Bob, we have lost a friend who inspired us every day. The entire clinical immunology community has lost a great researcher, teacher, and clinician. Bob arrived at the National Institutes of Health (NIH) in 1977 as a clinical associate and held key leadership positions there, including chief of the National Eye Institute Laboratory of Immunology, Clinical Director, Scientific Director, Deputy Director for Intramural Research, and an NIH Distinguished Investigator. He was a mentor who loved teaching and a clinician-scientist who focused on the bench to bedside path every day. At its heart, the book stems from patient discussions with Bob at the National Eye Institute (NEI). My hope is that the heart of the book remains.

I would like to thank a number of people who are important to this edition of the book. First, I would like to thank the other two contributors to the book, Dr. H. Nida Sen and Dr. Alan Palestine. Nida is the director of the Uveitis Fellowship Program at the NEI and Professor at the George Washington University School of Medicine. She is an accomplished researcher and clinician and is an integral part to this fifth edition. It is also great to have Alan involved in this 5th edition of the book. Dr. Palestine is currently the Chief of the Uveitis and Ocular Immunology Section and Director of Resident Research at the University of Colorado School of Medicine. Alan was involved with the early editions of the book and brings a wealth of practical experience to some key chapters of this edition. I also want to thank Chi-Chao Chan, Igal Gery, and Rachel Caspi, whose knowledge, inquisitiveness, and insight contributed to the evolution of this textbook. As a friend and colleague, I greatly appreciate that Dr. Rubens Belfort has both contributed many clinical photographs and written the foreword to the book. This edition has a new chapter on the use of OCT in uveitis, and I thank Elias Reichel for contributing a number of OCTs for the chapter and reviewing the text. I also must thank the staff of the NEI, including the technicians and photographers. Most importantly, I would like to thank our patients who have participated in clinical research and valued the opportunity to contribute to our understanding of uveitis in an attempt to help others.

Finally, I would like to thank family and friends for their support of this latest edition and again to Bob for his continued inspiration.

Scott M. Whitcup, MD

ACKNOWLEDGMENTS

We would like to thank our colleagues for their input over the years and for supplying many of the outstanding images that help bring our text to life. We especially want to thank Igal Gery and Chi-Chao Chan for their assistance with the basic science of the book, Elias Reichel for his review of the new chapter on ocular coherence tomography, and to Rubens Belfort Jr. for authoring the Foreword for our book. We also thank the photographers and ophthalmic technicians of the National Eye Institute for their assistance in obtaining photographs, angiograms, OCT images, and other materials for the book. We also would like to thank Julie Taylor, Louise Cook, and the staff at Elsevier for their expertise and assistance in putting the book together. Importantly, we thank our patients for their willingness to participate in clinical trials and contribute to our understanding of uveitis and its treatment in the quest to help others.

We dedicate this fifth edition of the book to
Robert B. Nussenblatt.
Bob was a founding leader in ocular immunology, an outstanding scientist, a caring physician, and a dedicated teacher. He treasured learning, valued scientific collaboration, and loved his family. Bob saw the importance of a uveitis textbook that combines the basic science of immunology and ocular inflammatory disease with clinical discussions focused on the patient. We hope that this edition of the book continues to educate and help improve the lives of our patients.

To our families, friends, colleagues, and patients.

1

Elements of the Immune System and Concepts of Intraocular Inflammatory Disease Pathogenesis

H. Nida Sen

KEY CONCEPTS

- T cells play an important role in the pathogenesis of uveitis.
- The eye is very active immunologically, with ocular resident cells interacting with the immune system.
- Uveitogenic antigens are expressed in the eye, and immunization of animals with these antigens induces experimental uveitis, which resembles human uveitis in many aspects.

In an ever-changing field, a review of the immune system is the subject of numerous books, courses, and scientific articles. However, certain principles have been established, and in the main, these have survived the test of time and rigorous scrutiny. The aim of this chapter is to provide the reader with the essentials needed to follow a discussion on the mechanisms proposed for intraocular inflammatory disease; therefore topics relevant to the understanding of that subject are addressed. In addition, selected themes thought to be important in understanding the unique ocular immune environment and pathogenesis are covered.

The development of the immune system is an extraordinary product of evolution. Its goal is to recognize what is different from self, so its initial role is to respond to foreign antigens with an innate immune response that is geared to rapidly clear the body of the foreign invader. "Innate immunity" is restricted to the non–antigen-specific immune response, including phagocytic cells that engulf and destroy invaders (macrophages and polymorphonuclear cells [PMNs]); populations of lymphocytes that include innate lymphoid cells [ILCs], i.e., natural killer [NK] cells and natural killer T cells (NKTCs); and humoral factors, such as the complement system, and the receptors on antigen-presenting cells, such as phagocytes, called *toll-like receptors* (TLRs), which interact with the invaders' molecules. This activates the antigen-presenting cell to initiate the "adaptive" immune response. Clearly, the invader may return, in which case the adaptive immune response is in place to respond. The adaptive immune response is antigen specific and deals with the invaders that escaped the innate immune mechanism or have returned. The adaptive immune response consists of both B and T cells, and portions of these populations acquire the properties of the memory cells of the secondary immune response. This adaptive immune response connotes an immune memory, hence the development of a complex way in which high-affinity molecules and cell-surface markers can distinguish between the invader and self. A given of this concept is that self-antigens are not attacked; that is, an immune tolerance exists. Part of our story deals with the immune system's appropriate response to outside invaders (e.g., *Toxoplasma*) and the other part deals with understanding (and trying to explain) the response to autoantigens. The dynamic is not as simple as outlined; in fact, it starts as an appropriate response to a foreign antigen and then changes to an abnormal response against the eye. Many mechanisms, such as molecular mimicry, have been proposed.

Achieving this complex but highly specific immune response requires multiple players. Some of these are reviewed in the first part of this chapter. In the second part, findings and theories of disease mechanisms relevant to ocular diseases are introduced and discussed.

ELEMENTS OF THE IMMUNE SYSTEM

The immune system consists of several cell types, including macrophages, dendritic cells, polymorphonuclear cells, and a variety of lymphocyte lines with specific functions. These components add up to a complex immune circuitry or "ballet," which, in the vast number of individuals, responds in a way that is beneficial to the organism. The interactions among these cells and their movements are mediated by several families of molecules, including cytokines, chemokines, and adhesion molecules.

Macrophages/Monocytes

Phagocytic cells originate in bone marrow. The concept that phagocytosis is important for the immunologic defense of the organism was proposed by Metchnikoff at the end of the nineteenth century. The macrophage, which is relatively large (15 μm), has an abundant smooth and rough endoplasmic reticulum. Lysosomal granules and a well-developed Golgi apparatus are also found. Several functional, histochemical, and morphologic characteristics of these cells can be noted (Table 1.1). In addition to the phagocytic characteristics already alluded to, these cells contain esterases and peroxidases and bear membrane markers that are typical of their cell line (i.e., OKM1 antigen

TABLE 1.1 Macrophage Characteristics

Histochemical	Surface Antigens	Receptors	Functions
5′-Nucleotidase	OKM1	Fc	Phagocytosis
Esterase	Class II antigens	Immunoglobulin M (IgM)	Pinocytosis
Alkaline phosphodiesterase		Lymphokine	Immune activation
Aminopeptidase		Lactoferrin	Secretory
Insulin			Microbicidal
		Cb3	Tumoricidal
		Fibrinogen	
		Lipoprotein	

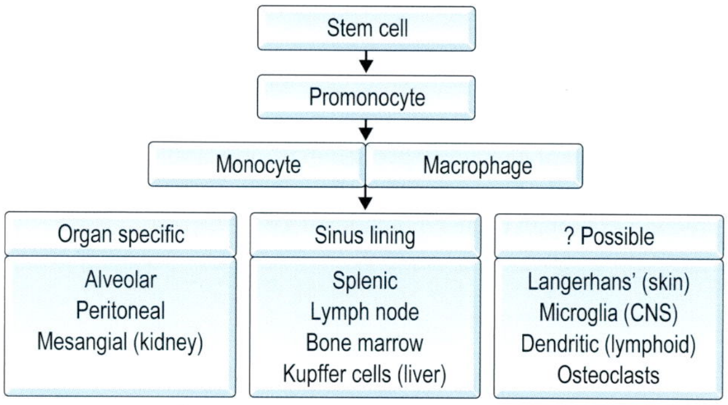

Fig. 1.1 Macrophage differentiation.

and F4/80). Other cell-surface markers are also present, such as class II antigens, Fc receptors (for antibody), and receptors (for complement). These enzymes and cell markers help identify this class of cells and their state of activation. The presence of esterase is a useful marker to distinguish macrophages from granulocytes and lymphocytes. Monocytes will leave the bloodstream because of either a predetermined maturational process or induced migration into an area as a result of chemotactic substances, often produced during inflammatory events. After taking up residence in various tissues, they become macrophages, which are frequently known by other names (Fig. 1.1). Dendritic cells, such as Langerhans' cells, are found in the skin and the cornea and play an important role in presenting antigens to lymphocytes.

Macrophages play at least three major roles within the immune system. The first is to directly destroy foreign pathogens and clear dying or diseased tissue. Killing of invading microbes is, in part, mediated by a burst of hydrogen peroxide (H_2O_2) activity by the activated macrophage. An example with ocular importance is the engulfment of the toxoplasmosis organism, with the macrophage often being a repository for this parasite if killing is inadequate. The second is to activate the immune system. Macrophages, dendritic cells, or other cells with similar characteristics are mandatory for antigen-specific activation of T lymphocytes. Internalizing and processing of the antigen by the macrophage are thought to be integral parts of this mechanism, and the macrophage or the dendritic cell is named *antigen-presenting cell* (APC). Other cells, such as B cells, can also serve this function. The macrophage and the lymphocyte usually need to be in close contact with each other for this transfer to occur. Another requirement is for the cells to have in common a significant portion of their major histocompatibility complex (MHC), genes that express various cell-surface membranes essential for cellular communication and function. Thus this MHC stimulation leads to the initiation of an immune response, ultimately with both T and B cells potentially participating. Other cell-surface markers are needed for activation. This "two signal" theory has centered on other cell-surface antigens, such as the B7–CD28 complex. The engagement of B7 (on the macrophage side) with CD28 enhances the transcription of cytokine genes. Third, the macrophage is a potent secretory cell. Proteases can be released in abundance, and this can degrade vessel surfaces and perivascular areas. Degradation products that result from these reactions are chemotactic and further enhance an immune response. Interleukin (IL)-1, a monokine with a molecular weight of 15 kilodaltons (kDa), is produced by the macrophage (and other cells) after interaction with exogenous pathogens or internal stimuli, such as immune complexes or T cells. IL-1 release directly affects T-cell growth and aids this cell in releasing its own secretory products. IL-1 is noted to act directly on the central nervous system (CNS), with a by-product being induction of fever. Still other macrophage products stimulate fibroblast migration and division, all of which have potentially important consequences in the eye.

Macrophages also produce IL-12, IL-18, IL-10, and transforming growth factor (TGF)-β. In a feedback mechanism, interferon (IFN)-γ can activate macrophages, and the production of IL-12 by the macrophage plays an important role in T-cell activation. The role of macrophages in the eye remains to be fully explored.

Dendritic Cells

Although macrophages play an important role, it is conjectured that dendritic cells are important macrophage-like cells in tissues. They are a subset of cells, perhaps of different lineage from macrophages, and they can be distinguished by lack of persistent adhesion and by the bearing of an antigen, 33D1, on their surface, features that macrophages do not possess. The major role of dendritic cells is to serve as APCs for both CD4+ and CD8+ cells. Like macrophages, dendritic cells produce IL-12, an important activator of T-cell responsiveness. They are rich in MHC II intracellular compartments, an important factor in antigen presentation. The MHC class II compartments move to the surface of the cell when the dendritic cell matures, stimulated by IFN-γ and the CD40 ligand. Dendritic cells are special in that they inhabit tissues where foreign antigens may enter. Experiments with painting of the skin brought seminal observations. Antigens painted on the skin are "brought" to the draining lymph nodes by the dendritic cells of the skin (Langerhans' cells) where T-cell activation can occur. What is interesting is the migratory nature of these cells: They constantly carry important information to the peripheral centers of the immune response. Whether dendritic APCs can activate T cells efficiently in the tissues themselves is an open question, and the answer is important to our understanding of immune responses in the eye. Dendritic cells are thought to be the APCs (or one of the major players) in corneal graft rejection. Thus the concept of removing dendritic cells from a graft has been proposed and used in experimental models. However, there is an opposing concept that peripheral immune tolerance, induced by antigens that foster programmed cell death (apoptosis), may depend on presentation of antigen by dendritic cells in the tissue.

T cells

T-cell responses to antigens provide the basis for a large part of the inflammatory process. They are generated in bone marrow and mature in the thymus, the first lymphoid organ to develop. The thymus consists of two compartments, the cortex and the medulla. In the cortex, immature thymocytes develop through a complex process; their T-cell receptors (TCRs; see later) then interact with thymic epithelium, a process that determines their becoming CD4 ("helping") or CD8 ("cytotoxic") T cells. Thymocytes that fail this process die by apoptosis ("positive selection"), whereas thymocytes that succeed in this selection migrate to the thymic medulla, where epithelial and dendritic cells express all the body's major autoantigens. Thymocytes

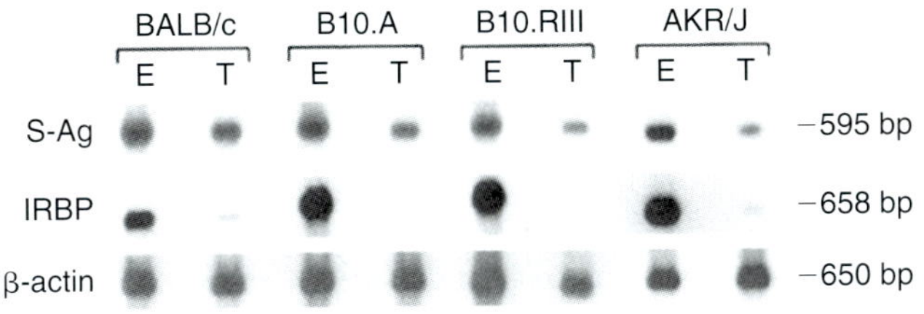

Fig. 1.2 Transcription of S-antigen (S-Ag) and interphotoreceptor retinoid-binding protein (IRBP) genes (uveitogenic antigens) in eyes and thymuses of mouse strains. S-Ag and IRBP are abundant in the eyes of all animals and S-Ag is found in the thymuses of all four strains tested. However, IRBP was seen only in thymuses of two strains – BALB/c and AKR/J – and not in those of B10.A or B10.RIII. The last two animals are susceptible to induction of uveitis with IRBP. (From Egwuagu CE, Charukamnoetkanok P, Gery I. Thymic expression of autoantigens correlates with resistance to autoimmune disease. *J Immunol.* 1997;159:3109–3112. Copyright 1997, The American Association of Immunologists, Inc.)

expressing TCRs with strong affinity to autoantigens are deleted ("negative selection"), and the remaining T cells enter the lymphoid system. Importantly, the negative selection is incomplete and T cells specific to autoantigens do escape the negative selection (see later).

A major component of the negative selection system is the autoimmune regulator (AIRE), a protein that is produced by medullary cells and that controls the expression of organ-specific antigens. Loss of the *AIRE* gene leads to autoimmunity,[1] which is known to occur in humans who develop autoimmune polyglandular syndrome (APS) type I, an autoimmune disease that is inherited in an autosomal recessive fashion. In addition to adrenal insufficiency, mucocutaneous infections, and hypoparathyroidism, these patients can have diabetes, Sjögren syndrome, vitiligo, and uveitis.[2]

The expression of ocular self-antigens in the thymus was investigated in both mice and humans. Egwuagu et al.[3] have shown in different mouse strains an inverted relationship between thymic expression of ocular-specific retinal antigens and the susceptibility to induction of experimental autoimmune uveitis (EAU): Thymic expression of retinal antigens causes lack of responsiveness to these antigens. An example of this phenomenon is shown in Fig. 1.2. Four inbred strains of mice were evaluated for the expression in their thymus of two uveitogenic antigens, interphotoreceptor retinoid-binding protein (IRBP) and S-antigen (S-Ag). All four strains were resistant to the induction of uveitis when S-Ag was used as the immunizing antigen, and all four expressed S-Ag in their thymus. However, two of the four strains, B10.A and B10.RIII, did not express IRBP in their thymuses and were susceptible to uveitis induction when IRBP was used as the immunizing antigen. These observations were extended to include other rodents and primates.[4] In the Lewis rat, which is susceptible to both antigens, neither message was found in the thymus. These observations may provide an insight into the propensity for the disease in humans. Takase et al.[5] evaluated 18 human thymus samples taken from patients undergoing surgery for congenital heart disease. They found that there was expression of the four antigens that can induce experimental uveitis (S-Ag, recoverin, RPE65, and IRBP) in the thymuses of the tested patients. However, the expression of the various antigens was very variable, with some thymus samples showing strong expression and others not. The implication of the findings from these studies is that expression of these antigens in the thymus is very variable in humans, similar to what is seen in the differences among various rodent strains.

T cells with specificity to ocular self-antigens that escape the negative selection are found in the circulation, but do not induce uveitis. This observation is explained by two mechanisms: (1) the inhibitory effect of T-regulatory (Treg) cells, which are normally present in the body; and (2) the retina being isolated from circulating cells by the blood–retina barrier. The normal presence of T cells is indicated by the finding of T cells specific to retinal antigens in healthy individuals with no eye disease.

One important quality possessed by T cells is their immunologic recall or anamnestic capacity after re-exposure to their specific target antigen. The exposure to the antigen increases the number of specific cells and changes them into a "memory" phenotype. A memory T cell to a particular antigen can retain this immunologic memory (see later) essentially for its lifetime. With a repeat encounter, this memory response leads to an immune response that is more rapid and more pronounced than the first. An example is the positive skin response seen after purified protein derivative (PPD) testing.

The central role of the T cell in the immune system cannot be overemphasized. T cells function as pivotal modulators of the immune response by helping production of antibody by B cells and augmenting cell-mediated reactions through the release of molecules, named *cytokines,* which activate immune-related and other cells. T cells also may downregulate or prevent immune reactions through active suppression. (i.e., Treg cells). The cytotoxic (CD8) T-cell subset plays a major role in transplantation rejection crises. Accumulated evidence supports the importance of T cells in many aspects of the intraocular inflammatory process – from the propagation of disease to its subsequent downregulation.

A state of suspended animation can be induced in T cells; this is termed *anergy.* For T cells to be activated, several signals need to be given: one through the TCR and the other through costimulatory receptors, such as CD28; the third is the costimulant B7 linking to CD28 (which is on the T cell). If the TCR is activated but the costimulant is not, a growth arrest can be seen in these cells: They simply stop functioning but do not die. A second way this can occur is when a weakly adherent peptide is linked to the TCR, even if costimulation occurs. It would seem to be a mechanism to prevent unwanted or nuisance immune responses. The full response takes place only if all the appropriate interactions have occurred.

T-cell Receptor

Much interest has focused on the TCR. T cells need to produce the TCR on their cell surface to recognize the target immunogenic peptide on the MHCs of APCs. This complex interaction involves either CD4 or CD8 and their TCRs. The TCR is similar in structure to an immunoglobulin, having both α and β chains. The more distal ends of these chains are variable, and the hypervariable regions are termed *V* (variable) and *J* (joining) on the α chain and *V* and *D* (diversity) regions on the β chain. Compared with the number of immunoglobulin genes, there are fewer *V* genes and more *J* genes in the TCR repertoire. It is logically assumed that the target peptide, which has a special shape and therefore fits specifically in a lock-and-key fashion into the groove between the MHC and the TCR, would be the "cement" of this union. It has been suggested that of all the possible combinations of gene arrangements that could possibly produce the variable region believed to cradle the peptide, certain genes within a family seem to be noted more frequently in autoimmune disease. One such group is the Vα family, with Vβ8.2 receiving much attention. A small number of cells have a TCR made up not of α and β chains but, rather, of γ and δ chains (detailed later). In addition to these physiologic mechanisms, T cells may also be activated by "superantigens," which are bacterial products, such as enterotoxins, or plant products, such as phytohemagglutinin. In addition, T cells may be activated by antibodies to certain surface antigens, mostly CD3 and CD28.

Major Populations of T Cells

The functions that have been briefly described are carried out by several subsets of CD4 T cells, identified by their products and functions. It was observed early on that T cells (and other cells) manifest myriad different molecules on their surface membranes, some of which are

TABLE 1.2 Selected human leukocyte Differentiation antigens (Incomplete list)

Cluster Designation	Main Cellular Distribution	Associated Functions
CD3	T cells, thymocytes	Signal transduction
CD4	Helper T (Th) cells	MHC class II coreceptor
CD8	Suppressor T cells, cytotoxic T cells	MHC class I receptor
CD11a	Leukocytes	LFA-1, adhesion molecule
CD11b	Granulocytes, MΦ	Mac-1, adhesion molecule
CD11c	Granulocytes, MΦ, T cells, B cells	α integrin, adhesion molecule
CD19	B cells	B-cell activation
CD20	B cells	B-cell activation
CD22	B cells	B-cell regulatory
CD25	T cells, B cells	—α chain of IL-2 receptor (Tac) activation
CD28	T cells	Costimulatory T-cell marker
CD45	Leukocytes	Maturation
CD54	Endothelial, dendritic, and epithelial cells; activated T and B cells	ICAM-1, adhesion molecule; ligand of LFA-1 and Mac-1
CD56	NK cells	N-CAM, adhesion molecule
CD68	Macrophages	
CD69	NK cells, lymphocytes	Signal transmission receptor
CX3CR1	Monocytes	Chemoattractant
CXCR3	T cells	Cell maturation
CCR7	T cells	Migration to inflammation
CCR5	T cells	Chemokine receptor

ICAM, intercellular adhesion molecule; *IL,* interleukin; *LFA,* lymphocyte function-associated molecule; *MHC,* major histocompatibility complex; *N-CAM,* neural cell adhesion molecule; NK, natural killer.

expressed uniquely at certain periods of cell activation or function. It was noted that certain monoclonal antibodies directed against these unique proteins bind to specific subsets of cells, thereby permitting a way to identify them (Table 1.2). The antibodies to the CD3 antigen in humans (e.g., OKT3) are directed against an antigen found on all mature human T cells in the circulation; approximately 70% to 80% of lymphocytes in the systemic circulation bear this marker. Antibodies to the CD4 antigen (e.g., OKT4) define the helper subgroup of human T cells (Th cells; about 60%–80% of the total T cells). These CD4+ cells respond to antigens complexed to MHCs of the class II type. The CD4 cells are particularly susceptible to human immunodeficiency virus (HIV) that causes acquired immunodeficiency syndrome (AIDS), with the percentage of this subset decreasing dramatically as this disease progresses. Furthermore, these helper cells are necessary components of the autoimmune response seen in the experimental models of ocular inflammatory disease induced by retinal antigens (see discussion of autoimmunity later in this chapter). Antibodies to the CD8 antigen (i.e., OKT8) distinguish a population that includes cytotoxic T cells, making up about 20% to 30% of the total number of T cells. Antibodies directed against the CD8 antigen block class I histocompatibility-associated reactions.

The two major populations of T cells (CD4 and CD8) are further divided into subpopulations that are detailed later. These subpopulations are generated by combinations of cytokines, which are products of other cells, and affect the immune system by the specific cytokines they produce.

T-cell Subsets

The population of Th cells has been further subdivided on the basis of their functional characteristics into several subsets. The major subsets are named Th1, Th2, and Th17. In normal conditions, Th1 cells defend against intracellular pathogens, Th2 cells defend against extracellular parasites and mediate antibody production, and Th17 cells defend against extracellular pathogens. Pathologically, Th1 and Th17 cells are responsible for initiation of "cell-mediated" immune responses, such as foreign tissue rejection and pathogenic autoimmune processes, whereas Th2 cells are involved in allergic responses and in immunoregulation. Th1 cells (Fig. 1.3) produce mostly IFN-γ, IL-2, and tumor necrosis factor-α

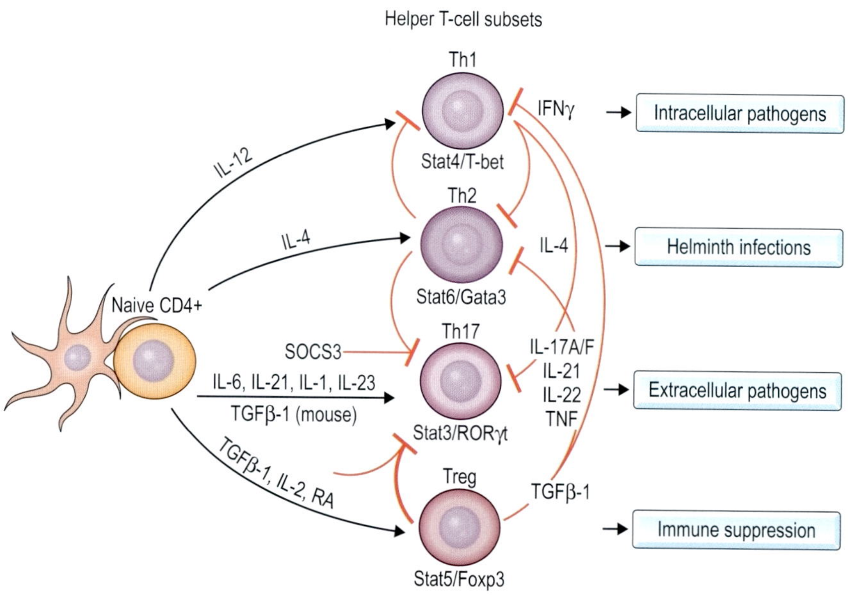

Fig. 1.3 Helper T-cell subsets now recognized. (From: Chen, Z, O'Shea JJ. Th17 cells: a new fate for differentiating helper T cells. *Immunol Res.* 2008;41:87, with permission.)

(TNF-α). The cytokine profile of Th2 cells consists of IL-4, IL-5, IL-10, IL-13, and perhaps TGF-β , and the major cytokines produced by Th17 cells are IL-17, IL-21, and IL-22. In many animal models of human diseases, Th1 and Th17 cells are associated with initiation of disease, whereas Th2 cells are associated with disease downregulation and allergy initiation.

Importantly, under experimental conditions, Th17 cells may switch to a Th1 phenotype, but Th1 cells maintain their phenotype and do not change.[6]

IL-22 is part of the IL-17 group of cytokines produced during an inflammatory response.[7] Albeit made by lymphocytes, its receptors are present on epithelial cells. Thus it has been suggested that one of its major roles is to be the cross-talk lymphokine between resident tissue cells and infiltrating inflammatory cells, particularly T cells. This proinflammatory cytokine is found in the synovia of patients with rheumatoid arthritis and is upregulated in both Crohn disease and ulcerative colitis[8,9] and in both the serum and intraocular fluids of patients with uveitis.[10,11]

Gamma Delta (γδ) T Cells

γδ T cells, which constitute a small fraction of peripheral T cells, play important roles in inflammatory processes, such as EAU.[12] Of particular importance is the involvement of γδ T cells in mucosal tissue inflammation in the conjunctiva, as shown by St Leger et al.,[13] where an inflammatory response to a commensal bacterium is mediated to a large extent by IL-17 produced by γδ cells.

T-regulatory Cells

It is now clear that just as the immune system needs cells to initiate a response, it needs cells to suppress or modify immune responses. One of the ways this need is met is with Treg cells.[14] These cells derive from a naive T-cell population under the influence of cytokines that are different from those involved in Th1, Th17, or Th2 cell development (see Fig. 1.3). Treg cells can be found in the thymus or in the peripheral circulation, where a large portion is "induced" (iTregs). An interesting report by Kemper et al.[15] described stimulating CD4+ cells with CD3 and CD46 (a complement regulator) and inducing Treg cells, that is, producing large amounts of IL-10, moderate amounts of TGF-β, and little IL-2. The literature is replete with information about different types of Treg cells, and these cells have been reported in several organs, such as the gut, where peripheral immune tolerance needs to be induced.[16] Certain Treg cells are characterized by their ability to produce IL-10 and TGF-β. They are capable of downregulating both CD4- and CD8-mediated inflammatory responses and apparently require cell-to-cell contact. The majority of Treg cells bear CD25 (the IL-2 receptor) on their cell surface and express the transcription factor forkhead/winged helix (FoxP3),[17] which is a reliable marker for the development and function of naturally occurring Treg cells.[18] When we evaluated the T cells of patients with ocular inflammatory disease, we found that the FoxP3 marker varied considerably among patients and was not a very good indicator of poor Treg cell function.[19] An interesting observation is the noted increase in a subset of NK cells (so-called CD56 "bright") after daclizumab therapy; this subset makes large amounts of IL-10, indicating the regulatory nature of these cells. The increase is seen when the patient's disease is well controlled, and it has also been seen in patients with multiple sclerosis receiving daclizumab therapy.

Lymphocytes of Innate Immune System

In addition to adaptive immunity cells and molecules, mentioned earlier, the protection against invasion of pathogenic agents is carried out by components of "innate" immunity that lack antigenic specificity but are capable of providing immunity. The cell populations of the innate immunity are discussed in the following sections.

Innate Lymphoid Cells

The recently discovered ILCs are lymphocytes that lack antigen specificity and are involved in the immune response by releasing cytokines or carry cytotoxic capacity (NK cells; see later). ILCs are mainly tissue resident and play major roles in keeping the homeostasis in these tissues.[20] Unlike T or B cells, ILCs react promptly to stimulations, such as pathogen invasion. ILCs are separated into three major groups (ILC1, ILC2, and ILC3) that selectively collaborate with Th1, Th2, and Th17 lymphocytes in the defense against intracellular pathogens and tumors, large extracellular pathogens and allergens, and extracellular pathogens, respectively.[20]

Natural Killer and Invariant Nature Killer T Cells

NK cells and invariant natural killer T (iNKT) cells are major components of the innate immune response, whose main function is to carry out the rejection by cytolytic activity of both tumors and virally infected cells. The main difference between NK cells and iNKT cells is their morphology, with NK cells being large granular lymphocytes, whereas iNKT cells express highly conserved TCRs. Both populations release large amounts of cytokines upon activation. NK cells seem to be involved in the pathogenesis of EAU because the disease was found to be diminished in mice with no NK cells.[21] Grajewski et al.[22] showed that similar to NK cells, iNKT cells ameliorate the EAU process. However, iNKT cells were also found to have a dual effect in the pathogenic process of EAU: The disease was enhanced in iNKT-deficient mice, but activation of these cells also exacerbated the pathologic process.[23]

Cytokines

Intercellular communication, which is crucial for active immune response, is mediated by cytokines, chemokines, and adhesion molecules. Cytokines are produced by lymphocytes, macrophages, and other cells. They are hormone-like proteins capable of amplifying an immune response and of suppressing it. With activation of a T lymphocyte, the production and release of various lymphokines will occur. One of the most important cytokines is IL-2, with a molecular weight of 15 kDa in humans. The release of this lymphokine stimulates lymphocyte growth and augments specific immune responses, including stimulation of Treg cells. Of particular interest are cytokines involved in the inflammatory process. They include proinflammatory cytokines, IFN-γ, IL-1, IL-17, and TNF-α and the anti-inflammatory IL-4, IL-5, IL-10, and TGF-β. Of interest, IFN-γ and TGF-β are active in both activation and suppression of immune responses. The number of lymphokines that have been purified and for which effects have been described continues to grow rapidly. An incomplete list is shown in Table 1.3 and a more recent list has been provided by Akdis et al.[24]

Chemokines

This family of chemoattractant cytokines is characterized by its ability to induce directional migration of movable cells. They direct cell adhesion, homing, and angiogenesis. There are four major subfamilies of chemokines: CXC (nine of which are found on chromosome 4); CC (11 of which are found on chromosome 17); C (only one well-defined member, lymphotactin, is found on chromosome 11); and CX3C (fractalkine is found on chromosome 16). The nomenclature is based on the cysteine molecules. The CC chemokines have two adjacent cysteines at their amino terminus; the CXC chemokines have their N-terminal cysteines separated by one amino acid; the C chemokines have only two cysteines, one at the terminal end and one downstream; the CX3C chemokines have three amino acids between their two N-terminal cysteines. Each chemokine family has special functions that affect different types of cells. An example of this fine specificity is seen with the CXC family. These chemokines, with a Glu–Leu–Arg sequence near the end

TABLE 1.3 Cytokines: An incomplete list

Type	Source	Target and Effect
IFN-γ	T cells	Antiviral effects; promotes expression of MHC II Antigens on cell surfaces; increases MΦ tumor killing; inhibits some T-cell proliferation
TGF-β	T cells, resident ocular cells	Suppresses generation of certain T cells; involved in ACAID and oral tolerance
Interleukin		
IL-1	Many nucleated cells, high levels in MΦ, keratinocyte, endothelial cells, some T and B cells	T- and B-cell proliferation; fibroblasts – proliferation, prostaglandin production; CNS – fever; bone and cartilage resorption; adhesion-molecule expression on endothelium
IL-2	Activated T cells	Activates T cells, B cells, MΦ, NK cells
IL-3	T cells	Affects hemopoietic lineage that is nonlymphoid eosinophil regulator; similar function to IL-5 GM-CSF
IL-4	T cells	Regulates many aspects of B-cell development; affects T cells, mast cells, and MΦ
IL-5	T cells, eosinophils	Affects hemopoietic lineage that is nonlymphoid, eosinophil regulator: similar function to IL-3 GM-CSF; induces B-cell differentiation into IgG- and IgM-secreting plasma cells
IL-6	MΦ T cells fibroblasts; endothelial cells, RPE	B cells – cofactor for Ig production; T cells – comitogen; proinflammatory in eye
IL-7	Stromal cells in bone marrow and thymus	Stimulates early B-cell progenitors; affects immature T cells
IL-8	NK cells, T cells	Chemoattractant of neutrophils, basophils, and some T cells; aids in neutrophils adhering to endothelium; induced by IL-1, TNF-α, and endotoxin
IL-9	T cells	Supports growth of helper T cells; may be enhancing factor for hematopoiesis in presence of other cytokines
IL-10	T cells, B cells, stimulated MΦ	Inhibits production of lymphokines by T helper 1 (Th1) cells
IL-11	Bone marrow stromal cells (fibroblasts)	Stimulates cells of myeloid, lymphoid, erythroid, and megakaryocytic lines; induces osteoclast formation; enhances erythrocytopoiesis, antigen-specific antibodies, acute-phase proteins, fever
IL-12	B cells, T cells	Induces IFN-γ synthesis; augments T-cell cytotoxic activity with IL-2; is chemotactic for NK cells and stimulates interaction with vascular endothelium; promotes lytic activity of NK cells; antitumor effects regulate proliferation of Th1 cells but not Th2 or Th0 cells
IL-13	T cells	Anti-inflammatory activity as IL-4 and IL-10; downregulates IL-12 and IFN-α production and thus favors Th2 T-cell responses; inhibits proliferation of normal αvδ leukemic human B-cell precursors; monocyte chemoattractant
IL-14	T cells	Induces B-cell proliferation, malignant B cells; inhibits immunoglobulin secretion
IL-15	Variety of cells	Stimulates proliferation of T cells; shares bioactivity of IL-2 and uses components of IL-2 receptor
IFN-α	Variety of cells	Antiviral
IFN-β	Variety of cells	Antiviral
IFN-γ	T and NK cells	Inflammation, activates MΦ
TNF-α	MΦ	Inflammation, tumor killing
TNF-β	T cells	Inflammation, tumor killing, enhanced phagocytosis

ACAID, anterior chamber acquired immune deviation; *CNS*, central nervous system; *GM-CSF*, granulocyte macrophage–colony-stimulating factor; *IFN*, interferon; *Ig*, immunoglobulin; *MΦ*, macrophage; MHC, major histocompatibility complex; *NK*, natural killer; *RPE*, retinal pigment epithelium; *TGF*, transforming growth factor; *TNF*, tumor necrosis factor.

of the N terminus, bind well to the CXCR2 on neutrophils. CXC chemokines not possessing that sequence are chemotactic for monocytes and lymphocytes. IL-8 can bind with either CXCR1 or CXCR2 chemokine receptors. Organisms have adapted to these chemokines as well. HIV gp120 binds to CCR5 and CCR3, aiding its entry into the lymphocyte. This area of knowledge is still evolving. Clearly, cell homing has importance in ocular inflammatory disease but probably in other conditions as well, such as diabetes and age-related macular degeneration (AMD), in which the immune components of the disease are just being explored but which may be important areas for therapeutic interventions.

Cell-Adhesion Molecules and Their Role in Lymphocyte Homing and in Disease

Cell-adhesion molecules (CAMs) are cell-surface glycoproteins important for the interaction between cells and for the interaction of cells with the extracellular matrix. CAMs play an integral role in the development of the inflammatory response. These adhesion molecules are especially important for directing leukocytes to areas of inflammation. The upregulation of CAM expression on the vascular endothelium and surrounding area allows inflammatory cells to home to inflamed tissues.[25] CAMs are also involved in the interaction of lymphocytes and APCs, important for lymphocyte stimulation.

CAMs are divided into three structural groups: selectins, integrins, and the immunoglobulin gene superfamily. The selectins are a group of CAMs that appear to mediate the initial adhesion of inflammatory cells to the vascular endothelium, leading to a rolling of the cells along the vascular wall.[26] The integrins and members of the immunoglobulin supergene family then interact to form a more firm adherence between the leukocytes and the vascular endothelium, leading to transendothelial migration of the cells into the inflamed tissue.[26]

E-selectin, also known as *endothelial leukocyte adhesion molecule-1* (ELAM-1, CD62E), mediates the attachment of polymorphonuclear leukocytes to endothelial cells in vitro and appears to be important in the recruitment of neutrophils in a local endotoxin response in the skin.[27] We investigated the expression of E-selectin in eyes with endotoxin-induced uveitis (EIU), a useful animal model for the study of acute ocular inflammation,[28] which is characterized by iris hyperemia, miosis, increased aqueous humor protein, and inflammatory cell infiltration into the anterior uvea and anterior chamber.[29,30] Inflammatory cells first enter the eye 6 hours after endotoxin injection, and the resultant uveitis peaks within 24 hours. EIU is thought to result from mediators released by activated cells, including macrophages, but the exact mechanism causing infiltration into the eye is not clearly defined. Recent data suggest that CAMs play an important role in the pathogenesis of this animal model of disease and that CAM expression is important for the recruitment of leukocytes into eyes with EIU.

ICAM-1 binds not only to Mac-1, but also to lymphocyte function-associated molecule-1 (LFA-1, CD11a/CD18), a second β_2-integrin expressed on all leukocytes predominantly involved in lymphocyte trafficking. A number of groups have studied how ICAM-1 and LFA-1 affect the development of EIU. In eyes with EIU in C3H/HeN mice, ICAM-1 is first expressed on the ciliary body epithelium 6 hours after endotoxin injection and, later, on the vascular endothelium of the ciliary body and iris and on the corneal endothelium.[31] Elner et al.[32] demonstrated the expression of ICAM-1 (CD54) on the corneal endothelium, and the expression of this cell adhesion molecule also appears to be important to the development of keratic precipitates. In experiments on Lewis rats, we have seen that EIU can be prevented by treating the animals with anti-ICAM-1 or anti-LFA-1 antibody at the time of endotoxin injection,[33] even when administered 6 hours after endotoxin injection when the eyes are already clinically inflamed. Rosenbaum and Boney[34] also showed that antibody to LFA-1 significantly reduced the cellular infiltrate associated with rabbit models of uveitis but that vascular permeability was less affected. An ICAM-neutralizing antibody can inhibit viral infection of the RPE by HTVL-1.[35]

The secretion of cytokines, particularly by infiltrating T lymphocytes, appears to regulate adhesion molecule expression. IFN-γ, IL-1, and TNF induce strong ICAM-1 expression at a transcriptional level, although the response to cytokines varies among cell types.[36-38] In vitro studies have shown that ICAM-1 expression on the cornea and the RPE is upregulated by cytokines, such as IL-1.[39,40] It is clear that one of the major effects of cytokines in the pathogenesis of EIU involves the upregulation of adhesion molecule expression.

CAMs have also been shown to play a critical role in the pathogenesis of EAU. We studied the expression of ICAM-1 and LFA-1 in B10.A mice with EAU.[41] ICAM-1 was first expressed on the vascular endothelium of the retina and ciliary body by 7 days after immunization, whereas infiltrating leukocytes expressing LFA-1 were not observed until 9 days after immunization, and clear histologic evidence of ocular inflammation did not occur until 11 days after immunization.

Treatment with monoclonal antibodies against ICAM-1 and LFA-1 inhibited the development of EAU, suggesting that antiadhesion molecule antibodies could inhibit EAU by interfering with immunization and antigen sensitization and/or by blocking leukocyte homing and migration into the eye. These data indicate that antibodies against ICAM-1 and LFA-1 inhibit EAU by interfering with both the induction and the effector phases of the disease. Adhesion molecules are also involved in the pathogenesis of lens-induced uveitis. Till et al.[42] showed that antibodies against adhesion molecules reduced ocular inflammation in lens-induced uveitis.

Recent studies in humans have shown that cell-adhesion molecules are important in the development of ocular inflammation. We have shown that ICAM-1 is expressed in the retina and choroid of human eyes with posterior uveitis.[43] In addition, we demonstrated increased expression of ICAM-1 in corneas with allograft rejection.[44] As indicated by animal data, clinical trials in 18 patients who received cadaver donor renal allografts showed that immunosuppression with anti-ICAM-1 antibody resulted in significantly less rejection.[45] These data showed not only that CAMs are involved in the pathogenesis of inflammation but also that treatment with drugs to block these adhesion molecules should provide effective therapy for inflammatory disease. We used efalizumab (Raptiva), a CD11a antibody that inhibits binding of LFA-1 to ICAM-1, in the treatment of patients with uveitis in a small pilot study, with positive therapeutic effects .[46]

B Cells

B cells make up the second broad arm of the lymphocyte immune response. Originating in mammals from the same pluripotent stem cells in bone marrow as T cells, the maturational process and role of B cells are quite different. The term *B cell* originates from the finding that in chickens, antibody-producing cells mature in the bursa of Fabricius, a uniquely avian structure. The mammal equivalent appears to be bone marrow. The role of the B cell is to function as the effector cell in humoral immunity. The unique characteristic of these cells is the presence of surface immunoglobulin on their cell membranes. There are two major subgroups of B cells. Innate-like B1 cells originate in the fetal liver, are long lived, and self-renew. They produce natural antibodies, mostly immunoglobulin M (IgM), in the absence of antigen stimulation. In contrast, B2 cells are crucial for adaptive immunity. They derive from bone marrow and produce high-affinity antibodies in response to exogenous stimuli. They produce immunoglobulins other than IgM (see next section). B2 cells also mediate the anamnestic, rapid, high-affinity antibody response to previously sensitizing antigens. When activated for antibody production B cells undergo morphologic change and are named "plasma cells" that are typical by having a round, eccentric nucleus with coarse clumps of heterochromatin and euchromatin.

The maturation process of B cells is complex and not fully understood. What is clear is that various gene regions that control the B cell's main product, that is, immunoglobulins, are not physically next to each other. Through a process of translocation, these genes align themselves next to each other, excising intervening genes. IL-7 is an important factor in this maturation process. B cells can be activated through their interaction with CD4+ T cells, which express class II MHC antigens and CD40 ligand on their surface. This process is promoted by T-cell cytokines, including IL-2, IL-4, IL-5, IL-6, and IL-17.

B cells initially express surface IgM and IgD simultaneously, with differentiation occurring only after appropriate activation. Five major classes of immunoglobulins are identified on the basis of the structure of their heavy chains: α, γ, μ, δ, and ε, corresponding to IgA, IgG, IgM, IgD, and IgE (Table 1.4). The structure of the immunoglobulin demonstrates symmetry, with two heavy chains and two light chains uniformly seen in all classes except IgM and IgA (Fig. 1.4). The production of immunoglobulins usually requires T-cell participation. Many "relevant" antigens are T cell dependent; that is, the addition of antigen to a culture of pure B cells will not induce immunoglobulin production. However, polyclonal B-cell activators, such as lipopolysaccharide, pokeweed mitogen, dextran, and certain viruses, such as Epstein-Barr virus, have the capacity to directly induce B-cell proliferation and immunoglobulin production. For a primary immune response, B cells will produce IgM, which binds complement. With time – and if they encounter these antigens again – B cells will switch immunoglobulin production to IgG, usually during the primary response. This immunoglobulin class switching, which requires a gene rearrangement, is inherent in the B cell and is partly controlled by lymphokines. IL-4 has been associated with a switch to express IgG (in mouse IgG_1, in human IgG_4) and IgE, whereas IFN-γ controls a switch to IgG_{2a} and TGF-β to IgA.

TABLE 1.4 Characteristics of human immunoglobulins

	IgG	IgA	IgM	IgE	IgD
Molecular weight (103)	150	150–300	900	190	180
Heavy chain	γ	α	μ	–	δ
Subclass	1,2,3,4	1,2	1,2	–	–
J chain	–	+	+	–	–
Crosses placenta	+	–	–	–	–
Serum half-life (days)	21	6	5	2	3
Complement activation	+	–	+	–	–
Serum concentration (mg/dL)	110	25	10	0.001	0.3
IN EYE					
Conjunctiva	Rich	Rich	Varies	Varies	Varies
Cornea	Moderate	Moderate	0	?	0
Aqueous	Low	Low	Low	?	0
Iris	Low	Low	Low	Varies	Varies
Choroid	Rich	Rich	Rich	Varies	Varies
Retina	Low	Low	Low	0	0
Vitreous	–	–	–	–	–

From Allansmith M. Unpublished data 1987. Used with permission.

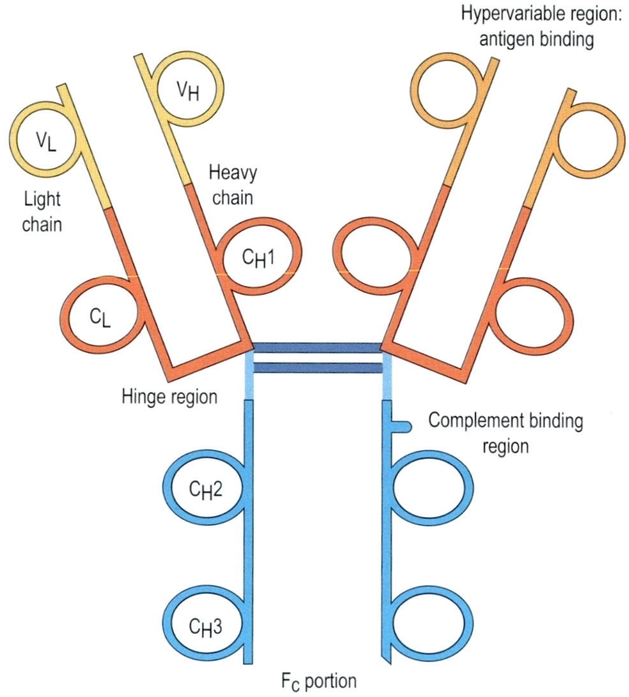

Fig. 1.4 Structure of human immunoglobulin G (IgG) molecule.

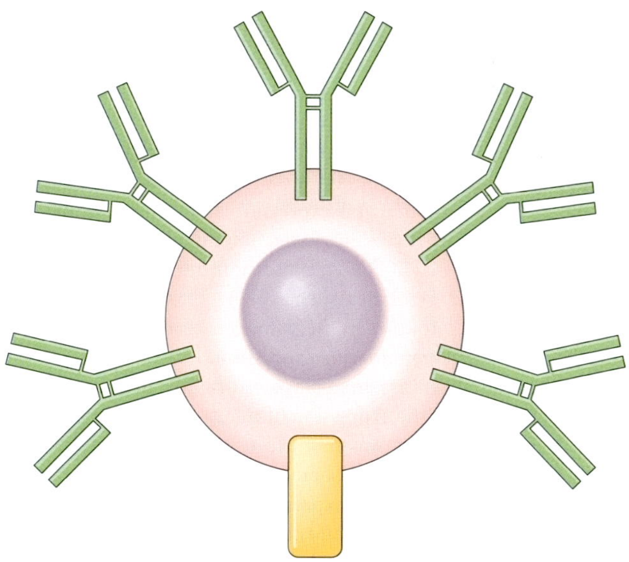

Fig. 1.5 Immunoglobulin M (IgM) pentamer with J chain.

Surprisingly, recent studies have revealed that B cells also function as immunoregulatory cells. Wang et al.[47] showed that the cytokine IL-35 induces B cells with immunoregulatory capacity ("Breg" cells), which release the immunosuppressive cytokines IL-10 and IL-35. Furthermore, Bregs were found to inhibit the development of EAU by inhibiting pathogenic Th1 and Th17 and promoting the expansion on Treg cells. Adoptive transfer of Breg cells was found to inhibit the development of EAU.[48]

Classes of Immunoglobulins

More IgA is made than any other immunoglobulin, most of it in the gut. IgG is the major circulating immunoglobulin class found in humans; it is synthesized at a very high rate and makes up about 75% of the total serum immunoglobulins. Plasma cells that produce IgG are found mainly in the spleen and the lymph nodes. Four subclasses of IgG have been identified in humans (G_1–G_4). G_1 and G_3 fix complement readily and can be transmitted to the fetus. The production of these subclasses is not random but reflects the antigen to which the antibody is being made. When doing tests in the serum or the chambers of the eye (aqueous or vitreous), we usually look at IgG production.

IgM is a pentamer made up of the typical antibody structure linked by disulfide bonds and J chains (Fig. 1.5). In conventional responses of B2 cells, IgM is produced in minute amounts. Because of its size, IgM generally stays within the systemic circulation and, unlike IgG, will not cross the blood–brain barrier or the placenta. This antibody is expressed early on the surface of B cells. Therefore initial antibody responses to exogenous pathogens, such as *Toxoplasma gondii,* are of this class. The observation of an IgM-specific antibody response helps confirm a newly acquired infection. IgM has a complement-binding site and can mediate phagocytosis by fixing C3b, a component of the complement system.

One major role of both IgG and IgM is to interact with both effector cells and the complement system to limit the invasion of exogenous organisms. These immunoglobulins help effector cells through opsonization, which occurs by the antibody coating an invading organism and assisting the phagocytic process. The Fc portion of the antibody molecule then can readily interact with effector cells, such as macrophages, thereby helping effectively resolve the infection. Persons with deficiencies in IgG and IgM are particularly prone to infections by pyogenic organisms, such as *Streptococcus* and *Neisseria* species. In addition, both these antibodies will activate the complement pathway, inducing cell lysis by that mechanism as well.

IgA is the major extravascular immunoglobulin, although it comprises only about 10% to 15% of the intravascular total. Two isotypes of IgA are

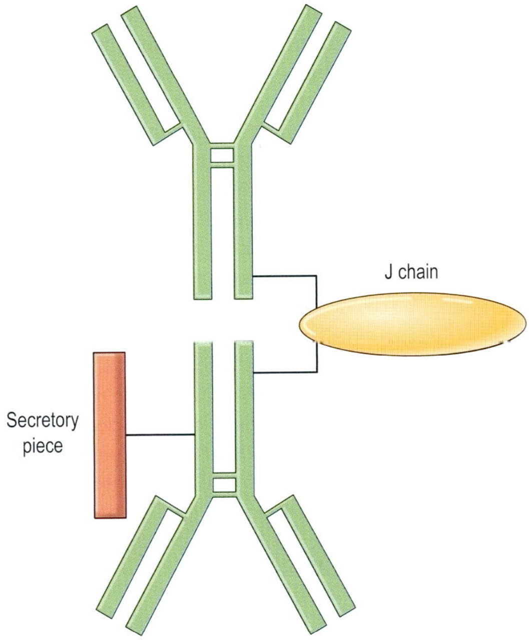

Fig. 1.6 Immunoglobulin A (IgA) dimer with J chain and secretory piece.

noted: IgA_1 is more commonly seen intravascularly, whereas IgA_2 is somewhat more prevalent in the extravascular space. The IgA-secreting plasma cells are found in the subepithelial spaces of the gut, respiratory tract, tonsils, and salivary and lacrimal glands. IgA is an important component to the defense mechanism of the ocular surface, being found in a dimer linked by a J chain, a polypeptide needed for polymerization. In addition, a secretory component, a unique protein with parts of its molecule having no homology to other proteins, is needed for the IgA to appear in the gut and outside vessels. The secretory component is produced locally by epithelial cells, which then form a complex with the IgA dimer/J chain (Fig. 1.6). This new complex is internalized by mucosal cells and then released on the apical surface of the cell through a proteolytic process. The amount of IgA within the eye is quite small. IgA can fix complement through the alternate pathway and can serve as an opsonin for phagocytosis. IgA appears to exert its major role by preventing entry of pathogens into the internal environment of the organism by binding with the infectious agent. It may also impede the absorption of potential toxins and allergens into the body. Furthermore, it can induce eosinophil degranulation.

IgE is slightly heavier than IgG because its heavy chain has an additional constant domain. Mast cells and basophils have Fc receptors for IgE, and IgE is thought to be one of the major mediators of the allergic or anaphylactoid reaction. It appears to be an important defense mechanism against parasites: one way IgE accomplishes this is to prime basophils and mast cells. Although its role in ocular surface disease has been well recognized, this has not been the case for intraocular inflammation.

IgD is found in minute quantities in the serum (0.5% of serum immunoglobulin). It is found simultaneously with IgM on B cells before specific stimulation. Little else is known about this antibody other than that it is a major B-cell membrane receptor for antigen.

Antibodies directed toward specific antigens, particularly cell-surface antigens of the immune system, have provided clinical and basic investigators with a powerful tool with which to identify various components of the immune system, as was described in the section on the T cell. The development of monoclonal antibodies by using hybridoma technology has allowed for the production of these immune probes in almost unlimited quantities. Immortalized myeloma cells can be fused with a B cell committed to the production of an antibody directed toward a relevant antigen. This is usually accomplished with the use of polyethylene glycol, which promotes cell membrane fusion. By careful screening, clones of these fused cells (i.e., hybrid cells or hybridomas) can be identified as producing the antibody needed. These can be isolated and grown, yielding essentially an unlimited source of the antibody derived from one clone of cells and directed against one specific determinant. Monoclonal antibodies have been raised against cell markers of virtually all cellular components of the immune system. Antibodies can now be "humanized" so that only small parts of the variable end remain of mouse origin. The advantage of this is the reduced probability of an immune response against the foreign protein.

Other Cells

Mast Cells

This large (15–20 μm) cell is intimately involved in type I hypersensitivity reactions (see next section). Its most characteristic feature is the presence of large granules in the cytoplasm. It is clear that there are subtypes of mast cells. In humans, mast cells are characterized by the presence or absence of the granule-associated protease chymase. It has been suggested that tryptase-positive, chymase-negative human mast cells are suggestive of mucosal mast cells found in the mouse. Mast cells contain a large number of biologically active agents, including histamine, serotonin, prostaglandins, leukotrienes, chemotactic factors of anaphylaxis, and cytokines and chemokines. Histamine is stored within the mast-cell granules. Once released into the environment, histamine can cause smooth muscle to contract and can increase small vessel permeability, giving the typical "wheal and flare" response noted in skin tests. Serotonin, in humans, appears to have a major effect on vasoconstriction and blood pressure, whereas in rodents, it may also affect vascular permeability. Prostaglandins, a family of lipids, are capable of stimulating a variety of biologic activities, including vasoconstriction and vasodilation. Leukotrienes are compounds produced de novo with antigen stimulation. Leukotriene B_4 is a potent chemotactic factor for both neutrophils and eosinophils, whereas leukotrienes C_4 and D_4, for example, enhance vascular permeability. At least two chemotactic factors of anaphylaxis attract eosinophils to a site of mast-cell degranulation, whereas other factors attract and immobilize neutrophils.

Mast-cell involvement in several external ocular conditions has been established. However, it is not yet clear what role this cell may play in intraocular inflammatory disorders. Mast cells are present in abundance in the choroid and appear to be related to the susceptibility of at least one experimental model for uveitis (see discussion on autoimmunity). Findings from human studies have supported the hypothesis that many cytokine-dependent processes are implicated in IgE-associated disorders. Many different cytokines and chemokines have been seen in mast cells. These include IL-4, IL-6, IL-8, TNF-α, vascular endothelial growth factor (VEGF), and macrophage inflammatory protein (MIP)-1α.

All of these findings link the mast cell to a whole variety of immune processes. It can be speculated that when a mast cell degranulates in the choroid, it also releases chemokines and lymphokines, which may be the initiating factors of what we describe as a T-cell–mediated disorder.

The role of mast cells in the pathogenesis of EAU has been noted in early studies. Mochizuki et al.[49] have noted that rat strain susceptibility to EAU induced with S-Ag was dramatically associated with the number of mast cells in the choroid, and de Kozak et al.[50] have shown that mast cells in the choroid degranulate just before the influx of T cells into the eye, suggesting that these cells "open the door" into the eye for the T cells. This concept is especially provocative because Askenase et al.[51] showed that mast-cell degranulation can be induced not only by IgE antibodies but also by T cells.

Eosinophils

These bilobed nucleated cells are about 10 to 15 μm in size and are thought to be terminally differentiated granulocytes. Their most morphologically unique characteristic is the approximately 200 granules that are highly acidophilic (taking up eosin in standard staining procedures) and which are found in the cytoplasm. The granules are almost entirely made up of major basic protein (molecular weight 9 kDa), but other toxic cationic granules include eosinophil-derived neurotoxia, eosinophil cationic protein, and eosinophil peroxidase. A minor percentage of these cells (5%–25%) have IgG receptors, and about half may have complement receptors on their surface membranes, although it is not clear whether receptors for IgE are present. Eosinophils contain an abundant number of enzymes, which are quite similar in nature to those contained in neutrophils. Both cells contain a peroxidase and catalase, both of which can be antimicrobial, but eosinophils lack lysozymes and neutrophils lack the major basic protein. Eosinophils also contain several anti-inflammatory enzymes, such as kininase, arylsulfatase, and histaminase. In addition, eosinophils produce growth factors, such as IL-3 and IL-5; chemokines, such as RANTES and MIP-1; and cytokines, such as TGF-α and TGF-β, VEGF, TNF-α, IL-1α, IL-6, and IL-8.

The eosinophil arises in bone marrow from a myeloid progenitor, perhaps from a separate stem cell than neutrophils. The time spent in the systemic circulation is probably quite short, and the number seen on a routine blood smear is usually very low (≤1% of nucleated cells). These cells can be attracted to an area in the body through the release of mast-cell products and, once localized to an inflammatory site, are capable of performing several functions. The eosinophil may play an immunomodulatory role in the presence of mast-cell and basophil activation.

As mentioned, the eosinophil contains the anti-inflammatory agents histaminase and arylsulfatase, which are capable of neutralizing the effect of histamine release and slow-reacting substance, both products of mast cells. Furthermore, basophil function may be inhibited by prostaglandins E_1 and E_2, both produced by eosinophils. An additional immunomodulatory mechanism is the capacity of the eosinophil to ingest immunoreactive granules released by mast cells. An extremely important role played by these cells is in the response of the immune system to parasitic organisms. Eosinophils are seen in high numbers at the site of a parasitic infiltration and are known to bind tightly to the organism through receptors. Furthermore, the release of the major basic protein granules or an eosinophil-produced peroxidase complexed with H_2O_2 and deposited on the parasite's surface membrane will lead to the death of the invading organism. Major basic protein may play a role in corneal ulceration in severe cases of allergy.

Neutrophils

Neutrophils are the most abundant type of white blood cells (WBCs), and it is clear that they play an important role in acute inflammation. They do not live as long as monocytes or lymphocytes and are attracted to inflammatory sites by IL-8, IFN-γ, and C5a. One of their main functions is phagocytosis, in particular killing microbes by using reactive oxygen species (ROS) and hydrolytic enzymes. Although their role in innate immunity seemed clear, some thought-provoking findings have suggested a relationship with IL-17. IL-17 is made by not only by T cells and macrophages but also by neutrophils. Furthermore, IL-17 appears to mobilize lung neutrophils after a bacterial challenge.[52] This would therefore suggest that neutrophils are responding to immune responses from both the innate and the acquired sides of the immune process.

Resident Ocular Cells

The interaction of the resident ocular cells with those of the immune system is an interesting concept. It is clear that several cells of the eye, including the RPE and Müller cells, either have functions similar to cells within the immune system or can be induced to bear markers that potentially permit them to participate in immune-mediated events; for example, Müller cells were found to inhibit lymphocyte stimulation.[53] There are microglia in the retina that are of hematopoietic origin. One can speculate that the initial priming of the immune system may occur through this interchange or that the continued recruitment of immune cells may be mediated through these mechanisms. Interestingly, microglia were recently found to be critical for the initiation of EAU by T cells.[54] The effects of immune cells and their products may also be important for certain ocular conditions, inasmuch as macrophages and T-cell products have a profound effect on fibrocyte growth and division, and the RPE and Müller cells may respond in like fashion. The RPE, when activated, can act as efficient APCs. Numerous lymphokines are found in the eye, many of which are produced by ocular resident cells. As mentioned earlier, it is not clear whether there can be antigen presentation in the eye, but in experimental models, these cells do modulate this process. We also know that resident ocular cells modulate the ocular environment by eliciting molecules that alter the immune process (anterior chamber associated immune deviation [ACAID]; see section on ACAID).

Complement System

The complement system is a cascade of soluble proteins that "complement" the function of antibodies in the immune system. Each complement protein is a proteolytic enzyme that acts as a substrate for the enzymes that precede it in the cascade, and which then acts as a part of a proteolytic complex for the next protein in the cascade. The classic complement pathway begins when C1q, C1r, and C1s (parts of the first component of complement) interact with membrane-bound antigen–antibody complexes to form an enzyme that cleaves C4 into C4a and C4b. C4b binds to the cell membrane, followed by C2, which is then split by C1s to yield a complex called *C4b,2a.* This complex splits C3 into C3a and C3b, which then joins the complex to make C4b,2a,3b. This complex cleaves C5 into C5a and C5b. C5b then binds to the cell membrane, and C6, C7, and C8 bind to it. The resulting C5b,6,7,8 complex then leads to C9 polymerization into the membrane of the target cell or a pathogen.

The alternate pathway of complement does not require antibody but can be activated directly by bacterial cell walls and is therefore a nonspecific defense mechanism. In this pathway, a small amount of pre-existing C3b cleaves factor B into Ba and Bb. The bacterial cell wall or other membranes assist in this step. The resulting C3b,Bb complex then cleaves more C3, forming a C3b,Bb,3b complex, which can then cleave C5, and the pathway proceeds as already described.

The result is the generation of chemotactic protein fragments (C5a), protein fragments that cause smooth muscle contraction (C3a and C5a), protein fragments that cause mast-cell degranulation (C5a), molecules that assist in neutrophil phagocytosis (C3b), and molecules that are capable of promoting cell lysis (C5b,6,7,8,9). The complement system is therefore involved in many of the effectors of the inflammatory response.

Complement has become an area of special focus because of its possible role in the pathogenesis of AMD. Complement factors have been found in the drusen of AMD eyes, suggesting that an immune response may have occurred after the activation of the complement cascade.[55] Several reports have appeared showing an association between a complement factor H variant and AMD.[56,57] These observations are thought provoking and remain functionally undefined. However, we felt that it may be part of a larger series of mechanisms that we collectively called the *downregulatory immune environment* of the eye.[58] Indeed, this concept is now supported by the report that the complement regulatory gene factor H (CFH) variant is associated with some forms of uveitis, hence an alteration not unique to AMD.[59]

Cellular Interactions: Hypersensitivity Reactions

Fig. 1.7 is a simplified version of the myriad interactions that have been identified in the immune system's repertoire in the eye. Although many exceptions and alternative (sometimes contradictory) mechanisms have been proposed or partially demonstrated, certain useful basic concepts can be of help to the observer. The initiation of a response leading to immune memory requires antigen to be presented to T cells. Classically, this is performed by dendritic cells and perhaps macrophages bearing the same class II (human leukocyte antigen [HLA]-DR) antigens as the T cells. Other cells, however, may also be equally competent in performing this task. Potential candidates in the eye include the vascular endothelium, RPE, and Müller cells. Macrophages release factors, such as IL-1, which are essential for the activation of the T cell. IL-1 also may be necessary as a cell-membrane component for antigen presentation to occur.

The subsets of T cells, discussed earlier, cover a wide range of functions, from aiding B cells to produce antibody, to cell-mediated killing, to modulation of the immune response. A point worth bearing in mind is that T-cell recruitment is very much dependent on the release of factors (cytokines) that help recruit and activate other initially uncommitted T cells. This seems to be a basic underlying mechanism for T-cell function.

Other cells also have a major impact on this T cell–B cell–macrophage axis. Mast-cell degranulation may assist the egress of immune cells into an organ, and the eosinophils and neutrophils will aid in killing and/or preparing pathogens for disposal by other parts of the immune system. T cells have a direct effect on mast-cell maturation in bone marrow by the release of IL-3, whereas the T cell and other immune components have similar effects on other cells of the nonlymphoid series by the release of colony-stimulating factors.

Classic Immune Hypersensitivity Reactions

Although it is not rare for any inflammatory response to involve several arms of the immune repertoire, it frequently appears that one arm of the system predominates. Inflammatory reactions were originally classified into four types or "hypersensitivity reactions" by British immunologists Philip Gell and Robin Coombs, with some recent additions.

Type I. This inflammatory reaction is mediated by antibodies, especially IgE. The binding of this antibody to mast cells or basophils results in the degranulation of these cells and the release of pharmacologically active products, as already mentioned. An ocular example of this reaction is hay fever. Typically, a large amount of edema without structural damage is noted. The role for this immune mechanism in intraocular inflammatory disease remains unclear. It is not inconceivable that mast cells could play an ancillary role in some cases, but hard evidence is still lacking.

Type II. This type of reaction is mediated by cytotoxic antibodies and is thought to mediate hemolytic disorders, such as blood mismatch reactions and the scarring seen in ocular pemphigoid. It is clear that in ocular pemphigoid, antibodies directed to the basement membrane of mucosal surfaces are present and may, indeed, be cytotoxic. One might consider the antibody effect of carcinoma- or melanoma-associated retinopathy to be a type II reaction. Intravitreal injections of human mixed antiglobulin reaction (MAR) IgG has been shown to alter retinal signaling.[60] Another ocular example may be the rare disorder acute annular outer retinopathy.[61] However, T cells can be noted to be infiltrating into the lesion in this disease. Some have suggested including reactions termed *antibody-dependent cell-mediated cytotoxicity* in this category, thereby making this category one that has a mixed mechanism.

Type III. This reaction is frequently referred to as an immune complex–mediated inflammatory response. The binding of antibody to an antigen – either fixed in tissue or free floating, which then deposits as a complex – can initiate the complement cascade, which, in turn, attracts cells capable of causing tissue damage. An example is the Arthus reaction, seen approximately 4 hours after the injection of antigen into the skin of a sensitized person or animal having substantial levels of circulating antibody directed to the antigen being injected locally. The role of immune complex–mediated tissue damage in the eye still needs to be defined. Immune complexes have been demonstrated in the aqueous humor of patients with uveitis.[61,62] Circulating immune complexes have been reported in patients with Behçet disease (see Chapter 27) and HLA-B27+ uveitis (see Chapter 20).[63,64] It is now believed, however, that this hypersensitivity reaction has a minor role in the pathogenesis of intraocular inflammatory disease, such as Behçet disease, but may play a major role in phacoanaphylaxis, a disorder that follows after damage to the lens and release of lens proteins and appears to be immune complex driven, at least partially.

Type IV. This category of immune response comprises those mediated solely by T cells. It is therefore termed a *cell-mediated immune mechanism,* rather than a humoral mechanism, as was the case for the other three types of hypersensitivity reactions. The positive skin test reaction noted 48 hours after a PPD skin test is an example of a type IV hypersensitivity reaction. Granulomatous responses, as seen in sarcoid and sympathetic ophthalmia, are mediated by this mechanism. In all of these cases, the humoral arm of the immune system is not thought to play a significant role in the inflammatory reaction. To date, evidence suggests that the pathogenic process is mediated by T cells sensitized against an ocular antigen. This notion is supported by similar pathologic changes in the eye seen in animals immunized against ocular-specific antigens. The animal disease EAU is discussed in detail later in the chapter.

Type V. This reaction has been added to the original four. In this reaction, an antibody can act as a stimulant to a target cell or organ. An example is long-acting thyroid stimulator (LATS) antibody, a feature of Graves' disease. The LATS antibody is directed toward a portion of the thyroid-stimulating hormone (TSH) receptor in the thyroid and mimics the function of TSH.

CONCEPTS OF DISEASE PATHOGENESIS

The potential mechanisms by which tissue damage is mediated by the immune system pose a question that has been hotly debated for some time. The debates are particularly vociferous because most arguments are difficult to support. However, recently these potential mechanisms have opened some of their secrets to observers, and the arguments of a previous generation are no longer acceptable. With our increased understanding of immune mechanisms comes the realization of the network's complexity: that the system has many alternative choices and that there is an extraordinary intertwining of events that appears to be necessary for the immune system to respond appropriately and inappropriately. It still is conceptually valid to simplify these potential mechanisms, and in the following sections we attempt to do that – to provide the reader with concepts rather than numerous specific details. The understanding of these mechanisms is certainly an intellectually stimulating undertaking. However, it has a practical aspect as well. Therapeutic interventions will be increasingly specific, tailored to the problem at hand. Therefore, in the not-too-distant future, an understanding of the mechanisms of ocular inflammatory disease will be invaluable in choosing the appropriate therapy for the patient.

Immune Characteristics of the Eye

It seems reasonable to begin a section on immune mechanisms that may be responsible for intraocular inflammatory disease by reviewing the characteristics of the eye that might influence these responses. For years, the eye was considered a "privileged" immune site. The implication of this was that the immune system somehow ignored or was tolerant of the antigens in the eye. We think it appropriate to consider the eye as being, indeed, immune privileged, but in a different way from that implied by the original notion. Although the characteristics to be reviewed are not always unique to the eye, the combination of all these factors does elevate this organ to a special relationship with the immune system.

Absence of Lymphatic Drainage

Like the brain, placenta, and testes, the eye has no direct lymphatic drainage, although in mice, submandibular nodes do collect antigen from the eye.[65] The environment in which antigen presentation occurs plays an important role in the type of immune response the organism may mount. Experimentally, for example, antigen placed in an area with good lymphatic drainage will elicit an excellent immune response, with a measurable antibody response and cell-mediated immune response. However, the same antigen given intravenously may elicit a very different immune response, the ultimate response being immune tolerance (or anergy). Therefore this anatomic phenomenon may have a profound effect on the types of immune response elicited in the eye.

Intraocular Microenvironment

It has been suggested that the eye has at least four ways to protect itself against unwanted or nuisance inflammatory processes. The first is having a barrier, such as the blood–ocular barrier. The second is the presence of soluble or membrane-bound inhibitors that block the function of invading organisms. The third strategy is to kill an invading organism or cell that may be inducing an unwanted inflammation (by perhaps speeding up apoptosis or programmed cell death), and the fourth is to devise a method by which a state of tolerance is induced.[66] All of these barriers appear to exist in the eye.

Anterior Chamber Associated Immune Deviation

This phenomenon could be seen as an example of the fourth strategy mentioned above. The immune response elicited by antigen placement into the anterior chamber has interested immunologists for some time.[67,68] Allogeneic tissue implants (i.e., tissue from the same species but not an identical twin) in the anterior chamber were noted to survive longer than those placed in other orthotopic sites.[69] The placement of alloantigens into the anterior chamber of the eye has been noted to elicit a transient depression of cell-mediated immunity but an intact humoral response.[70,71] The model has been further extended to include soluble antigen alone.[72] The capacity of the immune system to enhance or suppress tumor growth can be successfully manipulated by using this phenomenon. Good antibody responses and cytotoxic T cells directed against the intraocularly placed tumor (or antigen) develop. However, although cells that mediate delayed hypersensitivity reactions do not form, antigen-specific suppressor cells do. ACAID can be also induced in primates.[73]

Of prime importance in ACAID is the presence of an ocular–splenic axis. The induction of suppressor T cells is enhanced when antigen processing bypasses the lymphatic drainage system normally present. There appears to be a unique processing of antigen in the dendritic cells of the eye. Cells then carry the ACAID signal to the spleen for the activation of regulatory T cells.[74] It has been reported that this signal in blood was associated with F4/80+ macrophages, which populate the anterior uvea. Also of interest is the fact that in vitro exposure of APCs to aqueous humor – or TGF-β – confers ACAID-like properties on these cells. Indeed, TGF-β appears to play one of the important roles in ACAID.[75]

Physiologic Mechanisms for Inhibition of Ocular Inflammation: A Summary

The sight system is composed of numerous cell populations, many of which cannot be replaced, and the inflammatory process can cause damage to these cells and to vision. To protect against such damage, the eye is endowed with several anti-inflammatory preventive mechanisms. In addition, the potential development of damaging autoimmune processes is suppressed by two mechanisms: (1) the great majority of lymphocytes specific to ocular antigens are eliminated by the negative selection in the thymus; and (2) cells that escaped this process are inhibited by the population of Treg cells. On the latter immunosuppressive mechanisms see a recent review.[76]

Fas-Fas Ligand Interactions and Programmed Cell Death (Apoptosis)

Fas ligand (FasL) is a type II membrane protein that belongs to the TNF superfamily. It is found in the eye and can induce apoptotic cell death in cells that express Fas. Fas is part of the TNF receptor family and is found on lymphocytes. It is believed that apoptosis is one method of immune privilege in the eye.[77] Organs that appear to be able to limit immune responses, such as the eye, testes, and brain, express FasL. Other organs, such as the liver and the intestine, express this antigen only during severe inflammatory processes. Gene therapy experiments performed on other organs where FasL is transferred can confer immune privilege. It is clear that the Fas-FasL interaction works in concert with several factors. One cofactor appears to be TNF. Activated lymphocytes producing TNF will be more at risk to become apoptotic. Other mechanisms induce apoptosis through IL-2 activation of lymphocytes. These highly activated cells will ultimately die a programmed death. This raises the interesting question whether blockage of part of either the TNF system or the IL-2 circuitry, despite being beneficial on the one hand, could, on the other, prevent apoptosis of these cells, thereby leaving them at a site of inflammation longer or circulating longer.

Resident Ocular Cells and Immune System

Although communication between resident organ cells and the immune system is not unique to the eye, the number of cells potentially capable of fulfilling this role in the eye is, indeed, remarkable. The list begins at the cornea with Langerhans' cells and includes cells in the ciliary body that can express Ia antigens on their surfaces, the Müller cells, which are capable of profound effects on the immune response, and the RPE, with characteristics similar to those of macrophages. Finally, the vascular endothelium of the eye, as in other organs, may be of great importance in regulating immune system activity.

Müller cells have been shown to have a profound effect on T cells.[53] Isolated pure cultures of rat Müller cells downregulate the proliferative capabilities of S-Ag–specific T cells capable of inducing experimental uveitis. Cell-to-cell contact is needed to see this phenomenon. It is interesting to note that when Müller cells are killed with a specific poison, the disease induced by S-Ag immunization in rats appears to be worse than in rats with "intact" retinal Müller cells in the retina.[78] Such experiments would suggest that Müller cells play a role similar to that of ACAID – that is, as part of the protective mechanisms that downregulate "nuisance" inflammatory responses in the eye.

As mentioned, RPE cells have many of the characteristics of macrophages. These cells have the capacity to migrate and engulf particles and have characteristics that strongly suggest a capacity to participate in the local immune response. The RPE has been shown to produce cytokines, perhaps one of the most notable, to date, being IL-6,[79] a lymphokine capable of inducing intraocular inflammatory disease when injected into the eye. RPE cells, which express MHC class I antigens constitutively on their surface, can express class II antigens when

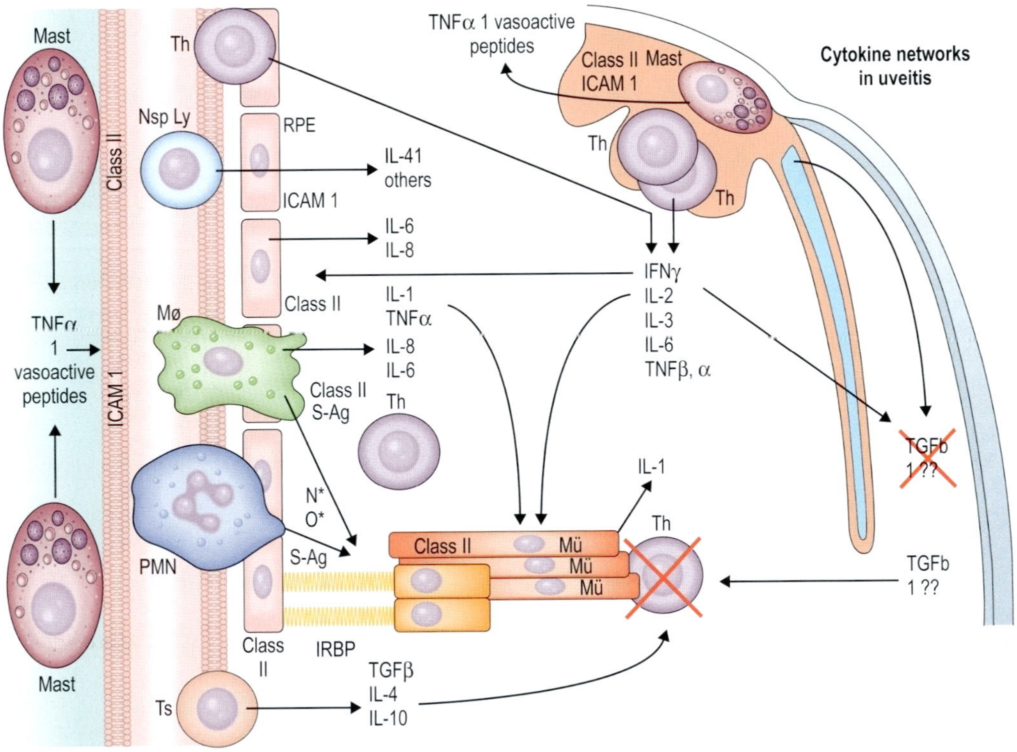

Fig. 1.7 Schematic representation of (1) numerous interactions in the eye of cells of the immune system, and (2) cells resident in the eye. (Courtesy Rachel Caspi, PhD.)

BOX 1.1 Cytokines

Proinflammatory Cytokines	
IL-1	TNF
IL-6	IL-2
IL-3	IL-8
IFN-γ	IL-4
IL-12	IL-17
Anti-inflammatory Cytokines	
TGF-β	IL-4 (systemic)
IFN-γ	IL-10

IFN, interferon; *IL*, interleukin; *TGF*, transforming growth factor; *TNF*, tumor necrosis factor.

activated[80] (see later discussion). Furthermore, RPE cells in culture can act as APCs for S-Ag–specific T cells. Here, then, it would appear that we have an example of an ocular resident cell capable of augmenting (or initiating?) an immune response in the eye, but there is no clinical proof to support this concept. However, we do have further experimental evidence that it could, indeed, happen. We have shown that the glucocorticoid-induced TNF-related receptor ligand (GITRL) is expressed constitutively at low levels on the RPE (and other ocular cells). When GITRL expression is upregulated on RPE cells, the suppressive effects of the RPE on T-cell proliferation is abrogated and so is the production of TGF-β, an important contributor to the downregulatory environment. GITRL upregulation also induced proinflammatory cytokines in T cells.[81] Interestingly, GITR serves as a negative regulator for NK cell activation.[82] Indeed, one may argue that there are so many APCs, such as macrophages and dendritic cells, in the eye that it really does not seem reasonable to think that these ocular resident cells would initiate an immune response.

Cytokines and Chemokines and the Eye

A large number of cytokines, some produced locally by ocular resident cells and others by cells of the immune system, have been implicated in the ocular immune response. In addition to cytokines, numerous neuropeptides and other factors have been cited as being involved in the ocular immune response (see Fig. 1.7, which shows the complex nature of this response). Cytokines can be termed "proinflammatory" or "immunosuppressive" in the intraocular milieu (Box 1.1). Some cytokines have been noted to both stimulate and suppress the immune response, depending on the environment in which the cytokine is found. Instead of considering it contradictory, this phenomenon should be viewed as evidence of the complex immune response we are studying. IL-6 (produced locally), IL-2, and IFN-γ are perhaps the most important cytokines to be considered when an intraocular inflammatory response occurs. Foxman et al.[83] evaluated the simultaneous expression of several cytokines, chemokines, and chemokine receptors in the eye during an inflammatory episode. Of interest were the relatively high levels of chemokine activity in noninflamed eyes. For experimental autoimmune uveitis, IL-1α, IL-1β, IL-1 receptor antagonist, IL-6, and TNF-α were highly expressed (Fig. 1.8). IFN-β is found in the serum of a large number of retinal vasculitis patients (including those with Behçet disease).[84] Importantly, in more recent studies, IL-17 was found to play a major role in most inflammatory eye conditions including Behçet disease.[85]

The ocular downregulatory immune environment (DIE) appears to be rich with many factors, as already noted: in addition to TGF-β,[86] which has been localized to trabecular cells,[87] α-melanocyte-stimulating hormone,[88] calcitonin gene-related peptide,[89] and vasoactive intestinal peptide are also found in the eye.[90] Other factors, such as hormones, may significantly affect the microenvironment. Sternberg et al.[91] have shown that rats not capable of mounting a major intrinsic cortisol response to trauma (or immunization with protein) are more prone to the development of autoimmune disorders. This observation is of

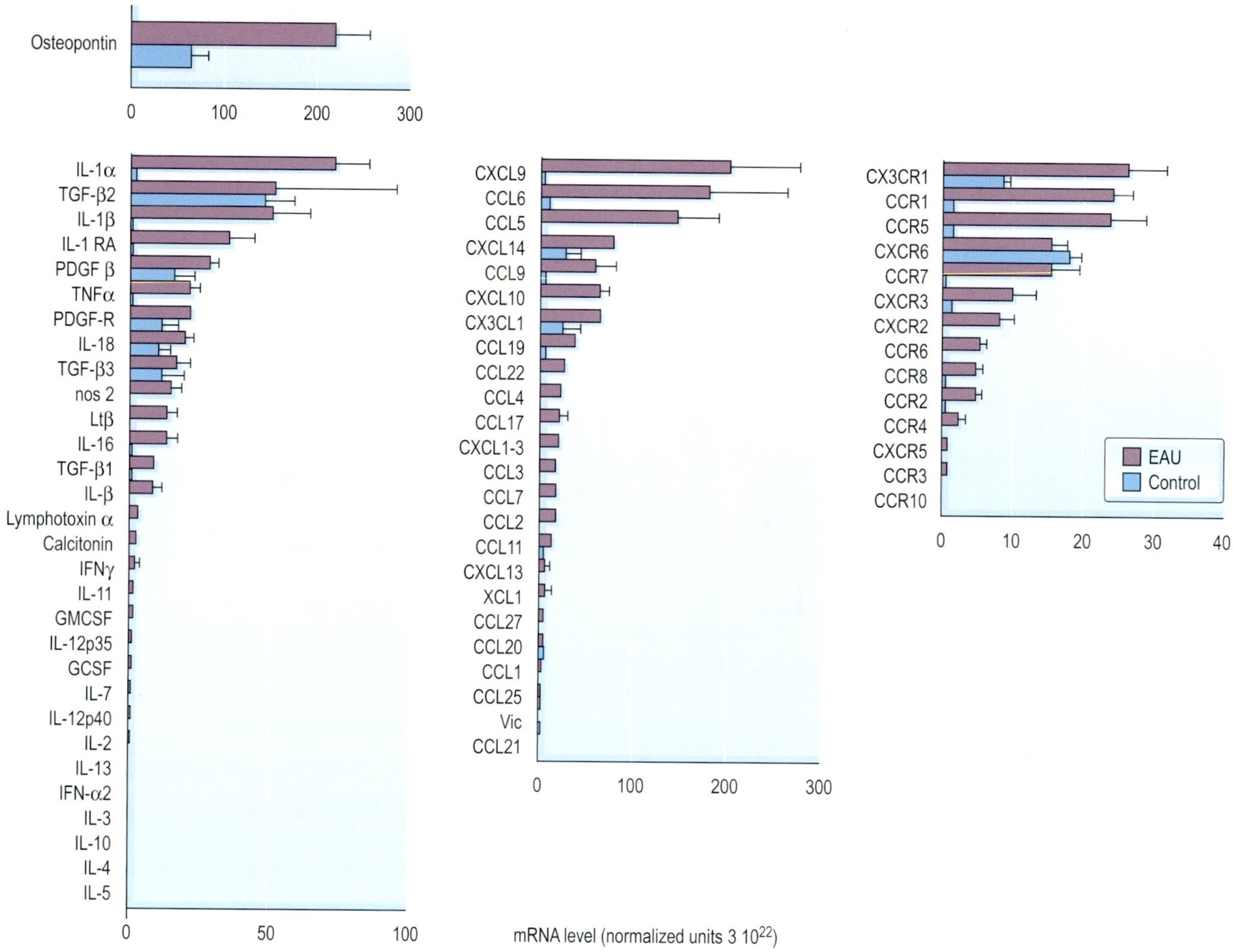

Fig. 1.8 Upregulation of cytokines, chemokines, and chemokine receptor messenger ribonucleic acid (mRNA) transcripts in eyes with experimental autoimmune uveitis (EAU). Animals were immunized with interphotoreceptor retinoid-binding protein (IRBP) to induce disease. (From Foxman EF, Zhang M, Hurst SD, et al. Inflammatory mediators in uveitis: differential induction of cytokines and chemokines in Th1- versus Th2-mediated ocular inflammation. *J Immunol.* 2002;168:2483–2492. Copyright 2002, American Association of Immunologists.)

further interest because the aqueous is deficient in cortisol-binding globulin; therefore this hormone could play a most important role in downregulating an immune response in the eye.[92]

Oral Tolerance

Oral tolerance has long been recognized as inducing systemic tolerance. It was first described in 1911 by Wells,[93] who prevented anaphylaxis in guinea pigs by feeding them egg protein. Information about positive mechanisms has been gained over the past few years.[94] Three possible immune mechanisms can be hypothesized: clonal deletion of autoaggressive cells, clonal anergy, and active suppression. Most information would suggest that active suppression is perhaps a predominant mechanism, but it is also clear that clonal anergy can be demonstrated under certain circumstances.[95,96] TGF-β appears to be the basic mediator of the active suppression seen after feeding. In studies using myelin basic protein, oral tolerance has been shown to markedly alter the expression of S-Ag–induced EAU.[97] Feeding S-Ag to Lewis rats before immunization with this antigen suppressed the expression of EAU. Feeding of S-Ag even after immunization with S-Ag still was capable of suppressing EAU. Furthermore, regulatory cells could be isolated from the spleen of fed animals. These are Th2 cells, cells that are capable of downregulating, as opposed to the pro–immune-augmenting Th1 cells. An intact spleen appears to be important in the development of this phenomenon.[98] It is of interest to note that nasal administration of retinal antigens can also suppress E.[99]

Because of these initial data and information being gathered from our collaborators working in the realm of other animal models and with patients having multiple sclerosis, we embarked on a pilot study, in which we fed S-Ag to two patients who had uveitis and were receiving immunosuppressive therapy for their disease. Feeding S-Ag could replace the suppressive therapy in reducing the inflammatory process. A double-masked study resulted from these initial findings (see Chapter 8). Feeding either the antigen itself, or an HLA peptide that cross-reacts with S-Ag, has shown promise.[100,101]

Choroidal Circulation and Anatomy

The choroid has a blood flow comparable only with that of the kidney. Therefore systemic influences can be assumed to rapidly affect this portion of the eye. Indeed, the relatively large blood flow and its anatomy would act as a sort of trap for many bloodborne problems, most notably fungal disorders. Therefore most fungal lesions begin as a choroiditis.[102] The choroid has the capacity to function as a repository

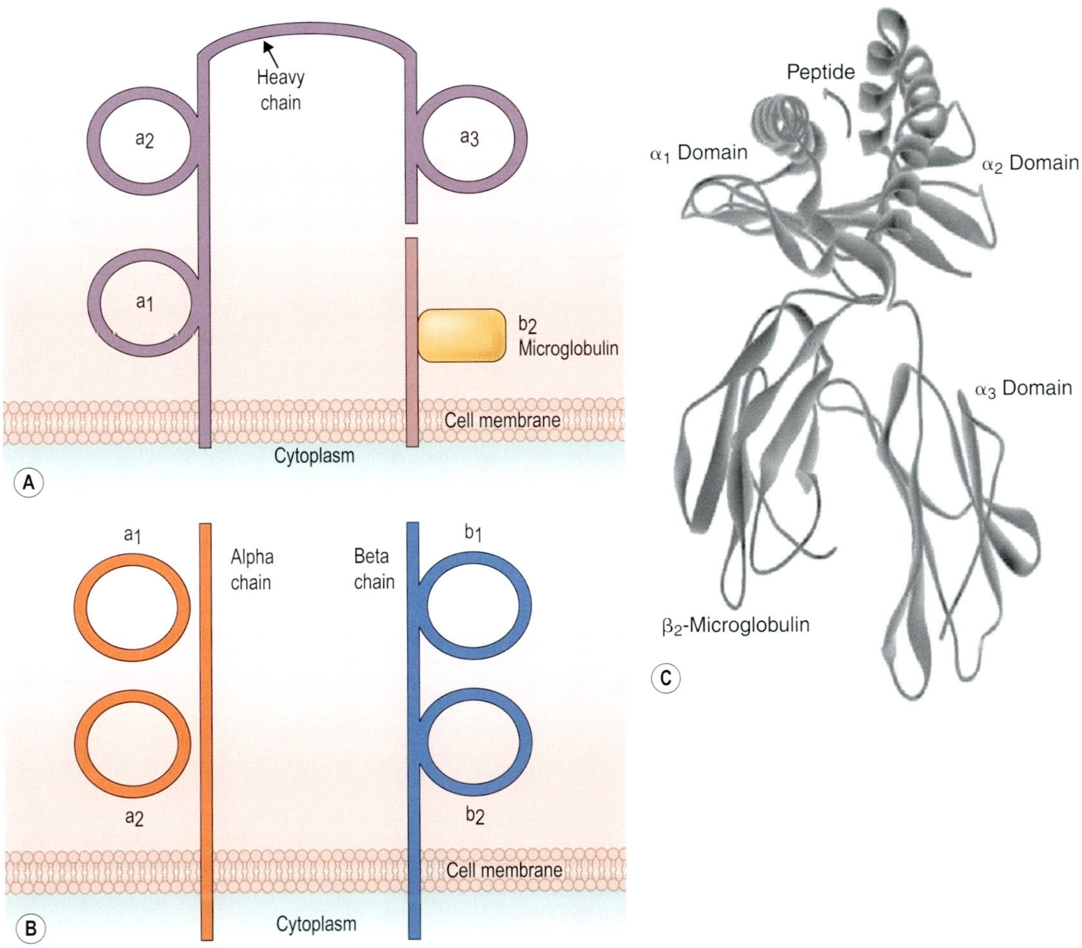

Fig. 1.9 (A) Structure of class I antigen. (B) Structure of class II antigen. (C) Three-dimensional view of class I antigen bound to peptide. (From Lopez-Larrea C, Gonzalez S, Martinez-Borra J. The role of HLA-B27 polymorphism and molecular mimicry in spondyloarthropathy. *Mol Med Today.* 1998;4:540–549.)

for immunoreactive cells, in the extreme taking on the anatomic structure of a lymph node (lymphoid hyperplasia). Therefore this organ can be the center for profound immune responses, as is the case in many disorders to be discussed. The high concentration of mast cells in the choroid may be one mechanism by which immunoreactive cells in the choroid could spread to other parts of the eye. The mast cell's release of immunoreactive factors could help T-cell egress and ingress from this compartment.

Retina

In addition to the uveitogenic antigens resident in its layers, the retina being an "extension of the brain" makes it particularly prone to certain neurotropic organisms. Examples include *T. gondii* and many viruses of the herpes family, which have a propensity for central nervous system tissue.

It is also important to remember that under normal circumstances, the retinal vasculature has tight junctions, thus being impermeable to cells and many molecules. Any perturbation that alters this permeability, such as inflammation, can result in a profound change in retinal functioning. Furthermore, it is interesting to speculate that because the retina maintains a high degree of oxidative metabolism, the potential for the generation of oxygen radicals may lead to autotoxicity.

IMMUNOGENETICS

The capacity to respond to a specific immune stimulant is genetically determined. It has been noted that various mouse strains are variably susceptible to the same bacterial infection.[103] Another example of such a variable response is that seen against an allograft – that is, tissue taken from the same species but from an animal of another inbred strain. The strength of the immune reaction against the allograft is, in large part, determined by antigens sitting on cell-surface membranes that are the products of genes classified as being in the MHC. The MHC region is termed the *H-2 region* in mice, and the HLA region in humans. Immune response *(IR)* genes were discovered by Benacerraf et al.[104] in their experiments evaluating the immune response of guinea pigs to amino acid polymers. Breeding and cross-breeding led to the realization that a genetic region was responsible for this responsiveness or nonresponsiveness.[105] McDevitt and Chinitz[106] showed that antibody responses in mice to synthetic polypeptides were, indeed, linked to the MHC region. The observation that one region appeared to be responsible for both transplantation and general immune responses evoked enormous interest and led to the realization of the importance of this region. The *HLA* gene loci are found on chromosome 6 in humans. Three major classes of antigen are controlled by these genes.

Class I Antigens

Class I antigens, which are proteins found on essentially all nucleated cells, are controlled by three loci in humans: A, B, and C. The class I molecule has a molecular weight of about 45 kDa, is a glycoprotein, and is noncovalently linked to a β_2-microglobulin (Fig. 1.9, A and C). The β_2-microglobulin molecule is not encoded within the MHC region but, rather, on chromosome 15 and is linked to the class I molecule at a later stage. A strong homology has been shown between moieties of the class I molecule and immunoglobulins, suggesting similar early evolutionary paths. Class I molecules are quite heterogeneous, and several cell-surface membrane antigens controlled by each of the loci are defined. Complement-fixing cytotoxic antibodies can be raised against each variation, and these antigens are determined by serologic methods. The class I molecule has an extracellular portion extending through the membrane into the cytoplasm of the cell. Although the precise mechanisms are still unknown, it is known that class I antigens participate in transplantation immunity by being the principal antigenic targets in allograft rejection. They also serve as recognition antigens for cytotoxic (CD8) T cells when they attack virally infected cells.

Class II and Class III Antigens

Class II antigens are produced by the HLA-D/DR locus. There has been considerable debate as to whether the D/DR systems are the same. Some discrepancies in typing by means of the two methods have been noted in some nonwhite populations. Numerous alleles have been identified in the DR system. The test is performed on B cells by means of a complement-dependent microcytotoxicity assay and use of sera from multiparous women. The HLA-D/DR loci are thought to be the equivalent of the *IR* gene region, as already discussed. Furthermore, expression of the cell-surface molecules controlled by these loci has been given the generic term *Ia antigens.* The class II molecule is different from that of the class I molecule. Here it is made up of an α chain with a molecular weight of 35 kDa and a β chain of about 28 kDa, which are noncovalently bound. No β_2-microglobulin is present (see Fig. 1.9, B).

The importance of the *MHC* gene products cannot be overstated because large components of the immune response are histocompatibility restricted; that is, immune cooperation will occur only if both components share identical D/DR antigens. B- and T-cell cooperation and T-cell cooperation with macrophages are examples. This means that macrophages from one individual cannot present antigen to T cells from another unless they express the same class II antigens. In the case of the eye, the appearance of DR (or Ia) antigens on the cell surface of resident ocular cells (not usually thought of as part of the immune system) may indicate the potential for their role as accessory immune cells. Forrester et al.[107] found that the posterior uveal tract is richly populated with classic dendritic cells that constitutively express high levels of MHC II antigens. Those authors further speculated about their important role in the interaction of resident ocular cells with the immune system and, by extension, their initiation of autoimmune responses in the posterior pole.

Class III antigens produced within the MHC region are components of the complement cascade. Control of the levels of C1, C2, and C4 may also be encoded in this region.

Histocompatibility Lymphocyte Antigens

A logical adjunct to the recognition of the critical role the MHC region plays in the organism's immune response was the attempt to correlate certain disease processes with HLA antigens. There are several loci determining class I and II antigens (HLA A, B, C, DR, DQ, etc.). Each human has the capacity to express many different alleles. In the early days testing could not reveal that number in many persons, either because they had yet undetermined antigens or because they were homozygote for a specific allele. Associations have been made with certain diseases and HLA antigens. Brewerton et al.[108] were among the first to observe that an extremely high percentage of white patients with ankylosing spondylitis showed HLA-B27 positivity. The testing of other racial groups could not demonstrate as strong a correlation. Khan et al.[109] demonstrated that HLA-B7 was, indeed, associated with ankylosing spondylitis in African Americans to a greater degree than was HLA-B27. One can infer from this and other studies that HLA associations may be different for various ethnic groups, and perhaps that different genes initiate responses that lead ultimately to a common pathway that we identify as disease. HLA allele distributions can vary dramatically from one ethnic group to another.[110] Therefore identifying an HLA association in patients with a specific disease requires testing a large group of persons from the same gene pool who do not have the disease in question. This is done to determine the normal distribution of HLA antigens in that ethnic group. Only with this approach can it be determined whether a specific HLA antigen is more prevalent in a disease entity.

An example of such an HLA distribution can be seen from our studies dealing with birdshot retinochoroidopathy (Table 1.5) (see Chapter 26). One can see from Table 1.5 the distribution of alleles in both the white control and the white patient populations. Although not perhaps apparent initially, certain antigens may appear together more frequently than estimated by chance. This phenomenon is termed *linkage disequilibrium.* It indicates that certain HLA antigens appear consistently together more often than chance would allow. Such examples are HLA-A1, which is in known linkage disequilibrium with HLA-B8 and HLA-DR3; another would be HLA-A3 with HLA-B7 and HLA-DR2. In Table 1.6, it is HLA-A29 and HLA-B44. The percentage of patients bearing specific antigens can be seen, and the relative risk is calculated as follows:

Relative risk = Antigen-positive patients ×
Antigen-negative control subjects/
Antigen-negative patients ×
Antigen-positive control subjects

The relative risk is an important indicator of the strength of the observation because it indicates the increased risk for development of a given disease in persons having the antigen relative to those not carrying it. For birdshot retinochoroidopathy, it tells the observer that a white person who has the HLA-A29 antigen has an almost 50 times greater potential risk for this disease. Others have even calculated a higher relative risk for this disorder. Relative risks that are three to five times or less are usually of little practical help in determining risk. Some studies have used historic HLA data – that is, results obtained by others, perhaps at different institutions, possibly with different anti-HLA sera. It is clear that the use of such control subjects should be avoided, if possible. Because of the great possible variation of HLA alleles in different groups, the use of control subjects of the same ethnic or racial group as that of patients in the disease group is essential. Although there are mathematic programs to mix information gained from different ethnic or racial groups, the data obtained from these attempts are quite suspect. The basic rule poses real problems for those doing this type of research in countries with large numbers of citizens who are of mixed racial and ethnic parentage, such as Brazil, where great regional differences in HLA distribution are seen. Such problems also exist in India where, because of a strict caste system, groups rarely intermarry, thereby creating a large number of "mini-gene pools" in a society that, to an outsider, may appear homogeneous.

Ocular diseases have been evaluated extensively for their HLA associations (see Table 1.6), some of which have large relative risks associated with them. The reader should always scrutinize the findings carefully, bearing in mind the aforementioned principles. Why should there be an association between HLA and certain diseases? The answer is that the reasons are unclear. The association may, indeed, reflect a specific immune response gene or one with which that gene is in linkage disequilibrium. Other concepts deal with HLA antigens and the exogenous environment. A provocative theory is one that was suggested by Bottazzo et al.[111] some years ago. The reasoning behind this hypothesis is the requirement of class II antigens for antigen presentation and the

TABLE 1.5 **Distribution of HLA haplotypes in patients with birdshot retinochoroidopathy and in control subjects**

	PHENOTYPE FREQUENCY (%)			
HLA-A	**Control Subjects (n = 418)**	**Patients (n = 20)**	**Exact *P* value**	**Relative Risk HLA-A**
1	24.4	20.0	0.7935	0.78
2	52.6	35.0	0.1687	0.49
3	27.3	15.0	0.3044	0.47
9	17.9	10.0	0.5493	0.51
10	13.9	10.0	1.0000	0.69
11	13.6	5.0	0.4955	0.33
23	2.6	5.0	0.4335	1.95
24	14.6	5.0	0.3337	0.31
25	5.5	0.0	0.6147	0.00
26	8.1	10.0	0.6751	1.26
28	8.4	5.0	1.0000	0.58
29	7.4	80.0	0.0000[a]	49.94
30	5.5	0.0	0.6147	0.00
31	4.3	0.0	1.0000	0.00
32	9.3	10.0	1.0000	1.08
33	1.4	0.0	1.0000	0.00
36	0.2	0.0	1.0000	0.00
HLA-B				
5	13.6	5.0	0.4955	0.33
7	20.1	30.0	0.2676	1.70
8	14.4	20.0	0.5133	1.49
12	27.5	50.0	0.0409[b]	2.64
13	4.8	0.0	0.6147	0.00
14	7.7	20.0	0.0719	3.02
15	13.6	0.0	0.0911	0.00
16	11.7	10.0	1.0000	0.84
17	10.5	10.0	1.0000	0.94
18	8.1	10.0	0.6751	1.26
21	9.3	10.0	1.0000	1.08
22	3.1	0.0	1.0000	0.00
27	8.9	0.0	3.978	0.00
35	19.4	15.0	0.7775	0.073
37	2.4	0.0	1.0000	0.00
38	7.4	5.0	1.0000	0.66
39	4.3	5.0	0.5964	1.17
40	12.0	10.0	1.0000	0.82
42	0.5	0.0	1.0000	0.00
44	25.4	45.0	0.6690	2.41
45	1.9	5.0	0.3460	2.70
47	0.7	0.0	1.0000	0.00
48	0.2	0.0	1.0000	0.00
49	5.7	5.0	1.0000	0.86
50	3.1	5.0	0.4855	1.64
51	6.0	5.0	1.0000	0.83
52	3.8	0.0	1.0000	0.00

Continued

TABLE 1.5 Distribution of HLA haplotypes in patients with birdshot retinochoroidopathy and in control subjects—cont'd

	PHENOTYPE FREQUENCY (%)			
HLA-A	Control Subjects (n = 418)	Patients (n = 20)	Exact *P* value	Relative Risk HLA-A
53	3.4	0.0	1.0000	0.00
54	1.0	0.0	1.0000	0.00
55	0.7	0.0	1.0000	0.00
HLA-C1				
1	8.4	5.0	1.0000	0.58
2	9.1	10.0	0.7028	1.11
3	25.4	10.0	0.1819	0.33
4	20.6	15.0	0.7769	0.68
5	5.7	10.0	0.3358	1.82
6	5.5	5.0	1.0000	0.90

[a]$P < 0.0001$.
[b]$P < 0.05$.
From Nussenblatt RB, Mittal KK, Ryan S, et al. Birdshot retinochoroidopathy – an association with HLA-A29 and immune responsiveness to retinal S-antigen. *Am J Ophthalmol.* 1982;94:147–158. Used with permission.
HLA, histocompatibility lymphocyte antigen.

TABLE 1.6 Selected ocular diseases and their HLA associations

Disease	Antigen	Relative Risk
Acute anterior uveitis	HLA-B27 (W)	10
	HLA-B8 (AA)	5
Ankylosing spondylitis	HLA-B27 (W)	100
	HLA-B7 (AA)	
Complex-mediated disease	HLA-B51 (O) (?W)	4–6
Birdshot retinochoroidopathy	HLA-A29 (W)	49
Ocular pemphigoid	HLA-B12 (W)	3–4
Presumed ocular histoplasmosis	HLA-B7	(W)
Reiter syndrome	HLA-B27 (W)	40
Rheumatoid arthritis	HLA-DR4 (W)	11
Sympathetic ophthalmia	HLA-A11 (M)	3.9
Vogt-Koyanagi-Harada disease	MT–3 (O)	74.5

AA, African American; *HLA,* histocompatibility lymphocyte antigen; *M,* mixed ethnic study; *O,* oriental; *W,* white.

initiation of the immune response. The inappropriate expression of class II coupled with other lapses of immune surveillance could lead to disease. A study that would support this notion was reported by Taurog et al.[112] In rats transgenic for HLA-B27 and β_2-microglobulin, these authors found that the B27 transgene was expressed in a copy number–dependent fashion, and inflammatory disease depended on the expression of B27 above a critical threshold. The implication of essentially all theories is that mechanisms to produce disease are multifactorial and that exogenous and endogenous immune factors are needed. If not, disease expression would be far more common. Caspi et al.[113] performed a long series of experiments in mice with experimentally induced uveitis, and their findings support this idea. From their observations, it is clear that the MHC plays a very important role in determining disease susceptibility. In mice, certain permissive MHC types would include the H-2^k. However, the genetic background of the experimental mice plays a very important role in determining the severity of disease such that a permissive MHC in a nonpermissive background will result in either very mild or no disease at all. Others have suggested that for some HLA antigens, it is a question of molecular mimicry, with clones that escaped the negative selection process in the thymus being activated by exogenous factors and ultimately attacking tissue when self-peptide is presented in the context of HLA-B27 (Fig. 1.10). Molecular mimicry is an often used hypothesis, in which sequences from one antigen, whether from the host or from an invading organism, are very similar to sequences found in the proteins of the body. An immune response directed against the first antigen may thus be misdirected against the second. Therefore an antigen derived from a pathogen may be similar to sequences of a structure in the eye, and the immune response initially directed against the pathogen will now be directed against the eye. This notion is supported by recent studies showing activation of naïve T cells by the gut microbiota (see discussion on the microbiome below).

Single-Nucleotide Polymorphisms

An area that has received much attention is the genetic variations found normally in genes that mediate the immune response as opposed to those that control it. Any two random genomes are essentially identical: perhaps only 0.1% of the sequences will vary. Although this variance is caused by several factors, the most common reason is single-nucleotide polymorphisms (SNPs), which are found throughout the genome, are stable, and are not considered mutations but, rather, (but relatively rare) variations from the norm. They are markers for different allelic forms of genes that can perform many different functions. For the purposes of this discussion, single-nucleotide changes can be found in genes whose products, such as the cytokines, play an important role in the immune response. Indeed, one cytokine may have several SNP variations. Some SNPs do not appear to change the functioning of the protein at hand, but others appear to do so. An example would be an SNP in the promoter region of a cytokine that when stimulated

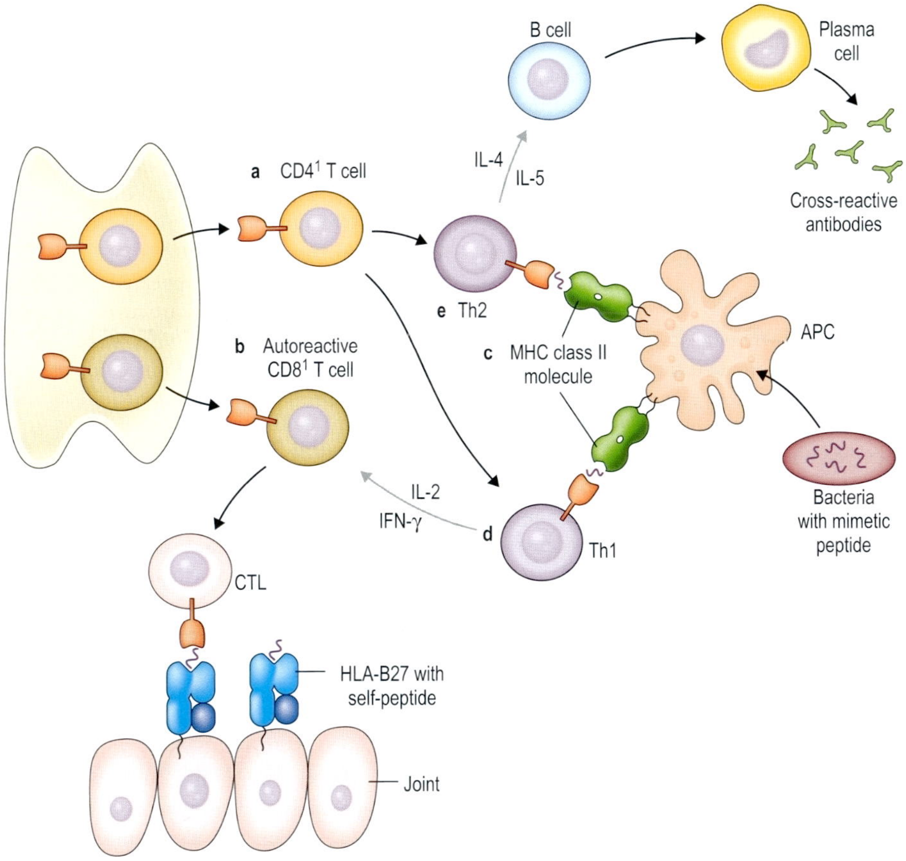

Fig. 1.10 Molecular mimicry concept of autoimmunity as it may apply to histocompatibility lymphocyte antigen (HLA)-B27. Clones of cells (a and b) escape positive and negative thymic selection described earlier in the chapter. They are capable of responding to autoantigens. These cells come into close contact with the antigen-processing cell (c), which has processed antigenic material from bacterium. Antigen mimics that of self-antigen. After antigenic information has been transferred, these cells are activated, becoming either Th1 or Th2 cells (e and d). They then elicit lymphokines, which produce a cell-mediated response against self-peptide linked to the HLA-B27 or a B-cell/plasma-cell response, with antibodies also directed against the self-peptide. (From Lopez-Larrea C, Gonzalez S, Martinez-Borra J, et al. The role of HLA-B27 polymorphism and molecular mimicry in spondyloarthropathy. *Mol Med Today*. 1998;4(12):540–549.)

produces either less or more of the given cytokine. One could imagine, then, that if population studies were performed as with HLA – that is, a disease group versus controls – SNPs might be identified more commonly in the disease group and hence possibly associated with disease. This is, indeed, what has been done and is actively being done for many disorders, some of which are autoimmune and some neoplastic.[114] As mentioned earlier, variants of the *CFH* gene have been associated with age-related macular degeneration and uveitis (multifocal choroiditis).

Epigenetics

The current definition of *epigenetics* is "the study of mechanisms that control somatically heritable gene expression status without changes in the underlying deoxyribonucleic acid (DNA) sequence,[115] including DNA methylation/demethylation; histone modification (acetylation/deacetylation); chromatin modification; and control of transcription by noncoding ribonucleic acids (RNAs: small interfering RNA [siRNA], micro-RNA [miRNA]). We are evaluating the involvement of DNA methylation in the immune system and the eye. DNA methylation has been shown to participate in the control of hematopoietic cell development. Comprehensive studies on DNA methylation in controlling cytokine expression in other immune cells (e.g., monocytes, NK cells and B cells) and genes with anti-inflammatory effect (e.g., *IL-10*), are still lacking. This will be an area that will be very actively studied. It is hoped that such studies will help us understand why one person with a particular gene sequence has the disease, whereas another with the same sequence does not.

Gene Expression Profiling

Technology now permits the analysis of up- or downregulation in many genes at once. We were interested in characterizing gene expression in monocytes from the blood of patients with uveitis. Using a pathway-specific complementary DNA (cDNA) microarray, we found that 67 inflammation- and autoimmune-associated gene products were differentially expressed in these cells. IL-22, IL-19, IL-20, IL-17, and IL-25 were highly expressed. We also found that there were four general patterns of gene expression, which were seen in related individuals but did not necessarily correlate with clinical entities. Clearly, multiple gene upregulation combinations can lead to the same clinical disease. This once again emphasizes how heterogeneous humans are.[116]

T-cell Responses and Autoimmunity

On the basis of current concepts of autoimmunity and their apparent relevance to the eye, it seems appropriate to discuss T-cell mechanisms here because they appear to be inextricably intertwined. T-cell mechanisms are mediated not by the humoral route but, rather, through the direct contact of the T cell to the target cell or other immune cells or through its release of lymphokines, thereby controlling the recruitment of other cells into the site of an immune response, these cells ultimately being effector cells. In addition, T cells play a major suppressive role, both specific and nonspecific. Therefore dysregulation of this exquisite balance leading to autoimmunity would logically need to involve T cells.

Autoimmunity is an immune response directed against the host. This phenomenon is common and, in the vast number of individuals, does not lead to obvious disease. It is when these initial autoimmune mechanisms lead to tissue damage that we denote the outcome as autoimmune disease.[117] The mechanisms for autoimmune disease may vary considerably, depending on the organ in question. Several mechanisms may lead ultimately to one final disease entity because of the relatively restricted way in which an organ is capable of responding to any immune response. Allison[118] theorized that although sensitization may occur, the expression of disease would not be seen as long as the effector T cell is rendered "tolerant" to the antigen in question. This notion is in line with more recent studies revealing the existence of T cells specific to autoantigens in the circulation of normal animals. Activation of these cells by TLR ligands (e.g., lipopolysaccharides [LPS]) was found by Fujimoto et al. to initiate pathogenic processes.[119] This hypothesis is also in line with findings of molecular mimicry (see discussion of the microbiome below).

T-CELL RECEPTOR AND THE EXPRESSION OF DISEASE

As mentioned earlier, much interest has centered on the antigen receptor expressed on the T-cell surface. The TCR has a complex structure, made up of several chains controlled by different genes. It has been suggested that a specific subfamily, the β chain of the TCR, is preferentially expressed on autoaggressive lymphocytes. In rats the Vβ8.2 subfamily epitope is expressed on a disproportionately large number of T cells capable of inducing EAU in naive animals.[120,121] Further work has refined this concept to a degree. It would appear that the Vβ8 family is expressed in these cells, but not necessarily exclusively. Egwuagu et al.[122] found that in rats, the T cells invading the retina in S-Ag–induced EAU preferentially express Vβ8.2, but IRBP-immunized animals had in their retinas, at an early stage of EAU, T cells bearing both the Vβ8.2 and Vβ8.3 phenotypes. Furthermore, in mice, Rao et al.[123] demonstrated a preferential usage of Vβ2, Vβ12, and Vβ15. These findings have both basic scientific and practical clinical implications. If it were true that one subfamily of Vβ8 was always expressed on T cells that are autoaggressive (i.e., induce autoimmune disease), then one could use this as a marker to identify such cells in the body, and, perhaps more importantly, these TCR peptide fragments could be used as a vaccinating agent to induce protection against all cells bearing this particular structure. Indeed, immunization (i.e., vaccination) with the Vβ8.2 fragments suppressed experimental autoimmune encephalomyelitis (EAE).[124] These results could not be reproduced, however, in the EAU model.[125] It is important to note that many questions still remain about the TCR–peptide–MHC complex. Structural biologic studies have not fully elucidated this relationship.[126] In one study,[127] in which the crystal structure of these relationships was evaluated, it was noted that the interface between the TCR and the peptide to which it is bound had minimal shape complementarity, and the β chain of the TCR, which is thought to determine the complementarity, had minimal interaction with the peptide. There was also a structural plasticity to the TCR once binding took place, suggesting a certain accommodation to different but similar proteins that it could or might bind with. In the evaluation of the crystal structure of an immunodominant sequence of myelin basic protein (which induces EAE, a model of multiple sclerosis), the binding of the antigen in the TCR groove was found to be weak, and only a portion of the groove was occupied by the disease-inducing antigen.[128]

Ocular Autoimmunity

The concept that the eye harbors autoimmune-inducing or uveitogenic materials has been suggested by many since the beginning of this century. It was the demonstration of autoantibody production to the lens by Uhlenhuth[129] that pioneered this whole area of investigation. Several investigators used homogenates from the eye which, when injected into an animal, appeared capable of inducing an intraocular inflammatory response. Particular tribute must be paid to Wacker et al.,[130] working in Louisville, Kentucky, and to Jean-Pierre Faure et al.,[131] working in Paris, France, for their zeal and scientific prowess in this area.

Experimental Autoimmune Uveitis

As repeatedly mentioned earlier, the investigation of inflammatory eye disease was mainly carried out in animals in which similar ocular diseases were induced. The most commonly used system is that of EAU, a disease that closely resembles the family of uveitic conditions, assumed to be mediated by pathogenic T lymphocytes.[132] EAU is inducible in several experimental animals, immunized with ocular-specific antigens, but the most commonly used is EAU in mice, induced by immunization with IRBP or with peptides derived from its sequence, emulsified in complete Freund adjuvant (CFA), along with treatment with *Pertussis* toxin. Ocular inflammation develops within approximately 2 weeks and can be measured by both funduscopy and histologic analysis. The two methods are detailed in the report by Horai et al.[133] Fig. 1.11 also demonstrates the similarity between the histopathologic changes in the mouse eye with EAU and the changes in a patient with sarcoidosis, namely, retinal detachment and accumulation of exudate in the subretinal space. Fig. 1.12 shows sections of typical EAU changes in monkeys and mice, with EAU induced by whole IRBP, or peptides 651 to 670, respectively. Many changes in the diseased animal eyes resemble those seen in human eyes with uveitis.

Uveitogenic Antigens

Several antigens that are capable of inducing ocular disease in rodents – in many respects similar to that seen in humans – have been isolated. This number of identifiable antigens capable of stimulating the immune system makes the eye unique and suggests that the old concept of autoimmunity may be an important factor in ocular disease.

Retinal S-antigen (arrestin). Wacker and colleagues[130] reported the isolation, partial characterization, and immunologic properties of the retinal S-Ag in 1977, with the French group (Jean-Pierre Faure et al.)[131] soon after adding important new dimensions to this most important observation. The retinal S-Ag is one of the most potent of the uveitogenic antigens defined to date. This 48-kDa intracellular protein is localized to the photoreceptor region of the retina and the pineal gland in some species. Preparations from various species demonstrate high levels of cross-reactivity, reflecting the fact that the molecule appears to be highly conserved through evolution. The function of S-Ag is to mediate rhodopsin-catalyzed adenosine triphosphate (ATP) binding and to quench cyclic guanosine monophosphate (cGMP) phosphodiesterase (PDE) activation. It binds to photoactivated phosphorylated rhodopsin, preventing the transducin-mediated activation of PDE.[134]

S-Ag is highly uveitogenic in rats,[135] guinea pigs,[130] and primates.[136] As mentioned earlier, most mouse strains, however, are resistant to the disease induced by this antigen because of its being highly expressed in the thymuses of these animals. Interestingly, Pennesi et al.[137] have created a transgenic mouse that has been humanized in terms of its HLA

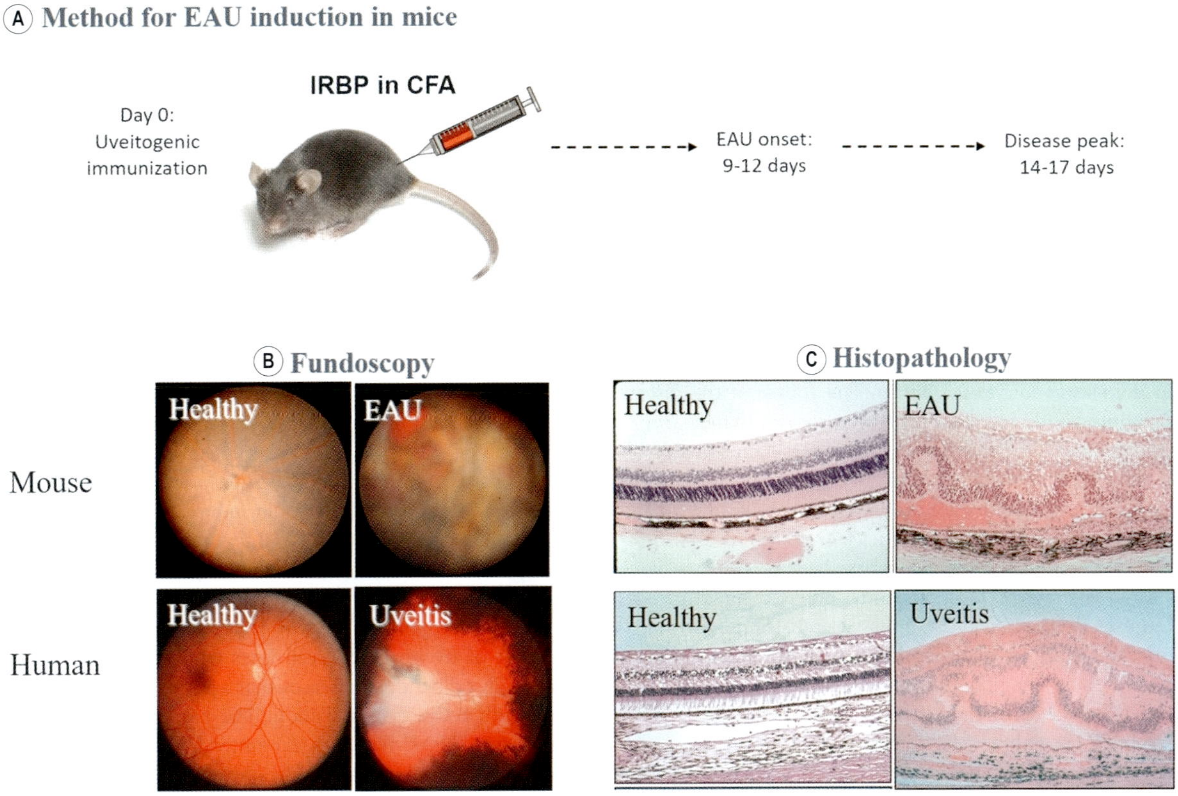

Fig. 1.11 (A) Induction of experimental autoimmune uveitis (EAU) in mice. (B) Funduscopic features of EAU with retinal infiltrates, edema, and disorganization and those of a human case with uveitis (sarcoidosis) with infiltrates and fibrosis. (C) Similar histopathological changes in a mouse with EAU and a patient with uveitis: retinal detachment and accumulation of exudate in the subretinal space. (Courtesy Drs. Igal Gery, Rachel Caspi, and Chi Chao Chan, National Eye Institute [NEI].)

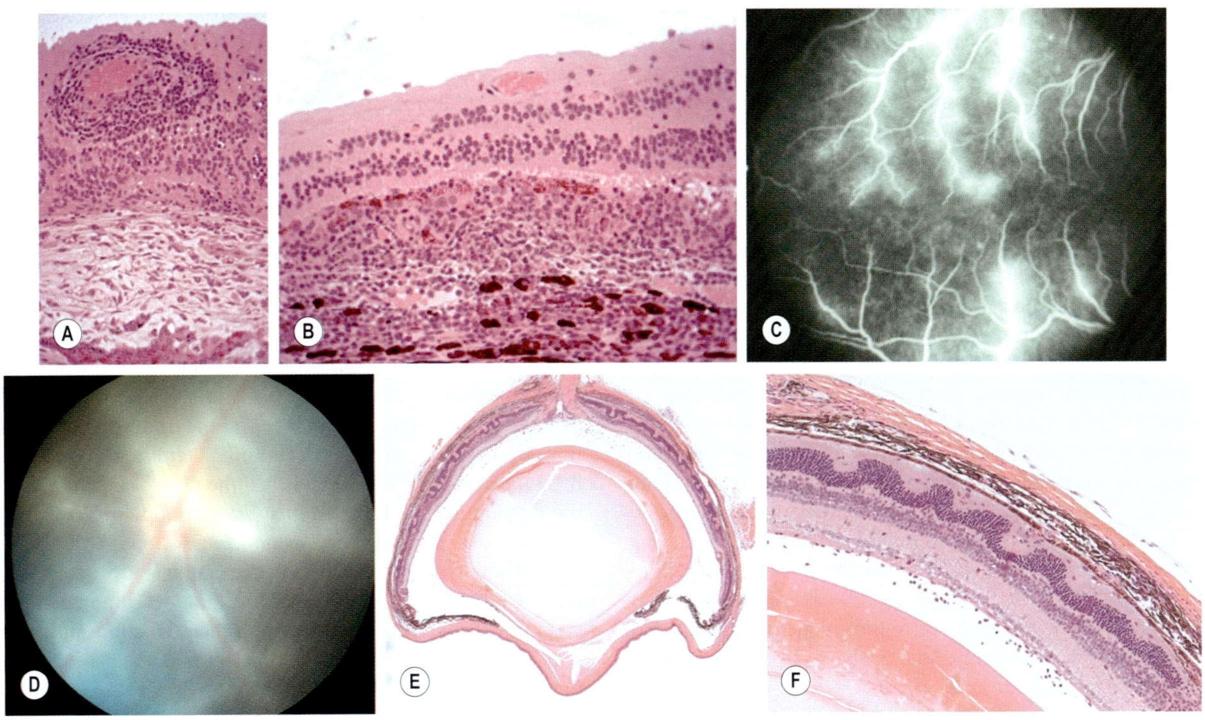

Fig. 1.12 Typical changes in experimental autoimmune uveitis (EAU) in monkeys and mice. Rhesus monkeys were immunized with whole bovine interphotoreceptor retinoid-binding protein (IRBP) and their eyes were collected 3 weeks after disease onset. (A) Retina, showing perivascular infiltration. (B) Granulomatous uveitis. (C) Fluorescein angiography showing retinal vascular leakage, indicating vascular inflammation. The mice, C57Bl/6, were immunized with peptide 651 to 670 of human IRBP, and their eyes were collected at the peak of the inflammatory process (day 15 after immunization). (D) Funduscopy showing typical vascular exudation caused by inflammation. Retinal exudation and folding at a low magnification (E) and at a higher magnification (F), with proteinaceous and cellular exudate in the subretinal space, and cellular infiltration throughout the retinal layers. (Courtesy Drs. Igal Gery, Rachel Caspi, and Chi Chao Chan, National Eye Institute [NEI].)

class II circuitry. This animal presented antigen using human HLA molecules and developed S-Ag–induced uveitis when it was resistant in the normal genotype.

Interphotoreceptor retinoid-binding protein. The second uveitogenic retinal antigen to be identified is IRBP. This 140-kDa molecule was identified, purified, and characterized by Wiggert and Chader.[138] The molecule has four homologous domains, and its function is to carry vitamin A derivatives between the photoreceptors and the RPE.[139] Fox et al.[140] demonstrated that IRBP, purified to homogeneity, has potent uveitogenic properties, with disease induction occurring at dosages as low as 0.3 μg/rat. The course of the disease in the IRBP-induced EAU in rats is somewhat shorter than that seen with S-Ag, and the meninges surrounding the pineal glands of animals immunized with IRBP showed inflammatory disease, whereas those receiving S-Ag did not. The disease induced in nonhuman primates with IRBP (see Fig. 1.12) shares similarities with that seen after S-Ag immunization.[141] Several IRBP fragments have been reported as being pathogenic for Lewis rats.[142,143] Importantly, unlike S-Ag, IRBP was found by Caspi et al. to be uveitogenic in several strains of mice.[144] More recently, this group used IRBP and its peptides to collect basic new information concerning the process of autoimmunity in the eye, and their system has become the universal tool to investigate many issues concerning EAU and the related immunologic processes.

Recoverin. Recoverin, a 23-kDa protein, is a calcium-binding protein that localizes to the retina and the pineal gland. This antigen has been shown to be the target of antibodies in the cancer-associated retinopathy syndrome.[145] Immunization of rats with as little as 10 μg of recoverin induced both uveitis and pinealitis.[146] The disease appears to be similar to that seen with S-Ag.

RPE 65. RPE 65 is a 61-kDa protein that is found specifically and abundantly in the RPE.[147] It is associated with the microsomal fraction of the RPE and appears to be highly conserved across vertebrates. It seems to play an important role in vitamin A metabolism. Mutations of RPE65 have been associated with Leber congenital amaurosis and retinitis pigmentosa.[148] RPE65 is unique to the eye, and immunization of rats with this antigen was shown to induce uveitis.[149] Although disease could be induced with the same dose of S-Ag (1 μg), the disease induced at higher doses was not as severe as that seen with S-Ag. Of interest was the fact that in this model pinealitis was not seen, unlike that seen with S-Ag immunization. Strains of rats that usually are resistant to S-Ag–induced disease, such as the Brown Norway rat, did develop disease after immunization with RPE65.

Bovine melanin protein. Bovine melanin protein is derived from choroid-containing remnants of adherent RPE. Broekhuyse et al.[150] reported that immunization was capable of inducing an autoimmune uveitis in rats. In the initial report, an anterior uveitis was the prominent aspect of the disease, with minimal choroidal involvement, and was therefore first called experimental autoimmune anterior uveitis.[150] However, Chan et al.[151] showed choroidal disease to be a more constant finding. Broekhuyse et al. and Chan et al. have thus proposed the term *experimental melanin protein-induced uveitis* to describe this disorder.

Tyrosinase. Tyrosine proteins are found in melanocytes. It has been hypothesized for some time that melanocytic antigens were associated with the Vogt-Koyanagi-Harada (VKH) syndrome (see Chapter 25). Two of these, tyrosinase-related proteins 1 (TRP1) and 2 (TRP2), have been isolated. TRP1 converts dihydroxyindole-2-carboxylic acid to Eu-melanin and TRP2 converts dopachrome to dihydoxyindol-2-carboxylic acid. Immunization with these antigens induced severe anterior and posterior uveitis 12 days later,[152] and this continued for longer than a month, with some animals experiencing severe serous detachment and even lesions that appeared to resemble Dalen-Fuchs nodules. Lymphocytes of patients with VKH syndrome respond strongly to this antigen (immune memory).[153,154]

Other uveitic antigens. Other ocular antigens with uveitogenic capacity are rhodopsin[155] and phosducin,[156] but their effect is apparent only at high concentrations.

The Role of T-lymphocytes in the Etiology of EAU

The S-Ag– and IRBP-induced models and the antigens themselves have been the ones best investigated to date.[157] The study of these immune-mediated models for human intraocular inflammatory disease has yielded information invaluable for our understanding of the human condition. Perhaps the most important observation was the dominant role of the T cell in this disorder. This was first reported when Salinas-Carmona et al.[135] noted that active immunization of nude rats (animals lacking an intact cell-mediated system) would not readily induce disease, whereas in the heterozygote nude, having an intact T-cell circuitry, the disease readily developed. Furthermore, transfer of splenic lymphocytes from S-Ag–immunized heterozygote animals to the nude rat (homozygote) did yield EAU.

Further support for the mandatory role of the T cell was the development of uveitogenic T-cell lines from Lewis rats[158] and mice.[159] These Th cells induce diseases that are similar histologically to those seen with active immunization. The participation of other immune pathways in EAU has been examined. Neither hyperimmune serum containing anti–S-Ag antibodies nor cobra venom resulted in EAU development. Cobra venom is a potent method by which the complement system is depleted.[160]

The changing patterns of cellular components and markers in the eye have given us a new understanding of this rapidly changing, finely orchestrated "ballet." Recent studies have revealed that the pathogenic process of EAU is initiated by activated CD4 lymphocytes specific to a retinal antigen, mostly S-Ag or IRBP. These cells are capable of crossing the retina–blood barrier, and upon exposure to their target antigen, they release cytokines that attract inflammatory cells, including other lymphocytes and other inflammatory cells. The pathogenic process is also promoted by the increased expression of class II antigens on several resident ocular cells. These observations thus support the notion that these ocular resident cells may be playing a role in the localized immunopathogenic process. The potential pathogenic processes are physiologically inhibited, however, by the population of Treg cells, described earlier in detail. More recent studies have revealed the existence of retina-specific Treg cells that bring about resolution and maintain remission of autoimmune uveitis, in addition to the circulating Treg cells.[161]

The Microbiome and Autoimmunity

Data collected in recent years provide evidence of the relationship between the intestinal microbiota and the immune system. This relationship has been observed in various systems and the elegant studies by Horai et al.[162,163] have established the role of the gut microbiome in the development of EAU. In this system, spontaneous EAU develops in mice in which transgenic T lymphocytes specific to a retinal antigen migrate into the retina and initiate the pathogenic process. The authors reported that the disease, however, did not develop in germ-free mice or in mice in which the gut microbiome was significantly reduced by antibiotics,[163] indicating that the gut microbiome plays a major role in the generation of the T cells responsible for the pathogenesis of the disease. It is assumed that cells specific to the retinal antigen that escaped the negative selection in the thymus are activated by the gut microbiome antigens, which mimic the uveitogenic retinal antigen, and initiate the pathogenic EAU process. Furthermore, it is conceivable that a similar phenomenon plays a role in the pathogenesis of certain cases of uveitis in humans. Indeed, several recent reports have shown the relationship between the microbiome and uveitis.[164]

Uveitis Induced by Endotoxin and Other Bacterial Antigens

Another experimental uveitic model (but not autoimmune) is induced by the injection into rats, at a site far from the globe, of the endotoxin LPS, a normal component of gram-negative bacterial cell walls. This induces a relatively fleeting anterior segment inflammatory response characterized mostly by an infiltration of polymorphonuclear cells[165] and cytokine release.[166] This model has potential relevance because patients with ankylosing spondylitis and uveitis[167] have been reported to have a higher incidence of *Klebsiella* organisms in their stool or infection with another gram-negative bacterium during or shortly before the active portion of their disease compared with the time when their disease is quiet or compared with control subjects. Although these observations have not been universally corroborated, the findings do bring into question the potential role these gram-negative organisms might play in the pathogenic process. These antigens may activate complement without the participation of antibody. However, it is known that LPS can cause B-cell clonal expansion, bypassing the normal T-cell circuitry present to control such responses. The abundant B-cell response could cause large amounts of antibody formation and possibly immune complex formation, leading to an immune response. Either mechanism may be playing a role in the induction of anterior uveitis. One observation was the demonstration of the homology of six consecutive amino acids between HLA-B27 and *Klebsiella pneumoniae* nitrogenase residues, with autoantibodies against this residue being found in HLA-B27–positive Reiter syndrome and in patients with ankylosing spondylitis.[168]

Toll-like Receptor Ligands

Microorganisms are identified by the host immune system by their specific antigenic markers. In addition, microorganisms, including bacteria, viruses, and fungi, express structurally conserved molecules that are recognized by various host cells, including macrophages, monocytes, dendritic cells, and B cells. These molecules on the host cells are named *Toll-like receptors* (TLR) and play a vital role in the modulation of the innate immune system by releasing inflammatory mediators, including IL-6, IL-12, IL-18, and TNF-α. TLRs can also bind to certain endogenous molecules called *damage-associated molecular patterns* (DAMPs) and activate the innate immune response.[169] Importantly, TLR ligands, such as LPS or *Pertussis* toxin, were found to activate pathogenic autoimmune processes by stimulating naïve T cells with specificity toward autoantigens to undergo maturation and initiate inflammation in tissues containing the target antigen.[119] This observation thus supports the notion that random common infections may play a significant role in initiating pathogenic ocular immune responses.[170]

Importance of Animal Studies

This short synopsis concerning noninfectious ocular inflammatory animal models may convince the reader just how powerful a tool these models can be. The diseases induced have many features also seen in humans, allowing us to dissect the ocular immune response and drawing attention to the potential role of ocular resident cells in the immune response. Many of the clinical and pathologic alterations seen in the animal models are also seen in human disease. These models (particularly S-Ag and IRBP EAU) have been excellent templates with which newer approaches to immunosuppression can be tested.[170]

Cyclosporin was first evaluated for ocular autoimmune disease with the use of the S-Ag–induced model of experimental uveitis. Experiments clearly demonstrated the efficacy of this agent in preventing the expression of disease in rats even if therapy was begun 1 week after immunization, at a time when immunocompetent cells capable of inducing disease are present.[171] Furthermore, treatment of rats with

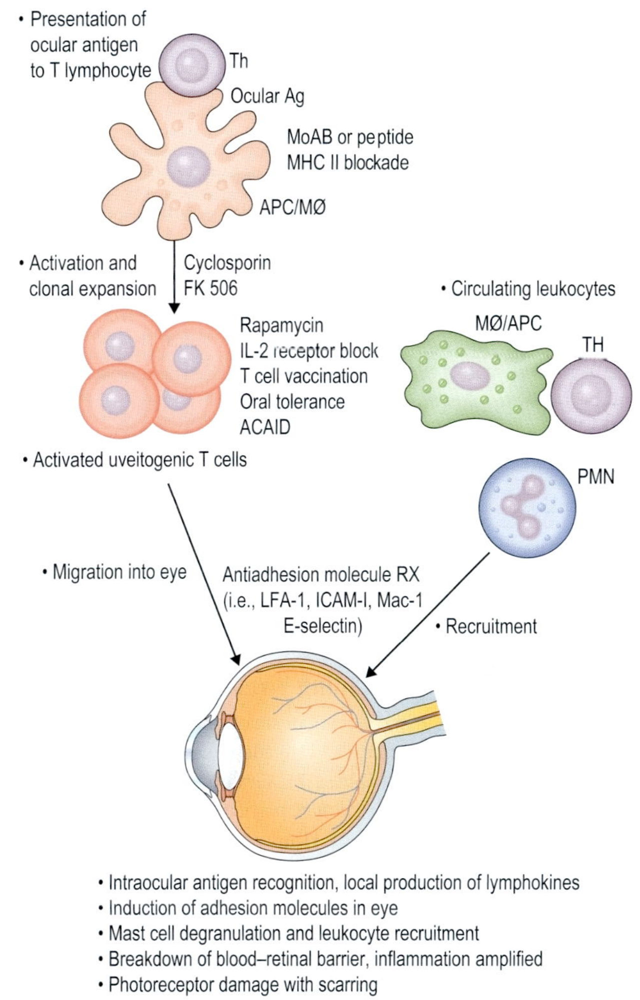

Fig. 1.13 Scheme showing induction of uveitis. Bullets (•) indicate what may be occurring on the basis of evaluation of S-antigen uveitis model. (Modified from Caspi RR, Nussenblatt RB. Natural and therapeutic control of ocular autoimmunity: rodent and man. In: Coutinho A, Kazatchkine MD, eds. *Autoimmunity: Physiology and Disease.* New York: Wiley-Liss; 1994.)

cyclosporin also reduced their lymphocyte response to the immunizing antigen.[172] These initial observations led to the use of cyclosporin in human disease.[173]

Tacrolimus (FK506) has been evaluated in a similar fashion and found to be quite effective in preventing EAU, as were rapamycin and oral administration of the retinal S-Ag for induction of tolerance (see Chapter 8).

The continued evaluation of immunomodulation in EAU will lead to a variety of new therapeutic approaches because this model is increasingly used as a template to evaluate new therapies. Some of these strategies are presented in Fig. 1.13. Here the reader can see that numerous points of the immune system can be delineated and appropriate strategies employed. Microarray technology is being applied to these models to gain insight into gene activation in a way that could not have been done before, that is, to observe hundreds and thousands of gene responses simultaneously.

What is the potential role of S-Ag or the other uveitogenic antigens found in the retina? This remains a matter of speculation. We have reported that patients with posterior and intermediate uveitis have exhibited in vitro cell-mediated proliferative responses to the S-Ag, not unlike those seen in the immunized animals.[174] It is certainly possible that the initial event was not initiated by S-Ag alone, but that

TABLE 1.7 Immune mechanisms involved in infectious disease

Infectious Agent	Mode of Defense
Bacteria, viruses	For neutralization, immunoglobulin G (IgG) with complement and neutrophils
Bacteria, viruses	Gastrointestinal and respiratory infections: immunoglobulin A (IgA), alternative complement pathway
Helminths	Intestinal immunoglobulin E (IgE) with mast cells
Pneumococci, encapsulated organisms	Immunoglobulin M (IgM), macrophages, and complement
Mycobacteria, viruses	Cytotoxic T cells and perforin
Mycobacteria, viruses, syphilis fungi	Macrophages and delayed-type hypersensitivity

the release of S-Ag followed an infectious process, whether viral or even toxoplasmic. It is also clear that the events leading to an "autoimmune" uveitis are multifactorial.

Immune Responses to Invading Viruses and Parasites

The host's response to invading organisms is critical to its survival. Essentially, all types of organisms can invade the eye, and the response of the immune system varies (Table 1.7). Viral infections are, of course, of great concern to the ophthalmologist, particularly to those with a special interest in the anterior segment. However, the immune response to a virus has taken on greater importance for those involved with intraocular inflammatory disease for both theoretical and practical reasons. Certain viruses have a particular propensity for retinal tissue, with herpes viruses, particularly cytomegalovirus, being of ever-increasing concern.

The invasion of a virus into the organism leads to the mobilization of several aspects of the immune response. Antibody responses are abundant and may directly kill the virus. More frequently, however, cellular immune mechanisms appear to play a crucial role in eliminating the invader. T-cell responses against an invading virus have been well documented. The T-cell response is MHC restricted. The T cell is required to respond to a dual signal, that of the viral antigen and that of class I antigens sitting on a target cell membrane. NK cell activity is also seen to be directed against viral invasion. Found in the systemic circulation, these spontaneously cytotoxic cells are known also as *large granular lymphocytes.* NK cell activity is not MHC restricted, and virus-infected cells seem to be particularly vulnerable to this cell's attack, but the mechanism of recognition still remains unclear, although the cells are known to recognize certain viral antigens. These cells are thought to participate in antibody-dependent cell-mediated cytotoxicity, in which a specific antibody binds to the cell to enhance its destruction by cytotoxic cells. Macrophages also have important antiviral activity and will kill some engulfed virus particles. Others can be removed if macrophage activation is adequate.

The immune system is rapidly activated to efficiently handle a viral infection largely through the production of IFN. In response to a viral infection, both IFN-α and IFN-β are produced. The effect of IFNs on a virally infected cell seems to be at least twofold: (1) the production of a protein kinase, which inhibits viral protein synthesis and (2) the production of 2′,5′-adenylate synthetase, which inhibits viral RNA synthesis. In addition to this direct effect on the virus, the IFNs, because of their immunomodulatory properties,[175] profoundly affect the immune response as well. The appearance of class II MHC on cell-surface membranes could have an important effect on the rapidity of the immune response.

Because the immune response to the virus is largely cell mediated, any damage to this system could have grave consequences. This is the case with HIV infection, the virus that causes AIDS. This RNA virus, which has a marked propensity for T(Th) cells, uses reverse transcriptase to effectively incorporate its genetic library into that of the host cell. As the T cell becomes activated through antigen presentation by macrophages or other cells, the virus genome is also stimulated. The assembling and release of HIV often lead to cell death. This virus then severely damages an important part of the immune system's mechanism for removing such infections. This has secondary repercussions in the body's attempt to clear other virus infections, such as cytomegalovirus.

Parasitic infections of the eye include many types of organisms, from helminths to protozoa. The classically described response to parasitic infections is eosinophilia. The release of the basic protein and other toxic products (see earlier discussion) from the eosinophil is thought to kill the organism. Certainly eosinophilia is characteristic of some forms of ocular parasitic infections, such as toxocariasis (see Chapter 17). However, for other infections, such as toxoplasmosis and onchocerciasis (see Chapters 15 and 18), this appears not to be the case. T cells seem to predominate in the eye in the more chronic forms of these diseases, and deficient T-cell functioning can lead to serious consequences. An example of this is the systemic and ocular toxoplasmic infection seen in patients with AIDS, in patients immunosuppressed because of neoplasms, or in those with iatrogenic suppression for graft survival.

Parasitic invaders have an additional capacity to evade immune surveillance. Immunosuppressive factors appear to be elaborated by the parasite, leading to a downgrading of macrophage and T-cell activity around it. Certain parasites cloak themselves in nonantigenic proteins, thereby avoiding immune attack. The cyst of *T. gondii* found in the eye is such an example, with the wall incorporating antigens from the host. Other parasites vary their antigenic appearance frequently to avoid the T-cell and macrophage-directed responses.

Acknowledgments

The author thanks Dr. Igal Gery for his extensive review of and input into this chapter.

SUGGESTED READINGS

Paul WE, ed. *Fundamental Immunology*. 7th ed. Philadelphia: Lippincott Williams & Wilkins; 2020.

Delves, PJ, et al. *Roitt's Essential Immunology*. 13th ed. New York: Wiley Blackwell.

REFERENCES

1. Anderson MS, Venanzt ES, Klein L, et al. Projection of an immunological self shadow within the thymus by the Aire protein. *Science.* 2002;298:1395–1401.
2. Meloni A, Furcas M, Cetani F, et al. Autoantibodies against type I interferons as an additional diagnostic criterion for autoimmune polyendocrine syndrome type I. *J Clin Endocrinol Metab*. 2008;93(11):4389–4397.
3. Egwuagu CE, Charukamnoetkanok P, Gery I. Thymic expression of autoantigens correlates with resistance to autoimmune disease. *J Immunol.* 1997;159:3109–3112.
4. Gery I, Egwuagu CE. Central tolerance mechanisms in control of susceptibility to autoimmune uveitic disease. *Int Rev Immunol.* 2002;21:89–100.
5. Takase H, Yu CR, Mahdi RM, et al. Thymic expression of peripheral tissue antigens in humans: a remarkable variability among individuals. *Int Immunol.* 2005;17(8):1131–1140.
6. Shi G, Cox CA, Vistica BP, et al. Phenotype switching by inflammation-inducing polarized Th17 cells, but not by Th1 cells. *J Immunol.* 2008;181(10):7205–7213.
7. Ouyang W, Kolls JK, Zheng Y. The biological functions of T helper 17 cell effector cytokines in inflammation. *Immunity*. 2008;28(4):454–467.

8. Andoh A, Zhang Z, Inatomi O, et al. Interleukin-22, a member of the IL-10 subfamily, induces inflammatory responses in colonic subepithelial myofibroblasts. *Gastroenterology*. 2005;129(3):969–984.
9. Brand S, Beigel F, Olszak T, et al. IL-22 is increased in active Crohn's disease and promotes proinflammatory gene expression and intestinal epithelial cell migration. *Am J Physiol Gastrointest Liver Physiol.* 2006;290(4):G827–G838.
10. Jawad S, Liu B, Agron E, Nussenblatt RB, Sen HN. Elevated serum levels of interleukin-17A in uveitis patients. *Ocul Immunol Inflamm.* 2013;21(6):434–439.
11. Kuiper JJ, Mutis T, de Jager W, de Groot-Mijnes JD, Rothova A. Intraocular interleukin-17 and proinflammatory cytokines in HLA-A29-associated birdshot chorioretinopathy. *Am J Ophthalmol.* 2011;152(2):177–182–e1.
12. Liang D, Shao H, Born WK, et al. Connection between γδT-cell and adenosine-mediated immune regulation in the pathogenesis of experimental autoimmune uveitis. *Crit Rev Immunol.* 2018;38:233–243.
13. St Leger AJ, Desai JV, Drummond RA. An ocular commensal protects against corneal infection by driving an interleukin-17 response from mucosal γδ T-cells. *Immunity*. 2017;47:148–158.
14. Shevyrev Tereshchenko V. Treg heterogeneity, function, and homeostasis. *Front Immunol.* 2020;10:3100.
15. Kemper C, Chan AC, Green JM, et al. Activation of human CD4+ cells with CD3 and CD46 induces a T-regulatory cell 1 phenotype. *Nature.* 2003;421:388–392.
16. Tsuji NM, Mizumachi K, Kurisaki J. Antigen-specific, CD4+ CD25+ regulatory T cell clones induced in Peyer's patches. *Int Immunol.* 2003;15:525–534.
17. Sakaguchi S, Ono M, Setoguchi R, et al. Foxp3+ CD25+ CD4+ natural regulatory T cells in dominant self-tolerance and autoimmune disease. *Immunol Rev*. 2006;212:8–27.
18. Yeh S, Li Z, Forooghian F, et al. CD4+ Foxp3+ T-regulatory cells in non-infectious uveitis. *Arch Ophthalmol.* 2009;127:407–413.
19. Li Z, Lim WK, Mahesh SP, et al. Cutting edge: in vivo blockade of human IL-2 receptor induces expansion of CD56 (bright) regulatory NK cells in patients with active uveitis. *J Immunol.* 2005;174(9):5187–5191.
20. Vivier E, Artis D, Colonna M, et al. Innate lymphoid cells: 10 years on. *Cell.* 2018;174:1054–1066.
21. Kitaichi N, Kotake S, Morohashi T, et al. Diminution of experimental autoimmune uveoretinitis (EAU) in mice depleted of NK cells. *J Leukoc Biol.* 2002;72:1117–1121.
22. Grajewski RS, Hansen A, Agarwal RK, et al. Activation of iNKT cells ameliorates experimental ocular autoimmunity by a mechanism involving innate IFN-gamma production and dampening of adaptive Th1 and Th17 responses. *J Immunol.* 2008;181:4791–4797.
23. Satoh M, Namba KI, Kitaichi N, et al. Invariant natural killer T cells play dual roles in the development of experimental autoimmune uveoretinitis. *Exp Eye Res.* 2016;153:79–89.
24. Akdis M, Aab A, Altunbulakil C, et al. Interleukins (from IL-1 to IL-38), interferons, transforming growth factor-beta, and TNF-alpha: receptors, functions, and roles in diseases. *J Allergy Clin Immunol.* 2016;138(4):984–1010.
25. Bevilacqua M, Stengelin S, Gimbrone M, et al. Endothelial leukocyte adhesion molecule-1: an inducible receptor for neutrophils related to complement regulatory proteins and lectins. *Science.* 1989;243:1160–1164.
26. Springer T. Traffic signals for lymphocyte recirculation and leukocyte emigration: the multistep paradigm. *Cell.* 1994;76:301–314.
27. Munro J, Pober J, Cotran R. Recruitment of neutrophils in the local endotoxin response: association with de novo endothelial expression of endothelial leukocyte adhesion molecule-1. *Lab Invest.* 1991;64: 295–299.
28. Whitcup S, Wakefield D, Li Q, et al. Endothelial leukocyte adhesion molecule-1 in endotoxin-induced uveitis. *Invest Ophthalmol Vis Sci.* 1992;33:2626–2630.
29. Rosenbaum J, McDevitt HO, Guss RB, et al. Endotoxin-induced uveitis in rats as a model for human disease. *Nature.* 1980;286:611–613.
30. Forrester J, Worgul B, Merriam GJ. Endotoxin-induced uveitis in the rat. *Albrecht von Graefes Arch Klin Ophthalmol.* 1980;213:221–233.
31. Whitcup S, Debarge L, Caspi R, et al. Monoclonal antibodies against ICAM-1 (CD54) and LFA-1 (CD11a/CD18) inhibit experimental autoimmune uveitis. *Clin Immunol Immunopathol.* 1993;67:143–150.
32. Elner V, Elner S, Pavilack M, et al. Intercellular adhesion molecule-1 in human corneal endothelium: modulation and function. *Am J Pathol.* 1991;138:525–536.
33. Whitcup S, Hikita N, Shirao M, et al. Effect of monoclonal antibodies against ICAM-1 (CD54) an LFA-1 alpha (CD11a) in the prevention and treatment of endotoxin-induced uveitis (EIU). *Invest Ophthalmol Vis Sci.* 1993;34:1143.
34. Rosenbaum J, Boney R. Efficacy of antibodies to adhesion molecules, CD11a or CD18, in rabbit models of uveitis. *Curr Eye Res.* 1993;12:827–831.
35. Liu B, Li Z, Mahesh SP, et al. HTLV-1 infection of human retinal pigment epithelial cells and inhibition of viral infection by an antibody to ICAM-1. *Invest Ophthalmol Vis Sci.* 2006;47(4):1510–1515.
36. Springer T. Adhesion receptors of the immune system. *Nature.* 1990;346:425–434.
37. Dustin M, Springer T. Lymphocyte function-associated antigen-1 (LFA-1) interaction with intercellular adhesion molecule (ICAM-1) is one of at least three mechanisms for lymphocyte adhesion to cultured endothelial cells. *J Cell Biol.* 1988;107:321–331.
38. Norris D. Cytokine modulation of adhesion molecules in the regulation of immunologic cytotoxicity of epidermal targets. *J Invest Dermatol.* 1990;95:11S–120S.
39. Kaminska G, Niederkom J, McCulley J. Intercellular adhesion molecule-1 (ICAM-1) expression in normal and inflamed human cornea: induction by recombinant interferon gamma and interleukin-1. *Ophthalmol Vis Sci.* 1991;32(Suppl):677.
40. Liversidge J, Sewell H, Forrester J. Interactions between lymphocytes and cells of the blood–retina barrier: mechanisms of T lymphocyte adhesion to human retinal capillary endothelial cells and retinal pigment epithelial cells in vitro. *Immunology.* 1990;71:390–396.
41. Whitcup SM, De Barge LR, Caspi RR, et al. Monoclonal antibodies against ICAM-1 (CD54) and LFA-1 (CD11a/CD18) inhibit experimental autoimmune uveitis. *Clin Immunol Immunopathol.* 1993;67:143–150.
42. Till G, Mulligan M, Lee S, et al. Adhesion molecules in experimental phacoanaphylactic endophthalmitis. *Invest Ophthalmol Vis Sci.* 1992;33(Suppl): 795.
43. Whitcup S, Mulligan M, Lee S. Expression of cell adhesion molecules in posterior uveitis. *Arch Ophthalmol.* 1992;110:662–666.
44. Whitcup S, Nussenblatt R, Price FJ, et al. Expression of cell adhesion molecules in corneal graft failure. *Cornea.* 1993;12:475–480.
45. Haug C, Colvin RB, Delmonico FL, et al. A phase I trial of immunosuppression with anti-ICAM-1 (CD54) mAb in renal allograft recipients. *Transplantation.* 1993;55:766–773.
46. Faia LJ, Sen HN, Li Z, Yeh S, Wroblewski KJ, Nussenblatt RB. Treatment of inflammatory macular edema with humanized anti-CD11a antibody therapy. *Invest Ophthalmol Vis Sci.* 2011;52(9):6919–6924.
47. Wang RX, Yu CR, Dambuza IM, et al. Interleukin-35 induces regulatory B cells that suppress autoimmune disease. *Nat Med.* 2014;20:633–641.
48. Dambuza IM, He C, Choi JK, et al. IL-12p35 induces expansion of IL-10 and IL-35-expressing regulatory B cells and ameliorates autoimmune disease. *Nat Commun.* 2017;8:719.
49. Mochizuki M, Kuwabara T, Chan C, et al. An association between susceptibility to experimental autoimmune uveitis and choroidal mast cell numbers. *J Immunol.* 1984;33:1699–1701.
50. de Kozak Y, Sainte-Laudy J, Benveniste J, et al. Evidence for immediate hypersensitivity phenomena in experimental autoimmune uveoretinitis. *Eur J Immunol.* 1981;11:612–617.
51. Askenase P, Rosenstein R, Ptak W. T-cells produce an antigen-binding factor with in vivo activity analogous to IgE antibody. *J Exp Med.* 1983;157:862–873.
52. Ferretti S, Bonneau O, Dubois GR, et al. IL-17, produced by lymphocytes and neutrophils, is necessary for lipopolysaccharide-induced airway neutrophilia: IL-15 as a possible trigger. *J Immunol.* 2003;170(4):2106–2112.
53. Caspi R, Roberge F, Nussenblatt R. Organ-resident, nonlymphoid cells suppress proliferation of autoimmune T-helper lymphocytes. *Science.* 1987;237:1029–1032.

54. Okunuki Y, Mukai R, Nakao T, et al. Retinal microglia initiate neuroinflammation in ocular autoimmunity. *Proc Natl Acad Sci U S A.* 2019;116:9989–9998.
55. Ng TK, Chen LJ, Liu DT, et al. Multiple gene polymorphisms in the complement factor H gene are associated with exudative age-related macular degeneration in Chinese. *Invest Ophthalmol Vis Sci.* 2008;49(8):3312–3317.
56. Tuo J, Ning B, Bojanowski CM, et al. Synergic effect of polymorphisms in ERCC6 5' flanking region and complement factor H on age-related macular degeneration predisposition. *Proc Natl Acad Sci USA.* 2006;103(24):9256–9261.
57. Hageman GS, Anderson DH, Johnson LV, et al. A common haplotype in the complement regulatory gene factor H (HF1/CFH) predisposes individuals to age-related macular degeneration. *Proc Natl Acad Sci U S A.* 2005;102(20):7227–7232.
58. Nussenblatt RB, Ferris 3rd F. Age-related macular degeneration and the immune response: implications for therapy. *Am J Ophthalmol.* 2007;144(4):618–626.
59. Ferrara DC, Merriam JE, Freund KB, et al. Analysis of major alleles associated with age-related macular degeneration in patients with multifocal choroiditis: strong association with complement factor H. *Arch Ophthalmol.* 2008;126(11):1562–1566.
60. Lei B, Bush RA, Milam AH, et al. Human melanoma-associated retinopathy (MAR) antibodies alter the retinal ON-response of the monkey ERG in vivo. *Invest Ophthalmol Vis Sci.* 2000;41(1):262–266.
61. Derchnouchamps J, Vaerman J, Michiels J, et al. Immune complexes in the aqueous humor and serum. *Am J Ophthalmol.* 1977;84:24–31.
62. Char D, Stein P, Masi R, et al. Immune complexes in uveitis. *Am J Opthalmol.* 1979;87:678–681.
63. Lehner T, Almedida J, Levinsky R. Damaged membrane fragments and immune complexes in the blood of patients with Behçet's syndrome. *Clin Exp Immunol.* 1978;34:206–212.
64. Vinje O, Miller P, Mellbye J. Immunological variables and acute phase reactants in patients with ankylosing spondylitis (Bechterew's syndrome) and their relatives. *Clin Rheumatol.* 1984;3:501–513.
65. Egan RM, Yorkey C, Black R, et al. Peptide-specific T cell clonal expansion in vivo following immunization in the eye, an immune privileged site. *J Immunol.* 1996;157:2262–2271.
66. Ferguson TA, Green JM, Griffith TS. Cell death and immune privilege. *Int Rev Immunol.* 2002;21:153–172.
67. Streilein-Stein J, Streilein JW. Anterior chamber associated immune deviation (ACAID): regulation, biological relevance, and implications for therapy. *Int Rev Immunol.* 2002;21:123–152.
68. Stein-Streilein J. Immune regulation and the eye. *Trends Immunol.* 2008;29:548–554.
69. Medawar P. Immunity to homologous grated skin. III. The fate of skin homografts transplanted to brain, to subcutaneous tissue and to the anterior chamber of the eye. *Br J Exp Pathol.* 1948;29:58–69.
70. Kaplan H, Streilein J. Immune response to immunization via the anterior chamber of the eye. I. F1-lymphocyte induced immune deviation. *J Immunol.* 1977;118:809–814.
71. Streilein J, Neiderkom J. Induction of anterior chamber-associated immune deviation requires an intact, functional spleen. *J Exp Med.* 1981;153:1058–1067.
72. Mizuno K, Clark A, Streilein J. Anterior chamber associate immune deviation induced by soluble antigens. *Invest Ophthalmol Vis Sci.* 1989;30:1112–1119.
73. Eichhorn M, Horneber M, Streilein JW, et al. Anterior chamber associated immune deviation elicited via primate eyes. *Invest Ophthalmol Vis Sci.* 1993;342:2926–2930.
74. Hara Y, Caspi R, Wiggert B, et al. Suppression of experimental autoimmune uveitis in mice by induction of anterior chamber associated immune deviation with interphotoreceptor retinoid binding protein. *J Immunol.* 1992;148:1685–1692.
75. Wilbanks G, Mammolenti M, Streilein J. Studies on the induction of anterior chamber-associated immune deviation (ACAID). III. Induction of ACAID depends upon intraocular transforming growth factor-beta. *Eur J Immunol.* 1992;22:165–173.
76. Gery I, Caspi RR. Tolerance induction in relation to the eye. *Front Immunol.* 2018;9:2304.
77. Green DR, Ferguson TA. The role of FAS ligand in immune privilege. *Nat Rev Mol Cell Biol.* 2001;2:917–924.
78. Chan C, Roberge F, Ni M, et al. Injury of Muller cells increases the incidence of experimental autoimmune uveoretinitis. *Clin Immunol Immunopathol.* 1991;59:201–207.
79. Planck S, Dang T, Graves D, et al. Retinal pigment epithelial cells secrete interleukin-6 in response to interleukin-1. *Invest Ophthalmol Vis Sci.* 1992;33(1):78–82.
80. Percopo C, Hooks J, Shinohara T, et al. Cytokine-mediated activation of a neuronal retinal resident cell provokes antigen presentation. *J Immunol.* 1990;145:4101–4107.
81. Mahesh SP, Li Z, Liu B, et al. Expression of GITR ligand abrogates immunosuppressive function of ocular tissue and differentially modulates inflammatory cytokines and chemokines. *Eur J Immunol.* 2006;36(8):2128–2138.
82. Liu B, Li Z, Mahesh SP, et al. Glucocorticoid-induced tumor necrosis factor receptor negatively regulates activation of human primary natural killer (NK) cells by blocking proliferative signals and increasing NK cell apoptosis. *J Biol Chem.* 2008;283(13):8202–8210.
83. Foxman EF, Zhang M, Hurst SD, et al. Inflammatory mediators in uveitis: differential induction of cytokines and chemokines in Th1- versus Th2-mediated ocular inflammation. *J Immunol.* 2002;168:2483–2492.
84. Lee MT, Zhang M, Hurst SD, et al. Interferon-beta and adhesion molecules (E-selectin and s-intracellular adhesion molecule-1) are detected in sera from patients with retinal vasculitis and are induced in retinal vascular endothelial cells by Toll-like receptor 3 signalling. *Clin Exp Immunol.* 2007;147(1):71–80.
85. Jawad S, Liu B, Agron E, et al. Elevated serum levels of interleukin-17A in uveitis patients. *Ocul Immunol Inflamm.* 2013;21(6):434–439.
86. Cousins S, McCabe M, Danielpour D, et al. Identification of transforming growth factor beta as an immunosuppressive factor in aqueous humor. *Invest Ophthalmol Vis Sci.* 1991;32:2201–2211.
87. Tripathi R, Li J, Borisuth N, et al. Trabecular cells of the eye express messenger RNA for transforming growth factor beta 1 and secrete this cytokine. *Invest Ophthalmol Vis Sci.* 1993;34:2562–2569.
88. Taylor A, Streilein J, Cousins S. Identification of alpha-melanocyte stimulating hormone as a potential immunosuppressive factor in aqueous humor. *Curr Eye Res.* 1992;11:1199–1206.
89. Wahlestedt C, Beding B, Ekman R, et al. Calcitonin gene-related peptide in the eye-release by sensory nerve stimulation and effects associated with neurogenic inflammation. *Regul Pept.* 1986;16:107–115.
90. Taylor A, Streilein J, Cousins S. Vasoactive intestinal peptide (VIP) contributes to the immunosuppressive activity of normal aqueous humor. *J Immunol.* 1994;153:1080–1086.
91. Sternberg E, Hill J, Chrousos G, et al. Inflammatory mediator-induced hypothalamic–pituitary–adrenal axis activation is defective in streptococcal cell wall arthritis-susceptible Lewis rats. *Proc Natl Acad Sci U S A.* 1989;153:2374–2378.
92. Knisely TL, Hosoi J, Nazareno R, et al. The presence of biologically significant concentrations of glucocorticoids but little or no cortisol binding globulin within aqueous humor: relevance to immune privilege in the anterior chamber of the eye. *Invest Ophthalmol Vis Sci.* 1994;35:3711–3723.
93. Wells H. Studies on the chemistry of anaphylaxis. III. Experiments with isolated proteins, especially those of hens' eggs. *J Infect Dis.* 1911;9:147–151.
94. Weiner H, Friedman A, Miller A, et al. Oral tolerance: immunologic mechanisms and treatment of animal and human organ specific autoimmune diseases by oral administration of autoantigens. *Ann Rev Immunol.* 1994;12:809–834.
95. Friedman A, Weiner H. Induction of anergy or active suppression following oral tolerance is determined by antigen dosage. *Proc Natl Acad Sci U S A.* 1994;91:6688–6692.
96. Gregerson D, Obritsch W, Donoso L. Oral tolerance in experimental autoimmune uveoretinitis. Distinct mechanisms of resistance are induced by low dose vs high dose feeding protocols. *J Immunol.* 1993;151:5751–5761.

97. Nussenblatt R, Caspi R, Mahdi R, et al. Inhibition of S-antigen induced experimental autoimmune uveoretinitis by oral induction of tolerance with S-antigen. *J Immunol.* 1990;144:1689–1695.
98. Suh E, Vistica B, Chan C, et al. Splenectomy abrogates the induction of oral tolerance in experimental autoimmune uveoretinitis. *Curr Eye Res.* 1993;12:833–839.
99. Dick A, Cheng Y, McKinnon A, et al. Nasal administration of retinal antigens suppresses the inflammatory response in experimental allergic uveoretinitis. A preliminary report of intranasal induction of tolerance with retinal antigens. *Br J Ophthalmol.* 1993;77:171–175.
100. Nussenblatt RB, Gery I, Weiner HL, et al. Treatment of uveitis by oral administration of retinal antigens: results of a phase I/II randomized masked trial. *Am J Ophthalmol.* 1997;123:583–592.
101. Thurau SR, Wildner G. Oral tolerance for treating uveitis – new hope for an old immunological mechanism. *Prog Retinal Eye Res.* 2002;21:577–589.
102. Cogan D. Immunosuppression and eye disease. First Vail lecture. *Am J Ophthalmol.* 1977;83:777–788.
103. Shutze H, Gorer P, Finlayson M. The resistance of four mouse lines to bacterial infections. *J Hyg.* 1936;36:37–49.
104. Benacerraf B, Green I, Paul W. The immune response of guinea pigs to hapten-poly-L-lysine conjugates as an example of the genetic control of the recognition of antigenicity. *Cold Spring Harbor Symp Quant Biol.* 1967;32:569–575.
105. Bluestein HG, Green I, Benacerraf B. Specific immune response genes of the guinea pig. II. Relationship between the poly-L-lysine gene and the genes controlling immune responsiveness to copolymers of L-glutamic acid and L-tyrosine in random bred Hartley guinea pigs. *J Exp Med.* 1971;134:471–481.
106. McDevitt H, Chinitz A. Genetic control of the antibody response: relationship between immune response and histocompatibility (H-2) type. *Science.* 1969;163:1207–1208.
107. Forrester J, McMenamin P, Holothouse I, et al. Localization and characterization of major histocompatibility complex class II-positive cells in the posterior segment of the eye: implications for induction of autoimmune uveoretinitis. *Invest Ophthalmol Vis Sci.* 1994;35:64–77.
108. Brewerton D, Hart, Nicholls FD, et al. Ankylosing spondylitis and HL-A27. *Lancet.* 1973;i:904.
109. Khan M, Kushner I, Braun WE. HLA-B7 and ankylosing spondylitis in American Blacks. *N Engl J Med.* 1977;297:513.
110. Terasaki P. *Histocompatibility testing 1980. UCLA Tissue Typing Laboratory.* Los Angeles: University of California Los Angeles; 1980.
111. Bottazzo G, Pujol-Borrell R, Hanafusa T, et al. Role of aberrant HLA-DR expression and antigen presentation in induction of endocrine autoimmunity. *Lancet.* 1983;ii:1115–1119.
112. Taurog JD, Maika SD, Simmons WA, et al. Susceptibility to inflammatory disease in B27 transgenic rat lines correlates with the level of B27 expression. *J Immunol.* 1993;150:4168–4178.
113. Caspi R, Grubbs B, Chan C, et al. Genetic control of susceptibility to experimental autoimmune uveoretinitis in the mouse model: concomitant regulation by MHC and non-MHC genes. *J Immunol.* 1992;148:2384–2389.
114. Shastry BS. SNP alleles in human disease and evolution. *J Hum Genet.* 2002;47:561–566.
115. van der Maarel SM. Epigenetic mechanisms in health and disease. *Ann Rheum Dis.* 2008;67(Suppl 3):97–100.
116. Li Z, Liu B, Maminishkis A, et al. Gene expression profiling in autoimmune noninfectious uveitis disease. *J Immunol.* 2008;181(7):5147–5157.
117. Rose N, Bona C. Defining criteria for autoimmune diseases (Wetebsky's postulates revisited). *Immunol Today.* 1993;14:426–430.
118. Allison A. Unresponsiveness to self antigens. *Lancet.* 1971;ii:1401–1403.
119. Fujimoto JI, Shi G, Gery I. Microbial products trigger autoimmune ocular inflammation. *Ophthalmic Res.* 2008;40:193–199.
120. Egwuagu C, Chow C, Beraud E, et al. T cell receptor beta-chain usage in experimental autoimmune uveoretinitis. *J Autoimmunol.* 1991;4:315–324.
121. Gregerson D, Fling S, Merryman C, et al. Conserved T cell receptor V gene usage by uveitogenic T cells. *Clin Immunol Immunopathol.* 1991;58:154–161.
122. Egwuagu C, Mahdi R, Nussenblatt R, et al. Evidence for selective accumulation of V beta 8+ T lymphocytes in experimental autoimmune uveoretinitis induced with two different retinal antigens. *J Immunol.* 1993;151:1627–1636.
123. Rao N, Naida Y, Bell R, et al. Usage of T cell receptor beta-chain variable gene is highly restricted at the site of inflammation in murine autoimmune uveitis. *J Immunol.* 1993;150:5716–5721.
124. Vandenbark A, Hashim G, Offner H. Immunization with a synthetic T-cell receptor V region peptide protects against experimental autoimmune encephalomyelitis. *Nature.* 1989;341:541–544.
125. Kawano Y, Sasamoto Y, Kotake S, et al. Trials of vaccination against experimental autoimmune uveoretinitis with a T cell receptor peptide. *Curr Eye Res.* 1991;10:789–795.
126. Bankovich AJ, Garcia KC. Not just any T cell receptor will do. *Immunity.* 2003;18:7–11.
127. Garcia KC, Degano M, Pease LR, et al. Structural basis of plasticity in T cell receptor recognition of a self peptide-MHC antigen. *Science.* 1998;279:1166–1172.
128. He XL, Radu C, Sidney J, et al. Structural snapshot of aberrant antigen presentation linked to autoimmunity: the immunodominant epitope of MBP complexed with I-A^u. *Immunity.* 2002;17:83–94.
129. Uhlenhuth P. *Zur Lehre von der Unterscheidung Verschiedener Eiweissarten mit Hilfe Spezifischer Sera. Festschrift zum 60 Geburstag von Robert Koch.* Jena, Germany: Fischer; 1903:49–74.
130. Wacker W, Donoso L, Kalsow C. Experimental allergic uveitis. Isolation, characterization, and localization of a soluble uveitopathogenic antigen from bovine retina. *J Immunol.* 1977;119:1949–1958.
131. Faure J. Autoimmunity and the retina. *Curr Topics Eye Res.* 1980;2:215–302.
132. Agarwal RK, Silver PB, Caspi RR. Rodent models of experimental autoimmune uveitis. *Methods Mol Biol.* 2012;900:443–469.
133. Horai R, Silver PB, Chen J. Breakdown of immune privilege and spontaneous autoimmunity in mice expressing a transgenic T cell receptor specific for a retinal autoantigen. *J Autoimmun.* 2013;44:21–33.
134. Pfister C, Chabre M, Plouet J, et al. Retinal S antigen identified as the 48K protein regulating light-dependent phosphodiesterase in rods. *Science.* 1986;228:891–893.
135. Salinas-Carmona M, Nussenblatt R, Gery I. Experimental autoimmune uveitis in the athymic nude rat. *Eur J Immunol.* 1982;25:481–484.
136. Nussenblatt RB, Kuwabara T, de Monasterio FM, et al. S-antigen uveitis in primates. A new model for human disease. *Arch Ophthalmol.* 1981;99:1090–1092.
137. Pennesi G, Mattapallil MJ, Sun SH, et al. A humanized model of experimental autoimmune uveitis in HLA class II transgenic mice. *J Clin Invest.* 2003;111:1171–1180.
138. Wiggert B, Chader GJ. Monkey interphotoreceptor retinoid-binding protein (IRBP): isolation, characterization, and synthesis. *Prog Clin Biol Res.* 1985;190:89–110.
139. Borst D, Redmond T, Elser J, et al. Interphotoreceptor retinoid-binding, protein. Gene characterization, protein repeat structure, and its evolution. *J Biol Chem.* 1989;264:1115–1123.
140. Fox G, Kuwabara T, Wiggert B, et al. Experimental autoimmune uveoretinitis (EAU) induced by retinal interphotoreceptor retinoid-binding protein (IRBP): differences between EAU induced by IRBP and by S-antigen. *Clin Immunol Immunopathol.* 1987;43:256–264.
141. Hirose S, Kuwabara T, Nussenblatt R, et al. Uveitis induced in primates by interphotoreceptor retinoid-binding protein. *Arch Ophthalmol.* 1986;143:79–83.
142. Kozhich AT, Caspi RR, Berzofsky JA, et al. Immunogenicity and immunopathogenicity of an autoimmune epitope are potentiated by increasing MHC binding through residue substitution. *J Immunol.* 1997;158:4145–4151.
143. Donoso LA, Merryman CF, Sery WT, et al. Human IRBP: characterization of uveitopathogenic sites. *Curr Eye Res.* 1988;7:1087–1095.
144. Caspi R, Grubbs BG, Chan CC, et al. Genetic control of susceptibility to experimental autoimmune uveoretinitis in the mouse model. Concomitant regulation by MHC and non-MHC genes. *J Immunol.* 1992;148:2384–2389.

145. Thirkill C, Tait R, Tyler N, et al. The cancer-associated retinopathy antigen is a recoverin-like protein. *Invest Ophthalmol Vis Sci*. 1992;33:2768–2772.
146. Gery I, Chanaud NI, Anglade E. Recoverin is highly uveitogenic in Lewis rats. *Invest Ophthalmol Vis Sci*. 1994;35:3342–3345.
147. Hamel CP, Tsilou E, Pfeffer BA, et al. Molecular cloning and expression of RPE65, a novel retinal pigment epithelium-specific microsomal protein that is post-transcriptionally regulated in vitro. *J Biol Chem*. 1993;268:15751–15757.
148. Morimura H, Fishman GA, Grover SA, et al. Mutations in the RPE65 gene in patients with autosomal recessive retinitis pigmentosa or Leber congenital amaurosis. *Proc Natl Acad Sci U S A*. 1998;95:3088–3093.
149. Ham DI, Gentleman S, Chan CC, et al. RPE65 is highly uveitogenic in rats. *Invest Ophthalmol Vis Sci*. 2002;43:2258–2263.
150. Broekhuyse R, Kuhlmann E, Winkens H. Experimental autoimmune anterior uveitis (EAAU), a new form of experimental uveitis. I. Induction by a detergent-insoluble, intrinsic protein fraction of the retina pigment epithelium. *Exp Eye Res*. 1991;52:465–474.
151. Chan C, Hikita N, Dastgheib K, et al. Experimental melanin-protein-induced uveitis in the Lewis rat. Immunopathologic processes. *Ophthalmology*. 1994;101:1275–1280.
152. Yamaki K, Kondo I, Nakmura H, et al. Ocular and extraocular inflammation induced by immunization of tyrosinase related protein 1 and 2 in Lewis rats. *Exp Eye Res*. 2000;71:361–369.
153. Yamaki K, Gocho K, Hayakawa K, et al. Tyrosinase family proteins are antigens specific to Vogt-Koyanagi-Harada disease. *J Immunol*. 2000;165:7323–7329.
154. Gocho K, Kondo I, Yamaki K. Identification of autoreactive T cells in Vogt-Koyanagi-Harada disease. *Invest Ophthalmol Vis Sci*. 2001;42:2004–2009.
155. Schalken J, Winkens H, Van Vugt A, et al. Rhodopsin-induced experimental autoimmune uveoretinitis: dose-dependent clinicopathological features. *Exp Eye Res*. 1988;47:35–145.
156. Dua H, Lee R, Lolley R, et al. Induction of experimental autoimmune uveitis by the retinal photoreceptor cell protein, phosducin. *Curr Eye Res*. 1992;11:107–111.
157. Caspi RR. Immune mechanisms in uveitis. *Springer Semin Immunopathol*. 1999;21:113–124.
158. Rozenszajn L, Muellenberg-Coulombre C, Gery I, et al. Induction of experimental autoimmune uveoretinitis (EAU) in rats by T cell lines. *Immunology*. 1986;57:559–565.
159. Rizzo LV, Silver P, Wiggert B, et al. Establishment and characterization of a murine CD4+ T cell line and clone that induce experimental autoimmune uveoretinitis in B10.A mice. *J Immunol*. 1996;156:1654–1660.
160. Marak GJ, Wacker W, Rao N, et al. Effects of complement depletion on experimental allergic uveitis. *Ophthalmol Res*. 1979;11:97–107.
161. Silver BP, Horai R, Chen J, et al. Retina-specific T regulatory cells bring about resolution and maintain remission of autoimmune uveitis. *J Immunol*. 2015;194:3011–3019.
162. Horai R, Zarate-Blades CR, Dillenburg-Pilla P, et al. Microbiota-dependent activation of an autoreactive T cell receptor provokes autoimmunity in an immunologically privileged site. *Immunity*. 2015;43:343–353.
163. Horai R, Caspi RR. Microbiome and autoimmune uveitis. *Front Immunol*. 2019;10:232.
164. Kodati S, Sen HN. Uveitis and the gut microbiota. *Best Pract Res Clin Rheumatol*. 2020;33(6):101500.
165. Rosenbaum J, McDevitt HO, Guss RB, et al. Endotoxin-induced uveitis in rats as a model for human disease. *Nature*. 1980;286:611–613.
166. De Vos A, Hoekzema R, Kijlstra A. Cytokines and uveitis, a review. *Curr Eye Res*. 1992;11:581–597.
167. Ebringer A, Cowdell D, Cowling P. Sequential studies in ankylosing spondylitis. *Ann Rheum Dis*. 1978;37:146–151.
168. Schwimmbeck P, Yu D, Oldstone M. Autoantibodies to HLA B27 in the sera of HLA B27 patients with ankylosing spondylitis and Reiter's syndrome. *J Exp Med*. 1987;166:173–181.
169. Kawai T, Akira S. TLR signaling. *Semin Immunol*. 2007;19:24–32.
170. Nussenblatt R, Lecture Proctor. Experimental autoimmune uveitis: mechanisms of disease and clinical therapeutic indications. *Invest Ophthamol Vis Sci*. 1991;32:3131–3141.
171. Nussenblatt R, Rodrigues M, Wacker W, et al. Cyclosporin A. Inhibition of experimental autoimmune uveitis in Lewis rats. *J Clin Invest*. 1981;67:1228–1231.
172. Nussenblatt R, Rodrigues M, Salinas-Carmona M, et al. Modulation of experimental autoimmune uveitis with cyclosporin A. *Arch Ophthalmol*. 1982;100:1146–1149.
173. Nussenblatt RB, Palestine AG, Rook AH, et al. Treatment of intraocular inflammatory disease with cyclosporin A. *Lancet*. 1983;2:235–238.
174. Nussenblatt R, Gery I, Ballintine E, et al. Cellular immune responsiveness of uveitis patients to retinal S-antigen. *Am J Ophthalmol*. 1980;89:173–179.
175. Hooks J, Detrick B. Immunoregulatory functions of interferon. In: Torrence P, ed. *Biological Response Modifiers*. New York: Academic Press; 1985:55–75.

2

Medical History in the Patient with Uveitis

Scott M. Whitcup

KEY CONCEPTS

- A detailed medical history is one of the keys to accurate diagnosis of uveitis in the majority of cases.
- Use of the uveitis medical history questionnaire provides a set of standardized information useful for diagnosis.
- Therapy should be targeted not only to address inflammation noted on examination but also to treat symptoms that affect function or quality of life.
- Quality-of-life questionnaires can be useful in assessing the effect of disease on patients and in determining appropriate therapy.
- The medical history is also important in assessing response to therapy and the side effects of medications.
- Use of electronic medical records and electronic collection of medical history information from patients outside of the office should improve the quality of data used to diagnose and treat patients.

The word *diagnosis* is derived from the Greek word *diagnosi* meaning "to distinguish and discern." Accurate diagnosis encompasses both data collection and analysis of the compiled clinical information. The facts used in diagnosis come from a detailed medical history, a thorough physical examination, and diagnostic tests and imaging, where indicated. In the case of patients with uveitis, one must look beyond the eye for important diagnostic clues because the rheumatologic, infectious, and oncologic diseases that cause uveitis are often easier to diagnose after a careful medical history has been taken and a detailed physical examination has been performed. The ophthalmologist who does not examine the skin or the joints of the patient with uveitis will miss the opportunity to correctly diagnose many cases. Observing the course of the disease and the patient's response to therapy can also provide insights into identifying the correct causes of the disease.

A careful and detailed medical history is one of the keys to accurate diagnosis of uveitis. It has been estimated that greater than 90% of diagnoses can be made on the basis of the medical history alone. Medical questionnaires have also been shown to improve the accuracy of diagnosis when used as part of an algorithm. For example, an algorithm employing a questionnaire designed to diagnose patients presenting with red eyes was accurate 72% of the time.[1] It helped correctly diagnose 100% of acute angle closure cases, 82% of iritis cases, and 50% of infective conjunctivitis cases. Clearly, standardization of nomenclature will also help improve the accuracy of data collected from medical questionnaires and the interpretation of this information. Both the International Uveitis Study Group (IUSG)[2] and the Standardization of Uveitis Nomenclature (SUN) Working Group[3] have begun the process of standardizing some of the terms used in the classification of uveitis.

It is important to not only obtain a series of medical facts but also form an impression about the overall course of the disease and its effect on the patient's quality of life. Are there defined disease episodes, or is the condition truly chronic? Is ocular inflammation accompanied by pain and redness or by floaters and visual loss? In chronic disease, the level of visual disability and discomfort that is tolerable for one patient is intolerable for another, and it is important to understand the patient's perspective before recommending therapy. In addition, some aspects of the disease can be modified by therapy, but others cannot. By determining what is really bothering the patient, the physician can attempt to focus therapy on the most troublesome aspect of the disease. For example, some patients are troubled by mild conjunctival erythema and request treatment. Other patients do not like to use medications and tolerate mild redness. Importantly, the perception of visual loss differs greatly among patients. Even mild distortion in vision related to inflammation may interfere with the activities of some patients and warrant aggressive anti-inflammatory therapy. Only by fully understanding the patient and the way the disease has an effect on his or her life can the physician put the disorder into proper perspective to best counsel the patient and recommend an individualized treatment plan.

Use of standardized vision-related quality-of-life questionnaires can help assess the effect of uveitis on patients and assist in determining therapy. A study using the National Eye Institute Visual Functioning Questionnaire (NEI VFQ-25) showed that patients with uveitis reported markedly poorer visual functioning and general health status compared with normal subjects.[4] These questionnaires have also been used to demonstrate that systemic therapy can be effectively used to control severe uveitis without a significant adverse effect on quality of life.[5] Disease-specific quality-of-life questionnaires are being developed and may be useful for managing certain ocular inflammatory diseases. Finally, depression may be an important, but often underrecognized, condition in patients with uveitis and vision impairment, and use of depression questionnaires, such as the Beck Depression Inventory-II, in addition to vision-related and overall health-related quality-of-life measures may be useful in managing patients with uveitis.[6]

Floaters and reduced vision are the two most common complaints of patients with inflammation of the vitreous, retina, and choroid. Most patients describe floaters as multiple small- or medium-sized spots that move as the eye moves. Other patients complain of blurred or reduced vision. In fact, when visual acuity is severely diminished, patients may be unable to visualize the floaters and may only complain of floaters as their vision starts to improve after therapy. A change in the pattern of floaters or visual impairment often signals a change in the underlying ocular disease, such as increased inflammation, the development of vitreous hemorrhage, or the condensation of the vitreous into a more organized opaque tissue. A careful history can also differentiate causes of brief visual impairment, such as vascular emboli, shifting subretinal fluid, or neurologic diseases (e.g., migraine) from visual disability caused by ocular inflammatory disease.

The medical history should include demographic details of the patient, including age, sex, race, and occupation. The chief complaint should be succinctly stated, including the reason for the visit and the duration of the problem. The history of the present illness should then be documented, with the major symptoms in chronologic order and a definition of what makes those symptoms better or worse. A detailed past medical history, including family history, social history, and sexual history, is frequently omitted from ophthalmologic evaluations but is critical to the assessment of the patient with uveitis. We find it extremely useful to have patients complete a uveitis medical history questionnaire before the examination; our questionnaire was developed in conjunction with Dr. C. Steven Foster at the Massachusetts Eye and Ear Infirmary (see Appendix). The questionnaire is then reviewed with the patient during the medical history, when answers can be clarified and additional questions can be asked. The survey helps guarantee that in all cases, core medical information is gathered and important medical questions are not neglected. However, the clinician should realize that completed questionnaires may contain errors. It is important to clarify patient responses and to ask the patient verbally about important aspects of the history, even if the patient denied a symptom on the questionnaire. A study by Seltzer and McDermott[7] showed that 66% of patients who completed the same medical history questionnaire twice made at least one significant omission in their history.

Although it is relatively uncommon for uveitis to occur in families, many forms of the disease, such as iritis associated with ankylosing spondylitis and birdshot retinochoroidopathy, have strong human leukocyte antigen (HLA) associations that suggest an important inherited component. Thus it is important to recognize that autoimmune diseases may run in a family and to document the occurrence of these diseases in other family members. Patients with uveitis may have relatives with such diseases as rheumatoid arthritis or systemic lupus erythematosus (SLE). Obtaining the social history is also important in the evaluation of the patient with uveitis. A patient's social situation can influence not only the type and severity of a disease he or she acquires but also the physician's ability to effectively treat the condition. Social problems can impede a patient's compliance with medical or surgical therapy. Furthermore, patients who are not able to take medication reliably or to comply with frequent laboratory monitoring of hematologic and renal status are not good candidates for immunosuppressive therapy that can impair the immune system.

Electronic medical records (EMRs), also known as electronic health records (EHRs), have been incorporated into many clinical practices. The EMR can help address issues, such as missing records, missing critical information in the medical records, and poor legibility, and promote more structured collection of data.[8] Some systems use speech recognition to assist in documenting the history. Computerized algorithms may help clinicians improve both diagnosis and subsequent therapy. Although the adoption of EMRs have historically been slow,[9] in 2014, 765 hospitals had adopted at least a basic EHR system.[10] Finally, the ability of patients to enter their medical history and symptoms into their own medical records electronically from home on personal devices, such as their mobile phones, should improve the accuracy of the data used to diagnose and treat patients.[11]

REFERENCES

1. Timlin H, Butler L, Wright M. The accuracy of the Edinburgh Red Eye Diagnostic Algorithm. *Eye (Lond)*. 2015;29:619–624.
2. Deschenes J, Murray PI, Rao NA, Nussenblatt RB. International Uveitis Study Group. International Uveitis Study Group (IUSG): clinical classification of uveitis. *Ocul Immunol Inflamm*. 2008;16:1–2.
3. Jabs DA, Nussenblatt RB, Rosenbaum JT. Standardization of Uveitis Nomenclature (SUN) Working Group. Standardization of uveitis nomenclature for reporting clinical data. Results of the First International Workshop. *Am J Ophthalmol*. 2005;140:509–516.
4. Schiffman RM, Jacobsen G, Whitcup SM. Visual functioning and general health status in patients with uveitis. *Arch Ophthalmol*. 2001;119:841–849.
5. Gui W, Marcus DM, Stowe MH, et al. Quality of life in patients with non-infectious uveitis treated with or without systemic anti-inflammatory therapy. *Ocul Immunol Inflamm*. 2015;2:135–143.
6. Qian Y, Glaser T, Esterberg E. Depression and visual functioning in patients with ocular inflammatory disease. *Am J Ophthalmol*. 2012;2:370–378.
7. Seltzer MH, McDermott JH. Inaccuracies in patient medical histories. *Compr Ther*. 1999;25:258–264.
8. Bleeker SE, Derksen-Lubsen G, van Ginneken AM, et al. Structured data entry for narrative data in a broad specialty: patient history and physical examination in pediatrics. *BMC Med Inform Decis Mak*. 2006;6:29.
9. Blumenthal D, Glaser JP. Information technology comes to medicine. *N Engl J Med*. 2007;356:2527–2534.
10. Charles D, Gabriel M, Searcy T. *Adoption of electronic health record systems among U.S. non-federal acute care hospitals: 2008-2014*. Office of the National Coordinator for Health Information Technology ONC Data Brief No. 23; April 2015. https://www.healthit.gov/sites/default/files/data-brief/2014HospitalAdoptionDataBrief.pdf.
11. Bousquet J, Caimmi DP, Bedbrook A, et al. Pilot study of mobile phone technology in allergic rhinitis in European countries. The MASK-Rhinitis Study. *Allergy*. 2017;72(6):857–865.

3

Clinical Examination of the Patient with Uveitis

Scott M. Whitcup

KEY CONCEPTS

- A thorough clinical ophthalmic examination is critical for both diagnosis and assessment of response to therapy.
- Use of standardized grading scales for assessing intraocular inflammation can improve patient management.
- Standard grading scales are available for assessment of anterior chamber cells and flare and vitreous cells and haze.
- A detailed examination of the peripheral retina can reveal pars plana exudates, signs of retinal vasculitis, Delen-Fuchs nodules, or other lesions suggesting active inflammation or infection.
- Use of ancillary tests, such as optical coherence tomography angiography (OCTA), should supplement, but not replace, careful clinical examination.

The ocular examination of patients with uveitis is important not only to diagnose the disease correctly but also to determine the appropriate therapy. The examination will provide information that enables the examiner to generate a differential diagnosis and will allow the patient's subjective complaints to be placed in the framework of objective clinical findings. In addition, the baseline examination findings become an important yardstick against which treatment success or failure will be measured. Many inflammatory diseases are chronic and require potentially toxic therapy. Therefore it is critical to accurately assess whether a patient is benefiting from treatment. This includes a thorough review of the patient's previous medical records and accurate assessment of disease status at each clinic visit. A complete review of the patient's medical records provides important information for planning new therapeutic approaches and guards against repeating therapies that were unsatisfactory in the past. Because a patient's medical record is valuable in assessing response to therapy, it is important to accurately record the presence or absence of important physical findings in a reproducible and standardized manner. Furthermore, because many of the ophthalmic findings in inflammatory disease, such as vitreous cells and haze, are evaluated only by subjective means, the examiner should strive to maintain internal consistency in grading the severity of the observations and to standardize these observations, whenever possible. Importantly, standard grading scales should be used, whenever possible. The use of standard scales ensures consistency when different ophthalmologists are involved in the care of the patient over time. This also allows for comparison of cases with those reported in the literature.

VISUAL ACUITY

Several factors can lead to reduced visual acuity in patients with uveitis or retinitis. A combination of corneal opacity, anterior chamber inflammation, cataract, and vitreous haze may exacerbate disturbance of retinal function caused by retinal edema, necrosis, or scarring. In addition, optic nerve function may be compromised after inflammation or glaucoma. It is important for the clinician to determine the cause of diminished vision because the therapeutic approach will vary, depending on the cause. For example, it would be inappropriate to increase the dose of prednisone to treat worsening vision caused by progressive posterior subcapsular cataract. Whatever type of visual acuity measurement is used, it must be performed under the same lighting conditions each time; otherwise the fluctuations induced by the testing environment will mask changes in vision caused by worsening disease or response to therapy. A best-corrected visual acuity measurement should be obtained either by refraction or, at the very least, with the use of a pinhole occluder. Near-vision measurement is also helpful because we have observed that improvement in near vision can precede improvement in distance vision by several weeks in patients with chronic macular edema.

The most common method to measure visual acuity is use of the Snellen eye chart. Like all eye charts, the Snellen chart helps assess a patient's ability to read high-contrast letters, and its use is satisfactory if the vision is good. Unfortunately, the chart does not have enough sensitivity for use in patients with poor vision. There are no lines between 20/100 and 20/200 or between 20/200 and 20/400. In addition, there are too few letters on the lines above 20/100. Although an improvement in visual acuity from 20/200 to 20/125 may not be significant to the patient, the ability to measure this improvement is an important indicator that the current therapeutic approach is working. Because many patients with macular edema have visual acuity less than 20/80, initial improvement might be missed when the standard Snellen chart is used.

For these reasons, we have used the ETDRS chart initially developed for the evaluation of patients in the Early Treatment for Diabetic Retinopathy Study (ETDRS) (Fig. 3.1).[1] This chart has five letters per line, starting with the 20/200 line, and every set of three lines represents a doubling of the visual angle. Therefore improving from 20/40 to 20/20 represents the same level of improvement in visual function as does 20/80 to 20/40. If patients cannot read the 20/200 line while sitting 4 m from the chart, they are moved to 1 m from the chart, and the acuities are recorded as 5 over the appropriate denominator, that is, 5/200. Because each line has five letters, visual acuity can be expressed as the total number of letters read. The 1- and 4-m scales can be made continuous by adding 30 letters to those read at 4 m. The scale of visual acuity is then linear and continuous from 5/200 (five letters) to 20/12.5 (95 letters).

A computerized method for testing visual acuity for clinical research has been developed as an alternative to the standard ETDRS

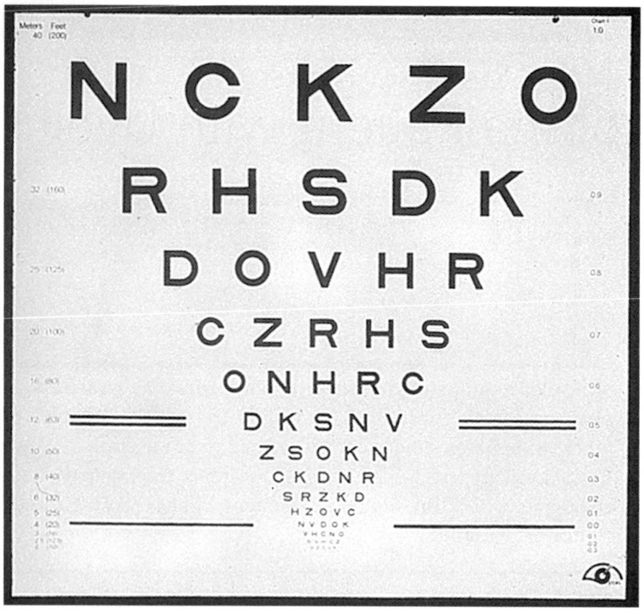

Fig. 3.1 Visual acuity chart from Early Treatment of Diabetic Retinopathy Study (ETDRS). (Courtesy Frederick Ferris, MD.)

testing protocol.[2] A multicenter study comparing this electronic visual acuity testing algorithm (E-ETDRS) with the standard testing protocol showed high test–retest reliability and good concordance of the electronic protocol with the standard ETDRS testing. This new method allows electronic capture of data, eliminates computational errors, reduces testing time, and may help reduce technician bias. Mobile technology is also being used to measure visual acuity, and some of these devices have demonstrated appropriate photometric characteristics, including luminance and contrast.[3] However, reliability and validity of self-administered visual acuity measurements need to be assessed. New visual acuity charts or assessment of reading speed may be useful in assessing patients with more severe vision loss or macular disease, but, again, it is critical to validate these methods for their widespread use.

EXTERNAL EXAMINATION

As stated earlier, a detailed examination of the skin can provide useful diagnostic clues to the astute clinician. Not only should the skin of the lids be closely examined, but the entire skin should also be evaluated for the presence of rashes, nodules, or vitiligo. We have diagnosed sarcoidosis on the basis of the presence of lid granulomas and of lesions on the extremities and the chest, and we have diagnosed Kaposi sarcoma on the basis of characteristic vascular lesions on the upper eyelid. If any skin findings are noted, photographs, a consultation with a dermatologist, and a skin biopsy should be considered.

PUPILS AND EXTRAOCULAR MUSCLES

Evaluation of the pupils is frequently difficult in the patient with uveitis because of synechiae or chronic cycloplegic therapy. The inflamed pupil, even without synechiae, may not move well as a result of iris atrophy, a parasympathetic nerve lesion caused by herpes infection, or because it is trapped by a displaced intraocular lens. When examination is possible, the status of the optic nerve can be assessed with the standard swinging flashlight test to detect an afferent pupillary defect.

Involvement of the extraocular muscles in intraocular inflammatory disease is unusual. Esotropia or exotropia resulting from long-standing visual loss may develop as a result of cataract, retinal disease, or optic nerve disease. The finding of new vertical tropia or internuclear ophthalmoplegia should alert the physician to underlying diseases of the central nervous system (CNS) that may be associated with causes of uveitis, such as multiple sclerosis, sarcoidosis, or non-Hodgkin lymphoma.

INTRAOCULAR PRESSURE MEASUREMENT

Either elevated intraocular pressure or hypotony can occur as a result of intraocular inflammation. Goldmann applanation tonometry is usually sufficient to measure intraocular pressure in patients with uveitis; however, fluorescein should not be instilled until slit-lamp examination and ophthalmoscopy are completed because fluorescein enters the eye and prevents accurate assessment of the amount of flare in the anterior chamber. In addition, fluorescein may obscure the view of the posterior segment if the pupil is small and may persist in the eye for longer than 24 hours, especially in eyes with hypotonia and reduced aqueous flow. Therefore applanation tonometry should be performed either with the patient under anesthesia, without using fluorescein, and with a pneumotonometer or, preferably, at the end of the examination.

CONJUNCTIVA

Conjunctival hyperemia is a common sign of acute anterior inflammation but is rare in chronic posterior segment disease. Usually, conjunctival injection is uniform in the perilimbal region and represents ciliary body inflammation. The conjunctival injection of uveitis can be differentiated from conjunctivitis by the lack of involvement of the fornix and the palpebral conjunctiva. Scleritis and episcleritis may occur in conjunction with some types of intraocular inflammation. Injected deep scleral vessels, a purple scleral hue, and severe pain distinguish true scleritis from more superficial inflammation. Scleritis associated with uveitis is often nodular and confined to a section of the globe, whereas ciliary body injection tends to involve the globe more diffusely. Some confusion may arise when a patient with intraocular inflammation develops an allergic reaction to topical medication. The eye becomes more painful and red during treatment, and this may be misinterpreted as worsening disease and failure of treatment. However, itching, dermatitis, and significant conjunctival injection affecting the palpebral conjunctiva often develop in patients with a superimposed allergic reaction.

CORNEA

Keratic Precipitates

Keratic precipitates (KPs) are the most commonly reported corneal finding in uveitis (Fig. 3.2). They are small aggregates of inflammatory cells that accumulate on the endothelial surface of the cornea. The presence of these deposits on the endothelium of the cornea provides useful diagnostic information and indicates the current level of inflammatory activity. Also, in an eye without active anterior segment inflammation manifesting as cells and flare, the presence of KPs tells the practitioner that the eye was previously inflamed.

KPs usually accumulate on the lower half of the cornea, often in a base-down triangle configuration; however, in some disorders, such as Fuchs iridocyclitis, KPs may be present superiorly. The precipitates vary in size from flecks that are the size of cornea guttata to 1 mm in diameter. Because cornea guttata may be present in patients with uveitis, very fine, small KPs can be distinguished by their inferior corneal location and slightly elongated shape. KPs can be easily seen with the slit lamp and direct or retroillumination. The small aggregates have been conventionally described as "nongranulomatous," whereas

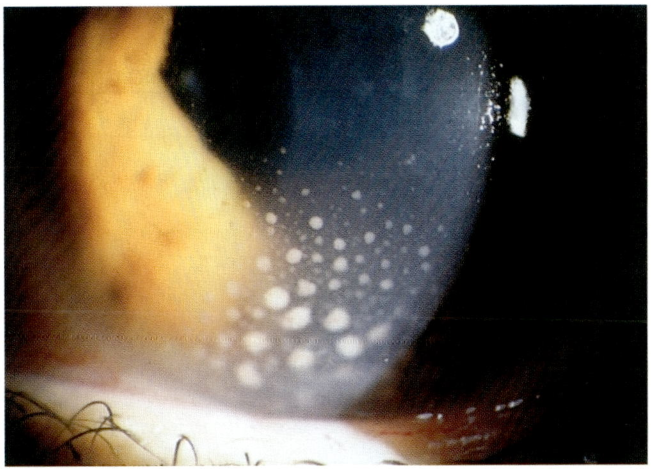

Fig. 3.2 Granulomatous keratic precipitates present in patient with sarcoidosis.

the larger, more greasy-appearing ones have been described as "mutton fat" or "granulomatous." These descriptions may be misleading because they imply a pathologic correlation that is rarely known. There is no objective way of defining granulomatous versus nongranulomatous KPs. Both types of precipitates can coexist in a patient at the same time or vary during the course of the disease or therapy. In general, the larger granulomatous aggregates are composed of macrophages and giant cells and occur in chronic inflammation, whereas the smaller nongranulomatous ones occur in acute inflammation and are more likely to be composed of neutrophils and lymphocytes. In a small study of 25 patients, corneal specular microscopy showed no significant difference in keratic precipitates in infectious and noninfectious uveitis.[4]

Nevertheless, there are a number of diseases typically associated with granulomatous KPs (see Box 4.3), and the presence of these precipitates can aid in making a differential diagnosis. In most inflammatory reactions, the neutrophil is the first cell present, and the transformed macrophages (epithelioid cells) and lymphocytes accumulate as the inflammation becomes more chronic. KPs therefore mimic the course of the inflammation in the tissue. For example, patients with documented pulmonary sarcoidosis may have acute anterior inflammatory episodes with small nongranulomatous KPs. If the inflammatory disease becomes chronic, the KP aggregates may become larger and more granulomatous. After the resolution of active inflammation, the KP aggregates may disappear completely or become smaller, translucent, or pigmented. KPs may also be washed away during intraocular surgery. Finally, the subtle appearance of fine KPs may be the first sign of inflammation,[5] and the posterior cornea should be examined closely in all patients with possible uveitis. Not only can the corneal endothelium be the first sign of ocular inflammation, central endothelial cell density can also be decreased in patients with anterior uveitis.[6]

Other Corneal Findings

Other corneal findings can provide clues to the correct diagnosis. For example, corneal dendrites may be seen with uveitis as a result of herpes simplex virus infection. Interstitial keratitis may be associated with syphilis or Cogan syndrome. The clinician should examine the cornea carefully because the presence of stromal ghost vessels extending more than several millimeters from the limbus may easily be overlooked. We have noted similar findings in the inferior cornea in patients with sarcoidosis. Finally, we have seen several patients with corneal grafts who were referred with conditions diagnosed as idiopathic uveitis. In a number of these, the uveitis was actually caused by early allograft rejection.

ANTERIOR CHAMBER

The anterior chamber is easily examined with the slit lamp for signs of ocular inflammation. Because inflammatory cells do not arise in the aqueous, the presence of cells or increased protein (flare) in the anterior chamber is evidence of spillover from the inflamed iris or ciliary body. Not infrequently, a patient with recurrent iritis comes to the ophthalmologist complaining of pain, but because of the lack of cells or flare on examination, the patient is told that there is no uveitis and that no therapy is needed. To the practitioner's dismay, the patient returns the next day with full-blown iritis. The explanation for this is that the inflammation begins in the iris and the ciliary body, and only when sufficient inflammatory cells accumulate within these tissues do the cells begin to enter the aqueous and become visible to the clinician. Therefore anterior chamber inflammation is a convenient, but somewhat indirect, measure of the inflammatory reaction in the iris and the ciliary body.

Anterior chamber cells are primarily lymphocytes in most episodes of anterior uveitis, but a significant number of neutrophils may be present early in the course of disease. Anterior chamber cells are best seen by directing the spillover beam obliquely across the eye and focusing posterior to the cornea. There is considerable variation among physicians on the grading of the number of cells. Because the cells represent an index of activity, but not a direct measure of the active inflammation, we do not believe that the grading system must discriminate between small increments of disease. Table 3.1 summarizes the system proposed by Hogan et al.,[7] the system proposed by Schlaegel that uses a wide beam with a narrow slit,[8] and our preferred system that uses a 1 × 1 mm slit beam. The smaller slit allows some resolution for more severe inflammation and less resolution at the milder end of the spectrum. We are most interested in quantifying anterior chamber cells during the early stages of acute inflammation when a change in cellularity may signal early response to therapy and when lack of response might dictate a change in therapy. The problem with most classification systems is that it is impossible for clinicians to remember how many cells are associated with a grade of trace, occasional, or rare cells. Therefore we have modified our grading system: for grades of trace cells (1–5) and 1+ cells (6–15 cells), we put the exact number of cells counted in parentheses after the grade, for example, 1+ (11) or trace (3). The grading scale we use was adopted at the First International Workshop discussing the standardization of uveitis nomenclature and published in 2005.[9] In many chronically inflamed eyes, it may be impossible to eliminate every last cell, and these rare cells may not require treatment. Nevertheless, persistence of more than a rare cell may place the patient at increased risk for inflammatory complications and worsen the prognosis after cataract extraction.

It is also our experience that the size of the individual cells in the anterior chamber will decrease as the inflammation begins to resolve. This may occur before the number of cells actually decreases. A change from large activated lymphocytes to smaller cells may account for this clinical observation. It is important to differentiate inflammatory cells from other types of cells in the anterior chamber. Red blood cells, iris pigment cells, and malignant cells may be mistaken for inflammatory cells. The differentiation is especially difficult if a lymphoid malignancy is present: monoclonal antibody staining of cells obtained by paracentesis may be critical in identifying the type of cell.

Increased protein content in the anterior chamber is a manifestation of a breakdown of the blood–ocular barrier. When the slit beam is obliquely aimed across the anterior chamber, the ability to visualize the path of the beam is termed *flare*. There are approximately 7 g of protein/100 mL of blood, but only 11 mg of protein/100 mL of aqueous. A faint amount of flare is normal if a bright light is used. The amount of light scattering is proportional to the concentration of protein in a solution, and hence more flare indicates increased protein in the anterior chamber fluid. Flare can be clinically graded on a scale

TABLE 3.1 Grading of Anterior Chamber Cells

SCHLAEGEL[a]		HOGAN ET AL.[b]		AUTHORS' APPROACH[b]		SUN WORKING GROUP	
Grade	Cells	Grade	Cells	Grade	Cells	Grade	Cells
–	–	0	0	0	0	0	<1
½+	Rare (normal)	Rare cells	1–2	–	–		
–	–	Occasional cell	3–7	–	–		
–	–	–	–	Trace[c]	1–5	Trace	1–5
1+	Occasional cell	1+	7–10	1+[c]	6–15	1+	6–15
1½+	2–7	1–2+	10–15	–	–		
2+	8–15	2+	15–20	2+	16–25	2+	16–25
2½+	16–30	–	–	–	–		
3+	Too many to count	3+	20–50	3+	26–50	3+	26–50
3½+	Too many to count	–	–	–	–		
4+	Most ever seen	4+	>50	4+	>50	4+	>50

[a]Using a wide beam with a narrow slit.
[b]Using a 1 × 1 mm slit.
[c]For grades of trace and 1+ the exact number of cells is recorded in parentheses, that is, 1+ (11).
Data from Schlaegel TF, Jr. *Essentials of Uveitis.* Boston, MA: Little, Brown; 1967:7; Hogan MJ, Kimura SJ, Thygeson P. Signs and symptoms of uveitis. I. Anterior uveitis. *Am J Ophthalmol.* 1959;47:155–170.

TABLE 3.2 Grading of Anterior Chamber Flare

Grade	Schlaegel	Hogan et al.	SUN Working Group
0	Complete absence		None
½+	Faint (normal)	–	
1+	Very slight (normal)	Very slight	Faint
1½+	Mild	–	
2+	Mild to moderate	Moderate (iris and lens clear)	Moderate (iris and lens details clear)
3+	Moderate	Marked flare (iris and lens hazy)	Marked (iris and lens details hazy)
4+	Severe	Intense (fibrin, plastic aqueous)	Intense (fibrin or plastic aqueous)

Data from Schlaegel TF, Jr. *Essentials of Uveitis.* Boston, MA: Little, Brown; 1967:7; Hogan MJ, Kimura SJ, Thygeson P. Signs and symptoms of uveitis. I. Anterior uveitis. *Am J Ophthalmol.* 1959;47:155–170.

of 0 to 4+ using a grading scale published by Hogan et al.[7] in 1959 (Table 3.2). This scale was adopted by the Standardization of Uveitis Nomenclature (SUN) Working Group with slight modification.[9] We have reserved the 4+ grade for leakage of protein so extensive that a fibrin clot is present. In addition to the subjective grading of flare, it is possible to more accurately measure the degree of light scattering and quantify the amount of protein. A technique described by Herman et al.[10] uses the principle that fluorescein in the anterior chamber will bind to albumin, and the amount of bound fluorescein will alter the polarization of fluorescein as measured by fluorophotometry. This method is able to quantify alterations in blood–ocular barrier leakage of albumin. A newer technique of objectively assessing aqueous flare measures the scattering of a laser beam projected across the anterior chamber. This laser flare meter is more fully described in Chapter 5.

Some disagreement exists as to whether the presence of flare by itself, without cells or other signs of active inflammation, should be treated. In our opinion, without objective quantification of a change in the leakage across the blood–ocular barrier, chronic flare alone is not a sign of active inflammation. Damaged blood vessels may be leaky for a long time after the active inflammation has resolved. Continued treatment with drugs, such as corticosteroids, may do little to alter the repair of these vessels in the absence of active inflammation. Although there is no evidence that small amounts of increased protein in the anterior chamber are detrimental to the eye, factors associated with worsening visual acuity in patients with uveitis included incident anterior segment flare.[11] Further studies are needed to determine whether continued therapy is useful in patients with persistent, stable levels of flare in the absence of other inflammatory signs. Specifically, children with juvenile rheumatoid arthritis with persistent flare but no cells may not require ocular anti-inflammatory therapy. Therefore flare should be considered a marker of inflammation but not necessarily a pathognomonic finding of active inflammation.

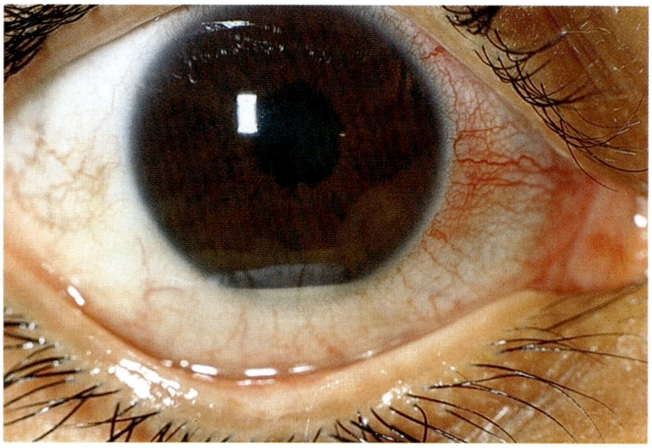

Fig. 3.3 Hypopyon in patient with Behçet disease.

A hypopyon (Fig. 3.3) is a collection of leukocytes that settle in the lower angle of the anterior chamber. The cause of a hypopyon is unclear and is not related solely to the number of cells in the anterior chamber. It is also related to the presence of sufficient fibrin to cause the cells to clump and settle. Hypopyon is a dramatic but short-lived finding in ocular

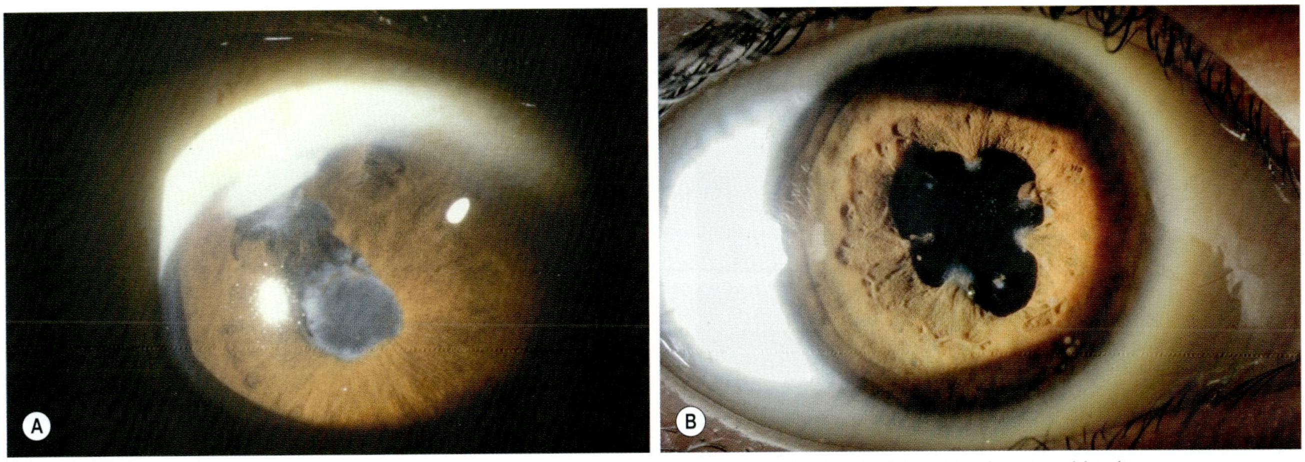

Fig. 3.4 Plate A: Posterior synechiae and closure of iridectomy. Plate B: Multiple posterior synechiae in a patient with Blau syndrome.

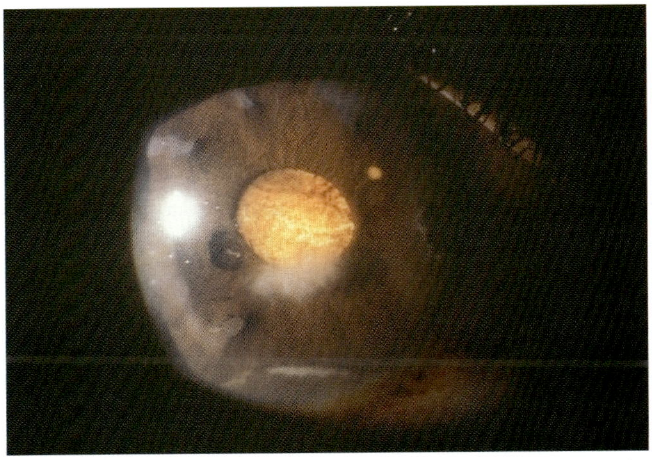

Fig. 3.5 Anterior synechiae in patient with sarcoidosis demonstrating iris–cornea adhesions.

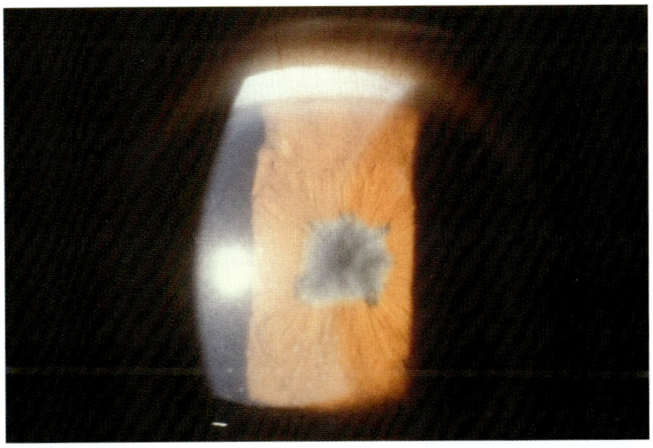

Fig. 3.6 Posterior synechiae with fibrin membrane and totally occluded pupil.

inflammation and has been associated with Behçet disease, endophthalmitis, and rifabutin toxicity in patients with acquired immunodeficiency syndrome (AIDS). A hypopyon may also occur sporadically in severe acute inflammation associated with many other types of uveitis.[12] Of course, a hypopyon frequently develops in patients with endophthalmitis, and infection should always be considered a potential etiology. This is especially true in patients who have had recent intraocular surgery. However, a sterile hypopyon can also occur after intraocular surgery. Severe exacerbation of uveitis can occur after ocular surgery in patients with uveitis, especially if appropriate anti-inflammatory therapy is not given. Retained lens fragments can also precipitate severe intraocular inflammation and hypopyon.[13] A pseudohypopyon, composed of tumor cells or hemorrhagic debris, can occur in some of the masquerade syndromes (see Chapter 31) after vitreous hemorrhage. Finally, a hyphema can occur in eyes with uveitis, often as a result of neovascularization of the iris. Interestingly, a case of a pink hypopyon was noted in a patient with *Serratia marcescens* endophthalmitis.[14] Cytologic examination revealed no erythrocytes, and the pink color was caused by the bacteria.

IRIS

A detailed examination of the iris can often provide important diagnostic clues to the clinician. Inflammation is often accompanied by the release of mediators that promote fibrin deposition, clotting, and fibroblast proliferation, which are the probable causes of synechiae. Synechiae are adhesions between the iris and the lens capsule (posterior synechiae) (Fig. 3.4) or the iris and the cornea near the anterior chamber angle (peripheral anterior synechiae [PAS]). The former are responsible for the development of pupillary block glaucoma, and the latter contribute to the development of obstruction of aqueous outflow. In general, the presence of synechiae indicates that the inflammation has been chronic or recurrent; however, these adhesions may occasionally develop within a few days in patients with severe inflammation. Although most peripheral anterior synechiae can be seen only by gonioscopy, some patients will develop more profound anterior adhesions (Fig. 3.5). Most posterior synechiae are located at the pupillary border, but in patients with severe chronic inflammation, adhesions of the entire posterior iris surface to the anterior lens capsule can develop. A fibrovascular membrane may develop in patients with long-standing and recurrent inflammation in whom the pupil size has been reduced to a few millimeters by posterior synechiae (Fig. 3.6). This membrane may be translucent and adherent to the surface of the lens and not apparent until cataract removal is attempted. The iris may also become atrophic in certain uveitic conditions. For example, iris transillumination defects (Fig. 3.7) can be a clue to herpetic uveitis, especially when associated with corneal disease and persistent anterior uveitis. Other causes or iris atrophy include trauma, pigment dispersion syndrome, pseudoexfoliation, angle closure glaucoma, and Vogt-Koyanagi-Harada (VKH) syndrome.

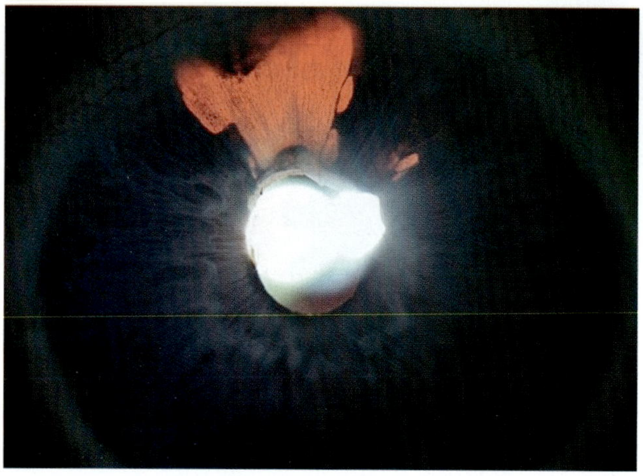

Fig. 3.7 Iris transillumination defect in a patient with herpes virus uveitis.

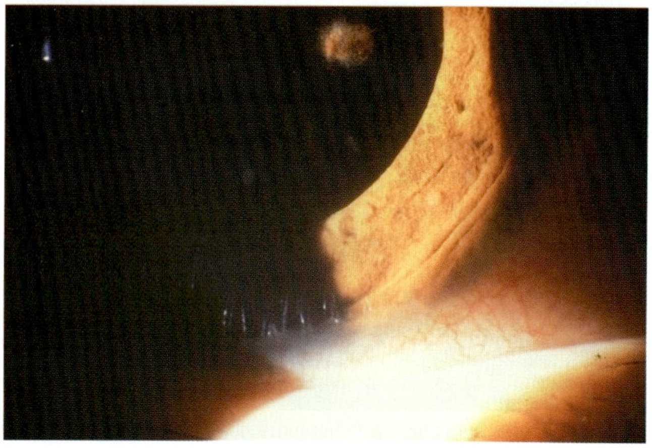

Fig. 3.8 Busacca nodules of iris in patient with Vogt-Koyanagi-Harada (VKH) syndrome.

Iris nodules are accumulations of inflammatory cells in the iris or on its surface. The Koeppe nodule, named after the German ophthalmologist Leonhard Koeppe, develops on the pupillary border, whereas the Busacca nodules, named after the Brazilian ophthalmologist Archimede Busacca, occur on the iris surface (Fig. 3.8). Iris nodules tend to be found in diseases that have been described as "granulomatous" and are more specific for these conditions than are granulomatous KPs.

ANTERIOR CHAMBER ANGLE

Because glaucoma is a frequent (and often the most severe) complication of uveitis, a thorough examination of the anterior chamber angle is indicated. The finding of neovascularization may indicate the need for panretinal photocoagulation or other therapy. In addition, in patients with a uniocular uveitis, examination of the angle may reveal an occult foreign body or ciliary body malignancy.

LENS

In many patients with uveitis, cataracts develop because of underlying inflammation and the use of corticosteroids to treat the disease. Posterior subcapsular opacities are commonly seen early (Fig. 3.9), but the advanced cataract in uveitis is frequently complicated, with nuclear, cortical, and capsular opacities. It is important to determine how much of the diminished vision of a patient with uveitis is the result of progressive cataract because the therapy for cataract is surgical extraction and not increased immunosuppressive therapy. Cataract can also obscure the view of the vitreous, retina, and optic nerve, making evaluation of patients with severe vision loss and dense cataracts difficult. In these patients, it is important to determine whether vision loss is caused by the cataract, reversible ocular inflammatory disease, or an untreatable problem, such as irreversible retinal or optic nerve atrophy. We have removed opaque cataracts in some patients in whom viewing the back of the eye was critical to determining whether systemic immunosuppressive therapy should be started. Electroretinography (ERG) can help determine whether the patient has residual visual function; however, dense cataract can affect ERG recording. Optical coherence tomography (OCT) can also be useful in assessing the posterior segment in eyes with media opacity and is discussed in detail in Chapter 6. Evaluation of lens opacity and reduced vision is discussed in greater depth in Chapter 5 on diagnostic testing.

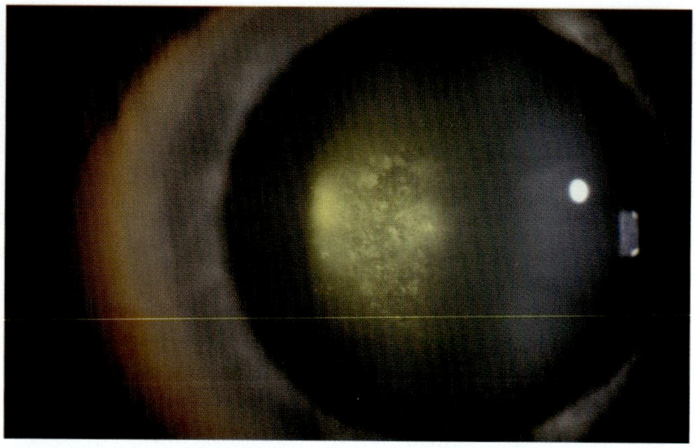

Fig. 3.9 Posterior subcapsular cataract in patient with chronic recurrent anterior uveitis.

VITREOUS

Inflammation in the vitreous, as in the anterior chamber, is characterized by increased cells and protein. The vitreous is rarely the source of inflammatory cells, which, instead, arise from the choroid, retina, and ciliary body. However, in certain infections, the focus of the inflammation may be in the vitreous. Both vitreous cells and haze are more difficult to quantify compared with aqueous cells and flare. The vitreous is larger, and cells or haze may be localized to only a part of it. Therefore quantification may depend on how the eye is examined. For example, the anteroposterior location of small numbers of cells in a relatively clear vitreous can be determined with the use of the slit lamp, but in the severely inflamed eye, the mid- and posterior areas of the vitreous may be obscured by anterior vitreous cells and haze. Small pupil size, corneal opacity, and cataract will also make the grading process more difficult.

The grading of vitreous cells described by Kimura et al.[15] uses the Hruby lens to view the cells in retroillumination. The cells appear as black dots, and in some eyes, it may be difficult to differentiate vitreal debris from active inflammatory cells. Debris is often pigmented and forms clumps that are larger than individual cells. We grade overall vitreous cells and opacities in a manner similar to the scale devised by Kimura et al. (Table 3.3). We then note whether the major accumulation of cells is immediately behind the lens, in the anterior or the posterior area of the vitreous, or adjacent to a retinal lesion. Location of the cells is a function of both the ocular disease and its severity. The location of the cells is important in classifying the inflammation, but we have noted, for example, that patients with pars planitis, who usually have cells in the anterior part of the vitreous, will develop many cells in the posterior area if the inflammation is more severe. In many diseases, but especially in sarcoidosis and pars planitis, vitreous cells tend to aggregate into clumps called *snowballs*. These snowballs settle in the inferior periphery near the retinal surface and are seen best with the indirect ophthalmoscope.

It is our strong opinion that vitreous haze is a better indicator of active inflammation compared with vitreous cells because it combines the optical effect of cellular infiltration and protein leakage. We have developed a grading scale based on the view of the optic disk and posterior retina with the use of the indirect ophthalmoscope and a 20-diopter lens (Fig. 3.10).[16] It is important to mentally correct for lens opacities, anterior segment inflammation, and corneal disease; however, the use of the indirect ophthalmoscope prevents mild media opacities from interfering with the grading. The use of photographic standards makes this system more reproducible compared with other subjective grading systems. In practice, it is useful to have the standard color photographs in the examining room. One can then examine the patient's eye and look at the grading chart to select the standard that best matches the degree of haze. This grading scale was used to quantify vitreous haze as a primary endpoint for U.S. Food and Drug Administration (FDA) approval for the dexamethasone intravitreal implant for uveitis.[17] This scale has been adapted by the SUN Working Group.[5] There are now other validated photographic scales for grading vitreous haze.[18,19] Automated methods of grading vitreous haze are also being developed.[20] The key is to use a scale consistently so that disease severity and response to therapy can be more accurately assessed.

Vitreous strands, membranes, and areas of vitreoretinal traction are not uncommon in intermediate and posterior uveitis. They are best seen with the indirect ophthalmoscope but may be studied in detail with a contact lens or a +90-diopter lens at the slit lamp. There is frequently posterior vitreous detachment in patients with long-standing vitreous inflammation as the fibrin in the vitreous contracts and pulls the posterior vitreous face forward. Some investigators have suggested that vitreous traction that causes an incomplete posterior vitreous detachment may be associated with the development of cystoid macular edema.[21]

TABLE 3.3 Grading of Vitreous Cells with Use of Hruby Lens

Cells in Retroilluminated Field	Description	Grade
0–1	Clear	0+
2–20	Few opacities	Trace
21–50	Scattered opacities	1+
51–100	Moderate opacities	2+
101–250	Many opacities	3+
>251	Dense opacities	4+

RETINA AND CHOROID

Examination of the retina in inflammatory disease is best done with a combination of the indirect ophthalmoscope, the Hruby lens, the +90-diopter lens, and a mirrored contact lens. A combination of careful clinical assessment with supplemental testing, such as OCT and fluorescein angiography, will provide the best information for correctly diagnosing and treating patients. Because of coexisting vitreous inflammation, each of these modalities has advantages and disadvantages. The indirect ophthalmoscope is ideal for defining the extent and height of retinal and choroidal lesions; it penetrates vitreous haze and other media opacities better than any other instrument. It is not good for defining the relative depth of a lesion within the retina or determining the presence of macular

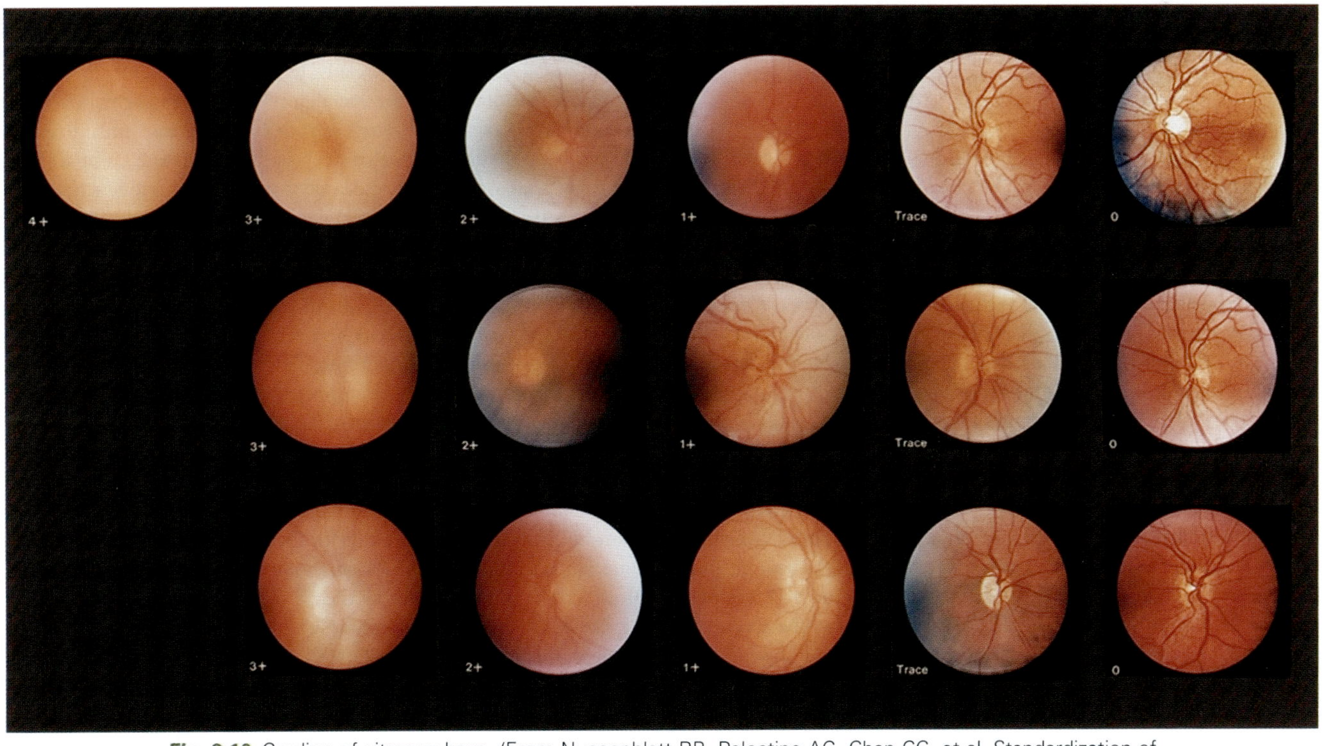

Fig. 3.10 Grading of vitreous haze. (From Nussenblatt RB, Palestine AG, Chan CC, et al. Standardization of vitreal inflammatory activity in intermediate and posterior uveitis. *Ophthalmology*. 1985;92:467–471.)

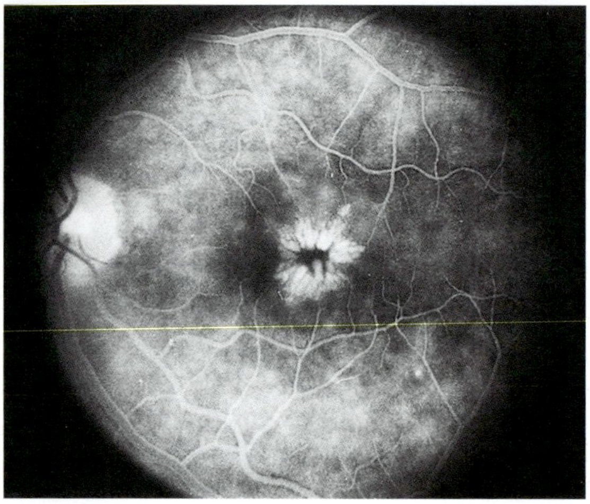

Fig. 3.11 Fluorescein angiogram demonstrating cystoid macular edema caused by pars planitis.

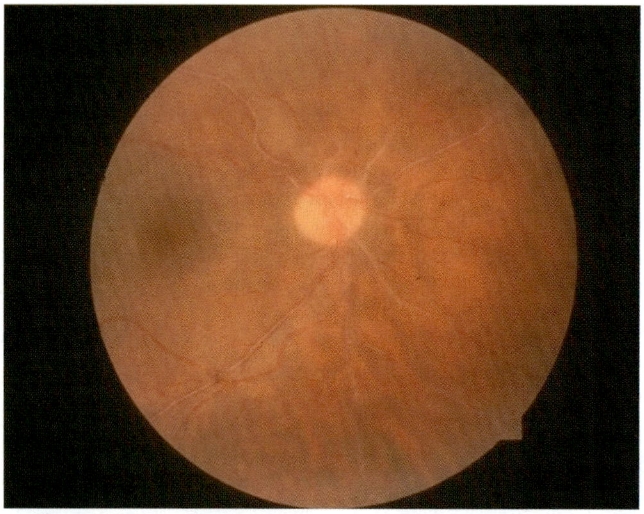

Fig. 3.12 Retinal vascular sheathing in patient with idiopathic retinal vasculitis.

edema. The Hruby lens is somewhat better at penetrating haze than the +90-diopter or +78-diopter lenses and is better for assessing macular edema. If the medium is reasonably clear, the +90-diopter or +78-diopter lens, which provides an inverted view of the fundus, is ideal for viewing vascular abnormalities, intraretinal lesions, and vitreoretinal traction in the posterior retina. The midperiphery of the retina also can be seen with this lens, but the mirrored contact lens is more useful for the detailed examination of peripheral chorioretinal lesions.

Cystoid macular edema is a common retinal finding in patients with uveitis (Fig. 3.11). Although fluorescein angiography can document the presence of macular edema more objectively, clinical examination with the Hruby lens is easier, is cost effective, and can be performed on each visit. Today, optical coherence tomography (OCT) is more frequently used to document the extent of macular edema, retinal thickening, and the response to therapy over time. In the absence of vitreous haze, cystoid macular edema is easily seen. However, macular edema may be obscured by overlying vitreous haze and is best observed by viewing the macula with the light directed slightly to one side of the fovea. Cystoid macular edema may then be visualized by indirect illumination and will "light up" in contrast to the surrounding retina. This technique also reduces light scattering from the vitreous. The surface of a cyst can sometimes

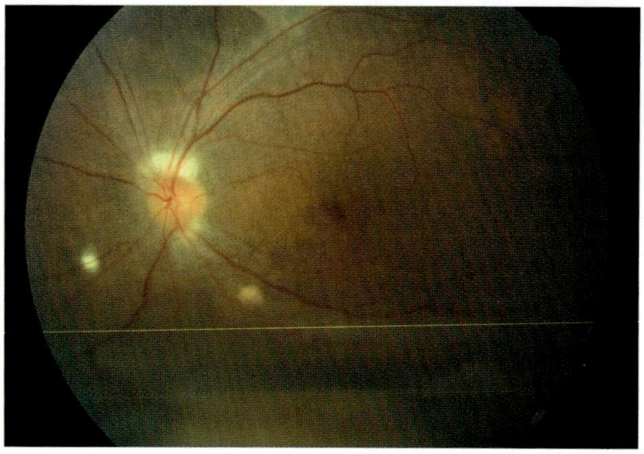

Fig. 3.13 Exudative retinal detachment in a patient with Vogt-Koyanagi-Harada (VKH) syndrome is seen inferior to the macula.

be visualized as a subtle surface elevation, distinguishing it from a true macular hole. If the pupil is small, the viewing aperture will be reduced, and only a faint glimpse of the macular cysts will be seen by this method. Macular holes, lamellar holes, and retinal pigment epithelial clumping are also commonly observed, and it is possible to see cloudy white areas of retinal edema without a classic cystoid pattern.

Retinal vascular alterations are also a common finding in patients with intermediate or posterior uveitis. Vascular sheathing of the arteries or veins, usually caused by infiltration of inflammatory cells around the vessels, is easily seen in the posterior pole (Fig. 3.12). Peripheral vascular sheathing is more subtle and may be missed if not specifically sought. Sheathing is often accompanied by vessel narrowing and sometimes by vascular obliteration. Peripheral vascular narrowing and obliteration are best evaluated with the indirect ophthalmoscope, manifesting as absence of small peripheral vessels. Acute vascular occlusion is accompanied by retinal edema, but old areas of vascular loss show only atrophic retina and retinal pigment epithelial stippling. Retinal neovascularization occurs in many patients with occlusive retinal vascular disease but can also occur as a result of inflammatory stimuli in some diseases, such as VKH syndrome and Behçet disease.

Retinal hemorrhages and cotton-wool spots frequently accompany retinal vasculitis, presumably related to the retinal ischemia produced by the inflammation. In addition, cellular retinal infiltrates can be observed in certain types of retinitis. These appear as white areas similar to cotton-wool spots but may be located deep within the retina compared with the superficial location of cotton-wool spots. In addition, active retinal infiltrates frequently have fuzzy edges, overlying vitreal cells, and surrounding retinal edema. Hard retinal exudates are relatively uncommon in inflammatory disease. It is possible that the retinal vessels do not leak large lipid-containing proteins from plasma. When hard exudates are observed, they frequently occur between an area of retinal ischemia and an area of essentially normal retina. The presence of a subretinal neovascular membrane should be suspected if hard exudates, retinal edema, hemorrhage, or gray-white elevated lesions are seen.

Careful examination with the Hruby, +90-diopter, or contact lens is crucial in distinguishing a lesion that involves the neurosensory retina from lesions at the level of the retinal pigment epithelium (RPE) or the choroid. Examination of the edge of the lesion is often helpful in determining its depth and cause. At times, it may still be difficult to know the location of an infiltrate without the aid of fluorescein angiography or the use of OCT. Although OCT can provide the clinician with extremely useful anatomic information, it should not replace a careful clinical examination. Many lesions will have associated subretinal fluid or be covered by increased cellularity in the vitreous, and this should be documented. Exudative retinal detachments can be associated with a number of ocular inflammatory diseases but are characteristic of specific conditions such as

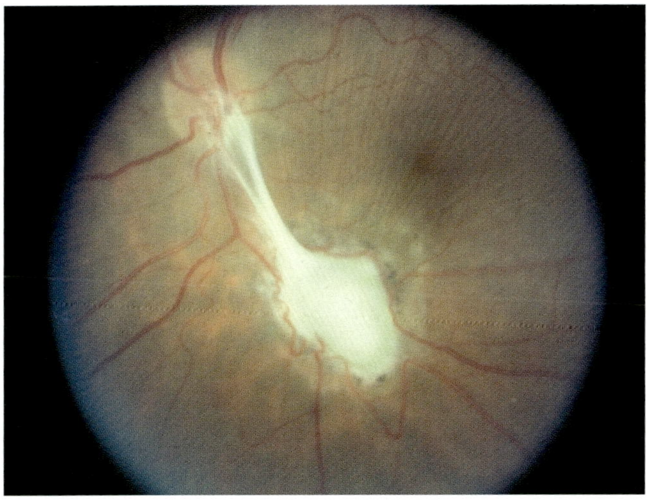

Fig. 3.14 Dense fibrotic band extends from the optic disc to the inferior vascular arcade.

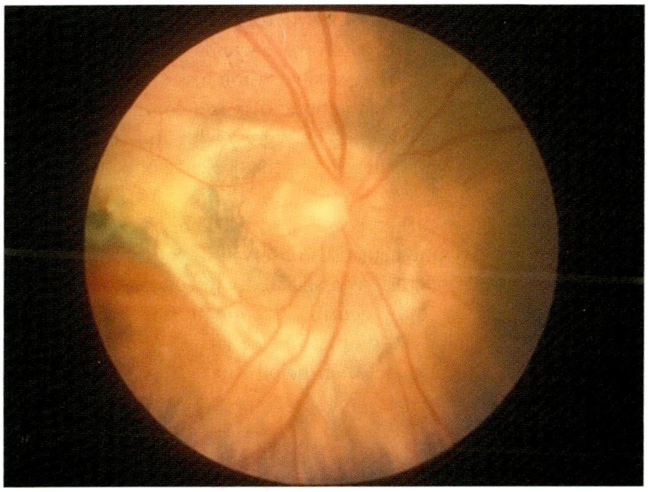

Fig. 3.15 Large choroidal granuloma around optic disc in a patient with sarcoidosis.

VKH syndrome (Fig. 3.13). The clinician, however, must carefully rule out a rhegmatogenous retinal detachment in these patients because treatment of rhegmatogenous detachment will require surgical repair.

In addition to subretinal fluid, the subretinal space can be infiltrated by glial and retinal pigment epithelial cells that have proliferated as a consequence of inflammation. These appear as plaques and bands of yellow-white tissue, which, for lack of a more specific term, are often referred to as *subretinal fibrosis.* The inflammatory process stimulates the growth of fibroblasts and the metaplasia of the retinal pigment epithelium and possibly Müller cells. The bands of this tissue, combined with epiretinal and vitreoretinal bands, produce retinal traction and distortion (Fig. 3.14).

Choroidal lesions, with or without retinal involvement, are common in posterior inflammatory disease. When inflammatory lesions are deep and isolated to the choroid, they often appear as grayish-yellow elevated masses (Fig. 3.15). They are best seen with the indirect ophthalmoscope but may be missed because they can be subtle in both elevation and pigmentary change. One or more choroidal nodules may be present and can vary in size from 50 μm to 500 μm in diameter. Atrophic chorioretinal lesions with surrounding hyperpigmentation are a striking sign of inflammatory disease in the patient with uveitis. However, these lesions do not represent areas of active inflammation,

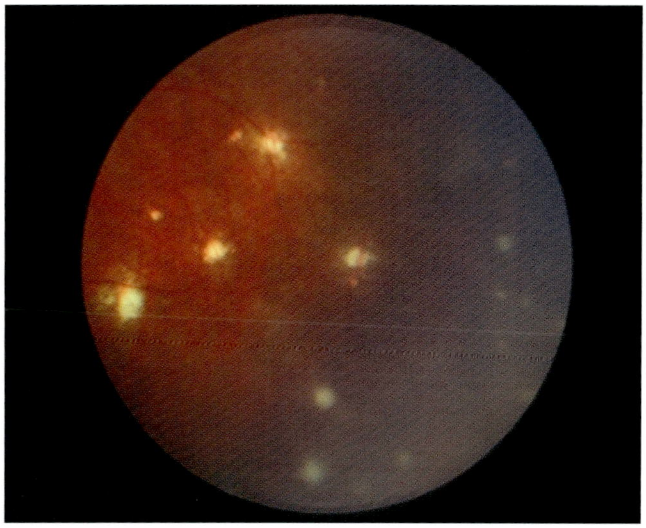

Fig. 3.16 Dalen-Fuchs nodules are small, fairly discrete, yellow-to-white lesions that most commonly occur in the retinal periphery. The lesions are composed of collections of inflammatory cells between the retinal pigment epithelium and the Bruch membrane.

and although they are the most prominent clinical feature of some diseases, they represent old, inactive disease. Only active inflammation, not residual scarring, can be treated by drugs that modulate the immune response. Thus therapy is not indicated in patients with multiple chorioretinal scars without infiltrative lesions of the retina or choroid or active vitritis. Although the appearance of inflammatory lesions of the retina and choroid can vary greatly, some lesions have a characteristic presentation and can aid in diagnosis. Dalen-Fuchs nodules tend to be small, discrete, deep, yellow-white chorioretinal lesions that may be associated with hyperpigmentation (Fig. 3.16). Dalen-Fuchs nodules are associated with sarcoidosis and sympathetic ophthalmia. The chorioretinal lesions associated with birdshot choroidopathy also have a characteristic appearance and distribution in the fundus, typically clustering nasal to the optic disk.

Examination of the retinal periphery and pars plana is an important part of the ocular examination of patients with uveitis. Pars plana snowbanking is the accumulation of a white fibroglial mass over the pars plana and adjacent retina (see Intermediate Uveitis, Chapter 22). It is usually restricted to the inferior pars plana but may extend superiorly. Scleral depression is usually required to see the pars plana exudate, but in some patients, the inflammatory mass may be large enough to be seen with the indirect ophthalmoscope without a lens (Fig. 3.17). Peripheral vitreous infiltrates lying on the retinal surface should not be interpreted as snowbanking. Peripheral neovascularization may be present within the snowbank, increasing the risk of vitreous hemorrhage. If the pars plana exudate is sparse and located only along the ora serrata, it may be difficult to identify unless immediate comparison is made with the ora serrata in other locations within the eye.

As stated earlier, advancements in technology, including OCT, fluorescein angiography, indocyanine green (ICG) angiography, wide-field photography, and electrophysiology, have improved the assessment of diseases involving the retina and choroid and are discussed in detail in Chapters 5 and 6.

OPTIC NERVE

The optic nerve is a frequently overlooked cause of vision loss in patients with uveitis. Uveitis may affect the optic nerve in several ways.

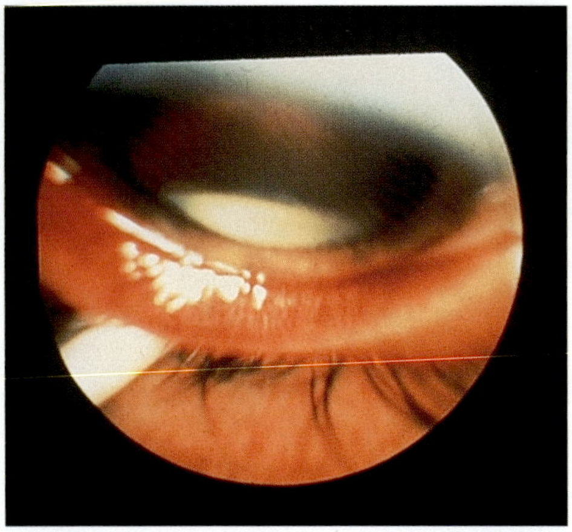

Fig. 3.17 Exudate on pars plana (snowbank) in a patient with pars planitis. (Courtesy Ronald Smith, MD.)

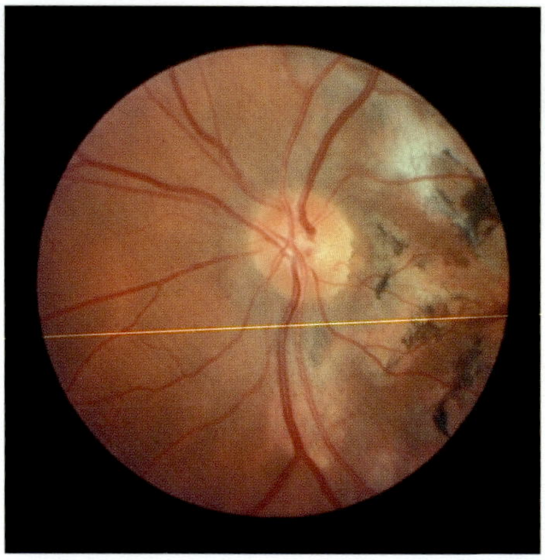

Fig. 3.20 Optic neuritis in a patient with chorioretinitis.

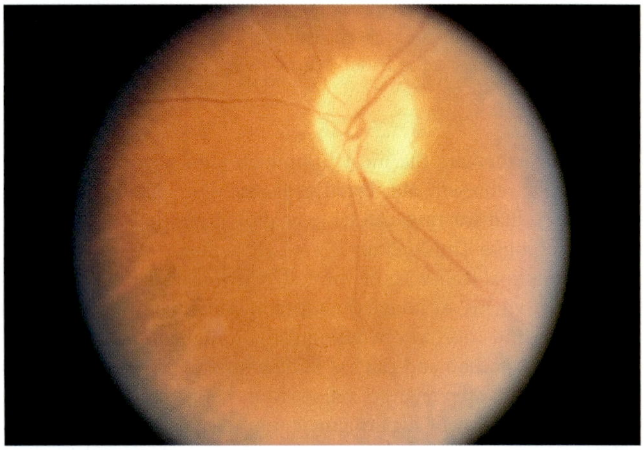

Fig. 3.18 Optic atrophy in a patient with posterior uveitis. Thinning and occlusion of the retinal vessels can also be seen.

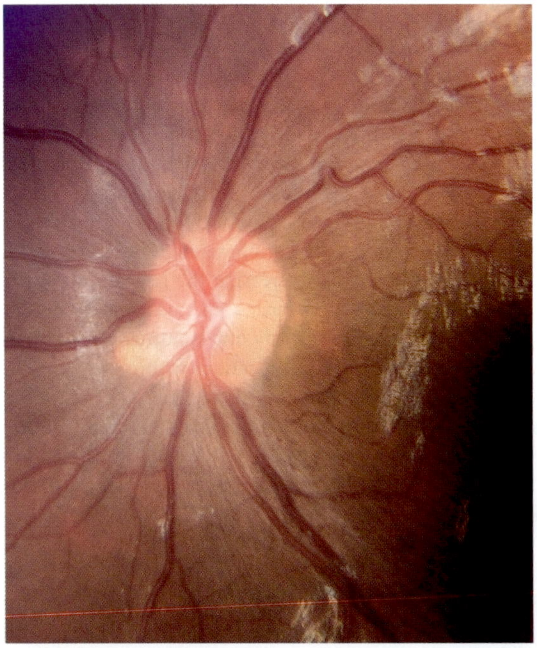

Fig. 3.19 Optic nerve granuloma in a patient with panuveitis.

Disk hyperemia, papillitis, or papilledema may be seen in a number of uveitic conditions. Disk hyperemia may persist even in an eye with little clinically active inflammation elsewhere. Prominent disk hyperemia is frequently noted with VKH syndrome. Secondary glaucoma is one of the most common causes of irreversible vision loss in the patient with uveitis. Neovascularization of the optic disk is a common finding in uveitis with retinal vasculitis and can regress with anti-inflammatory therapy. Optic atrophy may develop in the presence of ocular inflammation or after diffuse loss of retinal tissue (Fig. 3.18). Granulomas may impinge on the optic nerve and optic disc in diseases, such as sarcoidosis (Fig. 3.19). Optic neuritis is observed in patients with uveitis (Fig. 3.20). Multiple sclerosis is associated with intermediate uveitis and often manifests as optic neuritis. Examination of the optic disk with the Hruby lens or a +90-diopter lens, serial disk photographs, and electrophysiologic testing are often helpful in evaluating the patient with uveitis and visual loss.

REFERENCES

1. Ferris III FL, Kassoff A, Bresnick GH, et al. New visual acuity charts for clinical research. *Am J Ophthalmol*. 1982;94:91–96.
2. Beck RW, Moke PS, Turpin AH, et al. A computerized method of visual acuity testing: adaptation of the early treatment of diabetic retinopathy study testing protocol. *Am J Ophthalmol*. 2003;135:194–205.
3. Livingstone IA, Tarbert CM, Giardini ME, et al. Photometric compliance of tablet screens and retro-illuminated charts as visual acuity measurement devices. *PLoS One*. 2016;11:e0150676.
4. Oliveira Fd, Oliveira Motta AC, Muccioli C. Corneal specular microscopy in infectious and non-infectious uveitis. *Arq Bras Oftamol*. 2009;4:457–461.
5. Baydoun L, Livny E, Ham L, et al. 360-degree Scheimpflug imaging to predict allograft rejection after Descemet membrane endothelial keratoplasty. *Cornea*. 2016;11:1385–1390.
6. Alfawaz AM, Holland GN, Yu F, et al. Corneal endothelium in patients with anterior uveitis. *Ophthalmology*. 2016;8:1637–1645.
7. Hogan MJ, Kimura SJ, Thygeson P. Signs and symptoms of uveitis. I. Anterior uveitis. *Am J Ophthalmol*. 1959;47:155–170.
8. Schlaegel Jr TF. *Essentials of Uveitis*. Boston, MA: Little, Brown; 1967:7.
9. Jabs DA, Nussenblatt RB, Rosenbaum JT. Standardization of Uveitis Nomenclature (SUN) Working Group. Standardization of uveitis nomenclature for reporting clinical data. Results of the First International Workshop. *Am J Ophthlamol*. 2005;140:509–516.
10. Herman DC, McLaren JW, Brubaker RF. A method of determining concentration of albumin in the living eye. *Invest Ophthalmol Vis Sci*. 1988;29:133–137.

11. Kempen JH, Van Natta ML, Altaweel MM, et al. Factors predicting visual acuity outcome in intermediate, posterior and panuveitis: the Multicenter Uveitis Steroid Treatment (MUST) Trial. *Am J Ophthalmol.* 2015;6:1133–1141.
12. Muccioli C, Belfort Jr R. Hypopyon in a patient with presumptive diffuse unilateral subacute neuroretinitis. *Ocul Immunol Inflamm.* 2000;8:119–121.
13. Irvine WD, Flynn Jr HW, Murray TG, et al. Retained lens fragments after phacoemulsification manifesting as marked intraocular inflammation with hypopyon. *Am J Ophthalmol.* 1992;114:610–614.
14. al Hazzaa SA, Tabbara KF, Gammon JA. Pink hypopyon: a sign of *Serratia marcescens* endophthalmitis. *Br J Ophthalmol.* 1992;76:764–765.
15. Kimura SJ, Thygeson P, Hogan MJ. Signs and symptoms of uveitis. II. Classification of the posterior manifestations of uveitis. *Am J Ophthalmol.* 1959;47:171–176.
16. Nussenblatt RB, Palestine AG, Chan CC, et al. Standardization of vitreal inflammatory activity in intermediate and posterior uveitis. *Ophthalmology.* 1985;92:467–471.
17. Lowder C, Belfort Jr R, Foster CS, et al. for the HURON Study Group. Dexamethasone intravitreal implant for non-infectious intermediate or posterior uveitis. *Arch Ophthalmol.* 2011;129:545–553.
18. Madow B, Galor A, Feuer WJ, et al. Validation of a photographic vitreous haze grading technique for clinical trials in uveitis. *Am J Ophthalmol.* 2011;152:170–176.
19. Davis JL, Madow B, Cornett J, et al. Scale for photographic grading of vitreous haze in uveitis. *Am J Ophthalmol.* 2010;150:637–641.
20. Passaglia CL, Arvaneh T, Greenberg E, et al. Automated method of grading vitreous haze in patients with uveitis for clinical trials. *Transl Vis Sci Technol.* 2018;7:10.
21. Hikichi T, Trempe CL. Role of the vitreous in the prognosis of peripheral uveitis. *Am J Ophthalmol.* 1993;116:401–405.

4

Development of a Differential Diagnosis

Scott M. Whitcup

KEY CONCEPTS

- Diagnosis of uveitis is often challenging, and developing an erudite differential diagnosis is the key to success.
- Classification of uveitis is the first step and is guided by a series of questions that can be answered from both the medical history and clinical examination.
- Classification of uveitis and development of a list of potential diagnoses will help determine appropriate diagnostic testing, guide therapy, and help determine prognosis.
- Diagnostic tests should not be used to develop a differential diagnosis but instead to investigate diseases on the list.
- Associated symptoms and signs are important sources of information and require a systemic review of symptoms and a detailed physical examination. Examination of the skin can be extremely rewarding in diagnosing uveitis. Referral to an internist, primary care physician, rheumatologist, or other specialist is often required in the workup of uveitis.

Accurate diagnosis of uveitis is often challenging, not only for the general ophthalmologist but also for the uveitis specialist. Patients present with a plethora of ocular findings and associated systemic symptoms and signs. Ocular inflammation may be the initial presentation of an underlying systemic disease that, if undiagnosed and untreated, may lead to significant morbidity and even death. For example, we have seen a number of patients with intraocular lymphoma, which had been misdiagnosed and inappropriately treated as idiopathic uveitis. Even in patients with uveitis without an underlying systemic disease, misdiagnosis can lead to inappropriate therapy. A patient with fungal endophthalmitis who is thought to have sarcoidosis may be treated with corticosteroids, leading to exacerbation of the infection, when appropriate antifungal therapy could have been curative. In this chapter, we review our diagnostic approach to patients with uveitis and present two cases to illustrate our approach.

Diagnosis is based largely on recognition of patterns that include findings from the medical history, clinical examination, and ordered tests, including laboratory tests and medical imaging. Medical experts are much better at recognizing the patterns consistent with medical diagnoses than are novices. Studies on memory suggest that this pattern recognition can be learned and takes practice. It should therefore not be surprising that doctors with many years of clinical practice are often better diagnosticians compared with less experienced care providers.

Much of what we know about memory and pattern recognition comes from the study of chess. In the 1960s, de Groot[1,2] performed an intriguing study comparing the ability to recall chess patterns among players of varying abilities. A chessboard position, taken from a master game unknown to the subjects, was presented to participants for a short period varying from 2 to 15 seconds. Participants then had to reconstruct the board on the basis of their memory. The findings were dramatic. Grandmasters remembered board positions accurately, recalling an average of 93% of the pieces correctly after seeing the chess layout for only 2 to 5 seconds. The least experienced players only recalled about 50% of the pieces correctly. de Groot hypothesized that chess masters encode the positions of the pieces not as individuals but as groups. The data also suggest that the ability to recognize these patterns improves with experience and can be learned with appropriate teaching and a great deal of practice.

The goal of this chapter is to provide the framework for clinicians to start collecting the information needed to form patterns of diseases that aid in diagnosis. Knowing what questions to ask, what findings to look for, and what tests to order are all critical in seeing clear patterns from background noise. Every patient seen should help fine-tune the pattern recognition skills and allow clinicians to better diagnose diseases. First, the clinician needs to collect the pieces of the puzzle to create the disease pattern. Second, the clinician needs to start putting the pieces together in ways that form several disease patterns. This is known as *forming a differential diagnosis:* identifying pieces of a puzzle that, when assembled, can form a handful of disease pictures. Finally, a specific diagnosis is made, often by ordering a key test that rules out all but one disease pattern. Recognizing potential disease patterns and forming a good differential diagnosis is the key to success in achieving the final diagnosis.

FORMING A DIFFERENTIAL DIAGNOSIS

The first step in developing a differential diagnosis for patients with inflammatory eye disease is to classify uveitis in as detailed a fashion as possible. This can be achieved by systematically asking the eight questions listed in Box 4.1. Then a list of possible diagnoses can be generated by combining the data obtained from the answers. Some of the information, such as the age and demographics of the patient and associated systemic symptoms, is obtained from the history. Other data, such as the type and anatomic location of the inflammation, are obtained from the ocular examination. Again, the need for information about systemic and neurologic signs necessitates careful physical and neurologic examinations of the patient by the ophthalmologist or by a consulting internist, internal medicine subspecialist, neurologist, or general medical practitioner.

Once uveitis has been classified, a preliminary differential diagnosis should be generated. The answers to each of the questions in Box 4.1 will generate a list of possible diagnoses. One of the diagnoses that appear most frequently on these lists is then the most likely cause of the disorder. Of course, the lists provided here include many of the most common disorders, but the lists are not exhaustive. They do, however, illustrate the deductive diagnostic process. Once the initial lists of diagnoses are generated, ancillary examinations, including laboratory tests;

BOX 4.1 Classification of Uveitis

1. Is the disease acute or chronic?
2. Is the inflammation granulomatous or nongranulomatous?
3. Is the disease unilateral or bilateral?
4. Where is the inflammation located in the eye?
5. What are the demographics of the patient?
6. What associated symptoms does the patient have?
7. What associated signs are present on physical examination?
8. What is the time course of the disease and response to previous therapy?

specialized examinations (e.g., radiography electrophysiology); or a surgical procedure (e.g., diagnostic vitrectomy) can then be obtained to discern among the most likely diagnoses. In the next chapter on diagnostic testing, we show that the "shotgun approach" of ordering every diagnostic test available will mislead the clinician into making the wrong diagnosis.

Classifying Uveitis

1. Is the Disease Acute or Chronic?

Acute occurrences of uveitis usually have a sudden onset and last up to 6 weeks. The most common causes are listed in Box 4.2. Most occurrences of anterior uveitis, such as human leukocyte antigen (HLA)-B27–associated iritis and idiopathic anterior uveitis, fall into this category. Other diseases that typically cause acute uveitis include Vogt-Koyanagi-Harada (VKH) syndrome; postoperative bacterial infection; toxoplasmosis; many of the "white-dot syndromes," such as acute posterior multifocal placoid pigment epitheliopathy (APMPPE) and multiple evanescent white-dot syndrome (MEWDS); and traumatic iritis. Although many diseases can cause acute uveitis, the above-mentioned conditions should be considered first in the differential diagnosis. Chronic forms of uveitis have an insidious onset and typically last longer than 6 weeks. Other authors have defined a limited duration of uveitis as 3 months or less and persistent disease as lasting longer than 3 months.[3] Again, many diseases can cause uveitis that persists longer than 6 weeks; the uveitides that are characteristically chronic are listed in Box 4.2. Knowing whether a particular case of uveitis is acute or chronic is never sufficient to make a diagnosis, but it may aid in the diagnostic process.

2. Is the Inflammation Granulomatous or Nongranulomatous?

The ocular examination offers a unique opportunity to determine the type of infiltrating inflammatory cells involved in the disease process, without having to take a biopsy sample for histologic analysis. In anterior uveitis, inflammatory cells attach to the corneal endothelium in conglomerates called *keratic precipitates* (KPs). The appearance of KPs has been used to classify the inflammatory process as granulomatous or nongranulomatous. The more common nongranulomatous type of KP is characterized by fine, white collections of lymphocytes, plasma cells, and pigment. These precipitates can form in any disease and cause anterior uveitis; the finding of nongranulomatous KPs does not help tremendously in the formulation of a differential diagnosis other than to alert the clinician that anterior inflammatory disease has occurred in the eye. Granulomatous KPs are large, greasy-appearing collections of lymphocytes, plasma cells, and giant cells (see Fig. 4.2 later in the chapter). The finding of granulomatous KPs, also called "mutton fat" KPs, on slit-lamp examination can be a useful diagnostic clue. Patients with granulomatous KPs usually have a history of a chronic disease of an insidious onset and frequently have posterior segment disease in addition to their anterior segment inflammation. Other ocular findings suggestive of granulomatous inflammation are iris nodules and choroidal granulomas. Importantly, the finding of granulomatous inflammation in the eye suggests a unique set of diagnostic possibilities, which are listed in Box 4.3.

BOX 4.2 Causes of Acute and Chronic Uveitis

Acute Uveitis

Most cases of anterior uveitis: idiopathic, ankylosing spondylitis, Reiter syndrome, Fuchs heterochromic iridocyclitis
Vogt-Koyanagi-Harada syndrome
Toxoplasmosis
White-dot syndromes: acute posterior multifocal placoid pigment epitheliopathy and multiple evanescent white-dot syndrome
Acute retinal necrosis
Postsurgical bacterial infection
Trauma

Chronic Uveitis

Juvenile rheumatoid arthritis
Birdshot choroidopathy
Serpiginous choroidopathy
Tuberculous uveitis
Postoperative uveitis (*Propionibacterium acnes*, fungal)
Intraocular lymphoma
Sympathetic ophthalmia
Multifocal choroiditis
Sarcoidosis
Intermediate uveitis/pars planitis

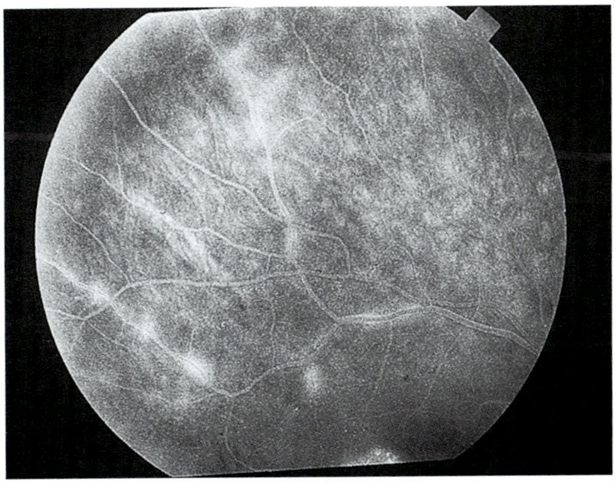

Fig. 4.1 Late phase of fluorescein angiography demonstrating staining of blood vessel walls and leakage of dye from peripheral retinal vasculature.

3. Is the Disease Unilateral or Bilateral?

Although one eye may be affected first, uveitis resulting from most causes involves both eyes within the first several months. Therefore the history of the disease being both chronic and unilateral can help in diagnosing the condition. Diseases that frequently involve a single eye, even after months or years of the disorder, are listed in Box 4.4. Parasitic disease typically involves one eye, although some of the diseases, such as toxoplasmosis, occur bilaterally. Uveitis after ocular surgery or the presence of an intraocular foreign body is almost exclusively unilateral. The one disease that most ophthalmologists

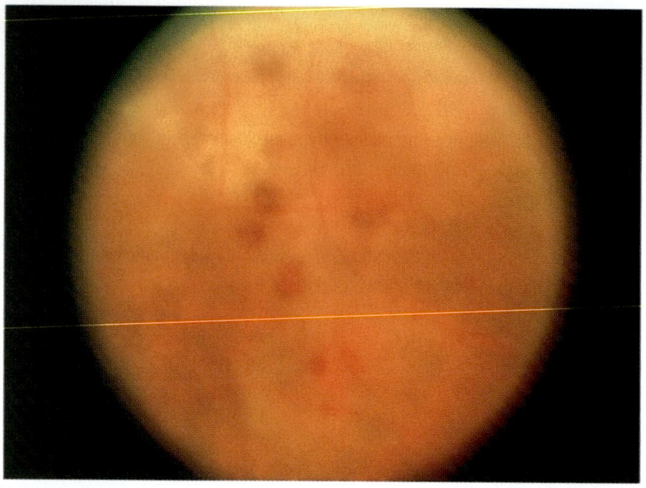

Fig. 4.2 Fundus photograph showing yellow subretinal infiltrates, retinal hemorrhage, and retinal edema in eye with 20/125 visual acuity and moderate vitritis.

BOX 4.3 Causes of Granulomatous Inflammation in the Eye

Sarcoidosis
Sympathetic ophthalmia
Uveitis associated with multiple sclerosis
Lens-induced uveitis
Intraocular foreign body
Vogt-Koyanagi-Harada syndrome
Syphilis
Tuberculosis
Other infectious agents

think of as a bilateral disease, but is seen involving a single eye in a number of patients, is sarcoidosis. Similarly, a number of patients, especially those of Asian descent, have Behçet disease involving a single eye.

4. Where is the Inflammation Located in the Eye?

It is important to determine the anatomic position of the inflammation within the eye. Table 4.1 delineates three similar methods for the anatomic classification of intraocular inflammatory disease. We based our anatomic classification on the scheme proposed by the International Uveitis Study Group.[4] This was modified by the Standardization of Uveitis Nomenclature (SUN) Working Group, which classified uveitis as anterior, intermediate, posterior, and panuveitis; this classification functions to both simplify and standardize the way the disease is described.[4] In addition to classifying uveitis as anterior, intermediate, or posterior uveitis or panuveitis, we note whether there is a predominant involvement of the cornea (keratouveitis), sclera (sclerouveitis), or retinal vasculature (retinal vasculitis) because these findings point to specific causes.

Anterior uveitis describes a disease limited predominantly to the anterior segment of the eye. Other terms used in the literature for anterior uveitis are *iritis, iridocyclitis,* and *anterior cyclitis.* The inflammation is characterized by conjunctival hyperemia, anterior chamber cell and flare, KPs, and iris abnormalities, including posterior synechiae and peripheral anterior synechiae. A mild cellular inflammatory response in the anterior vitreous is often seen. The common causes of anterior uveitis are listed in Box 4.5.

BOX 4.4 Causes of Unilateral Uveitis

Sarcoidosis
Postsurgical uveitis
Intraocular foreign body
Parasitic disease
Acute retinal necrosis
Behçet disease

TABLE 4.1 Anatomic Classification of Uveitis

IUSG[a]	Tessler[b]	SUN Working Group[c]
–	Sclerouveitis	
–	Keratouveitis	
Anterior uveitis	Anterior uveitis	Anterior uveitis
Iritis	Iritis	Iritis
Anterior cyclitis	Iridocyclitis	Iridocyclitis
Iridocyclitis		Anterior cyclitis
Intermediate uveitis (formerly known as pars planitis)	Intermediate uveitis	Intermediate uveitis
Posterior cyclitis	Cyclitis	Pars planitis
Hyalitis	Vitritis	Posterior cyclitis
Basal retinochoroiditis	Pars planitis	Hyalitis
Posterior uveitis	Posterior uveitis	Posterior uveitis
Focal, multifocal, or diffuse choroiditis	Choroiditis	Focal, multifocal, or diffuse choroiditis
Chorioretinitis or retinochoroiditis	Retinitis	Retinitis, chorioretinitis, or retinochoroiditis
Neuroretinitis	–	Neuroretinitis
Panuveitis	–	Panuveitis

[a]From Bloch-Michel E, Nussenblatt RB. International Uveitis Study Group recommendations for the evaluation of intraocular inflammatory disease. *Am J Ophthalmol.* 1987;103:234–235.
[b]From Tessler HH. Classification and symptoms and signs of uveitis. In: Duane TD, Jaeger EA, eds. *Clinical Ophthalmology.* Vol. 4. Philadelphia: JB Lippincott; 1987:1–10.
[c]From Jabs DA, Nussenblatt RB, Rosenbaum JT. Standardization of Uveitis Nomenclature (SUN) Working Group. Standardization of uveitis nomenclature for reporting clinical data. Results of the First International Workshop. *Am J Ophthlamol.* 2005;140:509–516.
IUSG, International Uveitis Study Group; *SUN,* Standardization of Uveitis Nomenclature.

Intermediate uveitis is the anatomic diagnosis that causes the most confusion among ophthalmologists. However, the proper classification of uveitis as intermediate is very important because an underlying cause for the disease can often be determined. Intermediate uveitis is characterized by inflammation that primarily affects the vitreous and the peripheral retina. Aggregates of inflammatory cells are frequently seen in the inferior vitreous and have been termed *vitreous snowballs.* In the same vein, accumulations of inflammatory cells and debris along the pars plana and ora serrata have been called *snowbanks.* Mild anterior uveitis often coexists, and cystoid macular edema is a frequent finding. The conditions associated with intermediate uveitis are listed in Box 4.6.

BOX 4.5 Causes of Anterior Uveitis

Idiopathic
Ankylosing spondylitis
Reiter syndrome
Inflammatory bowel disease
Psoriatic arthritis
Behçet disease
Human leukocyte antigen (HLA)-B27–associated disease
Juvenile rheumatoid arthritis
Fuchs heterochromic iridocyclitis
Sarcoidosis
Syphilis
Glaucomatocyclitic crisis
Masquerade syndromes

BOX 4.6 Causes of Intermediate Uveitis

Sarcoidosis
Inflammatory bowel disease
Multiple sclerosis
Lyme disease
Pars planitis[a]

[a]Not an etiologic diagnosis, but patients with intermediate uveitis of the pars planitis subtype tend to have a worse prognosis.

Disease limited to the posterior segment of the eye, particularly to the retina and choroid, is termed *posterior uveitis.* A large number of diseases cause posterior uveitis, so to further subdivide the disorders, posterior uveitis is classified as predominantly retinitis or choroiditis and as focal or multifocal disease. The disorders that cause focal and multifocal retinitis and choroiditis are listed in Box 4.7.

The term *panuveitis* is reserved for diseases that involve all segments of the eye, typically with a severe sight-reducing inflammatory response. The common causes of panuveitis are listed in Box 4.8.

Severe scleritis in association with uveitis is most frequently seen in patients with underlying connective tissue diseases, such as rheumatoid arthritis and ankylosing spondylitis. Inflammatory bowel diseases, such as Crohn disease and ulcerative colitis, also cause sclerouveitis. Finally, severe retinal vasculitis is associated with a subset of diseases that cause uveitis. Similar to scleritis, retinal vasculitis is often associated with underlying connective tissue disease. A full list of the disorders that cause retinal vasculitis can be found in Chapter 28.

5. What Are the Demographics of the Patient?

Demographic information can lead the ophthalmologist to suspect certain types of uveitis, although there are always patients with presentations varying from the age, sex, race, ethnic heritage, or social parameters characteristic of any particular disease. The age of the patient can be particularly useful in developing a differential diagnosis because certain causes of uveitis are more common among patients of specific age groups. A list of the diseases that occur more frequently in certain age groups is provided in Table 4.2. One must be careful, however, not to rigidly apply these guidelines to all cases. For example, although intraocular lymphoma is typically found in patients older than 65 years of age, we have seen patients in their 30s with this disease. Nevertheless, these guidelines are clearly useful, especially in diagnosing uveitis in children. Other demographic considerations in patients with uveitis are listed in Table 4.3.

BOX 4.7 Causes of Posterior Uveitis

Focal Retinitis
Toxoplasmosis
Onchocerciasis
Cysticercosis
Masquerade syndromes

Multifocal Retinitis
Syphilis
Herpes simplex virus
Cytomegalovirus
Sarcoidosis
Masquerade syndromes
Candidiasis
Meningococcus

Focal Choroiditis
Toxocariasis
Tuberculosis
Nocardiosis
Masquerade syndromes

Multifocal Choroiditis
Histoplasmosis
Sympathetic ophthalmia
Vogt-Koyanagi-Harada syndrome
Sarcoidosis
Serpiginous choroidopathy
Birdshot choroidopathy
Masquerade syndromes (metastatic tumor)

BOX 4.8 Causes of Panuveitis

Syphilis
Sarcoidosis
Vogt-Koyanagi-Harada syndrome
Infectious endophthalmitis
Behçet disease

6. What Associated Symptoms Does the Patient Have?

As stated in Chapter 2, a thorough medical history is often the key to accurate diagnosis. Specific symptoms, both those relating to the eye and those suggesting systemic disease, should lead the clinician to suspect certain types of uveitis. We find that carefully defining a patient's symptoms is the most important step in determining the correct diagnosis. Many of the symptoms that suggest specific diagnoses are listed in Table 4.4. However, the enthusiasm to classify a case within a diagnostic category may tempt the clinician to stretch the symptoms to fit a particular disease. For example, a patient who reports mild knee pain after playing basketball for the first time in 2 years should not be classified as having a chronic arthritis with symptoms consistent with rheumatoid arthritis. Similarly, ringing in the ears after a 4-hour rock concert does not qualify as tinnitus suggestive of VKH syndrome. Importantly, the clinician must be careful not to suggest symptoms to the patient. The clinician should avoid asking such questions as "You must have had some joint pain with this, haven't you?" Although it is important to interview patients for their medical history, the use of a standardized questionnaire helps ensure that symptoms are not missed or inappropriately suggested.

TABLE 4.2 Age Considerations in Patients with Uveitis[a]

Age (year)	Diagnostic Considerations
<5	Juvenile rheumatoid arthritis Toxocariasis Postviral neuroretinitis (Retinoblastoma) (Juvenile xanthogranuloma) Leukemia
5–15	Juvenile rheumatoid arthritis Pars planitis Toxocariasis Postviral neuroretinitis Sarcoidosis Leukemia
16–25	Pars planitis Ankylosing spondylitis Idiopathic anterior uveitis Toxoplasmosis Sarcoidosis Acute retinal necrosis
25–45	Ankylosing spondylitis Idiopathic anterior uveitis Fuchs heterochromic iridocyclitis Idiopathic intermediate uveitis Toxoplasmosis Behçet disease Idiopathic retinal vasculitis Sarcoidosis White-dot syndromes Vogt-Koyanagi-Harada syndrome Acquired immunodeficiency syndrome (AIDS), syphilis Serpiginous choroidopathy
45–65	Birdshot retinochoroiditis Idiopathic anterior uveitis Idiopathic intermediate uveitis Idiopathic retinal vasculitis Behçet disease Serpiginous choroidopathy Acute retinal necrosis
>65	Idiopathic anterior uveitis Idiopathic intermediate uveitis Idiopathic retinal vasculitis Serpiginous choroidopathy (Masquerade syndromes)

[a]Parentheses indicate noninflammatory diseases.

7. What Associated Signs Are Present on Physical Examination?

Most ophthalmologists rarely take a detailed medical history in the office, and a detailed physical examination performed in the office is almost unheard of. Unless the ophthalmologist is prepared to do a thorough physical examination, it is probably more practical to refer patients to their primary care physician for this part of the evaluation. Nevertheless, it is fruitful for the ophthalmologist to assess a few areas before making the referral. We have found that examination of the skin can be extremely rewarding in diagnosing uveitis. We have discovered sarcoid granulomas, rashes consistent with Lyme disease and syphilis, and Kaposi sarcoma. A brief examination of the joints for signs of inflammation is also useful, and a screening neurologic examination is warranted, especially in patients who may have intraocular lymphoma,

TABLE 4.3 Demographic Considerations in Uveitis

Factor	Disease Risks
Female	Pauciarticular juvenile rheumatoid arthritis, chronic anterior uveitis
Male	Ankylosing spondylitis, sympathetic ophthalmia
African American	Sarcoidosis
Native American	Vogt-Koyanagi-Harada (VKH) syndrome
Midwestern American	Presumed ocular histoplasmosis
Japanese[a]	VKH syndrome Behçet syndrome
Mediterranean ancestry	Behçet syndrome
Central American	Cysticercosis, onchocerciasis
South American	Cysticercosis, toxoplasmosis
West African	Onchocerciasis
Intravenous drug user	Fungal endophthalmitis, acquired immunodeficiency syndrome (AIDS)
Promiscuous sexual activity	AIDS, syphilis
Frequent hiking in wooded areas	Lyme disease

[a]Not in Americans of Japanese extraction.

sarcoidosis, or Behçet disease. Table 4.4 lists the systemic signs associated with specific uveitic conditions.

8. What Is the Time Course of the Disease and Response to Previous Therapy?

The time course of the disease and the response to therapy can provide useful information in determining the cause. Is the disease responsive to anti-inflammatory therapy? Does it require continued corticosteroid therapy? If so, how much corticosteroid is needed? Is the disease resistant to corticosteroid therapy? Answers to these questions can help the clinician determine the correct diagnosis. In general, infectious diseases may initially improve with anti-inflammatory therapy but worsen later. Postoperative endophthalmitis caused by *Propionibacterium acnes* typically improves temporarily with topical or systemic corticosteroid therapy but then recurs. A temporary and partial response to therapy also suggests that the ocular inflammation may be associated with a chronic systemic disease, such as sarcoidosis or a malignancy-like lymphoma. A long history of intermittent response to therapy tends to be more suggestive of a chronic noninfectious and nonmalignant disease because both infection and malignancy often become evident after several years.

The old adage "When you hear hoofbeats, think of horses and not zebras" also applies to the evaluation of the patient with uveitis. Common diseases are frequently the cause of uveitis, even in cases that are difficult to diagnose. Table 4.5 lists the most common causes of anterior and posterior uveitis from two published surveys of patients with uveitis.

Once the above questions are answered, lists of possible diagnoses are generated. By identifying the conditions that appear most frequently, a final list of the most likely ones responsible for the patient's uveitis is generated. The clinician can then order diagnostic studies to discern among them. The following cases illustrate the process of developing a differential diagnosis in the patient with uveitis.

TABLE 4.4 Systemic Signs and Symptoms in Uveitis

Symptom or Sign	Possible Associated Conditions
Headaches	Sarcoidosis, Vogt-Koyanagi-Harada (VKH) syndrome
Neurosensory deafness	VKH syndrome, sarcoidosis
Cerebrospinal fluid pleocytosis	VKH syndrome, sarcoidosis, acute posterior multifocal placoid pigment epitheliopathy, Behçet syndrome
Paresthesia, weakness	Intermediate uveitis associated with multiple sclerosis, Behçet syndrome, steroid myopathy
Psychosis	VKH syndrome, sarcoidosis, Behçet disease, steroid psychosis, systemic lupus erythematosus
Vitiligo, poliosis	VKH syndrome
Erythema nodosum	Behçet syndrome, sarcoidosis
Skin nodules	Sarcoidosis, onchocerciasis
Alopecia	VKH syndrome
Skin rash	Behçet syndrome, sarcoidosis, viral exanthem, syphilis, herpes zoster, psoriatic arthritis, Lyme disease
Oral ulcers	Behçet syndrome, inflammatory bowel disease
Genital ulcers	Behçet syndrome, Reiter syndrome, sexually transmitted diseases
Salivary or lacrimal gland swelling	Sarcoidosis, lymphoma
Lymphoid organ enlargement	Sarcoidosis, acquired immunodeficiency syndrome (AIDS)
Diarrhea	Whipple disease, inflammatory bowel disease
Cough, shortness of breath	Sarcoidosis, tuberculosis, malignancy
Sinusitis	Wegener granulomatosis
Systemic vasculitis	Behçet syndrome, sarcoidosis, relapsing polychondritis
Arthritis	Behçet syndrome, Reiter syndrome, sarcoidosis, juvenile rheumatoid arthritis, rheumatoid arthritis, Lyme disease, inflammatory bowel disease, Wegener granulomatosis, systemic lupus erythematosus, other connective tissue diseases
Sacroiliitis	Ankylosing spondylitis, Reiter syndrome, inflammatory bowel disease
Chemotherapy or other immunosuppression	Cytomegalovirus retinitis, *Candida* retinitis, other opportunistic organisms

TABLE 4.5 Common Causes of Anterior and Posterior Uveitis

Diagnosis	Perkins et al. (%)[a]	Henderly et al. (%)[b]
ANTERIOR UVEITIS		
Idiopathic anterior uveitis	32.7	12.1
Human leukocyte antigen (HLA)-B27–associated anterior uveitis	–	3.0
Juvenile rheumatoid arthritis	5.1	2.8
Fuchs heterochromic iridocyclitis	6.3	1.8
Ankylosing spondylitis	5.7	1.5
Reiter syndrome	5.2	1.0
Inflammatory bowel disease	2.9	0.3
Syphilis	1.2	0.8
Intraocular lens–related anterior uveitis	–	1.0
POSTERIOR UVEITIS		
Toxoplasmic retinochoroiditis	9.2	7.0
Idiopathic retinal vasculitis	4.6	6.8
Idiopathic posterior uveitis	6.9	3.7
Ocular histoplasmosis	–	3.5
Toxocariasis	2.9	2.6
Serpiginous choroidopathy	–	2.0
Acute posterior multifocal placoid pigment epitheliopathy	–	1.8
Acute retinal necrosis	–	1.3
Birdshot choroidopathy	–	1.2
Intraocular lymphoma	1.1	1.2

[a]Data from Perkins ES, Folk J. Uveitis in London and Iowa. *Ophthalmologica.* 1984;36:189.

[b]Data from Henderly DE, Genstler AJ, Smith RE, et al. Changing patterns of uveitis. *Am J Ophthalmol.* 1987;103:131–136.

COMPUTERS IN DIAGNOSIS

As the complexity of diagnostic information increases, the use of computers to analyze these data will become more commonplace. Machine learning has been employed to better analyze image data, including findings from optical coherence tomography (OCT). Artificial intelligence, employing an automated natural language processing system and using deep learning techniques, was able to extract clinically relevant information from electronic health records and accurately diagnose pediatric diseases in a study that included over a million patient visits.[5] Computer-assisted algorithms can be generated and refined to help clinicians collect and analyze clinical data to assist in generating initial differential diagnoses and suggesting diagnostic tests. Furthermore, machine learning can refine the analysis and interpretation of the diagnostic data with the significant increase in the quantity and complexity of image, laboratory, and genetic testing data. In the end, however, the clinician is responsible for making diagnostic and treatment decisions that incorporate their patients' wishes.

CASE 4.1

A 42-year-old white woman presented with a 10-year history of bilateral uveitis, which had been treated intermittently with topical and systemic corticosteroids, and the chief complaint of blurred vision that was worse in the left eye. A detailed medical history was significant for sinusitis and depression. On examination, her visual acuity was 20/50 in the right eye and 20/100 in the left eye. Slit-lamp biomicroscopy showed "mutton fat" KPs in the left eye. There were trace vitreous cells and haze in the right eye and 2+ vitreous cells and haze in the left eye. There were peripheral retinal vasculitis and cystoid macular edema in both eyes (Fig. 4.1). Physical examination revealed no rash, joint findings, or other abnormalities. Neurologic examination results were normal.

Most clinicians will find it difficult to derive an informed differential diagnosis by simply reading this case history; however, by classifying the patient's uveitis on the basis of the answers to the eight questions previously outlined, lists of possible diagnoses can be generated. By comparing these lists, the most likely diagnoses can then be identified. Question 1 asks whether the disease is acute or chronic. Because the patient has a 10-year history of disease, her uveitis is clearly chronic, and this is associated with the diseases listed in Box 4.2. The patient has "mutton fat" KPs, suggesting that the uveitis is granulomatous, and this suggests the diagnoses listed in Box 4.3. The disease is bilateral, which does not point to a specific set of diseases; however, with prominent vitritis and peripheral retinal vasculitis, the anatomic classification of an intermediate uveitis does suggest a specific set of possible diseases to the clinician (see Box 4.6). The patient is white and in the 24- to 45-year age range, suggesting the diagnoses listed in Table 4.2. As seen in Table 4.4, a complaint of sinusitis suggests a possible diagnosis of Wegener granulomatosis, but the patient had no specific findings on physical examination.

In summary, this patient's uveitis can be classified as chronic, granulomatous, bilateral, intermediate uveitis, found in a middle-aged white woman with intermittent response to topical and systemic corticosteroids. The lists containing possible diagnoses for this patient are shown in Box 4.9. When these lists are compared, the most frequently mentioned disorders are sarcoidosis; other causes of intermediate uveitis, such as multiple sclerosis and inflammatory bowel disease; and other chronic disorders, such as Behçet disease and Wegener granulomatosis. In this case, diagnostic tests were then ordered to discern among the most likely disorders. Results of diagnostic evaluations for sarcoidosis and Wegener granulomatosis, including a chest x-ray, serum angiotensin-converting enzyme (ACE) level, antineutrophil cytoplasmic antibody test, and computed tomography (CT) of the sinuses, were normal. However, magnetic resonance imaging (MRI) of the brain revealed lesions consistent with a diagnosis of multiple sclerosis. An episode of lower extremity weakness developed subsequently and was followed by a second episode of paresthesia, which extended to the level of the umbilicus and thus was diagnostic of multiple sclerosis.

BOX 4.9 Lists of Diagnoses Generated for Case 4.1

Chronic, granulomatous, bilateral, intermediate uveitis in a middle-aged white woman with intermittent response to topical and systemic corticosteroids

Chronic Uveitis

Juvenile rheumatoid arthritis
Birdshot choroidopathy
Serpiginous choroidopathy
Tuberculous uveitis
Postsurgical uveitis (*Propionibacterium acnes*, fungal)
Intraocular lymphoma
Sympathetic ophthalmia
Multifocal choroiditis
Sarcoidosis
Intermediate uveitis/pars planitis

Intermediate Uveitis

Sarcoidosis
Inflammatory bowel disease
Multiple sclerosis
Lyme disease
Pars planitis

Granulomatous Inflammation in Eye

Sarcoidosis
Sympathetic ophthalmia
Uveitis associated with multiple sclerosis
Lens-induced uveitis
Intraocular foreign body
Vogt-Koyanagi-Harada syndrome
Syphilis
Tuberculosis
Other infectious agents

Age 25 to 45 Years

Ankylosing spondylitis
Idiopathic anterior uveitis
Fuchs heterochromic iridocyclitis
Intermediate uveitis
Toxoplasmosis
Behçet disease
Idiopathic retinal vasculitis
Sarcoidosis
White-dot syndromes
Vogt-Koyanagi-Harada syndrome

AIDS

Syphilis
Serpiginous choroidopathy

Associated Symptoms and Signs

Sinusitis – Wegener granulomatosis

CASE 4.2

A 73-year-old white woman presented with bilateral blurred vision that had been present since the previous year. The patient first noted floaters in the left eye a year ago but did not see an ophthalmologist until 3 months earlier, when she was found to have a slight decrease in visual acuity in the left eye and bilateral mild vitritis. Over the next 3 months, her vision decreased in both eyes, and she was referred to the National Eye Institute. She had a history of type 2 diabetes mellitus, which was controlled with oral hypoglycemic agents, and a childhood history of rheumatic fever. She also complained of weight loss and unsteady gait. She lived in a wooded area in eastern New York.

On examination, visual acuity was 20/50 in the right eye and 20/125 in the left eye. The anterior segment examination result was normal, but there were 2+ vitreous cells and 1+ vitreous haze in both eyes. Funduscopic examination revealed punctate yellow subretinal infiltrates in both eyes and retinal hemorrhage and edema in the left eye (Fig. 4.2). Physical examination revealed ataxia.

Again, this patient's condition presents difficulty in diagnosis, but with use of the approach detailed in Case 4.1, a differential diagnosis can be readily developed. In this case, the disease was chronic and the inflammation nongranulomatous. The condition was classified as chronic, nongranulomatous, bilateral, multifocal retinitis. The patient was an older-adult white woman, and her history of residence in a wooded area suggests demographic susceptibility to Lyme disease. Her weight loss suggested the possibility of underlying malignancy, malnutrition, or possible gastrointestinal disease, and the unsteady gait alerts the clinician to the possibility of neurologic disease. The diagnoses generated by this classification are shown in Box 4.10. As you can see, the most frequently listed diagnoses include sarcoidosis, infectious diseases, and masquerade syndromes, most notably intraocular lymphoma.

Our first concern was the possibility of underlying malignancy. Systemic evaluation was unrewarding, and vitrectomy showed no malignant cells. However, two measurements of serum ACE levels were elevated at 81 units/L and 101 units/L (normal range 8–52 units/L), and bronchoscopy confirmed the diagnosis of sarcoidosis.

We hope that this chapter will provide the ophthalmologist with a pragmatic approach to generating a differential diagnosis, which will then help determine the appropriate tests to discern among the most likely possibilities. As you will see in Chapter 5 on diagnostic testing, the alternative, that is, the shotgun approach of indiscriminately ordering every test available, may be both expensive and misleading.

BOX 4.10 Lists of Diagnoses Generated for Case 4.2

Chronic, nongranulomatous, bilateral, multifocal retinitis in an older-adult white woman

Chronic Uveitis

Juvenile rheumatoid arthritis
Birdshot choroidopathy
Serpiginous choroidopathy
Tuberculous uveitis
Postsurgical uveitis (*Propionibacterium acnes*, fungal)
Intraocular lymphoma
Sympathetic ophthalmia
Multifocal choroiditis
Sarcoidosis
Intermediate uveitis/pars planitis

Granulomatous Inflammation in the Eye

Sarcoidosis
Sympathetic ophthalmia
Uveitis associated with multiple sclerosis
Lens-induced uveitis
Intraocular foreign body
Vogt-Koyanagi-Harada syndrome
Syphilis
Tuberculosis
Other infectious agents

Multifocal Retinitis

Syphilis
Herpes simplex virus
Cytomegalovirus
Sarcoidosis
Masquerade syndromes
Candida
Meningococcus

Age >65 Years

Idiopathic anterior uveitis
Idiopathic intermediate uveitis
Idiopathic retinal vasculitis
Serpiginous choroidopathy
Masquerade syndromes
Sarcoidosis

Demographic Considerations

Patient lives in an area endemic for Lyme disease

REFERENCES

1. de Groot AD. *Thought and Choice in Chess*. The Hague, The Netherlands: Mouton Publishers; 1965.
2. de Groot AD, Gobet F. *Perception and Memory in Chess. Studies in the Heuristics of the Professional Eye*. Assen, The Netherlands: Van Gorcum; 1966.
3. Jabs DA, Nussenblatt RB, Rosenbaum JT. Standardization of Uveitis Nomenclature (SUN) Working Group. Standardization of uveitis nomenclature for reporting clinical data. Results of the First International Workshop. *Am J Ophthlamol*. 2005;140:509–516.
4. Bloch-Michel E, Nussenblatt RB. International Uveitis Study Group recommendations for the evaluation of intraocular inflammatory disease. *Am J Ophthalmol*. 1987;103:234–235.
5. Liang H, Tsui BY, Ni H, et al. Evaluation and accurate diagnosis of pediatric diseases using artificial intelligence. *Nat Med*. 2019;25:433–438.

5

Diagnostic Testing and Imaging

Scott M. Whitcup

KEY CONCEPTS

- Mistakes in ordering and interpreting diagnostic tests can lead to misdiagnosis and inappropriate therapy.
- Diagnostic tests, including laboratory tests and imaging studies, should be ordered to narrow down the differential diagnosis.
- Clinicians must know the sensitivity and specificity of the diagnostic test to avoid misinterpretation of the results.
- A few diagnostic tests are both highly sensitive and highly specific and may therefore be useful as screening tests for patients with many forms of uveitis. The fluorescent treponemal antibody absorption (FTA-ABS) test for syphilis is an example of a diagnostic test often used as a general screening test in patients with uveitis.
- Assessing the likelihood of disease before the diagnostic test is crucial in determining the likelihood of disease after either a positive or a negative diagnostic test.
- New diagnostic tests for a number of infectious diseases have improved the diagnosis and treatment of infectious uveitis.
- Some tests, including fluorescein angiography and ocular coherence tomography (OCT), are helpful in assessing response to therapy.
- Advances in OCT, including OCT angiography, have improved the diagnosis and management of patients with uveitis and are now discussed in a separate chapter (Chapter 6).
- Some diagnostic tests, such as bone mineral density studies, help limit the side effects of therapy and are now part of the standard care of patients on systemic anti-inflammatory therapy.

What diagnostic tests should you order in the evaluation of the patient with uveitis? This is one of the most difficult questions we are asked. It is clear, however, that a nonselective approach to testing is costly and inefficient and provides information that is often irrelevant or, worse yet, that may lead to an incorrect diagnosis and inappropriate therapy. It is important to understand how to interpret diagnostic data because this information will help the clinician to order the appropriate tests. This chapter will discuss the approach to ordering and interpreting diagnostic tests. In addition, some of the more commonly ordered tests will also be reviewed here. Other tests will be reviewed in specific chapters on the relevant diseases.

Why does the clinician order diagnostic tests? Usually, diagnostic tests are ordered to help make the correct diagnosis. Unfortunately, many clinicians are overly influenced when positive or negative results of diagnostic tests come back from the laboratory. A clinical example will serve to illustrate this point. A 34-year-old African American woman from Texas presents with an intermediate uveitis in both eyes that has been present for the past 7 months. There is no history of rash, arthritis, or fever, but the patient does complain of wheezing and shortness of breath on exertion. The ophthalmologist orders a battery of diagnostic tests, including a serologic test for Lyme disease, which yields a positive result. Of course, the ophthalmologist is pleased to diagnose the patient's condition and treats her with a 2-week course of ceftriaxone. There are only three problems with this scenario: The patient probably does not have Lyme disease, does not need the expensive 2-week course of intravenous antibiotics, and more likely has sarcoidosis that is not being treated.

Before one can appropriately interpret the results of a diagnostic test, three pieces of information are needed. First, one needs to know the sensitivity of the diagnostic test (Fig. 5.1). This is calculated by dividing the number of patients who actually have the disease and who, upon being tested, have a positive result by the total number of patients with the disease who are tested. Another name given to patients who have a disease and have a positive test result is *true positives*: These patients have a positive test result and actually have the disease. Patients who have the disease but have a negative test result are called *false negatives.* Many of the commonly used serologic tests for Lyme disease have sensitivity of approximately 90%. What does that mean? It means that if 100 patients with Lyme disease were tested, 90 would have a positive result (true positives), but 10 would have a negative result (false negatives). Furthermore, many diagnostic tests have varying sensitivities, depending on the stage of the disease. For example, Lyme disease serologies are less sensitive during the acute stage of the disease.

The second piece of information you need to have to interpret a diagnostic test result is the specificity (see Fig. 5.1). The specificity of a diagnostic test is calculated by dividing the number of patients who do not have the disease in question and have had an appropriately negative test result by the total number of people without the disease who are tested. People who do not have the disease and have a negative test result are called *true negatives.* Similarly, people who do not have the disease but have a positive test result anyway are called *false positives.* In the case of the serologic test for Lyme disease, the specificity is also 90%. This means that if 100 patients without Lyme disease undergo this test, 90 will have an appropriately negative result, but 10 will have a misleading positive result.

PRETEST LIKELIHOOD OF DISEASE

The third and critical piece of information needed for test interpretation is often ignored by many doctors. This piece of information is called the *pretest likelihood of the disease* and is defined as the chance that the patient has a particular disease before the diagnostic test is ordered. The pretest likelihood can be based on a number of factors, such as the patient's history and physical examination findings and the incidence of a particular disease in that area. This is the figure that most depends on the clinician's prowess and ability: The more accurate the physician's calculation of the pretest likelihood of disease, the more accurate will be the subsequent interpretation of the test result.

	Disease present	Disease absent
Test positive	True positives (a)	False positives (b)
Test negative	False negatives (c)	True negatives (d)

Fig. 5.1 Sensitivity and specificity of diagnostic tests. Sensitivity = a/a + c. Specificity = d/b + d.

What is the pretest likelihood of Lyme disease in the case of the 34-year-old woman from San Antonio who has intermediate uveitis but no other symptoms and signs of Lyme disease and who does not live in an area endemic for the disease? The prevalence of Lyme disease in San Antonio, Texas, is probably less than 1 in 1000, and with no other evidence of the disease, the pretest likelihood of the disease would probably be less than this. But let us be generous and say that the pretest likelihood of this patient having Lyme disease is 1 in 1000 or 0.1%. How do we interpret her positive test result for Lyme disease?

The likelihood that the diagnosis of Lyme disease is correct in this patient can be calculated because we now have the sensitivity of the test (90%), the specificity of the test (90%), and the pretest likelihood of the disease (0.1%). This calculation of what is called the *posttest likelihood of disease* is carried out with the use of a formula derived by the mathematician Bayes and is called *Bayes' theorem*. The standard form of Bayes' theorem states the following:

$$\text{Posttest probability} = \frac{\text{Pretest probability} \times \text{sensitivity}}{(\text{Pretest probability} \times \text{sensitivity}) + (1 - \text{Pretest probability})(1 - \text{specificity})}$$

Bayes' theorem has been understood for two centuries but has only been applied to clinical reasoning over the past 30 years.[1-5] Although formulas may appear daunting to some clinicians, computer programs and nomograms have been developed to help the clinician interpret the data.[6,7] So what is the likelihood that our patient has Lyme disease, given her positive laboratory test result? With Bayes' theorem, the chance that she has Lyme disease is still only 0.9%, or a chance of 9 out of 1000. Although this represents an almost 10-fold increase in likelihood compared with the pretest likelihood because there was a very small chance that she had Lyme disease before the test, she still probably does not have the disease. Knowing that the posttest likelihood of the patient having Lyme disease is less than 1%, the clinician probably would not opt to treat her with antibiotics.

Diagnostic tests are also not as useful if there is a very strong likelihood that a patient has the disease before the test is ordered. If this same patient came from Lyme, Connecticut; had a history of a tick bite followed by an erythematous, round rash; and now presented with intermediate uveitis and arthritis, she would probably have a greater than 99% chance of having the disease, even without testing. Even if the result of her serologic test for Lyme disease was negative, on application of Bayes' theorem, the patient would still have about a 99% chance of having the disease.

Diagnostic tests are most helpful when the pretest likelihood of the disease is about 50%. For our patient with intermediate uveitis, if after our initial assessment we thought that her chance of having Lyme disease was 50%, a positive serologic test result would increase the posttest likelihood of the disease to 90%. So in this case, we start with a 50:50 chance of Lyme disease but end up with Lyme disease being, by far, the most likely diagnosis.

Receiver Operating Characteristic Curve

Many diagnostic tests involve establishing a numerical cut-off, above which a patient is felt to have a "positive" test result and hence is more likely to have the disease. Where you set that cut-off affects the sensitivity and the specificity of the test and determines the number of false-positive

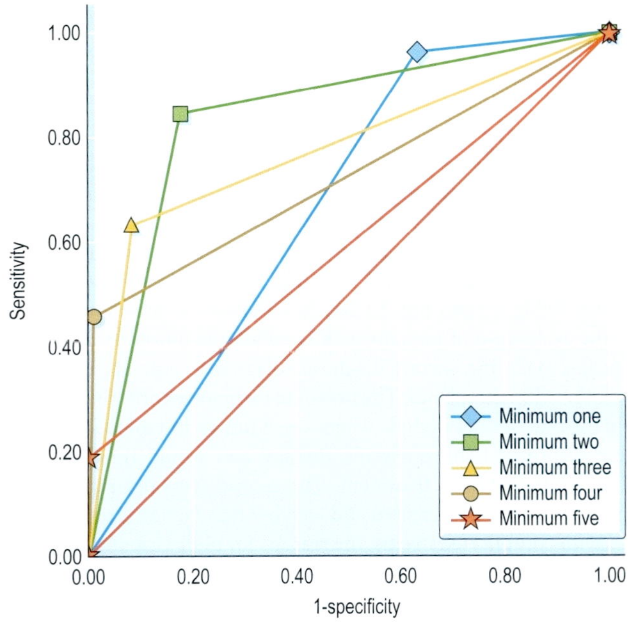

Fig. 5.2 Receiver operating characteristic (ROC) curve for the requirement for each additional number of ocular features required to make a diagnosis of ocular sarcoidosis. The area under the ROC curve is greatest (0.84) for requiring a minimum of two ocular features to make the diagnosis, with sensitivity of 84% and specificity of 83%. (From Asukata Y, Ishihara M, Hasumi Y, et al. Guidelines for the diagnosis of ocular sarcoidosis. *Ocul Immunol Inflamm*. 2008;16:77–81, with permission.)

and false-negative test results. Unless a test is 100% sensitive and 100% specific, the more sensitive it is, the more likely you are to get false-positive results. The sensitivity of a test can be graphed against the 1-specificity of the test to obtain what is called the *receiver operating characteristic* (ROC) curve (Fig. 5.2). The performance of a diagnostic test can be quantified by calculating the area under the ROC curve. Importantly, the ability of two continuous variables to diagnose a disease can be distinguished by comparing the two ROC curves and the area under these curves and determining whether this difference is statistically significant.[8,9] If so, the test with the greater area under the ROC curve may be more discriminating.

It is also important to critically assess the quality of the data underlying the sensitivity and the specificity numbers you use.[10] Data usually come from a number of clinical trials that have used the given test. A meta-analysis of these studies can be used to assess diagnostic test accuracy by graphing the results on the ROC curve.

So now that you have the knowledge to analyze data, it should be easy to interpret your patients' test data, right? Unfortunately, it is not that easy. It is difficult to obtain the sensitivities and the specificities of many of the common diagnostic tests we order. Many laboratories are considering providing a nomogram listing the posttest likelihood of a disease for differing pretest likelihoods because they already know the current sensitivity and specificity for that test. But how do we know the sensitivity or the specificity of chest x-ray for the diagnosis of sarcoidosis or that of diagnostic vitrectomy for intraocular lymphoma? These figures are difficult to obtain and may vary tremendously from institution to institution. More and more, however, articles are being published on the sensitivity and the specificity of diagnostic procedures and tests. In addition, the clinician can do the calculations on the basis of hypothetical numbers. For example, one might ask this question: Given 95% sensitivity and 95% specificity for a test in a patient with a 10% chance of having the disease, what is the posttest likelihood of the disease? It is surprising how much such calculations can help you to determine the diagnostic or therapeutic approach to patients with complicated conditions. Rosenbaum and Wernick[3] have published a review on how to apply Bayes' theorem to the evaluation of patients with uveitis, and this should be useful to many clinicians.

DIAGNOSTIC TESTS FOR UVEITIS

After the initial differential diagnosis is generated, diagnostic tests that help discern among the most likely disorders should be ordered. Remember that diagnostic tests will have the most utility in confirming or rejecting diagnoses that start with about a 50% chance of being correct. Table 5.1 and Box 5.1 list the common diagnostic tests useful for the evaluation of patients with uveitis. In addition to helping the clinician make the correct diagnosis, diagnostic tests are ordered in two other clinical settings. The first of these involves ordering tests that help the practitioner exclude diagnoses of tumor and infection because these disorders require specific therapy and would be exacerbated by anti-inflammatory treatment. The second is to determine why a patient's vision has decreased and whether this change is reversible. In eyes with complicated uveitis, the reasons for poor vision may be multifactorial, and the clinician needs as much information as possible.

Should all patients with uveitis undergo a standard set of diagnostic tests regardless of the presentation? Uveitis specialists have a high rate of use of laboratory testing in evaluating new patients. When presented with 13 patient scenarios, a group of uveitis specialists almost always ordered some testing for all scenarios, with an average cost of $282.80 per scenario.[11] It makes more sense to try to develop an initial differential diagnosis first; however, there are some tests with relatively low cost that can help rule out treatable diseases with potential adverse outcomes. Many uveitis specialists have a low threshold for ordering a complete blood count (CBC), chest radiography, and syphilis serology in many uveitis patients.

In this chapter, we will review some of the more commonly ordered diagnostic tests that may be useful in the diagnosis of uveitis. The number of diagnostic tests available to the ophthalmologist has increased tremendously over the past decade. Many tests are expensive and yet yield little useful information; others are critical for the appropriate management of patients. These tests can be arbitrarily grouped into laboratory tests, imaging techniques, skin testing, surgical specimens, and ancillary ophthalmic tests. Many of the tests listed in Table 5.1 and Box 5.1 are more thoroughly discussed in later chapters on specific diseases; however, several points for each group of diagnostic tests deserve comment here.

Laboratory Tests

Laboratory tests usually are the first diagnostic tests that most physicians order (see Table 5.1). Although we have emphasized that laboratory tests should not be routinely used to screen patients with uveitis for that disease and that tests should be ordered only to discern among likely diagnoses, there are exceptions. As stated previously, practically all patients with idiopathic uveitis should be tested for syphilis. There are many factors that support the use of laboratory tests to screen for syphilis in most patients with uveitis. Syphilis remains a common cause of uveitis and is easily treatable. Patients with untreated ocular syphilis often have devastating visual outcomes. Importantly, the fluorescent treponemal antibody absorption (FTA-ABS) test for syphilis is both extremely sensitive and specific. In patients with late syphilis, the stage of disease associated with uveitis, both sensitivity and specificity of the FTA-ABS test are 99%. With the combined presence of a treatable, common disease; poor outcome in untreated patients; and a highly sensitive and specific diagnostic test with little risk and moderate cost, screening becomes useful. Previous reports stated that the Venereal Disease Research Laboratory (VDRL) test has a sensitivity of only 70% for late syphilis. Therefore many uveitis specialists recommended a FTA-ABS test for evaluation of the patient with uveitis. More recently, the sensitivity of nontreponemal tests, including the VDRL and rapid plasma reagin (RPR) tests, is estimated to be 78% to 86% for detecting primary syphilis infection, 100% for detecting secondary syphilis infection, and 95% to 98% for detecting latent syphilis infection with specificity ranges between 85% and 99%.[12] A two-step process has been recommended with an initial nontreponemal test, followed by a treponemal test, such as FTA-ABS. However, because the sensitivity and specificity of nontreponemal tests may be less in patients with underlying autoimmune diseases and coinfection with human immunodeficiency virus (HIV), we believe it may be prudent to screen patients with uveitis for syphilis with both nontreponemal and treponemal tests. Additionally, the incidence of syphilis in patients with acquired immunodeficiency syndrome (AIDS) is increasing.[13,14] As a result, all patients who have syphilis and uveitis should also be tested for HIV infection, and vice versa.

A number of tests are primarily used for research purposes but are commercially available. Many practitioners order these tests but do not know what to do with the results when they come back. One example is testing for circulating immune complexes. Circulating immune complexes were first thought to be the mechanism underlying the destruction of the eye in various forms of uveitis. In the past, tests for circulating immune complexes were ordered, and if these complexes were present, they were assumed to be the cause of the disease. However, it is no longer clear whether immune complexes are the cause in many cases of uveitis.

Numerous laboratory tests can be useful in evaluating patients with possible rheumatologic disease.[15] Acute-phase reactants include a number of proteins produced by the liver in response to stress and signal underlying inflammation. The most commonly used tests for acute-phase reactants are the erythrocyte sedimentation rate (ESR) and cross-reactive protein (CRP). Rheumatoid factor (RF) is an autoantibody against the Fc portion of human immunoglobulin G (IgG). The test is relatively sensitive for rheumatoid arthritis (RA) and may also be positive in patients with other rheumatic diseases, including Sjögren syndrome and systemic lupus erythematosus (SLE). However, RF may also be positive in patients with chronic inflammatory diseases or malignancy and is seen in normal subjects as well. The antinuclear antibody (ANA) test is another test that can help detect underlying connective tissue diseases. These antibodies are extremely sensitive for SLE, and depending on the immunofluorescence pattern of the test, can indicate specific disorders, such as polymyositis, dermatomyositis, or CREST (calcinosis, Raynaud phenomenon, esophageal dysmotility, sclerodactyly, and telangiectasis) syndrome.

Rheumatologic Tests

Because rheumatologic and autoimmune disorders are common causes of uveitis, many patients undergo laboratory evaluation for these diseases. Again, these laboratory tests are most useful to confirm a clinically suspected diagnosis, rather than to screen for a less likely disease.[16] Some of the common laboratory tests ordered in the evaluation of rheumatologic diseases are discussed here.

Acute-phase Proteins

Inflammation is a core feature of the rheumatologic diseases, and acute-phase proteins are a class of proteins that can increase in response to the inflammatory response and can be detected in serum. As a result of increases in inflammatory proteins, such as fibrogen, the ESR is often increased in rheumatologic diseases (RA, SLE, and systemic vasculitis). However, the ESR can be elevated in a number of other nonrheumatologic conditions, including pregnancy, cancer, and infection. The levels of CRP can also increase during inflammation associated with rheumatologic diseases and can help differentiate osteoarthritis from RA. In addition, polymyalgia rheumatica is often accompanied by high levels of CRP.

TABLE 5.1 Laboratory Tests Commonly Ordered In Patients With Uveitis

Tests	Conditions/Comments
Angiotensin-converting enzyme	Sarcoidosis; may be elevated in children without sarcoidosis
Antiphospholipid Ab (lupus anticoagulant and anticardiolipin Ab)	Thrombosis, CNS disease, and spontaneous abortions in patients with systemic lupus erythematosus
Anti-CCP	Rheumatoid arthritis (60%–70% patients with RA, associated with erosive disease)
Antihistone	Specific for drug induced SLE and present in 50%–70% of SLE
Anti-RNP	SLE or other connective tissue diseases
Anti–double-stranded DNA (dsDNA)	Relatively specific for SLE
Anti-SS-A(Ro)	60%–70% of patients with Sjögren syndrome and 30%–40% with SLE
Anti-SS-B(La)	50%–60% with Sjögren syndrome and 10%–15% with SLE
Anti-Smith (Sm)	Relatively specific for SLE
ANA	Systemic lupus erythematosus and other rheumatic diseases
Antifungal Ab	Fungal disease
ANCA	Wegener granulomatosis cytoplasmic pattern ANCA (cANCA)
Peripheral pattern ANCA pANCA	Polyarteritis nodosa
Antitoxoplasma Ab	Toxoplasmosis
Antiviral Ab	Viral infection
Bartonella antibody	Bartonellosis
Calcium	Sarcoidosis
Complete blood count	Underlying systemic disease, such as malignancy or infection
Cross-reactive protein	Underlying inflammatory disease, such as rheumatic disease
Creatinine	Renal disease associated with autoimmune diseases, such as SLE
Cultures	Bacterial, fungal, mycobacterial, and viral diseases
Erythrocyte sedimentation rate	Underlying systemic diseases (such as rheumatic disease or malignancy)
FTA-ABS	Treponemal test for syphilis
HIV ELISA	HIV
HTLV-1	HTLV-1 infection
HLA typing	Specific HLA types associated with specific diseases (HLA-B27, HLA-A29, and HLA-B51)
Immune complexes	Rarely useful
Liver function tests	Sarcoidosis, hepatitis
Lumbar function for cell count	Infection, malignancy, VKH, APMPPE
Lumbar puncture for CSF VDRL	Syphilis
Lumbar puncture for culture and Gram stain	Infection
Lumbar puncture for cytology	CNS lymphoma
Lupus antibody	Lupus
Lyme antibody	Lyme disease (be aware of false-positive results)
Lysozyme	Sarcoidosis
QuantiFERON test	Tuberculosis
Rheumatoid factor (RF)	Rheumatoid arthritis; girls with JRA and uveitis often RF negative but ANA positive
Stool for ova and parasites	Parasitic disease
T-cell subsets	Low CD4+ count predisposes patient for opportunistic infections
Thyroid function tests	Increased incidence of thyroid disease in patients with uveitis
Toxocara antibody	Toxocariasis
Urinalysis	(Blood suggests rheumatic disease)
VDRL/RPR	Nontreponemal tests for syphilis
West Nile antibody	West Nile disease (serum or CSF)

Ab, Antibody; *ANA,* antinuclear antibody; *ANCA,* antineutrophil cytoplasmic antibody; *APMPPE,* acute posterior multifocal placoid pigment epitheliopathy; *Anti-CCP,* anti-cyclic citrullinated peptide; *anti-RNP,* antiribonucleoprotein; *CNS,* central nervous system; *CSF,* cerebrospinal fluid; *ELISA,* enzyme-linked immunosorbent assay; *HIV,* human immunodeficiency virus; *HTLV,* human T-cell leukemia/lymphoma virus; *JRA,* juvenile rheumatoid arthritis; *VDRL,* Venereal Disease Research Laboratory; *VKH,* Vogt-Koyanagi-Harada syndrome.

BOX 5.1 Other Diagnostic Tests In Uveitis

Imaging Tests
Computed tomography (CT) of the head
Magnetic resonance imaging (MRI) of the head
CT of sinuses
Gallium scan
Hand radiography
Sacroiliac radiography

Skin Testing
Allergy testing
Anergy testing
Histoplasmin
Pathergy
Purified protein derivative (PPD)

Ancillary Ophthalmic Testing
Color vision testing
Contrast sensitivity
Electroretinography
Electro-oculography
Fluorescein angiography
Indocyanine green angiography
Laser interferometry
Laser flare photometry
Manifest refraction
Optical coherence tomography
Optical coherence tomography angiography
Ultrasonography of the orbit
Ultrasonography of the retina
Visual evoked potentials
Visual field testing

Biopsy Specimens
Conjunctiva
Lacrimal gland
Aqueous humor
Vitreous
Choroid and retina
Skin

Autoantibodies

RF is an antibody against the Fc portion of immunoglobulins. It is positive in approximately 70% of patients with RA but can be positive in patients without disease and increases with age.[17] It is also elevated in other diseases, such as SLE and cryoglobulinemia, and in a number of infections. Unlike the ESR, which often decreases with anti-inflammatory therapy, RF is not a good measure of disease activity.

Anticitrullinated peptide antibodies (ACPAs) are autoantibodies directed against citrullinated peptides and proteins and are present in the majority of patients with RA. However, the sensitivity of these autoantibodies for RA is less than 80% with specificity of approximately 88% to 96%.[18]

Antibodies to Nuclear Antigens

ANAs, which are antibodies against nuclear antigens, including deoxyribonucleic acid (DNA), ribonucleic acid (RNA), centromeres, histones, nucleoli, and other nucleoproteins, are common in patients with rheumatologic disease. Currently, several methods are used to measure ANAs. The fluorescent ANA (FANA) test is highly sensitive for rheumatologic diseases, such as SLE (approximately 95%), but far less specific for any particular rheumatologic disease.

There are different types of ANAs. Autoantibodies against extractable nuclear antigens include antibodies to Smith antigen (Sm), ribonucleoproteins (RNPs), Scl-70, PM1, RoSSA, La/SSB, and histidyl-tRNA synthetase (Jo-1). Tests for these can be useful in confirming the diagnosis of specific rheumatologic diseases (see Table 5.1).

The antineutrophil cytoplasmic antibody (ANCA) test has been very helpful in the diagnosis of Wegener granulomatosis, a systemic vasculitis characterized by necrotizing granulomatous vasculitis of the upper and lower respiratory tracts, focal necrotizing glomerulonephritis, and systemic small vessel vasculitis involving a number of organ systems, and is found during follow-up of patients with Wegener granulomatosis. Ocular involvement, including uveitis, scleritis, and retinal vasculitis, occurs in about 16% of patients.[19-21] Young[22] described 98 patients with uveitis tested for the presence of ANCAs by using an indirect immunofluorescence method and obtained positive ANCA test results in patients with chronic uveitis resulting from various factors. A cytoplasmic pattern of staining (cANCA) is felt to be more specific for Wegener granulomatosis than is a peripheral pattern (pANCA). Soukasian et al.[23] reported that ANCA test results were positive in seven patients with scleritis caused by Wegener granulomatosis but negative in 54 patients with other ocular inflammatory diseases; this suggests that the test is both sensitive and specific. High specificity of the cANCA test for Wegener granulomatosis in patients with ocular inflammatory disease has been reported by other investigators as well.[24] The ANCA test may also be useful in guiding immunosuppressive therapy. Failure of ANCA levels to revert to normal levels may be associated with an increased risk of relapse.[25] These patients may benefit from more aggressive immunosuppressive therapy.

Radiography

Although newer techniques provide practitioners with high-resolution images, simple radiographic techniques, such as skull radiography to evaluate patients with suspected congenital toxoplasmosis for calcifications, should not be overlooked. Computed tomography (CT) or magnetic resonance imaging (MRI) of the brain is indicated for patients with possible intraocular lymphoma (see Chapter 31). Sinus radiography is frequently ordered as part of the evaluation of patients who have uveitis and symptoms or a history of sinus disease; however, it is not clear that this test is helpful on a routine basis. Patients with a history of sinus disease and uveitis may have an underlying systemic vasculitis, such as Wegener granulomatosis, but in these patients the ANCA test, consultation with an otolaryngologist, and possibly CT of the sinuses may be more appropriate and useful than sinus radiography.

Chest radiography should be considered in patients with uveitis suspected of having pulmonary involvement by such diseases as tuberculosis (Fig. 5.3). It remains unclear whether chest radiography should be routinely ordered in patients suspected of having sarcoidosis. In a retrospective study, chest images for 200 patients with new-onset uveitis were reviewed.[26] Eleven percent of the patients had biopsy-confirmed sarcoidosis. Findings of chest radiographic abnormalities that are typical of sarcoidosis were specific (91%) but not sensitive (64%) for biopsy-proven sarcoidosis. Sensitivity increased to 79% when combined with an elevated serum angiotensin-converting enzyme level. Chest CT may be warranted if sarcoidosis is suspected.

Skin Testing

Skin testing is often neglected by practitioners, but these simple tests can provide a large amount of information. The purified protein derivative (PPD) and histoplasmin skin tests are easily performed and yield important clinical data. The PPD test is important in the evaluation of

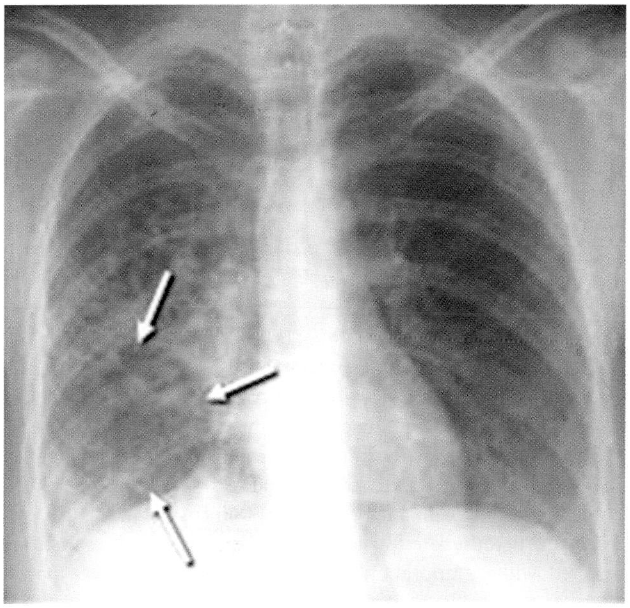

Fig. 5.3 Chest radiograph from a patient with tuberculosis showing a lower lobe cavity *(arrows)*. (From Diagnosis of tuberculosis disease. Core curriculum on tuberculosis: what the clinician should know. https://www.cdc.gov/tb/education/corecurr/index.htm)

the patient who has uveitis and a history suggesting tuberculosis.[27] In addition, patients should undergo a PPD test before immunosuppressive therapy because if the PPD test result is positive, these patients will require antituberculosis therapy before immunosuppressive therapy is begun. Patients with a history of possible tuberculosis or a positive reaction to the tuberculosis skin test should be tested with a lower-strength PPD, such as a 1-unit test dose, instead of the usual 5-unit test dose. If these test results are negative, then a higher test dose can be given. The histoplasmin skin test is useful in evaluating patients with presumed ocular histoplasmosis syndrome; however, the test may activate an old, inactive histoplasmosis lesion and should be avoided in patients with macular lesions.

Skin testing can also be used to document anergy. Patients with sarcoidosis are typically anergic and should have depressed responses to skin testing with control antigens, such as tetanus. Systemic corticosteroid administration sometimes reverses anergy in these patients, whereas cyclosporin may prevent type IV hypersensitivity reactions in the skin and yield a negative result to the skin test. In the past, the Kveim test was commonly performed for sarcoidosis, but the result was very dependent on the batch of Kveim antigen that was used. Currently, Kveim antigen cannot be obtained, and the test is no longer used. The pathergy skin test is also infrequently performed. In this test, patients with suspected Behçet disease are stuck with a sterile needle, and the skin is observed or biopsy samples are obtained for evidence of a type IV reaction. The hypothesis is that patients with Behçet disease will display a positive delayed hypersensitivity response to the needlestick (pathergy). Although the test is rarely performed, a history of skin reactions to phlebotomy draws or intravenous line placements may suggest pathergy and the diagnosis of Behçet disease.

Allergy testing was once a very important component in the evaluation of the patient with uveitis. The relevance of atopy or a specific allergy to uveitis is not clear. Hard evidence showing that type I hypersensitivity reactions are a major underlying force in intraocular inflammatory disease is lacking: Only anecdotal information suggests a possible secondary role.[28] As a result, we only occasionally order allergy testing for our patients.

BOX 5.2 Analysis of Aqueous Humor for Antibody

A = Inverse titer of specific immunoglobulin G (IgG) in aqueous
B = Total IgG in aqueous
X = Inverse titer of specific IgG in serum
Y = Total IgG in serum

If $(A/B)/(X/Y) < 1$, then there is local antibody production within the eye, suggesting intraocular infection

EXAMPLE:

Aqueous titer to toxoplasmosis = 1:200; aqueous IgG = 0.1 g/dL
Serum titer to toxoplasmosis = 1:400; serum IgG = 3 g/dL
Therefore: A/B = 60, suggesting that uveitis is caused by toxoplasmosis

Tissue Samples

The diagnosis of many forms of uveitis is based on the history and the typical appearance of the ocular disease. Nevertheless, the definitive diagnosis of many occurrences of uveitis requires histologic confirmation. No oncologist or radiation therapist would agree to treat a patient with presumed intraocular lymphoma without a tissue diagnosis. Similarly, the definitive diagnosis of sarcoidosis also requires histologic confirmation. In many other instances, analysis of ocular fluid or tissue can provide a wealth of information to the clinician. The information is, however, only as good as the evaluation of the specimen. It is imperative that the tissue is processed expeditiously by a person experienced in a variety of histologic and immunologic techniques, including immunohistochemical staining.

The evaluation of intraocular fluid is potentially of great value. Assays for antibody titers were used to diagnose ocular infections; however, the use of real-time polymerase chain reaction (PCR) has improved diagnostic accuracy and thus the utility of obtaining intraocular fluids to diagnose intraocular infectious disorders. A condition for which the analysis of intraocular fluids has aided the clinician in diagnosis is toxoplasmosis. Problems arise when atypical lesions are noted in a patient with low levels of circulating antitoxoplasma antibody. Desmonts[29] proposed that local (i.e., intraocular) production of specific antitoxoplasmosis antibody strongly suggests an active ocular lesion as a result of toxoplasmosis. To demonstrate local production of antibody, the specific antibody in the eye is measured relative to the total amount of globulin in the eye. This led Desmonts to calculate the antibody coefficient (C). The formula for determining this value is:

$$C = \text{Antibody titer}\frac{\text{Aqueous humor}}{\text{Serum}} \times \text{Immunoglobulin}\frac{\text{Serum}}{\text{Aqueous humor}}$$

Ideally, the antibody coefficient should be 1.0. A coefficient of 2.0 to 7.0 is compatible with local production of specific antibody, but a coefficient greater than 8.0 is considered highly suggestive of local production. An example of the use of this formula is presented in Box 5.2. With the increasing availability of PCR-based tests for common infections, the quantification of antibody titers has been relegated to testing for infections when no PCR tests are available (see section on PCR).

Historically, similar evaluations have been performed to look for local antibody production to virus.[30] Timsit et al.[31] detected herpes simplex virus (HSV) antibodies in the aqueous of half the patients with clinically confirmed herpes keratouveitis. Kaplan et al.[32] found antibodies against either HSV or vesicular stomatitis virus in the aqueous of four of 20 with idiopathic uveitis. Samples may, however, be contaminated by peripheral serum. Furthermore, local production of specific antibody may be related to polyclonal B-cell activation totally unrelated to the virus in question. Diagnostic vitrectomy is mostly used to evaluate the possibility of either infection or malignancy. Intraocular inflammation as a result of autoimmune disease may look similar to inflammation after infection. In patients with a history of postsurgical uveitis, diagnostic vitrectomy and anterior chamber tap are often warranted. Recently, some slow-growing bacteria have been identified as causes of chronic insidious postsurgical uveitis. One of these organisms, *Propionibacterium acnes,* is described in detail in the chapter on postsurgical uveitis (see Chapter 19) and the chapter on masquerade syndromes (see Chapter 31). Davis et al.[33] reported on 84 eyes in 78 patients who underwent pars plana vitrectomy for diagnostic purposes. The preoperative diagnosis was either infection or malignancy. Vitreous testing led to a diagnosis in 48 of 78 patients. When the preoperative indication was compared with the final clinical diagnosis, the efficiency rates of the diagnostic procedure of cytologic evaluation, flow cytometry, and bacterial or fungal culture were 67%, 79%, and 96%, respectively. Margolis et al.[34] reviewed 45 eyes of 44 consecutive patients who had posterior segment inflammation and underwent pars plana vitrectomy for diagnostic purposes. The vitreous analysis, which included culture, cytologic analysis, and flow cytometry, identified a specific cause in nine (20%) of the 45 eyes. In addition, visual acuity improved in 60%.

Many clinicians routinely obtain samples for biopsy from the conjunctiva and lacrimal gland in their search for histologic evidence of sarcoidosis. Most studies, however, report disappointing results with random "blind biopsies."[35] We suggest obtaining a biopsy sample from the conjunctiva only if a specific lesion is noted and from the lacrimal glands only if they are clinically enlarged or show increased uptake on gallium scanning. We have, however, found that biopsy of skin lesions can be extremely helpful to the clinician. We have made the diagnosis of sarcoidosis in numerous patients on the basis of a noncaseating granuloma found on skin biopsy.

Finally, we have performed chorioretinal biopsy in patients with severe posterior uveitis that caused severe visual loss in one eye and threatened vision in the other eye despite therapy. This technique is more fully described in the chapter on the role of surgery in the diagnosis and treatment of uveitis (see Chapter 9).

OPHTHALMIC IMAGING

Fundus Photographs

Fundus photographs remain important in the diagnosis and management of uveitis. They allow for a more detailed examination of retinal lesions and for more accurate assessment of disease progression and response to therapy. Wide-field retinal photographs can be particularly useful in assessing peripheral lesions and vasculitis. They are particularly beneficial in documenting disease progression and response to therapy over time.

Fluorescein Angiography

Fluorescein angiography is an invaluable aid in evaluating the numerous changes in uveitic eyes. The alterations seen are variable and frequently require the observer to evaluate the angiogram for some time before a satisfactory interpretation can be made. Some of the more frequently noted ocular changes that are highlighted with fluorescein angiography are listed in Box 5.3. Corresponding stereoscopic photographs may be helpful in establishing the level at which the pathologic condition in the eye is occurring, although use of OCT has made the detailed analysis of stereoscopic photographs and angiograms less critical.

Macular edema is one of the major causes of reduced vision in many types of intraocular inflammatory disease. The cause of this is not absolutely known. We assume, logically, that it results from swelling of the retinal layers, which disrupts the intimate association of the retinal elements that aids in crisp vision or distorts the alignment of the photoreceptors. However, we know that patients with angiographic evidence of mild or moderate macular edema can have good visual acuity. Furthermore, we have been most struck by the finding that patients can experience improvement of vision after therapeutic intervention, although the fluorescein angiogram shows no change in the leakage of fluorescein. Because late leakage seen on angiography is not strongly correlated with deterioration in vision, we explored other possible alterations that might be evaluated with fluorescein angiography. We hypothesized that retinal thickening, not the leakage of fluorescein into the retina, was one of the major causes of the deterioration in vision. We measured the amount of retinal thickening with the use of standard photos taken early during angiography (Fig. 5.4).[36] We noted a strong correlation between retinal thickening and the visual acuity of these eyes (Figs 5.5 and 5.6). The amount of dye leakage in the late phase of angiography did not, however, correlate well with visual acuity. More recently, OCT has been used to assess macular edema in patients with uveitis. Nevertheless, useful information about the vascular morphology and the presence of vasculitis can be best assessed with fluorescein angiography.

BOX 5.3 Major Fluorescein Angiographic Findings In Uveitis

- Cystoid macular edema
- Subretinal neovascular membranes
- Disk leakage
- Late staining of retinal vessels
- Neovascularization of retinal vessels
- Retinal vascular capillary dropout and reorganization
- Retinal pigment epithelium perturbations

In reading the angiogram, it is important to look at the early frames to best visualize the microvasculature surrounding the fovea. Many inflammatory eye diseases are thought to be associated with abnormalities in choroidal blood flow. Unfortunately, the excitation and fluorescence of fluorescein dye are absorbed and scattered by the retinal pigment. In addition, the fluorescein dye rapidly leaks from the fenestrated vessels of the choriocapillaris, leading to a diffuse background choroidal fluorescence. Both these factors combine to obscure any detailed analysis of the choroidal blood flow with fluorescein angiography. Wide-field fluorescein angiography can be useful in detecting peripheral disease activity and lead to changes in therapy.[37]

The use of OCT has decreased the use of fluorescein angiography in the assessment of uveitis. However, subtle vascular changes are still best assessed with angiography. The use of OCT angiography will be discussed in the chapter on OCT in uveitis (Chapter 6).

Indocyanine Green

Indocyanine green (ICG) is a water-soluble tricarbocyanine dye that was first used to measure cardiac output.[38] Unlike fluorescein, ICG is almost completely bound to plasma proteins and does not leak from normal retinal or choroidal vessels. Importantly, the pigment of the retinal pigment epithelium (RPE) and of the neurosensory retina does not significantly block the choroidal fluorescence when the ICG dye is illuminated with infrared light. ICG fluorescence is also more easily detected through hemorrhage. As a result, ICG angiography, which is recorded on either infrared photography or video angiography, is a useful tool for demonstrating abnormalities of choroidal blood flow, including choroidal neovascular membranes.[39-42]

ICG angiography is now being used to study patients with a number of uveitic conditions. In patients with serpiginous choroiditis, ICG angiography has demonstrated blockage of choroidal fluorescence in active areas

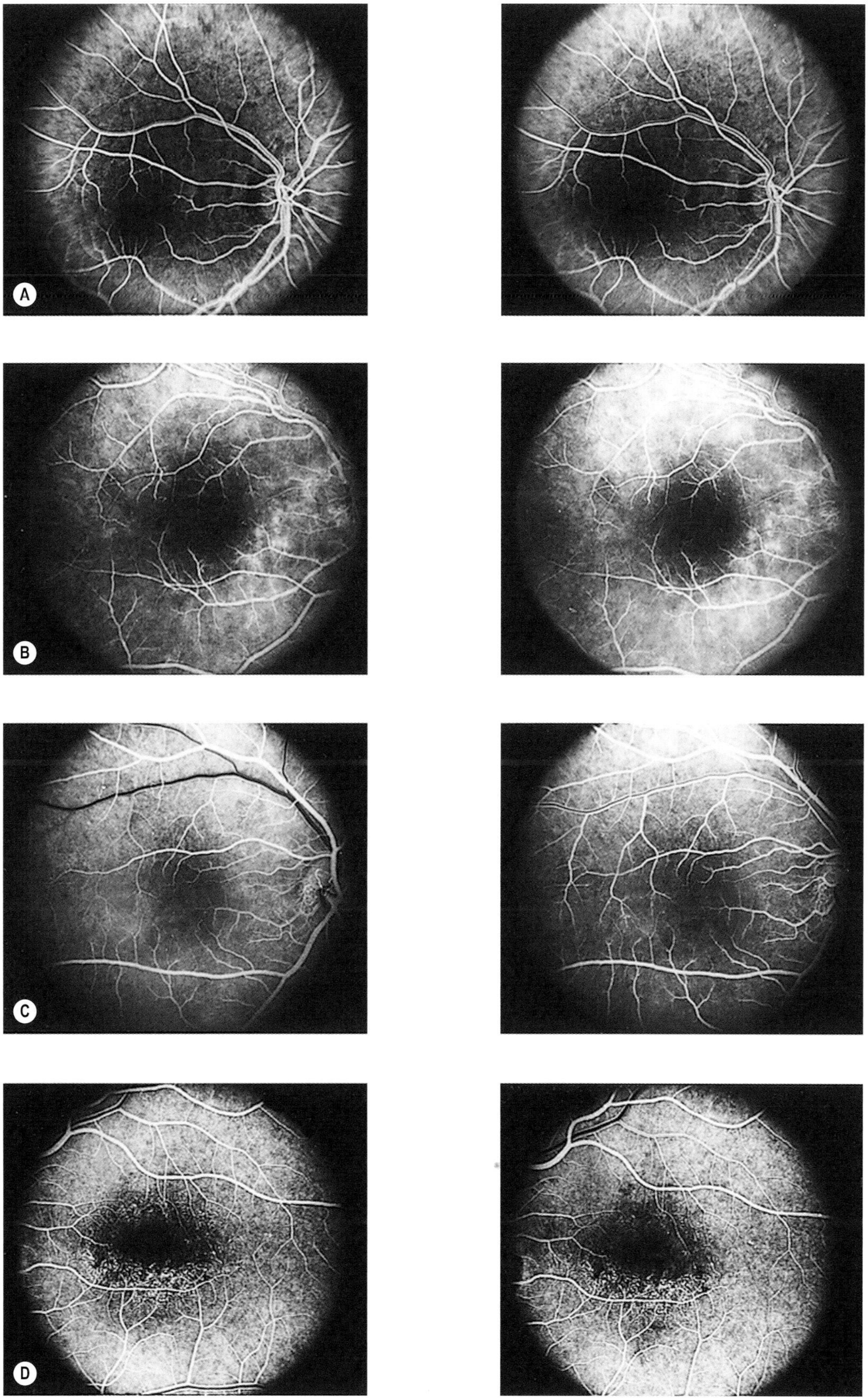

Fig. 5.4 Standard stereoscopic fluorescein angiographic photographs showing varying degrees of macular thickening. A, "Normal." B–D, In order of increasing macular thickening. A strong light source should be placed under photographs, and macular thickening can be best evaluated using "map reader" (Air Photo Supply, model PS-2 stereo viewer), which will yield maximum stereopsis. (From Nussenblatt RB, Kaufman SC, Palestine AG, et al. Macular thickening and visual acuity. *Ophthalmology.* 1987;94:1134–1139.)

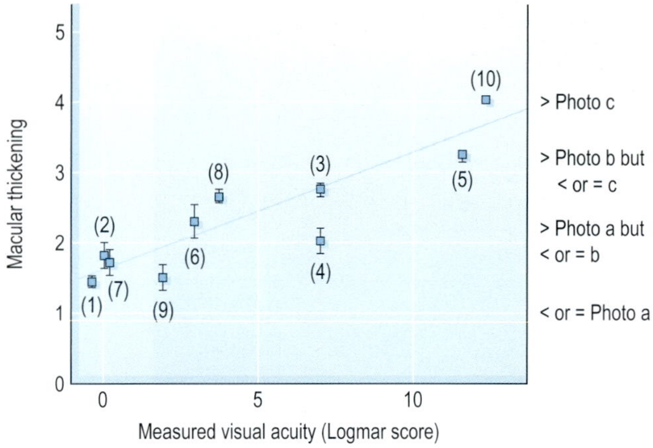

Fig. 5.5 Mean (±1 standard error) of 13 gradings of macular thickening for eyes with cystoid macular edema (11 because of uveitis, two because of diabetes). Simple linear regression showed significant relationship between mean thickening and actual visual acuity. (From Nussenblatt RB, Kaufman SC, Palestine AG, et al. Macular thickening and visual acuity. *Ophthalmology.* 1987;94:1134–1139.)

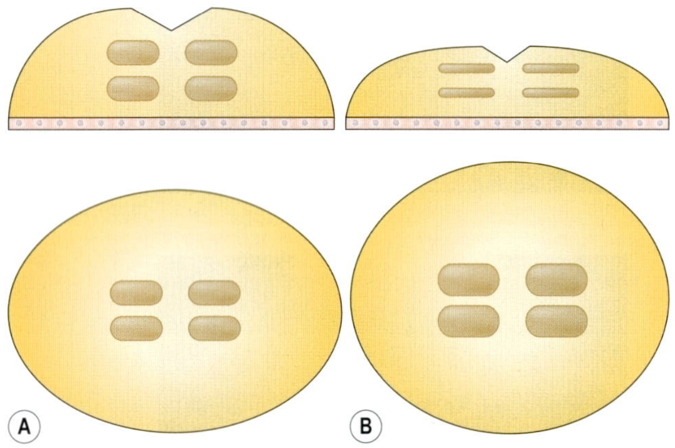

Fig. 5.6 Proposed scheme as to why fluorescein leakage may appear to be the same but macular thickening may have decreased, resulting in improvement in visual acuity. (A) During an acute episode of uveitis, cystic spaces are filled with fluid and the macula is thickened. (B) With therapy there is a reduction in macular thickening but the amount of leakage will appear to be the same if the angiogram is reviewed in standard fashion. (From Nussenblatt RB, Kaufman SC, Palestine AG, et al. Macular thickening and visual acuity. *Ophthalmology.* 1987;94:1134–1139.)

of lesions, with return of the normal choroidal fluorescence as the inflammation subsides.[43] In addition, the chorioretinal lesions associated with birdshot choroiditis are often difficult to observe clinically or to document with fluorescein angiography. However, Krupsky et al.[44] showed that ICG angiography was superior to fluorescein angiography in demonstrating these lesions that appeared as hypofluorescent areas, suggesting loss of the choriocapillaris. Herbort et al.[45,46] used ICG angiography to assess disease activity in several forms of uveitis, including Vogt-Koyanagi-Harada (VKH) syndrome and Behçet disease. Researchers are also using ICG angiography to compare active and quiescent chorioretinal lesions in patients with uveitis, and it is hoped that this technique will provide new insight into the pathophysiology of a number of uveitic disorders.

Optical Coherence Tomography

OCT initially allowed clinicians to noninvasively assess retinal thickness. With improved resolution of retinal and choroidal architecture and the advent of OCT angiography, OCT has become an integral diagnostic and management tool for the uveitis specialist and is discussed in greater detail in Chapter 6. This technique may be useful in assessing retinal edema in patients with uveitis and response to therapy. In a recent study, Antcliff et al.[47] compared OCT and fluorescein angiography in 58 patients with uveitis and suspected cystoid macular edema (CME). One hundred and eight eyes had similar results from both OCT and fluorescein angiography: 67 eyes had CME and 41 eyes had no CME. In 10 eyes, subretinal fluid was detected by OCT but not by fluorescein angiography. Five of these eyes had CME detected by fluorescein angiography but not by OCT. Three other eyes had CME detected by fluorescein angiography but not by OCT. The authors concluded that OCT is as effective as fluorescein angiography in detecting CME but is superior in demonstrating axial distribution of fluid. Similar to fluorescein angiography, the accuracy of the measurements is affected by small pupil size and media opacity.

There have been improvements in OCT technology and a number of new studies assessing its use in uveitis. OCT is useful for detecting macular edema and assessing response to therapy.[48] Reductions in macular thickness in patients with uveitic CME can be clearly detected on OCT after treatment with corticosteroid therapy. OCT may be useful in detecting retinal pathology in other forms of posterior uveitis.[49] Finally, spectral-domain OCT may provide additional information and be useful in assessing uveitic eyes, especially when hazy media obscures clinical examination.[50]

High-Frequency Ultrasound Biomicroscopy and Multifrequency Ultrasonography

High-frequency ultrasound biomicroscopy (UBM) allows for detailed imaging of the anterior segment of the eye, ciliary body, pars plana, and peripheral vitreous. Because many patients with uveitis have severe media opacity, which impairs the clinician's ability to examine these structures clinically, UBM can allow for assessment of inflammatory lesions not otherwise visible. In our experience, UBM is useful in selected patients with uveitis. UBM also can help in assessing inflammation in patients with severe media opacity, in assessing the placement of an intraocular lens to see whether it may be contributing to inflammation, and in evaluating causes of hypotony because it can provide detailed information on the anatomy of the ciliary body. Recently, Tran et al.[51] retrospectively reviewed UBM findings from 111 eyes in 77 patients with uveitis. They noted that UBM findings contributed to the diagnosis or influenced treatment in 43% of patients. In a study of seven eyes in five patients with intermediate uveitis, ultrasound examination with both 50- and 20-MHz frequency probes were able to detect snowbanks; this modality may be useful in eyes with small pupils or dense vitritis to assess disease activity.[52]

Fundus Autofluorescence

Liebman and Leigh, in an article in *Nature* in 1969, described autofluorescence of visual receptors.[53] Fundus autofluorescence occurs when fluorophores within the retina are induced to emit light when stimulated with specific light frequencies. Accumulation of lipofuscin in the retina is thought to be the main cause of fundus autofluorescence. Fundus autofluorescence has been used to assess pathologic changes in the RPE that are thought to be associated with clinically relevant changes in function, and, importantly, it may be useful in assessing changes to the RPE that may be missed with other imaging modalities. The technique has been used to assess patients with a number of retinal conditions, including age-related macular degeneration and uveitis. For example, focal accumulation of autofluorescent material was shown at the level of the RPE in patients with central serous chorioretinopathy.[54] Autofluorescence may also indicate disease progression

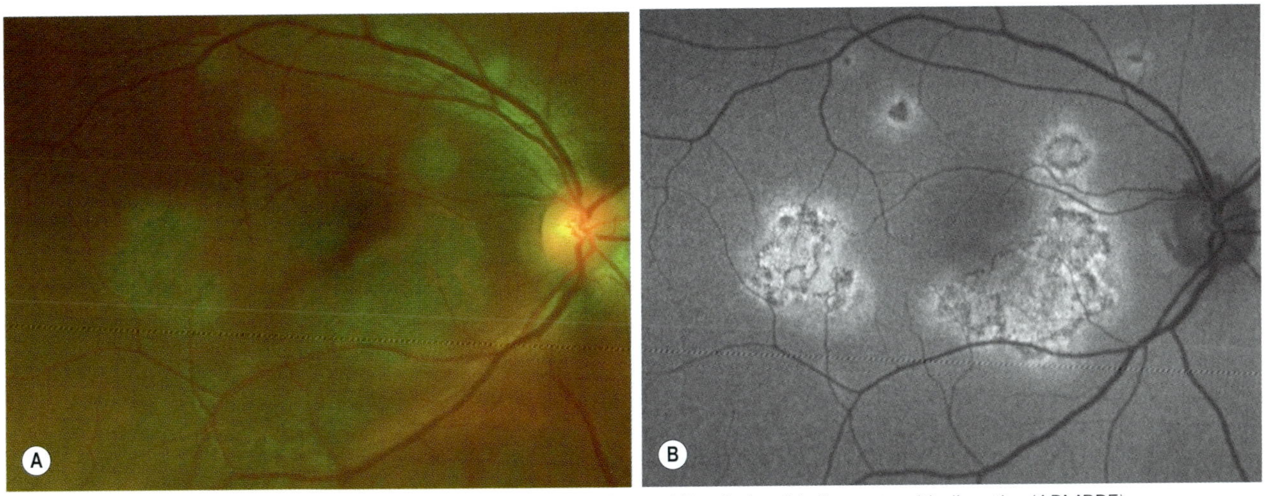

Fig. 5.7 Right eye of a patient with acute posterior multifocal placoid pigment epitheliopathy (APMPPE). (A) Fundus photograph showing multiple white-yellow colored plaques at the level of the retinal pigment epithelium. (B) Fundus autofluorescence shows hyperautofluorescent borders with central areas of hypo-autofluorescence.

and resolution. In acute posterior multifocal placoid pigment epitheliopathy (APMPPE), retinal lesions have autofluorescent borders (Fig. 5.7), which become more hypoautofluorescent as the lesions heal.[55] Autofluorescence can also show more widespread involvement of the RPE than previously documented in patients with multifocal choroiditis and panuveitis.[56] A number of abnormal autofluorescence patterns have been described for specific uveitic diseases including serpiginous choroidopathy, acute posterior multifocal placoid pigment epitheliopathy, the white dot syndromes, and birdshot choroidopathy.[57,58]

ANCILLARY OPHTHALMIC TESTS

Electrophysiology

Electrophysiologic testing can help determine the cause of visual loss in some patients with uveitis but, in general, rarely leads to a specific diagnosis. Both the electroretinography (ERG) and the electro-oculography (EOG) results can be altered in many of the inflammatory disorders of the retina and of the choroid. Experiments in the 1960s showed that ERG results were altered in animals with experimental uveitis.[59] Clinical studies also showed altered ERG results in patients with uveitis.[60] Because of the general lack of specificity, ERG will only tell the observer if significant widespread damage has occurred, and to date, we are not aware of changes noted on the ERG or on EOG that are specific for entities within the broad category of posterior uveitis. Feurst et al.[61] reported that the ERG results of patients with birdshot retinochoroidopathy show loss of blue cone responses in the dark-adapted state (see Chapter 26). We have noted loss of blue cone responses not only in birdshot retinochoroidopathy[62] but also in other posterior uveitis entities. This may reflect a general effect of the immune response on the retina's electrophysiologic responsiveness. Because it is difficult to assess the clinical response to therapy in some patients with birdshot retinochoroidopathy, a number of uveitis specialists use ERG monitoring to assess the progression of disease and response to therapy.[63-65]

One problem with the use of electrophysiology in assessing some forms of uveitis is that the pathology is limited to the macula. As a result, the ERG result may be relatively normal. The use of multifocal ERG allows for assessment of function in the central retina.[66,67] Multifocal ERG may also be used to assess changes with therapy.[68]A review of the literature concluded that the use of electrophysiologic examination in uveitis can be used to both diagnose disease and monitor disease progression and response to therapy and is most useful in patients with white dot syndromes, acute posterior multifocal placoid pigment epitheliopathy, birdshot chorioretinopathy, VKH disease, Behçet disease, ocular syphilis, and Fuchs heterochromic cyclitis.[69]

Laser Interferometry

With the widespread use of imaging techniques, most notably OCT, laser interferometry visual acuity is not routinely used to predict the visual prognosis. However, previous studies on the use of laser interferometry in predicting clinical outcomes in uveitis highlight an important principle: It is important to assess the viability of the retina and that of the optic nerve before patients are exposed to systemic immunosuppressive agents to treat uveitis and improve vision. Early in our therapeutic studies, we wanted to know whether we could predict which patients with uveitis might improve with immunosuppressive therapy. We had noted that there was a discrepancy between the visual acuity obtained with the standard Snellen chart and later the Early Treatment Diabetic Retinopathy Study (ETDRS) eye chart and the laser interferometer. Measurements of visual acuity obtained with the laser interferometer are often better than those obtained with eye charts. We hypothesized that these differences might be caused by potentially reversible macular changes as a result of the ongoing inflammatory disease. In a prospective study of 26 patients treated with cyclosporin for endogenous intermediate and posterior uveitis, we noted improvement in 86% of patients in whom the laser interferometer predicted a three-line or better improvement in vision compared with the standard measurement of visual acuity. In contrast, only 52% of cases where laser interferometry showed less than a three-line improvement later showed improvement with cyclosporin therapy. There was moderate correlation between the predicted number of lines of improvement with the laser interferometer and the number of lines actually improved with therapy ($R = 0.59$, $P < 0.001$). Thus, although laser interferometry is not routinely used in assessing visual potential in patients with uveitis, it is still important to assess visual potential in all patients before determining a therapeutic approach.

Laser Flare Photometry

Although standardized schemes for assessing anterior chamber cells and flare have been described in the literature, grading differs significantly among clinicians and even for the same grader over time. A laser device has been developed to assess flare in the anterior chamber of the eye and should standardize the grading of anterior chamber inflammation; objective grading of flare is extremely useful in determining response to therapy.[70,71] Furthermore, it is difficult to detect the induced flare caused by small amounts of protein in the aqueous humor resulting from early breakdown of the blood–aqueous barrier. After cataract surgery, for example, it would be useful to predict which eyes were at risk of developing uveitis and cystoid macular edema. The laser flare photometer is more sensitive than the eye in detecting flare and may be useful in predicting which eyes are at risk for developing worsening inflammatory disease, and possibly identifying eyes that require more aggressive anti-inflammatory therapy. In one study of 30 patients with uveitis, outflow facility was significantly reduced in patients with elevated flare photometry results.[72] An association between laser flare photometry values and the complications of uveitis has also been reported.[73] However, randomized clinical trials have not demonstrated that increasing therapy to decrease laser flare photometry values improves clinical outcomes compared with basing therapy on clinical assessment.[74]

BOX 5.4 FDA-approved PCR Tests for Infectious Agents Associated With Uveitis*

Adenovirus
Candida tropicalis, Candida albicans, Candida parapsilosis, Candida glabrata, Candida krusei
Clostridium difficile
Chlamydia trachomatis
Ebola virus
Neisseria gonorrhoeae
Cytomegalovirus
Dengue virus
Hepatitis virus
HIV-1
Leishmania species
Mycobacterium tuberculosis
Zika virus

*Some of these tests are authorized only for emergency use.
FDA, U.S. Food and Drug Administration; *HIV*, human immunodeficiency virus; *PCR*, polymerase chain reaction.

OTHER DIAGNOSTIC TESTS

Polymerase Chain Reaction

Since its initial description by Saiki et al.,[75] PCR has become one of the most commonly used techniques in biomedical research. It provides a simple way to amplify a specific fragment of DNA, and this technique has proved useful for the study of genetic diseases and the detection of infectious agents. Pertinent to the field of uveitis, PCR has also been used to detect viruses, bacteria, and parasites in the eye.[76]

To start PCR, four components are combined: (1) target DNA; (2) primers (short strands of DNA that tag the section of target DNA to be copied); (3) polymerase (the enzyme that catalyzes gene replication); and (4) nucleotides. PCR is based on the consecutive repetition of three reactions. First, the target DNA is denatured by heating the test tube to 95° C. Second, primers are annealed to a targeted strip of DNA as the temperature of the test tube is reduced. Finally, in the third step of the PCR, polymerase triggers the synthesis of a new DNA molecule between the primers. These three steps of the reaction are then repeated consecutively during 30 to 40 cycles and controlled by the raising and lowering of the temperature of the test tube.

At the end of PCR, the amount of target DNA is increased by 1 million to 1 billion times. However, the extreme sensitivity of the technique requires very strict laboratory procedures to prevent carryover of positive substrate between samples that could lead to false-positive results. PCR can be used to detect DNA fragments in many types of specimens, including cells, body fluids, and paraffin-embedded sections. PCR is currently being used to identify the DNA of infectious agents in the eye because, as has been seen, the interpretation of serologic tests is often misleading. Before PCR can be carried out, the sequence of the target DNA (specific for the organisms in question) must be available, and the appropriate primers must then be synthesized. Viral DNA has been identified by PCR in eyes with a number of disorders, including acute retinal necrosis.[77] We currently use PCR in our laboratory to diagnose ocular toxoplasmosis.[78,79]

The U.S. Food and Drug Administration (FDA) has approved nucleic acid amplification tests for the detection of a number of infectious agents that can also cause uveitis (Box 5.4). Tests are listed on the FDA website and regularly updated. PCR tests are now available for *Mycobacterium tuberculosis*.[80] Initially, these tests were only indicated for use in patients with respiratory specimens that produced negative results on acid-fast bacilli (AFB) smears. These tests are now thought to be reasonable adjunctive tests in all patients with presumed tuberculosis. Of course, these tests should not replace the standard AFB smear or mycobacterial cultures and should only be interpreted in the context of other clinical information. Unfortunately, these commercial tests have not been well studied for the diagnosis of tuberculosis from ocular specimens, although there are studies showing that PCR can detect *M. tuberculosis* from the vitreous in some patients.[81,82] There are now commercially available PCR tests for detecting other infectious agents that can cause uveitis. FDA-approved tests to detect *Neisseria gonorrhoeae, Chlamydia trachomatis,* HIV, hepatitis C virus, and *Aspergillus* can now be ordered. Importantly, noncommercial PCR testing can be useful in elucidating infectious causes of uveitis. *Tropheryma whipplei* was identified by PCR from the vitreous of a patient with uveitis associated with Whipple disease.[83] New qualitative multiplex real-time PCR assays have been developed for detecting a number of infections, including HSV-1, HSV-2, varicella-zoster virus, cytomegalovirus, and *Toxoplasma gondii.*[84]

The use of PCR in diagnosing infections is increasing; however, although these tests are exquisitely sensitive, false-positive results can occur. In addition, a small piece of DNA found in the eye of a patient may represent a remnant from an infection that occurred long ago and may be totally unrelated to the patient's current illness. Nevertheless, the development of additional PCR assays for infections will continue to proliferate and will be available clinically to aid clinicians in the diagnosis of infectious uveitis.

Rapid Tests for Herpes Simplex and Herpes Zoster

Biopsy specimens, including cells obtained from anterior chamber taps, are tested for herpesvirus with the use of a direct fluorescent antibody test after 48 hours and 5 days of growth. Enzyme-linked immunosorbent assays, which give almost immediate diagnostic information, are available. However, problems with sensitivity and specificity arise and need to be thoroughly investigated before these tests can be used routinely in clinical practice.

Bone Mineral Density Studies

Historically, clinical tests, including laboratory tests and imaging studies, were performed to make a diagnosis or to assess the efficacy of therapy. Diagnostic tests are now used to monitor treatment toxicity. As we have stated, corticosteroids remain the mainstay of therapy for uveitis. Unfortunately, researchers have found that corticosteroids can promote osteoporosis. One study showed that patients receiving prednisone at a dose greater than 7.5 mg/day lost 10% to 15% of trabecular bone in the lumbar spine within 1 year.[85] At prednisone doses greater than 30 mg/day, bone loss increased to 30% to 50%. In one study of corticosteroid-induced osteoporosis in patients with uveitis, seven symptomatic fractures occurred in 129 patients during treatment.[86] Bone mineral density studies can accurately assess bone loss in patients treated with corticosteroids. If there is a reasonable chance for chronic steroid use, bone mineral density studies should be performed within 3 months of the start of systemic corticosteroid therapy and annually thereafter. If these studies show osteoporosis, patients may benefit from antiresorptive agents, such as calcitonin, alendronate, etidronate, or risedronate.

Genetic Testing for Steroid-Induced Glaucoma

Glaucoma is a major cause of visual loss in patients with uveitis. Glaucoma occurs in many patients with uveitis in the presence of active inflammation. In addition, glaucoma can occur as a side effect of corticosteroid use. To date, it has not been possible to predict which patients with uveitis are at greatest risk for glaucoma. Stone et al.[87] analyzed sequence-tagged site content and haplotype sharing between families affected by chromosome 1q-linked open-angle glaucoma to prioritize candidate genes for mutation screening. These researchers identified a gene encoding a trabecular meshwork protein (TIGR) associated with glaucoma. Polansky et al.[88] showed that glucocorticoids and oxidative stress stimuli induced TIGR in cultures of human trabecular meshwork cells, suggesting a mechanism of action for both corticosteroid-induced glaucoma and uveitic glaucoma. Clinical testing for genes associated with glaucoma, such as TIGR, may help clinicians predict which patients are at greatest risk for developing glaucoma, but to date, it is not routinely used in clinical practice.

Neurologic Tests

The eye is a part of the brain, and many forms of uveitis have associated central nervous system involvement. Because the eye can be a window to the brain and provide insight into neurologic disease, evaluation of the brain and cerebrospinal fluid can give important clues to the underlying cause of ocular inflammatory disease. For example, lumbar puncture is useful in evaluating patients with possible VKH syndrome or intraocular lymphoma.

REFERENCES

1. Griner PF, Mayewski RJ, Mushlin AL, et al. Selection and interpretation of diagnostic tests and procedures: principles and applications. *Ann Intern Med.* 1981;94:553–600.
2. Rembold CM, Watson D. Posttest probability calculation by weights: a simple form of Bayes' theorem. *Ann Intern Med.* 1988;108:115–120.
3. Rosenbaum JT, Wernick R. The utility of routine screening of patients with uveitis for systemic lupus erythematosus or tuberculosis. *Arch Ophthalmol.* 1990;108:1291–1293.
4. Warner HR, Toronto AF, Veasey LG, et al. A mathematical approach to medical diagnosis: application to congenital heart disease. *JAMA.* 1961;177:177–183.
5. Warner HR, Toronto AF, Veasy LG. Experience with Bayes' theorem for computer diagnosis of congenital heart disease. *Ann NY Acad Sci.* 1964;115:558–567.
6. Fagan TJ. Nomogram for Bayes' theorem. *N Engl J Med.* 1975;293:257.
7. Gorry GA, Barnett GO. Sequential diagnosis by computer. *JAMA.* 1968;205:849–854.
8. Cassoux N, Giron A, Bodaghi B, et al. IL-10 measurement in aqueous humor for screening patients with suspicion of primary intraocular lymphoma. *Invest Ophthalmol Vis Sci.* 2007;48:3253–3259.
9. Asukata Y, Ishihara M, Hasumi Y, et al. Guidelines for the diagnosis of ocular sarcoidosis. *Ocul Immunol Inflamm.* 2008;16:77–81.
10. Leeflang MMG, Deeks JJ, Gatsonis C, et al. on behalf of the Cochrane Diagnostic Test Accuracy Working Group. Systematic reviews of diagnostic test accuracy. *Ann Intern Med.* 2008;149:889–897.
11. Lee CS, Randhawa S, Lee AY, et al. Patterns of laboratory testing utilization among uveitis specialists. *Am J Ophthalmol.* 2016;170:161–167.
12. U.S. Preventive Services Task Force. Screening for syphilis infection: recommendation statement. *Ann Fam Med.* 2004;2:362–365.
13. Passo MS, Rosenbaum JT. Ocular syphilis in patients with human immunodeficiency virus infection. *Am J Ophthalmol.* 1988;106:1–6.
14. Tramont EC. Syphilis in the AIDS era. *N Engl J Med.* 1987;316:1600–1601.
15. Quan T, Kan I, Craft JE. Diagnostic tests in rheumatic diseases. In: Goldman L, Ausiello D, eds. *Cecil Textbook of Medicine.* Philadelphia: WB Saunders; 2004:1627–1630.
16. Birtane M, Yavuz S, Tastekin N. Laboratory evaluation in rheumatic diseases. *World J Methodol.* 2017;7:1–8.
17. Castro C, Gourley MN. Diagnostic testing and interpretation of tests for autoimmunity. *J Allergy Clin Immunol.* 2010;125:S238–S247.
18. Coenen D, Verschueren P, Westhovens R, et al. Technical and diagnostic performance of 6 assays for the measurement of citrullinated protein/peptide antibodies in the diagnosis of rheumatoid arthritis. *Clin Chem.* 2007;53:498–505.
19. Fauci AS, Haynes BF, Katz P, et al. Wegener's granulomatosis: prospective clinical and therapeutic experience with 85 patients for 21 years. *Ann Intern Med.* 1983;98:76–85.
20. Nolle B, Specks U, Ludemann J, et al. Anticytoplasmic autoantibodies: their immunodiagnostic value in Wegener's granulomatosis. *Ann Intern Med.* 1989;111:28–40.
21. Cohen-Tervaert MD, van der Woude FJ, Fauci AS, et al. Association between active Wegener's granulomatosis and anticytoplasmic antibodies. *Arch Intern Med.* 1989;149:2461–2465.
22. Young DW. The antineutrophil antibody in uveitis. *Br J Ophthalmol.* 1991;75:208–211.
23. Soukasian SH, Foster CS, Niles JL, et al. Diagnostic value of anti-neutrophil cytoplasmic antibodies in scleritis associated with Wegener's granulomatosis. *Ophthalmology.* 1992;99:125–132.
24. Nolle B, Coners H, Guncker G. ANCA in ocular inflammatory disorders. *Adv Exp Med Biol.* 1993;336:305–307.
25. Power WJ, Rodriguez A, Neves RA, et al. Disease relapse in patients with ocular manifestations of Wegener granulomatosis. *Ophthalmology.* 1995;102:154–160.
26. Groen F, van Laar JAM, Rothova A. Chest radiographic screening for sarcoidosis in the diagnosis of patients with active uveitis. *Ann Am Thorac Soc.* 2017;14:912–918.
27. Morimura Y, Okada AA, Kawahara S, et al. Tuberculin skin testing in uveitis patients and treatment of presumed intraocular tuberculosis in Japan. *Ophthlamology.* 2002;109:851–857.
28. Bloch-Michel E, Timsit JC. Uveitis with allergy to candidin. *Ophthalmologica.* 1985;191:102–106.
29. Desmonts G. Definitive serological diagnosis to ocular toxoplasmosis. *Arch Ophthalmol.* 1966;76:839–853.
30. Kijlstra A, Breebaart AC, Baarsma GS, et al. Aqueous chamber taps in toxoplasmic chorioretinitis. *Doc Ophthalmol.* 1986;64:53–58.
31. Timsit JC, Fortier B, Pontet F, et al. Value of the immunoenzyme method (ELISA) in determining serum and aqueous humor antiherpes immunoglobulin levels (apropos of 155 cases). *J Fr Ophthalmol.* 1982;5:669–674.
32. Kaplan HJ, Lee FK, Waldrep JC, et al. Viral antibodies in the aqueous humor in idiopathic uveitis. In: Saari KM, ed. *Uveitis Update.* Amsterdam: Excerpta Medica; 1984:437–442.
33. Davis JL, Miller DM, Ruiz P. Diagnostic testing of vitrectomy specimens. *Am J Ophthalmol.* 2005;140:822–829.
34. Margolis R, Brasil OF, Lowder CY, et al. Vitrectomy for the diagnosis and management of uveitis of unknown cause. *Ophthalmology.* 2007;114:1893–1897.
35. Weinreb RN, Tessler H. Laboratory diagnosis of ophthalmic sarcoidosis. *Surv Ophthalmol.* 1984;28:653–664.
36. Nussenblatt RB, Kaufman SC, Palestine AG, et al. Macular thickening and visual acuity. *Ophthalmology.* 1987;94:1134–1139.
37. Campbell JP, Leder HA, Sepah YI. Wide-field retinal imaging in the management of non-infectious posterior uveitis. *Am J Ophthalmol.* 2012;154:908–911.
38. Fox IJ, Wood EH. Indocyanine green: physical and physiologic properties. *Proc Mayo Clin.* 1960;35:732–744.

39. Kogure K, David NJ, Yamanouchi U, et al. Infrared absorption angiography of the fundus circulation. *Arch Ophthalmol.* 1970;83:209–214.
40. Flower RW, Hocheimer BF. A clinical technique and apparatus for simultaneous angiography of the separate retinal and choroidal circulations. *Invest Ophthalmol.* 1973;12:248–261.
41. Flower RW, Hochheimer BF. Indocyanine green dye fluorescence and infrared absorption choroidal angiography performed simultaneously with fluorescein angiography. *Johns Hopkins Med J.* 1976;138:33–42.
42. Destro M, Puliafito CA. Indocyanine green videoangiography of choroidal neovascularizations. *Ophthalmology.* 1989;96:846–853.
43. Bischoff P. Bedeutung der infrarotangiographie fur die differentialdiagnostik der aderhauttumoren. *Klin Mbl Augenheilkd.* 1985;186:187–193.
44. Krupsky S, Friedman E, Foster CS, et al. Indocyanine green angiography in choroidal diseases. *Invest Ophthalmol Vis Sci.* 1992;33(Suppl):723.
45. Herbort CP, Mantovani A, Bouchenaki N. Indocyanine green angiography in Vogt–Koyanagi–Harada disease: angiographic signs and utility in patient follow-up. *Int Ophthalmol.* 2007;27:173–182.
46. Klaeger AJ, Tran VT, Hiroz CA, et al. Use of ultrasound biomicroscopy, indocyanine green angiography and HLA-B51 testing as adjunct methods in the appraisal of Behçet's uveitis. *Int Ophthamol.* 2004;25:57–63.
47. Antcliff RJ, Stanford MR, Chauhan DS, et al. Comparison between optical coherence tomography and fundus fluorescein angiography for the detection of cystoid macular edema in patients with uveitis. *Ophthalmology.* 2000;107:593–597.
48. Sivaprasad S, Ikeji F, Xing W, et al. Tomographic assessment of therapeutic response to uveitis macular oedema. *Clin Exp Ophthalmol.* 2007;35:719–723.
49. Gallagher MJ, Yilmaz T, Cervantes-Castaneda RA, et al. The characteristic features of optical coherence tomography in posterior uveitis. *Br J Ophthalmol.* 2007;91:1680–1685.
50. Gupta V, Gupta P, Singh R, et al. Spectral-domain cirrus high-definition optical coherence tomography is better than time-domain stratus optical coherency tomography for evaluation of macular pathologic features in uveitis. *Am J Ophthalmol.* 2008;145:1018–1022.
51. Tran VT, LeHoang P, Herbort CP. Value of high-frequency ultrasound biomicroscopy in uveitis. *Eye.* 2001;15:23–30.
52. Doro D, Manfre A, Deligianni V, et al. Combined 50- and 20-MHz frequency ultrasound imaging in intermediate uveitis. *Am J Ophthalmol.* 2006;141:953–955.
53. Liebman PA, Leigh RA. Autofluorescence of visual receptors. *Nature.* 1969;221:1249–1251.
54. von Ruckmann A, Schmidt KG, Fitzke FW, et al. Serous central chorioretinopathy. Acute autofluorescence of the pigment epithelium of the eye. *Ophthalmologe.* 1999;96:6–10.
55. Haen SP, Spaide RF. Fundus autofluorescence in multifocal choroiditis and panuveitis. *Am J Ophthalmol.* 2008;145:847–853.
56. Spaide RF. Autofluorescence imaging of acute posterior multifocal placoid pigment epitheliopathy. *Retina.* 2006;26:479–482.
57. Takata H. Electroretinographic studies of experimental uveitis. (III). Characteristics of B- and C-potential of "inflammation type ERG." *Nippon Ganka Kiyo.* 1963;14:409–415.
58. Meleth AD, Sen HN. Use of fundus autofluorescence in the diagnosis and management of uveitis. *Int Ophthalmol Clin.* 2012;52:45–54.
59. Lee CS, Forooghian F, Bergstrom C, Yan J, Yeh S. Fundus autofluorescence features in the inflammatory maculopathies. *Clin Ophthalmol.* 2014;8:2001–2012.
60. Ourgaud AG, Haudiquet G, Tassy AF. Clinical study and ERG (oscillatory potential) in Vogt–Koyanagi–Harada syndrome. *Bull Soc Ophthalmol Fr.* 1966;66:470–475.
61. Feurst DJ, Tessler HH, Fishman GA, et al. Birdshot retinochoroidopathy. *Arch Ophthalmol.* 1984;102:214–219.
62. Gasch AT, Smith JA, Whitcup SM. Birdshot retinochoroidopathy. *Br J Ophthalmol.* 1999;83:241–249.
63. Zacks DN, Samson CM, Lowenstein J, et al. Electroretinograms as an indicator of disease activity in birdshot retinochoroidopathy. *Graefes Arch Clin Exp Ophthalmol.* 2002;240:601–607.
64. Holder GE, Robson AG, Pavesio C, et al. Electrophysiological characterisation and monitoring in the management of birdshot chorioretinopathy. *Br J Ophthalmol.* 2005;89:709–718.
65. Sobrin L, Lam BL, Liu M, et al. Electroretinographic monitoring in birdshot chorioretinopathy. *Am J Ophthalmol.* 2005;140:52–64.
66. Kretschmann U, Schlote T, Stubiger N, et al. Multifocal electroretinography in acquired macular dysfunction. *Klin Monatsbl Augenheilkd.* 1998;212:93–100.
67. Kretschmann U, Bock M, Gockeln R, et al. Clinical applications of multifocal electroretinography. *Doc Ophthalmol.* 2000;100:99–113.
68. Stubiger N, Besch D, Deuter CM, et al. Multifocal ERG changes in patients with ocular Behçet's disease during therapy with interferon alpha 2a. *Adv Exp Med Biol.* 2003;528:529–532.
69. Shah SM, Spalton DJ, Taylor JC. Correlations between laser flare measurements and anterior chamber protein concentrations. *Invest Ophthalmol Vis Sci.* 1992;33:2878–2884.
70. Moschos MM, Gouliopoulos NS, Kalogeropoulos C. Electrophysiological examination in uveitis: a review of the literature. *Clin Ophthalmol.* 2014;8:199–214.
71. Guex-Crosier Y, Pittet N, Herbort CP. Evaluation of laser flare-cell photometry in the appraisal and management of intraocular inflammation in uveitis. *Ophthalmology.* 1994;101:728–735.
72. Ladas JG, Yu F, Loo R, et al. Relationship between aqueous humor protein level and outflow facility in patients with uveitis. *Invest Ophthalmol Vis Sci.* 2001;42:2584–2588.
73. Gonzales CA, Ladas JG, Davis JL, et al. Relationships between laser flare photometry values and complications of uveitis. *Arch Ophthalmol.* 2001;119:1763–1769.
74. Davis JL, Dacanay LM, Holland GN, et al. Laser flare photometry and complications of chronic uveitis in children. *Am J Ophthalmol.* 2003;135:763–771.
75. Saiki RK, Gelfand DH, Stoffel S, et al. Primer-directed enzymatic amplification of DNA with a thermostable DNA polymerase. *Science.* 1988;239:487–491.
76. Van Gelder RN. Applications of polymerase chain reaction to diagnosis of ophthalmic disease. *Surv Ophthalmol.* 2001;46:248–258.
77. Forster DJ, Dugel PU, Frangieh GT, et al. Rapidly progressive outer retinal necrosis in the acquired immunodeficiency syndrome. *Am J Ophthalmol.* 1990;110:341–348.
78. Chan CC, Palestine AG, Li Q, et al. Diagnosis of ocular toxoplasmosis by the use of immunocytology and the polymerase chain reaction. *Am J Ophthalmol.* 1994;117:803–805.
79. Brezin AP, Egwuagu CE, Burnier M Jr, et al. Identification of *Toxoplasma gondii* in paraffin-embedded sections by the polymerase chain reaction. *Am J Ophthalmol.* 1990;110:599–604.
80. Update: nucleic acid amplification tests for tuberculosis, *MMWR Morbid Mortal Wkly Rep.* 2000;49:593–594.
81. Therese KL, Jayanthi U, Madhavan HN. Application of nested polymerase chain reaction (nPCR) using MPB 64 gene primers to detect *Mycobacterium tuberculosis* DNA in clinical specimens from extrapulmonary tuberculosis patients. *Indian J Med Res.* 2005;122:165–170.
82. Matos K, Muccioli C, Belfort R Jr, et al. Correlation between clinical diagnosis and PCR analysis of serum, aqueous, and aqueous and vitreous samples in patients with inflammatory eye disease. *Arq Bras Oftalmol.* 2007;70:109–114.
83. Rickman LS, Freeman WR, Green WR. Brief report: uveitis caused by *Tropheryma whippelii* (Whipple's bacillus), *N Engl J Med.* 1995;332:363–366.
84. Bispo PJM, Davoidi S, Sahm ML, et al. Rapid detection and identification of uveitis pathogens by qualitative multiplex real-time PCR. *Invest Ophthalmol Vis Sci.* 2018;59:582–589.
85. Lukert BP, Raisz LG. Glucocorticoid-induced osteoporosis. *Rheum Dis Clin North Am.* 1994;20:629–650.
86. Jones NP, Anderton LC, Cheong FM, et al. Corticosteroid-induced osteoporosis in patients with uveitis. *Eye.* 2002;16:587–593.
87. Stone EM, Fingert JH, Alward WL, et al. Identification of a gene that causes primary open angle glaucoma. *Science.* 1997;275:668–670.
88. Polansky JR, Fauss DJ, Chen P, et al. Cellular pharmacology and molecular biology of the trabecular mesh-work inducible glucocorticoid response gene product. *Ophthalmologica.* 1997;211:126–139.

6

Optical Coherence Tomography in Uveitis

Scott M. Whitcup

KEY CONCEPTS

- Optical coherence tomography (OCT) using low-coherence, long-wavelength light can produce high-resolution images of all layers of the retina as well as the choroid and vitreous.
- Two types of OCT devices are most commonly used in ophthalmology today: spectral-domain OCT (SD-OCT) and swept-source OCT (SS-OCT). Current SS-OCT devices allow better imaging of deeper structures like the choroid.
- OCT is frequently used to detect, document, and quantify macular edema in patients with uveitis and can be used to objectively assess the response to treatment.
- OCT is also useful in diagnosing epiretinal membranes and choroidal neovascular membranes in patients with uveitis.
- Specific OCT findings are being described for a number of uveitic conditions such as Vogt-Koyanagi-Harada disease and masquerade syndromes like intraocular lymphoma.
- OCT angiography is a useful alternative to fluorescein angiography and can be used to diagnose vascular leakage and inflammatory lesions.

Although a complete patient medical history followed by detailed clinical examination remains the cornerstone of the diagnosis and management of patients with uveitis, certain technologic advances have contributed to improvements in patient care. Optical coherence tomography (OCT) is one technology that is being increasingly used in the diagnosis and treatment of uveitis. More recently, the development of optical coherence tomography angiography (OCTA) has given clinicians a less invasive and prompt tool to assess the retinal and choroidal vasculature.

OCT uses low-coherence light to obtain high-resolution images of ocular tissues, including the retina and the optic nerve head. The use of long-wavelength light that penetrates into tissues allows imaging of all layers of the retina and of the choroid by detecting light reflectance in the Fourier domain. OCT of the normal retina can image individual layers of the retina and the overlying vitreous and the underlying choroid. Experts have worked to develop a consensus nomenclature for the classification of the retinal and choroidal layers and bands visible on OCT images of the normal eye.[1] Fig. 6.1 shows an OCT image of a normal retina obtained by using a spectral domain (SD)-OCT machine. OCT is not only used in ophthalmology but also in other areas of medicine (e.g., in cardiology to image the coronary arteries and in dermatology).

OCT images are created from the interference pattern created as scattered light from the tissue is compared with a reference wave. First-generation OCT machines used time-domain technology characterized by low-coherence, near-infrared light from a superluminescent diode light source split to a reference mirror and to the retina.[2] Today, two types of OCT devices are most commonly used in ophthalmology: SD-OCT and swept-source OCT (SS-OCT). SD-OCT machines are more prevalent in clinical practices and use a broadband light source, a spectrometer, and a high-speed line-scan camera to measure the interference patterns. The newer SS-OCT machines use a light source with a wavelength around 1 μm that sweeps across a narrow band of wavelengths and a simpler point photodetector. Current SS-OCT devices allow better imaging of deeper structures, such as the choroid, but are more expensive and have less ideal axial resolution and less normative data compared with SD-OCT. However, the technology continues to improve, and comparisons of state-of-the-art devices will change over time.

OCTA allows assessment of the retina and vasculature. Analysis of successive OCT B-scans at the same cross-sectional area of the retina allows detection of motion caused by flow through the retinal vessels. Although OCTA is less invasive and has a higher resolution compared with fluorescein angiography, it is susceptible to motion and projection artifacts, making some images difficult to interpret. That said, the technology continues to improve, with faster scanning speeds and better software algorithms resulting in better images for analysis.

MACULAR EDEMA

The most common use of OCT in diagnosing and managing uveitis centers on the detection, characterization, and quantification of macular edema. Before the introduction of OCT, macular edema was primary diagnosed and monitored clinically with slit-lamp examination or fluorescein angiography. However, these methods were variable and affected by the presence of not only media opacity but also by retinal hemorrhage, pigment, or lipid exudation in the retina.[3] Compared with angiography, OCT is a highly sensitive (96%) and sensitive (100%) test for the presence of macular edema in uveitic eyes.[4] SD-OCT has been shown to be better at detecting macular edema compared with time-domain OCT (TD-OCT) in patients with uveitis; this is not surprising, given the better resolution with SD-OCT.[5] Importantly, as a result of its reproducibility in measuring retinal thickness, OCT can reliably be used to assess therapeutic response for uveitic macular edema.[6]

In addition to quantifying macular edema, OCT can detect two different patterns of macular edema: cystic macular edema and a more diffuse pattern of macular edema.[7] In a study of SD-OCT, in a single eye from 500 consecutive patients with anterior, intermediate, posterior, or panuveitis, cystoid macular edema was seen in 25% of eyes, and diffuse macular edema was seen in 11% of eyes.[8] Cystoid macular edema was most frequent in intermediate uveitis (40%) and panuveitis (36%), and diffuse macular edema was most frequent in panuveitis (18%) and posterior uveitis (17%). Furthermore, the junction between the inner and outer segments of the photoreceptors (the IS/OS junction) and the external limiting membrane can be readily

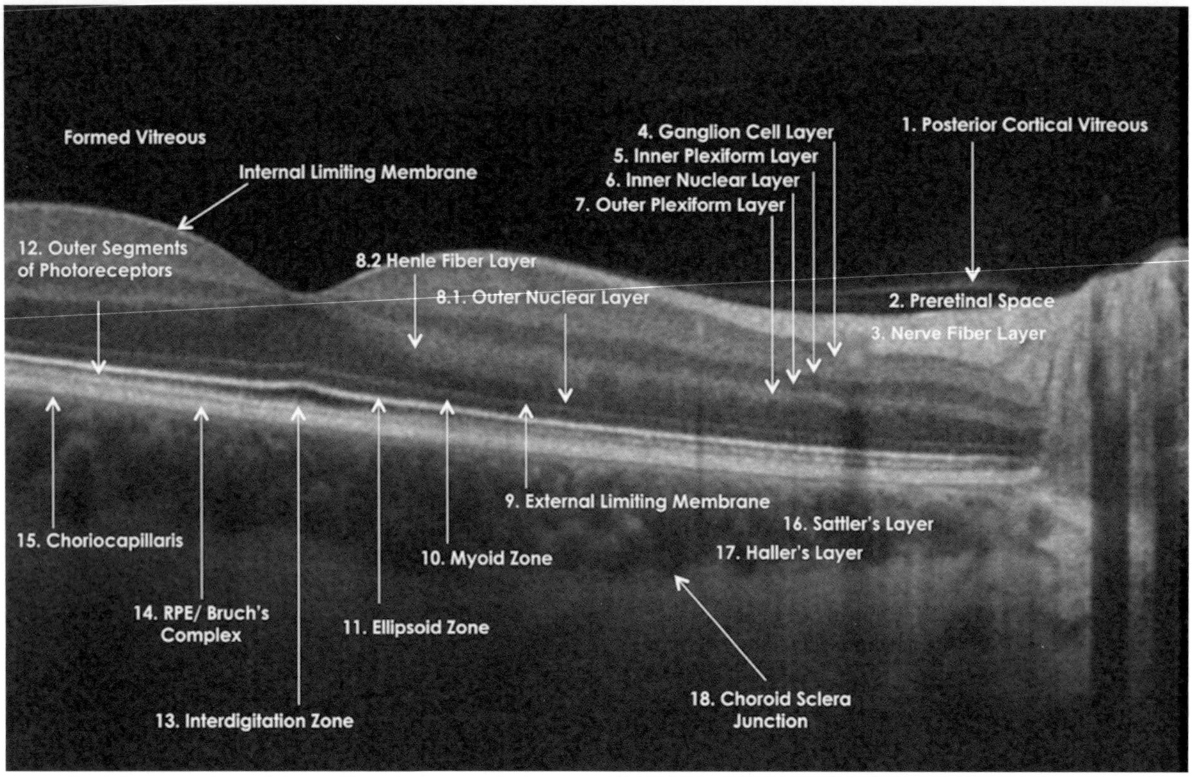

Fig. 6.1 Nomenclature for normal anatomic landmarks seen on spectral domain optical coherence Tomography Panel. Healthy retina imaged using Heidelburg Spectralis. *RPE,* Retinal pigment epithelium. (From Staurenghi G, Sadda S, Chakravarthy U, Spaide RF, for the International Nomenclature for Optical Coherence Tomography (IN.OCT) Panel. Proposed lexicon for anatomic landmarks in normal posterior segment spectral-domain optical coherence tomography. *Ophthalmology.* 2014;121:1572–1578.)

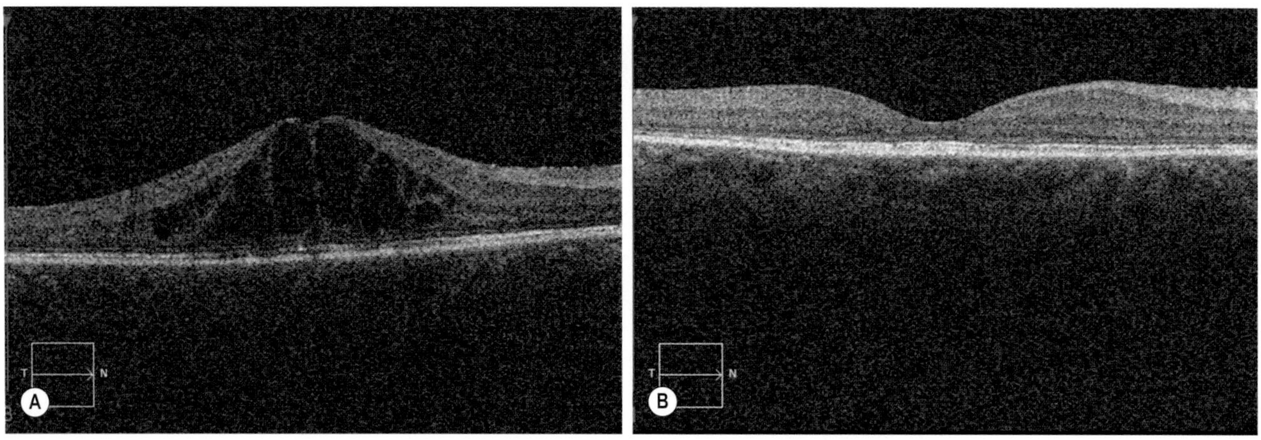

Fig. 6.2 Optical coherence tomography (OCT) of a patient with uveitis and cystoid macular edema before and after therapy with corticosteroids. (A) Massive cystoid edema in the macula with large intraretinal cystic spaces. (B) Resolution of cystoid macular edema 2 months after treatment with a sustained-release dexamethasone implant.

identified with SD-OCT. The integrity of the IS/OS junction may predict improvement in visual acuity after treatment of macular edema or epiretinal membrane removal.[3]

Importantly, OCT is used to more precisely monitor response to therapy and can guide therapy. Resolution of cystoid macular edema after treatment with intravitreal corticosteroid therapy is nicely demonstrated with OCT (Fig. 6.2). Collapse of the cystic spaces and complete resolution of retinal fluid and thickness occurred by 2 months after therapy (see Fig. 6.2B).

RETINAL AND CHOROIDAL PATHOLOGY

Uveitis frequently causes structural damage to the retina and the choroid. Epiretinal membranes can cause impaired vision in patients with uveitis and can also be detected with OCT, appearing as corrugated hyperreflective lines adherent to the inner retina (Fig. 6.3). Serous retinal detachments are common in a number of inflammatory eye diseases and can be diagnosed and monitored with OCT. Choroidal neovascularization also occurs in patients with uveitis and can be more difficult to diagnose in patients with extensive posterior segment inflammation. OCT can be useful in diagnosing choroidal neovascular membranes in uveitis patients (see Fig. 6.7A, later in the chapter) and in monitoring response to therapy. In addition, as the clinical use of OCT increases, descriptions of OCT findings in a number of specific forms of uveitis are being reported in the literature.

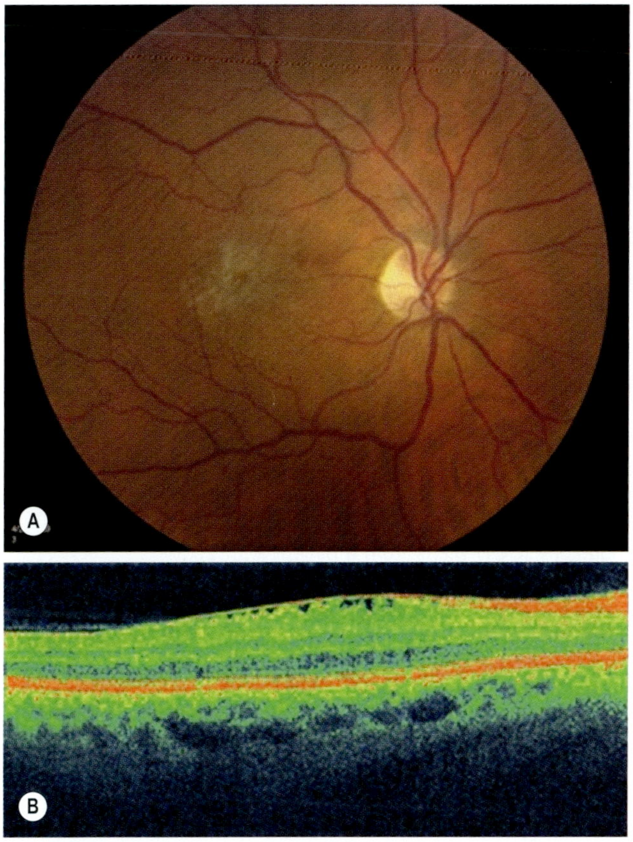

Fig. 6.3 Patients with uveitis and an epiretinal membrane. (A) Color photograph showing epiretinal proliferative changes consistent with fibrosis. (B) Optical coherence tomography (OCT) scan showing a corrugated appearance of the inner retina with an overlying hyperreflective epiretinal membrane. Retinal thickening with cystic changes in the outer retina is also seen.

EXAMPLES OF OPTICAL COHERENCE TOMOGRAPHY IN SPECIFIC UVEITIC DISEASES

OCT has also been useful in assessing a number of forms of posterior uveitis, including Vogt-Koyanagi-Harada (VKH) syndrome and birdshot chorioretinopathy. Fong et al. demonstrated significant loss of focal hyperreflectivity in the inner choroid of patients with VKH syndrome compared with controls in both the acute and convalescent stages of disease, which may represent permanent structural change to the small choroidal vessels.[9] In addition to detecting and delineating subretinal fluid in VKH syndrome, OCT can also show subretinal fibrosis in patients with VKH (Fig. 6.4). Importantly, OCT can be used to demonstrate and quantify treatment response to inflammatory retinal disease. Dastiridou et al. showed higher choroidal reflectivity and lower choroidal thickness in patients with inactive birdshot retinopathy compared with those with active disease and controls; this may be useful in monitoring disease activity.[10] Fig. 6.5 shows decreased retinal edema in response to treatment in another patient with VKH.

The white-dot syndromes are another group of disorders where OCT has improved our understanding and management of uveitis. Cho et al. reported abnormal reflectivity in the inner layer of the retinal pigment epithelium (RPE) on SD-OCT in all 18 eyes with acute retinal pigment epitheliitis.[11] Iu et al. later noted that early examination with SD-OCT showed an inflammatory lesion in the photoreceptor outer segment layer displacing the external limiting membrane in patients with the disease.[12] They also noted that recovery occurred in a sequence of the external limiting membrane, the ellipsoid zone, and then the interdigitation zone and that vision improved when the interdigitation zone was restored.

Finally, OCT can be especially useful in investigating potential masquerade syndromes. Diagnosis of primary central nervous system (CNS) lymphoma involving the eye can be challenging, and the early clinical signs and symptoms are frequently subtle. OCT can be useful in illustrating tumor infiltration into the retina and also helpful in assessing response to therapy.[13] We have seen many patients at the National Eye Institute who were referred with vitritis, minimal retinal changes on clinical examination, and good visual acuity and were diagnosed with intraocular lymphoma. Lymphoma cells can collect between the Bruch membrane and the RPE and can be difficult to recognize. A patient was seen with subtle changes in the outer retina with some stippling of the RPE (Fig. 6.6A). Although the changes seen on the photograph are subtle, OCT clearly showed

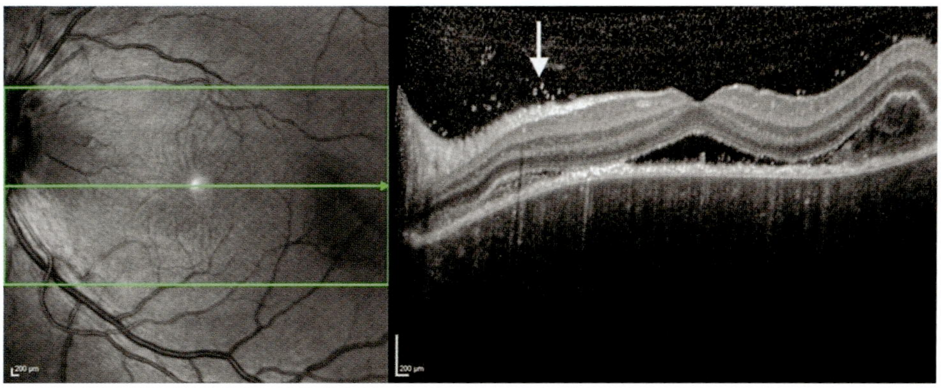

Fig. 6.4 Infrared retinal image and corresponding optical coherence tomography (OCT) showing subretinal fibrosis in a patient with Vogt-Koyanagi-Harada syndrome. Subretinal fluid is observed as a hyporeflective space underneath the fovea in the line scan. Temporal to this area of fluid is a pocket of more hyperreflective material consistent with fibrin containing subretinal fluid. Hyperreflective foci in the vitreous are consistent with inflammatory cells *(arrow)*.

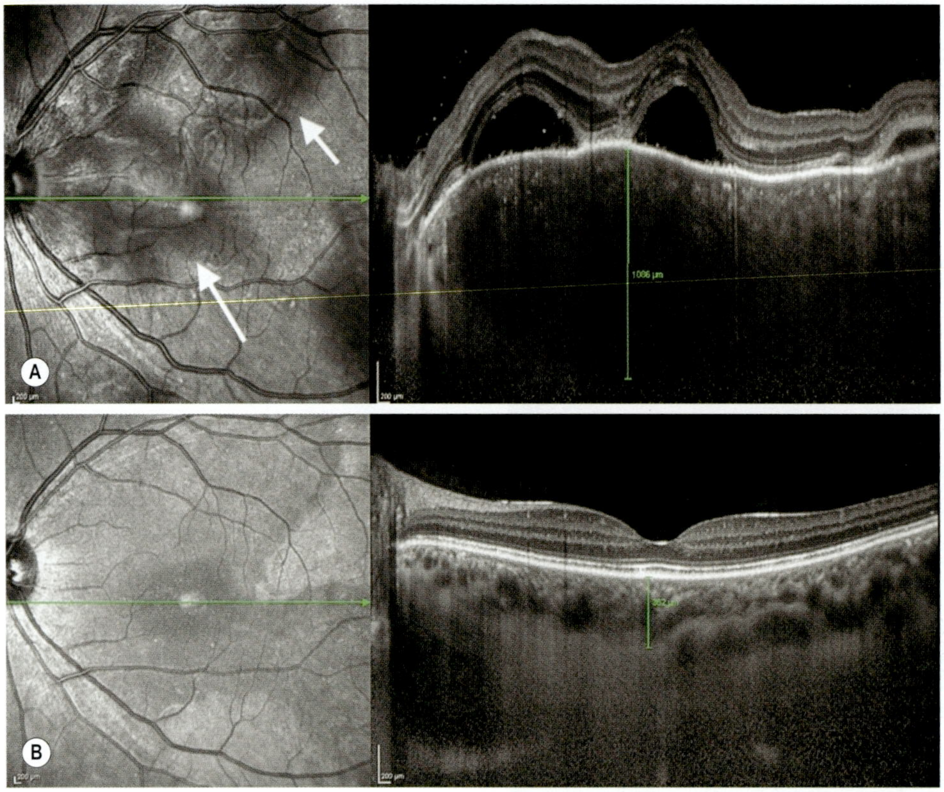

Fig. 6.5 Infrared retinal images and optical coherence tomography (OCT) scans from a patient with Vogt-Kayanagi-Harada syndrome. (A) Subretinal fluid accumulation and thickening of choroid observed on line scan *(right)*. Extensive lobular darkening on the infrared image *(left)* consistent with fluid accumulation can be seen *(white arrows)*. (B) Resolution of subretinal fluid and more normal appearance to the choroid after anti-inflammatory therapy. Lobular changes on the infrared image *(left)* are less dark and consistent with resolution of retinal and choroidal changes.

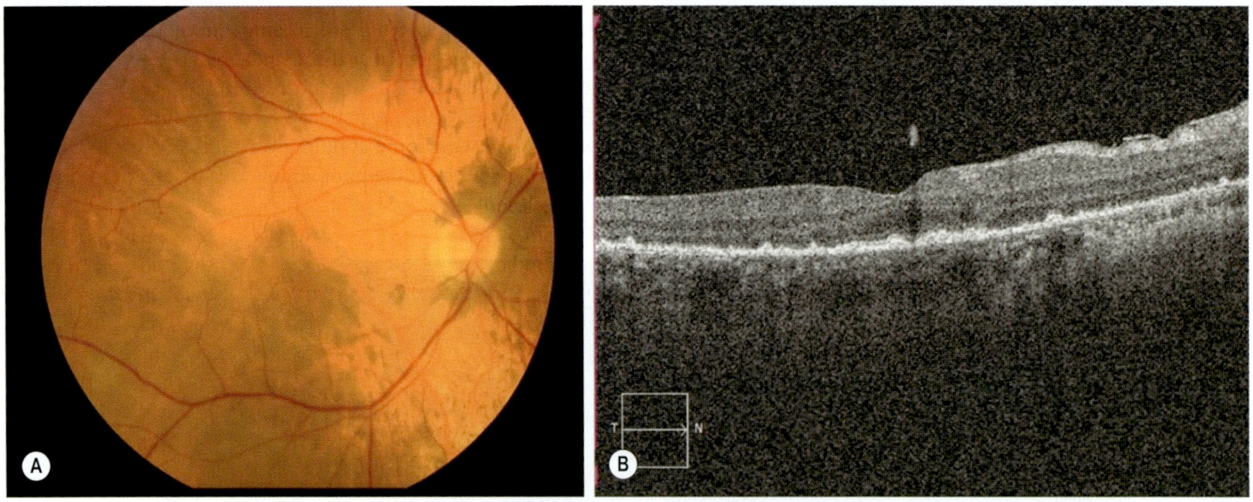

Fig. 6.6 Patient with intraocular lymphoma. Retinal photograph shows mild changes in the outer retina and retinal pigment epithelium in the macula and inferior to the disc (A). The optical coherence tomography (OCT) scan shows multiple areas of hyperreflective sub–retinal pigment epithelium (RPE) material consistent with tumor infiltration (B). Additional information can be found in Chapter 31.

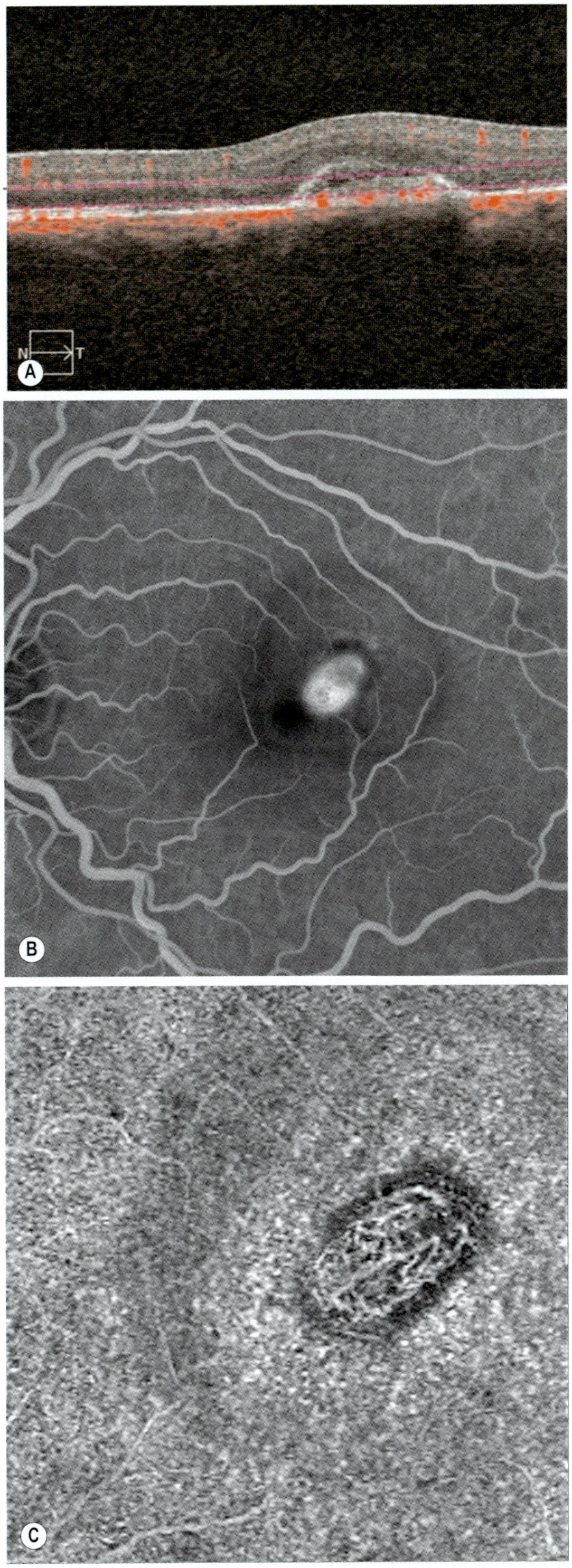

Fig. 6.7 Retinal imaging from a patient with multifocal choroiditis. (A) Horizontal line scan optical coherence tomography (OCT) showing the choroidal neovascular membrane with overlying retinal elevation. Retinal blood flow is shown as red pixels. (B) Midphase fluorescein angiography image showing lacy hyperfluorescence in the area of filling of the vascular complex. (C) Optical coherence tomography (angiography (OCTA) image detailing the vascular structure of the membrane. (Images courtesy of Elias Reichel, MD.)

sub-RPE hyperreflective material consistent with tumor infiltration (see Fig. 6.6B), and the patient was diagnosed with primary intraocular lymphoma.

Anterior Uveitis

Although OCT is rarely used clinically for diagnosing or treating patients with anterior uveitis, there has been interest in developing more automated and standardized techniques for measuring anterior segment inflammation, especially for use in clinical trials. There are non-OCT devices that can measure and quantify anterior chamber inflammation. A flare meter (Kowa Pharmaceuticals, Montgomery, AL) useful in detecting aqueous humor flare has been developed, but the device is not available to quantify anterior chamber cells. More recently, anterior segment OCT has been used to image and grade the degree of anterior chamber inflammation and correlates with clinical grades of anterior chamber cell counts.[14] This technique may be useful in the future, particularly for clinical trials where accurate and reproducible measurements across patients at different clinical sites are needed.

OPTICAL COHERENCE TOMOGRAPHY ANGIOGRAPHY

OCTA is also being used more frequently in patients with uveitis as an alternative to fluorescein angiography. In addition to demonstrating vascular leakage and inflammation, OCTA is demonstrating disease-specific findings that may help in the management of these conditions. For example, Klufas et al. used both OCT and OCTA to study patients with acute posterior multifocal placoid pigment epitheliopathy (APMPPE), persistent placoid maculopathy, or relentless placoid chorioretinitis.[15] OCTA demonstrated decreased choroidal blood flow, suggesting that the inner choroid is the primary site of disease.

OCTA is also useful in diagnosing and managing choroidal neovascular membranes in patients with uveitis. Fig. 6.7 shows an OCT scan, a fluorescein angiogram, and an OCTA angiography from a patient with multifocal choroiditis.

SUMMARY

OCT is a useful technique for assessing eyes with uveitis. It is especially helpful in detecting, characterizing, and quantifying macular edema. OCT findings can help guide clinicians during therapy. However, there are some limitations to this imaging technology. Media opacity can lead to signal attenuation and artifacts. OCT is also adversely affected by motion. Finally, because OCTA detects motion, it is less useful for detecting small amounts of blood flow. Despite these limitations, OCT has been a beneficial tool in both the diagnosis and the management of uveitis. The benefits of OCT in managing uveitis should only increase as the technology improves and our clinical experience grows.

REFERENCES

1. Staurenghi G, Sadda S, Chakravarthy U, Spaide RF, for the International Nomenclature for Optical Coherence Tomography (IN.OCT) Panel. Proposed lexicon for anatomic landmarks in normal posterior segment spectral-domain optical coherence tomography. *Ophthalmology*. 2014;121:1572–1578.
2. Herbort CP Jr, Tugal-Tutkun I, Neri P, et al. Failure to integrate quantitative measurement methods of ocular inflammation hampers clinical practice and trials on new therapies for posterior uveitis. *J Ocul Pharmacol Ther*. 2017;33:263–277.

3. Regatieri CV, Alwassia A, Zhang JY, et al. Use of optical coherence tomography in the diagnosis and management of uveitis. *Int Ophthalmol Clin.* 2012;52:33–43.
4. Antcliff RJ, Stanford MR, Chauhan DS, et al. Comparison between optical coherence tomography and fundus fluorescein angiography for the detection of cystoid macular edema in patients with uveitis. *Ophthalmology.* 2000;107:593–599.
5. Gupta V, Gupta P, Singh R, et al. Spectral-domain Cirrus high-definition optical coherence tomography is better than time-domain Stratus optical coherence tomography for evaluation of macular pathologic features in uveitis. *Am J Ophthalmol.* 2008;145:1018–1022.
6. Iannetti L, Pesci FR, Spinucci G, et al. Reproducibility of retinal thickness measurements in eyes with uveitic macular oedema using Spectralis optical coherence tomography. *Acta Ophthalmol.* 2012;90:e490–e491.
7. Markomichelakis NN, Halkiadakis I, Pantelia E, et al. Patterns of macular edema in patients with uveitis: qualitative and quantitative assessment using optical coherence tomography. *Ophthalmology.* 2004;111:946–953.
8. Grajewski RS, Boelke AC, Adler W, et al. Spectral-domain optical coherence tomography findings of the macula in 500 consecutive patients with uveitis. *Eye.* 2016;30:1415–1423.
9. Fong AH, Li KK, Wong D. Choroidal evaluation using enhanced depth imaging spectral-domain optical coherence tomography in Vogt-Koyanagi-Harada disease. *Retina.* 2011;31:502–509.
10. Dastiridou AI, Bousquet E, Kuehlwein L, et al. Choroidal imaging with swept-source optical coherence tomography in patients with birdshot chorioretinopathy: choroidal reflectivity and thickness. *Ophthalmology.* 2017;124:1186–1195.
11. Cho HJ, Han SY, Cho SW, et al. Acute retinal pigment epitheliitis: spectral-domain optical coherence tomography findings in 18 cases. *Invest Ophthalmol Vis Sci.* 2014;55(5):3314–3339.
12. Iu LPL, Lee R, Fan MCY, et al. Serial spectral-domain optical coherence tomography findings in acute retinal pigment epitheliitis and the correlation to visual acuity. *Ophthalmology.* 2017;124:903–909.
13. Liu TYA, Ibrahim M, Bittencourt M, et al. Retinal optical coherence tomography manifestations of intraocular lymphoma. *J Ophthalmic Inflamm Infect.* 2012;2:215–218.
14. Sharma S, Lowder CY, Vasanji A, et al. Automated analysis of anterior chamber inflammation by spectral-domain optical coherence tomography. *Ophthlamology.* 2015;122:1464–1470.
15. Klufas MA, Phasukkijwatana N, Iafe NA, et al. Optical coherence tomography angiography reveals choriocapillaris flow reduction in placoid chorioretinitis. *Ophthalmol Retina.* 2016;1:77–91.

7

Evidence-Based Medicine in Uveitis

Scott M. Whitcup

KEY CONCEPTS

- All published literature does not have equal import.
- All medical literature, including this book, must be read critically.
- Whenever possible, treatment decisions should be based on evidence-based medicine. The practice of evidence-based medicine is defined as the conscientious, explicit, and judicious use of current best evidence in making decisions about the care of individual patients.
- The best evidence usually comes from well-conducted, randomized clinical trials, but even the data from these studies should be assessed critically.
- It is important to understand the strength or level of evidence supporting treatment decisions.

The practice of medicine is based on applying what we have learned from our medical training, in addition to the knowledge gained by reading books and articles and attending scientific conferences. It is our hope, for example, that the book you are reading will assist you in the care of patients with uveitis. However, all medical literature, including our book, must be read critically. Much of the information that appears to be irrefutable scientific dogma is actually based on inconclusive data derived from a handful of patients. Because the recommendations are in print and stated by seemingly reputable authorities, they are often followed blindly. It is useful to thoroughly review the original references on which various therapeutic approaches are based; what you find may surprise you.

There is a growing movement to base treatment decisions on evidence-based medicine. The practice of evidence-based medicine is defined as the conscientious, explicit, and judicious use of current best evidence in making decisions about the care of individual patients.[1] Evidence-based medicine has been divided into two types: evidence-based guidelines and evidence-based individual decision making. In each case, the goal is to base therapy on the best evidence available. A number of classifications for the quality of evidence have been proposed. Many of these classifications are derived from a rating system described in a report by the Canadian Task Force on the Periodic Health Examination in 1979.[2] One commonly used stratification was proposed by the U.S. Preventive Services Task Force[3] and is detailed in Table 7.1. An assessment of the quality of the information in the literature is critical in determining the best treatment for our patients.

When treatment recommendations are made in published guidelines or in the literature, they can be graded based on the strength of the data and used to provide suggestions for clinical practice. The U.S. Preventive Services Task Force updated its grade definitions in 2012, and they are listed in Table 7.2.[4]

When you read the medical literature, it is important to determine the experimental methods used in the various studies. Sometimes this information can be discerned from the title of the paper; at other times, the Methods section must be read. Occasionally, the study method is not stated in the paper: if this is the case, the article is probably not worth reading. Many of the clinical studies in the literature are retrospective; that is, the data reported by the study were collected from past patient visits. Retrospective studies can provide valuable information but are usually limited by the quality and thoroughness of patient records. A patient's symptoms and clinical findings, although present, are often not recorded. For example, if there is no comment in a patient's record about vitreous haze, does this mean that vitreous haze was absent or that it was present but not recorded in the note? Fortunately, most ophthalmic notes contain a core of data, including visual acuity, intraocular pressure, and results of anterior segment and retinal examination. Nevertheless, prospective studies are less prone to errors when specific data are collected during patient visits on specifically designed case report forms.

STUDY DESIGN

There are four basic clinical studies: case series, case-control studies, cohort studies, and randomized clinical trials.[5] The case report or case series are probably the weakest methods of deriving clinical data. Case series are usually retrospective reviews that list the clinical findings of patients with a specific disease. Case series can illustrate the variety of clinical manifestations of diseases and provide information about diagnosis, management, and prognosis. However, in addition to the problem of data missing from patient records, the reader should be aware of other pitfalls that may jeopardize the value of the report. First, the disease or condition may not be adequately defined. If patients with sympathetic ophthalmia are inadvertently included in a series of patients with Vogt-Koyanagi-Harada (VKH) syndrome, the findings and conclusions may be altered. Second, the patient population reported may be dissimilar from that in the clinician's practice. Frequently, uveitis specialists see patients with more severe diseases because these are the patients referred to their practice. Therefore a uveitis specialist may report that the visual prognosis for a given disease, such as sarcoidosis, is poor. If this report is based on a series of patients composed of referred patients with end-stage disease, it may be biased. One should be especially wary of retrospective reviews that make global dogmatic statements on the basis of a few patients. Finally, case series do not have a control group for comparison. If a report states that depression was found in 35% of patients with uveitis, it is not clear that this represents a causal relationship. Visual loss, not uveitis, may be the cause of depression. It would be important to know how many patients with other ocular diseases that cause visual loss (a control group) have

TABLE 7.1 U.S. Preventive Services Task Force Classification for the Quality of Scientific Information in the Literature

Level I	Evidence obtained from at least one properly designed randomized controlled trial.
Level II–1	Evidence obtained from well-designed controlled trials without randomization.
Level II–2	Evidence obtained from well-designed cohort or case-control analytic studies, preferably from more than one center or research group.
Level II–3	Evidence obtained from multiple time series with or without the intervention. Dramatic results in uncontrolled trials might also be regarded as this type of evidence.
Level III	Opinions of respected authorities, based on clinical experience, descriptive studies, or reports of expert committees.

TABLE 7.2 U.S. Preventive Services Task Force Classification for Treatment Recommendations

Level A	The USPSTF recommends the service. There is high certainty that the net benefit is substantial.
Level B	The USPSTF recommends the service. There is high certainty that the net benefit is moderate or there is moderate certainty that the net benefit is moderate to substantial.
Level C	The USPSTF recommends selectively offering or providing this service to individual patients based on professional judgment and patient preferences. There is at least moderate certainty that the net benefit is small.
Level D	The USPSTF recommends against the service. There is moderate or high certainty that the service has no net benefit or that the harms outweigh the benefits.
Level I	The USPSTF concludes that the current evidence is insufficient to assess the balance of benefits and harms of the service. Evidence is lacking, of poor quality, or conflicting, and the balance of benefits and harms cannot be determined.

depression. For example, the same percentage of patients with visual loss from retinal degenerations may also be depressed.

The case-control study is a second type of clinical study in which the investigator compares a group of patients with a given condition with a control group without the condition. The records of both groups are then compared to see whether certain factors were more likely to occur in one group than in the other. The classic example of a case-control study would be a study examining patients with lung cancer and a group without the disease and determining their smoking history. It is then possible to compute an odds ratio that determines the relative risk for a given condition, such as lung cancer, given a specific factor, such as smoking. Case-control studies, albeit more powerful than case series, are prone to bias, many relying on a retrospective review of patients' records to determine the differences between cases and controls in a number of clinical parameters. Additional bias arises from the method of choosing the case and the control subjects. Despite the potential bias, case-control studies are more commonly reported in the literature because they are easy to carry out, especially with computerization of clinical records. In addition, they are often the only feasible method available to study rare disorders.

A cohort study identifies two groups or "cohorts" of patients, for example, one cohort that receives a certain treatment and one cohort that does not. The groups are then followed up prospectively for the development of a specific outcome. However, because the treatments are not assigned randomly, it is possible that the two groups differ in important parameters. For example, if you followed up two groups of patients with glaucoma, one treated with medications and one treated surgically, you may falsely conclude that surgical therapy is inferior for treating glaucoma because these patients had a worse visual outcome. However, it may be that the patients treated medically had milder disease and better initial visual acuity compared with patients who received surgical therapy.

Pharmaceutical drug development includes a number of clinical studies, but the final determination of safety and efficacy is based predominantly on pivotal randomized controlled trials (RCTs). Clinical studies during the development of a new medication are divided into four phases. Phase I clinical trials are the initial safety trials of a new medicine and are usually conducted in normal volunteers. The trials can be open-label ones, for which patients and investigators are unmasked to the treatment allocation. Multiple doses may be tested in a phase I trial, often starting with the lowest dosage and escalating to higher dosages, if tolerated. Phase II trials are designed to study the safety and efficacy of a new medication. These trials are often double-masked, in which neither patients nor investigators know what treatment is being administered. Classically, these are called *double-blind studies;* however, in ophthalmology, we prefer the term *double-masked* because it is difficult to get a patient with an eye disease to enroll in a study with "double-blind" in the title. Phase II trials typically have more patients compared with phase I trials and are conducted in patients with the disease but still may examine several dosages or treatment regimens. The phase III clinical trial is the pivotal clinical trial for the approval of the medication. These are almost always larger RCTs comparing the new medication to the standard treatment or to placebo. The U.S. Food and Drug Administration (FDA) almost always requires two phase III trials with corroborative findings before approving a new drug. Studies conducted after a medicine is approved and marketed are called phase IV trials. These are conducted in patient populations for which the medicine is intended and may compare the medicine to other currently available therapies.

The RCT provides the most powerful evidence about the value of a new therapy or a diagnostic approach.[6] Because patients enrolled in the study are randomly assigned to specific groups, if there are sufficient numbers of patients, the groups are usually equivalent clinically. From an ethical standpoint, RCTs should compare treatments when the investigator is not sure which therapy is better. The situation where both treatment approaches have equivalent merits is termed *clinical equipoise.*[7,8]

Even RCTs need to be designed appropriately and well conducted to ensure meaningful results. Key issues in the design and conduct of RCTs are listed in Box 7.1. The investigators should have performed previous studies in the area and include researchers with appropriate training in the conduct and analysis of the study. The primary outcome of the study should be clearly stated, even if multiple outcomes are examined. The procedure for enrolling patients should be clearly delineated, including the inclusion and exclusion criteria. In addition, the therapy to be employed should be clearly stated, and the control group should be clinically appropriate. For example, if one were designing a trial to study the efficacy and safety of a new medication for newly diagnosed glaucoma, it would be inappropriate to use pilocarpine as the medication for the control group because this drug is rarely used as initial therapy for this disease.

It is extremely important that the report include a discussion of sample size calculation. Sample size is based not only on the event rate

BOX 7.1 Components of a Randomized Clinical Trial

- Study approved by Institutional Review Board (IRB) and appropriate informed consent obtained from patients
- Disease well defined with specific diagnostic criteria
- Patient population well defined with specific inclusion and exclusion criteria
- Patients randomly assigned to new treatment and control treatment according to standardized and documented procedures
- Patients and investigators appropriately masked from treatment assignment
- Sample size accurately determined to control for type I and type II errors
- Outcome measures specified and details of minimum differences to be considered as clinically important provided
- Procedures for the conduct of the trial described in detail
- Timing of study visits and collection of data strictly specified and monitored
- Statistical analysis plan specified before locking of the database and unmasking of treatment assignments
- Results of an intent to treat analysis, in which all randomly assigned patients are included in the analysis provided, even if additional analyses performed

expected in the two groups but also on the level of protection against type I and type II errors. A type I error occurs when the study falsely concludes that the therapies tested are different when, in fact, they are the same. A type II error occurs when the study falsely concludes that there is no difference between the therapies when, in fact, a difference exists. Many RCTs reported in the literature are underpowered. This means that the potential for a type II error is high: sometimes 30% or higher. In these studies, a conclusion that there was no statistically significant difference between the two study groups is meaningless: There could, in fact, be a big difference between the two groups, but not enough patients were tested to show that difference. Here is an example of an underpowered study. If we wanted to test the hypothesis that the two sides of a quarter are different, we could flip the coin a number of times and record the results. If we flipped the coin three times (similar to enrolling three patients) and got heads each time, we might falsely conclude that the two sides were the same: that both sides had heads. The chance that we would reach this wrong conclusion would, however, diminish if we increased the number of times we flipped the coin! We would then have more power to show a difference between the two sides of the coin and thus have more protection against a type II error. Remember that studies can never definitively prove that two treatments are the same. No matter how many times we flip a coin and only see heads, there is still some chance that there was a tail on the other side that did not come up. Nevertheless, if we flip the coin enough times, or enroll enough patients in a trial, the chance of this type II error becomes increasingly unlikely.

In RCTs, data should be appropriately collected, and patients should have a reasonably high level of adherence to protocol procedures, with few missed data or loss of patients to follow-up. Observers should be masked to the treatments that patients receive. Statistical methods should be appropriate for the data and the tables and figures easy to read. Finally, it is important that the authors' conclusions are supported by the data and do not go beyond the evidence. There are many examples in the literature where results in a narrowly defined patient population are inappropriately generalized to broader patient groups.

The reader should also be cautious in assessing subset analyses or secondary analyses from RCTs. In most instances, these analyses should be used for hypothesis generation, and not to prove a hypothesis. If the analyses were prespecified in the original study protocol and statistical plan, the data may have greater validity; however, caution in interpretation of results is still warranted. Meta-analyses, where a number of studies meeting specific study criteria are analyzed together, can be useful in assessing diagnosis and therapy. The Cochrane Database of Systematic Reviews has been a useful resource for these types of reviews. One of the earliest uses of the Cochrane Controlled Trials Register assessing treatment of uveitis reviewed pharmacotherapy for Behçet syndrome.[9]

UVEITIS CLINICAL TRIALS

Unfortunately, much of the uveitis literature is composed of case series and case reports. As stated earlier, these studies can provide useful information but are highly prone to bias and lack a control population for comparison of the findings. Despite their superior strength as a clinical design, few case-control studies or cohort studies of patients with uveitis have been conducted. Even rarer are RCTs of therapies for patients with uveitis.[10] Historically, most of the published RCTs in uveitis focus on postoperative inflammation. Relatively few RCTs have studied therapies for other forms of uveitis. Part of the explanation is the difficulties that arise when patients with this disorder are studied. Many forms of uveitis are rare; therefore it is difficult to recruit enough patients to fulfill the sample size requirements. It is important that the observers are masked to the therapy, which may be difficult if surgical treatment is compared with medications. Patients with uveitis often have underlying systemic diseases that make it difficult for them to follow a predetermined therapeutic protocol because their other diseases often require systemic therapy.

Nevertheless, RCTs can be conducted in patients with uveitis. In these trials, it is important to collect data in a standardized fashion. We record visual acuity according to a standard protocol by using the Early Treatment Diabetic Retinopathy Study (ETDRS) charts.[11] Inflammatory activity is similarly recorded with standardized methods, such as grading scales for vitreous haze or laser interferometry for anterior chamber haze.[12] Well-conducted RCTs are not only important in illustrating the safety and efficacy of new treatments but also in better defining the natural history of the disease. We will undoubtedly learn more about the underlying natural history of inflammatory eye disease through analysis of data from RCTs.

Many large RCTs are conducted as part of the drug approval process. Unfortunately, relatively few medications have been developed specifically for the treatment of intermediate and posterior uveitis, and as a result, most of the therapies administered in clinical practice were off-label ones. More recently, there has been an interest in obtaining regulatory approval of medications for noninfectious intermediate and posterior uveitis, and this has led to the performance of larger RCTs as part of the approval process. Sustained-release fluocinolone acetonide intravitreal implants were shown to significantly reduce uveitis recurrences in patients with noninfectious posterior uveitis.[13] A biodegradable, dexamethasone intravitreal implant was shown to improve intraocular inflammation and visual acuity in patients with noninfectious intermediate or posterior uveitis.[14] Subcutaneous injections of adalimumab was associated with a lower risk of uveitis flare or visual impairment in patients with active noninfectious intermediate, posterior, or panuveitis.[15]

The National Eye Institute (NEI) conducted several small RCTs in patients with uveitis. In one study, cyclosporin was compared with prednisolone for the treatment of endogenous uveitis.[16] In this trial, 28 patients were randomly assigned to treatment with cyclosporin, and 28 were randomly assigned to treatment with prednisolone. Although no statistically significant difference was found between the primary outcomes of visual acuity or vitreous haze in patients in the two groups, because of the small numbers, it would be wrong to conclude that the two therapies were the

BOX 7.2 Examples of National Institutes of Health–Funded Randomized Controlled Trials on Inflammatory Eye Diseases

1. Argon laser photocoagulation for ocular histoplasmosis. Results of a randomized clinical trial. *Arch Ophthalmol.* 1983;101:1347–1357.
2. Endophthalmitis Vitrectomy Study Group. Results of the Endophthalmitis Vitrectomy Study. A randomized trial of immediate vitrectomy and of intravenous antibiotics for the treatment of postoperative bacterial endophthalmitis. *Arch Ophthalmol.* 1995;113:1479–1496.
3. Wilhelmus KR, Gee L, Jauck WW, et al. for the Herpetic Eye Disease Study Group. Herpetic Eye Disease Study (HEDS). A controlled trial of topical corticosteroids for herpes simplex stromal keratitis. *Ophthalmology.* 1994;101:1883–1896.
4. Herpetic Eye Disease Study Group. A controlled trial of oral acyclovir for iridocyclitis caused by herpes simplex virus. *Arch Ophthalmol.* 1996;114:1065–1072.
5. Nussenblatt RB, Gery I, Weiner HL, et al. Treatment of uveitis by oral administration of retinal antigens. Results of phase I/II randomized masked trial. *Am J Ophthalmol.* 1997;123:583–592.
6. Nussenblatt RB, Palestine AG, Chan CC, et al. Randomized, double-masked study of ciclosporin compared to prednisolone in the treatment of endogenous uveitis. *Am J Ophthalmol.* 1991;112:138–146.
7. Whitcup SM, Csaky KG, Podgor MJ, et al. A randomized, masked, cross-over trial of acetazolamide for cystoid macular edema in patients with uveitis. *Ophthalmology.* 1996;103:1054–1063.
8. Beck RW, Cleary PA, Anderson MM Jr., et al. for the Optic Neuritis Study Group. A randomized, controlled trial of corticosteroids in the treatment of acute optic neuritis. *N Engl J Med.* 1992;326:581–588.
9. Buggage RR, Levy-Clarke G, Sen HN, et al. A double-masked, randomized study to investigate the safety and efficacy of daclizumab to treat the ocular complications related to Behçet's disease. *Ocul Immunol Inflamm.* 2007;15:63–70.
10. Smith JA, Thompson DJ, Whitcup SM, et al. A randomized, placebo-controlled, double-masked clinical trial of etanercept for the treatment of uveitis associated with juvenile idiopathic arthritis. *Arthritis Rheum.* 2005;53:18–23.
11. Multicenter Uveitis Steroid Treatment (MUST) Trial Research Group, Kempen JH, Altaweel MM, Holbrook JT, et al. Randomized comparison of systemic anti-inflammatory therapy versus fluocinolone acetonide implant for intermediate, posterior, and panuveitis: the multicenter uveitis steroid treatment trial. *Ophthalmology.* 2011;118:1916–1926.

same. The authors were careful not to state that the study proved that the two therapies were equivalent and, instead, suggested that because similar outcomes were achieved, cyclosporin could be considered an alternative to corticosteroid therapy. The RCT is often the best source of useful clinical information; therefore some of the RCTs on uveitis or other inflammatory eye diseases sponsored by the National Institutes of Health are listed in Box 7.2. Many important RCTs have also been conducted on the ocular complications of acquired immunodeficiency syndrome (AIDS), and these trials are described in Chapter 12.

More recently, the NEI sponsored a multicenter uveitis steroid treatment (MUST) trial.[17] The purpose of the trial was to compare the relative effectiveness of systemic therapy consisting of corticosteroids plus immunosuppression, when indicated, versus the fluocinolone acetonide implant for noninfectious intermediate, posterior, or panuveitis. The primary endpoint of the study was change in best-corrected visual acuity from baseline, and 255 patients were randomized in the trial. At 24 months, improvement in visual acuity was not statistically significantly different between treatment groups: +6.0 letters with implant therapy and +3.2 letters with the steroid implant. Implant therapy was associated with a statistically significantly greater improvement in vision-related quality of life and less residual active uveitis. Implant-assigned eyes had a higher risk of cataract surgery and treatment for elevated intraocular pressure and glaucoma. Patients assigned to systemic therapy had more prescription-requiring infections but without noted long-term health consequences.

Finally, clinically important information can also be obtained from large epidemiologic studies of patients with uveitis. For example, the association between cigarette smoking and uveitis was examined in a retrospective, population-based, case control study.[18] Smoking in 100 confirmed incident uveitis cases was compared with 522 randomly selected controls from the general Kaiser Hawaii population and 528 randomly selected controls from the Kaiser Hawaii Ophthalmology Clinic. Current smokers had 1.63 and 2.33 times greater odds of developing uveitis compared with those who never smoked, using the general and ophthalmology control groups, respectively. This association could not be easily obtained with an RCT because it would be unethical to randomize nonsmokers to a smoking group and because the length of time for uveitis to develop would make this study design unfeasible.

REFERENCES

1. Sackett DL, Rosenberg WM, Gray JA, et al. Evidence based medicine: what it is and what it isn't. *Br Med J.* 1996;312:71–72.
2. The periodic health examination. Canadian Task Force on the Periodic Health Examination. *Can Med Assoc J.* 1979 Nov 3;121(9):1193–1254.
3. Guide to clinical preventative services: *Report of the U.S. Preventive Services Task Force.* DIANE Publishing; 1989:24.
4. https://epss.ahrq.gov/ePSS/gradedef.jsp#after2012.
5. Sackett DL, Haynes RB, Tugwell P. *Clinical Epidemiology: A Basic Science for Clinical Medicine.* Boston, MA: Little, Brown; 1985:224–229.
6. Meinert CL, Tonascia S. *Clinical Trials Design, Conduct, and Analysis.* New York: Oxford University Press; 1986:274–275.
7. Freedman B. Equipoise and the ethics of clinical research. *N Engl J Med.* 1987;317:141–145.
8. Johnson N, Lilford RJ, Brazier W. At what level of collective equipoise does a clinical trial become ethical? *J Med Ethics.* 1991;17:30–34.
9. Saenz A, Ausejo M, Shea M, et al. Pharmacotherapy for Behçet's syndrome. *Cochrane Database Syst Rev.* 2000;2:CD001084.
10. Okada AA. Noninfectious uveitis: a scarcity of randomized clinical trials. *Arch Ophthalmol.* 2005;123:682–683.
11. Ferris FL III, Kassoff A, Bresnick GH, et al. New visual acuity charts for clinical research. *Am J Ophthalmol.* 1982;94:91–96.
12. Nussenblatt RB, Palestine AG, Chan CC, et al. Standardization of vitreal inflammatory activity in intermediate and posterior uveitis. *Ophthalmology.* 1985;92:467–471.
13. Jaffe GJ, Martin D, Callanan D, et al. Fluocinolone Acetonide Uveitis Study Group. Fluocinolone acetonide implant (Retisert) for noninfectious posterior uveitis: thirty-four-week results of a multicenter randomized clinical study. *Ophthalmology.* 2006;113:1020–1027.
14. Lowder C, Belfort R Jr, Lightman S, et al. Dexamethasone intravitreal implant for non-infectious intermediate or posterior uveitis. *Arch Ophthlamol.* 2011;129:545–553.
15. Jaffe GJ, Dick AD, Brezin AP, et al. Adalimumab in patients with active non-infectious uveitis. *N Engl J Med.* 2016;375:932–943.
16. Nussenblatt RB, Palestine AG, Chan CC, et al. Randomized, double-masked study of cyclosporine compared to prednisolone in the treatment of endogenous uveitis. *Am J Ophthalmol.* 1991;112:138–146.
17. Multicenter Uveitis Steroid Treatment (MUST) Trial Research Group, Kempen JH, Altaweel MM, Holbrook JT, et al. Randomized comparison of systemic anti-inflammatory therapy versus fluocinolone acetonide implant for intermediate, posterior, and panuveitis: the Multicenter Uveitis Steroid Treatment Trial. *Ophthalmology.* 2011;118:1916–1926.
18. Yuen BG, Tham VM, Browne EN, et al. Association between smoking and uveitis. Results from the Pacific Ocular Inflammation Study. *Ophthalmology.* 2015;122:1257–1261.

8

Approaches to Medical Therapy

H. Nida Sen

KEY CONCEPTS

- Therapy is guided by the etiology of the inflammation (infectious versus noninfectious), severity, and anatomic location.
- Corticosteroid therapy can be used to quiet acute inflammation, but steroid-sparing therapies must be added if systemic corticosteroids cannot be tapered successfully by 3 months.
- It is important to establish goals of therapy and consider further workup or altering therapy if goals of therapy are not achieved.
- Patients should be counseled about the goals and side effects of and expectation from immunomodulatory therapy and the need for regular monitoring for potential side effects.

Choosing the best therapy is difficult and should be guided not only by etiology, laterality, associated systemic disease, anatomic location, and disease severity, but also the patient's general health, concomitant medical problems, current medications, and personal preferences. The decision as to which medications to use, whether it should be local treatment options (e.g., injections or implants) or systemic immunomodulatory agents, is a responsibility shared between the physician and the patient. It is truly a partnership. The more informed the patient is about the goals and potential side effects of treatment, the more likely it is that the individual will be compliant. It is fair to say that enormous advances have occurred in our understanding of how to use many of the drugs under discussion. There has been a shift to the use of intraocular therapy and also to more specific therapies, such as the use of monoclonal antibodies that target specific parts of the immune cascade. Translational studies and animal models have helped improve our understanding of the underlying mechanisms, which has led to a more rational decision-making process.[1] Furthermore, pharmacology is a burgeoning area, with real hope for the future; indeed, other, yet untapped, sources may also provide new immunosuppressive drugs to the growing armamentarium.[2] At present, there may not be any one ideal drug, but treating physicians have some latitude in their choices. However, each of the agents discussed in this chapter is a powerful medication, which must be evaluated with care and expertise.

GOALS AND PHILOSOPHY

In the treatment of uveitis, the decision to intervene by using any therapeutic agent should be based on both a thorough clinical evaluation and philosophic guidelines. In general, the approach to therapy should take into account at least the considerations discussed in the following sections.

Pain, Photophobia, and Discomfort

Symptom relief is an important goal for several reasons. The first and foremost is, of course, the ethical imperative of the physician. However, practical considerations should not be overlooked. Pain relief helps in the establishment of a good patient–physician relationship, which is of primary importance in what is frequently a long therapeutic course with ups and downs. A second practical reason is that once pain relief is obtained, the patient is able to cooperate more readily. The ability to examine the patient's ocular condition in greater detail and to obtain more reliable test results, particularly visual acuity, is of immeasurable help to the physician.

Degree and Location of Inflammatory Disease

The type and frequency of administration of any therapeutic choice depend on the physician's evaluation of how "serious" the inflammatory disease is and what ocular structures are being affected. For instance, if the sequela of an intraocular inflammation is limited to the posterior synechiae, then the use of topical mydriatics and corticosteroids may be a reasonable approach to therapy. However, disease that is more posteriorly located would need to be approached by means of quite different strategies. If alternative therapies are available, the physician needs to decide which one to start with. In addition, if vital structures, such as the macula, are involved, more aggressive immunosuppressive therapy may need to be used, even though the potential for side effects may be greater.

Evaluation of Visual Acuity and Prospect of Reversibility

In most cases of inflammatory disease involving the posterior segment, decreased visual acuity is the reason for therapeutic intervention. It is also the major reason that the patient consults the physician, in the hope that therapy will improve vision. It is therefore imperative that the physician attempt to define as clearly as possible why the vision has decreased. On this decision will hinge the therapeutic approach. Patients frequently have multifactorial reasons for vision changes; common causes are macular edema and cataract. The use of various tests in the clinic can aid in this evaluation.

Before embarking on any therapy that has a significant risk for the patient, the physician must weigh this inherent risk against any benefits. It is therefore necessary to decide whether any or all of the visual alterations are caused by irreversible changes. It is difficult to justify starting therapy if no reasonable hope for visual improvement exists. The decision to start therapy is always based on the physician's belief that the side effects of the therapeutic intervention are outweighed by the potential benefit. It is the physician's duty to desist from inappropriate therapy as much as it is to institute beneficial treatment.

Follow-Up Procedures and Standardization of Observations

It is imperative that a reasonable time be allotted to evaluate whether a specific therapy is effective. For most medications, up to 3 months is a reasonable period in which to evaluate whether an acute problem will improve. One should remember that ocular changes caused by uveitis may resolve slowly, and the observer must use changes sometimes subtle in the ocular examination to determine whether to continue therapy. The patient should adhere to a regular follow-up schedule and should know who to contact if an emergency arises. Depending on the severity of disease, initially frequent—as frequent as weekly—visits may be needed both to ensure improvement and to evaluate potential side effects from therapy. The physician needs to preset the definition of a therapeutic "success" and adhere to these criteria. Just as it is unwise to stop or alter therapy too soon, it is not reasonable to continue therapy if the minimal criteria for success are not met. Such criteria may include symptoms and/or findings, such as an increase in vision, a decrease in the amount of vitreous haze, a decrease in the number of cells in the anterior chamber, or a decrease in the photophobia the patient is experiencing.

With regard to the criteria that determine successful treatment, there is a presupposition that tests are performed in a standard manner and that test results reflect a change in the ocular status rather than the variability inherent in the test. Standardization of observations is critical to the successful evaluation of the condition in these patients.

Disease Laterality

In patients with unilateral uveitis and no underlying systemic disease, use of local therapy is preferred over systemic drugs. In our experience, it is rare that unilateral disease justifies long-term therapy, but it certainly happens. In the patient with sight remaining in only one eye, a judgment as to the use of local therapy before systemic therapy needs to be made.

General Health and Age of Patient

The very basic considerations of patient health and age must play a role in deciding what sort of therapy to use. We thoroughly evaluate all patients and examine all therapeutic alternatives before starting systemic therapy, especially in children. The secondary effects of systemic immunosuppressive agents, such as steroids, can have a major and lifelong effect on a growing child. A diagnosis of diabetes may be a relative contraindication for systemic corticosteroid therapy, whereas uncontrolled hypertension or renal disease may make cyclosporin a poor therapeutic choice. The physician must be always aware that most of these therapies can have significant systemic and local effects.

Patient Reliability, Preferences, and Understanding

Sufficient time should be spent with the patient, who deserves an explanation of ocular (and systemic) findings, the seriousness of these findings, the type of therapy warranted, and the possible positive and adverse effects. A fully informed patient provides invaluable aid to the treating physician. Obtaining informed written consent may be a requirement under certain circumstances, such as with experimental therapies. Patients with uveitis usually require long-term care, and the more the patient understands the medical concerns, uncertainties, and possible therapeutic alternatives early on, the easier is the treating physician's task.

NONSURGICAL THERAPEUTIC OPTIONS

Corticosteroids

The corticosteroid family of medications has been the mainstay of therapy for ocular inflammatory disease since its introduction by Gordon in the early 1950s.[3] Its use in ophthalmology began soon after its introduction into the medical armamentarium.[4] The synthetic compounds usually used by the physician are variations of the compounds normally found in the body, and they profoundly affect many aspects of the organism's physiology. The synthetic preparations available to the physician were developed because of their particularly effective mediation of one aspect of these hormones' effects: immunosuppression. The treating physician should be totally at ease with the various therapeutic strategies available.

Mode of action. In humans, corticosteroids are not considered to be cytotoxic agents. Human immune cells are not susceptible to lysis by corticosteroid administration, even at the higher dosages usually employed, unlike some of the other agents covered in this chapter. Mice, rats, and rabbits are considered to be corticosteroid-sensitive animals, with their lymphocytes showing a marked tendency toward lysis after the administration of corticosteroids. Therefore extrapolation from animal experiments must take place only after careful evaluation.

The mechanism of entry into the cell by steroids has been evaluated by means of several systems. The underlying point for the action of all the steroid hormones is a need for cellular receptors. The steroid is met at the cell surface by the appropriate receptor and then complexes with it in the cytoplasm of the cell. This complex then migrates to the nucleus, where it exerts its effect on deoxyribonucleic acid (DNA) transcription, leading to changes in ribonucleic acid (RNA) production. These RNA alterations result in changes in protein production and cell function. In steroid-sensitive animals, such as rats, cells with steroid receptors will be lysed. However, this is not the case in humans.

The effects of steroids on the immune system are both local and systemic. Essentially, all cellular components are affected. On the systemic level, a profound change is seen particularly with neutrophils and lymphocytes (Fig. 8.1). Clamen[5] and Fauci[6] showed that a large number of the lymphocytes in the intravascular space continuously recirculate with the extravascular lymphocyte pool in organs, such as bone marrow, the spleen, and lymph nodes. The addition of steroids induces a change in the recirculation pattern, with a large number of T cells, particularly the helper T (Th cells) subset, sequestered out of the intravascular circulation. This phenomenon results in a break in the recruitment of immunoreactive cells to the site of the inflammatory reaction. The effect on neutrophils appears to be quite striking as well. Steroid therapy induces a larger number of neutrophils to be produced by bone marrow. In addition to this increased production, the circulating half-life of these cells on reaching the intravascular space is prolonged. Concomitant with these effects is an impeding of neutrophil migration from this space to the site of inflammation. Decreases in the number of circulating monocytes, eosinophils, and basophils have also been observed.

Glucocorticoids	
Antiinflammatory effects	
Neutrophils	Inhibit neutrophil migration ↓ Neutrophil adherence to vascular endothelium ↓ Bactericidal activity of neutrophils
Immunosuppressive effects	
Mononuclear phagocytes	↓ Chemotaxis ↓ Clearance of antibody coated particles ↓ Production of Il-1 and TNFα
Lymphocytes	Redistribution of T lymphocytes (CD4.CD8) Inhibit T lymphocyte activation → ↓ proliferation and lymphokine production Inhibit Ig production by B cells (high dose)

Fig. 8.1 Anti-inflammatory effects of corticosteroids.

Although the changes in the immune system are profound, it is important to remember that they are temporary. Fauci[7] demonstrated that T-cell subsets return to essentially the presteroid ingestion state after about 24 hours. This observation is most important in developing a strategy for the treatment of an acutely active inflammatory condition, whether in the eye or elsewhere.

Profound effects on cell function have been noted with the addition of a steroid. The effects on the various immune cell populations include a decrease in bactericidal activity, delayed hypersensitivity reactions, lymphokine production, and changes in immediate hypersensitivity reactions. In addition, steroid administration has a profound effect on local resident cells in an organ, particularly the vascular endothelium. A reduction in the leakage of fluid during an inflammatory episode from the capillary endothelium results from steroid administration, thereby reducing tissue swelling. Furthermore, during an inflammatory response, there is a decrease in the amount of intracellular fluid taken in by cells, thereby reducing cell swelling and avoiding the resultant decrease in function and ultimate lysis. The effect of steroids on lysosome membranes, thought at one time to be an important stabilizing factor, now remains unclear.

Preparations, dosage schedules, and complications. Many steroid preparations are available and they have varying potencies. Therefore the dosages to be used are different for each (Table 8.1 and Fig. 8.2).

Topical application of corticosteroids is an excellent way to treat certain uveitides. Prednisolone acetate formulations have been commonly used for anterior uveitis. Although studies do show differences in corneal penetration between phosphate and acetate preparations of steroids, it is not clear whether there is any difference in clinical efficacy between the two preparations in treating active inflammation. When the diagnosis is made, it is imperative that initial treatment of uveitis be aggressive. In severe cases, hourly administration (while the patient is awake) and even beginning therapy with administration of a drop every 15 minutes for the first hour, as a "loading dose," could be considered. Once a dosing schedule has been found to be effective, as evidenced by a reduction in the flare and cells in the eye, we then see the patient often (every 2–3 days to once a week) and begin a very slow tapering of the drops. The schedule for tapering is unique to each patient, but persons who have had numerous attacks may need to continue one or two drops a day for weeks or even months.

The newer topical corticosteroid preparation 0.05% difluprednate (Durezol) is indicated for the treatment of inflammation and pain associated with ocular surgery and the treatment of endogenous anterior uveitis. It is considered twice as potent as prednisolone acetate 1% ophthalmic suspension and is started typically at a dosage of four times a day and tapered based on clinical response. Durezol was found to be as effective as 1% prednisolone acetate ophthalmic suspension in treating subjects with endogenous anterior uveitis in two randomized, double-masked active controlled trials, in which patients were treated with either Durezol four times daily or 1% prednisolone acetate ophthalmic suspension eight times daily for 14 days. The mean intraocular pressure (IOP) values in both groups remained less than 21 mm Hg throughout the study. A high rate of steroid-induced IOP elevation and cataract formation has been observed in pediatric uveitis cases[8,9]

A second option is to inject the corticosteroids periocularly. This method, which permits a relatively high concentration of the drug to be given rapidly, is an effective way to treat particularly severe inflammatory conditions. There is the general choice between long-acting preparations (in a depot vehicle) and shorter-acting soluble preparations. These injections can be given as frequently as every 1 to 2 weeks for short periods. In addition to treatment of severe anterior segment inflammation in general, this is a useful approach for unilateral disease, for perioperative management of a uveitic eye, and for patients in whom the systemic steroids are contraindicated. It is an effective way to treat both active inflammation and cystoid macular edema (CME), even in children, although the procedure may require general anesthesia in young children.

Several approaches to periocular injections have been suggested, and it probably is best to use the approach that one feels the most comfortable with. The approach from the superotemporal aspect of

TABLE 8.1 Relative Potencies of Corticosteroids

Preparation	Systemic Equivalent (mg)	Anti-inflammatory Potency
Hydrocortisone	20	1.0
Cortisone	25	0.8
Prednisolone	5	4.0
Prednisone	5	4.0
Dexamethasone	0.75	26
Methylprednisolone	4	5
Triamcinolone	4	5
Betamethasone	0.6	33

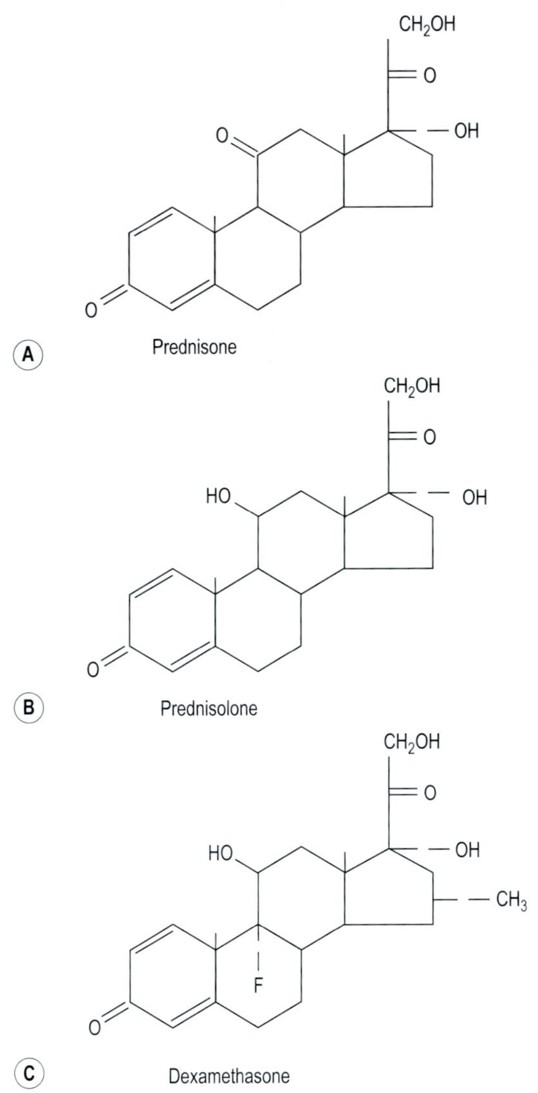

Fig. 8.2 Structures of more commonly used corticosteroids.

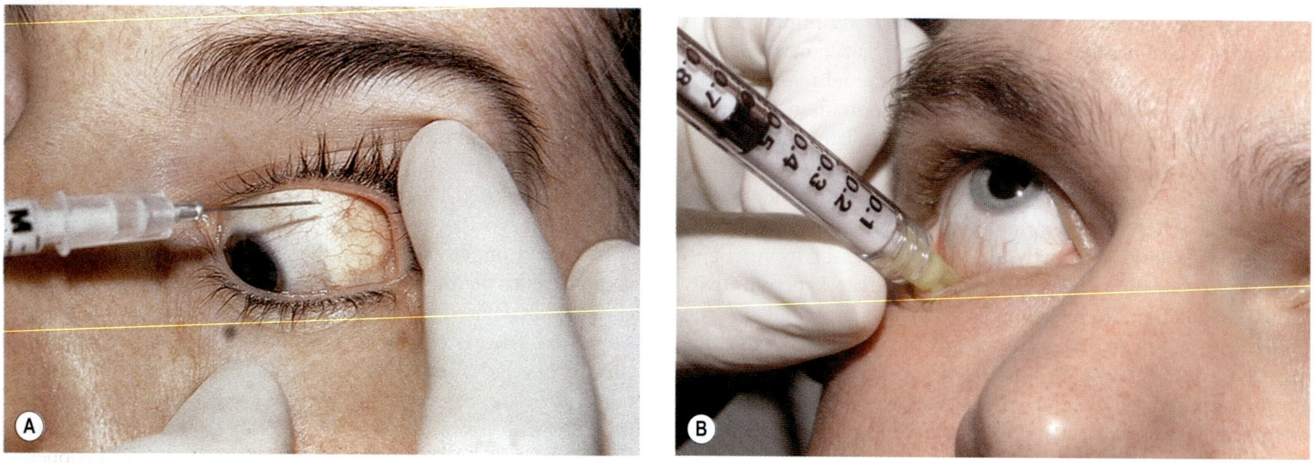

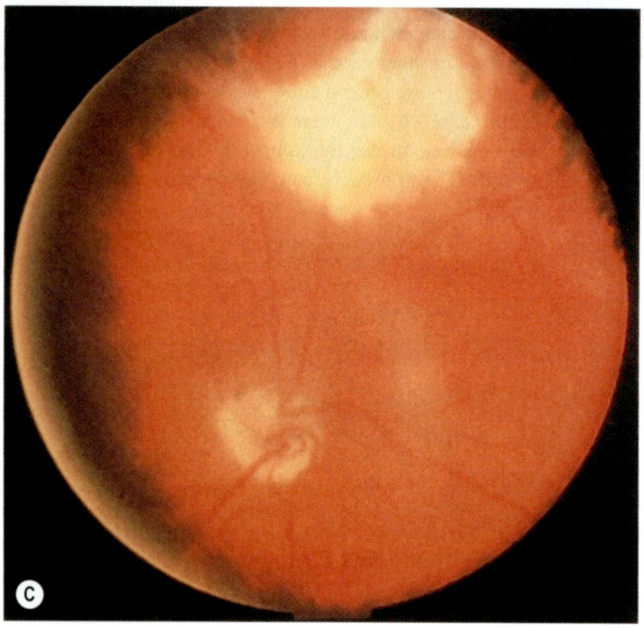

Fig. 8.3 (A) Temporal approach to giving periocular injection. (B) Inferior fornix approach. (Courtesy Dr. Roxana Ursea.) (C) Although the possibility is markedly reduced if precautions are taken, perforation of the globe can occur, as seen here.

the globe, as described by Schlaegel,[10] is thought to reduce the possibility of penetration of the globe and to place the medication under the Tenon capsule and in the region of the macula. Freeman et al.[11] demonstrated that the temporal approach is efficient for injecting the steroid close to the macula. Topical anesthetics are liberally used, and the area in which the injection is to be given (e.g., superotemporal aspect of the globe) is further anesthetized with a cotton swab soaked in topical anesthetic (either 4% lidocaine or cocaine). Triamcinolone 40 mg in 1 mL injectable suspension is the preferred depot steroid formulation (preservative-free formulation used for intraocular injection). An alternative approach is to inject the steroid preparation directly through the lower lid or the inferior fornix (using a 25-gauge needle) while the patient looks upward and is known as the *orbital floor injection*. Periocular injections can be performed in 4- to 12-week intervals, in a series of two to four injections before considering this method ineffective (Fig. 8.3).

Periocular injection of corticosteroids has been shown to be effective in treating active intraocular inflammation and CME. In a large retrospective cohort study of greater than 900 patients, 73% of eyes achieved complete control of inflammation, and 50% showed improvement in vision. Within 12 months, ocular hypertension was seen in 15% to 34%, glaucoma surgery was performed in 2.4%, and cataract surgery was performed in 13.8% of eyes.[12] An additional local approach is the intraocular administration of corticosteroids. To date, this route of administration has been achieved by using several approaches. The most common is direct injection, usually of preservative-free triamcinolone suspension (Triesence) (2–4 mg), into the vitreous fluid. There are newer intravitreal corticosteroid formulations in the form of 0.7 mg dexamethasone intravitreal implant (Ozurdex), 0.18 mg fluocinolone acetonide intravitreal implant (Yutiq), and 0.59 mg fluocinolone intravitreal implant (Retisert); the last is implanted surgically, whereas others are injectable. These sustained release formulations are discussed in more detail below. Surgical or in-office placement of a slow-release fluocinolone acetonide-containing implant into the eye is another option.

Intravitreal steroid injections have been reported to be effective in treating many intraocular problems, including choroidal neovascularization, CME secondary to uveitis, diabetes, central vein occlusion, and pseudophakia (Fig. 8.4).[13-15] In a 40-patient randomized study,[16] which compared orbital floor injection of steroid and intravitreal injections for CME, foveal thickness increased with orbital floor injections; however, it decreased with intravitreal injections, with CME improving in 50% of patients. However, at 6 months, there was no difference in the best corrected vision (BCVA) between the two groups. This perhaps underlines the issue that repeat injections are necessary for a sustained effect.

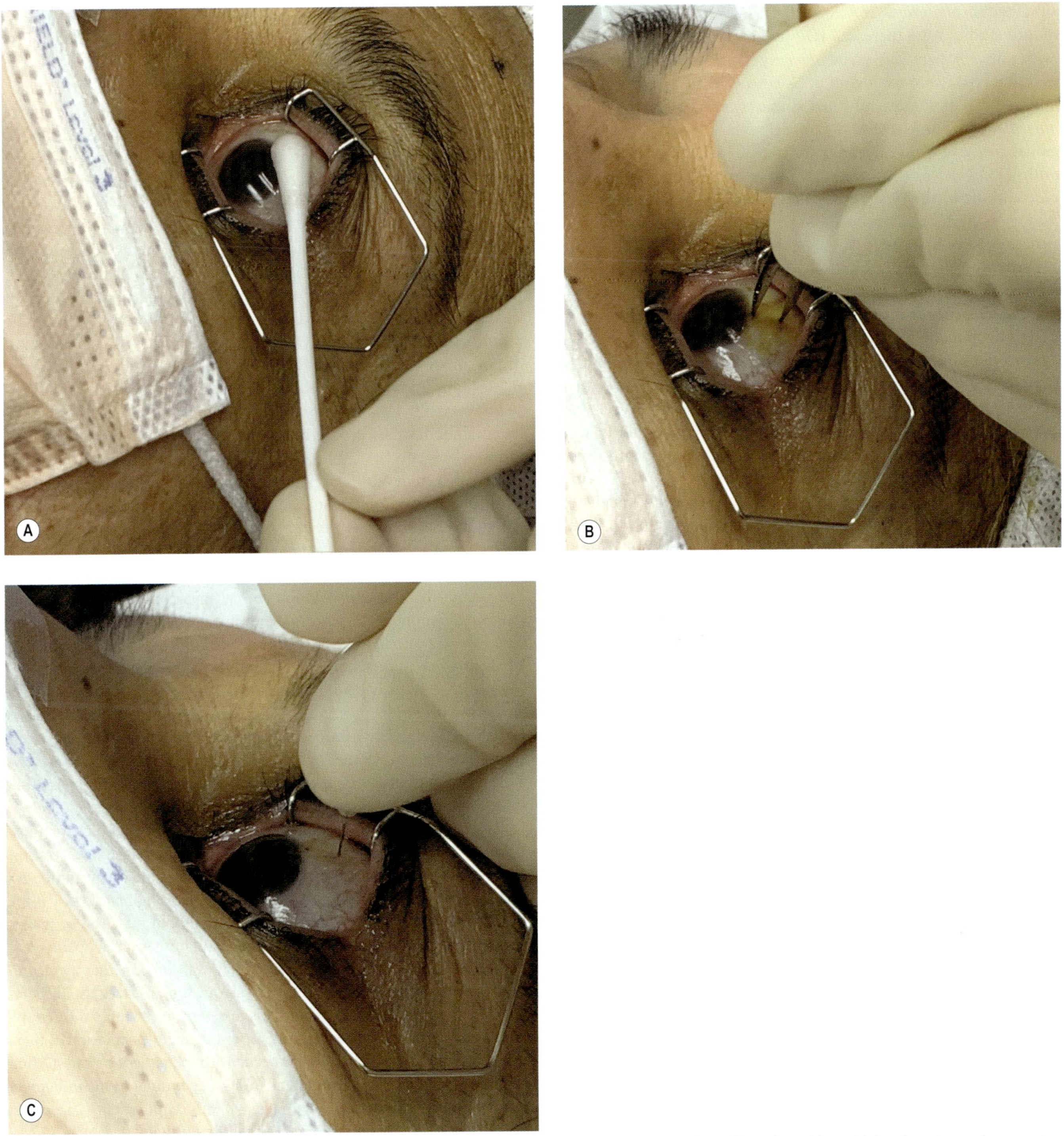

Fig. 8.4 Intravitreal injection in a phakic patient. Following topical anesthesia, betadine application, (A) and marking of injection site at 4 mm using calipers, (B) intravitreal injection is performed at 90 degrees to the sclera aiming the center of the globe (C).

Since 2009 longer-acting slow-release formulations of injectable intravitreal corticosteroids have become available. A 0.7 mg dexamethasone in a solid polymer drug delivery system (Ozurdex) is currently approved by the U.S. Food and Drug Administration (FDA) for treating posterior segment uveitis. The implant is placed in the vitreous fluid by using a 22-gauge applicator, and the biodegradable polymers break down into water (H_2O) and carbon dioxide (CO_2) as dexamethasone is released over a period of approximately 6 months. The efficacy of dexamethasone implant was assessed in a masked randomized study of 153 patients with noninfectious posterior segment uveitis receiving a single injection. By 8 weeks, 47% of patients receiving the implant reached a vitreous haze score of 0 versus 12% of those receiving the sham treatment. There was a significant improvement in central macular thickness in the dexamethasone implant treated eyes compared with sham. The percent of patients achieving a 3-line improvement from baseline vision was 43% for patients receiving implant versus 7% for those receiving the sham treatment. Overall, the response peaked at week 8 and was maintained through week 26.[17] Side effects in initial sham-controlled 6-month studies were increased IOP in 25%, and it peaked at week 8, with only 1% requiring glaucoma surgery, and cataract in 5% of eyes. Cataract rates were higher at 54% to 68% in 2-year observational and 3-year sham-controlled studies (package insert). A randomized controlled trial (RCT) comparing the effectiveness of three regional corticosteroid injections for uveitic macular edema over 6 months (POINT Trial) showed that intravitreal triamcinolone acetonide and the intravitreal dexamethasone implant (Ozurdex) were superior to periocular triamcinolone acetonide. The intravitreal approaches were associated with higher incidence of IOP increase compared with periocular injection.[18] In our group, we prefer periocular injection for mild, injection naive cases and intravitreal steroid injections-triessence or ozurdex-for more severe or recalcitrant cases.

The fluocinolone acetonice 0.18 mg implant (Yutiq) is a sterile nonbioerodible intravitreal implant that releases drug over 36 months; it is preloaded into a single-dose applicator and is designed to release fluocinolone acetonide at an initial rate of 0.25 μg/day. In a 3-year double-masked RCT of patients with chronic recurrent posterior segment uveitis, 6-month and 12-month uveitis recurrence rates were significantly lower with the fluocinolone acetonide insert (28% and 38%) and the sham treatment (91% and 98%), respectively. Incidence of 15-letter decrease or greater in BCVA and adjunctive systemic treatment was reduced by 50% among eyes injected with fluocinolone acetonide. IOP increase and cataract were more common in eyes that received 0.18 mg fluocinolone intravitreal implant (Yutiq) injection; by 12 months 33% versus 5% of eyes receiving fluocinolone acetonide versus the sham injection required cataract surgery.[19] We typically use Yutiq for long term management.

The 0.59 mg fluocinolone acetonide sterile implant (Retisert) is designed to release fluocinolone acetonide between 0.3 and 0.6 μg/day over approximately 30 months and is FDA approved for treating posterior segment uveitis. It is surgically implanted into the posterior segment of the eye through a pars plana incision. 0.59 mg fluocinolone acetonide implant has been evaluated in mainly two multicenter RCTs. In a 3-year, multicenter, randomized, historically controlled trial of the 0.59-mg fluocinolone acetonide intravitreous implant in 110 patients and the 2.1-mg fluocinolone acetonide intravitreous implant in 168 patients, uveitis recurrence was reduced from 62% in the preimplantation period to 4%, 10%, and 20% during the 1-, 2-, and 3-year postimplantation periods for the 0.59-mg implant.[20] An improvement in vision occurred more in implanted eyes than in nonimplanted eyes. As indicated by the results of clinical trials with 0.59 mg fluocinolone acetonide implant, during the 3-year postimplantation period, nearly all phakic eyes are expected to develop cataracts and require cataract surgery. IOP-lowering medications to lower IOP were required in approximately 77% of patients; filtering surgeries were required to control IOP in 37% of patients. The Multicenter Uveitis Steroid Treatment (MUST) trial was a phase IV RCT comparing the fluocinolone acetonide implant and standard systemic therapy in patients with vision-threatening noninfectious intermediate uveitis, posterior uveitis, or panuveitis. The results of the MUST trial at 2 years showed that among the 255 patients (479 eyes with uveitis) randomized to implant or systemic therapy, both the implant and the systemic therapy groups had an improvement in visual acuity (+6.0 and +3.2 letters, respectively), and there was no difference between the treatment groups. However, fluocinolone acetonide implant therapy was associated with faster and more frequent control of inflammation and a greater quantitative improvement in central macular thickness. Long-term results also showed that spontaneous dissociation of the implant occurred in 22 of the 250 implanted eyes between 4.8 and 8.6 years. The cumulative risk of dissociation over 6 years was 4.8%, and the risk of both spontaneous dissociation and surgery-related dissociation increased with longevity of the implants.[21] Therefore it is recommended that the physician periodically monitor the integrity of the implant by visual inspection.

A novel suprachoroidal injection platform that delivers triamcinolone acetonide suspension (CLST-TA) has been shown to be effective in treating uveitic macular edema in a phase 3 randomized clinical trial (PEACCHTREE Trial). Among the 160 patients visual acuity improvement by 15 or more ETDRS letters was seen in 47% of patients that received the suprachoroidal injection versus 16% in the control arm ($P < 0.001$). As of late 2020 an NDA filing for triamcinolone acetonide ophthalmic suspension for Suprachoroidal Injection (Xipere) based on the results of the PEACHTREE trial was accepted by the FDA.[22]

Secondary effects. The topical application of steroid induces an increase in IOP in a significant number of patients. This should be monitored closely. The reactivation of corneal herpes simplex infection can occur with topical steroid therapy.

Regional injection of steroid has secondary effects unique to the procedure as well: (1) Although steroid injections are an effective therapy for childhood uveitis, general anesthesia may be required, with potential inherent side effects. (2) Possible penetration of the globe during periocular (sub-Tenon or orbital floor) injection is a concern.[23] (3) Repeated periocular injections can induce orbital problems, such as proptosis of the globe and fibrosis of the extraocular muscles. (4) Retinal and choroidal vascular occlusions after posterior sub-Tenon injections given to treat CME have been reported.[24] (5) Severe or intractable glaucoma can occur after periocular or intravitreal injections. This can become particularly problematic when a depot injection has been used. In such cases, the depot may need to be removed surgically, and this is sometimes a major undertaking. (6) Reactions to the vehicle in which the steroid injection was placed can also occur; this is, however, less of a concern with newer preservative-free triamcinolone formulations. (7) In patients with scleritis and ocular toxoplasmosis, periocular injections can be problematic. (8) Endophthalmitis is a rare, but potentially severe, complication of intravitreal steroid injections and has been reported in 0.13% of patients receiving intravitreal steroid injections.[25]

Systemic corticosteroids remain the initial drug of choice for most patients with severe bilateral endogenous sight-threatening uveitis. When initiating systemic steroid therapy, one should keep in mind several considerations. It is imperative that the treating physician (to the best of his or her ability) rule out the possibility of infection or malignant disease as a cause of the intraocular inflammation. Uppermost is the clinical impression, based on the ocular examination, that there is an inflammatory response that requires systemic therapy. It is also important for the practitioner to set standards to determine whether the therapy is successful or not. A detailed discussion that includes duration of therapy, goals, and side effects should occur with the patient before starting therapy. The duration of treatment varies, depending on the individual patient and the clinical scenario. Each patient's requirements, capacities, and willingness to undergo treatment are very unique.

We generally find it advisable to begin therapy with prednisone 1 mg/kg/day or 60 mg/day, whichever is lower (Table 8.2). The high doses of corticosteroids should be maintained until a clinical effect is seen or for 4 weeks. If it is determined that the corticosteroids are having a beneficial effect, then a slow reduction of the therapeutic dose needs to be established. As a general tapering schedule, if the dose of prednisone is greater than 40 mg/day, then the daily dose can be reduced by 10 mg/day every 1 to 2 weeks; if the dose is between 20 and 40 mg/day, the dose can be reduced by 5 mg/day every 1 to 2 weeks; if the dose is between 10 and 20 mg/day, the dose can be reduced by 2.5 mg/day every 1 to 2 weeks; and if the dose is less than 10 mg, the dose can be reduced by 1 to 2.5 mg/day every 1 to 2 weeks.[26] As soon as it is clear that long-term (i.e., >3 months) therapy will be needed, addition of a second agent should be considered.

TABLE 8.2 Common Agents Used to Control Intraocular Inflammatory Disease

Agent	Usual Dosage[a]
Prednisone	Oral: 1–2 mg/kg/day
Methylprednisolone	Intravenous pulse: 1 g over 1–2 hours
Intraocular triamcinolone[b]	Intravitreal: 2–4 mg
Periocular triamcinolone	Subtenon or periorbital injection: 20–40 mg
Fluocinolone acetonide intravitreal implant (Retisert)	0.59 mg (sustained release for 30 months; surgical implantation)
Fluocinolone acetonide intravitreal implant (Yutiq)	0.18 mg (sustained release for 36 months; in office injection)
Dexamethasone intravitreal implant (Ozurdex)	0.7 mg (sustained release for 6 months; in office injection)
Antimetabolites	
Methotrexate	Oral: 7.5–25 mg weekly; can be given intramuscularly
Azathioprine	Oral: 50–150 mg daily, 1–1.5 mg/kg/day, but up to 2.5 mg/kg/day
Mycophenolate mofetil	Oral: 1 g twice per day
Alkylating Agents	
Cyclophosphamide	Oral: 50–100 mg daily, up to 2.5 mg/kg body weight/day
	Intravenous pulse: 750 mg/m^2 (adjusted to kidney function and white blood cell count)
Chlorambucil	Oral: 0.1–0.2 mg/kg/day
Calcineurin Inhibitors	
Cyclosporin	Oral: Up to 5 mg/kg/day, usually given with prednisone, 10–20 mg/day
Tacrolimus	Oral: 0.15–0.30 mg/kg/day
Biologics	
Adalimumab[c]	Subcutaneous: 40 mg per injection
Infliximab	Intravenous: 3–10 mg/kg, usually 5 mg/kg per infusion given at 4–8 week intervals
Interferon-α	Subcutaneous: 3–6 × 10^6 units four times daily × 1 month, then every 6 hours; 3 × 10^6 units three times per week

[a]It is important to note that the dosages should ultimately be determined by a treating physician with experience using these medications on the basis of the medical state of the patient in question. Furthermore, not all of these medications (or the route of therapy indicated) have been approved by various governmental agencies (i.e., U.S. Food and Drug Administration [FDA]) for use in patients with uveitis. Therefore the physician needs to inquire about their specific use.

[b]For intraocular administration preservative free Triesence is used.

[c]Adalimumab is currently the only biologic approved for the treatment of uveitis at the following dose schedule: Induction dose is 80 mg followed by 40 mg 1 week later. Maintenance dosing is 40 mg every 2 weeks.

Antacids or proton pump inhibitors can be considered on a case-by-case basis. Calcium and vitamin D supplements should be prescribed to patients, particularly those receiving long-term therapy. We recommend 800 units of vitamin D and 1500 mg of calcium daily to minimize the risk of steroid-induced osteoporosis, which mostly occurs in the first 6 months of treatment.[27]

Intravenously administered "pulse" corticosteroid therapy can also be employed. This approach is typically used in patients who have a severe bilateral process that needs to be treated as rapidly as possible with 1 g methylprednisolone intravenously and repeated daily for 3 days. It is not yet clear whether this method, indeed, renders better results compared with a high dose of oral prednisone, such as 80 mg/day, but in our experience, it certainly reverses an acute process very rapidly. This approach has been used to treat imminently vision-threatening manifestations of Vogt-Koyanagi-Harada (VKH) syndrome and Behçet disease.[28]

Those administering the medications should be familiar with the potential side effects of corticosteroids. Notable side effects are hyperglycemia and diabetes mellitus, osteoporosis, hyperlipidemia, weight gain, hypertension, and mood and sleep changes. Avascular necrosis of weight-bearing joints is a rare, but well-recognized, complication.[29] Some of the more common secondary problems are listed in Box 8.1. Other adverse reactions have included nonketotic hyperosmolar coma, in young patients without diabetes receiving systemic corticosteroids for a short time,[30] and central serous retinopathy.[31]

The effects of long-term corticosteroid administration are a constant concern, particularly in children. Polito et al.[32] studied growth in 10 boys with glomerulonephritis who received prednisone (1.2 mg/kg) every other day for at least 2 consecutive years. They found that in six patients, the peak growth velocity was delayed after age 15 years. However, after age 16 years, growth velocity was significantly higher than expected, permitting these patients to reach their genetic height potential.

A question that must be constantly asked is whether the desired effect warrants the potential or real side effects. There is no easy answer, and a dialogue between the patient and the physician is the only way this question can be addressed. Although corticosteroids remain the mainstay of therapy for uveitis, in some patients, the condition is resistant to steroids. For those receiving long-term steroid therapy, the risk of unacceptable side effects at the dosages that need to be given to control the disease are real. In those patients, other immunomodulatory agents are added as steroid-sparing agents so that lower steroid doses (≤10 mg daily) can be used or none at all. When needed, a daily maintenance dose of 10 mg or less of steroid is considered acceptable.[26] The combination of steroids with these agents provides reasonable and effective regimens for some patients and is discussed next. Although we may often begin therapy with corticosteroids, we add a steroid-sparing agent if significant amounts of steroids (>10 mg) for longer than 3 to 4 months are needed to control the ocular inflammation.

Cytotoxic Agents

Although mustard gas was synthesized earlier, its use during World War I, with the resultant lymphopenia and lymphoid aplasia, led to the evaluation of this family of agents for therapeutic purposes. On a practical basis, two major categories of cytotoxic agent are used in the treatment of ocular inflammatory disease: alkylating agents, such as chlorambucil and cyclophosphamide (Fig. 8.5), and antimetabolites, such as azathioprine and methotrexate (see Fig. 8.8 later in the chapter). They have been used by physicians for several decades, but their true efficacy in many ocular disorders remains unclear; however, more knowledge has been gained with regard to their use for other putative autoimmune diseases. The physician treating severe sight-threatening diseases should be aware of these agents and how they may fit into the general scheme of nonsurgical therapy for uveitis. Although, when viewed as a group, cytotoxic agents are associated with serious side effects, the role they play as steroid-sparing or steroid-replacing agents cannot be denied.[33,34]

Alkylating Agents

Mode of action. Alkylating agents have the ability to undergo reactions that result in the formation of covalent links (alkylation) of

BOX 8.1 Secondary Effects of Corticosteroid Therapy

Fluids, Electrolytes
Sodium retention, potassium loss
Fluid retention
Hypokalemic alkalosis
Hyperosmolar coma

Musculoskeletal
Muscle weakness
Steroid myopathy
Osteoporosis
Aseptic necrosis of femoral and humeral heads
Tendon rupture

Gastrointestinal
Nausea
Increased appetite
Peptic ulcer
Perforation of small and large bowel
Pancreatitis

Dermatologic
Poor wound healing
Easy bruisability
Increased sweating

Neurologic
Convulsions
Headaches
Hyperexcitability
Moodiness
Psychosis

Endocrine
Menstrual irregularities
Cushingoid state
Suppression of growth in children
Hirsutism
Suppression of adrenocortical pituitary axis
Diabetes

Ophthalmic
Cataracts
Glaucoma
Central serous retinopathy
Activation of herpes (topical)

Other
Weight gain
Thromboembolism

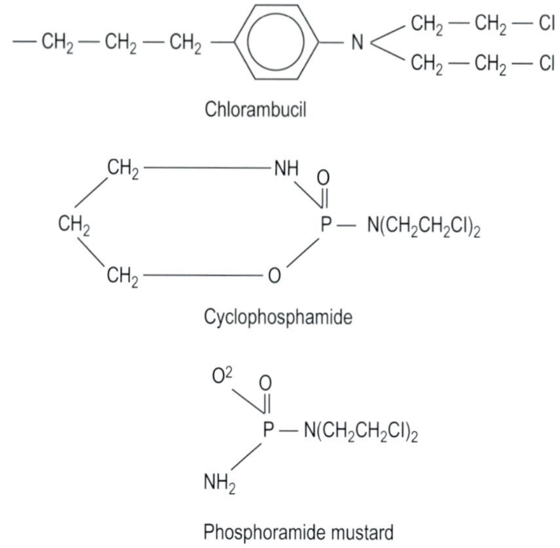

Fig. 8.5 Structure and active moiety of the two most-used alkylating agents.

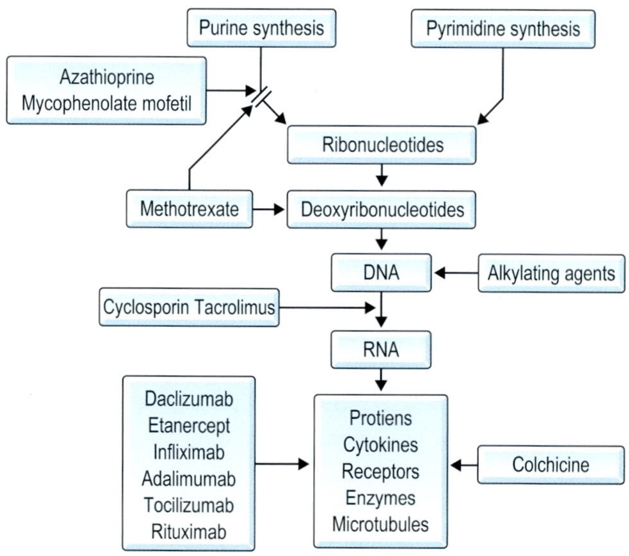

Fig. 8.6 Site of action of several agents used to treat ocular inflammatory disease.

neutrophilic substances. In interacting with DNA strands, alkylating agents are thought to interact with the 7-nitrogen guanine (Fig. 8.6).[35] This cross-linking of DNA would result in the inability of the cell's DNA to properly separate during division, ultimately leading to the death of the cell.

An aromatic modification of mustard gas is chlorambucil (Leukeran) (see Fig. 8.5), a compound stable enough to be given orally. Cyclophosphamide (Cytoxan, Neosar) is yet another modification, with the addition of a cyclic phosphamide group. For cyclophosphamide to become an active agent, it must be metabolized in the liver's microsomal system. It is theorized that phosphoramide mustard (see Fig. 8.5) is the most active of the metabolites.

The effect of alkylating agents on the immune system is rather profound. Higher doses are thought to affect B-cell function more acutely than T-cell function, but long-term lower dosages may have an equal or even greater effect on T-cell function. Alkylating agents are thought to be more potent in inducing a response compared with antimetabolites. However, with greater efficacy comes higher risk for adverse secondary effects. These agents are thought to control ocular inflammatory disease through the killing of clones of cells that are causing damage in the eye. This may be occurring at some central location (e.g., lymph node or bone marrow) or at the end organ itself. The response is not specific and will theoretically affect any actively dividing cell.

Indications and dosages. Buckley and Gills[36] reported the efficacy of cyclophosphamide therapy in the treatment of intermediate uveitis. In addition, alkylating agents have been frequently used in the treatment of Behçet disease.[37] The recommendations of the International Uveitis Study Group for the use of cytotoxic agents were decided upon in the early 1980s. Although somewhat dated, their basic concepts still seem to hold true. Treatment of Behçet disease was one absolute recommendation because corticosteroid therapy was not thought to adequately control the retinal/retinal vascular disease frequently observed in these patients. In general, alkylating agents are indicated for severe bilateral sight-threatening endogenous uveitis. Again, it cannot be overly stressed that the treating physician must be confident that the disease being treated does not have an infectious component. Furthermore, the physician should consider therapy only if there is some vision that can be saved because the potential side effects of these agents call for a good reason for their administration. The patient must be well informed of the physician's intentions and expectations and of any possible side effects, including risk for malignancy. Although this therapeutic approach is used in generalized life-threatening autoimmune diseases in children, it is not typically used in children with uveitis. If these drugs are used in younger persons, the physician should discuss the side effects in depth. One important consideration is the possibility that the medication may induce sterility, so banking of sperm or eggs before the initiation of therapy may need to be considered.

For cyclophosphamide, adult patients can start at about 2 mg/kg/day orally, with the usual starting dose for a rapid effect being 150 to 200 mg/day (see Table 8.2). The drug should be taken on an empty stomach because it can be activated in the gastrointestinal tract if taken with food. The white blood cell (WBC) count with differential must be monitored closely, and the dose should be titrated on the basis of the WBC count and the clinical effect. A drop in the WBC count may be seen within a few days to a week. Once this occurs, the dosage may be reduced by 25 to 50 mg, the objective being WBC count stabilizing at a level not lower than 3000/mm^3. The total neutrophil count should not fall to less than 1500 to 2000/mm^3.

Pulse cyclophosphamide (see Table 8.2) has been widely used in the treatment of systemic collagen vascular disease, such as lupus nephritis. This approach to therapy is thought to carry fewer risks compared with daily oral therapy; however, its efficacy has also been questioned.[38,39] Systemic steroids can be administered along with the alkylating agent. This permits the use of lower dosages of both, thus avoiding some of the side effects of both.

Godfrey et al.[40] have used chlorambucil to treat several disorders, including Behçet disease and sympathetic ophthalmia. This medication can be administered on an outpatient basis. The total dose is usually between 6 and 12 mg/day. We generally give a lower initial dose (2 mg) to ensure that there are no idiosyncratic responses and then increase the dose. As with cyclophosphamide, the WBC count and differential must be closely monitored.

A somewhat different approach was discussed by Tessler and Jennings,[41] who reported the use of high-dose short-term chlorambucil in the treatment of Behçet disease and sympathetic ophthalmia. These authors believed that remission was induced in all patients with the use of an average total dose of 2.2 g over 23 weeks in the patients with Behçet disease and a total of 0.9 g over 11 weeks for the patients with sympathetic ophthalmia.

Secondary effects. A wide range of side effects of alkylating agents has been reported.[42] Leukopenia is a major effect of these particular agents, resulting in immunosuppression. Thrombocytopenia and anemia also occur. An increased incidence of infection, particularly viral infections, is another great concern. Interstitial fibrosis of the lungs, testicular atrophy, and hemorrhagic cystitis are associated with cyclophosphamide therapy, the last being a relative indication for discontinuation of the drug. Renal toxicity has been attributed to the metabolites of alkylating agents,[43] and visual disturbances have been reported with high doses of cyclophosphamide.[44] Teratogenicity is a major concern, and cyclophosphamide is excreted in breast milk.

Because sterility is a real concern in those receiving alkylating agents, sperm can be banked and oocytes cryopreserved.

Perhaps the most disquieting adverse effects seen with these agents are those that may occur after long-term therapy. The first is the potential for secondary malignancy.[42] Secondary urinary bladder cancer seems to occur in patients who have hemorrhagic cystitis. Of course, the underlying disorder being treated may also predispose some patients to these disorders, particularly myeloproliferative and lymphoproliferative neoplasms. In a longitudinal cohort study in patients with rheumatoid arthritis with a 20-year follow-up, 119 patients treated with cyclophosphamide between 1968 and 1973 were compared with 119 patients who did not receive cyclophosphamide. An increased risk of malignancy was seen in the cyclophosphamide group (relative risk 1.5%).[45] Of interest were the nine bladder malignancies seen in the cyclophosphamide group versus none in the group not receiving cyclophosphamide. A large retrospective cohort study showed no increase in overall mortality in uveitis patients receiving alkylating agents compared with the average population and showed a nonsignificantly increased risk for cancer related mortality.[46]

It should be added that in the past few years, because of the aforementioned complications and because of the availability of effective biologic agents, alkylating agent therapy has been used less and less. However, anecdotal evidence certainly suggests a positive therapeutic effect of these agents in curtailing severe intraocular inflammatory disease recalcitrant to standard treatment. For life-threatening systemic vasculitis or in some patients with sight-threatening retinal vasculitis, cyclophosphamide may be the most effective medication. Also, in resource limited countries, two very important considerations are the ready availability and the relatively low cost. As with many other problems encountered in medicine, this class of drugs represents a double-edged sword, and their use should be considered only after long reflection.

The ophthalmologist should have someone well versed in this therapeutic approach actively involved in the care of the patient, should set strict goals in terms of the therapeutic effect that must be reached, and should avoid using these agents in children.

Antimetabolites

In this category of medications, azathioprine and mycophenolate mofetil, which alter purine metabolism, and methotrexate, a folate analogue, are the three most widely used (Fig. 8.7).

Azathioprine

Mode of action. Azathioprine (Imuran) is thought to be a prodrug. Upon metabolism, it is converted into the active agent 6-mercaptopurine. Azathioprine is better absorbed, causes less gastrointestinal disturbance, and is less likely to be inactivated by liver enzymes compared with 6-mercaptopurine. Once converted to its active form, it is thought to affect DNA and RNA metabolism by being converted to 6-thioinosine-5-phosphate (T-IMP) by the enzyme hypoxanthine guanine phosphoribosyltransferase. T-IMP is probably incorporated into nucleic acids, leading to false codes being generated. It appears that azathioprine has a greater effect on the afferent arm of the immune response when it is given before the antigenic challenge.

Indications and dosages. For putative autoimmune diseases, such as rheumatoid arthritis, the suggested dosage of azathioprine is about 1 to 2.5 mg/kg/day,[47,48] the average dose being 50 to 100 mg daily, given as one dose or in divided doses[49] (see Table 8.2). The combination of azathioprine with low-dose steroid has been used in the treatment of uveitis by Andrasch et al.[50] Others have used the drug for the treatment of sympathetic ophthalmia, VKH syndrome, serpiginous choroiditis, and

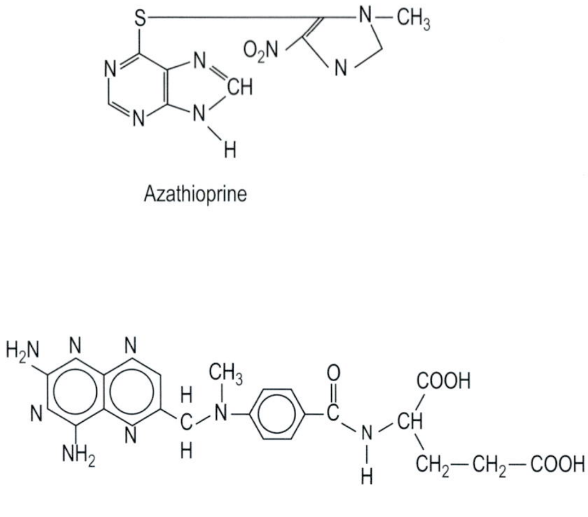

Azathioprine

Methotrexate

Fig. 8.7 Structures of two antimetabolites.

pars planitis.[51,52] Yazici et al.[53] showed, in a double-masked study, that azathioprine (2.5 mg/kg/day) was superior to placebo in the prevention of new eye disease associated with Behçet disease. Certain drugs, such as allopurinol, can interfere with the metabolism of 6-mercaptopurine, and the dosage of the agent must be reduced accordingly.

In a subgroup analysis of the SITE (Systemic Immunosuppressive Therapy for Eye Diseases) study (see the last paragraph of this chapter), 145 patients were who were treated with azathioprine as a sole immunosuppressive agent were evaluated.[54] Azathioprine was noted to be moderately effective as a single steroid-sparing agent for control of disease (complete control of disease in 40%–62%), and its steroid-sparing value (allowed for prednisone tapering to ≤ 10 mg daily in 32%–47%). It required months to achieve the treatment goal and was tolerated by most patients. It appeared particularly useful in patients with intermediate uveitis.

Secondary effects. Antimetabolites can have serious side effects,[43] but in the past few years, the use of lower doses has prevented these effects from occurring or has made them more tolerable. For azathioprine, perhaps the most problematic acute adverse effects are leukopenia, thrombocytopenia, and gastrointestinal disturbances. Of great long-term concern is chronic immunosuppression increasing the risk of neoplasia. Connell et al.[55] studied the risk of neoplasia in 755 patients with inflammatory bowel disease treated with azathioprine at a dosage of 2 mg/kg/day for a median of 12.5 months, and no cases of non-Hodgkin lymphoma were reported. It appears that the risk of neoplasia is lower in those treated for autoimmune disorders, such as rheumatoid arthritis, than in those receiving therapy for the prevention of transplant rejection. Similarly, the results of the SITE study indicated no increased overall or cancer-related mortality among patients with uveitis using azathioprine.[46]

Mycophenolate Mofetil

Mycophenolate mofetil (CellCept) is frequently used in uveitis treatment.[56] It has a molecular weight of 433.5 Da and metabolizes to mycophenolic acid, which reversibly inhibits inosine monophosphate dehydrogenase, inhibiting a pathway of guanosine nucleotide synthesis without incorporation into DNA. It affects both T and B cells and interferes with cellular adhesion to the vascular endothelium. This agent has been used in preventing experimental autoimmune uveitis (EAU) (30 mg/kg/day) even after immunization, but at higher doses (60 mg/kg/day).[57] It was first used in humans in combination with corticosteroids and cyclosporin for the prevention of organ rejection after allogeneic renal transplantation. Mycophenolate mofetil is taken on an empty stomach and has high oral bioavailability. It is a reasonable alternative to either azathioprine or methotrexate. Several small studies have reported good results with mycophenolate mofetil.[58,59] It has also been found effective in treating scleritis.[59-61] As a single agent, mycophenolate mofetil was found to control inflammation in 53% to 73% of 236 patients with uveitis and provided successful prednisone taper (≤ 10 mg daily) in 41% to 55%; only 2% discontinued mycophenolate mofetil in the first year because of side effects.[62]

The dose of mycophenolate mofetil is usually 1 g orally twice daily. Some patients have received up to 3 g/day (1.5 g twice daily). The most common adverse event (AE) appears to be gastrointestinal effects, with as many as 31% of patients reporting this problem. In addition to nausea, myalgia, fatigue, headache, anemia, leukopenia, malignancy, and opportunistic infections can occur. Mycophenolate mofetil has been associated with embryofetal toxicity, and it can decrease the effectiveness of oral contraceptives. Therefore women with childbearing potential need to be particularly counseled about the use of additional contraceptive methods.

Methotrexate

Mode of action. Methotrexate (Otrexup, Rasuvo, Rheumatrex, Trexall) is a folate analogue, differing from folic acid only in that a hydrogen atom and the hydroxyl group have been replaced by a methyl and amino group. Folate analogues are known to have profound effects on cellular metabolism by inhibiting dihydrofolate reductase activity. This enzyme is imperative for the production of tetrahydrofolate, an important coenzyme in cell metabolism. Tetrahydrofolate is needed for the production of thymidylate, an essential component of DNA, and mediates the production of purine nucleotides, also needed for RNA metabolism. Methotrexate demonstrates time-specific characteristics in that under certain experimental conditions, an augmented immune response may be noted if the drug is given before antigenic challenge. Methotrexate has been shown to have an antiproliferative effect on endothelial cells,[63] can reduce the synthesis of leukotriene B4 in neutrophils,[64] has been shown to reduce the concentration of interleukin (IL)-1β in synovial fluid,[65] and can suppress cell-mediated immunity.[66] An added action of methotrexate is inhibition of histamine release.

Indications and dosages. Several dosage schedules have been suggested, with a weekly oral or intramuscular dose of 7.5 to 25 mg given until a therapeutic response is noted (see Table 8.2). Patients need to be told to abstain from all alcohol consumption. Cyclitis and sympathetic ophthalmia have been reported to improve with the administration of this agent, but Behçet disease and iridocyclitis have not.[67] Methotrexate is well tolerated in children and is used extensively. In a subgroup analysis of the SITE study (see the final conclusions of this chapter), methotrexate was evaluated in 384 patients with uveitis and found to provide sustained control of inflammation in 66% and steroid-sparing effect in 58%. Adding methotrexate to an anti-inflammatory regimen was often effective in the management of anterior uveitis, sometimes effective for scleritis, but less often effective for intermediate, posterior, or panuveitis; 42% discontinued methotrexate within the first year because of ineffectiveness or side effects.[68] In a randomized clinical trial, methotrexate was found to be equally effective as mycophenolate mofetil as a first-line steroid-sparing therapy in posterior segment uveitis[69] and elevated liver enzymes were the most common side effect for both methotrexate and mycophenolate mofetil (13% and 7.4%, respectively).

Methotrexate has been shown to be equally effective as Mycophenolate Mofetil in controlling inflammation in posterior segment uveitis in The First-line Antimetabolites as Steroid-sparing Treatment (FAST) uveitis trial.[69]

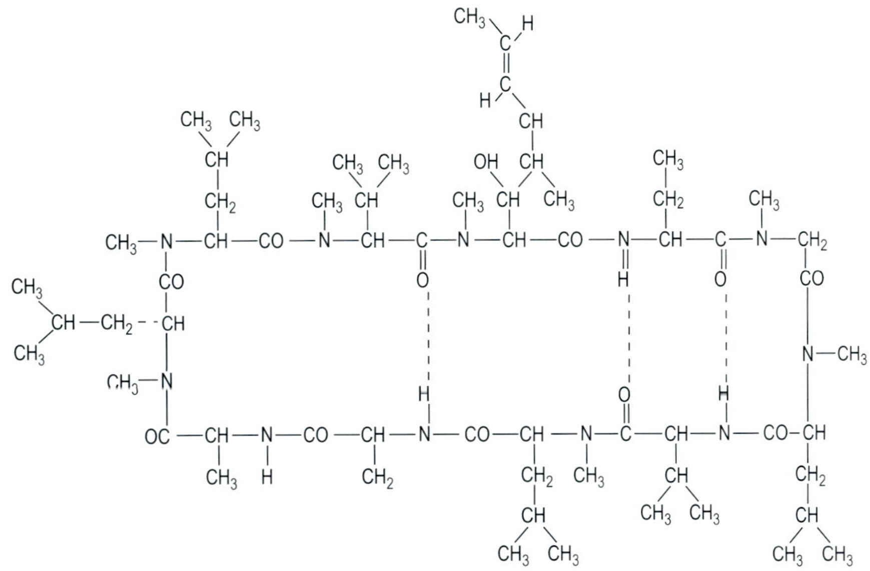

Fig. 8.8 Structure of cyclosporin (Sandimmune).

Methotrexate has been used intravitreally to treat intraocular B-cell lymphoma.[70] Good responses have been seen using 400 μg/0.1 mL. It has also been used to treat intraocular inflammation or macular edema.[71] A clinical trial comparing its effectiveness against intravitreal anti–vascular endothelial growth factor (VEGF) and corticosteroids for the treatment of macular edema is currently ongoing (NCT02623426). These injections can be repeated, but care must be taken because reflux at the side of the intravitreal injection can damage limbal stem cells.

Secondary effects. The secondary effects of methotrexate are legion,[26,42] but more recent use of lower doses has invested this agent with new therapeutic possibilities. Marked depression of the WBC count and thrombocytopenia can occur at high doses. Hepatotoxicity is one of the most worrisome side effects.[72] Up to one-third of those receiving long-term weekly doses of methotrexate will have elevated serum aminotransferase levels.[73] Liver enzyme levels twice normal warrant withholding or stopping the medication; the levels usually return to normal rapidly. Liver biopsy should also be considered during therapy if elevated liver function test results persist or a decrease in the serum albumin concentration is seen.[34]

Another concern is acute pneumonitis that can be accompanied by fever, progressive shortness of breath, and cough in 1% to 5% of patients treated with methotrexate.[74-76] This appears to be caused by a drug hypersensitivity reaction, and it can occur early or late in the course of therapy. In most patients, the reaction disappears with discontinuation of therapy.

Patients should be closely monitored for bone marrow suppression and liver, lung, and kidney toxicities. Dosage needs to be adjusted in patients with impaired renal function. Mild to moderate liver enzyme elevations are seen frequently but often resolve with dose adjustments.

Methotrexate is teratogenic and has been reported to cause fetal death and/or congenital anomalies. Therefore appropriate steps should be taken to avoid conception during methotrexate therapy. It is contraindicated in pregnancy and during nursing. Pregnancy should be avoided if either partner is receiving methotrexate: during and for a minimum of 3 months for male partners and for at least one ovulatory cycle for women.

Cyclosporin

Mode of action. Cyclosporin (Gengraf, Neoral, Sandimmune) is a natural product of several fungi. It was first investigated because of its potential antibiotic qualities and, indeed, has antibacterial effect but with a very limited spectrum. It was its unique immunomodulatory properties, first observed by Jean Borel at Sandoz Ltd. that altered immunotherapy principles and therapeutics in a profound way. Cyclosporin A, now termed *cyclosporin* (Sandimmune), is a neutral lipophilic cyclic undecapeptide with a unique amino acid side chain at the C1 position (Fig. 8.8). It is one of a large family of cyclosporins, some naturally occurring and some synthesized. This uncharged molecule, with a molecular weight of 1202 Da, is insoluble in water. The original preparation for human use was an olive oil solution with 12.5% ethanol, which had variable bioavailability.[77,78] Cyclosporin is now available in tablet form.

The parent structure appears to be the most active form. The agent is metabolized in the liver by the cytochrome P450 microsomal enzyme system. Drugs that interfere with cytochrome P450 activity will slow cyclosporin metabolism and will affect cyclosporin levels. Ketoconazole is one such agent, permitting reduction of the oral dose of cyclosporin by up to 90%.[79] Other medications that inhibit cyclosporin metabolism, thus increasing plasma concentrations of cyclosporin, include oral contraceptives, androgens, and erythromycin.

Cyclosporin has been demonstrated to have a far more restricted effect on the immune system compared with any other immunosuppressive agent or other monoclonal antibodies. Although, theoretically, cyclosporin would affect any cell with its binding protein, its major clinical effect is actively directed against the factors that promote T-cell activation and recruitment. The exact point at which cyclosporin intervenes in this scheme is still being debated (Fig. 8.9). It appears that cyclosporin enters the cell and is bound to an immunophilin (cyclophilin), meeting it at the cell membrane, similar to the action seen with corticosteroids. It then is escorted into the nucleus, where it affects messenger ribonucleic acid (mRNA) production and ultimately protein synthesis. Although the mechanism still remains to be definitively shown, much has been elucidated.[80] Cyclosporin blocks the activation of genes in T cells.[81] One intriguing notion is that cyclosporin binds to proteins binding to the IL-2 enhancer (e.g., nuclear factor of activated T cell [NF-AT] and octamer-associated protein), which helps in the activation of the transcription of the *IL-2* gene. These sites have been shown to be sensitive to cyclosporin.[82-86] Cyclosporin is unique in mediating its action through the T-cell circuitry.

Dosages and indications. The dosage schedule for cyclosporin administration has undergone much change.[87] In initial studies[88] on the use of cyclosporin in patients with ocular inflammatory disease, patients were given an initial dose of 10 mg/kg/day, which was thought to be rather modest at the time but led to dose-induced renal

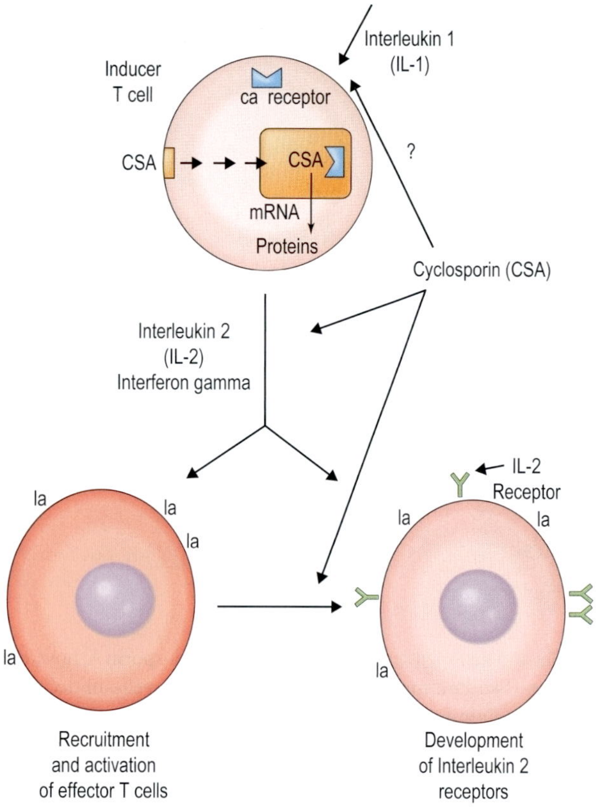

Fig. 8.9 Proposed mechanisms of cyclosporin on T-cell circuitry.

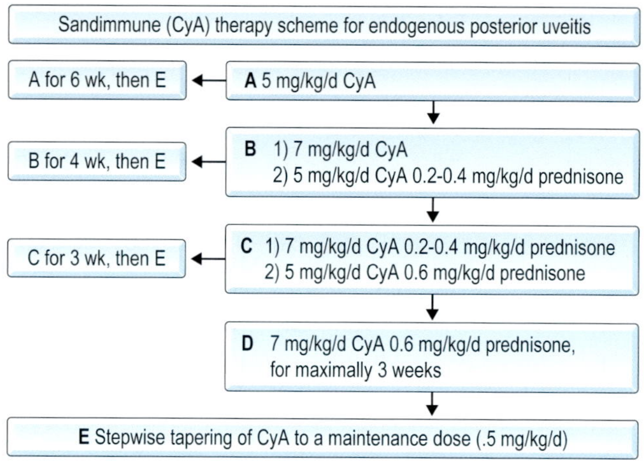

Fig. 8.10 Therapeutic scheme for treatment of sight-threatening bilateral endogenous uveitis with cyclosporin. (Reproduced with permission from Ben Ezra D, Nussenblatt RB, Timonen P. *Optimal Use of Sandimmune in Endogenous Uveitis*. With kind permission of Springer Science & Business Media.)

alterations. It is usually suggested that cyclosporin be given at a starting dose of 2.5 to 5 mg/kg/day[26] (Fig. 8.10; see also Table 8.2), as a twice-daily regimen. The twice-daily regimen is more commonly employed to avoid large spikes in serum cyclosporin levels, which may predispose the patient to renal toxicity. A recommended maximum dose of 7 mg/kg/day can be considered in special cases, such as children or patients with documented low trough cyclosporin serum levels. Cyclosporin is often used in combination with prednisone, usually at 10 to 20 mg/day, but for short periods at even higher levels.

A relative contraindication for the initiation of therapy is poorly controlled hypertension, a history of renal disease accompanied by reduced creatinine clearance, or both. In addition, older patients (older than 55 years of age) must be monitored particularly closely because they lack an adequate renal reserve. The ocular response to cyclosporin may be relatively slow (weeks to months), but preset goals should be established and should be met by about 3 months of therapy. The serum creatinine level should not be permitted to rise to 30% over baseline. Optimal decreases in cyclosporin dosages are usually 50 to 100 mg/day at a time. Stopping the medication may lead to rebound of the ocular disease.

The question regarding the length of treatment with cyclosporin is somewhat open ended. It appears that an immunologically tolerant state is not induced with this medication, and therefore an extended therapeutic course is indicated in most patients.

On the basis of our group's early observations,[88-90] cyclosporin was used in patients with active bilateral sight-threatening noninfectious uveitis.[91] Of special interest was the particularly positive clinical effect seen in patients with Behçet disease who were treated with this medication.[92] This finding was supported by a randomized, masked study in Japan[93] and a study by Diaz-Llopis et al.,[94] who used a dose of 5 mg/kg/day and a maintenance dose of 2 mg/kg/day, and found a good response in 86% of patients, with disappearance of attacks in 43%.

Several reports support the use of cyclosporin in various types of intraocular inflammatory diseases. Cyclosporin is now usually used in conjunction with another immunosuppressive agent, probably most frequently with corticosteroids. Cyclosporin is well tolerated by children,[95] with Walton et al. reporting improvement in 64% or stabilization in 75% of eyes treated in children and adolescents with uveitis. A subgroup analysis of the SITE study evaluated 373 patients starting cyclosporin monotherapy.[96] As was noted in our randomized study, 33% gained sustained, complete control of inflammation by 6 months and about 50% gained sustained complete control of their inflammation by 1 year. We felt that, along with corticosteroid therapy, cyclosporin was modestly effective in controlling ocular inflammation. Adult doses, ranging from 150 to 250 mg/day, were more likely to be effective than lower doses. Approximately 10% discontinued therapy because of toxicity within 1 year, and patients older than 55 years of age were more than three times more likely to discontinue therapy.

Like corticosteroids, cyclosporin has been placed into slow-release implants. Gilger et al.[97] reported that cyclosporin implants decreased the severity of experimental uveitis in horses. A pilot study at the National Eye Institute (NEI) was initiated to evaluate the safety of such a device and to elicit observations to determine its effectiveness. The implants were tolerated in the small number of patients treated, but a marked therapeutic effect was not seen.[98] Most patients continued to have CME and required systemic immunosuppressive therapy. Thus, the implant was not further developed and is not commercially available.

A topical preparation of cyclosporin (Restasis) is now commercially available and has been shown to be effective in treating moderate to severe dry eye.[99] Although perhaps important for treatment of immune diseases involving the ocular surface, this method of application does not result in significant amounts of drug entering the eye because of the physical properties of the medication. Therefore topical application does not appear to a useful therapeutic approach for treating uveitis in the formulations currently available.

Secondary effects. At lower doses, the secondary effects of cyclosporin noted by patients with uveitis diminish considerably. However, the two secondary problems that cause the most concern in the treating physician are hypertension and renal toxicity. Depending on the definition of renal toxicity, it develops in as many as 75% to

100% of patients treated with cyclosporin.[100,101] It is not clear what the incidence rate of irreversible renal toxicity is likely to be with the lower dosage of cyclosporin now recommended. At a higher dosage, the alterations we noted on renal biopsy, after an average of 2 years of therapy, were renal tubular atrophy and interstitial fibrosis, with the glomeruli remaining mainly intact. Renal vascular alterations can also appear[101] (Fig. 8.11). These alterations were noted histologically when the mean serum creatinine level of the patients undergoing biopsy was 1.5 mg/dL, which was within the upper limits of normal. It would appear that there are reversible and irreversible components to the renal toxicity induced by cyclosporin. However, more recent reports from investigators treating autoimmune conditions (other than uveitis) with lower starting and maintenance doses of cyclosporin have been encouraging because little to no alteration in renal function associated with this agent has been noted.[102] Feutren and Mihatsch[98] reviewed 192 renal biopsy specimens from patients treated with cyclosporin for a variety of conditions, including diabetes mellitus, Sjögren syndrome, and uveitis. It was found that three independent variables distinguished the 41 patients with cyclosporin-induced nephropathy from those free of nephropathy: a higher initial dose of cyclosporin, a larger maximal increase in the serum creatinine concentration above baseline, and age. Therefore it has been suggested that to reduce the risk of nephropathy, a dose of 5 mg/kg/day should be used, and serum creatinine levels should not rise to greater than 30% over the patient's baseline level. Also, a retrospective analysis of 1663 patients who had undergone renal transplantation and were receiving long-term cyclosporin therapy demonstrated that progressive toxic nephropathy did not occur.[103] Cyclosporin interacts with many agents, and one must be very cognizant of this. The concomitant use of nonsteroidal anti-inflammatory drugs (NSAIDs) with cyclosporin will almost ensure decreased renal function. Other medications that can interact with cyclosporin are listed in Box 8.2.

We and others[104,105] have reported that cyclosporin can be found in the anterior chamber of patients receiving systemic medication, and in cerebrospinal fluid (CSF) as well.

Opportunistic infections have not been a major problem in patients with uveitis treated with cyclosporin. Certainly, some risk is present if patients receive other immunosuppressive agents combined with cyclosporin. A trend toward less renal toxicity was observed in patients who received combined cyclosporin/steroid therapy rather than cyclosporin alone.[106] We have noted that patients with uveitis treated with cyclosporin demonstrate appropriate immune responses both to new antigens and to old ones requiring a "recall" response.[107] Therefore vaccination can apparently be performed on patients treated with this medication, but pre- and postimmunization titers should be checked. Cyclosporin may cause central nervous system (CNS) changes: the most common ones we have seen are tremors (at higher dosages). Cyclosporin has been reported to cause headache; mood alterations; rarely, leukoencephalopathy, seizures, visual disturbances, and psychiatric problems; and motor and speech disturbances.[108] The incidence of lymphoma observed in graft recipients treated with cyclosporin was 0.3%.[101] In the SITE study, patients who received cyclosporine had overall and cancer mortality rates similar to those of patients who never took immunosuppressive drugs.[46]

Tacrolimus

Mode of action. Tacrolimus (Prograf), an immunosuppressive agent with molecular weight of 822 Da, was isolated from the broth of *Streptomyces tsukubaensis*[109,110] (Fig. 8.12) and is believed to have essentially the same mechanism of action as cyclosporin.[80] One difference is that the immunophilin that binds with tacrolimus is FK506-binding protein (FKBP) instead of cyclophilin. It suppresses the formation of mRNA for IL-2, as does cyclosporin, but at an effective in vitro therapeutic concentration about 100 times less than that of cyclosporin.[110] Using a dose 10 to 30 times less than that of cyclosporin, tacrolimus was found to be effective in preventing the development of EAU in rats[111] and in monkeys.[112] It is metabolized by the cytochrome P450 system.

Indications and dosages. An open-label clinical trial to evaluate the use of tacrolimus was performed in Japan; 53 patients (most with Behçet disease) were treated with varying doses, and about three-quarters were thought to have benefited.[109] A review of patients with Behçet disease alone[113] confirmed these initial observations. A daily dose of 0.10 to 0.15 mg/kg body weight/day has been suggested to be appropriate. Sloper et al.[114] reported their experience with tacrolimus, treating six patients with uveitis refractory to cyclosporin. Five of the six patients had a two-line or more improvement. Kilmartin et al.[115]

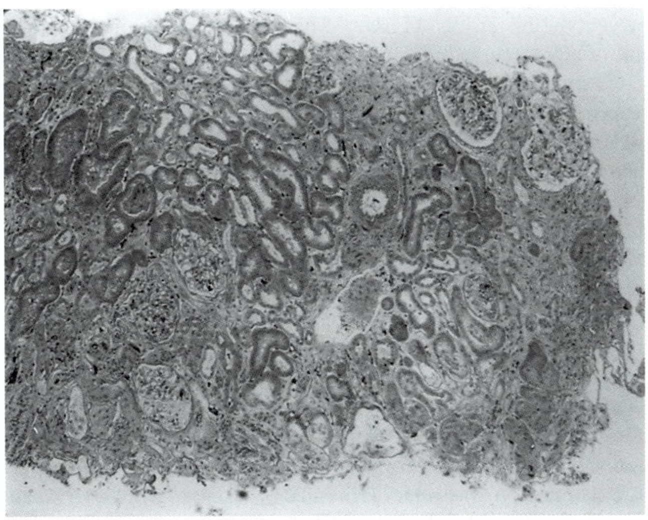

Fig. 8.11 Renal biopsy from patient receiving cyclosporin for uveitis. Interstitial fibrosis and marked patchy loss of renal tubules suggest toxicity caused by this agent. Serum creatinine level was within normal limits at the time of biopsy.

BOX 8.2 Medications That May Interact Pharmacokinetically With Cyclosporin

Amiodarone
Carbamazepine
Clarithromycin
Corticosteroid
Diltiazem
Doxycycline
Erythromycin
Fluconazole
Itraconazole
Ketoconazole
Nicardipine
Nifedipine
Phenytoin
Protease inhibitors
Rifampin
Verapamil
Theophylline

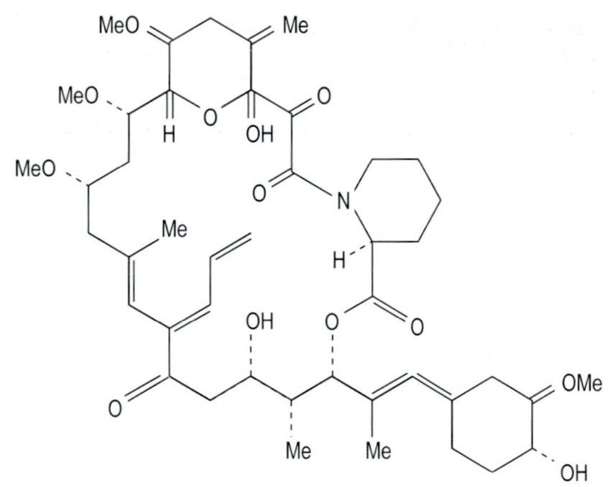

Fig. 8.12 Structure of tacrolimus (FK506). (From Schreiber SL, Crabtree GR. The mechanism of action of ciclosporin A and FK506. *Immunol Today.* 1992;13:136.)

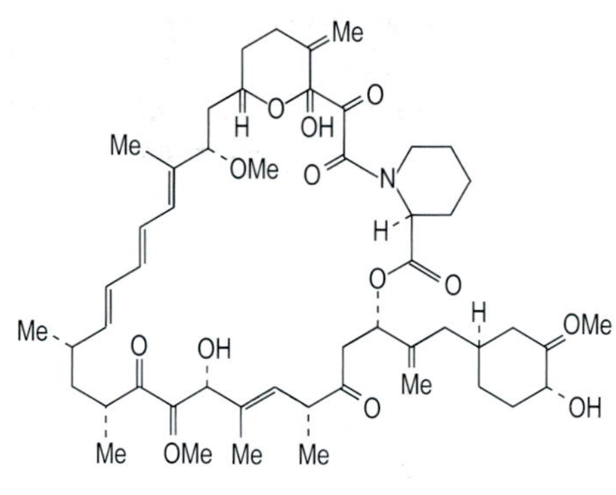

Fig. 8.13 Structure of rapamycin. (From Schreiber SL, Crabtree GR. The mechanism of action of ciclosporin A and FK506. *Immunol Today.* 1992;13:136.)

reported on seven patients with uveitis treated with tacrolimus, with two being withdrawn from therapy and the other five continuing. An initial dose of 0.05 mg/kg/day has generally been used in the treatment of uveitis, whereas for use in transplant recipients doses of 0.10 to 0.15 mg/kg/day have been used. Concentrations in blood need to be monitored.

In retrospective studies, tacrolimus was effective in patients with chronic posterior segment uveitis. In a cohort of 62 patients with posterior segment uveitis with various etiologies, tacrolimus therapy resulted in success in steroid sparing (< 10 g/day) in 85% and visual acuity improved significantly, although this improvement was mostly experienced by those who continued using tacrolimus for 2 years. Tacrolimus was well tolerated overall, renal toxicity was uncommon, and the discontinuation rate was approximately 25% by 2 years.[116] In a separate cohort of 25 patients with birdshot retinopathy, 64% success was observed when tacrolimus was used as monotherapy or in combination with steroids or mycophenolate mofetil; and 84% of patients tolerated tacrolimus well.[117] Additionally, tacrolimus has been found to be effective in posterior segment uveitis in an open-label RCT as a monotherapy or in combination with corticosteroids.[118]

Secondary effects. With essentially the same mechanism of action as that of cyclosporin, one might assume similar secondary effects for tacrolimus. Adverse effects include renal impairment, noted in 28% of patients reported by Mochizuki and colleagues.[109] Neurologic symptoms, including tremors, headache, ophthalmoplegia, and meningitis-like symptoms, have been noted. Gastrointestinal symptoms, usually manifested as nausea, loss of appetite, and abdominal pain, can occur. Hyperglycemia was reported by Mochizuki et al.[109] in 13% of patients.

Rapamycin

Mode of action. Rapamycin (Rapamune, Sirolimus) is a macrolide immunosuppressant purified from isolates of *Streptomyces hygroscopicus* collected on Rapa Nui (Easter Island).[119] It blocks the proliferative signals of transduction in T cells[120,121] (Fig. 8.13). Rapamycin inhibits the mammalian target of rapamycin (mTOR). This blockage has been shown to prevent the expression of IL-2, IL-4, and IL-6. Of great interest and potential therapeutic importance is the fact that rapamycin's effect occurs much later in the cell cycle (G1- to S-phase transition) than that of either cyclosporin or tacrolimus. Rapamycin appears not to inhibit the expression of IL-2 receptors and IL-2 production, but may interfere with the cell's ability to respond to interleukins, such as IL-2 and IL-4.[120,122] Rapamycin is bound in the cytoplasm to the same immunophilin as tacrolimus (FKBP), and therefore these two agents will competitively inhibit each other if placed in the same environment.

Indications and dosages. Rapamycin has been used at a dose of 2 mg/day in a small number of patients with uveitis and in those undergoing renal transplantation.[123,124] A comprehensive review of mTOR-inhibiting drugs and their use in uveitis found no RCTs on systemic sirolimus. There were several case series and reports, the largest of which had 8 patients. The dose ranged from 2 to 12 mg/day, and the effectiveness of systemic sirolimus was limited in uveitis, with 50% to 63% achieving desired outcomes, and there was a high rate of side effects even at lower doses.[125] Because it is bound by the same cytoplasmic receptor as tacrolimus, the two agents should not be given together. Rapamycin has been shown to be very effective in inhibiting the induction of EAU in Lewis rats[126] and in completely inhibiting the transfer of EAU[127] at a dose of 0.1 mg/kg/day given as a continuous intravenous infusion. Studies have shown that cyclosporin and rapamycin may have a synergistic effect in vitro on T lymphocytes.[128] The combination of cyclosporin 2 mg/kg/day (one-fifth the normal dose) plus intravenously administered rapamycin 0.01 mg/kg/day (one-tenth the normal therapeutic dose) will act synergistically to prevent the expression of EAU.[129] There is great interest in the possible role of rapamycin in inducing peripheral immune tolerance.

Toxicity. At a therapeutic dosage of 0.1 mg/kg/day, animals have been reported to lose weight.[121] Of concern have been reports of myocardial toxicity in rats.[130] However, these have occurred at relatively high doses of the drug. Gastrointestinal vasculitis has been noted in dogs.[131] In some patients, diarrhea and pneumonitis have been associated with the administration of the drug. In two studies, one with a retrospective cohort of 8 patients and one an open-label prospective study of 8 patients, AEs, such as abdominal pain, abnormal liver function, sclerodermatous-like skin changes, DVT, excessive nausea and vomiting, and, in one case, thrombocytopenia, were reported.[125,132]

Systemic Immunosuppressive Therapy for Eye Diseases (SITE) cohort studies have investigated the effectiveness of various immunosuppressive agents when used as a single agent in the treatment of noninfectious uveitis. One year after starting therapy sustained control of inflammation was achieved in 62.2%, 66.0%, 73.1%, 51.9%, and 76.3% of patients taking azathioprine, methorexate, mycophenolate mofetil, cyclosporine, and cyclophosphamide, respectively.[133]

Comparison of effectiveness of each imunosuppressive agent by anatomical location can be seen in Table 8.3.

TABLE 8.3 Comparative effectiveness of antimetabolites and cyclosporine in uveitis based on Systemic Immunosuppressive Therapy for Eye Diseases (SITE) study.

	Azathioprine	MMF	MXT	CsA	Chi-Square[+]
Age (Median) [range in years]	50.6 [9.2-86.4]	47.1 [8.1-84.2]	46.9 [0.4-93.5]	36.1 [5.5-81.5]	
Female (%)	67.6	63.6	72.9	62.7	0.0153
Caucasian (%)	76.6	66.9	73.2	73.7	0.157
# of patients (n)*	145	236	384	373	
Complete control at 6/12 months (%)					
- Total	40.8/62.2	53.1/73.1	49.4/66.0	33.4/51.9	<0.0001/<0.0001
- Anterior	23.7/34.6	55.2/72.4	55.6/67.2	30.4/54.3	<0.0001/<0.0001
- Intermediate	69.3/89.8	65.0/76.7	47.4/74.9	39.3/51.8	<0.0001/<0.0001
- Posterior/Pan	44.2/59.7	50.6/70.9	38.6/52.1	29.2/51.7	<0.0001/<0.0001
Inactive or slightly active at 6/12 months (%)					
- Total	56.8/72.7	77.5/91.2	62.8/74.3	60.8/76.4	<0.0001/<0.0001
- Anterior	28.2/42.6	84.9/100	69.7/71.6	52.8/85.8	<0.0001/<0.0001
- Intermediate	87.5/100	83.1/100	62.8/89.4	73.7/80.2	<0.0001/<0.0001
- Pan/Posterior	72.0/83.2	86.5/93.2	53.9/66.2	56.6/75.2	<0.0001/<0.0001
Steroid-sparing success at 6/12 months (%)					
Total					
- Prednisone ≤10 mg	32.2/46.9	40.7/55.0	37.3/58.4	22.1/36.1	<0.0001/<0.0001
- Prednisone ≤5 mg	20.6/40.6	27.3/43.7	32.6/52.9	18.1/30.0	<0.0001/<0.0001
- Off prednisone	05.2/09.5	04.4/12.1	05.1/18.8	03.6/08.2	0.629/0.0002
Anterior (n)	21	48	126	75	
- Prednisone ≤10 mg	16.6/24.9	47.2/53.1	46.1/62.6	28.5/42.4	0.0038/0.0017
- Prednisone ≤5 mg	11.5/19.5	46.4/51.3	41.8/59.4	26.9/40.4	0.0041/0.0013
- Off prednisone	00.0/08.3	05.8/18.4	06.2/17.6	08.8/14.9	0.61^/0.756
Intermediate (n)	18	28	38	99	
- Prednisone ≤10 mg	47.0/68.2	39.0/49.2	41.3/68.8	24.1/38.0	0.0915/0.0060
- Prednisone ≤5 mg	29.9/64.9	26.0/43.6	31.8/57.0	19.0/32.5	0.454/0.0068
- Off prednisone	00.0/00.0	00.0/13.8	07.4/15.0	03.7/09.2	0.443^/0.264^
Posterior/Pan (n)	52	94	82	171	
- Prednisone ≤10 mg	36.3/44.0	41.2/60.3	20.7/39.1	16.2/32.3	<0.0001/0.0001
- Prednisone ≤5 mg	16.6/42.9	21.3/41.7	20.2/32.0	12.7/23.6	0.251/0.0064
- Off prednisone	07.1/09.9	02.6/09.1	03.0/11.9	00.7/03.9	0.0259^/0.105

MMF, mycophenolate mofetil; MXT, methotrexate; CsA, cyclosporine A; D/c, discontinued; SE, side effects; GI, gastrointestinal; HTN, hypertension
[+]p values calculated by comparison of proportions unless noted otherwise.
*Total # of patients includes patients with scleritis, ocular cicatricial pemphigoid, and other ocular inflammatory diseases not otherwise included in this table.
^p value calculated by Fisher's exact test because of small sample size.
From Knickelbein JE, Kim M, Argon E, Sen HN. Comparative efficacy of steroid-sparing therapies for non-infectious uveitis. Expert Review of Ophthalmology. 2017;12(4):313-319

Antibodies and Monoclonal Antibodies

Antibodies and monoclonal antibodies directed against various parts of the immune cascade have been used more and more extensively in the treatment of uveitis in humans[134,135] (see Table 8.2). These antibodies have been used for some time in other areas of medicine. Anti–T-cell monoclonal antibodies, such as OKT3, have been recognized as effective immunosuppressive agents,[136] and their use to prevent renal graft rejection has become well established.[137] Many regimens for the prevention of graft rejection call for OKT3 monoclonal antibody therapy, followed by other immunosuppressive therapy. It was reported that two patients who underwent renal transplantation suffered marked visual loss after OKT3 therapy.[138] In the one patient tested, the amplitudes of electroretinography were extinguished.

More and more antibodies directed against specific receptors to lymphokines on T cells and other players in the immune system have been developed and evaluated. Other biologic agents, such as alemtuzumab and anakinra, have been used in limited case reports for ocular inflammatory diseases, although other agents have been used more extensively. Initial problems dealt with immune reactions against a foreign protein (i.e., mouse-produced antibody), but current technology now allows for "humanizing" these antibodies (Fig. 8.14), so

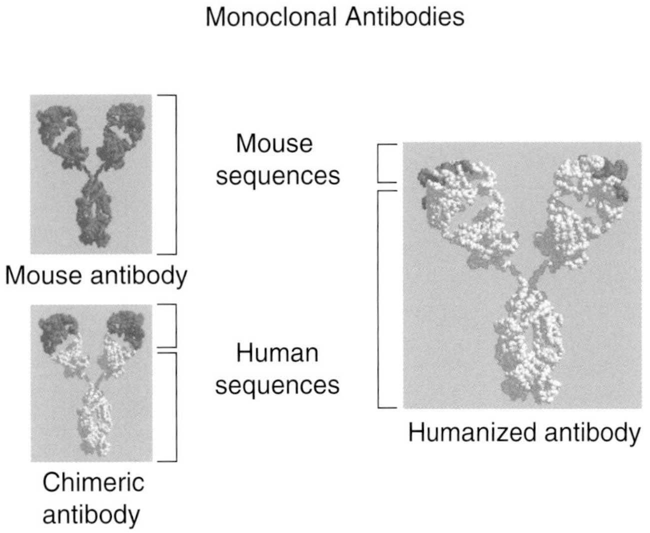

Fig. 8.14 Monoclonal antibodies are usually derived in mice. Giving such an antibody to humans induces an immune response against it because it is seen as foreign. Some antibodies are chimeras, which reduces the foreign antigen load to some degree. Most antibodies now are "humanized," with very few of the original amino acids left, allowing the necessary conformational integrity of the antibody. (Courtesy Protein Design Laboratories.)

that, essentially, they are not recognized as "foreign."[139] There are also several monoclonal antibodies targeting IL-17 (secukinumab) or IL-1 (gevokizumab) that failed to meet their primary endpoints in phase III trials.

Daclizumab

Daclizumab (Zybrinta) is an IL-2R inhibitor. IL-2 receptor (IL-2R) system is a well-characterized lymphokine receptor system that plays a central role in the induction of immune responses. High-affinity IL-2R complexes are expressed on activated lymphoid cells. They consist of three subunits (α, β, and γ), each capable of binding IL-2. The 70-kDa IL-2R and 64-kDa IL-2R subunits are normally expressed on most resting T, B, natural killer (NK), and lymphokine-activated killer cells, which mediate signaling and receptor internalization. The 55-kDa IL-2 (p55, Tac, or CD25) subunit, however, is expressed by most T, B, and NK cells only after they have been activated by interaction with an antigen or with IL-2. The Tac subunit associated with the IL-2R β-γ subunits forms the high-affinity IL-2R complex. Thus expression of the Tac subunit marks a critical step in the activation of all T cells that are major contributors to both allograft destruction and autoimmune disorders. Caspi et al.[140] demonstrated the presence of high-affinity IL-2 receptors in animal models of uveitis (see Chapter 1). Additionally, IL-2 receptors can be demonstrated on the surface of human cells in patients with uveitis. The humanized anti-Tac monoclonal antibody (daclizumab [Zybrinta]) is a recombinant monoclonal immunoglobulin of the human immunoglobulin (Ig)G1 isotype. The recombinant genes encoding daclizumab are a composite of human (90%) and murine (10%) antibody sequences. Therefore the antibody is "humanized" by combining the complementarity-determining regions and other selected residues of the murine anti-Tac antibody with the framework and constant regions of the human IgG1 antibody. It is hoped that daclizumab can suppress the autoreactive T cells, which play a critical role in the development of intraocular inflammation in patients with uveitis. There are no known toxicities specific to daclizumab, although administration of such a foreign protein could cause an allergic or anaphylactic reaction. Some of the reactions that may have been associated with daclizumab in a small number of patients were shortness of breath and low blood pressure.

A trial of daclizumab at the NEI, which has been going on for several years,[141,142] suggests that there is benefit from daclizumab therapy for noninfectious uveitis. This observation is based on outcomes in a small group of patients. In the original study, in nine of 10 participants with uveitis treated with daclizumab infusions every 4 weeks, the doses were successfully tapered off the standard immunosuppressive regimens, and the patients subsequently continued to receive daclizumab, with maintenance or improvement of their visual acuity. After 4 years, seven of these 10 patients continued to receive the drug. Patients initially received infusions and currently receive a subcutaneous preparation of the medication once a month. Adverse effects possibly, but not clearly, related to daclizumab recorded in this study included cutaneous lesions; edema; upper extremity neuralgia; upper respiratory tract infections, such as colds and bronchitis; and herpes zoster. One patient in this study, after 4 years of monthly daclizumab therapy, was found to have a small, low-grade renal cell carcinoma that was surgically removed. This patient was initially withdrawn from further daclizumab treatments, but subsequently the treatment was restarted. One of the subsequent studies was a small multicenter study examining the possibility of treatment with subcutaneously administered daclizumab without an infusion as induction therapy. Preliminary data suggested that de novo subcutaneous daclizumab therapy yields very good serum levels for an extended period, permitting tapering of other immunosuppressive agents. It would appear that this approach is useful in treating disease that is controlled: that is, daclizumab is given when patient's disease is controlled with "standard" immunosuppression, which then can be tapered, leaving daclizumab as the only agent. Papaliodis et al.[143] have reported that daclizumab was an effective therapeutic agent for some of their patients. We noted that patients with active intraocular inflammatory disease did not respond and those with quiet disease did not respond, and they were then switched to daclizumab therapy. We performed a small study in which patients with active intermediate and posterior uveitis initially received 8 mg/kg of daclizumab, followed 2 weeks later by 4 mg/kg, after which a standard dose of daclizumab was administered monthly. By 4 weeks, four of the five patients showed a two-step decrease in vitreous haze, with the fifth patient meeting that goal at week 20. Vision at enrollment was 69.2 ETDRS letters, and after treatment was 78.2 letters ($P < 0.12$).[144] Daclizumab was approved by the FDA for the treatment of multiple sclerosis in 2016. However, in 2018, it was voluntarily withdrawn from the market after reports of encephalitis in Europe.

Etanercept

Etanercept (Enbrel) is engineered to contain two identical soluble tumor necrosis factor (TNF) receptors that have been fused with the Fc domain of human IgG1. This molecule binds to and inactivates TNF. In support of the use of this medication in the treatment of human disease is the finding that TNF-α is found during the acute phase of experimental autoimmune uveoretinitis.[145] Additionally, TNF-α levels are higher in both the aqueous humor and the serum of patients with uveitis compared with those of control subjects.[146] Interestingly, the serum levels were significantly higher than the aqueous humor levels and correlated with recurrent uveitis. In the clinical realm, etanercept has been used extensively in the treatment of patients with rheumatologic disorders. In one randomized study, patients with rheumatoid arthritis that was persistently active despite methotrexate therapy did significantly better when etanercept was added to their regimen (25 mg subcutaneously twice weekly).[147] In a study treating children with polyarticular juvenile rheumatoid arthritis, patients' joints responded statistically far better to etanercept (0.4 mg/kg subcutaneously twice weekly) than to placebo.[148] No differences in adverse effects were noted. The effect of this medication and the next (infliximab) seems not to be as clear. Smith et al.[149] evaluated 16 patients, 14 receiving etanercept and two receiving infliximab for either eye inflammation or joint disease. Eight patients had rheumatoid arthritis, three had juvenile rheumatoid arthritis, and three had uveitis without joint disease. All of the 12 with articular disease saw benefits with either medication; however, only six of 16 (38%) of those with uveitis had any benefit. It was the conclusion of the authors that other TNF inhibitors, particularly Remicade, may be better at controlling associated inflammatory arthritis than uveitis. Since the initial observation, multiple studies have reported either new-onset uveitis while using etanercept for rheumatologic indications or failure of control of the existing uveitis with etanercept. A study from the United Kingdom[150] evaluated the risk of new-onset uveitis among 2294 patients with juvenile idiopathic arthritis (JIA) receiving methotrexate (n = 943), adalimumab/infliximab (n = 304), etanercept (n = 1047) and observed that new-onset uveitis was most common among methotrexate users followed by etanercept, whereas it was uncommon among infliximab or adalimumab users. The authors noted the younger age of some of the methotrexate users, which was an inherent risk factor for uveitis. Overall, uveitis was significantly less likely to develop in patients on biologics.[150] A registry-based study from Germany indicated that the rate of new-onset uveitis was similar in etanercept and methotrexate users.[151]

In spite of ongoing debate regarding etanercept being associated with a higher risk of new-onset uveitis, it appears that etanercept is less effective for uveitis than for arthritis, and therefore current guidelines for inflammatory ocular disease strongly recommend the use of TNF inhibitors other than etanercept for the treatment of uveitis.[152]

The major concern associated with this agent is infection. Serious infections, including sepsis, have developed in patients who have received etanercept, and several have died as a result of their infections within 2 to 16 weeks of initiation of therapy. Etanercept should not be used in patients with active infections, whether chronic or acute, localized or generalized, and it should be discontinued if a serious infection develops. Live vaccines should not be given. The most frequent AEs reported in clinical trials were injection site reactions (37%), infections (35%), and headaches (17%). Malignancies were rare[153]; autoantibody development has been reported, although clinical symptoms of a lupus-like syndrome are rare. As with infliximab, there is concern regarding the possible reactivation of tuberculosis. Fonollosa et al.[154] reported that tuberculous uveitis appeared in a patient receiving etanercept for rheumatoid arthritis. A study in the United Kingdom by Davies et al. reported significantly higher rates of medically significant infections among etanercept-treated children compared with methotrexate-treated children with JIA (2.13 times higher risk in the etanercept cohort).[155]

Infliximab

Infliximab (Remicade) is a mouse-derived chimeric monoclonal antibody directed against TNF-α. It interferes with the binding of TNF to the two known receptors: TNFr1, which binds to soluble TNF, and TNFr2, which binds membrane-bound TNF. Sfikakis et al.[156] reported administering one infliximab infusion to five patients with Behçet disease, resulting in marked resolution of disease within 24 hours and "complete" suppression by 7 days (see also the review by Sfikakis[157]). It is difficult to assess the value of this treatment because the authors reported that the ocular inflammatory disease went into remission after 7 days, which is what could occur during the natural course of Behçet disease. Only a comparison of the number of attacks could really help assess the value of this approach (see Chapter 27). However, there have been more reports strongly suggesting that these initial observations may be valid. Indeed, the criteria for the use of infliximab in Behçet disease have been published, suggesting its use if first-line agents are not effective.[158] Pipitone et al.[159] reported the usefulness of this agent in treating neuro-Behçet disease. Seven patients with human leukocyte antigen (HLA)-B27–associated anterior uveitis were treated with infliximab (10 mg/kg);[160] six of the seven responded, but relapses were seen in four after a median 5 to 6.4 months. It has been used for active scleritis with good results.[161] There have been numerous reports on the use of this medication in childhood uveitis, other types of intermediate and posterior uveitis, and retinal vasculitis. As with many studies, the authors claimed success (we do that, too!). It is clear from the number of articles that a real therapeutic effect does exist. However, the caveat is always that without a controlled trial, we just cannot measure the real effect of a treatment in either the short term or the long term.

As with etanercept, the major concern with infliximab is an increased risk of infection, particularly tuberculosis[162] (including its unmasking), with one calculation being a risk of 70 in 147,000 cases. Ten instances of life-threatening *Histoplasmosis capsulatum* infection have also been reported, nine in patients receiving infliximab and one in a patient receiving etanercept.[163] It has been suggested that signaling through the TNF2 receptor may be crucial in host defenses against intracellular pathogens, such as *Mycobacterium tuberculosis.* In addition, the use of infliximab may exacerbate brain lesions associated with multiple sclerosis. These changes were noted on magnetic resonance imaging (MRI).[164] Aseptic meningitis, lupus-like syndromes, and retrobulbar optic neuritis have been reported.[165] Although methotrexate-associated pneumonitis is seen in 1% of patients, Kramer et al.[166] reported pulmonary toxicity in 3 of 50 patients (6%) receiving a stable dose of methotrexate and infliximab. Malignancies are rare.[153]

Infliximab is currently FDA approved for the treatment of Crohn's disease, ulcerative colitis, rheumatoid arthritis, psoriatic arthritis and psoriasis, and ankylosing spondylitis but is not approved for uveitis. Nevertheless, there are numerous anecdotal reports in the literature that support the use of infliximab in birdshot chorioretinitis, Behçet disease, and many other noninfectious uveitides.[167] It has been suggested to be effective also for uveitic macular edema.[168] In these uncontrolled studies, success rates in corticosteroid sparing was quite high at 80%, but relapses were common upon cessation. Use of a second agent, an antimetabolite, has been recommended to reduce the risk of anti–drug antibody formation. The dosage for FDA-approved indications range from 3 to 5 mg/kg and interval ranges from every 4 weeks to every 8 weeks for maintenance with varying regimens of induction.[169] For uveitis, the starting dose is commonly 5 mg/kg given 2 weeks apart as an induction dose followed by every 4 to 8 weeks as a maintenance regimen, although doses higher than 5 mg/kg can often be required to treat uveitis.[167] An expert panel review of the use of TNF inhibitors in ocular inflammatory disorders recommended infliximab and adalimumab as second-line immunomodulatory agents for the treatment of severe posterior and panuveitis and severe uveitis associated with seronegative spondyloarthropathies.[152] The panel also recommended the use of the same TNF inhibitors for the treatment of severe scleritis that is recalcitrant to standard immunosuppressives or with patient intolerance. The panel recommended that infliximab or adalimumab be used as a first- or second-line steroid-sparing agent for Behçet disease and as a second-line steroid-sparing agent after methotrexate use (Fig. 8.15). More recently, the American College of Rheumatology (ACR)/Arthritis Guidelines, published in 2019, recommended monoclonal TNF inhibitors, such as infliximab and adalimumab, as first-line biologic treatment for JIA-associated uveitis.[170] In case of poor response, the experts also conditionally recommended escalating the dose and/or frequency of the monoclonal TNFi to above the standard.

Adalimumab

Adalimumab (Humira) is a fully human anti–TNF-α monoclonal antibody (IgG1) that blocks the interaction of TNF-α with p75 and p55 cell surface receptors. Adalimumab has been evaluated in several trials in rheumatoid arthritis, including studies where it was combined with methotrexate. It has been licensed for use in rheumatoid arthritis, Crohn disease, ulcerative colitis, psoriasis and psoriatic arthritis, ankylosing spondylitis, hidradenitis suppurativa, and JIA. Adalimumab was approved for the treatment of uveitis by the FDA in 2016 after the successful completion of the VISUAL trials, making adalimumab the first

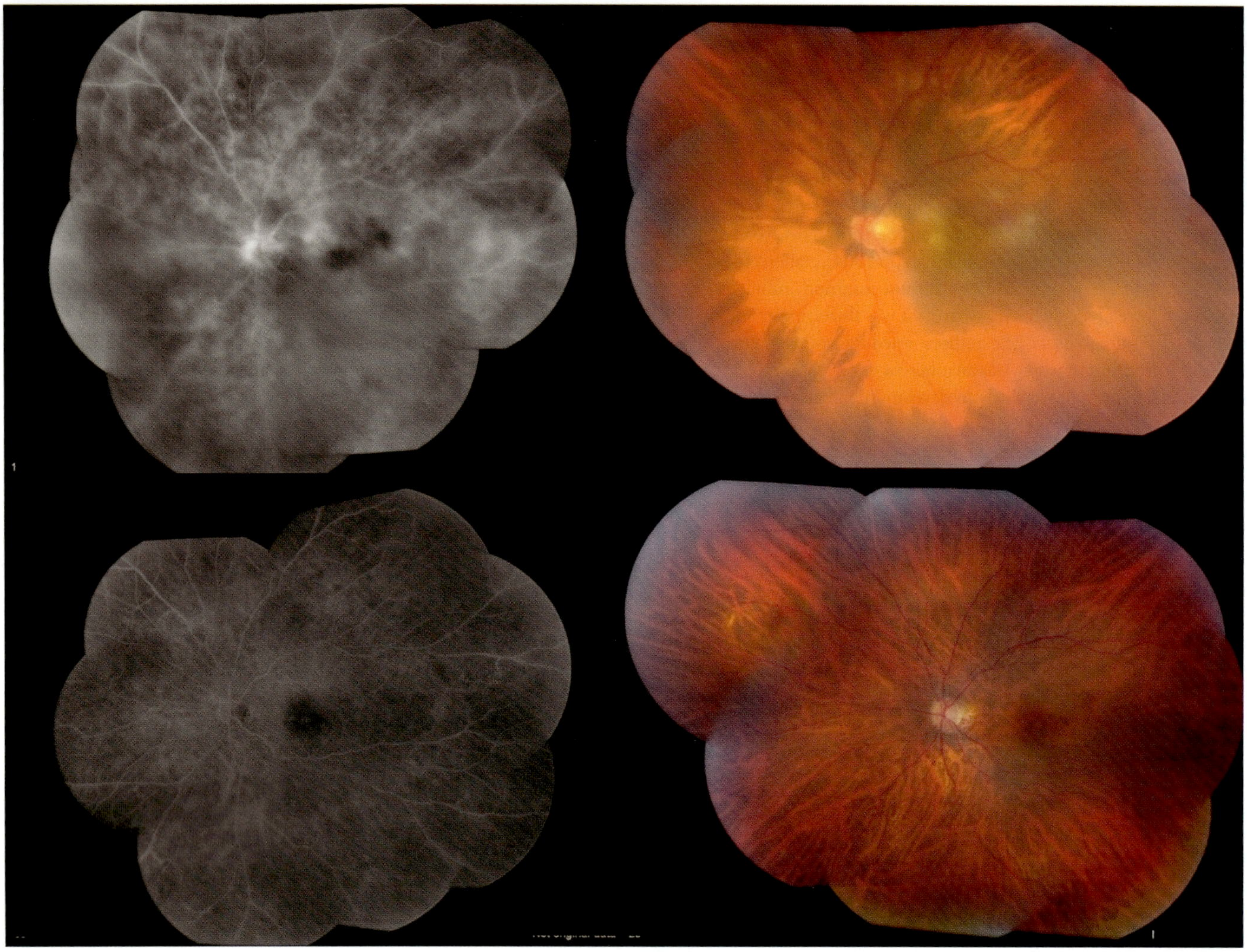

Fig. 8.15 Necrotizing retinitis and extensive retinal vasculitis in the left eye of a patient with Behcet's disease (upper panel) showed significant improvement with infliximab therapy (lower panel). Note the resolution of macular retinitis, vitritis and vasculitis.

biologic to be approved for the treatment of uveitis. Both the VISUAL-I (Efficacy and Safety of Adalimumab in Patients With Active Uveitis) and the VISUAL-II (Efficacy and Safety of Adalimumab in Subjects With Inactive Uveitis) trials were randomized, placebo-controlled, double-masked clinical trials, which enrolled patients with posterior segment uveitis.[171,172] In both studies, patients received placebo or adalimumab (80-mg loading dose and 40-mg dose every 2 weeks starting at week 1). VISUAL-I enrolled patients with active uveitis, and these patients received an initial 60-mg prednisone burst, and the dose was tapered to 0 mg corticosteroids by week 15; the primary outcome measure was time to treatment failure (TTF), which was defined as the inability to achieve anterior chamber cell grade or a vitreous haze grade of 0 to 0.5; worsening of anterior chamber or vitreous inflammation; new chorioretinal or retinal vasculitis lesion; or worsening of BCVA. Adalimumab reduced treatment failure by 50% and resulted in longer time to treatment failure (24 weeks versus 13 weeks). VISUAL-II enrolled patients with quiet but steroid-dependent chronic uveitis who needed 10 to 35 mg/day prednisone as a maintenance dose. Adalimumab reduced the risk of treatment failure by 43% and lengthened the time to treatment failure (18 versus 8.3 months in the adalimumab and placebo arms, respectively). AEs were more common in the adalimumab group compared with the placebo group in VISUAL-I, but similar rates of AEs were observed in VISUAL-II as well. In an open-label extension of both studies (N=424 patients) to assess the long-term safety and efficacy of adalimumab (VISUAL-III Trial), adjustments to the dosages of corticosteroids and other medications were permitted while all patients continued to receive 40 mg adalimumab every 2 weeks.[173] At 78 weeks, 80% of patients had quiet disease, with no or minimal corticosteroids. Those who entered the study with active uveitis showed improvement in visual acuity, and those who entered with quiet disease maintained their visual acuity. There were 36 severe AEs (3.8 events/100 person-years) possibly related to adalimumab, 38 serious infections, 12 malignancies, 1 active tuberculosis, and 15 latent tuberculosis. Importantly, no new safety signals were identified in the extension study or in comparison with other diseases.

Adalimumab, in combination with methotrexate, was also shown to be effective and superior to methotrexate alone in a randomized placebo-controlled trial in 90 patients with JIA-associated uveitis (a randomised controlled trial of the clinical effectiveness, SafetY and Cost-effectiveness of Adalimumab in Combination with MethOtRExate for the treatment of juvenile idiopathic arthritis associated uveitis: SYCAMORE trial).[174] Adalimumab reduced treatment failure by 75% in this study and resulted in decreased daily dose of topical corticosteroids. In a small, randomized, double-masked clinical trial, which enrolled 31 patients with early-onset JIA-associated uveitis (Effect of Adalimumab for the Treatment of Uveitis in Juvenile Idiopathic Arthritis: ADJUVITE Trial), 2 months of adalimumab treatment was effective in controlling inflammation and reduced anterior chamber inflammation by 30%, as determined by a laser flare photometer.[175]

Prior to its approval, adalimumab was reported to be useful in the treatment of Behçet disease, VKH, sarcoidosis, and childhood uveitis.[176-182] The dose for uveitis treatment is similar to that for plaque psoriasis: 80 mg initial dose, followed by 40 mg every other week starting 1 week after the initial dose.[183] Humanized monoclonal antibodies are theoretically superior to those that are chimeric and has the advantage of being less immunogenic. Whether adalimumab has therapeutic effectiveness equal to that of infliximab is still being debated. Studies on nonocular immune-mediated diseases, such as Crohn disease, showed that although the two most commonly used TNF inhibitors, infliximab and adalimumab, were in general comparable in their efficacy, infliximab was more likely to be used in more severe disease forms. They also noted that combination of infliximab with nonbiologic immunosuppressive drugs provided additional benefit; but it was not the case with adalimumab. This is largely explained by the improved pharmacokinetics of the biologic by the addition of the nonbiologic immunomodulator.[184] Two large studies in Europe investigated the comparative effectiveness of infliximab and adalimumab. A large retrospective multicenter study by the French Uveitis Network, which included 160 patients with uveitis of various etiologies, such as Behçet disease, JIA, and others, did not find any differences between infliximab and adalimumab in terms of effectiveness or side effects.[185] In a separate retrospective study of 107 patients in Italy, infliximab and adalimumab were shown to have comparable effectiveness overall; however, infliximab appeared better in terms of corticosteroid-sparing effect and resolution of macular edema. In contrast, Lejoyeux et al. showed that both adalimumab and infliximab improved macular edema at similar rates in a retrospective cohort of 25 patients from France.[186] As in the case of other TNF inhibitors, adalimumab use should also be avoided in patients with active tuberculosis or multiple sclerosis because it can cause serious infections, allergic reactions, reactivation of hepatitis B infection, heart failure, and lymphoma and other malignancies.[153] Screening patients with intermediate uveitis to rule out multiple sclerosis before starting TNF inhibitors has also been suggested.[135]

Other TNF inhibitors, such as golimumab (Simponi), a fully human monoclonal antibody, and certolizumab pegol (Cimzia), a humanized PEGylated monoclonal antibody, have also been used in the treatment of uveitis, albeit less often. Both certolizumab and golimumab have been found to be effective in 50% to 55% of patients, most of whom were previously treated with (and failed or were intolerant to) another TNF inhibitor.[187] Both agents have been used in Behçet disease–associated uveitis, spondyloarthropathy, or JIA-associated anterior uveitis.[188] Certolizumab, because of being PEGylated, is considered to have better bioavailability. In a phase III RCT evaluating its efficacy in the treatment of ankylosing spondylitis uveitis, flares were observed to be significantly lower in the certolizumab arm compared with the placebo arm.[189]

Rituximab

Rituximab (Rituxan) is a genetically engineered chimeric murine/human monoclonal IgG1 κ antibody directed against the CD20 antigen. The Fab domain of rituximab binds to the CD20 antigen on B lymphocytes, and the Fc domain recruits immune effector functions to mediate B-cell lysis in vitro, leading to B-cell depletion. Rituximab has an approximate molecular weight of 145 kDa. It has been used to treat a number of hematologic processes, including B-cell lymphoma and primary CNS lymphoma.[190,191] It will certainly be used for the treatment of primary intraocular lymphoma because preliminary reports have suggested its usefulness. There are also studies reporting its use in ocular adnexal lymphomas.[192,193] Rituximab has been reported to have a positive therapeutic effect in rheumatoid arthritis and other autoimmune diseases.[194] The recommended dose is 375 mg/m^2 as an intravenous infusion, weekly for four to eight doses for non-Hodgkin lymphoma and two 1000-mg intravenous infusions separated by 2 weeks for rheumatoid arthritis (for rheumatoid arthritis, it is given intravenously at days 0 and 15 and is combined with methotrexate 10–25 mg/week). Glucocorticoids, administered as methylprednisolone 100 mg intravenously or its equivalent 30 minutes before each infusion, are recommended to reduce the incidence and severity of infusion reactions. In rheumatoid arthritis, treatment with rituximab induced depletion of peripheral B lymphocytes, with all patients demonstrating near complete depletion within 2 weeks after receiving the first dose of Rituxan. The majority of patients showed peripheral B-cell depletion for at least 6 months, followed by subsequent gradual recovery after that time. A small proportion of patients (4%) had prolonged peripheral B-cell depletion lasting longer than 3 years after a single course of treatment. In rheumatoid arthritis studies, total serum immunoglobulin levels and IgM, IgG, and IgA levels were reduced at 6 months, with the greatest change observed in IgM levels. However, mean immunoglobulin levels remained normal over the 24-week period. Small numbers of patients experienced reductions in IgM (7%), IgG (2%), and IgA (1%) levels, below the lower limit of normal. The clinical consequences of a reduction in immunoglobulin levels in patients with rheumatoid arthritis treated with rituximab are unclear.

This raises a very interesting question with regard to the mechanism of rituximab because anti–T-cell therapy has been the predominant approach in the past. B cells may be acting at multiple sites in the autoimmune/inflammatory process, including through the production of rheumatoid factor (RF) and other autoantibodies, antigen presentation, T-cell activation, and/or proinflammatory cytokine production; alternatively, it may be inducing peripheral immune tolerance. Rituximab has been used in the treatment of anterior uveitis, Behçet disease, granulomatosis with polyangiitis (previously known as Wegener granulomatosis), scleritis, and orbital inflammation, with success rates ranging from 75% to greater than 90%. In most cases, rituximab was initiated as the third- or fourth-line immunosuppressive agent.[195-201]

Anakinra

Anakinra (Kineret) is a recombinant human IL-1 receptor antagonist (IL-1RA) that binds to IL-1 type 1 receptors. In doing so, it downregulates the proinflammatory effects of IL-1. It has been shown to effectively treat the clinical expression of experimentally induced uveitis in mice.[202] Reports of its use in patients with ocular inflammation have been published. This includes pediatric patients with uveitis and CINCA (chronic infantile neurologic, cutaneous, and articular) syndrome[203] and Blau syndrome, a pediatric granulomatous arthritis associated with the *NOD2* gene.[204]

Alemtuzumab

Alemtuzumab (Campath) is an anti-CD52 monoclonal antibody that targets T and B lymphocytes. It has been used to treat a variety of hematologic disorders, including myelodysplastic syndrome, aplastic anemia, chronic lymphocytic leukemia, and T-cell leukemias/lymphomas.[205-207] Dick et al.[208] reported its use for severe ocular inflammation in 10 patients with a variety of ophthalmic inflammatory diseases, including Wegener granulomatosis, retinal vasculitis, sympathetic ophthalmia, and Behçet disease. All patients showed initial improvement, and remission was seen in eight. No serious AEs were noted during a short follow-up period.[208] Alemtuzumab was found to induce remission in greater than 80% of patients with Behçet disease and in a case of multiple sclerosis–associated uveitis.[209,210] This finding is certainly intriguing and thought-provoking and needs further investigation.

Abatacept

Abatacept (Orencia) medication is a fusion protein that consists of the extracellular domain of the human cytotoxic T-lymphocyte–associated antigen 4 (CTLA-4) and a modified Fc portion of an IgG1 molecule. It binds to the ligand of CTLA-4 and is used in the treatment of rheumatoid arthritis and JIA. Its use, to date, in the treatment of uveitis has been very limited, with one report published so far.[211] It can be used alone or in conjunction with disease-modifying antirheumatic drugs (DMARDs), such as methotrexate, but not with a TNF-α inhibitor. Studies have shown that patients receiving abatacept and infliximab (Remicade) had considerably higher rates of infection compared with controls. Abatacept is also not recommended in patients with chronic obstructive pulmonary disease (COPD), again because of the risk of infection. It may increase the risk of lymphoma and possibly lung carcinoma. Studies investigating the effectiveness of abatacept in uveitis have been limited to small retrospective cohorts and have yielded mixed results. However, it should be noted that in most cases, abatacept has been used in TNF-inhibitor refractory disease. In a retrospective study by Tappeiner et al., which included 21 patients with JIA-associated refractory uveitis, abatacept was found to be minimally effective. Initial inflammation control was achieved in 11 of 21 patients, in 8 of whom the inflammation was later reactivated.[212] However, there have also been case series suggesting the contrary, with findings of sustained improvement in uveitis regardless of whether it is used as a first- or second-line biologic in JIA-associated uveitis.[213,214]

Tocilizumab

Tocilizumab (Actemra) is a monoclonal antibody directed against the IL-6 receptor. It is approved by the FDA for the treatment of JIA, rheumatoid arthritis, and giant cell arteritis. There have been many reports of tocilizumab use in various types of uveitis, including JIA-associated uveitis, Behçet disease–associated uveitis, birdshot chorioretinopathy, pediatric intermediate uveitis and panuveitis, and uveitic macular edema. Most of these reports were of cases that were refractory to TNF inhibitors and where tocilizumab was used as a second- or sometimes a third-line biologic. Response rates ranged from 63% to 75%.[215-221] Tocilizumab has been found particularly effective in uveitic macular edema. [216,222,223] In a retrospective multicenter study that included 25 patients with various uveitis subtypes recalcitrant to corticosteroids and at least one immunomodulatory agent, Vegas-Revenga et al. found tocilizumab to be effective in reducing macular edema and improving visual acuity.[216] The same group also investigated the effectiveness of tocilizumab in patients with recalcitrant JIA-associated uveitis and found that 76% of 25 patients achieved complete remission; significant improvement in macular edema and visual acuity and significant reduction in concomitant corticosteroids were also observed.[223] We have also found that tocilizumab can be effective in chronic retinal vasculitis and macular edema (Fig. 8.16). The ACR/Arthritis Guidelines, published in 2019, also conditionally recommended tocilizumab for patients who have already failed methotrexate and monoclonal TNF inhibitors.[170]

A phase II RCT using intravenous tocilizumab 4 mg/kg and 8 mg/kg every 4 weeks showed significant reduction in vitreous haze among patients with posterior segment uveitis, 60% of whom were treatment naive. Vitreous haze improved in approximately 45% of patients with grade 2 or greater vitreous haze at baseline.[224]

Ustekinumab

Ustekinumab (Stelara) is a monoclonal antibody that targets the p40 subunit of both IL-12 and IL-23. It is currently FDA approved for the treatment of Crohn disease, psoriasis, and psoriatic arthritis. There are three case reports of successful treatment of uveitis in patients with Crohn disease or psoriasis.[225,226] Ustekinumab is currently being evaluated for the treatment of uveitis in two phase II trials, one at the NEI and another in France (Clinicaltrials.gov).

Interferon-α

IFN-α (Intron® A, Roferon®-A) is used for its antitumor and antiviral actions, but the exact mechanism for either is not known, except that it inhibits tumor growth and viral replication. One report has suggested that IFN-α may inhibit the inflammatory processes by enhancing IL-10 production, which may be an AE in a patient with acquired immunodeficiency syndrome (AIDS) but very beneficial in one with an excessive sterile inflammatory response.[227] It has been used in the treatment of the ocular complications of Behçet disease and multiple sclerosis.[230] Several reports have suggested that treatment with IFN-α will diminish or completely stop all attacks (see Chapter 27). Both IFN-α2a and IFN-α12b and IFN-β have been used to treat uveitis, mostly Behçet uveitis, multiple sclerosis–associated uveitis, or uveitic macular edema.[229-233] Kötter et al.[234] used an initial dose of 6 × 106 units subcutaneously daily and then 3 × 106 units every day for 1 month, followed by 3 × 106 units subcutaneously every other day. This group saw an improvement in all seven patients treated. Pivetti-Pezzi et al.[235] and Wechsler et al.[236] used a dose of 3 × 106 units three times a week. Pivetti-Pezzi et al.[235] saw a 50% reduction in ocular relapses. Fardeau et al. showed, in an RCT with 48 patients, that IFN-α2a was superior to placebo in reducing macular edema.[237] A similar benefit was observed in patients with multiple sclerosis–associated uveitis and macular edema with the use of IFN-β.[238] There have been numerous reports suggesting the usefulness of this approach, from treating nerve-head neovascularization[239] in Behçet disease to performing intraocular surgery under IFN-α therapy.[240] All patients had a flu-like illness during therapy, and a Behçet disease–like retinopathy has been associated with IFN-α. It is interesting that the use of IFN for Behçet disease is far more common in Europe than in North America. The FDA further warns that IFN-α could cause or aggravate fatal or life-threatening neuropsychiatric, autoimmune, ischemic, and infectious disorders. RCTs are needed to resolve this difference and see whether the potential advantages of IFN-α outweigh the potential risks.

Intravenous Immunoglobulin Therapy

Intravenous immunoglobulin (IVIg) therapy has been used in the treatment of a few patients with ocular inflammatory disease, including ocular cicatricial pemphigoid, VKH syndrome, and birdshot retinopathy[241-243] and in patients with cancer-associated retinopathy.[244] IVIg was initially intended for the treatment of patients with immunodeficiency. It is a preparation that is almost completely intact IgG, including all IgG subclasses as seen in normal human plasma. It is a pooled material made up from 7 to 10,000 donors[241] and has slowly found a place in the treatment of putative immune-mediated disorders, such as Guillain-Barré syndrome, Kawasaki disease, and juvenile dermatomyositis. The mechanism of its action is speculative (Fig. 8.17),[245] and several, such as blockage of B-cell responses, inhibition of phagocytosis, and alteration of cytokine production, have been suggested.[246] It has been suggested that immunoglobulins may neutralize C3a and C5a of the complement cascade, also known as *anaphylotoxins.*[247] It has been reported to prevent the expression of experimental autoimmune uveitis.[248] Rosenbaum et al.[243] treated 10 patients with IVIg, five of whom appeared to have a clear clinical benefit. Patients received a dosage of 0.5 g/kg body weight/day (infused over 4 hours) for 3 consecutive days on a monthly basis, which was ultimately changed to an every-3-month schedule. Guy and Aptsiauri[244] reported using IVIg in three patients with carcinoma-associated retinopathy. One patient had improved visual acuity within 24 hours of the first dose, one had an improvement in visual fields but no increase in vision, and one had no improvement. Some concerns that have been raised include the

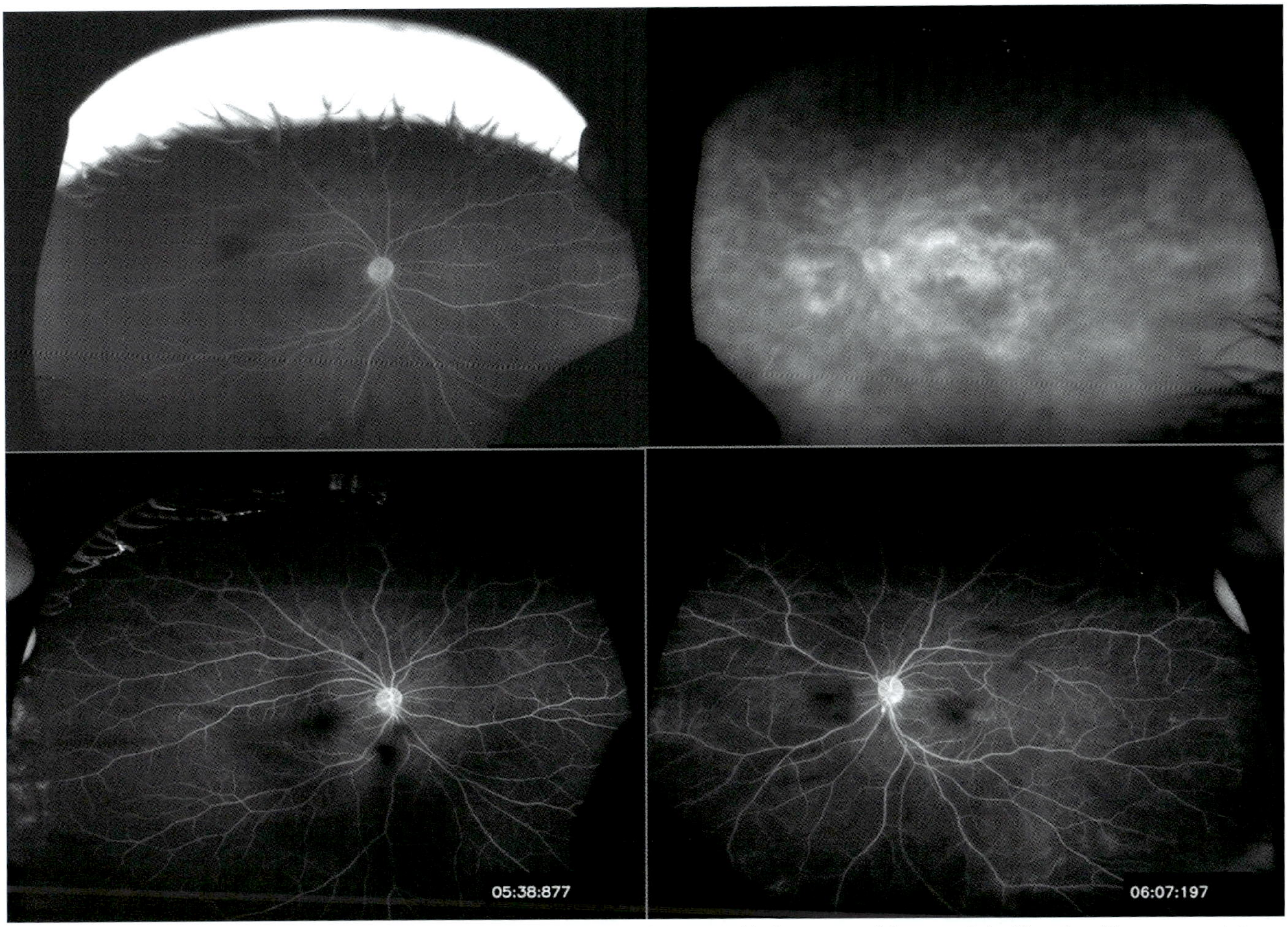

Fig. 8.16 Significant chronic vascular leakage in the left eye of a patient with panuveitis (upper panel) improved significantly with near complete resolution following intravenous tocilizumab therapy (lower panel). Note that this patient previously failed methotrexate, mycophenolate, cyclosporine, and two TNF inhibitors.]

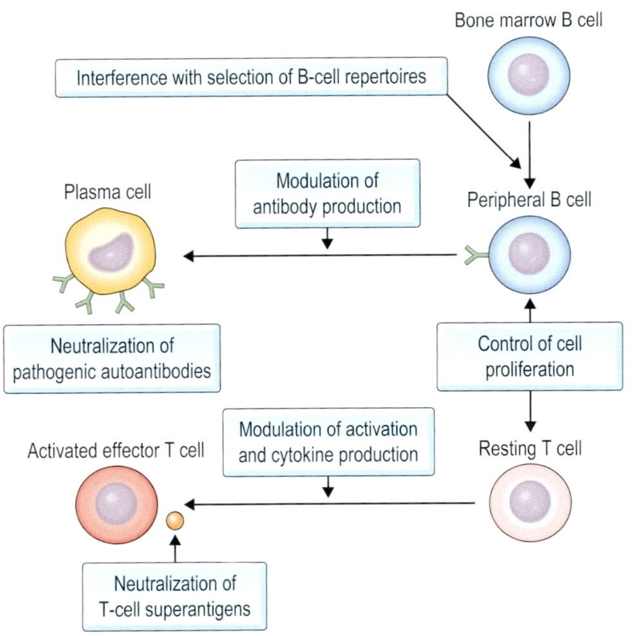

Fig. 8.17 Effects of intravenous immunoglobulin (IVIg) on the immune system. (Reproduced with permission from Kazatchkine MD, Kaveri SV. Immunomodulation of autoimmune and inflammatory diseases with intravenous immune globulin. *N Engl Med J.* 2001;345(6):747–755. Copyright 2001 Massachusetts Medical Society. All rights reserved.)

problem of infection despite surveillance. Hepatitis C infection was ascribed to this form of therapy, and we still are concerned about disorders caused by prions. Uveitis has been described in patients after IVIg infusions for immune-mediated (nonocular) disorders,[249] and there is a risk of thrombosis, including retinal vein thrombosis. Finally, IVIg should not be given to patients with isolated IgA deficiency because they develop allergic responses to preparations that contain IgA.

OTHER THERAPEUTIC APPROACHES

Janus Kinase Inhibitors

Janus kinases (JAKs) are intracellular cytoplasmic tyrosine kinases and the Janus kinase/signal transducers and activator of transcription (JAK-STAT) pathway mediates responses to cytokines (e.g., IL-6) and growth factors. JAK inhibitors are a new target for the treatment of immune-mediated diseases, including uveitis. Tofacitinib (Xeljanz; Pfizer Inc., New York, NY), a JAK1, -2, -3 inhibitor, is currently approved for the treatment of rheumatoid arthritis, psoriatic arthritis, ulcerative colitis, and ankylosing spondylitis. There are anecdotal reports suggesting that tofacitinib may be effective in refractory uveitis, scleritis, and JIA-associated uveitis.[250-252]

Another novel selective JAK1 inhibitor, filgotinib (GLPG0634/GS-6034; Galapagos NV/Gilead, Mechelen, Belgium; Foster City, CA) is currently under investigation in a phase II RCT for the treatment of uveitis. FDA approval is pending for the treatment of rheumatoid arthritis after successful completion of phase III trials in over 3000 patients with rheumatoid arthritis.

Plasmapheresis

The removal from the bloodstream of toxic products is a concept that originated in the study performed by Abel et al. in 1914.[253] The first therapeutic success with the use of plasmapheresis was for macroglobulinemia.[254] The rationale for this approach is that soluble products in blood could be readily removed, and so it was tried in such diseases as systemic lupus erythematosus (SLE), in which immune complexes were thought to play an important role in pathogenesis. The exact mechanism of action of plasmapheresis remains speculative. It is possible that even if humoral mechanisms are less important in intraocular inflammatory disease, this approach could remove cytokines important for the propagation or perpetuation of disease. The role of plasmapheresis in uveitis still is not clear. It has been reported as being effective in treating the acute attacks of Behçet disease,[255] but its continued use is unwieldy, and although initial success may be seen, a rebound of the disease may occur with time. Therefore to maintain a more prolonged clinical effect, most studies have resorted to adding corticosteroids or cytotoxic agents.[254]

Nonsteroidal Anti-inflammatory Agents

Prostaglandin inhibitors are well known to the ophthalmic community. They have been suggested to be therapeutically helpful in treating various ocular conditions, including aphakic macular edema.[256] Some reports have suggested that indomethacin reduces the severity and recurrences of anterior uveitis when used in conjunction with corticosteroids. Although isolated reports discussed the use of these agents in the treatment of uveitis,[257] they have not been demonstrated to be effective as sole agents in the treatment of endogenous intraocular inflammatory disease. Herbort,[258] however, has looked extensively at the use of diclofenac in the treatment of capsulotomy inflammatory responses after neodymium:yttrium–aluminum–garnet (Nd:YAG) laser treatment. He reported that an effective therapeutic endpoint could be achieved with a combination of dexamethasone acetate 0.1% (Maxidex drops), diclofenac drops 0.1% (Voltaren-Ophtha), and systemic diclofenac (Voltaren). Diclofenac may be useful as a sole agent in treating postoperative cataract inflammation.

Oral Tolerance

Oral tolerance is an approach that has received much clinical interest. A discussion of some of the basic mechanisms leading to the clinical application mentioned here can be found in Chapter 1. Feeding of antigens has been reported to be effective in the treatment of multiple sclerosis and rheumatoid arthritis.[259,260] In a pilot study, this approach was applied to two patients with uveitis, one with pars planitis and one with the ocular complications of Behçet disease.[261] The patients who entered into this study had lymphocytes demonstrating in vitro proliferative responses to the retinal S-antigen (S-Ag). The patient with pars planitis had been treated with prednisone and was able to stop his medication completely once administration of 30 mg of S-Ag three times a week was initiated. Of interest is the fact that because of the maintenance of good visual acuity with this approach, continued oral dosing of the retinal S-Ag was stopped, in the hope that long-standing tolerance had been achieved. However, the patient experienced reactivation of his disease. He was treated with systemic steroids and S-Ag was begun again; the patient ultimately needed no further medication because his disease abated, and he was left with a visual acuity of 20/20 and 20/25 in each eye. After these observations, a phase I/II masked RCT was undertaken to evaluate the effect and safety of the oral administration of retinal antigens.[263] Patients with uveitis were randomly assigned to receive either bovine retinal S-Ag alone, a mixture of soluble retinal antigens alone, retinal S-Ag and retinal soluble antigens, or placebo. Although the time to the primary endpoint (time to ocular inflammatory disease) was not statistically significant for any of the groups, in the group that received the purified S-Ag alone, it appeared that their immunosuppressive medication could be tapered off more successfully compared with either the placebo group ($P = 0.08$) or the two groups receiving multiple soluble antigens. No toxic effects attributable to any treatment were observed.[263] Thurau and Wildner[264] used as an antigen for uveitis a 14–amino acid sequence of HLA-B antigens that was seen to mimic retinal S-Ag. The underlying logic for this choice is different from using the retinal S-Ag found in the eye. Here, it is hypothesized that because of low avidity, T cells that can bind to this antigen sequence escape the normal clearing mechanisms in the thymus and enter the systemic circulation. Under certain circumstances, these cells can enter the eye and are then activated by antigens that mimic the original antigen in the eye, perhaps S-Ag, thereby producing uveitis. Thurau and Wildner suggested that this could explain the association between HLA class I antigens and uveitis. This approach has been used in a limited number of patients,[265] but its role in uveitis treatment has yet to be explored.

Immune tolerance inducing treatments are currently not commercially available for the treatment of uveitis. However, Glatiramer Acetate (Copaxone), a synthetic protein that simulates myelin basic protein, is approved by the U.S. Food and Drug Administration (FDA) for relapsing forms of multiple sclerosis. It is believed to work by inducing immune tolerance and blocking myelin-targeting T-cells. Additionally, in late 2020 ANK-700, an antigen-specific drug candidate that aims to treat multiple sclerosis (MS) by restoring immune tolerance was granted investigational new drug status by the FDA (https://anokion.com).

Colchicine

Mode of action. Colchicine, or acetyltrimethylcolchicinic acid, has poorly understood anti-inflammatory characteristics. Colchicine suppresses lactic acid production in leukocytes and reduces phagocytosis. In addition, it also reduces polymorphonuclear cell migration.

Indications and dosages. Heightened polymorphonuclear cell migration is a characteristic of patients with Behçet disease (see Chapter 27) and may be a cause of the repeated ocular attacks seen in that disorder. Colchicine has been used in the treatment of Behçet disease. It should be stressed that this agent is not employed to treat the active inflammatory condition but, rather, is used prophylactically in the person with multiple ocular attacks to reduce the frequency of these attacks, which can lead to blindness. This approach has not met with universal approval, being more popular in Japan than in other countries with a high incidence of this disease, such as Turkey. Many believe that this agent is not effective in treating white patients. Its use might be considered in those fairly rare patients with Behçet disease who have unilateral involvement and in whom one may not feel fully justified in using more powerful immunosuppressive agents. The average dose of oral colchicine is 0.6 mg twice daily. Some clinicians have suggested that higher dosages may be helpful, but this is based on anecdotal information. Its effect on Behçet disease has been, at best, marginal in our experience.

Secondary effects. Gastrointestinal reactions, such as abdominal pain, diarrhea, nausea, and vomiting, are quite common. Prolonged administration may cause bone marrow depression, with thrombocytopenia and aplastic anemia. Colchicine is contraindicated in pregnant women because it can harm the fetus.

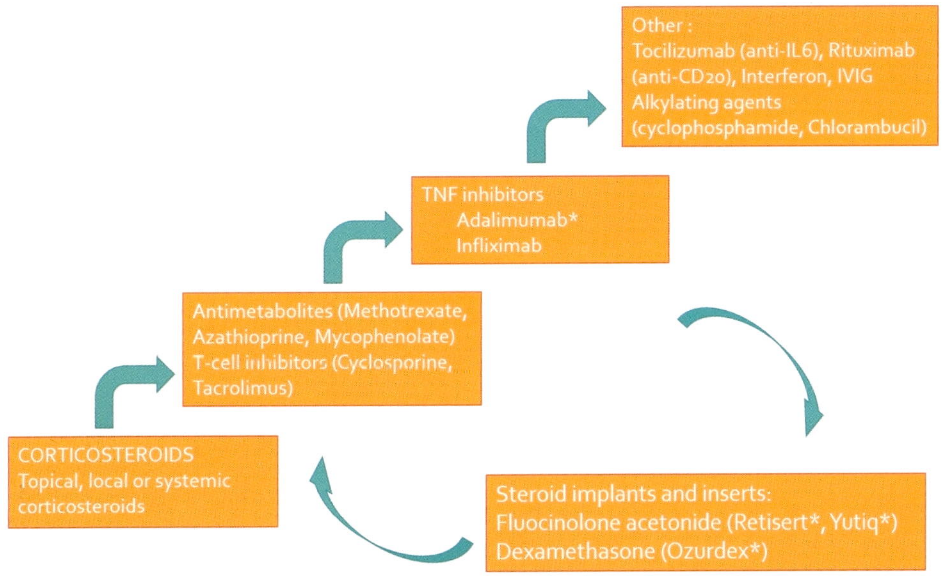

Fig. 8.18 Overall approach to management of noninfectious uveitis. Local sustained release corticosteroids can be used as adjunct or primary treatment option depending on the case. *These agents are FDA approved for the treatment of uveitis

Mydriatic and Cycloplegic Agents

The use of mydriatic and cycloplegic agents is an important adjunct to anti-inflammatory or immunosuppressive therapy. The major indication for the use of dilating agents is the presence of a "significant" anterior chamber inflammatory response. In those patients, the addition of mydriatics helps prevent the development of posterior synechiae and, in the extreme, iris bombé. Furthermore, cycloplegia will make the patient more comfortable and helps ensure that the treating physician has an unhindered view of the media and the fundus. We generally do not use long-term dilating agents, such as atropine, except postoperatively. Use of the shorter-acting agents, such as tropicamide (Mydriacyl), helps keep the iris moving and thus reduces the possibility of posterior synechiae. One medication possibly to be avoided in patients with uveitis is cyclopentolate (Cyclogyl) because this has been shown to be an effective chemoattractant for leukocytes.[266] Therefore the addition of this medication to the therapeutic regimen may prove problematic.

In summary, the general approach to the use of immunosuppressive agents is to choose the smallest amount historically considered effective for the anatomic area affected. However, it is important to establish control of the disease early with sufficient medication and to taper the medication after the inflammation resolves. Topical steroids for anterior segment disease can be most effective if given frequently. Periocular administration of steroids is often overlooked, but it is effective for the patient with unilateral disease or cystoid macular edema. The use of intraocular steroid (injection, insert or implant) changed our therapeutic paradigm significantly, particularly with newer options such as Ozurdex and Yutiq. Intravitreal administration of corticosteroids tends to be more effective in general than periocular administration in POINT Trial.[18] Suprachoroidal administration of triamcinolone (Xipere) appears promising for the treatment of uveitic macular edema.[22] Systemic corticosteroid administration is still the mainstay of therapy in sight-threatening bilateral posterior segment uveitis, but a second (and sometimes third) agent needs to be started once it is clear that immunosuppressive therapy needs to be continued for an extended period. Both antimetabolites (methotrexate, mycophenolate mofetil,. azathiopprine) and calcineurin inhibitors (cyclosporin, tacrolimus) are good first line steroid-sparing agents (Fig. 8.18). Methotrexate and mycophenolate mofetil are equally effective in adult posterior segment uveitis, though methotrexate is the preferable first line immunosuppressive in childhood uveitis. Monoclonal antibody therapies, particularly TNF inhibitors, have revolutionized the treatment of uveitis. TNF inhibitors have become the first or second line immunosuppressive agents in various adult and childhood uveitides. Our overall approach, as is seen in Figure 8.18, is to reserve cytotoxic agents for therapeutic failures with the aforementioned agents. Their use has declined with the invent of monoclonal antibody therapy. We would not use alkylating agents in children except under the most exceptional of circumstances. The safety of long term use of immunosuppressives have been supported by the MUST and SITE studies. MUST Trial 7 year results showed acceptable safety profile and better visual outcomes with systemic therapy compared to fluocinolone acetonide implant. However it is possible that low re-implantation rates in the implant arm and high rates of loss to follow-up may have led to underestimation of success with implant therapy.[267] The Systemic Immunosuppressive Therapy for Eye Diseases study (SITE) was able to evaluate the use of immunosuppressive agents in uveitis by collecting data from several centers with long-term experience in the use of these agents in the treatment of these patients.[46] With over 66 000 person-years of data the results suggested that the use of azathioprine, methotrexate, mycophenolate mofetil, cyclosporin, dapsone, and systemic corticosteroids did not increase the overall incidence of death nor cancer mortality.[268] Cyclophosphamide was not seen to increase overall mortality but did tend to increase overall cancer mortality, although its use can be justified short term in difficult-to-treat sight-threatening conditions. A second phase of the SITE study, SITE-2 confirmed these findings in 15,938 uveitis patients by showing that commonly used immunosuppressive agents including TNF inhibitors were not associated with increased overall or cancer mortality.[269] Majority of our patients are treated with systemic therapy with approximately 20-25% using biologic therapy. We often use local steroid therapy as a bridging or adjunct therapy and reserve the use of local treatment for long term management to select patients such as those with systemic medical problems that preclude the safe use of systemic therapy, those who plan to conceive or those with recent history of cancer. It is certainly reassuring to see that long term use of systemic treatments are associated with good visual outcomes and do not appear to be associated with increased risk of cancer mortality.

Newer treatment options that are in development as of late 2020 such as JAK/STAT pathway inhibition with Filgotinib (NCT03207815), intravitreal sirolimus (NCT03711929), non-viral gene therapy using plasmids encoding TNF inhibitor proteins (pEYS606) (NCT03308045) are promising approaches. Future approaches may include regulatory T cell therapy, advances on gene therapy, exosomes and bispecific antibodies.[270] It is imperative that the therapeutic approach be reevaluated if the patient's clinical course worsens. What is clear is that we now have many more options to offer our patients needing immunosuppressive therapy, and I am sure that these will increase dramatically in the next few years.

CAUTION

The drugs discussed in this chapter may have an important role in the treatment of various types of intraocular inflammatory diseases. The reader should be reminded that most of the drugs described here have been approved by the FDA for use in the treatment of uveitis. Others may be available under study protocols. It is the practitioner's duty to inquire as to the status of any medication and how the drug can be used within an accepted framework as well as the most updated information on dosing and route of administration. It is also important to remember that some agents have been reported to induce uveitis. Below are some examples of drugs that have been associated with uveitis, though this is not an exhaustive list (Box 8.3).

BOX 8.3 Medications Reported to Cause Uveitis (According to Micromedex)

Brimonidine
Bisphosphonates
Cidofovir
Demecarium
Deserpidine
Diethylcarbamazine
Echothiophate
Fomivirsen
Ganciclovir
Gentian violet
Immunoglobulin
Indinavir
Influenza vaccine
Isoflurophate
Latanoprost
Metipranolol
Pamidronate
Pyrethrum extract/piperonyl butoxide
Rescinnamine
Rifabutin
Ritonavir
Streptokinase
Terbinafine
Trimethoprim
Varicella vaccine
Bacille Calmette-Guérin (BCG)
Immune Checkpoint Inhibitors (Nivolumab, Ipilumumab, Pembrolizumab and others)

It is important to remember that many of the agents listed have a single or very few case reports associated with the event(s). Others seem more commonly associated with uveitis.

REFERENCES

1. Nussenblatt RB. Bench to bedside: new approaches to the immunotherapy of uveitic disease. *Int Rev Immunol.* 2002;21(2–3):273–289.
2. Wen S, Gao R, Hu Z. Comparison of Chinese traditional therapy combined with Western medicine and Western medicine alone in the treatment of uveitis. *Yen Ko Hsueh Pao.* 1991;7:205–208.
3. Gordon D. Prednisone and prednisolone in ocular disease. *Am J Ophthalmol.* 1956;41:593–600.
4. Hench P, Kendall E, Slocumb C. The effect of a hormone of the adrenal cortex (17-hydroxy-11-dehydrocorticosterone: compound E) and of pituitary adrenocorticotropic hormone on rheumatoid arthritis. *Proc Staff Meet Mayo Clin.* 1949;24:181–197.
5. Clamen H. Anti-inflammatory effects of corticosteroids. *Clin Immunol Allergy.* 1984;4:317–329.
6. Fauci AS, Dale DC, Balow JE. Glucocorticosteroid therapy: mechanisms of action and clinical considerations. *Ann Intern Med.* 1976;84(3):304–315.
7. Fauci A. Alternate-day corticosteroid therapy. *Am J Med.* 1978;64:729–731.
8. Slabaugh MA, Herlihy E, Ongchin S, van Gelder RN. Efficacy and potential complications of difluprednate use for pediatric uveitis. *Am J Ophthalmol.* 2012;153(5):932–938.
9. Sheppard JD, Toyos MM, Kempen JH, Kaur P, Foster CS. Difluprednate 0.05% versus prednisolone acetate 1% for endogenous anterior uveitis: a phase III, multicenter, randomized study. *Invest Ophthalmol Vis Sci.* 2014;55(5):2993–3002.
10. Schlaegel TJ. *Essentials of Uveitis.* Boston, MA: Little, Brown and Company; 1969:41–42.
11. Freeman W, Green R, Smith R. Echographic localization of corticosteroids after periocular injection. *Am J Ophthalmol.* 1987;103:281–288.
12. Sen HN, Vitale S, Sapna SG, et al. Periocular corticosteroid injections in uveitis: effects and complications. *Ophthalmology.* 2014;121(11):2275–2286.
13. Cunningham MA, Edelman JL, Kaushal S. Intravitreal steroids for macular edema: the past, the present, and the future. *Surv Ophthalmol.* 2008;53(2):139–149.
14. Martidis A, Duker JS, Puliafito CA. Intravitreal triamicinolone for refractory cystoid macular edema secondary to birdshot retinochoroidopathy. *Arch Ophthalmol.* 2001;119:1380–1383.
15. Antcliff RJ, Spalton DJ, Stanford MR, et al. Intravitreal triamcinolone for uveitic cystoid macular edema: an optical coherence tomography study. *Ophthalmology.* 2001;108:765–772.
16. Roesel M, Tappeiner C, Heinz C, et al. Comparison between intravitreal and orbital floor triamcinolone acetonide after phacoemulsification in patients with endogenous uveitis. *Am J Ophthalmol.* 2008;147:406–412.
17. Lowder C, Belfort R Jr, Lightman S, et al. Dexamethasone intravitreal implant for noninfectious intermediate or posterior uveitis. *Arch Ophthalmol.* 2011;129(5):545–553.
18. Thorne JE, Sugar EA, Holbrook JT, et al. Periocular triamcinolone vs. intravitreal triamcinolone vs. intravitreal dexamethasone implant for the treatment of uveitic macular edema: the periocular vs. intravitreal corticosteroids for uveitic macular edema (POINT) Trial. *Ophthalmology.* 2019;126(2):283–295.
19. Jaffe GJ, Foster CS, Pavesio CE, Paggiarino DA, Riedel GE. Effect of an Injectable Fluocinolone Acetonide Insert on Recurrence Rates in Chronic Noninfectious Uveitis Affecting the Posterior Segment: Twelve-Month Results. *Ophthalmology.* 2019 Apr;126(4):601–610. https://doi.org/10.1016/j.ophtha.2018.10.033. Epub 2018 Oct 25. PMID: 30367884.
20. Callanan DG, Jaffe GJ, Martin DF, et al. Treatment of posterior uveitis with a fluocinolone acetonide implant: three-year clinical trial results. *Arch Ophthalmol.* 2008;126(9):1191–1201.
21. Holbrook JT, Sugar EA, Burke AE, et al. Dissociations of the fluocinolone acetonide implant: the Multicenter Uveitis Steroid Treatment (MUST) trial and follow-up study. *Am J Ophthalmol.* 2016;164:29–36.
22. Yeh S, Khurana RN, Shah M, Henry CR, Wang RC, Kissner JM, Ciulla TA, Noronha G, PEACHTREE Study Investigators. Efficacy and Safety of Suprachoroidal CLS-TA for Macular Edema Secondary to Noninfectious Uveitis: Phase 3 Randomized Trial. *Ophthalmology.* 2020 Jul;127(7):948–955. https://doi.org/10.1016/j.ophtha.2020.01.006. Epub 2020 Jan 10. PMID: 32173113.

23. Piccolino FC, Pandolfo A, Polizzi A, et al. Retinal toxicity from accidental intraocular injection of Depo-Medrol. *Retina.* 2001;22:117–119.
24. Moshfeghi DM, Lowder CY, Roth DB, et al. Retinal and choroidal vascular occlusion after posterior sub-Tenon triamcinolone injection. *Am J Ophthalmol.* 2002;134:132–134.
25. VanderBeek BL, Bonaffini SG, Ma L. The association between intravitreal steroids and post-injection endophthalmitis rates. *Ophthalmology.* 2015;122(11):2311–2315. e1.
26. Jabs DA, Rosenbaum JT, Foster CS, et al. Perspective. Guidelines for the use of immunosuppressive drugs in patients with ocular inflammatory disorders: recommendations of an expert panel. *Am J Ophthalmol.* 2000;130:492–513.
27. American College of Rheumatology Task Force on Osteoporosis Guidelines. Recommendations for the prevention and treatment of glucocorticoid-induced osteoporosis. *Arthritis Rheum.* 1996;39:1791–1801.
28. Reed JB, Morse LS, Schwab IR. High-dose intravenous pulse methylprednisolone hemisuccinate in acute Behcet retinitis. *Am J Ophthalmol.* 1998;125:410–411.
29. Smith WM, Larson TA, Meleth AD, Krishnadev N, Nussenblatt RB, Sen HN. Corticosteroid-associated osteonecrosis: a rare, but serious, complication in uveitis. *Ocul Immunol Inflamm.* 2013;21(2):102–107.
30. Fujikawa L, Meisler D, Nozik R. Hyperosmolar hyperglycemic nonketotic coma. A complication of short-term systemic corticosteroids. *Ophthalmology.* 1983;90:1239–1242.
31. Wakakura M, Ishikawa S. Central serous chorioretinopathy complicating systemic corticosteroid treatment. *Br J Ophthalmol.* 1984;68:329–331.
32. Polito C, La Manna A, Papale MR, et al. Delayed pubertal growth spurt and normal adult height attainment in boys receiving long-term alternate-day prednisone therapy. *Clin Pediatr.* 1999;38:279–285.
33. Hemady R, Tauber J, Foster C. Immunosuppressive drugs in immune and inflammatory ocular disease. *Surv Ophthalmol.* 1991;35:369–385.
34. Cash J, Klippel J. Second-line drug therapy for rheumatoid arthritis. *N Engl J Med.* 1994;330:1368–1375.
35. Dorr R, Fritz W. *Cancer Chemotherapy Handbook.* New York: Elsevier; 1980.
36. Buckley CI, Gills JJ. Cyclophosphamide therapy of peripheral uveitis. *Arch Intern Med.* 1969;124:29–35.
37. Mamo J, Azzam S. Treatment of Behcet's disease with chlorambucil. *Arch Ophthalmol.* 1970;84:446–450.
38. Hoffman G, Kerr G, Leavitt R, et al. Treatment of Wegener's granulomatosis with intermittent high-dose intravenous cyclophosphamide. *Am J Med.* 1990;89:403–410.
39. Rosenbaum J. Treatment of severe refractory uveitis with intravenous cyclophosphamide. *J Rheumatol.* 1994;21:12–125.
40. Godfrey W, Epstein W, O'Connor GR, et al. The use of chlorambucil in intractable idiopathic uveitis. *Am J Ophthalmol.* 1974;78:415–428.
41. Tessler H, Jennings T. High-dose short-term chlorambucil for intractable sympathetic ophthalmia and Behcet's disease. *Br J Ophthalmol.* 1990;74:353–357.
42. Nashel D. Mechanisms of action and clinical applications of cytotoxic drugs in rheumatic disorders. *Med Clin North Am.* 1985;69:817–840.
43. DeFronzo R, Braine H, Colvin OM, et al. Water intoxication in man after cyclophosphamide therapy. *Ann Intern Med.* 1973;78:861–869.
44. Kende G, Sirkin S, Thomas PR, et al. Blurring of vision, a previously described complication of cyclophosphamide therapy. *Cancer.* 1979;44:69–71.
45. Radis CD, Kahl LE, Baker GL, et al. Effects of cyclophosphamide on the development of malignancy and on long-term survival of patients with rheumatoid arthritis. *Arthritis Rheum.* 1995;38:1120–1127. A 20-year follow-up study.
46. Kempen JH, Daniel E, Dunn JP, et al. Overall and cancer related mortality among patients with ocular inflammation treated with immunosuppressive drugs: retrospective cohort study. *BMJ.* 2009;339:b2480.
47. Urowitz M, Hunter T, Bookman M, et al. Azathioprine in rheumatoid arthritis: a double-blind study comparing full dose to half dose. *J Rheumatol.* 1974;1:274–281.
48. Woodland J, Chaput-de-Saintonge D, Evans SJ, et al. Azathioprine in rheumatoid arthritis: double-blind study of full versus half doses versus placebo. *Ann Rheum Dis.* 1981;40:355–359.
49. O'Reilly T. Azathioprine in the treatment of refractory rheumatoid arthritis. *J Ir Med Assoc.* 1977;70:344–346.
50. Andrasch R, Pirofsky B, Burns R. Immunosuppressive therapy for severe chronic uveitis. *Arch Ophthalmol.* 1978;96:247–251.
51. Newell F, Krill A, Thomson A. The treatment of uveitis with 6-mercaptopurine. *Am J Ophthalmol.* 1966;61:1250–1255.
52. Hooper PL, Kaplan HJ. Triple agent immunosuppression in serpiginous choroiditis. *Ophthalmology.* 1991;98:944–950.
53. Yazici H, Pazarli H, Barnes CG, et al. A controlled trial of azathioprine in Behcet's syndrome. *N Engl J Med.* 1990;322:281–285.
54. Pasadhika S, Gerald AF, Rando A, et al. Azathioprine for ocular inflammatory diseases. *Am J Ophthalmol.* 2009;148(4):500–509.
55. Connell W, Kamm M, Dickson M, et al. Long-term neoplasia risk after azathioprine treatment in inflammatory bowel disease. *Lancet.* 1994;343:1249–1252.
56. Zierhut M, Stubiger N, Siepmann K, et al. MMF and eye disease. *Lupus.* 2005;14(Suppl 1):s50–s54.
57. Chanaud NPI, Vistica BP, Eugui E, et al. Inhibition of experimental autoimmune uveoretinitis by mycophenolate mofetil, an inhibitor of purine metabolism. *Exp Eye Res.* 1995;35:429–434.
58. Kilmartin DJ, Forrester JV, Dick AD. Rescue therapy with mycophenolate mofetil in refractory uveitis. *Lancet.* 1998;352:35–36.
59. Larkin G, Lightman S. Mycophenolate mofetil. A useful immunosuppressive in inflammatory eye disease. *Ophthalmology.* 1999;106:370–374.
60. Sen HN, Suhler EB, Al-Khatib SQ, et al. Mycophenolate mofetil for the treatment of scleritis. *Ophthalmology.* 2003;110:1750–1755.
61. Baltatzis S, Tufail F, Vredeveld BA, et al. Mycophenolate mofetil as an immunomodulatory agent in the treatment of chronic ocular inflammatory disorders. *Ophthalmology.* 2003;110(5):1061–1065.
62. Daniel E, Thorne JE, Newcomb CW, et al. Mycophenolate mofetil for ocular inflammation. *Am J Ophthalmol.* 2010;149(3):423–432. e1-2.
63. Cronstein B. Molecular mechanism of methotrexate action in inflammation. *Inflammation.* 1992;16:411–423.
64. Sperling R, Benincaso A, Anderson RJ, et al. Acute and chronic suppression of leukotriene B4 synthesis ex vivo in neutrophils from patients with rheumatoid arthritis beginning treatment with methotrexate. *Arthritis Rheum.* 1992;35:376–384.
65. Thomas R, Carroll G. Reduction of leukocyte and interleukin-1 beta concentrations in the synovial fluid of rheumatoid arthritis patients treated with methotrexate. *Arthritis Rheum.* 1993;36:1244–1254.
66. Olsen N, Murray L. Antiproliferative effects of methotrexate on peripheral blood mononuclear cells. *Arthritis Rheum.* 1989;32:378–385.
67. Wong V. Immunosuppressive therapy of ocular inflammatory diseases. *Arch Ophthalmol.* 1969;81:628–637.
68. Gangaputra S, Newcomb CW, Liesegang TL, et al. Methotrexate for ocular inflammatory disease. *Ophthalmology.* 2009 Nov;116(11):2188–2198. e1.
69. Rathinam SR, Gonzales JA, Thundikandy R, et al. Effect of corticosteroid-sparing treatment with mycophenolate mofetil vs methotrexate on inflammation in patients with uveitis: a randomized clinical trial. *JAMA.* 2019;322(10):936–945.
70. Smith JR, Rosenbaum JT, Wilson DJ, et al. Role of intravitreal methotrexate in the management of primary central nervous system lymphoma with ocular involvement. *Ophthalmology.* 2002;109:1709–1716.
71. Taylor SR, Habot-Wilner Z, Pacheco P, Lightman SL. Intraocular methotrexate in the treatment of uveitis and uveitic cystoid macular edema. *Ophthalmology.* 2009;116:797–801.
72. Rothenberg S, Iqbal M, da Costa M. Effect of folate compounds on the accumulation of methotrexate and the activity of dihydrofolate reductase in liver, kidney, and small intestine of the mouse. *J Pharmacol Exp Ther.* 1982;223:631–634.
73. Furst D, Erikson N, Clute L, et al. Adverse experience with methotrexate during 176 weeks of a long-term prospective trial in patients with rheumatoid arthritis. *J Rheumatol.* 1990;17:1628–1635.

74. Hargreaves M, Mowat A, Benson M. Acute pneumonitis associated with low dose methotrexate treatment for rheumatoid arthritis: report of five cases and review of published reports. *Thorax.* 1992;47:628–633.
75. Carroll G, Thomas R, Phatouros CC, et al. Incidence, prevalence and possible risk factors for pneumonitis in patients with rheumatoid arthritis receiving methotrexate. *J Rheumatol.* 1994;21:51–54.
76. Cannon GW, Finck BK, Simpson KM, et al. Methotrexate induced pulmonary disease during treatment of rheumatoid arthritis in large clinical trials (abstract). *Arthritis Rheum.* 2000;43(Suppl 9):341.
77. Beveridge T, Gratwohl A, Michot F, et al. Cyclosporin A: pharmacokinetics after a single dose in man and serum levels after multiple dosing in recipients of allogeneic bone-marrow grafts. *Curr Ther Res.* 1981;30:5–18.
78. Beveridge T. Pharmacokinetics and metabolism of cyclosporin A. In: White D, ed. *Cyclosporin A.* New York: Elsevier Biomedical Press; 1982:35–44.
79. de Smet M, Rubin BI, Whitcup SM, et al. Combined use of cyclosporine and ketoconazole in the treatment of endogenous uveitis. *Am J Ophthalmol.* 1992;113:687–690.
80. Schreiber S, Crabtree G. The mechanism of action of cyclosporin A and FK506. *Immunol Today.* 1992;13:136–142.
81. Cross S, Halden NF, Lenardo MJ, et al. Functionally distinct NF-kappa B binding sites in the immunoglobulin kappa and IL-2 receptor alpha chain genes. *Science.* 1989;244:466–469.
82. Granelli-Piperno A, Nolan P, Inaba K, et al. The effect of immunosuppressive agents on the induction of nuclear factors that bind to sites on the interleukin 2 promoter. *J Exp Med.* 1990;172:1869–1872.
83. Larsson E. Cyclosporin A and dexamethasone suppress T-cell responses by selectively acting at distinct sites of the triggering process. *J Immunol.* 1980;124:2828–2833.
84. Bunjes D, Hardt C, Röllinghoff M, et al. Cyclosporin A mediates immunosuppression of primary cytotoxic T cell responses by impairing the release of interleukin 1 and interleukin 2. *Eur J Immunol.* 1981;11:657–661.
85. Kaufman Y, Chang AE, Robb RJ, et al. Mechanism of action of cyclosporin A: inhibition of lymphokine secretion studied with antigen-stimulated T-cell hybridomas. *J Immunol.* 1984;133:3107–3111.
86. DosReis G, Shevach E. Effect of cyclosporin on T-cell function in vitro: the mechanism of suppression of T cell proliferation depends on the nature of the T cell stimulus as well as the differentiation state of the responding T cell. *J Immunol.* 1982;129:2360–2367.
87. Nussenblatt R. The expanding use of immunosuppression in the treatment of non-infectious ocular disease. *J Autoimmun.* 1992;5(Suppl A):247–257.
88. Nussenblatt R, Palestine A, Chan C. Cyclosporin A therapy in the treatment of intraocular inflammatory disease resistant to systemic corticosteroids and cytotoxic agents. *Am J Ophthalmol.* 1983;96:275–282.
89. Nussenblatt R, Palestine AG, Rook AH, et al. Treatment of intraocular inflammatory disease with Cyclosporin A. *Lancet.* 1983;ii:235–238.
90. Nussenblatt R, Palestine A, Chan C. Cyclosporine therapy for uveitis: long term follow-up. *J Ocul Pharmacol.* 1985;1:369–381.
91. de Smet M, Nussenblatt R. Clinical use of cyclosporine in ocular disease. *Int Ophthalmol Clin.* 1993;33:32–45.
92. Nussenblatt R, Palestine A, Chan C, et al. Effectiveness of cyclosporin therapy for Behçet's disease. *Arthritis Rheum.* 1985;28:671–679.
93. Masuda K, Nakajima A, Urayama A, et al. Double-masked trial of cyclosporin versus colchicine and long-term open study of cyclosporin in Behcet's disease. *Lancet.* 1989;1(8647):1093–1096.
94. Diaz-Llopis M, Cervera M, Menezo J. Cyclosporin A treatment of Behçet's disease: a long-term study. *Curr Eye Res.* 1990;9(Suppl):17–23.
95. Walton RC, Nussenblatt RB, Whitcup SM. Cyclosporine therapy for severe sight-threatening uveitis in children and adolescents. *Ophthalmology.* 1998;105:2028–2034.
96. Kacmaz R, Austin H, Balow J, et al. Cyclosporine for ocular inflammation. *N Engl J Med.* 1986;314:1293–1298.
97. Gilger BC, Malok E, Stewart T, et al. Effect of an intravitreal cyclosporine implant on experimental uveitis in horses. *Vet Immunol Immunopathol.* 2000;76:239–255.
98. Feutren G, Mihatsch M. Risk factors for cyclosporine-induced nephropathy in patients with autoimmune diseases. International Kidney Biopsy Registry of Cyclosporine in Autoimmune Diseases. *N Engl J Med.* 1992;326:1654–1660.
99. Sall K, Stevenson OD, Mundorf TK, et al. Two multicenter, randomized studies of the efficacy and safety of cyclosporine ophthalmic emulsion in moderate to severe dry eye disease. CsA Phase 3 Study Group. *Ophthalmology.* 2000;107(4):631–639.
100. Nussenblatt R, Palestine A. Cyclosporine: immunology, pharmacology, and therapeutic uses. *Surv Ophthalmol.* 1986;31:159–169.
101. Palestine A, Austin HA 3rd, Balow JE, et al. Renal histopathologic alterations in patients treated with cyclosporine for uveitis. *N Engl J Med.* 1986;314:1293–1298.
102. Miescher P, Favre H, Chatelanat F, et al. Combined steroid-cyclosporin treatment of chronic auto-immune diseases. Clinical results and assessment of nephrotoxicity by renal biopsy. *Klin Wochenschr.* 1987;65(15):727–736.
103. Burke JJ, Pirsch JD, Ramos EL, et al. Long-term efficacy and safety of cyclosporine in renal-transplant recipients. *N Engl J Med.* 1994;331:358–363.
104. Tabbara KF, Gee SS, Alvarez H. Ocular bioavailability of cyclosporine after oral administration. *Transplant Proc.* 1988;20(2 Suppl 2):656–659.
105. Palestine AG, Nussenblatt RB, Chan CC. Cyclosporine penetration into the anterior chamber and cerebrospinal fluid. *Am J Ophthalmol.* 1985;99(2):210–211.
106. Whitcup SM, Salvo ECJ, Nussenblatt RB. Combined cyclosporine and corticosteroid therapy for sight-threatening uveitis in Behcet's disease. *Am J Ophthalmol.* 1994;118:39–45.
107. Palestine A, Roberge F, Charous BL, et al. The effect of cyclosporine on immunization with tetanus and keyhole limpet hemocyanin (KLH) in humans. *J Clin Immunol.* 1985;5:115–121.
108. Chang SH, Lim CS, Low TS, et al. Cyclosporine-associated encephalopathy: a case report and literature review. *Transplant Proc.* 2001;33(7–8):3700–3701.
109. Mochizuki M, Masuda K, Sakane T, et al. A clinical trial of FK506 in refractory uveitis. *Am J Ophthalmol.* 1993;115:763–769.
110. Tocci M, Matkovich DA, Collier KA, et al. The immunosuppressant FK506 selectively inhibits expression of early T cell activation genes. *J Immunol.* 1989;143:718–726.
111. Kawashima H, Fujino Y. Mochizuki M. Effects of a new immunosuppressive agent, FK506, on experimental autoimmune uveoretinitis in rats. *Invest Ophthalmol Vis Sci.* 1988;29:1265–1271.
112. Fujino Y, Mochizuki M, Chan CC, et al. FK506 treatment of S-antigen induced uveitis in primates. *Curr Eye Res.* 1991;10:679–690.
113. Mochizuki M, Japanese-FK506-Study-Group. Refractory uveitis in Behcet's disease. In: Wechsler B, Godeau P, eds. *Proceedings of the 6th International Conference on Behcet's Disease.* Amsterdam: Excerpta Medica; 1993:655–660.
114. Sloper CML, Powell RJ, Dua HS. Tacrolimus (F506) in the treatment of posterior uveitis refractory to cyclosporine. *Ophthalmology.* 1999;106:723–728.
115. Kilmartin DJ, Forrester JV, Dick AD. Tacrolimus (FK506) in failed cyclosporin A therapy in endogenous posterior uveitis. *Ocul Immunol Inflamm.* 1998;6:101–109.
116. Hogan AC, McAvoy CE, Dick AD, Lee RW. Long-term efficacy and tolerance of tacrolimus for the treatment of uveitis. *Ophthalmology.* 2007;114(5):1000–1006.
117. Islam F, Westcott M, Rees A, et al. Safety profile and efficacy of tacrolimus in the treatment of birdshot retinochoroiditis: a retrospective case series review. *Br J Ophthalmol.* 2018;102(7):983–990.
118. Lee RW, Greenwood R, Taylor H, et al. A randomized trial of tacrolimus versus tacrolimus and prednisone for the maintenance of disease remission in noninfectious uveitis. *Ophthalmology.* 2012;119(6):1223–1230.
119. Sehgal S, Baker H, Vezina C. Rapamycin (AY-22,989), a new antifungal antibiotic. II. Fermentation, isolation, and characterization. *J Antibiotics.* 1975;28:727–732.
120. Dumont F, Staruch MJ, Koprak SL, et al. Distinct mechanisms of suppression of murine T cell activation by the related macrolides FK-506 and rapamycin. *J Immunol.* 1990;144:251–258.

121. Bierer E, Mattila PS, Standaert RF, et al. Two distinct signal transmission pathways in T lymphocytes are inhibited by complexes formed between immunophilin and either FK506 or rapamycin. *Proc Natl Acad Sci U S A.* 1990;87:9231–9235.
122. Henderson D, Naya I, Bundick RV, et al. Comparison of the effects of FK-506, cyclosporin A and rapamycin on IL-2 production. *Immunology.* 1991;73:316–321.
123. Gonwa TA, Hricik DE, Brinker K, et al. Improved renal function in sirolimus-treated renal transplant patients after early cyclosporine elimination. *Transplantation.* 2002;74:1560–1567.
124. Nussenblatt RB, Coleman H, Jirawuthiworavong G, et al. The treatment of multifocal choroiditis associated choroidal neovascularization with sirolimus (rapamycin). *Acta Ophthalmol Scand.* 2007;85(2):230–231.
125. Blair J, Barry R, Moore DJ, Denniston AK. A comprehensive review of mTOR-inhibiting pharmacotherapy for the treatment of non-infectious uveitis. *Curr Pharm Des.* 2017;23(20):3005–3014.
126. Roberge F, Xu D, Chan CC, et al. Treatment of autoimmune uveoretinitis in the rat with rapamycin, an inhibitor of lymphocyte growth factor signal transduction. *Curr Eye Res.* 1993;12:197–203.
127. Roberge F, Kozhich A, Chan C-C, et al. Inhibition of cellular transfer of experimental autoimmune uveoretinitis by rapamycin. *Ocul Immunol Inflamm.* 1993;1:269–273.
128. Kahan B, Gibbons S, Tejpal N, et al. Synergistic interactions of cyclosporine and rapamycin to inhibit immune performances of normal human peripheral blood lymphocytes in vitro. *Transplantation.* 1991;51:232–239.
129. Martin D, DeBarge LR, Nussenblatt RB, et al. Synergistic effect of rapamycin and cyclosporin A in the treatment of experimental autoimmune uveoretinitis. *J Immunol.* 1995;154:922–927.
130. Whiting P, Woo J, Adam BJ, et al. Toxicity of rapamycin – a comparative and combination study with cyclosporine at immunotherapeutic dosage in the rat. *Transplantation.* 1991;52:203–208.
131. Calne R, Collier DS, Lim S, et al. Rapamycin for immunosuppression in organ allografting. *Lancet.* 1989;2:227–232.
132. Shanmuganathan VA, Casely EM, Raj D, et al. The efficacy of sirolimus in the treatment of patients with refractory uveitis. *Br J Ophthalmol.* 2005;89(6):666–669.
133. Knickelbein JE, Kim M, Argon E, Sen HN. Comparative efficacy of steroid-sparing therapies for non-infectious uveitis. *Expert Review of Ophthalmology.* 2017;12(4):313–319.
134. Jap A, Chee SP. Immunosuppressive therapy for ocular diseases. *Curr Opin Ophthalmol.* 2008;19(6):535–540.
135. Bhatt N, Tucker W, Sen HN, Nussenblatt RB. Biologic Therapies: Anti-Tumor Necrosis Factor-α, Anti-Interleukins, Rituximab and Others. In: Nguyen QD, Rodrigues EB, Farah ME, Mieler WF, Do DV (eds): Retinal Pharmacotherapeutics. Dev Ophthalmol. Basel, Karger, 2016, vol 55, pp 252–264.
136. Chatenoud L, Bach J-F. Anti-T-cell monoclonal antibodies as immunosuppressive agents. In: Rugstad H, Endresen L, Forre O, eds. *Immunopharmacology in Autoimmune Diseases and Transplantation.* New York: Plenum Press; 1992:189–203.
137. O'Connell P, Corpier C, Steele A, et al. Monoclonal antibody therapy. In: Thomson A, ed. *Immunology in Renal Transplantation.* London: Edward Arnold; 1993.
138. Dukar O, Barr C. Visual loss complicating OKT3 monoclonal antibody therapy. *Am J Ophthalmol.* 1993;115:781–785.
139. Queen C, Schneider WP, Selick HE, et al. A humanized antibody that binds to the interleukin 2 receptor. *Proc Natl Acad Sci U S A.* 1989;86:10029–10033.
140. Caspi RR, Roberge FG, Nussenblatt RB. Organ-resident, nonlymphoid cells suppress proliferation of autoimmune T-helper lymphocytes. *Science.* 1987 Aug 28;237(4818):1029–1032.
141. Nussenblatt RB, Fortin E, Schiffman R, et al. Treatment of noninfectious intermediate and posterior uveitis with the humanized anti-Tac mAb: a phase I/II clinical trial. *Proc Natl Acad Sci U S A.* 1999;96:7462–7466.
142. Nussenblatt RB, Thompson DJ, Li Z, et al. Humanized anti-interleukin-2 (IL-2) receptor alpha therapy: long term results in uveitis patients and preliminary safety and activity data for establishing parameters for subcutaneous administration. *J Autoimmun.* 2003;21(3):283–293.
143. Papaliodis GN, Chu D, Foster CS. Treatment of ocular inflammatory disorders with daclizumab. *Ophthalmology.* 2003;110(4):786–789.
144. Yeh S, Wroblewski K, Buggage R, et al. High-dose humanized anti-IL-2 receptor alpha antibody (daclizumab) for the treatment of active, non-infectious uveitis. *J Autoimmun.* 2008;31(2):91–97.
145. Kim HS, Yoon SK, Joo C. The expression of multiple cytokines and inducible nitric oxide synthase in experimental melanin-protein-induced uveitis. *Ophthalmic Res.* 2001;33:329–335.
146. Santos Lacomba M, Marcos Martín C, Gallardo Galera JM, et al. Aqueous humor and serum tumor necrosis factor-alpha in clinical uveitis. *Ophthalmic Res.* 2001;33:251–255.
147. Weinblatt M, Kremer JM, Bankhurst AD, et al. A trial of etanercept, a recombinant tumor necrosis factor receptor:Fc fusion protein, in patients with rheumatoid arthritis receiving methotrexate. *N Engl J Med.* 1999;340:253–259.
148. Lovell DJ, Criannini EH, Reiff A, et al. Etanercept in children with polyarticular juvenile rheumatoid arthritis. Pediatric Rheumatology Collaborative Study Group. *N Engl J Med.* 2000;342:763–769.
149. Smith JR, Levinson RD, Holland GN, et al. Differential efficacy of TNF inhibition in the management of uveitis and associated rheumatic disease. *Arthritis Rheum.* 2001;45:252–257.
150. Davies R, Cock D, Kearsley-Fleet L, et al. The risk of uveitis in patients with JIA receiving etanercept: the challenges of analysing real-world data. *Rheumatology (Oxford).* 2020;59(6):1391–1397.
151. Foeldvari I, Becker I, Horneff G. Uveitis events during adalimumab, etanercept, and methotrexate therapy in juvenile idiopathic arthritis: data from the Biologics in Pediatric Rheumatology Registry. *Arthritis Care Res (Hoboken).* 2015;67(11):1529–1535.
152. Levy-Clarke G, Jabs DA, Read RW, et al. Expert panel recommendations for the use of anti-tumor necrosis factor biologic agents in patients with ocular inflammatory disorders. *Ophthalmology.* 2014;121:785–796. e3.
153. Brown SL, Greene MH, Gershon SK, et al. Tumor necrosis factor antagonist therapy and lymphoma development. *Arthritis Rheum.* 2002;46:3151–3158.
154. Fonollosa A, Segura A, Giralt J, et al. Tuberculous uveitis after treatment with etanercept. *Graefes Arch Clin Exp Ophthalmol.* 2007;245(9):1397–1399.
155. Davies R, Southwood TR, Kearsley-Fleet L, et al. Medically significant infections are increased in patients with juvenile idiopathic arthritis treated with etanercept: results from the British Society for Paediatric and Adolescent Rheumatology Etanercept Cohort Study. *Arthritis Rheumatol.* 2015;67(9):2487–2494.
156. Sfikakis PP, Theodossiadis PG, Katsiari CG, et al. Effect of infliximab on sight-threatening panuveitis in Behcet's disease. *Lancet.* 2001;358:295–296.
157. Sfikakis PP. Behcet's disease: a new target for anti-tumour necrosis factor treatment. *Ann Rheum Dis.* 2002;61(Suppl 2):ii51–ii53.
158. Sfikakis PP, Markomichelakis N, Alpsoy E, et al. Anti-TNF therapy in the management of Behcet's disease – review and basis for recommendations. *Rheumatology (Oxford).* 2007;46(5):736–741.
159. Pipitone N, Olivieri I, Padula A, et al. Infliximab for the treatment of neuro-Behcet's disease: a case series and review of the literature. *Arthritis Rheum.* 2008;59(2):285–290.
160. El-Shabrawi Y, Hermann J. Anti-tumor necrosis factor-alpha therapy with infliximab as an alternative to corticosteroids in the treatment of human leukocyte antigen B27-associated acute anterior uveitis. *Ophthalmology.* 2002;109:2342–2346.
161. Sen HN, Sangave A, Hammel K, et al. Infliximab for the treatment of active scleritis. *Can J Ophthalmol.* 2009;44:e9–e12.
162. Liberopoulos EN, Drosos AA, Elisaf MS. Exacerbation of tuberculous enteritis after treatment with infliximab. *Am J Med.* 2002;113:615.
163. Lee J-H, Slifman NR, Gershon SK, et al. Life-threatening histoplasmosis complicating immunotherapy with tumor necrosis factor alpha antagonists infliximab and etanercept. *Arthritis Rheum.* 2002;46:2565–2570.
164. van Oosten BW, Barkhof F, Truyen L, et al. Increased MRI activity and immune activation in two multiple sclerosis patients treated with the monoclonal anti-tumor necrosis factor antibody cA2. *Neurology.* 1996;47:1531–1534.

165. Foroozan R, Buono LM, Sergott RC, et al. Retrobulbar optic neuritis associated with infliximab. *Arch Ophthalmol.* 2002;120:985–987.
166. Kramer N, Chuzhin Y, Kaufman LD, et al. Methotrexate pneumonitis after initiation of infliximab therapy for rheumatoid arthritis. *Arthritis Rheum.* 2002;47:670–671.
167. Jabs DA. Immunosuppression for the uveitides. *Ophthalmology.* 2018;125(2):193–202.
168. Markomichelakis NN, Theodossiadis PG, Papaefthimiou S, et al. Infliximab for chronic cystoid macular edema associated with uveitis. *Am J Ophthalmol.* 2004;138:648–650.
169. http://www.janssenlabels.com/package-insert/product-monograph/prescribing-information/REMICADE-pi.pdf.
170. Angeles-Han ST, Ringold S, Beukelman T, et al. 2019 American College of Rheumatology/Arthritis Foundation Guideline for the Screening, monitoring, and treatment of juvenile idiopathic arthritis-associated uveitis. *Arthritis Rheumatol.* 2019;71(6):864–877.
171. Jaffe GJ, Dick AD, Brezin AP, Nguyen QD, Thorne JE, Kestelyn P, et al. Adalimumab in patients with active noninfectious uveitis. *N Engl J Med.* 2016;375:932–943.
172. Nguyen QD, Merrill PT, Jaffe GJ, Dick AD, Kurup SK, Sheppard J, et al. Adalimumab for prevention of uveitic flare in patients with inactive non-infectious uveitis controlled by corticosteroids (VISUAL II): a multicentre, double-masked, randomised, placebo-controlled phase 3 trial. *Lancet.* 2016;388:1183–1192.
173. Suhler EB, Adan A, Brezin AP, Fortin E, Goto H, Jaffe GJ, et al. Safety and efficacy of adalimumab in patients with noninfectious uveitis in an ongoing open-label study: VISUAL III. *Ophthalmology.* 2018;125:1075–1087.
174. Ramanan AV, Dick AD, Jones AP, McKay A, Williamson PR, Compeyrot-Lacassagne S, et al. Adalimumab plus methotrexate for uveitis in juvenile idiopathic arthritis. *N Engl J Med.* 2017;376:1637–1646.
175. Quartier P, Baptiste A, Despert V, Allain-Launay E, Kone-Paut I, Belot A, et al. ADJUVITE: a double-blind, randomised, placebo-controlled trial of adalimumab in early onset, chronic, juvenile idiopathic arthritis-associated anterior uveitis. *Ann Rheum Dis.* 2018;77(7):1003–1011.
176. Mushtaq B, Saeed T, Situnayake RD, et al. Adalimumab for sight-threatening uveitis in Behcet's disease. *Eye.* 2007;21(6):824–825.
177. van Laar JA, Missotten T, van Daele PL, et al. Adalimumab: a new modality for Behcet's disease? *Ann Rheum Dis.* 2007;66(4):565–566.
178. Diaz-Llopis M, García-Delpech S, Salom D, et al. Adalimumab therapy for refractory uveitis: a pilot study. *J Ocul Pharmacol Ther.* 2008;24(3):351–361.
179. Tynjala P, Kotaniemi K, Lindahl P, et al. Adalimumab in juvenile idiopathic arthritis-associated chronic anterior uveitis. *Rheumatology (Oxford).* 2008;47(3):339–344.
180. Vazquez-Cobian LB, Flynn T, Lehman TJ. Adalimumab therapy for childhood uveitis. *J Pediatr.* 2006;149(4):572–575.
181. Bhatt N, Tucker W, Sen HN, Nussenblatt RB. Biologic therapies: anti-tumor necrosis factor-α, anti-interleukins, rituximab and others. *Dev Ophthalmol.* 2016;55:252–264.
182. Erckens RJ, Mostard RL, Wijnen PA, Schouten JS, Drent M. Adalimumab successful in sarcoidosis patients with refractory chronic non-infectious uveitis. *Graefes Arch Clin Exp Ophthalmol.* 2012;250(5):713–720.
183. *Humira Package Insert: HUMIRA (adalimumab). Full Prescribing Information.* Chicago, IL: AbbVie Inc.; 2016. North.
184. Benmassaoud A, Al-Taweel T, Sasson MS, et al. Comparative effectiveness of infliximab versus adalimumab in patients with biologic-naïve Crohn's disease. *Dig Dis Sci.* 2018;63(5):1302–1310.
185. Vallet H, Seve P, Biard L, et al. Infliximab versus adalimumab in the treatment of refractory inflammatory uveitis: a multicenter study from the French Uveitis Network. *Arthritis Rheumatol.* 2016;68(6):1522–1530.
186. Lejoyeux R, Diwo E, Vallet H, et al. Infliximab and adalimumab in uveitic macular edema. *Ocul Immunol Inflamm.* 2018;26(7):991–996.
187. Tosi GM, Sota J, Vitale A, et al. Efficacy and safety of certolizumab pegol and golimumab in the treatment of non-infectious uveitis. *Clin Exp Rheumatol.* 2019;37(4):680–683.
188. Thomas AS. Biologics for the treatment of noninfectious uveitis: current concepts and emerging therapeutics. *Curr Opin Ophthalmol.* 2019;30(3):138–150.
189. Rudwaleit M, Rosenbaum JT, Landewé R, et al. Observed incidence of uveitis following certolizumab pegol treatment in patients with axial spondyloarthritis. *Arthritis Care Res (Hoboken).* 2016;68:838–844.
190. Hoang-Xuan K, Camilleri-Broet S, Soussain C. Recent advances in primary CNS lymphoma. *Curr Opin Oncol.* 2004;16(6):601–606.
191. Bosly A, Keating MJ, Stasi R, et al. Rituximab in B-cell disorders other than non-Hodgkin's lymphoma. *Anticancer Drugs.* 2002;13(Suppl 2):S25–S33.
192. Rigacci L, Nassi L, Puccioni M, et al. Rituximab and chlorambucil as first-line treatment for low-grade ocular adnexal lymphomas. *Ann Hematol.* 2007;86(8):565–568.
193. Ferreri AJ, Ponzoni M, Martinelli G, et al. Rituximab in patients with mucosal-associated lymphoid tissue-type lymphoma of the ocular adnexa. *Haematologica.* 2005;90(11):1578–1579.
194. Gurcan HM, Keskin DB, Stern JN, et al. A review of the current use of rituximab in autoimmune diseases. *Int Immunopharmacol.* 2009;9(1):10–25.
195. Tappeiner C, Heinz C, Specker C, et al. Rituximab as a treatment option for refractory endogenous anterior uveitis. *Ophthalmic Res.* 2007;39(3):184–186.
196. Onal S, Kazokoglu H, Koc A, et al. Rituximab for remission induction in a patient with relapsing necrotizing scleritis associated with limited Wegener's granulomatosis. *Ocul Immunol Inflamm.* 2008;16(5):230–232.
197. Sadreddini S, Noshad H, Molaeefard M, et al. Treatment of retinal vasculitis in Behcet's disease with rituximab. *Mod Rheumatol.* 2008;18(3):306–308.
198. Ahmed A, Foster CS. Cyclophosphamide or rituximab treatment of scleritis and uveitis for patients with granulomatosis with polyangiitis. *Ophthalmic Res.* 2019;61(1):44–50.
199. Joshi L, Tanna A, McAdoo SP, et al. Long-term outcomes of rituximab therapy in ocular granulomatosis with polyangiitis: impact on localized and nonlocalized disease. *Ophthalmology.* 2015;122(6):1262–1268.
200. Suhler EB, Lim LL, Beardsley RM, et al. Rituximab therapy for refractory scleritis: results of a phase I/II dose-ranging, randomized, clinical trial. *Ophthalmology.* 2014;121(10):1885–1891.
201. Miserocchi E, Pontikaki I, Modorati G, Gattinara M, Meroni PL, Gerloni V. Anti-CD 20 monoclonal antibody (rituximab) treatment for inflammatory ocular diseases. *Autoimmun Rev.* 2011;11(1):35–39.
202. Lim WK, Fujimoto C, Ursea R, et al. Suppression of immune-mediated ocular inflammation in mice by interleukin 1 receptor antagonist administration. *Arch Ophthalmol.* 2005;123(7):957–963.
203. Teoh SC, Sharma S, Hogan A, et al. Tailoring biological treatment: anakinra treatment of posterior uveitis associated with the CINCA syndrome. *Br J Ophthalmol.* 2007;91(2):263–264.
204. Arostegui JI, Arnal C, Merino R, et al. NOD2 gene-associated pediatric granulomatous arthritis: clinical diversity, novel and recurrent mutations, and evidence of clinical improvement with interleukin-1 blockade in a Spanish cohort. *Arthritis Rheum.* 2007;56(11):3805–3813.
205. Nabhan C. The emerging role of alemtuzumab in chronic lymphocytic leukemia. *Clin Lymphoma Myeloma.* 2005;6(2):115–121.
206. Osterborg A, Mellstedt H, Keating M. Clinical effects of alemtuzumab (Campath-1H) in B-cell chronic lymphocytic leukemia. *Med Oncol.* 2002;19(Suppl):S21–S26.
207. Dearden C. The role of alemtuzumab in the management of T-cell malignancies. *Semin Oncol.* 2006;33(2 Suppl 5):S44–S52.
208. Dick AD, Meyer P, James T, et al. Campath-1H therapy in refractory ocular inflammatory disease. *Br J Ophthalmol.* 2000;84(1):107–109.
209. Mohammad AJ, Smith RM, Chow YW, Chaudhry AN, Jayne DR. Alemtuzumab as remission induction therapy in Behçet disease: a 20-year experience. *J Rheumatol.* 2015;42(10):1906–1913.
210. Willis MD, Pickersgill TP, Robertson NP, Lee RWJ, Dick AD, Carreño E. Alemtuzumab-induced remission of multiple sclerosis-associated uveitis. *Int Ophthalmol.* 2017;37(5):1229–1233.
211. Angeles-Han S, Flynn T, Lehman T. Abatacept for refractory juvenile idiopathic arthritis-associated uveitis—a case report. *J Rheumatol.* 2008;35(9):1897–1898.
212. Tappeiner C, Miserocchi E, Bodaghi B, et al. Abatacept in the treatment of severe, longstanding, and refractory uveitis associated with juvenile idiopathic arthritis. *J Rheumatol.* 2015;42(4):706–711.

213. Birolo C, Zannin ME, Arsenyeva S, et al. Comparable efficacy of abatacept used as first-line or second-line biological agent for severe juvenile idiopathic arthritis-related uveitis. *J Rheumatol.* 2016;43(11):2068–2073.
214. Zulian F, Balzarin M, Falcini F, et al. Abatacept for severe anti-tumor necrosis factor alpha refractory juvenile idiopathic arthritis-related uveitis. *Arthritis Care Res (Hoboken).* 2010;62(6):821–825.
215. Wennink RAW, Ayuso VK, de Vries LA, Vastert SJ, de Boer JH. Tocilizumab as an effective treatment option in children with refractory intermediate and panuveitis. *Ocul Immunol Inflamm.* 2020:1–5.
216. Vegas-Revenga N, Calvo-Río V, Mesquida M, et al. Anti-IL6-receptor tocilizumab in refractory and noninfectious uveitic cystoid macular edema: multicenter study of 25 patients. *Am J Ophthalmol.* 2019;200:85–94.
217. Atienza-Mateo B, Calvo-Río V, Beltrán E, et al. Anti-interleukin 6 receptor tocilizumab in refractory uveitis associated with Behçet's disease: multicentre retrospective study. *Rheumatology (Oxford).* 2018;57(5):856–864.
218. Eser Ozturk H, Oray M, Tugal-Tutkun I. Tocilizumab for the Treatment of Behçet uveitis that failed interferon alpha and anti-tumor necrosis factor-alpha therapy. *Ocul Immunol Inflamm.* 2018;26(7):1005–1014.
219. Mesquida M, Molins B, Llorenç V, et al. Twenty-four month follow-up of tocilizumab therapy for refractory uveitis-related macular edema. *Retina.* 2018;38(7):1361–1370.
220. Silpa-Archa S, Oray M, Preble JM, Foster CS. Outcome of tocilizumab treatment in refractory ocular inflammatory diseases. *Acta Ophthalmol.* 2016;94(6):e400–e406.
221. Papo M, Bielefeld P, Vallet H, et al. Tocilizumab in severe and refractory non-infectious uveitis. *Clin Exp Rheumatol.* 2014; 32(4 Suppl 84):S75–S79.
222. Mesquida M, Molins B, Llorenç V, Sainz de la Maza M, Adán A. Long-term effects of tocilizumab therapy for refractory uveitis-related macular edema. *Ophthalmology.* 2014;121(12):2380–2386.
223. Calvo-Río V, Santos-Gómez M, Calvo I, et al. Anti-interleukin-6 receptor tocilizumab for severe juvenile idiopathic arthritis-associated uveitis refractory to anti-tumor necrosis factor therapy: a multicenter study of twenty-five patients. *Arthritis Rheumatol.* 2017;69(3):668–675.
224. Sepah YJ, Sadiq MA, Chu DS, et al. Primary (month-6) outcomes of the STOP-Uveitis Study: evaluating the safety, tolerability, and efficacy of tocilizumab in patients with noninfectious uveitis. *Am J Ophthalmol.* 2017;183:71–80.
225. Chateau T, Angioi K, Peyrin-Biroulet L. Two cases of successful ustekinumab treatment for non-infectious uveitis associated with Crohn's disease. *J Crohns Colitis.* 2020;14(4):571.
226. Mugheddu C, Atzori L, Del Piano M, et al. Successful ustekinumab treatment of noninfectious uveitis and concomitant severe psoriatic arthritis and plaque psoriasis. *Dermatol Ther.* 2017;30(5).
227. Curreli S, Romerio F, Secchiero P, et al. IFN-alpha2b increases interleukin 10 expression in primary activated human CD8(+) T cells. *J Interferon Cytokine Res.* 2002;22:1167–1173.
228. Mackensen F, Max R, Becker MD. Interferon therapy for ocular disease. *Curr Opin Ophthalmol.* 2006;17(6):567–573.
229. Hasanreisoglu M, Cubuk MO, Ozdek S, et al. Interferon alpha-2a therapy in patients with refractory Behçet uveitis. *Ocul Immunol Inflamm.* 2017;25:71–75.
230. Diwo E, Gueudry J, Saadoun D, et al. Long-term efficacy of interferon in severe uveitis associated with Behçet disease. *Ocul Immunol Inflamm.* 2017;25:76–84.
231. Becker MD, Heiligenhaus A, Hudde T, et al. Interferon as a treatment for uveitis associated with multiple sclerosis. *Br J Ophthalmol.* 2005;89:1254–1257.
232. Deuter CM, Koetter I, Guenaydin I, et al. Interferon alfa-2a: a new treatment option for long lasting refractory cystoid macular edema in uveitis? A pilot study. *Retina.* 2006;26:786–791.
233. Butler NJ, Suhler EB, Rosenbaum JT. Interferon alpha 2b in the treatment of uveitic cystoid macular edema. *Ocul Immunol Inflamm.* 2012;20:86–90.
234. Kotter I, Eckstein AK, Stübiger N, et al. Treatment of ocular symptoms of Behcet's disease with interferon alfa 2a: a pilot study. *Br J Ophthalmol.* 1998;82:488–494.
235. Pivetti-Pezzi P, Accorinti M, Pirraglia MP, et al. Interferon alpha for ocular Behcet's disease. *Acta Ophthalmol Scand.* 1997;75:720–722.
236. Wechsler B, Bodaghi B, Huong DL, et al. Efficacy of interferon alfa-2a in severe and refractory uveitis associated with Behcet's disease. *Ocul Immunol Inflamm.* 2000;4:293–301.
237. Fardeau C, Simon A, Rodde B, et al. Interferon-alpha2a and systemic corticosteroid in monotherapy in chronic uveitis: results of the randomized controlled BIRDFERON Study. *Am J Ophthalmol.* 2017;177:182–194.
238. Mackensen F, Jakob E, Springer C, et al. Interferon versus methotrexate in intermediate uveitis with macular edema: results of a randomized controlled clinical trial. *Am J Ophthalmol.* 2013;156:478.e1-486.e1.
239. Tugal-Tutkun I, Onal S, Altan-Yaycioglu R, et al. Neovascularization of the optic disc in Behcet's disease. *Jpn J Ophthalmol.* 2006;50(3):256–265.
240. Krause L, Altenburg A, Bechrakis NE, et al. Intraocular surgery under systemic interferon-alpha therapy in ocular Adamantiades-Behcet's disease. *Graefes Arch Clin Exp Ophthalmol.* 2007;245(11):1617–1621.
241. Tellier Z. Human immunoglobulins in intraocular inflammation. *Ann NY Acad Sci.* 2007;1110:337–347.
242. Cassoux N, Haroun O, George F, et al. Effect of intravenous immunoglobulin (IVIg) in the treatment of birdshot retinochoroidopathy (Abstract). *Invest Ophthalmol Vis Sci.* 1996;37. S369.
243. Rosenbaum JT, George RK, Gordon C. The treatment of refractory uveitis with intravenous immunoglobulin. *Am J Ophthalmol.* 1999;127:545–549.
244. Guy J, Aptsiauri N. Treatment of paraneoplastic visual loss with intravenous immunoglobulin: report of 3 cases. *Arch Ophthalmol.* 1999;117:471–477.
245. Kazatchkine MD, Kaveri SV. Immunomodulation of autoimmune and inflammatory diseases with intravenous immune globulin. *N Engl J Med.* 2001;345(10):747–755.
246. Dalakas MC. Intravenous immune globulin therapy for neurologic diseases. *Ann Intern Med.* 1997;126:721–730.
247. Basta M, Van Goor F, Luccioli S, et al. F(ab)'2-mediated neutralization of C3a and C5a anaphylatoxins: a novel effector function of immunoglobulins. *Nat Med.* 2003;9(4):431–438.
248. Saoudi A, Hurez V, de Kozak Y, et al. Human immunoglobulin preparations for intravenous use prevent experimental autoimmune uveoretinitis. *Int Ophthalmol.* 1993;5:1559–1567.
249. Ayliffe W, Haeney M, Roberts SC, et al. Uveitis after antineutrophil cytoplasmic antibody contamination of immunoglobulin replacement therapy. *Lancet.* 1992;339:558–559.
250. Miserocchi E, Giuffrè C, Cornalba M, Pontikaki I, Cimaz R. JAK inhibitors in refractory juvenile idiopathic arthritis-associated uveitis. *Clin Rheumatol.* 2020;39(3):847–851.
251. Bauermann P, Heiligenhaus A, Heinz C. Effect of Janus kinase inhibitor treatment on anterior uveitis and associated macular edema in an adult patient with juvenile idiopathic arthritis. *Ocul Immunol Inflamm.* 2019;27(8):1232–1234.
252. Paley MA, Karacal H, Rao PK, Margolis TP, Miner JJ. Tofacitinib for refractory uveitis and scleritis. *Am J Ophthalmol Case Rep.* 2018;13:53–55.
253. Abel JJ, Rowntree LG, Turner BB. Plasma removal with return of corpuscles. *J Pharm Exp Ther.* 1914;5:920–925.
254. Skoog W, Adams W. Plasmapheresis in a case of Waldenström's macroglobulinemia. *Clin Res.* 1959;7:96.
255. Saraux H, Hoang Le, Audebert A-A, et al. Interet de la plasmapherese dans le traitement du syndrome de Behcet. *Bull Soc Ophthalmol Fr.* 1982;82(1):41–44.
256. Yanuzzi L. A perspective on treatment of aphakic cystoid macular edema. *Surv Ophthalmol.* 1984;28(Suppl):540–553.
257. Monthey K. Nonsteroid anti-inflammatory drugs in the treatment of intermediate uveitis. *Dev Ophthalmol.* 1992;23:158–162.
258. Herbort C. Uveoscleritis after excessive neodymium:YAG laser posterior capsulotomy. *J Cataract Refract Surg.* 1994;20(1):80–81.
259. Weiner H, Mackin GA, Matsui M, et al. Double-blind pilot trial of oral tolerization with myelin antigens in multiple sclerosis. *Science.* 1993;259(5099):1321–1324.
260. Trentham D, Dynesius-Trentham RA, Orav EJ, et al. Effects of oral administration of type II collagen on rheumatoid arthritis. *Science.* 1993;261(5129):1727–1730.

261. Nussenblatt R, de Smet M, Weiner HL, et al. The treatment of the ocular complications of Behcet's disease with oral tolerization. In: Wechsler B, Godeau P, eds. *Behcet's Disease. Proceedings of the 6th International Conference on Behcet's Disease*. Amsterdam: Excerpta Medica; 1993:641–646.
262. Nussenblatt RB, Gery I, Weiner HL, et al. Treatment of uveitis by oral administration of retinal antigens: results of a phase I/II randomized masked trial. *Am J Ophthalmol*. 1997;123:684–687.
263. Faria AM, Weiner HL. Oral tolerance: therapeutic implications for autoimmune diseases. *Clin Dev Immunol*. 2006;13(2–4):143–157.
264. Thurau SR, Wildner G. An HLA-peptide mimics organ-specific antigen in autoimmune uveitis: its role in pathogenesis and therapeutic induction of oral tolerance. *Autoimmun Rev*. 2003;2(4):171–176.
265. Thurau SR, Fricke H, Burchardi C, et al. Long-term follow-up of oral tolerance induction with HLA-peptide B27PD in patients with uveitis. *Ann NY Acad Sci*. 2004;1029:408–412.
266. Tsai E, Till G, Marak GJ. Effects of mydriatic agents on neutrophil migration. *Ophthalmic Res*. 1988;20:14–19.
267. Tomkins-Netzer O, Lightman SL, Burke AE, Sugar EA, Lim LL, Jaffe GJ, Altaweel MM, Kempen JH, Holbrook JT, Jabs DA; Multicenter Steroid Treatment Trial and Follow-up Study Research Group. Seven-Year Outcomes of Uveitic Macular Edema: The Multicenter Uveitis Steroid Treatment Trial and Follow-up Study Results. *Ophthalmology*. 2020 Sep 10:S0161-6420(20)30884-8. https://doi.org/10.1016/j.ophtha.2020.08.035. Epub ahead of print. PMID: 32918964.
268. Kempen JH, Gangaputra S, Daniel E, et al. Long-term risk of malignancy among patients treated with immunosuppressive agents for ocular inflammation: a critical assessment of the evidence. *Am J Ophthalmol*. 2008;146(6):802–812. e1.
269. Kempen JH, Newcomb CW, Foster CS, et al. Risk of overall and cancer mortality after immunosuppression of patients with noninfectious ocular inflammatory diseases. *Invest. Ophthalmol. Vis. Sci*. 2019;60(9):3854.
270. Sandhu HS, Kaplan HJ. Novel therapies in the treatment of noninfectious uveitis. *Expert Review Ophthalmology*. 2018;13(3):139–147.

9

Role of Surgery in the Patient with Uveitis

H. Nida Sen

KEY CONCEPTS

- Inflammatory disease needs to be clinically quiescent for at least 3 months before elective surgery is considered.
- Adequate immunosuppressive therapy perioperatively is very important.
- Surgery needs to be considered when there is something to save, not when the disease is at the end stage.

Despite even optimal medical therapy, structural damage will develop in many eyes with chronic inflammation, which can be repaired only by surgical intervention. In the past, surgery was often attempted hesitantly because of a high incidence of complications, including uncontrolled inflammation, hypotony, and phthisis. Two advances have contributed to safer surgical intervention in these eyes. The first is improved control of inflammation with steroids or other drugs, and the second is the rapid advancement in microsurgical techniques that has improved our ability to operate on the anterior segment, vitreous, and retina.[1] In this chapter, the principles of ophthalmic surgery as they apply to the inflamed eye, both for therapy and for diagnosis, are discussed. However, the anatomic alterations in eyes with severe uveitis are unique, and the approach to each eye often must be determined individually.

CONSIDERATIONS

In general, the indications for proceeding with surgery need to be more carefully considered in eyes with uveitis. Because of the possible increased risks, surgery is frequently not justified for eyes with slightly reduced, but functional, vision, which are not in danger of visual loss from a surgically repairable problem. However, we have observed many eyes in which surgery was delayed for so long that potentially treatable problems became hidden behind cataract or vitreous haze. Vision was then permanently lost because of the attempt to use surgery conservatively; vision might have been saved if the inflammatory disease and its complications could have been directly viewed and treated. There is a tendency to not operate on an eye with dense opacities and light-perception vision, but unseen and untreated inflammation causes further permanent damage to the retina. In addition to visual rehabilitation, surgical procedures in eyes with uveitis are performed as part of a diagnostic evaluation. The relative risks versus the potential benefits are considered here.

Except for the few situations in which it is necessary to operate on an acutely inflamed eye, surgery should be performed when the inflammation is quiescent. However, in some patients, it is impossible to clear every cell from the anterior chamber or vitreous. Furthermore, in patients with dense cataracts and primarily vitreoretinal inflammation, it is impossible accurately to assess the activity of the disease behind the opacity. Therefore an attempt should be made to reduce the inflammation as much as possible, but surgery should not be delayed while the patient endures a long-term visual handicap because the inflammation never becomes completely quiescent. If the inflammatory activity cannot be fully assessed, the eye may be treated prophylactically as though active inflammation were present.

In our opinion, corticosteroids are still the best drugs for control of inflammation in the perioperative period. In a small study of 20 patients randomly selected to receive prednisone or cyclosporin before cataract surgery, we found that 3 of 10 patients treated with cyclosporin, but none of the steroid-treated patients, had severe postoperative inflammation that necessitated a change in medication to the other drug. Corticosteroids work at multiple points in the inflammatory process, as described in Chapter 8, and are able to affect inflammation mediated by neutrophils and macrophages and that by lymphocytes. Therefore they may prevent nonspecific postoperative inflammation that may occur in a previously inflamed eye and inhibit the more specific pathways of inflammation. We prefer to begin steroid therapy on the day before or on the day of surgery if the patient is not already receiving the drug, and if there is no evidence of active inflammatory disease. Some practitioners prefer to start steroid therapy several days before the scheduled surgical intervention. If there is no strong contraindication this may not be unreasonable in some patients. Usually, a steroid dose of 1 mg/kg/day or 60 mg/day (whichever is lower) is adequate. Preoperative subconjunctival or intravitreal corticosteroid injection can also be considered as an alternative. If the patient has a history of severe intraocular inflammation, an intravenous dose of corticosteroids, such as 50 to 100 mg of methylprednisolone, can also be given at the time of surgery. The goal is clearly to prevent severe postoperative inflammation.

The surgeon should be aware that with the aforementioned perioperative therapy, the eye may appear relatively quiet for the first few days after surgery, but the inflammation may increase a few days later. It is therefore critical to monitor patients with uveitis closely during the first 5 to 7 days after surgery. It is also important to remember that this perioperative corticosteroid regimen is administered in addition to the immunomodulatory regimen that the patient has already been receiving. In young patients, marked postoperative flares of inflammation, accompanied by significant fibrin and protein within the eye, can occur. Tissue plasminogen activator can be used to clear severe fibrin accumulation in the anterior chamber (Fig. 9.1). After surgery, these eyes frequently have hypotony, and although they appear to be in imminent danger of phthisis, aggressive and continued treatment with steroids and other immunomodulators usually results in marked improvement.

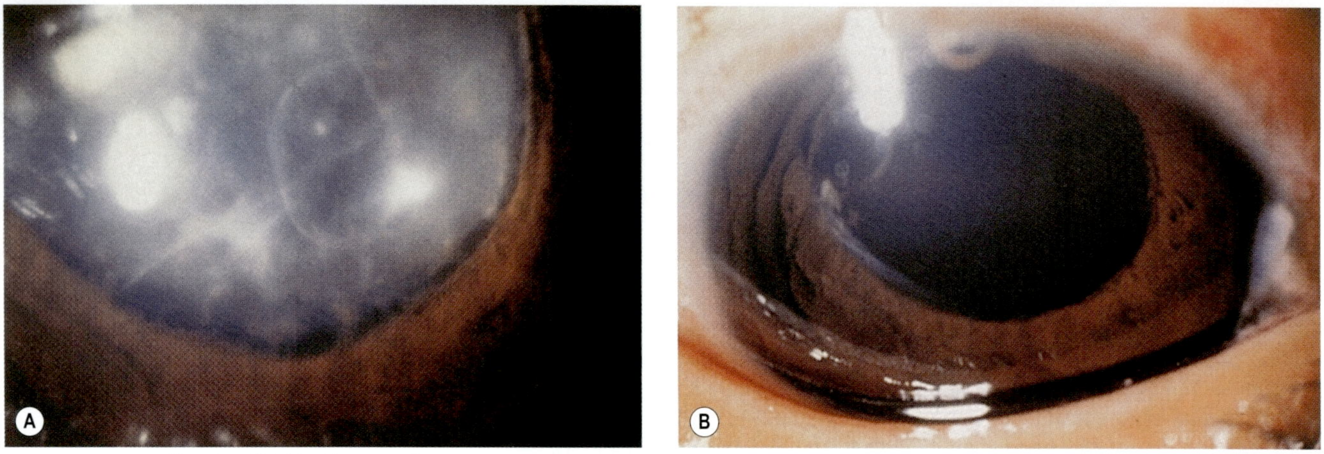

Fig. 9.1 (A) Uveitic eye after extracapsular cataract extraction (phacoemulsification) and intraocular lens placement. The postoperative inflammatory response was severe, with the development of fibrin in the anterior chamber. (B) Clinical improvement occurred 24 hours after injection with tissue plasminogen activator. (Courtesy Rubens Belfort, Jr., MD, Sao Paulo, Brazil.)

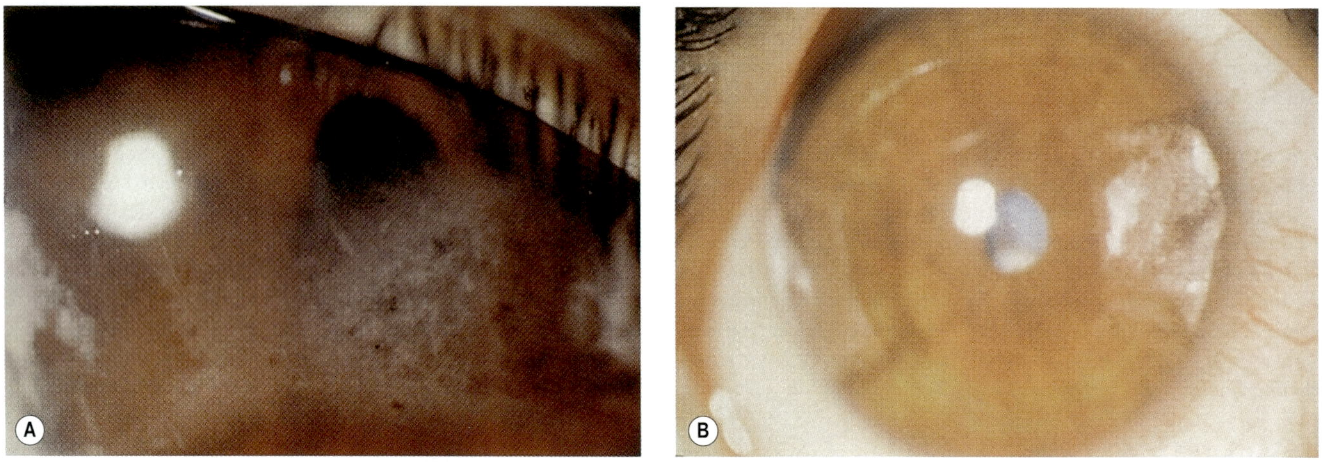

Fig. 9.2 (A) Band keratopathy in 6-year-old boy with bilateral uveitis. (B) Same eye 2 days after excimer laser surgery performed under topical anesthesia. (Courtesy Rubens Belfort, Jr., MD, Sao Paulo, Brazil.)

REMOVAL OF BAND KERATOPATHY

Calcium hydroxyapatite accumulates in the Bowman membrane of the cornea in some patients with sarcoidosis or juvenile rheumatoid arthritis (JRA) and occasionally in younger patients with chronic uveitis, such as pars planitis. Its location may be related to the local pH of the interpalpebral cornea. It can be removed by chelation if it is located centrally and interferes with vision because of opacity or glare or if it is the cause of recurrent corneal erosions. Although chelation with 1% to 2% ethylenediaminetetraacetic acid (EDTA) can be performed under local anesthesia, the young age of most patients with this condition makes general anesthesia necessary. Our procedure is to use a sterile 1.7% solution of EDTA in water or saline applied to the cornea with cotton or a cellulose applicator. Gentle pressure and movement of the applicator result in removal of the corneal epithelium and gradual solubilization of the calcium deposits. This procedure can take up to 30 minutes and often must be performed before intraocular surgery. Occasionally, resistant deposits must be gently removed with a spatula or a Tooke knife, but this may cause scarring of the Bowman membrane and should be avoided in the visual axis. The eye is then patched until the epithelial defect heals. Band keratopathy has also been removed with the excimer laser[2] (Fig. 9.2). It should be remembered that eyes with uveitis may have recurrences of the band even years after the removal of the calcium.[3] Further, the procedure may very rarely induce a severe inflammatory response, as was reported in one patient.[4]

CORNEAL TRANSPLANTATION

Although keratic precipitates involve the corneal endothelial surface, in our experience, endothelial decompensation is rare in patients with chronic uveitis. Thus corneal transplantation is rarely performed in this group because of corneal edema, but it may be necessary in patients with corneoscleral melting in association with systemic inflammatory disease and intraocular inflammation or in patients with herpetic keratouveitis. If the intraocular inflammation has been severe, there may be coexisting glaucoma or cataract. The primary goal before corneal transplantation in these patients is to control the immune process, or the newly grafted tissue will melt as well. The ongoing inflammatory response suggests that the risk for rejection of a cornea transplant in any patient with active uveitis is high because there are already large numbers of cells in the eye that could present corneal antigens to the immune system and participate in the rejection event. Certain severe manifestations of immune-mediated ocular surface disease, such as vernal

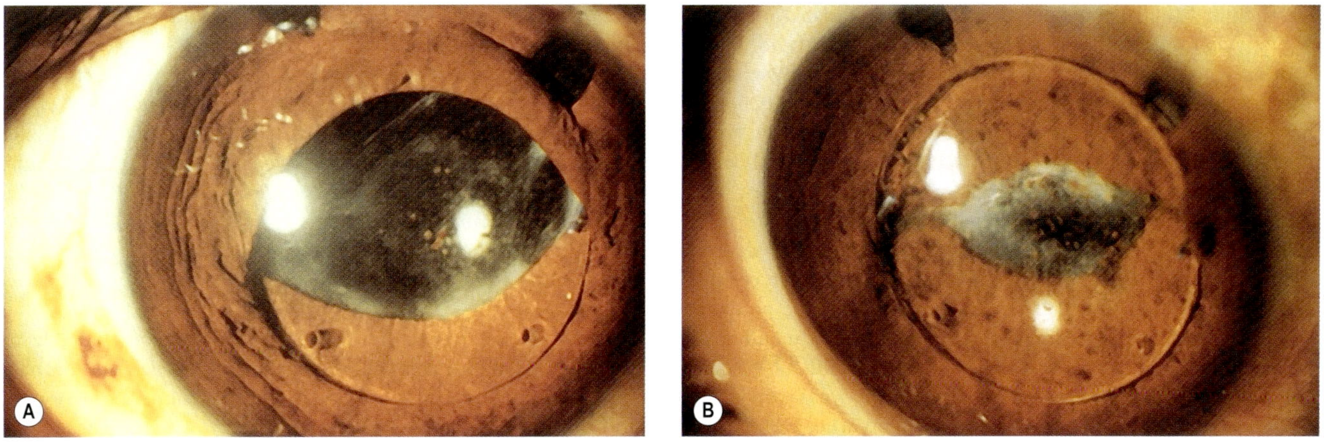

Fig. 9.3 Uveitic eye that underwent cataract surgery and posterior chamber intraocular lens (IOL) placement. (A) Inferior portion of lens has migrated anterior to lens plane. (B) The whole lens is now forward. This "iris capture" occurred without marked inflammatory disease. (Courtesy Rubens Belfort, Jr., MD, Sao Paulo, Brazil.)

keratoconjunctivitis, can lead to limbal stem cell deficiency, and before penetrating keratoplasty is considered, the ocular surface environment needs to be addressed. The treating physician should be aware of the drugs being given for other indications that may induce uveitis and risk graft survival. Richards et al.[5] described such a case of a patient receiving alendronate sodium for osteoporosis. The uveitis resolved after cessation of the drug. More recently, advanced endothelial keratoplasty techniques, such as deep lamellar endothelial keratoplasty (DLEK), Descemet stripping endothelial keratoplasty (DSEK), and Descemet membrane endothelial keratoplasty (DMEK), have resulted in improved visual outcomes and reduced rejection.[6]

CATARACT SURGERY

More information concerning cataract extraction in uveitic eyes has been acquired in recent years.[7,13] Individual patients and various disorders often require different approaches. Summaries of procedures performed 20 to 30 years ago suggested that the outcome of cataract surgery in eyes with uveitis was poor and that phthisis occurred frequently. This is clearly no longer the case, thanks largely to new technologies and approaches.

Extracapsular extraction with phacoemulsification is now the standard approach. This approach has the advantage of smaller incisions and less manipulation of the iris and, hence, less postoperative inflammation.[8-11] Postoperative complications include formation of posterior synechiae to the capsule, pupillary block glaucoma, the inability to remove vitreous debris, haze and vitreoretinal traction, and possible opacification of the posterior capsule. Neodymium:yttrium–aluminum–garnet (Nd:YAG) laser capsulotomy can also lead to exacerbation of inflammation. Herbort[12] reported the case of a patient in whom severe and recurrent scleritis and uveitis developed after Nd:YAG capsulotomy was performed 18 months after cataract extraction. Also, laser-induced iris punctures often close off readily in inflamed eyes. In all patients undergoing surgery, we wish to see the ocular inflammatory process well controlled with a stable treatment regimen for at least 3 months

The surgeon may encounter challenging technical problems. Various types of iris retractors can be used to overcome the issue of small pupils with synechiae. Posterior synechiae not only may be present at the pupillary border but also may extend over the entire surface of the lens.

It is imperative to reiterate that one needs to use any means necessary to bring the eye's inflammatory disease under strict control. In a meta-analysis, patients with uveitis with 2- to 3-month control had better visual outcomes compared with those who were active at the time of surgery, regardless of the type of surgery or the subtype of uveitis.[13] They also found that eyes with Fuchs uveitis, a disease with low-grade inflammation and now known to be associated with rubella infection, had the best outcomes, whereas posterior uveitis had worse visual outcomes. Sen et al.[14] found that cataract surgery outcomes were similar among patients receiving systemic immunosuppressive therapy compared with those who had fluocinolone acetonide implant as part of a randomized clinical trial with an overall gain of 23 letters postoperatively. Although longer duration of uveitis and preoperative hypotony was associated with poorer visual outcomes, there was still visual gain.[14] It is also important to note that in patients with chronic macular edema, this should be minimized with maximum therapy prior to cataract surgery. Bélair et al.[15] investigated postoperative cystoid macular edema (CME) incidence in uveitic and nonuveitic eyes in a prospective cohort study and found that CME, as determined with OCT, was higher (12% and 8%) among uveitic eyes compared with nonuveitic eyes (4% and 0%) at postoperative months 1 and 3. Eyes treated with perioperative oral corticosteroids and were quiet 3 months before cataract surgery had significantly less risk of CME.[15] The patient should be informed about the possible need for continued and even more aggressive immunosuppressive therapy to control the disease postoperatively. Phacoemulsification with placement of the intraocular lens (IOL) in the bag is the preferred approach.[16] Iris capture (Fig. 9.3)[17] is seen less with modern surgical approaches and better inflammation control, and patients with posterior synechiae have a greater risk for occurrence of this problem and capsule contraction syndrome postoperatively.[18]

Much interest has been shown in surface-modified lenses and the possibility of their ability to reduce the postoperative inflammatory response in the past. Alio et al.,[19] in a prospective study of cataract surgery in uveitic eyes, compared four different types of IOLs. Using hydrophobic acrylic, silicone, polymethylmethacrylate (PMMA), and heparin surface-modified PMMA lenses, they concluded that the acrylic IOLs had a better visual outcome and lower complication rate, whereas both acrylic and heparin surface-modified PMMA lenses had the lowest relapse rates. Multiple studies support the finding that acrylic IOLs and heparin-surface-modified (HSM) PMMA IOLs show slightly better visual outcomes compared with non-HSM PMMA or silicone IOLs.[13] Angle-supported lenses have been associated with anterior and intermediate uveitides.[20]

The eyes of patients with juvenile idiopathic arthritis (JIA) deserve particular attention.[21] Historically, these eyes have not been considered good candidates for IOLs. The reason for this is the potential of the lens to act as a scaffold for the development of membranes in eyes with low-grade chronic disease that is often difficult to control. Kotaniemi et al.[22] reported that 64% of 36 JIA eyes receiving an implant had visual acuities of 20/40 or better. Woreta et al.[23] reported on the risk factors for ocular complications in 75 patients with JIA undergoing surgery and found that 67% had ocular complications. Eyes with more than 1+ flare, a history of previous intraocular surgery, and posterior synechiae all had a higher risk of poorer vision postoperatively. Mehta et al., in their meta-analysis, evaluated 16 articles that focused on JIA-associated uveitis and found that among eyes with quiet or mostly quiet uveitis, 71% gained visual acuity of 20/40 or better, whereas only 22% of active eyes showed visual gain of 20/40 or better.[13] It would seem that the degree of activity, control of disease, and secondary structural complications caused by uveitis are important considerations.

Results from the literature support the notion that IOL placement in uveitic eyes can result in a positive outcome.[10,24] Pleyer et al.,[25] in their report of a 5-year series, stated that 71% of 28 eyes receiving an IOL had postoperative visual acuity of 0.5 or better, compared with 54% of the 24 eyes that were aphakic. Similarly, Foster et al. also reported 60% of 20 patients achieving 20/100 or better.[26] Because these were not randomized studies it is difficult to compare the relative "success" rates. A meta-analysis of cataract surgery in uveitis found that active uveitis at the time of surgery was associated with worse visual outcomes and that uveitic eyes that underwent cataract surgery with IOL placement did better than those without IOL placement. Their subgroup analysis also indicated that IOL use was preferable for the average case.[13]

Complications from cataract surgery or sequelae from the ongoing inflammation must be expected.[27,28] CME is the most common complication of cataract surgery in the general population. Among eyes with uveitis, CME has been reported to occur in up to 33% of eyes and can be particularly more common in intermediate uveitis.[29] However, preoperative inflammation control and perioperative corticosteroids have been associated with much lower CME incidence.[15] Posterior capsule opacification is seen frequently. When Dana et al.[30] compared rates of posterior capsule opacification between 78 patients with uveitis and 106 patients without uveitis undergoing cataract surgery, the rates were comparable when an adjustment was made for the younger age of the patients with uveitis. Estafanous et al.[9] reported that of the 39 uveitic eyes needing surgery, posterior capsular opacification was seen in 24 eyes (62%), with 12 of these (31%) needing Nd:YAG capsulotomy. Of these patients, 41% experienced recurrence of disease. If CME was present before surgery, it will most probably be there after the surgery and will need to be addressed. Epiretinal membrane formations can be seen. Lenses do need to be explanted, even after the best preoperative consideration by the surgeon. In a report by Foster et al.,[31] of 19 patients whose lenses were explanted, perilental membrane was the reason in eight, low-grade inflammation in eight, a cyclitic membrane leading to hypotony in one, retinal detachment in one, and vitreous hemorrhage in one.

Pars plana lensectomy, usually combined with vitrectomy, has been used by several authors to remove a cataract, reshape the pupil, and remove vitreous opacities and vitreoretinal traction in one operation.[32-36] The operation can be performed by using the standard technique: three 1-mm incisions 3 or 3.5 mm posterior to the limbus. Trauma to the trabecular meshwork is avoided. Removal of the vitreous can reduce the accumulation of cells and haze during an episode of inflammation, but vision will still be affected by a new inflammatory episode.

Results for cataract surgery have been reported to be favorable with the anterior chamber approach and with entry through the pars plana. Results depend more on previous damage from the inflammation than on the surgical technique. Praeger et al.[37] reported excellent improvement after extracapsular surgery in patients with JRA. Mackensen and Loeffler[38] reported that in 86 patients with chronic iridocyclitis who underwent extracapsular surgery, inflammation was reduced by 70% and recurrences by 94%. Vision improved in most patients. In a study by Smith et al.[32] 12 patients with chronic uveitis who underwent pars plana lensectomy/vitrectomy had improved vision, but CME impaired the acuity in most of them. Girard et al.[33] reported that 5-year remissions of uveitis occurred in all of their 23 patients, and 21 had improved vision after pars plana surgery. In the 39 patients Petrelli et al.[34] studied after pars plana surgery, 23% had vision better than 20/40, 56% had vision worse than 20/100, and 18% had CME. Other authors have reported similar experiences.[35,36]

Hypotony is often mentioned as a contraindication for cataract removal in these patients. However, visual gain after cataract surgery has been reported in patients with preoperative hypotony.[14] In many eyes with posterior inflammation, there is dense anterior hyaloid that may be associated with ciliary body traction. Removal of this traction may result in improved ciliary body function.

We have seen that removal of these tractional forces will cause an increase in intraocular pressure (IOP), not enormous, but enough to achieve a more reassuring pressure. Yu et al.[39] reported similar results in patients with JIA.

Although phthisis may result, we have observed five eyes with preoperative hypotony in which there was an increase in IOP of several millimeters of mercury (mm Hg) after pars plana lensectomy/vitrectomy.

GLAUCOMA SURGERY

Secondary glaucoma that cannot be controlled with medical therapy is sometimes a consequence of severe anterior segment inflammation, or it can be the result of corticosteroid therapy. It is important to differentiate between pupillary block glaucoma and secondary angle closure by peripheral anterior synechiae. The two processes may coexist in the eye with uveitis. Active inflammation may suppress ciliary body function and also reduce trabecular filtration. Thus IOP in the actively inflamed eye may be higher or lower than that in the uninflamed eye. Although patients with long-standing chronic inflammation have poor outflow, increased inflammation will lead to reduced aqueous production and a pressure decrease.

It may be difficult to distinguish pupillary block glaucoma in a patient with chronic inflammation and posterior synechiae that involve the entire lens surface. These patients do not show the classic iris bombé pattern but may have a subtle shallowing of the anterior chamber with a low, peripheral iris bombé. The iris elevation may be localized only to areas where the iris and the lens do not

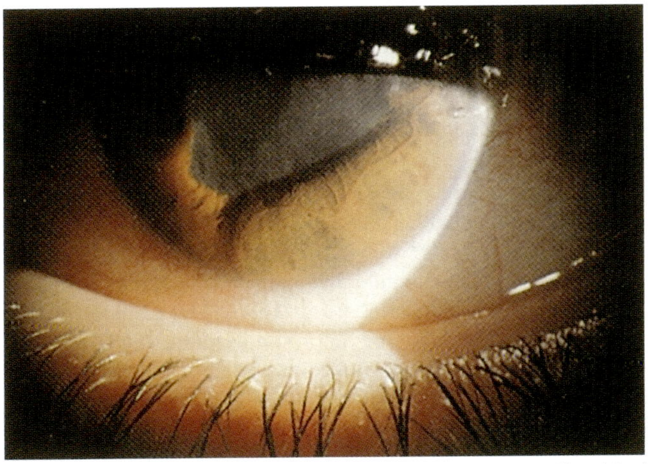

Fig. 9.4 Slit-lamp photograph of patient with uveitis and pupillary block glaucoma. Iris bombé, caused by broad iris–lens synechiae, localized from the 3- to the 6-o'clock position.

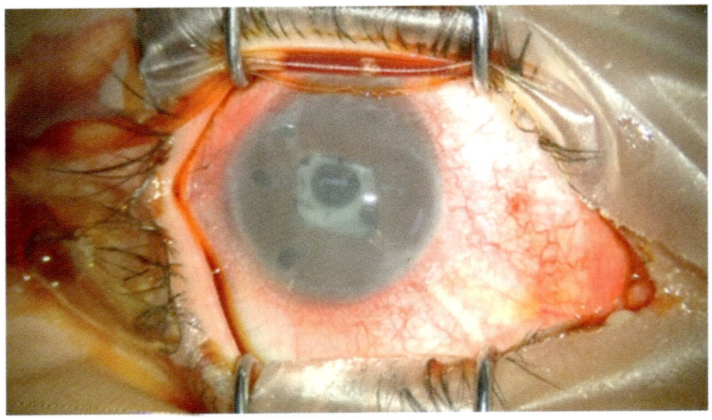

Fig. 9.5 Uveitic eye with secondary glaucoma with a failed superotemporal Ahmed glaucoma valve (AGV) placement, now with the second inferonasal AGV in the right eye. Note the patient is pseudophakic with pupillary membrane and multiple surgical iridectomies (see Case 9.3). (Courtesy Dr. Mehmet Yakin.)

adhere (Fig. 9.4). If the diagnosis is suspected but unclear, laser iridectomy will confirm it and also be therapeutic. If the laser iridectomy fails to lower the IOP, pupillary block can be ruled out as a mechanism.

Filtering surgery, such as a trabeculectomy, is less successful in patients with ongoing uveitis because of the younger age of such patients and because the inflammatory mediators promote fibrous tissue growth and closure of the filtering bleb. An alternative surgical approach, that is, deep sclerectomy using various implants, has been reported to be useful in treating uveitic glaucoma.[40] A normal response on the part of the treating physician is frequently to practice restraint because of the problems inherent in operating on patients with uveitis. An insidious loss of visual function caused by the glaucoma can ensue even with excellent control of the uveitis. If not clinically urgent, glaucoma surgery should be performed when the eye is quiet at a site where surgery has not previously been performed. Because these eyes frequently need repeat surgical procedures, combining a filtering operation (often with mitomycin C) with cataract removal, if appropriate, seems justified to reduce the number of possible interventions.[41] The rates of IOP control appear to be comparable between patients with uveitic glaucoma and those with primary open angle glaucoma after phacotrabeculectomy.[42]

5-fluorouracil (5-FU) and mitomycin C are some of the drugs used to improve the success of filtering surgery by slowing the growth of fibrous tissue. Patitsas et al.[43] used 5-FU combined with filtering surgery to treat patients with both uveitis and glaucoma. They found that IOP was controlled in 71% of 21 eyes over a median of 35 months. Control was better achieved in phakic eyes (90%) than in aphakic or pseudophakic (55%) eyes. Complications associated with 5-FU use have occurred. Towler et al.[44] reported their experience with 50 uveitic glaucomatous eyes in 43 consecutive patients. They observed an 82% success rate at 1 and 2 years and a 67% success rate at 5 years by applying 5-FU (25 mg/mL) for 5 minutes to the area of the bleb. In another report by Ceballos et al.[45] 44 eyes in 44 patients were treated with local application of either mitomycin C or 5-FU. "Complete success" was defined as IOP of 21 mm Hg or less in a patient taking no other antiglaucoma medication. In this study,[45] the success rates at 2 years were 39% in men and 71% in women, and 74% in whites but only 55% in black individuals. Over half of the patients developed cataracts or saw their cataracts progress, and 25% needed repeat surgery. Although 5-FU therapy may keep the bleb open during the initial few weeks, months, or years after surgery, recurrent inflammation could still threaten to destroy a functional filtering bleb.

Alternative approaches in children include modified goniotomy or trabeculodialysis. Kanski and McAllister[46] reported on 23 such operations, with a 60% success rate in patients with JRA. However, in only five patients could control be achieved without additional antiglaucoma medication. Williams et al.[47] reported success in 56% of 25 uveitic eyes undergoing trabeculodialysis, with aphakic eyes doing no worse than those that were phakic. Ultrasonic filtering surgery has not yet been used in an adequate number of patients with uveitis to determine whether this approach may be helpful.

The approach that has been most beneficial in patients with uveitis is the use of an aqueous draining device. There are several such devices, including nonvalved implants, such as the Molteno (Fig. 9.5), Baerveldt, Schocket, and Eagle vision implants. Valved or flow-restrictive implants allow unidirectional flow from the anterior chamber to the subconjunctival space. The most commonly used valved implant is the Ahmed glaucoma valve. These devices reduce acute postoperative hypotony and improve IOP control. Hill et al.[48] reviewed the cases of 45 patients with both uveitis and glaucoma and found that an aqueous drainage device was more likely to control IOP in those who had significant, immediate, or chronic postoperative inflammation. However, those authors believed that trabeculectomy produced surprisingly good results as well. Freedman and Rubin[49] have also reported good results with a single-plate Molteno implant. Long-term results with the Ahmed valve in patients with uveitis have been reported.[51] Success rates at 4 years ranged between 39%-65.7%[50,51] and the complication rate was 12% per person-year. Visual acuity loss was 4% per person-year. Several studies have suggested that the Ahmed valve implant is safe, especially in adult patients, but it appears that the Ahmed valve alone is moderately effective in controlling IOP.[52-54] Thus a significant number of patients may still need antiglaucoma medications over the long term. With its incorporated valve mechanism, the Ahmed valve tends to have less postoperative hypotony–related complications, whereas the Baerveldt implant, with its large surface area, has the advantage of better long-term IOP control.[55] Similar to trabeculectomy, good perioperative control of inflammation appears to improve the success rates of glaucoma drainage devices.[56]

If the aforementioned surgical approaches fail, an attempt can be made to reduce aqueous formation. Cyclocryotherapy and laser destruction are both possible methods for achieving this. Cryotherapy is now very rarely used for this purpose, particularly in uveitis. Cyclocryotherapy is performed in sequential treatments 4 to 8 weeks apart. Treatment begins from the 6- to the 8-o'clock positions with 1-minute freezes. If this fails to lower IOP after several weeks, six more clock-hour positions are treated, with three of the clock hours overlapping the first treatment. Further treatments may be required, but these need to be approached cautiously. The operation is accompanied by significant postoperative pain and does not offer immediate resolution. Laser destruction of the ciliary processes allows for more careful titration of the destructive process, particularly with the use of endoscopic cyclophotocoagulation. However, both approaches carry the risk of postprocedure inflammation.[57]

Although trabeculectomy is still the gold standard for the surgical management of many types of glaucoma and although both trabeculectomy and tube shunt surgeries are usually very effective in controlling IOP, around one-third of the patients develop long-term complications after both surgical procedures.[58,59] Thus there is a need for less invasive, but effective, surgical alternatives. A relatively new approach is microinvasive glaucoma surgery (MIGS). Although the pressure reduction does not match that achieved with traditional glaucoma surgeries, MIGS has significantly fewer adverse events.[60] Various types of MIGS have been developed so far, but very little is known about their safety and efficacy in uveitic glaucoma. Swamy et al. reported 91% success rate after ab interno trabeculectomy with the use of a trabectome in patients with uveitic glaucoma at the 12-month follow-up.[61] However, Sng et al. reported a 79.2% success rate after XEN-45 collagen implant at the 12-month follow-up.[62] Although these studies reported promising short-term results for uveitic glaucoma, long-term studies on the safety and efficacy of MIGS, especially for patients with different uveitis types and disease activity, are needed.

TREATMENT OF VITREORETINAL DISEASE

Significant vitreous opacities, areas of vitreoretinal traction, or epiretinal membranes sometimes develop in patients who have severe posterior inflammation, and newer techniques have permitted these problems to be approached with a reasonable hope of success.[63] Lens fragments persisting after cataract surgery can be a source of ongoing inflammation and should be promptly removed.[64] If the opacities and membranes appear to be the major source of a decrease in vision or if there is a significant tractional retinal detachment, then vitrectomy without lensectomy is indicated. In general, the surgical management of these eyes does not differ from that of eyes with vitreous opacities or traction from other causes. Vitrectomy is now often combined with phacoemulsification, and, in addition, there has been growing interest in using 27-gauge vitrectomy units, with many studies reporting good results.[65]

The value of vitrectomy alone as a therapeutic tool for intraocular inflammatory disease remains debatable.[66] Bacskulin and Eckardt[68] reported that in 13 children with uveitis who underwent vitrectomy, either alone or combined with lensectomy, the disease was easier to treat and that in some, there was resolution of macular edema. We have found that vitrectomy is useful to observe the posterior pole and thus to monitor the course of disease, and the procedure appears to make it easier for steroid to penetrate intraocularly. Kaplan[68] and Stavrou et al.[69] found that in 44% of 43 eyes, there was improvement in the course of intermediate uveitis. Bovey et al.[70] performed vitrectomy, cataract extraction, or both in 30 eyes and reported improvement in visual acuity, although no decrease in the inflammatory process; Nolle and Eckardt[71] also reported the same findings in nine patients with multifocal chorioretinitis who underwent vitrectomy. Gutfleisch et al.[72] performed pars plana vitrectomy coupled with intravitreal injections of triamcinolone to treat CME. CME improved in 58% of patients in the first 6 weeks, but the effect was transient, with 85% of patients showing cataract progression and increases in IOP seen in over one-quarter of the 19 patients treated. Indeed, a small, randomized controlled trial comparing vitrectomy (n = 12) with medical therapy (n = 11) for CME showed that in the vitrectomy group, CME improved in four patients, remained unchanged in seven, and worsened in one.[73] In a very good review of 44 interventional case series involving 1575 patients, Becker and Davis[74] found that in 39 reports, after vitrectomy of uveitic eyes, visual acuity improved in 68% of cases, was unchanged in 20%, and was worse in 12%. The CME findings in these patients halved. A systematic review of the literature by Henry et al.[75] included 627 patients and 708 total eyes undergoing pars plana vitrectomy for uveitis and found that vision improved in 69% of eyes and the proportion of eyes with CME decreased from 52% preoperatively to 37% postoperatively. Concomitant use of systemic corticosteroids and immunosuppressives also decreased.[75] However, lack of standardization in outcomes and reporting and lack of prospective data make it hard to draw definitive conclusions from these studies.

Epiretinal membrane is a common complication of uveitis, occurring in up to 41% of uveitic eyes, and intermediate uveitis is most commonly associated with epiretinal membrane compared with other anatomic locations.[76] The prognosis for visual improvement after removal of the epiretinal membrane has been reported to be worse in eyes with uveitis than in eyes with idiopathic membranes.[77] Retinal detachment is surprisingly not that uncommon in these patients. In one review of 1387 patients,[78] 43 (46 eyes) had a retinal detachment (3.1% of the total). It was most frequently associated with panuveitis and eyes with infectious disease. The uveitis was active in almost one-half of the patients studied. In addition, after repair of rhegmatogenous retinal detachment by using standard scleral buckling procedures, there is probably a higher risk of proliferative vitreoretinopathy (PVR) in eyes with ongoing chronic inflammation because inflammatory mediators stimulate fibrous tissue proliferation. It was seen in 30% of the patients in a study by Kerkhoff et al.[78] The development of PVR usually necessitates additional surgery with membrane stripping and gas–fluid exchange. After this procedure, control of inflammation is critical, or the membranes may form again.[78] However, a report on a small cohort of patients with uveitis with well-controlled preoperative inflammation indicated that the results and recurrence rates of epiretinal membrane removal in eyes with uveitis were similar to those for eyes without uveitis.[79]

Serous detachment is a commonly encountered problem in uveitis and is almost always treated medically. However, there are stubborn cases that may not respond to therapy, either for mechanical reasons, such as traction, or for reasons that are unclear. Surgical drainage can be contemplated, often with reattachment being successful.[80]

The repair of giant retinal tears that may complicate viral retinitis, such as acute retinal necrosis or cytomegalovirus retinitis, is not always best managed with scleral buckling. The retina in these diseases has become necrotic, and some areas may be ischemic. The use of a high buckle might increase this ischemia, leading to retinal neovascularization. An alternative solution has been to perform pars plana vitrectomy and to reattach the retina with gas or silicone oil tamponade and laser photocoagulation.[81]

LASER TREATMENT

Lasers can be used to perform peripheral iridectomies and posterior capsulotomies, to cut pupillary membranes, to clear deposits off the anterior surface of an IOL, and to treat retinal or subretinal neovascularization. The use of the laser, however, does not eliminate the possibility of induction of inflammation.

In the anterior segment either the YAG or the argon laser can be used to perform iridotomy. Although the procedure is probably technically easier with the YAG laser, there is the theoretic possibility that the incidence of hyphema from the vascular, inflamed iris may be greater after YAG laser treatment than after argon laser treatment because the YAG laser does not coagulate tissue. Posterior capsulotomy is easily performed with the YAG laser unless there has been a significant fibrous reaction or calcification as a result of the inflammation. Pupillary membranes can occasionally be so dense that the laser procedure becomes very long, necessitates the use of high energies, or cannot be successfully performed at all (Fig. 9.6). In addition, although an uncomplicated capsulotomy can be performed with only a few bursts of laser energy, and at the time of the procedure it appears that little has been disrupted within the eye, the energy delivered by the YAG laser does alter the blood–aqueous barrier.[82] In rabbits, the application of the YAG laser to the iris induced intraocular production of interleukin (IL)-6, IL-8, and tumor necrosis factor-α as well as nitric oxide.[83] Timolol seemed to reduce the production of all these mediators of inflammation, except for nitric oxide. Therefore use of the YAG laser in patients with severe inflammatory disease should be considered with the same care as that of an invasive surgical procedure; the procedure should be avoided in active eyes, and the patient should be pretreated with topical corticosteroids to prevent recurrence of inflammation.

Photocoagulation of the retina for surface or subretinal neovascularization may also be accompanied by bouts of inflammation. Panretinal or sector argon photocoagulation for surface neovascularization is indicated if the new vessels have not regressed with antiinflammatory therapy. Patients with sarcoidosis and neovascularization of the optic disk often show regression of the vessels with steroid therapy. In contrast, patients with retinal neovascularization caused by Behçet disease rarely experience resolution because retinal ischemia persists even when the eye is quiet. These eyes usually respond to panretinal photocoagulation. Retinal laser therapy may lead to increased intraocular inflammation, not only because of the alterations in the blood–retina barrier related to the laser energy but also because there may be significant amounts of retinal antigens released during destruction of the retina.

Subretinal neovascular membranes are seen in uveitis, as in presumed ocular histoplasmosis syndrome, punctate inner choroidopathy, multifocal choroiditis, and serpiginous choroidopathy. Because alterations in the Bruch membrane are widespread in some types of uveitis, these membranes can occur in a variety of locations. Historically, neovascular membranes at the posterior pole have been treated with the argon laser or with photodynamic therapy (PDT).[84,85] Anti-VEGF (vascular endothelial growth factor) therapy has become the standard in treating choroidal neovascularization. Invernizzi et al. investigated the benefits of anti-VEGF injections of drugs, including bevacizumab, ranibizumab, and aflibercept, in inflammatory choroidal neovascularization in 82 eyes and noted two- to three-line visual acuity gain after an average of 3 to 4 repeated treatments over 24 months.[86] Anti-VEGF therapy can have a significant effect on the membrane, but it is important to control the underlying inflammation by using immunosuppressive therapy first or together with the anti-VEGF therapy. In the case of extramacular lesions, the clinician must balance the potential visual loss resulting from the membrane with the potential risks of the therapy or the procedure.

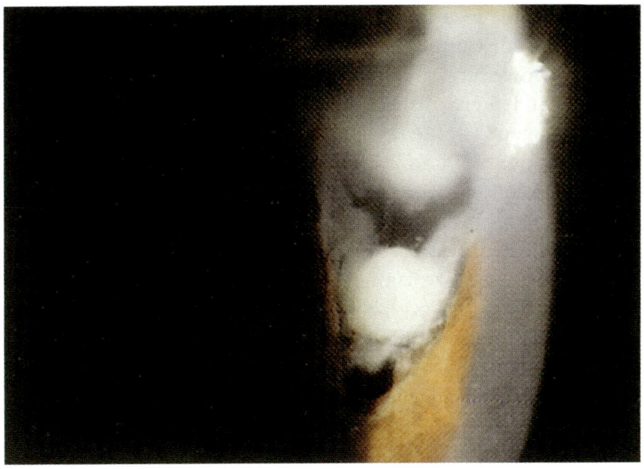

Fig. 9.6 Yttrium–aluminum–garnet (YAG) laser membrane disruption in a patient with dense pupillary membrane after cataract surgery.

DIAGNOSTIC SURGERY

Surgical procedures are frequently the only method for distinguishing a disease of presumed autoimmune etiology from an infectious or a malignant ocular process. The clinical appearances of many ocular infections and some malignant conditions are not always diagnostic. For example, a patient with cytomegalovirus retinitis may have lesions that are consistent with those of Behçet disease during a certain period in the disease course. The overall courses of the two diseases are different, but at the time the clinician examines the patient, the two may appear similar. In this example, a careful history would probably suggest that if the patient were immunosuppressed, viral retinitis was more likely than an autoimmune disease. Infection with *Propionibacterium acnes* (see Chapter 10) and large cell lymphoma of the vitreous (see Chapter 31) are other examples of diseases that are not autoimmune diseases but whose clinical manifestations may appear similar. In addition, if an infectious or a malignant process is suspected, the appropriate therapy usually cannot begin until the diagnosis is confirmed with histologic or microbiologic examination or molecular techniques.

The indication for any intraocular diagnostic procedure in an inflamed eye is that, in the clinician's experience, the course of uveitis or its appearance is not typical of the suspected autoimmune disease and that an infectious or a malignant process is suspected. This suspicion can be strong at the time of the first examination or if the patient's disease fails to respond to therapy in an expected manner. Once these alternative diagnoses are proposed, the appropriate diagnostic surgical procedure may be the only way to reliably rule out these possibilities.

Anterior Chamber Paracentesis

Anterior chamber paracentesis is an easily performed technique and yields a small amount of fluid for analysis. The procedure can be performed with the patient under local anesthesia. The eye can be fixed by a forceps firmly holding the limbus and is then entered with a 30-gauge needle on a tuberculin syringe; at least 200 to 250 μL of fluid can usually be obtained. A small hyphema may occur if the eye is actively inflamed, but this will resolve as the anterior chamber rapidly re-forms. This small amount of fluid must be handled carefully by using a plan established for handling the specimen before the procedure is begun. In general, we spin the fluid, separate the cells, and prepare slides for immunohistologic examination. The supernatant can then be analyzed for antibodies and cytokines, and PCR is now commonly performed. Serum should be obtained for comparison on the same day if antibodies are to be compared. However, if an infectious organism is suspected, the unspun fluid must be cultured. Because of the small amount of fluid, only one or two types of culture can be set up, and the clinician must select the tests that will be most helpful. If too many tests are attempted, the amount of fluid may produce negative results because of inadequate sample size.

We generally use samples of the aqueous for PCR and cytokine studies, in case of suspicion of infectious or malignant etiology, respectively. The IL-10-to-IL-6 ratios have proven to be useful screening tests when primary intraocular lymphoma is suspected.[87-89] PCR has become a very widely used test, particularly for deoxyribonucleic acid (DNA) viruses and other infectious organisms, such as bacteria (using 16S) and fungi (using internal transcribed spacer [ITS]). It is important to understand the strengths and weaknesses of PCR in the appropriate clinical context. In one report, evaluating PCR performed on both the aqueous and vitreous for a possible infectious process in the posterior segment, the predictive value of a positive test was 98.7% and that of a negative test was 67.9%.[90] The utility of anterior chamber tap for the diagnosis of anterior uveitis was much lower.[91]

If an infection is suspected, the vitreous provides more material for culture. In addition, even in postoperative endophthalmitis, the vitreous has a higher yield of positive culture results, and more types of cultures can be set up with the material. However, if you need to use an aqueous specimen, it should be cultured in its entirety if an infectious organism is suspected and if there is no other sample. Otherwise, it should be centrifuged at approximately 1000 revolutions per minute (rpm) and the supernatant carefully removed. The cells that remain can be resuspended in 50 to 100 μL of buffered saline, and samples of 10 to 15 μL can be placed on gelatinized glass slides. This provides a sufficient number of slides for monoclonal antibody studies or other special stains. In pseudophakia or aphakia and after vitrectomy, a communication between the vitreous cavity and the anterior chamber exists, and the aqueous specimen may show positive results for lymphomatous cells.

Vitreous specimens may be obtained either by vitrectomy or by direct aspiration. Vitreous aspiration has been reported by others to be adequate for diagnostic purposes in the majority of patients considered, except for a few in whom other tests needed to be performed.[92] In some situations, it is useful to obtain an undiluted vitreous sample. This can be accomplished by aspirating the vitreous directly with a syringe and needle or by using the vitrectomy instrument on low suction without turning on the infusion until 0.5 to 1 mL of fluid is obtained. This latter method prevents pulling on the vitreous base and prevents prolonged hypotony in the eye. The sample can be aspirated directly into a syringe. If lymphoma is suspected, we put a small amount of culture fluid (e.g., RPMI medium [Roswell Park Memorial Institute medium] 1640) into the vitrectomy cassette. This is immediately sent to the laboratory before the surgical procedure has been completed. When one uses the vitreous fluid that is diluted with irrigating solution, it is sometimes useful to pass a portion through a Millipore filter. The Millipore filter can be cut up to culture for fungi or can be studied by the cytologist. Direct application onto gelatinized slides is also useful for cytologic study and monoclonal antibody staining. If the cells are trapped in cut pieces of dense vitreous, a portion of the sample can be incubated with hyaluronidase to digest the vitreous and free the cells. The cells can be also cultured or typed by immunohistologic or cell-sorting techniques. The fluid can be analyzed for antibodies or cytokines,[93] and as mentioned earlier, PCR can be performed. These findings can be a valuable diagnostic aid in adjusting therapy.[90,94]

Chorioretinal Biopsy

Occasionally, neither the aqueous nor the vitreous specimens will provide a useful answer. Certain pathogens may not "spill over" into the vitreous if the disease involves the retina or the choroid only. For example, cytomegalovirus, which is difficult to culture from the vitreous, can be cultured from or seen on electron microscopic examination of the retina. In diseases in which vision is threatened and where the clinician is sure that continuation of the present therapy will not be effective, it may be reasonable to consider chorioretinal biopsy.[95,96] This procedure provides a small piece of tissue which, if handled carefully, can provide a diagnosis. This procedure is probably useful only when the diagnostic possibilities include diseases for which specific therapies are available. In general, it has been performed in patients with progressive chorioretinal lesions of unknown cause.[97] The indications for the biopsy include macula-threatening lesions unresponsive to therapy or suspicion of either a malignant process or an infection that could not be diagnosed with less invasive methods.

Careful handling of ocular specimens obtained for diagnostic purposes is essential if they are to be useful. Advance planning and notification of the laboratories that will be involved in processing the specimens are useful in ensuring that the specimens are expected and will be processed correctly.

SUBRETINAL SURGERY

Interest has centered on the development of new surgical and diagnostic techniques for subretinal (submacular) surgery (Fig. 9.7). The implications of these techniques would seem to go beyond the surgery itself and will also influence future work in RPE transplantation. The removal of subfoveal neovascular membranes[98] in the eyes of patients with presumed ocular histoplasmosis syndrome paved the way for an exciting new area of therapy (Fig. 9.8). This is in contrast to patients with age-related maculopathy, who have not consistently had such an improvement in vision. Thomas et al.[99] found that after subretinal surgery in eyes with ocular histoplasmosis syndrome, visual acuity stabilized or improved in 56 eyes (83%), whereas 20/40 or greater was achieved in 21 eyes (31%) (mean follow-up period 10.5 months). The results are quite different in eyes with age-related maculopathy, in which visual acuity improved in five of the eyes operated on (12%) and 20/40 or better visual acuity occurred in two (5%), with a mean follow-up period of 15 months. Of interest is the Gass hypothesis,[100] which states that membranes removed from patients with histoplasmosis grew in the subsensory retinal space and not under the RPE, as did those from patients with age-related maculopathy. In addition, the membranes from patients with histoplasmosis are covered with a redundant layer of RPE, and therefore removal may aid in the normal apposition of the retinal elements. The question that remains is how widely applicable subretinal surgery will be for patients with uveitis in general. Recurrence rates of membranes still need to be determined. However, removal of the membrane alone may not be sufficient to restore vision, as defective RPE cells and damaged or lost photoreceptors may be the major problem. This may then represent just the first step of a whole series of rehabilitation measures that will be needed.

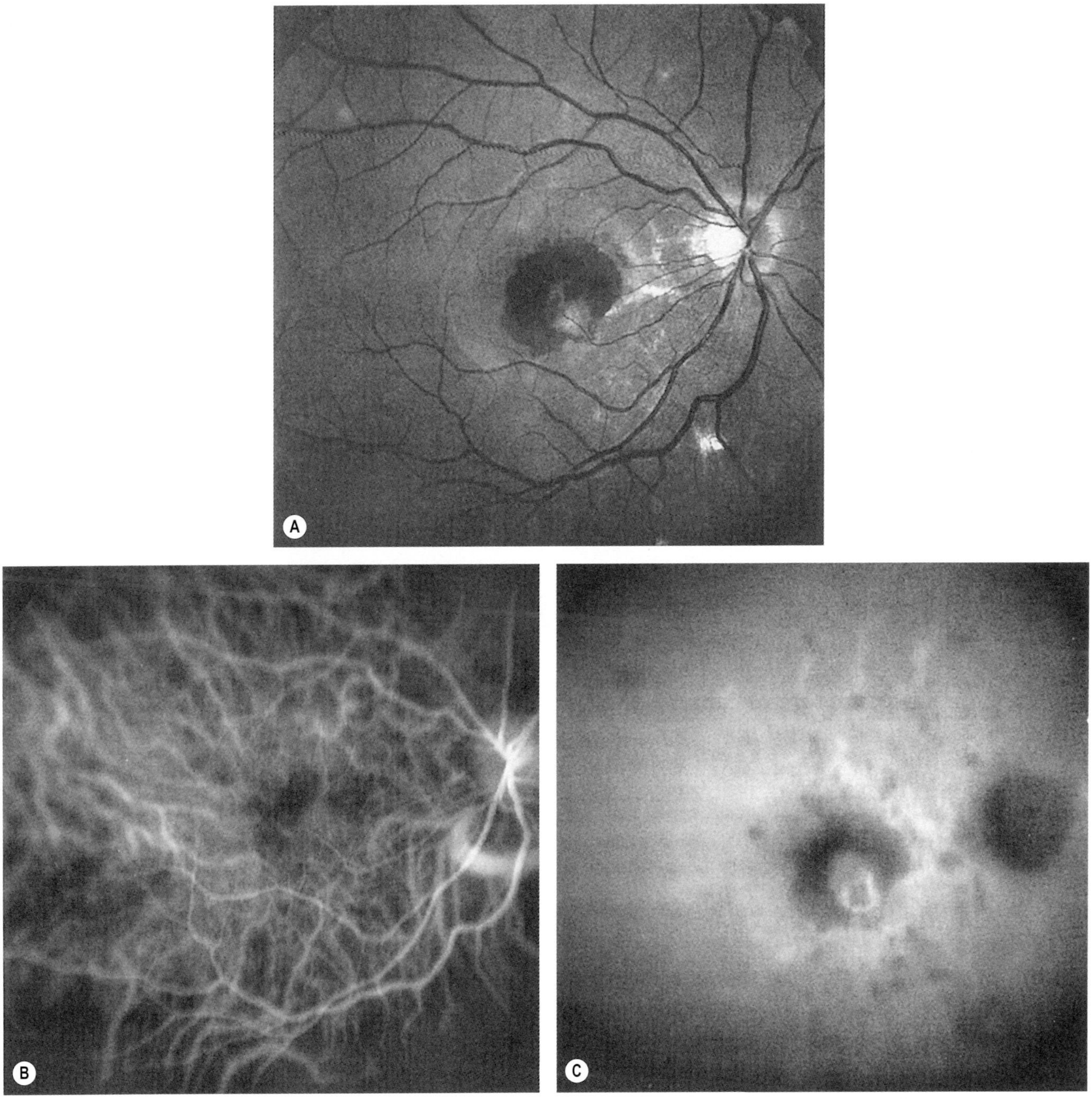

Fig. 9.7 Indocyanine green (ICG) angiogram showing position of submacular neovascular net. (A) Fundus photograph showing submacular hemorrhage with marked reduction in visual acuity. Because of the presence of blood, the fluorescein angiogram was difficult to interpret. (B) ICG early photograph shows feeder vessel to net. (C) Later photograph outlines the extent of the net, which was successfully treated with laser photocoagulation and not removed by surgery.

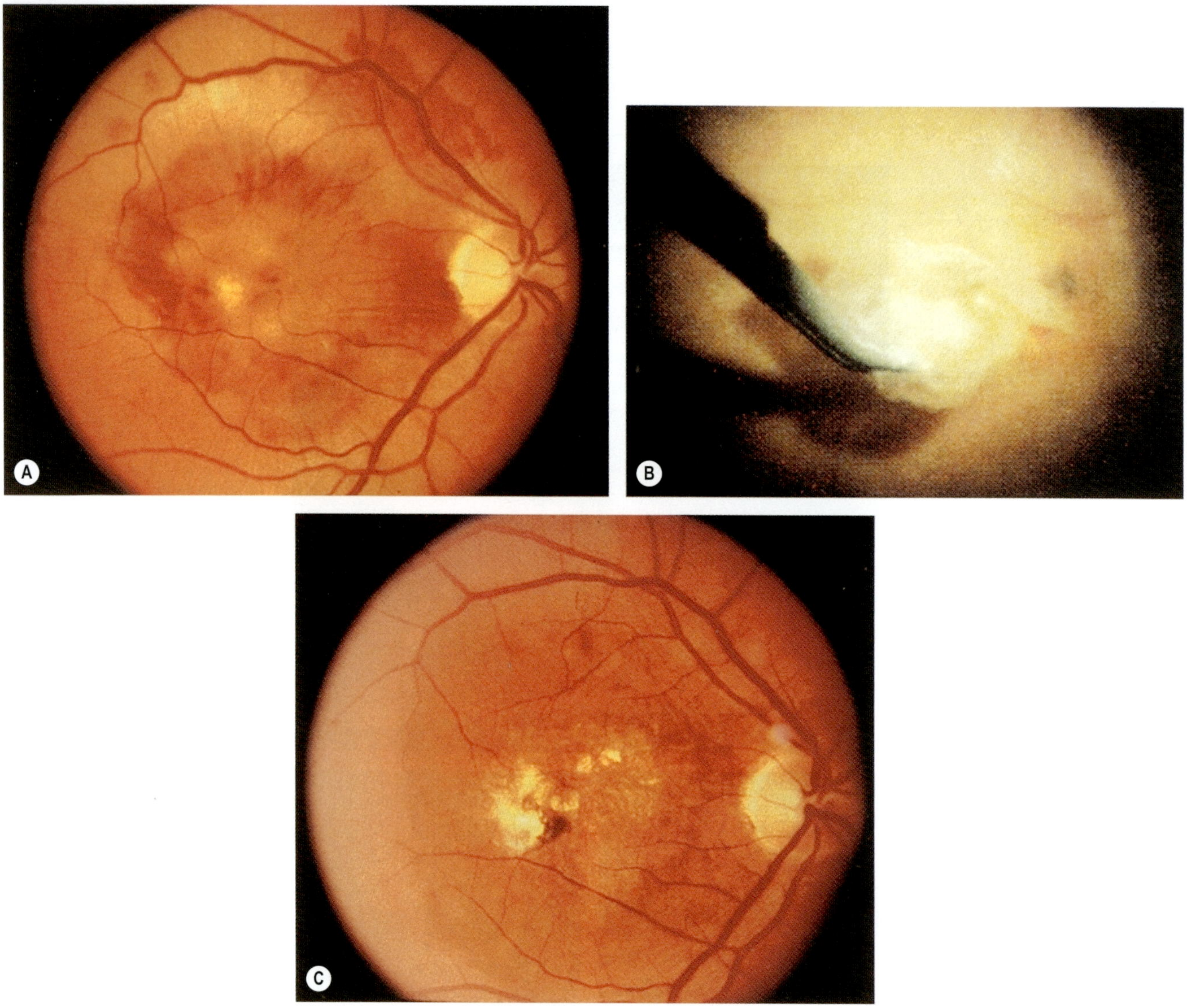

Fig. 9.8 (A) Subretinal neovascular lesion in the macular region. (B) Removal of lesion with special subretinal forceps. (C) Fundus as it appears after surgery. (Courtesy Antonio Capone, Jr., MD and Daniel Martin, MD, Emory University, Atlanta, GA.)

CASE 9.1

A 61-year-old man was referred for unilateral granulomatous anterior uveitis. Slit-lamp examination revealed a large vascularized iris nodule in the inferior angle. Ultrasound biomicroscopy showed that the mass extended from the ciliary body to the iris. An anterior chamber tap and 30-gauge needle biopsy of the lesion revealed atypical mucin–producing cells with large nuclei, prominent nucleoli, and abundant vacuolated cytoplasm intermixed with macrophages. Immunohistochemistry showed positive labeling for cytokeratin, an epithelial marker, and negative labeling for HBM45, a marker for melanocytes and neural crest–derived tumors, suggestive of metastasis of primary carcinoma to the iris.

For a more detailed description of this case, see Sen HN, Chan CC, Nussenblatt RB, Buggage RR. Occult primary carcinoma metastatic to the iris. *Acta Ophthalmol Scand.* 2004;82(6):746–747.

CASE 9.2

A 56-year-old Caucasian woman with a history of bilateral macular drusen was referred for chronic intermediate uveitis. She had undergone diagnostic vitrectomy prior to referral, and it had shown polyclonal mononuclear cells. Examination showed +1 vitreous cells in both eyes, with 20/20 vision in the right eye and 20/25 in the left eye and numerous small subretinal yellowish infiltrates in both eyes and a large lobulated subretinal mass in the left eye. Brain magnetic resonance imaging (MRI) was normal, and lumbar puncture showed reactive lymphocytes only. The patient underwent repeat diagnostic vitrectomy, along with fine-needle aspiration biopsy (FNAB) of the large subretinal lesion in the left eye. The specimen was immediately transferred to a vial containing RPMI [Roswell Park Memorial Institute] medium. The vitreous specimen showed reactive lymphocytes and a few atypical lymphoid cells and was not diagnostic. However, the FNAB sample showed numerous atypical large lymphoid cells with scant basophilic cytoplasm and an increased nuclear-to-cytoplasmic ratio. Atypical cells were positive for CD20 and kappa light-chain antibodies. The patient was diagnosed with primary intraocular (vitreoretinal) lymphoma.

For a more detailed description of this case, see Levy-Clarke GA, Byrnes GA, Buggage RR, et al. Primary intraocular lymphoma diagnosed by fine needle aspiration biopsy of a subretinal lesion. *Retina.* 2001;21(3):281–284.

CASE 9.3

A 23-year-old woman with a history of chronic bilateral nongranulomatous idiopathic anterior uveitis since childhood presented with complicated cataract and glaucoma and underwent cataract surgery, followed by two failed trabeculectomies. Subsequently, she underwent Ahmed glaucoma valve (AGV) implantation in the superotemporal quadrant of the right eye with stable intraocular pressure (IOP) for 8 years. She required a second AGV implantation in the inferonasal quadrant of the right eye because of rising IOP despite maximum tolerated medical therapy and because of progressing optic neuropathy. After the second AGV implantation, her IOP was stable, but tube exposure developed in the superotemporal quadrant, in the area of the first failed AGV. This was repaired by using amniotic membrane and pericardial tissue twice; however, tube exposure developed several weeks after surgery. A decision was made to remove the failed AGV implant. Intraoperatively, widespread perilimbal conjunctival scarring was noted. After the conjunctiva and the Tenon capsule were dissected, a very thick, fibrotic capsule surrounding the plate was identified. After removal of the fibrotic capsule and the AGV implant, the patient did well, with stable IOP and resolution of discomfort caused by the exposed tube (Fig. 9.9).

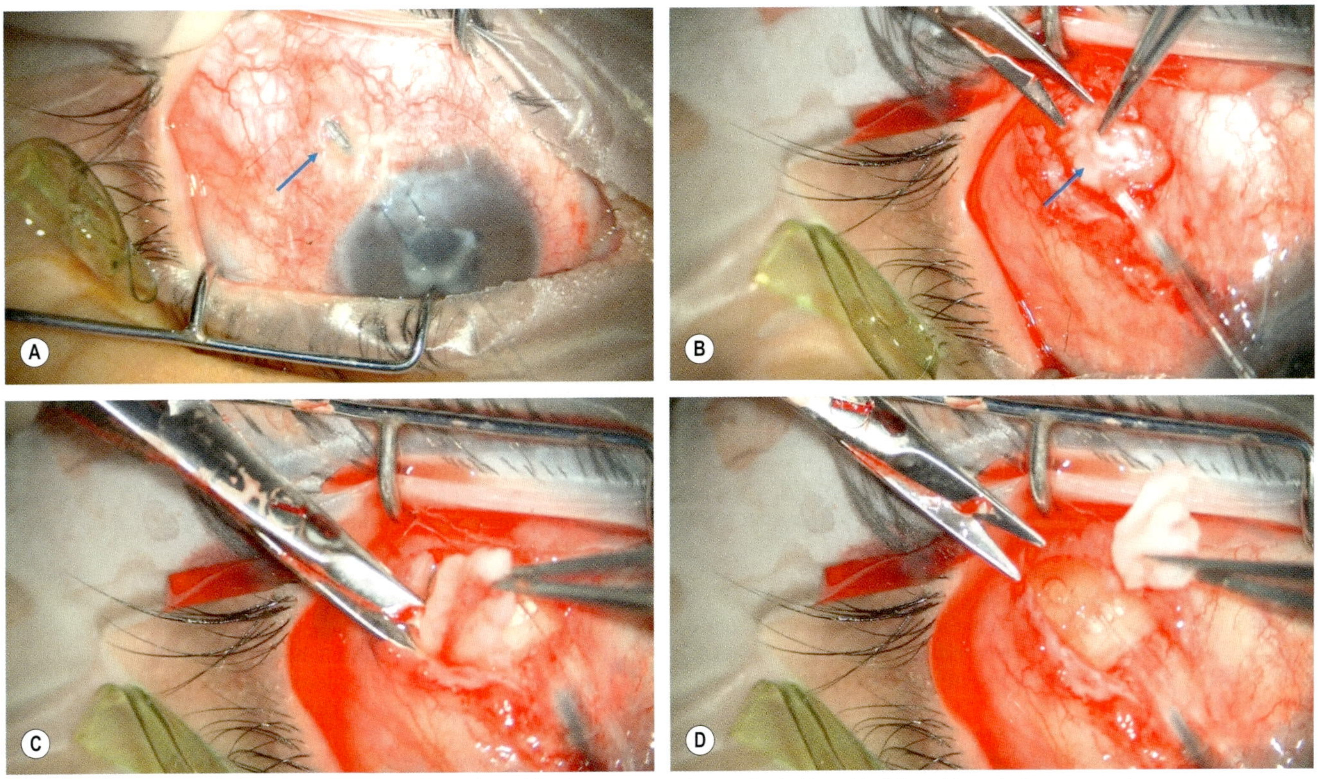

Fig. 9.9 Patient with complicated uveitic glaucoma and pseudophakia with failed Ahmed glaucoma valve (AGV) placement in the superotemporal quadrant of the right eye. Cornea is cloudy because of chronic endothelial insufficiency. The tube of the AGV was exposed (A, *blue arrow*) and a decision to remove the failed AGV was made. After dissecting the conjunctiva and the Tenon capsule, a very thick fibrotic capsule surrounding the plate was identified (B, *blue arrow*). The fibrotic capsule was successfully removed. The fibrotic capsule was noted to be as thick as sclera by the surgeon. (Courtesy Dr. Mehmet Yakin.)

REFERENCES

1. Arevalo JF, Garcia-Amaris RA. The role of vitreo-retinal surgery in children with uveitis. *Int Ophthalmol Clin*. 2008;48:153–172.
2. Kollias AN, Spitzlberger GM, Thurau S, Grüterich M, Lackerbauer CA. Phototherapeutic keratectomy in children. *J Refract Surg*. 2007;23(7):703–708.
3. Najjar DM, Cohen EJ, Rapuano CJ, et al. EDTA chelation for calcific band keratopathy: results and long-term follow-up. *Am J Ophthalmol*. 2004;137(6):1056–1064.
4. Babu K, Murthy KR. Hypopyon uveitis following band keratopathy removal in ankylosing spondylitis – a case report. *Ocul Immunol Inflamm*. 2006;14:57–58.
5. Richards JC, Wiffen SJ. Corneal graft rejection precipitated by uveitis secondary to alendronate sodium therapy. *Cornea*. 2006;25:1100–1101.
6. Rice MO, Gupta P, Lass J, Price FW, Jr . EK (DLEK, DSEK, DMEK): new frontier in cornea surgery. *Annu Rev Vis Sci*. 2017;3:69–90.
7. Foster C, Rashid S. Management of coincident cataract and uveitis. *Curr Opin Ophthalmol*. 2003;14:1–6.
8. Ram J, Kaushik S, Brar GS, et al. Phacoemulsification in patients with Fuchs' heterochromic uveitis. *J Cataract Refract Surg*. 2002;28:1372–1378.
9. Estafanous MF, Lowder CY, Meisler DM, et al. Phacoemulsification cataract extraction and posterior chamber lens implantation in patients with uveitis. *Am J Ophthalmol*. 2001;131:620–625.
10. Meier FM, Tuft SJ, Pavesio CE. Cataract surgery in uveitis. *Ophthalmol Clin North Am*. 2002;15:365–373.

11. Chee SP, Ti SE, Sivakumar M, et al. Postoperative inflammation: extracapsular cataract extraction versus phacoemulsification. *J Cataract Refract Surg*. 1999;25:1280–1285.
12. Herbort CP. Uveoscleritis after excessive neodynium YAG laser posterior capsulotomy. *J Cataract Refract Surg*. 1994;20:80–81.
13. Mehta S, Linton MM, Kempen JH. Outcomes of cataract surgery in patients with uveitis: a systematic review and meta-analysis. *Am J Ophthalmol*. 2014;158:676–692.
14. Sen HN, Abreu FM, Louis TA, et al. Cataract surgery outcomes in uveitis: the Multicenter Uveitis Steroid Treatment Trial. *Ophthalmology*. 2016;123(1):183–190.
15. Bélair ML, Kim SJ, Thorne JE, et al. Incidence of cystoid macular edema after cataract surgery in patients with and without uveitis using optical coherence tomography. *Am J Ophthalmol*. 2009;148(1):128–135.e2.
16. Kamoi K, Mochizuki M. Phaco-dislocation technique in young patients with uveitis. *J Cataract Refract Surg*. 2008;34:1239–1241.
17. Belfort R, Nussenblatt RB. Surgical approaches to uveitis. *Int Ophthalmol Clin*. 1990;30:314–317.
18. Davison JA. Capsule contraction syndrome. *J Cataract Refract Surg*. 1993;19:582–589.
19. Alio JL, Chipont E, BenEzra D, et al. Comparative performance of intraocular lenses in eyes with cataract and uveitis. *J Cataract Refract Surg*. 2002;28:2096–2108.
20. Leccisotti A. Iridocyclitis associated with angle-supported phakic intraocular lenses. *J Cataract Refract Surg*. 2006;32:1007–1010.
21. Zaborowski AG, Quinn AG, Dick AD. Cataract surgery in pediatric uveitis. *J Pediatr Ophthalmol Strabismus*. 2008;45:270–278.
22. Kotaniemi K, Penttila H. Intraocular lens implantation in patients with juvenile idiopathic arthritis-associated uveitis. *Ophthalmic Res*. 2006;38:318–323.
23. Woreta F, Thorne JE, Jabs DA, et al. Risk factors for ocular complications and poor visual acuity at presentation among patients with uveitis associated with juvenile idiopathic arthritis. *Am J Ophthalmol*. 2007;143(4):647–655.
24. Foster CS, Fong LP, Singh G. Cataract surgery and intraocular lens implantation in patients with uveitis. *Ophthalmology*. 1989;96:281–288.
25. Pleyer U, Pawlikowska J, Zierhut M, et al. Clinical aspects, follow-up and results of cataract extraction in uveitis. *Ophtalmologie*. 1992;89:295–300.
26. Foster RE, Lowder CY, Meisler DM, et al. Combined extracapsular cataract extraction, posterior chamber intraocular lens implantation, and pars plana vitrectomy. *Ophthalmic Surg*. 1993;24:446–452.
27. Carlson AN, Stewart WC, Tso PC. Intraocular lens complications requiring removal or exchange. *Surv Ophthalmol*. 1998;42:417–440.
28. Harper SL, Foster CS. Intraocular lens explantation in uveitis. *Int Ophthalmol Clin*. 2000;40:107–116.
29. Llop SM, Papaliodis GN. Cataract surgery complications in uveitis patients: a review article. *Semin Ophthalmol*. 2018;33(1):64–69.
30. Dana MR, Chatzistefanou K, Schaumberg DA, et al. Posterior capsule opacification after cataract surgery in patients with uveitis. *Ophthalmology*. 1997;104:1387–1393.
31. Foster C, Stavrou P, Zafirakis P, et al. Intraocular lens removal from patients with uveitis. *Am J Ophthalmol*. 1999;128:31–37.
32. Smith RE, Kokoris N, Nobe JR, et al. Lensectomy-vitrectomy in chronic uveitis. *Trans Am Ophthalmol Soc*. 1983;81:261–275.
33. Girard LJ, Rodriguez J, Mailman ML, et al. Cataract and uveitis management by pars plana lensectomy and vitrectomy by ultrasonic fragmentation. *Retina*. 1985;5:107–114.
34. Petrelli AM, Belfort Jr R, Abreu MT, et al. Ultrasonic fragmentation of cataract in uveitis. *Retina*. 1986;6:61–65.
35. Diamond JG, Kaplan HJ. Uveitis: effect of vitrectomy combined with lensectomy. *Ophthalmology*. 1979;86:1320–1328.
36. Dangel ME, Stark WJ, Michels RG. Surgical management of cataract associated with chronic uveitis. *Ophthalmic Surg*. 1983;14:145–152.
37. Praeger DL, Schneider HA, Sakowski AD Jr, et al. Kelman procedure in the treatment of complicated cataract of the uveitis of Still's disease. *Trans Am Ophthalmol Soc UK*. 1976;96:168–172.
38. Mackensen G, Loeffler K. Cataract extraction in chronic iridocyclitis: long term follow-ups. *Klin Monatsbl Augenheilkd*. 1983;183:7–9.
39. Yu EN, Paredes I, Foster CS. Surgery for hypotony in patients with juvenile idiopathic arthritis-associated uveitis. *Ocul Immunol Inflamm*. 2007;15:11–17.
40. Al Obeidan SA, Osman EA, Al-Muammar AM, et al. Efficacy and safety of deep sclerectomy in uveitic glaucoma. *Int Ophthalmol*. 2009;29(5):367–372.
41. Park UC, Ahn JK, Park KH, et al. Phacotrabeculectomy with mitomycin C in patients with uveitis. *Am J Ophthalmol*. 2006;142(6):1005–1012.
42. Wadke V, Lingam V, George R, et al. Phacotrabeculectomy in eyes with uveitic glaucoma: a retrospective case-control study. *J Glaucoma*. 2019;28(7):606–612.
43. Patitsas CJ, Rockwood EJ, Meisler DM, et al. Glaucoma filtering surgery with postoperative 5-fluorouracil in patients with intraocular inflammatory disease. *Ophthalmology*. 1992;99:594–599.
44. Towler HMA, McCluskey P, Shaer B, et al. Long-term follow-up of trabeculectomy with intraoperative 5-fluorouracil for uveitis related glaucoma. *Ophthalmology*. 2000;107:1822–1828.
45. Ceballos EM, Beck AD, Lynn MJ. Trabeculectomy with antiproliferative agents in uveitis glaucoma. *J Glaucoma*. 2002;11:189–196.
46. Kanski JJ, McAllister JA. Trabeculodialysis for inflammatory glaucoma in children and young adults. *Ophthalmology*. 1985;92:927–930.
47. Williams RD, Hoskins HD, Shaffer RN. Trabeculodialysis for inflammatory glaucoma: a review of 25 cases. *Ophthalmic Surg*. 1992;23:36–37.
48. Hill RA, Nguyen QH, Baerveldt G, et al. Trabeculectomy and Molteno implantation for glaucomas associated with uveitis. *Ophthalmology*. 1993;100:903–908.
49. Freedman J, Rubin B. Molteno implants as a treatment for refractory glaucoma in black patients. *Arch Ophthalmol*. 1992;109:1417–1420.
50. Papadaki TG, Zacharopoulos IP, Pasquale LR, et al. Long-term results of Ahmed glaucoma valve implantation for uveitic glaucoma. *Am J Ophthalmol*. 2007;144(1):62–69.
51. Bao N, Jiang ZX, Coh P, Tao LM. Long-term outcomes of uveitic glaucoma treated with Ahmed valve implant in a series of Chinese patients. *Int J Ophthalmol*. 2018;11(4):629–634.
52. Yakin M, Eksioglu U, Sungur G, Satana B, Demirok G, Ornek F. Short-term to long-term results of Ahmed glaucoma valve implantation for uveitic glaucoma secondary to Behcet disease. *J Glaucoma*. 2017;26(1):20–26.
53. Sungur G, Yakin M, Eksioglu U, Satana B, Ornek F. Assessment of conditions affecting surgical success of Ahmed glaucoma valve implants in glaucoma secondary to different uveitis etiologies in adults. *Eye*. 2017;31(10):1435–1442.
54. Eksioglu U, Yakin M, Sungur G, et al. Short- to long-term results of Ahmed glaucoma valve in the management of elevated intraocular pressure in patients with pediatric uveitis. *Can J Ophthalmol*. 2017;52(3):295–301.
55. Chow A, Burkemper B, Varma R, Rodger DC, Rao N, Richter GM. Comparison of surgical outcomes of trabeculectomy, Ahmed shunt, and Baerveldt shunt in uveitic glaucoma. *J Ophthalmic Inflamm Infect*. 2018;8(1):9.
56. Chaku M, Bajwa A, Lee JK, Netland PA. Treatment of uveitis and outcomes of glaucoma drainage implant surgery: a meta-analysis. *Ocul Immunol Inflamm*. 2020;28(5):833–838.
57. Edmiston AM, SooHoo JR, Seibold LK, Kahook MY, Palestine AG, Pantcheva MB. Postoperative inflammation after endoscopic cyclophotocoagulation: racial distribution and effect on outcomes. *J Glaucoma*. 2018;27(3):266–268.
58. Gedde SJ, Schiffman JC, Feuer WJ, et al. Treatment outcomes in the Tube Versus Trabeculectomy (TVT) study after five years of follow-up. *Am J Ophthalmol*. 2012;153:789–803.e2.
59. Gedde SJ, Herndon LW, Brandt JD, et al. Postoperative complications in the Tube Versus Trabeculectomy (TVT) study during five years of follow-up. *Am J Ophthalmol*. 2012;153:804–814.e1.
60. Wong SH, Panarelli JF. Update on microinvasive glaucoma surgery. *Int Ophthalmol Clin*. 2018;58(3):101–115.
61. Swamy R, Francis BA, Akil H. Clinical results of ab interno trabeculotomy using the trabectome in patients with uveitic glaucoma. *Clin Experiment Ophthalmol*. 2020;48:31–36.
62. Sng CC, Wang J, Hau S, Htoon HM, Barton K. XEN-45 collagen implant for the treatment of uveitic glaucoma. *Clin Exp Ophthalmol*. 2018;46(4):339–345.
63. Freeman WR. Application of vitreoretinal surgery to inflammatory and infectious disease of the posterior segment. *Int Ophthalmol Clin*. 1992;32:15–33.

64. Chen CL, Wang TY, Cheng JH, et al. Immediate pars plana vitrectomy improves outcome in retained intravitreal lens fragments after phacoemulsification. *Ophthalmologica*. 2008;222(4):277–283.
65. Lubiński W, Gosławski W, Podborączyńska-Jodko K, Mularczyk M, Post M. Comparison of 27-gauge versus 25-gauge vitrectomy results in patients with epiretinal membrane: 6-month follow-up. *Int Ophthalmol*. 2020;40(4):867–875.
66. Rothova A. Inflammatory cystoid macular edema. *Curr Opin Ophthalmol*. 2007;18:487–492.
67. Bacskulin A, Eckardt C. Results of pars plana vitrectomy in chronic uveitis in childhood. *Ophthalmologie*. 1993;90:434–439.
68. Kaplan HJ. Surgical treatment of intermediate uveitis. In: Boke WRF, Manthey KF, Nussenblatt RB, eds. *Intermediate Uveitis*. Basel, Switzerland: Karger; 1992:185–189.
69. Stavrou P, Baltatzis S, Letko E, et al. Pars plana vitrectomy in patients with intermediate uveitis. *Ocul Immunol Inflamm*. 2001;9:141–151.
70. Bovey EH, Gonvers M, Herbort CP. Pars plana vitrectomy in uveitis. *Klin Monatsbl Augenheilkd*. 1992;200:464–467.
71. Nolle B, Eckardt C. Vitrectomy in multifocal chorioretinitis. *Ger J Ophthalmol*. 1993;2:14–19.
72. Gutfleisch M, Spital G, Mingels A, et al. Pars plana vitrectomy with intravitreal triamcinolone: effect on uveitic cystoid macular oedema and treatment limitations. *Br J Ophthalmol*. 2007;91(3):345–348.
73. Tranos P, Scott R, Zambarakji H, et al. The effect of pars plana vitrectomy on cystoid macular oedema associated with chronic uveitis: a randomised, controlled pilot study. *Br J Ophthalmol*. 2006;90(9):1107–1110.
74. Trittibach P, Koerner F, Sarra GM, et al. Vitrectomy for juvenile uveitis: prognostic factors for the long-term functional outcome. *Eye*. 2006;20(2):184–190.
75. Henry CR, Becker MD, Yang Y, Davis JL. Pars plana vitrectomy for the treatment of uveitis. *Am J Ophthalmol*. 2018;190:142–149.
76. Nicholson BP, Zhou M, Rostamizadeh M, et al. Epidemiology of epiretinal membrane in a large cohort of patients with uveitis. *Ophthalmology*. 2014;121(12):2393–2398.
77. Michels RG. Vitrectomy for macular pucker. *Ophthalmology*. 1984;91:1384–1388.
78. Kerkhoff FT, Lamberts QJ, van den Biesen PR, et al. Rhegmatogenous retinal detachment and uveitis. *Ophthalmology*. 2003;110:427–431.
79. Rao P, Todorich B, Yonekawa Y, Wang J, Sobrin L, Faia LJ. Surgical outcomes of epiretinal membranes in patients with a history of well-controlled preoperative uveitis. *Ophthalmol Retina*. 2018;2(3):192–196.
80. Galor A, Lowder CY, Kaiser PK, et al. Surgical drainage of chronic serous retinal detachment associated with uveitis. *Retina*. 2008;28(2):282–288.
81. Freeman WR, Henderly DE, Wan WL, et al. Prevalence, pathophysiology, and treatment of rhegmatogenous retinal detachment in treated cytomegalovirus retinitis. *Am J Ophthalmol*. 1987;103:527–536.
82. Forster RK, Zachary IG, Cottingham AJ Jr, et al. Further observations on the diagnosis, cause and treatment of endophthalmitis. *Am J Ophthalmol*. 1976;81:52–56.
83. Er H, Doganay S, Evereklioglu C, et al. Effects of L-NAME and timolol on aqueous IL-1beta, IL-6, IL-8, TNF-alpha, and NO levels after Nd:YAG laser iridotomy in rabbits. *Eur J Ophthalmol*. 2002;12:281–286.
84. Parodi MB, Iacono P, Spasse S, Ravalico G. Photodynamic therapy for juxtafoveal choroidal neovascularization associated with multifocal choroiditis. *Am J Ophthalmol*. 2006;141:123–128.
85. Gerth C, Spital G, Lommatzsch A, et al. Photodynamic therapy for choroidal neovascularization in patients with multifocal choroiditis and panuveitis. *Eur J Ophthalmol*. 2006;16(1):111–118.
86. Invernizzi A, Pichi F, Symes R, et al. Twenty-four-month outcomes of inflammatory choroidal neovascularisation treated with intravitreal anti-vascular endothelial growth factors: a comparison between two treatment regimens. *Br J Ophthalmol*. 2020;104(8):1052–1056.
87. Cassoux N, Giron A, Bodaghi B, et al. IL-10 measurement in aqueous humor for screening patients with suspicion of primary intraocular lymphoma. *Invest Ophthalmol Vis Sci*. 2007;48(7):3253–3259.
88. Kuo DE, Wei MM, Armbrust KR, et al. Gradient boosted decision tree classification of endophthalmitis versus uveitis and lymphoma from aqueous and vitreous IL-6 and IL-10 levels. *J Ocul Pharmacol Ther*. 2017;33(4):319–324.
89. Wang Y, Shen D, Wang VM, Sen HN, Chan CC. Molecular biomarkers for the diagnosis of primary vitreoretinal lymphoma. *Int J Mol Sci*. 2011;12(9):5684–5697.
90. Harper TW, Miller D, Schiffman JC, et al. Polymerase chain reaction analysis of aqueous and vitreous specimens in the diagnosis of posterior segment infectious uveitis. *Am J Ophthalmol*. 2009;147(1):140–147. e2.
91. Anwar Z, Galor A, Albini TA, Miller D, Perez V, Davis JL. The diagnostic utility of anterior chamber paracentesis with polymerase chain reaction in anterior uveitis. *Am J Ophthalmol*. 2013;155(5):781–786.
92. Lobo A, Lightman S. Vitreous aspiration needle tap in the diagnosis of intraocular inflammation. *Ophthalmology*. 2003;110:595–599.
93. Davis JL, Solomon D, Nussenblatt RB, et al. Immunocytochemical staining of vitreous cells: indications, techniques, and results. *Ophthalmology*. 1992;99:250–256.
94. Baarsma GS, Luyendijk L, Kijlstra A, et al. Analysis of local antibody production in the vitreous humor of patients with severe uveitis. *Am J Ophthalmol*. 1991;112:147–150.
95. Martin DF, Chan CC, de Smet MD, et al. The role of chorioretinal biopsy in the management of posterior uveitis. *Ophthalmology*. 1993;100:705–714.
96. Lim LL, Suhler EB, Rosenbaum JT, et al. The role of choroidal and retinal biopsies in the diagnosis and management of atypical presentations of uveitis. *Trans Am Ophthalmol Soc*. 2005;103:84–91. Discussion 91–92.
97. Lafaut BA, Hanssens M, Verbraeken H, et al. Chorioretinal biopsy in the diagnosis of intraocular lymphoma: a case report. *Bull Soc Belge Ophtalmol*. 1994;252:67–73.
98. Thomas MA, Kaplan HJ. Surgical removal of subfoveal neovascularization in the presumed ocular histoplasmosis syndrome. *Am J Ophthalmol*. 1991;111:1–7.
99. Thomas MA, Dickinson JD, Melberg NS, et al. Visual results after surgical removal of subfoveal choroidal neovascular membranes. *Ophthalmology*. 1994;101:1384–1396.
100. Gass JDM. Biomicroscopic and histopathologic considerations regarding the feasibility of surgical excision of subfoveal neovascular membranes. *Am J Ophthalmol*. 1994;118:285–298.

10

Bacterial and Fungal Diseases

Scott M. Whitcup

KEY CONCEPTS

- Infection remains a common cause of uveitis. Better diagnostic tests are helping to identify specific bacteria as the cause of a number of uveitic conditions, such as bartonellosis as the cause of cat scratch disease.
- Prompt diagnosis is critical so that appropriate anti-infective therapy can be started.
- Clinicians should know the sensitivity and specificity of the diagnostic tests ordered for the infectious causes of uveitis. Clinicians must also know the pretest likelihood of disease to adequately interpret results (see Chapter 5). Otherwise, diagnostic tests for the infectious causes of uveitis can misinform the clinician and lead to inappropriate therapy.
- Ocular involvement from tuberculosis occurs in about 1% to 2% of patients but remains difficult to diagnose. Active tuberculosis can occur as a complication of immunosuppressive therapy with anticytokine therapy.
- Histoplasmosis is the fungal disease most commonly associated with uveitis.
- Risk factors for fungal infections of the eye include ocular surgery, immunosuppression, systemic mycotic infections, intravenous drug use, and ocular trauma.

INTRODUCTION

The next two chapters will focus on uveitis resulting from ocular infections caused by bacteria or fungi. Although a number of infectious agents can invade the eye and lead to ocular inflammation, we will concentrate on the most common systemic bacterial and fungal causes of uveitis, including leprosy, tuberculosis, syphilis, and other related spirochetal diseases; Lyme disease; relapsing fever; leptospirosis; bartonellosis; brucellosis; candidal infections; and aspergillosis. Spirochetal diseases, as a group, are discussed in detail in Chapter 11. Postsurgical bacterial and fungal endophthalmitis are also discussed in Chapter 19.

Half a century ago, bacterial diseases, such as tuberculosis (TB) and syphilis, were thought to cause the majority of cases of uveitis. Despite improvements in the diagnosis and treatment of infectious diseases, ocular infections are still important causes of uveitis. Because specific antimicrobial therapy can be curative and prevent long-term visual sequelae, early diagnosis of infectious causes of uveitis should be a priority for all practitioners. Furthermore, as immunosuppressive therapy can exacerbate an underlying infection, leading to blindness and rarely even to death, diagnosing and treating an infectious cause of uveitis can be both sight saving and lifesaving.

Infections may cause uveitis through a number of pathogenic mechanisms. Direct infection of ocular tissues, usually as a result of trauma or surgery, leads to an inflammatory response manifesting as signs and symptoms of uveitis. Injection of bacterial endotoxins at sites far from the eye will also elicit intraocular inflammation in the absence of ocular infection. Endotoxins generate a number of harmful biologic effects, including fever, hypotension, disseminated coagulation, and shock. In the same year that Murray Shear elucidated the basic structure of endotoxin, Ayo[1] demonstrated that a single intravenous injection of endotoxin could induce ocular inflammation, and this inflammatory response was ascribed to "Schwartzman toxins." Although this endotoxin-induced uveitis (EIU) was easily elicited in dogs, cats, and rabbits, smaller laboratory animals were resistant to development of the disease. In 1980, Rosenbaum et al.[2] demonstrated EIU in Lewis rats after intravenous, intraperitoneal, or intrafootpad injections of lipopolysaccharide (LPS), and Forrester et al.[3] showed EIU after intraocular LPS injection in Columbia–Sherman rats. EIU has since been described in C3H/HeN mice.[4] EIU is now a useful animal model for the study of acute ocular inflammation and is characterized by iris hyperemia, miosis, increased aqueous humor protein concentration, and inflammatory cell infiltration into the anterior uvea and anterior chamber (Fig. 10.1). Inflammatory cell infiltration into the vitreous in the area of the optic nerve head also occurs. As you will see in the chapter on anterior uveitis (Chapter 20), uveitis can occur after bacterial infections, such as bacterial dysentery, and the mechanism of some of these occurrences may be the result of an immunologic response to endotoxin.

LEPROSY

Leprosy was the first documented bacterial infection in humans and was described in Indian texts from the sixth century B.C. The etiologic agent of leprosy, *Mycobacterium leprae,* is a gram-positive, acid-fast intracellular bacillus, first identified by Hansen[5] in 1874; however, the disease has been a scourge of society for thousands of years. It is found predominantly in developing countries, but it is estimated that from 10 to 15 million people have leprosy[6] and that from 500,000 to 700,000

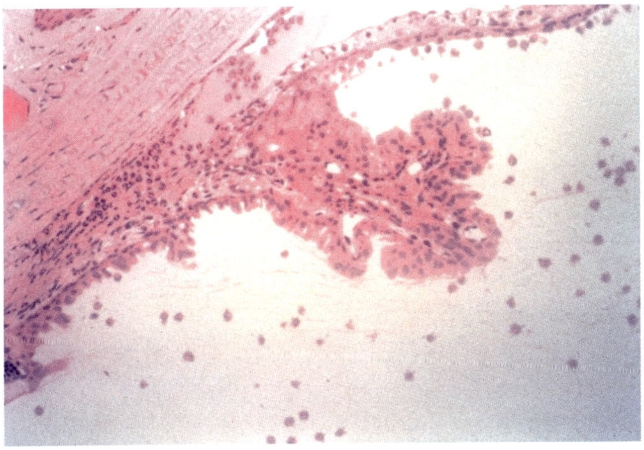

Fig. 10.1 Histologic section of anterior chamber of mouse with endotoxin-induced uveitis shows infiltration with neutrophils, macrophages, and occasional lymphocytes. (Hematoxylin and eosin, ×200.)

persons have been blinded by this condition.[7] Most of the cases come from a small number of countries, including India, China, Myanmar, Indonesia, Brazil, Nigeria, Madagascar, and Nepal.[8] The organisms have a tropism for parts of the body with low temperatures, particularly organs of ectodermal origin, such as the skin, peripheral nerves, nasal mucosa, and eyes. The mode of transmission of leprosy remains unclear. Although most of the population is exposed to the bacillus in endemic areas, greater than 90% are immune to the disease and do not develop symptoms. Leprosy is often divided into two major subtypes: tuberculoid and lepromatous. In patients with tuberculoid leprosy, the organism induces a strong cell-mediated immune response, and few organisms are found invading organ tissues. Little immunity follows the infection in patients with lepromatous leprosy, and a plethora of organisms are found throughout the body. Borderline forms of the disease also exist in some classification systems.[9]

Clinical Findings and Prognosis

From 50% to 70% of patients with leprosy have the tuberculoid form, which tends to be localized to the skin and nerves.[10] The disease in these patients is characterized by granuloma formation and the absence of a large number of bacilli because of their active cell-mediated immune response. The skin test with lepromin is highly positive (Mitsuda reaction). The lepromatous form of the disease is characterized by a severe generalized condition with massive bacterial infection. In contrast to patients with tuberculoid leprosy, these patients have a poor cellular immune response, and macrophages are predominantly found on histologic examination. Intraocular inflammatory disease occurs more commonly in lepromatous leprosy. In addition, severe disfiguring changes of the limbs and face are associated with lepromatous leprosy. In patients with borderline forms of leprosy, a sudden shift to the lepromatous state can occur. The differential diagnosis in patients with uveitis associated with suspected leprosy includes other disorders with similar skin lesions, including sarcoidosis, lymphoma, syphilis, and yaws.

A list of the ocular complications of leprosy is given in Box 10.1. In one study, over half the patients with multibacillary leprosy had ocular involvement.[11] Structural damage to the eyelids, poor lid closure as a result of facial nerve involvement, and impaired corneal sensation often lead to exposure of the cornea. Loss of the temporal portion of the eyebrows (madarosis) is a typical finding and a stigma in those affected. It is important to remember, however, that trachoma can exist in the same population with leprosy and can compound the external disease in these patients.[12] The keratitis associated with leprosy starts superiorly and first appears as subepithelial chalky infiltrates surrounded by gray stromal opacifications.[13] Corneal exposure predisposes patients to development of corneal ulcers (Fig. 10.2) that are often difficult to manage.

Intraocular inflammatory disease is a known complication of leprosy. In a retrospective study of 531 patients with leprosy, 4% had iritis.[14] The organisms can directly invade the iris and the ciliary body, and chronic anterior uveitis is commonly seen in these patients. If uveitis is not aggressively treated, cataract and hypotony frequently result. Less frequently, patients present with acute anterior uveitis. In a study of 100 patients with leprosy in Brazil, 72 had ocular complications.[15] Seventeen had a chronic anterior uveitis, whereas only two had acute anterior uveitis. In a study in Nepal, 8% of patients with tuberculoid leprosy had uveitis, whereas 16% of patients with lepromatous leprosy had anterior chamber inflammatory disease.[16] Spaide et al.[17] found that uveitis was uncommon in patients with leprosy in the United States, possibly

BOX 10.1 Ocular Manifestations of Leprosy

- Prominent corneal nerves
- Decreased corneal sensitivity
- Madarosis
- Ectropion
- Entropion
- Episcleritis/scleritis
- Trichiasis
- Glaucoma
- Cataract
- Blocked nasolacrimal ducts
- Pterygium
- Conjunctivitis
- Granulomatous anterior uveitis
- Iris pearls
- Iris atrophy
- Facial nerve palsy (tuberculoid leprosy)
- Ptosis
- Exposure keratitis
- Orbicularis oculi weakness
- Lagophthalmos
- Trigeminal nerve involvement
- Corneal anesthesia
- Lid lesions and deformities (lepromatous leprosy)
- Choroidal lesions

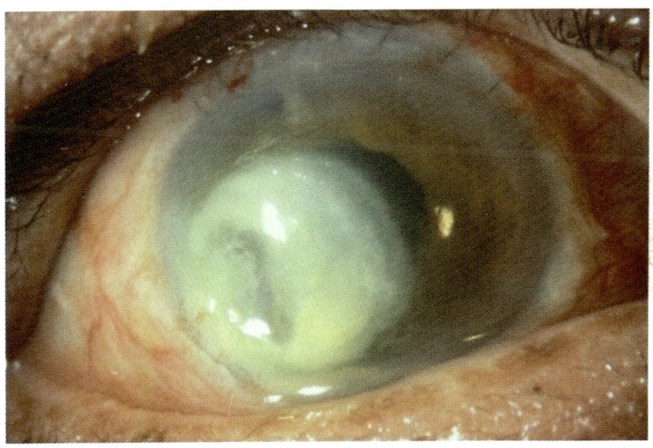

Fig. 10.2 Severe bacterial corneal ulcer in a patient with leprosy. (Courtesy R. Christopher Walton, MD.)

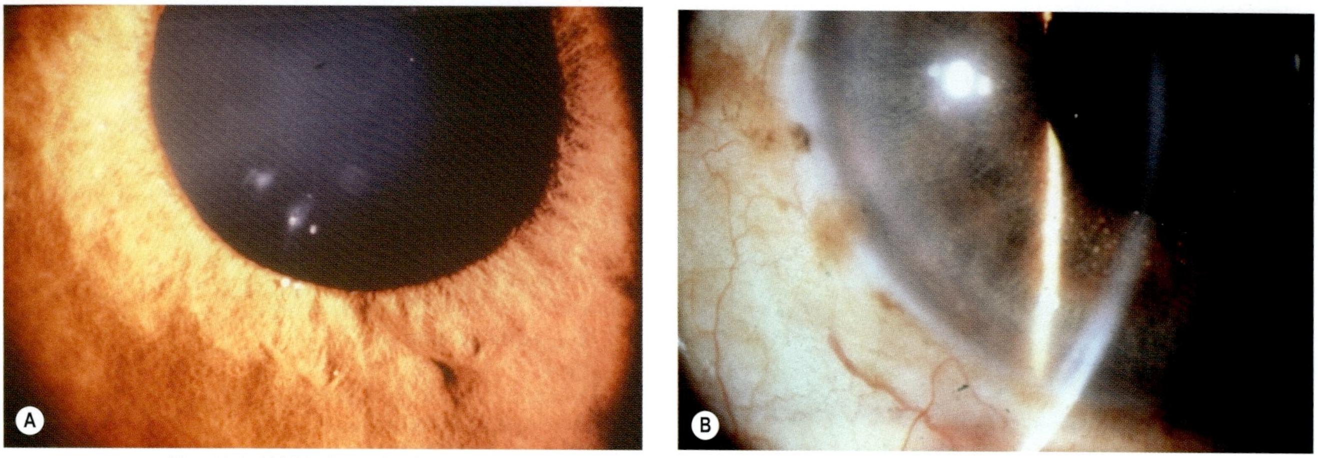

Fig. 10.3 (A) Iris "pearl" of leprosy seen as a small white object on iris edge. (B) Many of these objects can be seen just right of the slit beam. (Courtesy Khalid Tabbara, MD.)

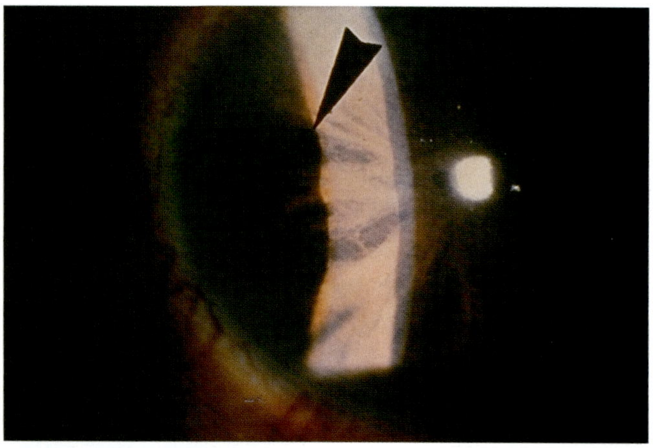

Fig. 10.4 Multiple areas of iris atrophy *(arrowhead)* in patient with iritis caused by leprosy. (Courtesy Fernando Orefice, MD.)

reflecting the results of more aggressive treatment with antilepromatous and anti-inflammatory agents. Granulomas form in the iris and appear as iris "pearls" on the anterior surface (Fig. 10.3). Iris atrophy also occurs in many patients but can be more subtle (Fig. 10.4) compared with the iris atrophy observed with herpes infection (see Fig. 3.7).

Although less common, changes to the retina have been described in patients with leprosy. Patients with long-standing lepromatous leprosy can have large numbers of organisms that invade not only the anterior segment but also the adjoining peripheral pars plana and retina. Pars planitis has been reported in patients with leprosy.[18] Chovet et al.[19] demonstrated segmental vasculitis in the posterior pole on fluorescein angiography in patients with lepromatous disease. Blindness can occur from a number of the ocular complications of leprosy. In a series of patients treated for multibacillary Hansen disease, unilateral or bilateral blindness occurred in almost 10% of patients.[20]

Immunology and Pathology

Humans are the only natural host for *M. leprae.* After entering the host, the organism reproduces in mononuclear cells, particularly skin histiocytes. The doubling time for the organisms is extraordinarily long, about 20 days, and attempts to culture the organism in a cell-free environment have not been successful. Some work has centered on the use of the nine-banded armadillo as an experimental model.[21] This animal has a low basal temperature that seems to permit large numbers of *M. leprae* to propagate.

The immune characteristics of patients with this disorder have been extensively studied. Imbalances in T cells,[22] antigen-specific suppressor T cells,[23] and defective production of monocyte-activating cytokines have all been described.[24] CD4+ T cells predominate in tuberculoid lesions, but CD8+ T cells are almost exclusively found in lepromatous lesions.[25] Family studies with human leukocyte antigen (HLA) typing have suggested that there is an HLA-linked recessive gene that may predispose patients to the tuberculoid form of the disease.[26]

The reactional states of leprosy have been divided into two categories: type I and type II. The type I reaction is also known as the *reversal reaction* and is a delayed hypersensitivity response directed against bacillary antigens. The type II reaction is also known as *erythema nodosum leprosum* and is an immune-complex reaction. Patients with the reversal reaction (type I) may be more likely to present with orbicularis oculi weakness and lagophthalmos.[27]

Therapy

Although a number of drugs to treat leprosy are available, treatment regimens remain somewhat controversial. The World Health Organization (WHO) recommends multidrug treatment regimens because of the existence of dapsone-resistant strains of *M. leprae.*[28] The WHO developed consensus guidelines for a multidrug therapy with dapsone and rifampin for 6 to 12 months for paucibacillary leprosy with the addition of clofazamine and longer duration of treatment for multibacillary disease.[29] Although a number of treatment regimens for leprosy have been proposed, a systematic review and meta-analysis failed to show better regiments that those implemented by WHO.[29] The use of thalidomide was reported to be useful in patients with recurring and persistent erythema nodosum leprosum.[30] Vaccination at birth with Bacille Calmette-Guérin (BCG) has variable efficacy in preventing disease. Despite efforts to eradicate the disease, long-term recurrences remain high. Ocular care of patients with leprosy requires careful management of the external disease, including surgical management of eyelid deformities and judicial use of ocular lubrication. If intraocular surgery is planned, great care must be taken to be sure that the eye has no active inflammation.

TUBERCULOSIS

Guyton and Woods identified TB as the most common underlying disease in the vast majority of patients with granulomatous uveitis seen by them in the 1940s.[31] It is now clear that many of these patients actually had other conditions, such as ocular histoplasmosis, that caused the

BOX 10.2 Ocular Manifestations of Tuberculosis

Tubercle formation of eyelids
Conjunctivitis
Interstitial keratitis
Anterior uveitis
Scleritis
Choroidal granulomas
Posterior uveitis
Retinal vasculitis

uveitis. Nevertheless, globally, tuberculosis kills more people than any other infection, and in the United States, tuberculosis is still an important cause of other diseases, including uveitis. Although the rates of incidence, mortality, and morbidity from TB have declined since the 1940s, 25,000 to 30,000 new cases are still reported annually in the United States.[32] For a time, reported cases of TB increased, predominantly because of acquired immunodeficiency syndrome (AIDS) and immigration from endemic countries.[33] However, 25,313 cases of TB (9.8 cases per 100,000 population) were reported to the Centers for Disease Control and Prevention (CDC) in 1993, a 5.1% decrease from 1992.[34] Since then, the number of cases has continued to decline, and in 2018, a total of 9029 new tuberculosis cases were reported in the United States.[35] Active tuberculosis has been associated with the use of anticytokine therapy, including anti–tumor necrosis factor (TNF) treatments.[36] As patients with uveitis with associated autoimmune disease are more commonly treated with anti-TNF drugs, tuberculosis may again return as a more common cause of uveitis, even in countries with lower prevalence of TB.

Disease Pathogenesis and Systemic Disease

The disease is caused by mycobacteria from the family Mycobacteriaceae and the order Actinomycetales. There are eight distinct subgroups from the *M. tuberculosis* complex; *Mycobacterium tuberculosis sensu stricto* is the most important agent causing human disease. Infection in the United States is transmitted predominantly via aerosolized droplets. The *M. tuberculosis* bacilli enter the alveoli, and infection develops and spreads from phagocytosis of the bacteria by macrophages, which circulate in blood and lymph.

In most patients, asymptomatic, self-limiting pneumonia develops and usually heals with granuloma formation. Sensitization develops 2 to 10 weeks after infection and is seen on the skin test as a positive reaction to an extract of the tuberculous bacillus (purified protein derivative [PPD]). The granulomas usually calcify and remain inactive. However, onset of symptoms can occur after a breakdown of the patient's immune system associated with age, disease, or the use of immunosuppressive therapy for other conditions. TB is classified as pulmonary TB, extrapulmonary TB, or both. Extrapulmonary TB most commonly involves the lymph nodes, genitourinary tract, bones, joints, peritoneum, pericardium, meninges, and pleura. Miliary or disseminated TB is caused by hematologic spread of the bacteria.

Ocular Disease

Ocular involvement occurs in about 1% to 2% of patients with TB.[37] The ocular manifestations of TB are listed in Box 10.2. TB can involve both the anterior and posterior segments of the eye and the ocular adnexa and the orbit. In miliary TB, tubercles can be seen in the choroid, giving the impression of unifocal or multifocal choroiditis (Fig. 10.5). Whether at least some cases of serpiginous choroiditis may be caused by tuberculosis has been an area of debate.[38,39] Choroidal tubercles have also been associated with the development of subretinal neovascularization.[40] More rarely, tubercles occur in the anterior chamber and may elicit a severe inflammatory response (Fig. 10.6). In addition, tubercle formation of the lids, conjunctiva, cornea, and sclera have been reported.[41] Granulomatous iritis is the inflammatory condition most often associated with TB.[42] Coles[43] stated that TB should be suspected not only in cases of granulomatous uveitis but also in cases of intense nongranulomatous anterior uveitis of short duration, mild relapsing uveitis, or chronic smoldering inflammatory disease.

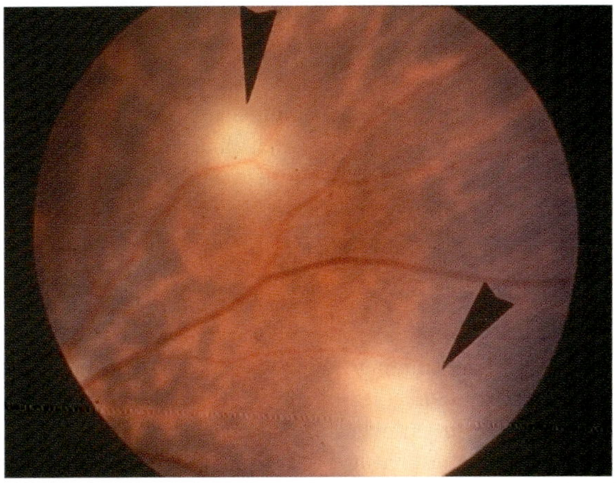

Fig. 10.5 Two large choroidal lesions *(arrowheads)* caused by miliary tuberculosis. (Courtesy Fernando Orefice, MD.)

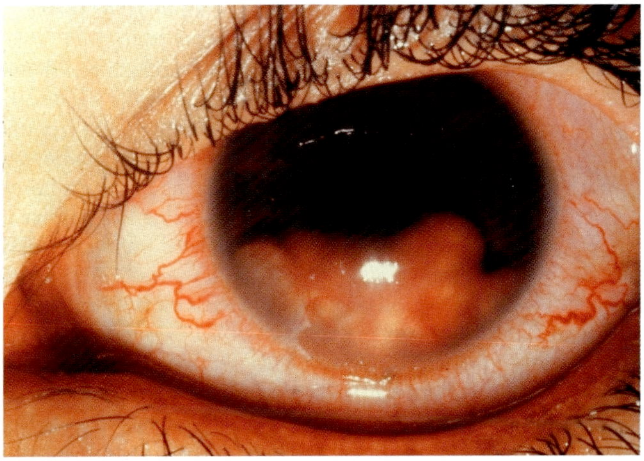

Fig. 10.6 Patient with systemic tuberculosis who presented with a large floccular mass in the anterior chamber. (Courtesy Roberto Neufeld, MD.)

Interstitial keratitis and phlyctenular keratoconjunctivitis are common findings in patients with ocular TB; however, these conditions are not thought to result from direct invasion of organisms but, instead, to represent an immunologic response to the mycobacteria. Eales disease, a disorder characterized by retinal vasculitis and vitreous hemorrhage, is also associated with TB (see Chapter 28). Finally, optic nerve involvement and cataracts have also been reported in patients with ocular TB.[37,41] A number of infectious and noninfectious disorders may cause ocular disease similar to that associated with TB. For example, the retinal periphlebitis that results from TB can mimic the ocular disease associated with sarcoidosis and syphilis. TB choroiditis can also mimic serpiginous choroiditis but more commonly is unilateral with more substantial cellular infiltration of the aqueous and vitreous. An underlying immunosuppressive state, such as AIDS, should always be considered in patients with ocular TB.

Diagnosis

The diagnosis of ocular TB is usually difficult to make. We have spent countless hours debating the diagnostic approach to patients with possible TB-associated uveitis. As with many infections, the key to diagnosis is suspecting the disease when clinical signs and symptoms suggest the disease. Definitive diagnosis requires the identification of *M. tuberculosis* organisms in ocular tissues or fluids, but samples are often difficult to obtain, and biopsy may be hard to justify in a patient who has only a small chance of having the disease. Patients with suspected ocular TB should have a systemic evaluation for evidence of the disease. A chest x-ray should be obtained and tuberculin skin tests performed. If the clinical findings support a diagnosis of TB, a complete course of antituberculosis therapy should be considered. In a study in Japanese patients with intraocular inflammation, 26 of 126 had a positive tuberculin skin test result.[44] Ten of these 26 patients had clinical findings consistent with TB and had a favorable response to antituberculosis therapy.

An intermediate-strength tuberculin skin test should be used in most patients. However, if a patient has a history of TB or has had a positive PPD test result in the past, an intermediate-strength PPD may cause a severe dermatologic response, so a lower-strength one should be used. The PPD test is not 100% sensitive or specific for the disease. One patient with numerous tubercle bacilli in the eye was reported to have a negative PPD test result and no systemic manifestations of disease.[45] The use of routine tuberculosis screening in county hospitals in patients with uveitis showed that TB screening was positive in 21.1%. Six patients were diagnosed with TB-related uveitis: one definite, four presumed, and one systemic TB with uveitis.[46] The posttest probabilities of a positive PPD in these higher-risk patients with uveitis showed a 17.2% overall risk of ocular TB or a 30.3% risk in foreign-born patients. Importantly, a positive PPD test result in a patient with uveitis does not mean that the uveitis was caused by TB because TB is a very rare cause of inflammatory eye disease in low-risk patients. In fact, without other signs of TB, a positive PPD test result in a patient with uveitis is probably more misleading than helpful.

Two interferon (IFN)-γ-release assays performed on blood have been approved by the U.S. Food and Drug Administration (FDA) for the diagnosis of TB infection. These new assays, the QuantiFERON-TB Gold In Tube (QFT-GIT) test and the T-SPOT.TB test, have excellent specificity and are unaffected by BCG vaccination; however, conflicting results from the two tests have been reported.[47,48] One study suggested that the QFT-GIT assay was more specific and slightly less sensitive overall, but more accurate in identifying true-positive tuberculous uveitis cases among discordant cases compared with the T-SPOT.TB assay.[49] Additional studies are needed to define the role of specific tests in the evaluation of patients with suspected tuberculous uveitis.

In general, testing use of both the TB skin test and TB blood test is not recommended. The IFN-γ-release assays are preferred for individuals who have received a TB vaccine (BCG) or who are unlikely to return for a second skin test. Finally, use of real-time polymerase chain reaction (PCR) with the Xpert MTB/RIF assay is recommended as an alternative to microscopy, culture, and histopathology, especially for analysis of cerebral spinal fluid (CSF) and in diagnosing human immunodeficiency virus (HIV)–associated TB. The test, by using the same sample, also demonstrates rifampicin resistance, which can be useful in determining therapy.

Although many patients with ocular TB will have evidence of systemic disease, TB infection limited to specific organs, including the eye, may occur. Microscopic examination of ocular tissues or fluids may show bacilli; however, culture is more sensitive. The PCR assay has also been used to diagnose TB infection,[50] but in most laboratories, this approach has been considered experimental. In 2017 the Xpert MTB/RIF assay has been used to diagnose intraocular tuberculosis from vitreous samples.[51] In a study of eyes with multifocal serpiginous choroiditis, PCR test results for tuberculosis were positive with use of one of three assays in 10 of 11 eyes.[52]

Therapy

Because of the development of treatment-resistant TB, recommended treatment regimens have become more aggressive. Historically, the recommended treatment was regimens of isoniazid and ethambutol for 1.5 to 2 years. Since the late 1960s, however, a number of studies have demonstrated that short-course treatment regimens can be effective. There are several goals of therapy, including treating the underlying disease to prevent morbidity and mortality, preventing the development of drug resistance, and limiting the spread of disease. Four drugs that are currently considered first-line agents for the treatment of TB are isoniazid, rifampin, pyrazinamide, and ethambutol. Standard treatment now consists of a 2-month induction phase, with at least isoniazid, rifampin, and pyrazinamide, followed by a 4-month consolidation phase with at least isoniazid and rifampin.[53] Although in many patients shorter regimens are effective in treating TB, overall treatment failures remain high, and this may be attributed to sequestered bacteria in inaccessible tissue compartments. Furthermore, because of the emergence of multidrug-resistant (MDR) TB, more intensive therapy is required in these patients and should include four drugs, selected based on drug susceptibility analysis performed on the patient's isolate whenever possible.[54] Intensified regimens have also been suggested in patients with HIV infection and in patients with more severe disease. A randomized controlled trial (RCT), however, showed that intensified antituberculosis therapy was not associated with a higher rate of survival among patients with tuberculous meningitis compared with standard treatment and suggested that additional studies were warranted.[55] Clearly, therapy should be administered by a practitioner well versed in the current treatment recommendations.

The difficult decision is whether antituberculosis therapy is warranted for the patient with uveitis and a presentation and clinical examination consistent with tuberculosis, no evidence of systemic disease, and a positive PPD test result. It is not surprising that there is lack of consensus on both the diagnosis and treatment of ocular tuberculosis among uveitis specialists.[56] Schlaegel and Weber[57] recommended performing the isoniazid therapeutic test in these patients. This involves giving isoniazid at 300 mg/day and examining the patient every week. If ocular inflammation improves after 1 to 2 weeks of therapy, the patient is considered to have a positive test response. Schlaegel and Weber suggested that these patients should then receive a full course of therapy. There are several problems with this test, however. From a practical point of view, many patients with presumed tuberculous uveitis are concomitantly treated with corticosteroids, which makes it difficult to determine whether the antituberculosis therapy or the anti-inflammatory therapy exerted the principal effect. The disease course may wax and wane; therefore improvement may result from the natural course of the disorder and be unrelated to antituberculosis drugs. Importantly, a randomized double-masked study of isoniazid in the treatment of uveitis showed no significant difference between the treated and placebo groups.[58]

Our current recommendation is to treat patients with uveitis and a positive PPD test result when there are other findings to support the diagnosis of TB or if there has been variable response to previous anti-inflammatory therapy. A retrospective cohort study of 801 patients (1272 eyes) with tubercular uveitis reported treatment failures greater than 20% at 2 years in patients with risk factors, including panuveitis and vitreous and choroidal involvement.[59]

BOX 10.3 Ocular Manifestations of Brucellosis

Disk edema
Optic neuritis
Keratitis
Corneal ulcers
Conjunctivitis
Episcleritis
Dacryoadenitis
Eyelid edema
Chronic anterior uveitis
Intermediate uveitis
Posterior uveitis
Multifocal choroiditis
Discrete white retinal or choroidal lesions
Branch retinal vein occlusion
Retinal vasculitis
Endophthalmitis
Retinal detachment
Cranial nerve palsies

The addition of antituberculosis therapy to corticosteroids in patients with uveitis with underlying latent or manifest TB appears to reduce the recurrences of uveitis.[60] Additionally, corticosteroid therapy, for example, with intravitreal steroids, is effective in treating inflammatory ocular disease associated with TB infection, including cystoid macular edema, vitritis, and choroidal lesions,[61] but it is critical that patients be adequately treated for their TB. Although hematogenous seeding of organisms from the lung is the most common mode of ocular infection, results on chest x-ray may be normal, and disease is occasionally limited to a specific organ. A history of exposure to TB, a history of inadequately treated TB, a positive PPD skin test result, or positive blood tests or culture results all greatly increase the likelihood of disease. Once a decision to treat is made, the patient should receive a full course of antituberculosis therapy before a decision about efficacy is made.

OTHER BACTERIAL INFECTIONS

Brucellosis

Brucellosis is a bacterium that infects the genitourinary tract of cattle (*Brucella abortus*) and pigs (*Brucella suis*). Humans become infected after exposure to infected animals or contaminated meat or dairy products. The disease in humans is characterized by fever, chills, headache, arthralgias, lymphadenopathy, and splenomegaly. Diagnosis can be difficult but is based on positive results on culture of blood or of usually sterile fluids. Serologic tests are available for brucellosis and aid in making the diagnosis.

In two case series, ocular manifestations associated with brucellosis were reported in 21% to 26% of the patients.[62,63] In another study of 1551 patients with brucellosis, only 52 (3.4%) had ocular involvement.[64] The organism has been reported to affect all the ocular structures, but optic nerve involvement appears to be the most serious ocular manifestation.[65] Box 10.3 lists the ocular manifestations of brucellosis. Anterior uveitis may be the most frequently reported manifestation and appears to occur in the acute stage of the disease. Recurrent iritis, localized thickening of the iris, and multiple irregular choroidal exudates associated with little inflammation, retinal hemorrhages, and retinal detachment have all been ascribed to brucellosis and are typically seen in the chronic stage of disase.[66,67] Walker et al.[68] published the case of a patient with brucellosis who had well-circumscribed lesions in the periphery of the choroid (Fig. 10.7). In uveitis, *Brucella* organisms have rarely been cultured from the eye, although high *Brucella* agglutination titers have been more commonly reported in the vitreous of eyes with ocular brucellosis.[69,70] With current health measures, including pasteurization, the incidence of this disease has declined dramatically.

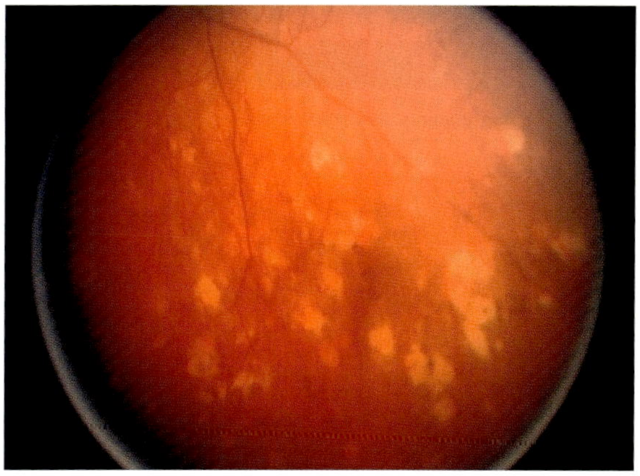

Fig. 10.7 Well-circumscribed lesions in periphery of choroid in patient with brucellosis. (Courtesy Narsing A. Rao, MD.)

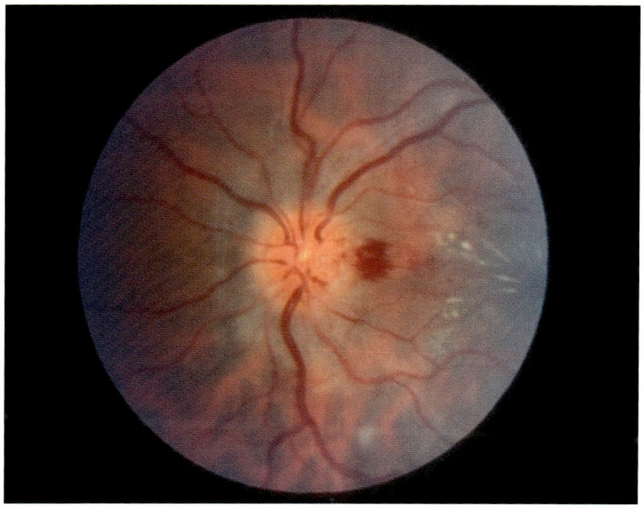

Fig. 10.8 Retinal photograph from a patient with neuroretinitis characterized by optic disk edema and hard exudate in the macula ("macular star").

Antimicrobial therapy for brucellosis is aimed at eradicating active infection, treating symptoms, and preventing recurrence. TB must also be excluded. The standard treatment for brucellosis in adults involves two antimicrobial agents, often intramuscular streptomycin (0.75–1 g daily for 14–21 days) with doxycycline (100 mg twice daily for 6 weeks). Rifampin and doxycycline are also used. Although there are no RCTs to guide therapy for ocular brucellosis, patients appear to respond well to systemic antibiotic treatment along with topical or systemic corticosteroid treatment.[63]

Bartonellosis

We now know that bartonellosis can cause uveitis with multiple clinical manifestations, but the association between *Bartonella* infection and ocular disease was made on the basis of findings from investigations of the links among neuroretinitis, cat scratch disease, and infectious disease. Neuroretinitis is an optic neuropathy with optic disk edema associated with peripapillary or macular hard exudates often described as a "macular star" (Fig. 10.8).

BOX 10.4 Infectious Causes of Neuroretinitis

Bartonella henselae infection
Hepatitis B
Herpes simplex
Herpes zoster
Histoplasmosis
Lyme disease
Leptospirosis
Mumps
Salmonella infection
Toxocariasis
Toxoplasmosis
Tuberculosis
Typhus

BOX 10.5 Ocular Manifestations of Bartonellosis

- Anterior segment
  - Conjunctivitis (usually as part of Parinaud oculoglandular syndrome)
  - Anterior uveitis
- Posterior segment
  - Optic edema
  - Macular star
  - Discrete focal retinal or choroidal lesions
  - Vitritis
  - Multifocal choroiditis
  - Serous retinal detachment
  - Retinal vascular occlusion
  - Intermediate uveitis
  - Epiretinal membrane

The condition was initially described in healthy patients by Leber in 1916 and has been called *Leber stellate neuroretinitis.*[71] Although the condition remains idiopathic in 50% of patients, neuroretinitis has been associated with autoimmune diseases, including sarcoidosis, and infections, including cat scratch disease.[72] The condition is usually unilateral and characterized by a single attack; however, both bilateral disease and recurrent episodes have been described. With improved diagnostic techniques, a number of possible infectious causes of neuroretinitis have been identified; these are listed in Box 10.4. Because they are one of the more common causes of neuroretinitis, *Bartonella* infections, including cat scratch disease, are discussed in more detail.

***Bartonella* infections.** *Bartonella* species are fastidious, intracellular, slow-growing, gram-negative bacteria, which have been associated with a wide range of systemic disease manifestations, including uveitis. The infection is transmitted usually after a cat scratch or bite. Dogs and ticks can also be disease reservoirs. *Bartonella henselae* and *Bartonella quintana* have both been identified as causative agents of uveitis. In the United States, the estimated disease incidence is four to 10 cases per 100,000 population.[73]

Most patients have what is classified as "typical" disease. The primary lesion is a small, painless, erythematous papule or pustule at the inoculation site. Lymphadenopathy then develops and can be associated with fever, malaise, and anorexia. Atypical disease, which occurs in 10% to 15% of patients, is described as "extranodal" or "complicated" disease and includes Parinaud oculoglandular syndrome, and *B. henselae* has been identified, by using PCR assay, in the conjunctiva of a patient with this condition.[74]

Bartonella infection can cause a plethora of ophthalmic signs and symptoms, although some patients with ocular bartonellosis can be asymptomatic. The ophthalmic findings of bartonellosis are listed in Box 10.5. In some series, optic disk edema, which can be identified clinically or by fluorescein leakage on angiography, was present in all patients[75] but may represent diagnostic bias because clinicians are more likely to consider the diagnosis of bartonellosis and cat scratch disease in patients with neuroretinitis. In a series of 14 patients with *Bartonella* infection, intermediate uveitis was present in seven eyes; vitritis in two eyes; neuroretinitis, a focal retinochoroiditis, branch retinal vein occlusion caused by vasculitis, disk edema with a peripapillary serous retinal detachment, and iridocyclitis in one eye each.[76] In a larger, multicenter retrospective cohort study of 107 eyes with cat scratch disease, optic nerve head lesions were found in 40%, uveitis in 36%, optic neuropathy in 33%, and retinal vessel occlusion in 7% (Fig. 10.9B).[77] In one study of the posterior segment manifestations of cat scratch disease, discrete white retinal or choroidal lesions, 50 to 3000 microns in diameter, were the most common posterior segment finding (see Fig. 10.9A).[78] Vision at presentation can be variable and range from normal to NLP (no light perception).[79]

Diagnosis is based on characteristic signs, history of a cat scratch, and enzyme immunoassay serology to *Bartonella.* In a study of 13 patients with presumed ocular bartonellosis, immunoglobulin G (IgG) levels were greater than 1:900 in eight patients, and IgM levels were greater than 1:250 in five patients.[75]

Treatment and Prognosis. There are limited data to guide treatment regimens for cat scratch disease. Suppurative nodes should be drained by using large-bore needles. Interestingly, the value of systemic antibiotics for some manifestations of bartonellosis, including cat scratch disease, remains controversial, and antibiotic treatment is not recommended by some for uncomplicated disease. However, most recommend antibiotic treatment for disease associated with uveitis, especially when vision is affected. In these cases, doxycycline (100 mg orally two times daily) plus rifampin (300 mg orally two times daily) for 4 to 6 weeks has been suggested.[80] Local and systemic corticosteroids have been used to treat ocular inflammatory disease, although its impact on visual outcome is unclear.[75] Although most patients with ocular bartonellosis could achieve good visual acuity, in one case series, visual acuity at 6 months was less than 20/100 in 17% of affected eyes,[75] and in another small case series, five of six eyes had final visual acuity of less than 20/40, and 50% had a final visual acuity of 20/400 or less.[79]

Whipple disease

Whipple disease, first described by George Whipple in 1907, is a chronic infectious disease caused by *Tropheryma whipplei.* This uncommon disorder is characterized by malabsorption that causes chronic diarrhea. Anterior uveitis, vitritis, retinitis, retrobulbar neuritis, optic disk edema, keratitis, ophthalmoplegia, and nystagmus have been rarely reported in patients with Whipple disease.[81,82] However, because antibiotic therapy can effectively treat Whipple disease, it is important to diagnose this disease in patients with uveitis who have gastrointestinal symptoms. *T. whipplei* DNA has been found in the stool and saliva of patients with the disease by using PCR analysis and may be of value in analyzing other specimens, including the aqueous humor,[83,84] and the development of PCR-based tests for *T. whipplei* has improved our ability to diagnose the disease.

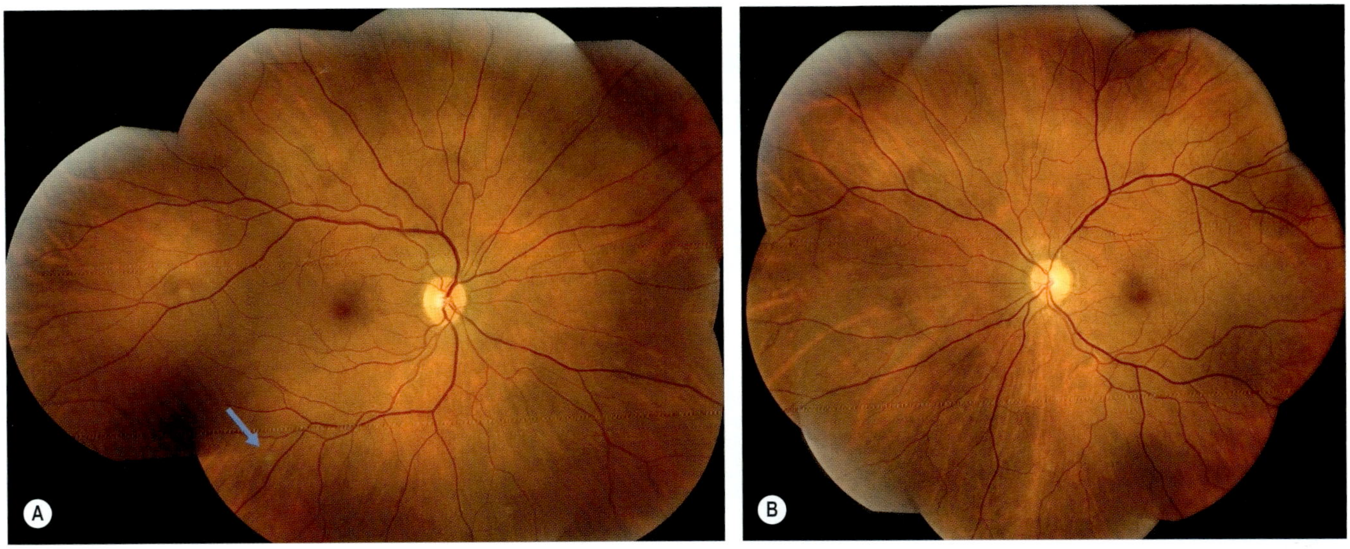

Fig. 10.9 Retinal montage from a patient with *Bartonella henselae* infection. (A) Discrete, small chorioretinal lesions are predominantly in the retinal periphery of the right eye *(arrow)*. (B) A branch retinal artery occlusion is present superiorly in the left eye.

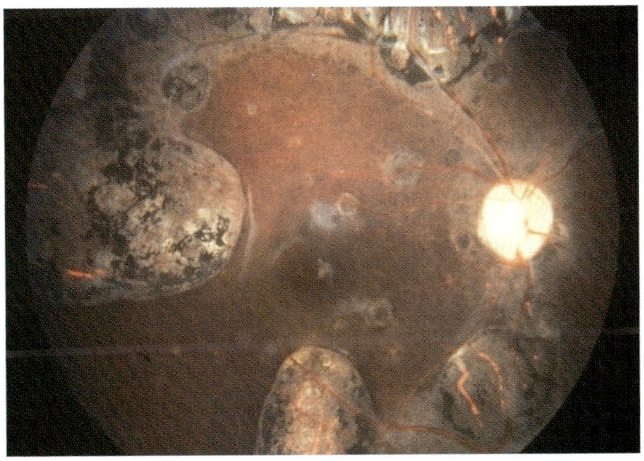

Fig. 10.10 Chorioretinal lesions in young patient with chronic granulomatous disease. Macular involvement resulted in decreased visual acuity.

Treatment and Prognosis

Before treatment with antibiotics was possible, Whipple disease was a fatal disorder. Antibiotics that cross the blood–brain barrier are felt to have lower recurrence rates, and many recommend oral administration of trimethoprim-sulfamethoxazole twice a day for 1 to 2 years.[85] This therapy is often preceded by intravenous administration of penicillin G or ceftriaxone. The prognosis is usually good if the disease is diagnosed promptly and treated appropriately. Patients with a neurologic recurrence, however, have a poor prognosis and may require additional antibiotic and anti-inflammatory therapies.[86]

CHRONIC GRANULOMATOUS DISEASE

Chronic granulomatous disease (CGD) is an inherited disorder that predisposes affected children to pyogenic infections. Currently, an X-linked recessive form and an autosomal recessive form of the disease have been identified. A number of ocular findings are associated with this disease, including blepharokeratoconjunctivitis with pannus formation and inflammatory chorioretinal lesions that lead to extensive scarring (Fig. 10.10).[87] We found chorioretinal lesions in seven of 19 patients (37%) with X-linked CGD but in none of six patients with autosomal recessive disease. Three of the patients with chorioretinal lesions had visual acuity less than 20/400 and abnormal electrooculography results. Usually, by the time these lesions are discovered in young children, who rarely complain of problems with their vision, there is no active inflammatory disease. It is unclear whether treatment with corticosteroids or antibiotics alters the course of the lesions; however, therapy is probably indicated if acute inflammatory disease is noted. In any event, sight-threatening disease is a frequent complication of CGD and appears to be associated with the X-linked form of the disease; periodic eye examinations are warranted in these patients.[88,89]

FUNGAL DISEASE

The most common fungal disease associated with uveitis is histoplasmosis. Ocular histoplasmosis and presumed ocular histoplasmosis syndrome are described in Chapter 16 on ocular histoplasmosis. In general, fungal infections of the choroid, retina, and vitreous occur in several types of patients: postoperative patients, immunosuppressed patients with systemic mycotic infections, immunocompetent patients with systemic mycotic infection, intravenous drug users, and patients with ocular trauma. In one case series, risk factors for fungal endophthalmitis included septicemia caused by intravenous drug use (78%), the presence of indwelling lines (9%), postocular surgery (9%), and trauma (4%).[90] Occasionally, a patient without a known risk factor may develop fungal endophthalmitis. Postsurgical causes of fungal endophthalmitis are discussed in Chapter 19.

Fungal endophthalmitis usually presents as chronic panuveitis. Fluffy, deep yellow-white retinal or choroidal lesions are frequently present, and the vitreous often contains "fluff balls" (Fig. 10.11). Posttraumatic cases of fungal endophthalmitis are easily differentiated from other forms of uveitis because of the clear history of trauma and the presence of uniocular disease, in contrast to sympathetic ophthalmia, which would be bilateral uveitis after trauma. Postsurgical fungal endophthalmitis may, however, mimic chronic idiopathic uveitis and is also discussed more fully in the chapter on postsurgical uveitis (see Chapter 19). This chapter will focus on endogenous fungal infections that cause uveitis. In cases of endogenous fungal endophthalmitis, the choroid is often initially involved because the eye is seeded through blood in this highly vascularized tissue. Because systemic signs and symptoms are often subtle or absent in many patients and culture results may be negative, the clinician must have a high degree of suspicion for the disease.

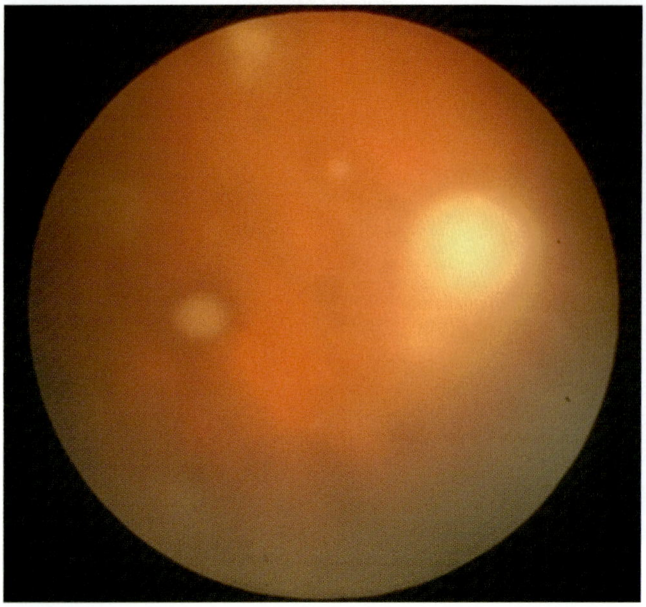

Fig. 10.11 Fundus of eye of known intravenous drug abuser who complained of floaters and decrease in vision. Multiple small choroidal lesions were present in addition to a large white fluffy mass in vitreous that contained *Candida* sp.

Candida species are the fungal organisms that most frequently cause fungal endophthalmitis.[91] *Candida albicans* is the most common of the *Candida* organisms, but others, such as *C. tropicalis, C. parapsilosis,* and *C. stellatoidea,* also cause fungal diseases in humans. *Candida* endophthalmitis usually occurs in chronically ill patients who have an indwelling catheter and are receiving antibiotics or immunosuppressive agents, including corticosteroids.[92] The disorder is also a frequent complication of intravenous drug use,[93] with outbreaks of fungal endophthalmitis reported in drug users.[94,95]

Patients with fungal endophthalmitis may complain of floaters. However, the disease is sometimes asymptomatic and detected only on ophthalmologic screening of patients with positive fungal culture results or fever of unknown origin, although the diagnostic yield from these examinations is not well established. Later in the course of the disease, redness, pain, reduced vision, hypopyon, dense vitritis, and dense retinal and choroidal lesions may occur. Chorioretinitis may precede the development of substantial vitreous inflammation. The diagnosis of *Candida* endophthalmitis is usually straightforward in a chronically ill patient with positive blood culture results. The usual assumption is that the same organisms in blood are responsible for the ocular disease. Nevertheless, multiple organisms may be present in the blood and eyes of severely immunocompromised patients. In addition, some intravenous drug users with candidal infection from emboli do not experience systemic infection. In these patients, multiple yellow-white deep retinal or choroidal lesions associated with vitreous fluff balls and retinal hemorrhage develop frequently (see Fig. 10.11).

Histopathologic examination of a vitreous specimen from patients with *Candida* endophthalmitis shows neutrophils, macrophages, and lymphocytes, along with either yeast forms or pseudohyphae consistent with *Candida.* Culture of the vitreous or aqueous confirms the diagnosis. The cellular infiltrate of the vitreous can be influenced by the patient's immune status, and patients with AIDS frequently have a diminished inflammatory response, especially when their CD4+ T-cell counts are severely diminished. In addition to cultures of intraocular fluids, including the vitreous humor and the aqueous humor, PCR assay of intraocular fluids can assist in making the diagnosis, although performance of these tests are predominantly limited to research laboratories.

The optimal treatment of *Candida* endophthalmitis remains controversial. Animal studies have shown that ocular infection spreads from the blood vessels in the retina and the choroid and suggests that with breakdown of the blood–retina barrier, intravenously administered antibiotics should adequately penetrate the eye.[96] Some experts have suggested that vitrectomy should only be performed in patients with dense vitreous opacities.[97] If vitrectomy is performed, 5 to 10 μg of amphotericin B or voriconazole should be injected into the vitreous at the end of the procedure.[98] The Infectious Diseases Society of America has published guidelines for the management of candidiasis.[99] Echinocandin (micafungin, caspofungin, or anidulafungin) or fluconazole were strongly recommended as initial therapy. Transition of all therapy to fluconazole for most patients with fluconazole-susceptible strains has also been recommended. Voriconazole was recommended for fluconazole-resistant but voriconazole-susceptible strains. Miconazole appears to penetrate the eye well but may not be useful in treating ocular disease until a dose of 2400 mg/day is used.[97] Patients with fungal ocular disease have been treated with systemic imidazoles, including ketoconazole and fluconazole, usually in combination with other antifungal agents.[100] Posaconazole is another new antifungal agent, but data regarding use for endophthalmitis are scarce,[101] although the agent has been effective in the management of fungal keratitis.[102] Initiation of therapy early in the course of the disease before macular involvement occurs improves the prognosis.[97]

Aspergillosis is the second most common disseminated fungal infection.[91] It has been reported as a cause of endophthalmitis in immunosuppressed patients and intravenous drug users.[103,104] *Aspergillus* infection of the eye presents as vitritis with fluff balls and yellow-white lesions in the retina, similar to those seen with candidal infections. Also similar to *Candida* endophthalmitis, redness, pain, hypopyon, retinal hemorrhages, and reduced vision can also occur. *Aspergillus* may be difficult to culture from blood.[105] In one case report, there was no evidence of systemic infection in an intravenous drug user with *Aspergillus* endophthalmitis.[104] This patient was successfully treated with vitrectomy, intravitreal and subconjunctival amphotericin B, and oral flucytosine. In a 15-day-old infant without any risk factors for infection, bilateral *Aspergillus* endophthalmitis was diagnosed after enucleation of one eye. Systemic amphotericin B resulted in good visual outcome in the other eye.[106] Unfortunately, many patients with ocular involvement caused by *Aspergillus* species have had poor visual outcomes.

Endogenous fungal endophthalmitis can be caused by a variety of these organisms, including *Coccidioides immitis,*[107] *Cryptococcus neoformans,*[108] *Histoplasma capsulatum,*[109] *Sporotrichum schenckii,*[110] and *Blastomyces dermatitidis.*[111] The risk factors and ocular characteristics of endogenous fungal infections are listed in Table 19.1. These infections are all less common than those caused by either *Candida* or *Aspergillus* and therefore represent a diagnostic challenge to the clinician. It is interesting to note that histopathologic examination of an eye with coccidioidomycosis showed both choroidal and retinal granulomatous lesions that did not overlap anatomically, suggesting hematogenous spread through both the retinal and choroidal circulations.[107] *Nocardia asteroides* is a weakly acid-fast bacterium that causes a disease that appears similar to fungal ocular infections. This disease, however, is resistant to antifungal agents but sensitive to antibiotic therapy, which makes prompt and accurate diagnosis imperative, especially because the visual outcome is poor when the presenting vision already has substantially diminished.[112] Advances in therapies for cancer, autoimmune disease, other chronic diseases, and organ transplantation have increased the number of chronically immunosuppressed patients. In addition, HIV infection has led to an increase in immunosuppressed patients prone to opportunistic infections. It is therefore of increasing importance that clinicians become well versed in the diagnosis and treatment of endogenous fungal diseases.

REFERENCES

1. Ayo C. A toxic ocular action: new property of Schwartzman toxins. *J Immunol.* 1943;46:113–132.
2. Rosenbaum JT, McDevitt HO, Guss RB, et al. Endotoxin-induced uveitis in rats as a model for human disease. *Nature.* 1980;286:611–613.
3. Forrester JV, Worgul BV, Merriam GR Jr. Endotoxin-induced uveitis in the rat. *Albrecht von Graefes Arch Klin Exp Ophthalmol.* 1980;213:221–233.
4. Tanouchi Y, Kogiso M, Miki S, et al. Endotoxin-induced uveitis in LPS-susceptible C3H/HeN mice. *Invest Ophthalmol Vis Sci.* 1991;32(Suppl):792.
5. Hansen GHA. Investigations concerning the etiology of leprosy. *Norsk Magazin Laegevidenskaben.* 1874;4:76–79.
6. Binford C, Meyers W, Walsh G. *Leprosy. JAMA.* 1982;247:2283–2292.
7. Blindness in leprosy [Editorial]. *Br J Ophthalmol.* 1981;65:221–222.
8. Gelber RH. Leprosy. In: *Harrison's Principles of Internal Medicine.* 20th ed. New York: McGraw-Hill Education; 2018: 1260
9. Ridley DS, Jopling WH. Classification of leprosy according to immunity, a five group system. *Int J Lepr Other Mycobact Dis.* 1966;34:255–273.
10. Sansonetti P, LaGrange PH. The immunology of leprosy: speculations on the leprosy spectrum. *Rev Infect Dis.* 1981;3:422–469.
11. Nepal BP, Shrestha UD. Ocular findings in leprosy patients in Nepal in the era of multidrug therapy. *Am J Ophthalmol.* 2004;137:888–892.
12. Schwab IR, Nassar E, Malaty R, et al. Leprosy in a trachomatous population. *Arch Ophthalmol.* 1984;102:240–244.
13. Hornblass A. Ocular leprosy in South Vietnam. *Am J Ophthalmol.* 1973;75:478–480.
14. Sharma N, Koranne RV, Mendiratta V, et al. A study of leprosy reactions in a tertiary hospital in Delhi. *J Dermatol.* 2004;31:898–903.
15. Shields JA, Waring GO III, Monte LG. Ocular findings in leprosy. *Am J Ophthalmol.* 1974;77:880–890.
16. Brandt F, Malla OK. Ocular findings in leprous patients: a report of a survey in Malunga/Nepal. *Albrecht von Graefes Arch Klin Exp Ophthalmol.* 1981;217:27–34.
17. Spaide R, Nattis R, Lipka A, et al. Ocular findings in leprosy in the United States. *Am J Ophthalmol.* 1985;100:411–416.
18. Vedy J, Graveline J. *Précis D'ophtalmologie Tropicale.* Marseille, France: Diffusion Generale de Librairie; 1979:125.
19. Chovet M, Metge P, Fauxpoint B, et al. Uvéite posté lépreuse. *Bull Soc Ophtalmol Fr.* 1976;12:1215–1217.
20. Parikh R, Thomas S, Parikh S, et al. Ocular manifestation in treated multibacillary Hansen's disease. *Ophthalmology.* 2009;116:2051–2057.
21. Kircheimer WF, Storrs EE. Attempts to establish the armadillo (*Drasypus novemcentus* Linn.) as a model for study of leprosy. *Int J Lepr.* 1971;39:693–702.
22. Wallach D, Cottenot F, Bach M-A. Imbalances in T-cell subpopulations in lepromatous leprosy. *Int J Leprosy.* 1982;50:282–290.
23. Stoner GL, Atlaw T, Touw J, et al. Antigen-specific suppressor cells in subclinical leprosy infection. *Lancet.* 1981;2:1372–1377.
24. Horwitz MA, Levis WR, Cohn ZA. Defective production of monocyte-activating cytokines in lepromatous leprosy. *J Exp Med.* 1984;159:666–678.
25. Van Voorhis WC, Kaplan G, Nunes Sarno E, et al. The cutaneous infiltrates of leprosy: cellular characteristics and the predominant T-cell phenotypes. *N Engl J Med.* 1982;307:1593–1597.
26. De Vries RRP, van Eden W, van Rood JJ. HLA-linked control of the course of *M. leprae* infection. *Leprosy Rev.* 1981;52(Suppl):109–119.
27. Daniel E, Koshy S, Rao GS, et al. Ocular complications in newly diagnosed borderline lepromatous and lepromatous leprosy patients: baseline profile of the Indian cohort. *Br J Ophthalmol.* 2002;86:1336–1340.
28. World Health Organization (WHO) Study Group. Chemotherapy of leprosy for control programmes. *WHO Tech Rep Ser.* 1982;675.
29. Lazo Porras M, Prutsky GJ, Barrionuevo P, et al. World Health Organization (WHO) antibiotic regimen against other regiments for the treatment of leprosy: a systematic review and meta-analysis. *BMC Infect Dis.* 2020;20(1):62. https://doi.org/10.1186/s12879-019-4665-0.
30. Walker SL, Waters MF, Lockwood DN. The role of thalidomide in the management of erythema nodosum leprosum. *Lepr Rev.* 2007;78:197–215.
31. Guyton JS, Woods AC. Etiology of uveitis: a clinical study of 562 cases. *Arch Ophthalmol.* 1941;26:986–1018.
32. Glassroth J, Robins AG, Snider DE. Tuberculosis in the 1980s. *N Engl J Med.* 1980;302:1441–1450.
33. Barnes PF, Bloch AB, Davidson PT, et al. Tuberculosis in patients with human immunodeficiency virus infection. *N Engl J Med.* 1991;324:1644–1650.
34. Centers for Disease Control and Prevention. Expanded tuberculosis surveillance and tuberculosis morbidity, United States 1993. *MMWR Morbid Mortal Wkly Rep.* 1994;43:361–366.
35. Talwar A, Tsang CA, Price SF, et al. Tuberculosis – United States, 2018. MMMR. 2019;68:257–262.
36. Giles JT, Bathon JM. Serious infections associated with anticytokine therapies in the rheumatic diseases. *J Intens Care Med.* 2004;19:320–334.
37. Donahue HC. Ophthalmologic experience in a tuberculosis sanatorium. *Am J Ophthalmol.* 1967;64:742–748.
38. Ustinova EI, Zhuravleva LV, Bataev VM, et al. Experience in the differential diagnosis of peripapillary 'geographic' choroid disease and tuberculous chorioretinitis. *Vestn Oftalmol.* 1990;106:43–46.
39. Mackensen F, Backer MD, Wiehler U, et al. QuantiFERON TB-Gold – A new test strengthening long-suspected tuberculous involvement in serpiginous-like choroiditis. *Am J Ophthlamol.* 2008;146(5):761–766.
40. Massaro D, Katz S, Sachs M. Choroidal tubercles: a clue to hematogenous tuberculosis. *Ann Intern Med.* 1964;60:231–241.
41. Helm CJ, Holland GN. Ocular tuberculosis. *Surv Ophthalmol.* 1993;38:229–256.
42. Darrell RW. Acute tuberculous panophthalmitis. *Arch Ophthalmol.* 1967;78:51–54.
43. Coles RS. Uveitis associated with systemic disease. *Surv Ophthalmol.* 1963;8:377–392.
44. Morimura Y, Okada AA, Kawahara S, et al. Tuberculin skin testing in uveitis patients and treatment of presumed intraocular tuberculosis in Japan. *Ophthalmology.* 2002;109:851–857.
45. Smith RE. Tuberculoma of the choroid, discussion. *Ophthalmology.* 1980;87:257–258.
46. Hong BK, Khanamiri HN, Bababeygy SR, et al. The utility of routine tuberculosis screening in county hospital patients with uveitis. *Br J Ophthalmol.* 2014;98:1091–1095.
47. Pai M, Zwerling A, Menzies D. Systemic review: T-cell-based assays for the diagnosis of latent tuberculosis infection: an update. *Ann Intern Med.* 2008;149:177–184.
48. Tanabe M, Nakamura A, Arai A, et al. The direct comparison of two interferon-gamma release assays in the tuberculosis screening of Japanese healthcare workers. *Intern Med.* 2017;56:773–779.
49. Ang M, Wong WL, Kiew SY, et al. Prospective head-to-head study comparing 2 commercial interferon gamma release assays for the diagnosis of tuberculous uveitis. *Am J Ophthalmol.* 2014;157:1306–1314.
50. Musial CE, Tice LS, Stockman L, et al. Identification of mycobacteria from culture by using the Gen-Probe Rapid Diagnostic System for *Mycobacterium avium* complex and *Mycobacterium tuberculosis* complex. *J Clin Microbiol.* 1988;26:2120–2123.
51. Sharma K, Gupta V, Sharma A, et al. Gene Xpert MTB/RIF assay for the diagnosis of intra-ocular tuberculosis from vitreous fluid samples. *Tuberculosis.* 2017;102:1–2.
52. Bansal R, Sharma K, Gupta A, et al. Detection of *Mycobacterium tuberculosis* genome in vitreous fluid of eyes with multifocal serpiginoid choroiditis. *Ophthlamology.* 2015;122:840–850.
53. Horsburgh CR Jr, Barry CE, Lange C. Treatment of tuberculosis. *N Engl J Med.* 2015;373:2149–2160.
54. Ahuja SD, Ashkin D, Avendano M, et al. Multidrug resistant pulmonary tuberculosis treatment regimens and patient outcomes: an individual patient data meta-analysis of 9,153 patients. *PLoS Med.* 2012;9(8). e1001300.
55. Dorothee-Heemskerk A, Bang ND, Mai NTH, et al. Intensified antituberculosis therapy in adults with tuberculous meningitis. *N Engl J Med.* 2015;374:124–134.
56. Lou SM, Larkin KL, Winthrop K, et al. Uveitis Specialists Study Group. Lack of consensus in the diagnosis and treatment for ocular tuberculosis among uveitis specialists. *Ocul Immunol Inflamm.* 2015;23:25–31.

57. Schlaegel TF Jr, Weber JC. Double-blind therapeutic trial of isoniazid in 344 patients with uveitis. *Br J Ophthalmol.* 1969;53:425–427.
58. Oksala A, Salminen A. Leptospiral uveitis. *Acta Ophthalmol.* 1956;34:185–194.
59. Agarwal R, Gunasekeran DV, Grant R, et al. Clinical features and outcomes of patients with tubercular uveitis treated with antitubercular therapy in the collaborative ocular tuberculosis study (COTS)-1. *JAMA Ophthalmol.* 2017;135(12):1318–1327.
60. Bansal R, Gupta A, Gupta V, et al. Role of anti-tubercular therapy in uveitis with latent/manifest tuberculosis. *Am J Ophthalmol.* 2008;146(5):772–779.
61. Agarwal A, Handa S, Aggarwal K, et al. The role of dexamethasone implant in the management of tubercular uveitis. *Ocul Immunol Inflamm.* 2018;26:884–892.
62. Gungur K, Bekir NA, Namiduru M. Ocular complications associated with brucellosis in an endemic area. *Eur J Ophthalmol.* 2002;12:232–237.
63. Sungur GK, Hazirolan D, Gurbuz Y, et al. Ocular involvement in brucellosis. *Can J Ophthalmol.* 2009;44:598–601.
64. Rolando I, Olarte L, Vilchez G, et al. Ocular manifestations associated with brucellosis: a 26-year experience in Peru. *Clin Infect Dis.* 2008;1:1338–1345.
65. Puig-Solanes M, Heatley J, Arenas F, et al. Ocular complications in brucellosis. *Am J Ophthalmol.* 1953;36:675.
66. Tabbara KF, al Kassimi H. Ocular brucellosis. *Br J Ophthalmol.* 1990;74:249.
67. Rolando I, Carbone A, Haro D, et al. Retinal detachment in chronic brucellosis. *Am J Ophthalmol.* 1985;99:733.
68. Walker J, Sharma OP, Rao NA. Brucellosis and uveitis. *Am J Ophthalmol.* 1992;114:374–375.
69. Akduman L, Or M, Hasanreisoglu B, et al. A case of ocular brucellosis: importance of vitreous specimen. *Acta Ophthalmol (Copenhagen).* 1993;71:130–132.
70. Rolando I, Vilchez G, Olarte L, et al. Brucellar uveitis: intraocular fluids biopsy studies. *Int J Infect Dis.* 2009;13:206–211.
71. Harnard P, Hamard H, Nghou S. Leber's idiopathic stellate neuroretinitis: apropos of 9 cases. *J Fr Ophthahlmol.* 1994;17(2):116–123.
72. Shoari M, Katz B. Recurrent neuroretinitis in an adolescent with ulcerative colitis. *J Neuro-ophthalmol.* 2005;25:286–288.
73. Giladi M, Ephros M. *Bartonella* infections, including cat-scratch disease. In: Jameson JL, Fauci AS, Kasper DL, et al., eds. *Harrison's Principles of Internal Medicine.* 20th ed. New York: McGraw-Hill Education; 2018:1209.
74. Grando D, Sullivan LJ, Flexman JP, et al. *Bartonella henselae* associated with Parinaud's oculoglandular syndrome. *Clin Infect Dis.* 1999;28:1156–1158.
75. Kerkhoff FT, Ossewaarde JM, de Loos WS, et al. Presumed ocular bartonellosis. *Br J Ophthalmol.* 1999;83:270–275.
76. Kalogeropoulos C, Koumpoulis J, Mentis A, et al. *Bartonella* and intraocular inflammation: a series of cases and review of literature. *Clin Ophthalmol.* 2011;5:817–829.
77. Habot-Wilner Z, Trivizki O, Goldstein M, et al. Cat-scratch disease: ocular manifestations and treatment outcome. *Acta Ophthalmol.* 2018;96:e524–e532.
78. Solley WA, Martin DF, Newman NJ, et al. Cat scratch disease: posterior segment manifestations. *Ophthlamology.* 1999;106:1546–1553.
79. Barros S, de Andrade GC, Cavalcanti C, et al. Cat scratch disease: not a benign condition. *Ocul Immunol Inflamm.* 2018;26:1115–1122.
80. Rolain JM, Brouqui P, Koehler JE, et al. Recommendations for treatment of human infections caused by Bartonella species. *Antimicrob Agents Chemother.* 2004;48:1921–1933.
81. Selsky EJ, Knox DL, Maumanee AE, et al. Ocular involvement in Whipple's disease. *Retina.* 1984;4:103–106.
82. Lisboa M, Domingues I, Paplona J, et al. Bilateral panuveitis associated with Whipple disease – case report. *GMS Ophthalmol Cases.* 2014;4:1–5.
83. Fenollar F, Laouira S, Lepidi H, et al. Value of *Tropheryma whipplei* quantitative polymerase chain reaction assay for the diagnosis of Whipple disease: usefulness of saliva and stool specimens for first-line screening. *Clin Infect Dis.* 2008;47:659–667.
84. Nubourgh I, Vandergheynst F, Lefebvre P, et al. An atypical case of Whipple's disease: case report and review of the literature. *Acta Clin Belg.* 2008;63:107–111.
85. Fenollar F, Puechal X, Raoult D. Whipple's disease. *N Engl J Med.* 2007;356:55–66.
86. Schneider T, Stallmach A, von Herbay A, et al. Treatment of refractory Whipple disease with interferon-gamma. *Ann Intern Med.* 1998;129:857–877.
87. Palestine AG, Meyers SM, Fauci AS, et al. Ocular findings in patients with neutrophil dysfunction. *Am J Ophthalmol.* 1983;95:598–604.
88. Parks DJ, Walton RC, Cheung MK, et al. Sight-threatening complications of chronic granulomatous disease. *Ophthalmology.* 1994;101(Suppl):132.
89. Goldblatt D, Butcher J, Thrasher AJ, et al. Chorioretinal lesions in patients and carriers of chronic granulomatous disease. *J Pediatr.* 1999;134:780–783.
90. Narndran N, Balasubramaniam B, Johnson E, et al. Five-year retrospective review of guideline-based management of fungal endophthalmitis. *Acta Ophthalmol.* 2008;86:525–532.
91. Abe F, Tateyama M, Shibuya H, et al. Disseminated fungal infection. *Acta Pathol Jpn.* 1984;34:1201–1208.
92. Edwards JE, Foos RY, Montgomerie JZ, et al. Ocular manifestations of *Candida* septicemia: review of seventy-six cases of hematogenous *Candida* endophthalmitis. *Medicine (Baltimore).* 1974;53:47–75.
93. Gallo J, Playfair J, Gregory-Roberts J, et al. Fungal endophthalmitis in narcotic abusers. *Med J Aust.* 1985;142:386–388.
94. Tirpack AR, Duker JS, Baumal CR. An outbreak of endogenous fungal endophthalmitis among intravenous drug abusers in New England. *JAMA Ophthalmol.* 2017;135:534–540.
95. Relhan N, Schwartz SG, Flynn HW Jr. Endogenous fungal endophthalmitis: an increasing problem among intravenous drug users. *JAMA.* 2017;318:741–742.
96. Cohen M, Edwards JE Jr, Hensley TJ, et al. Experimental hematogenous *Candida albicans* endophthalmitis: electron microscopy. *Invest Ophthalmol Vis Sci.* 1977;16:498–511.
97. Blumenkranz MS, Stevens DA. Therapy of endogenous fungal endophthalmitis. *Arch Ophthalmol.* 1980;98:1216–1220.
98. Durand ML. Bacterial and fungal endophthalmitis. *Clin Rev Microbiol.* 2017;30:597–613.
99. Pappas PG, Kauffman CA, Andes DR, et al. Clinical practice guideline for the management of candidiasis: 2016 update by the Infectious Diseases Society of America. *Clin Infect Dis.* 2016;62:e1–e50.
100. Goodman DF, Stern WH. Oral ketoconazole and intraocular amphotericin B for treatment of postoperative *Candida parapsilosis* endophthalmitis. *Arch Ophthalmol.* 1987;105:172–173.
101. Riddell JIV, Comer GM, Kauffman CA. Treatment of endogenous fungal endophthalmitis: focus on new antifungal agents. *Rev Anti-Infect Agents.* 2011;52:648–653.
102. Shah KB, Wu TG, Wilhelmus KR, et al. Activity of voriconazole against corneal isolates of *Scedosporium apiospermum*. *Cornea.* 2003;22:33–36.
103. Naidoff MA, Green WR. Endogenous *Aspergillus* endophthalmitis occurring after kidney transplant. *Am J Ophthalmol.* 1975;79:502–509.
104. Roney P, Barr CC, Chun CH, et al. Endogenous *Aspergillus* endophthalmitis. *Rev Infect Dis.* 1986;8:955–958.
105. Young RC, Bennett JE, Vogel CL, et al. Aspergillosis: the spectrum of the disease in 98 patients. *Medicine (Baltimore).* 1970;49:147–173.
106. Sihota R, Agarwal HC, Grover AK, et al. *Aspergillus* endophthalmitis. *J Ophthalmol.* 1987;71:611–613.
107. Glasgow BJ, Brown HH, Foos RY. Miliary retinitis in coccidioidomycosis. *Am J Ophthalmol.* 1987;104:24–27.
108. Hiles DA, Font RL. Unilateral intraocular cryptococcosis with unilateral spontaneous regression. *Am J Ophthalmol.* 1968;65:98–108.
109. Goldstein BG, Buellner H. Histoplasmic endophthalmitis: a clinicopathologic correlation. *Arch Ophthalmol.* 1983;101:774–777.
110. Font RL, Jakobiec FA. Granulomatous necrotizing retinochoroiditis caused by *Sporotrichum schenkii*. *Arch Ophthalmol.* 1976;94:1513–1519.
111. Font RL, Spaulding AG, Green WR. Endogenous mycotic panophthalmitis caused by *Blastomyces dermatitidis*. *Arch Ophthalmol.* 1967;77:217–222.
112. Dave VP, Pathengay A, Sharma S, et al. Diagnosis, clinical presentations, and outcomes of *Nocardia* endophthalmitis. *Am J Ophthalmol.* 2019;197:53–58.

11

Spirochetal Diseases

Scott M. Whitcup

KEY CONCEPTS

- Spirochetal diseases that cause uveitis include a gamut of historical and clinical infections, including syphilis, endemic syphilis, Lyme disease, relapsing fever, and leptospirosis.
- Syphilis remains a common and frequently missed, but treatable, cause of uveitis. Ocular findings can occur in primary, secondary, latent, and tertiary syphilis.
- The Venereal Disease Research Laboratory (VDRL) test can yield false–negative results, especially in the later stages of the disease, and a more sensitive test, such as the fluorescent treponemal antibody absorption (FTA-ABS) test, should be considered when evaluating patients with possible syphilitic uveitis.
- Patients with ocular syphilis should be treated with the recommended regimen for neurosyphilis.
- Lyme disease serology should be ordered in patients with a history or findings consistent with the disease. False-positive results are common when the test is ordered in patients with an extremely low likelihood of Lyme disease.
- Antibiotic regimens for spirochetal disease change frequently. Consulting a physician well versed in treating these diseases is important to ensure the appropriate drug, its dose and route of administration, and length of treatment.

SPIROCHETAL INFECTIONS AND THE EYE

This chapter focuses on uveitis caused by spirochetes. This comprises a variety of infectious diseases with ocular manifestations, including syphilis, bejel, pinta, yaws, Lyme disease, relapsing fever, and leptospirosis. The ocular manifestations of syphilis have been known for well over a century, whereas Lyme disease was first described only in the 1970s. The first section of this chapter is devoted to treponemal infections, of which syphilis is, by far, the most common and important infection to the practicing ophthalmologist. Syphilis remains an important cause of eye disease and blindness in the United States and is diagnosed with increasing frequency in patients with acquired immunodeficiency syndrome (AIDS). Sections on endemic syphilis (bejel) and nonvenereal treponemal infections (yaws and pinta) are also included.

The second part of the chapter contains sections on two infections caused by spirochetes of the genus *Borrelia* and a section on leptospirosis. Although the cause of syphilis was identified at the beginning of the twentieth century, the causative agent for Lyme disease was not discovered until 1982. Interestingly, Lyme disease and syphilis share many clinical features and should be considered together in the differential diagnosis of infectious diseases with ophthalmic involvement. The chapter also reviews relapsing fever, an additional infection caused by *Borrelia* that is often misdiagnosed. Leptospirosis is discussed at the end of the chapter and may be an important cause of uveitis of unknown etiology.

SPIROCHETES

Definition

Spirochetes are a phylum of bacteria characterized by long, helically coiled cells. These bacteria have lengthwise flagella, called *axial filaments,* which allow the spirochetes to move. There are three groups of spirochetes implicated in human disease: *Treponema,* which causes syphilis and the nonvenereal treponematoses; *Borrelia,* which causes relapsing fever and Lyme disease; and *Leptospira,* which causes leptospirosis.

Venereal Treponemal Diseases

Syphilis

Etiology. Syphilis was originally called the *great pox,* but it acquired its current name from the title character of a poem written in 1530 by the Veronese physician and poet Girolamo Fracastoro. Syphilis has also been called the *great imitator* because of the myriad symptoms and signs in its repertoire and its ability to mimic numerous other illnesses. Although clinical descriptions of syphilis date back at least half a millennium, it was not until 1905 that Schaudin and Hoffman[1] isolated the spirochete *Treponema pallidum* from the skin lesions of patients with syphilis.

After initial infection, there is both a humoral immune response and a cellular immune response. In 1910, Wasserman introduced a complement fixation test to detect nonspecific antibodies that react against cardiolipins, and these antibodies are commonly found in patients with syphilis. The next milestone in the history of syphilis was the use of arsenic derivatives to treat the disease. The *coup de grâce* in the war against syphilis came in 1943 with the discovery of penicillin, which is the mainstay of therapy even today.[2]

Epidemiology. In the late 1980s, there was a substantial increase in the rates of primary and secondary syphilis and an increased incidence of congenital syphilis, especially in the inner cities.[3] In 1986, only 57 cases of congenital syphilis were reported in New York City, but in 1989, more than 1000 cases were documented.[4] With focused efforts to reduce syphilis in the United States, in 2000, the rate of primary and secondary syphilis was 2.1 cases per 100,000 population, the lowest since reporting began in 1941.[5] From 2001 to 2004, the rate increased to 2.7 cases per 100,000 population. Approximately 84% of cases occurred in men. The incidence of primary and secondary syphilis

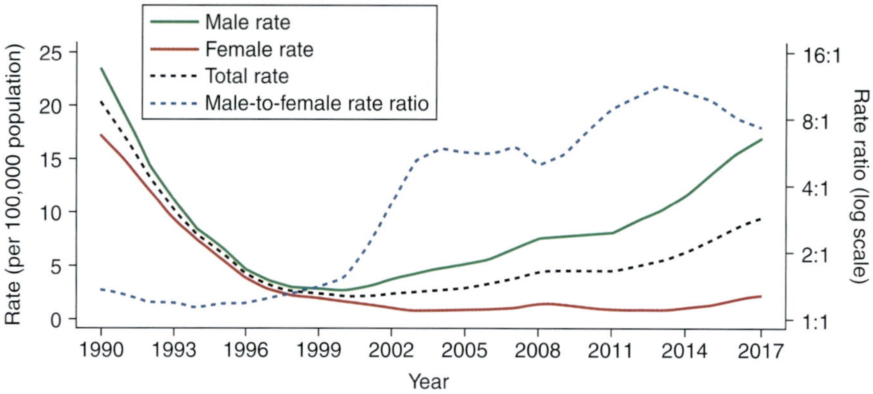

Fig. 11.1 Primary and secondary syphilis – rates of reported cases by sex and male-to-female rate ratios, United States, 1990–2017. (Sexually Transmitted Disease Surveillance 2017. https://www.cdc.gov/std/stats17/2017-STD-Surveillance-Report_CDC-clearance-9.10.18.pdf.)

also varied by race/ethnicity. The incidence of primary and secondary syphilis in 2004 was 9 per 100,000 among black, 1.6 among white, 3.2 among Hispanic, 1.2 among Asian/Pacific Islander, and 3.2 among American Indian/Alaska Native populations. Since reaching a low in 2000, the number of cases of syphilis in the United States has continued to increase, predominantly in men (Fig. 11.1). With an estimated 11 million new cases annually, syphilis remains a common infection globally, especially in resource-limited countries, where it is the second leading cause of stillbirths. Syphilis is also a problem in patients coinfected by human immunodeficiency virus (HIV). These patients may not mount a serologic response to the treponemal infection and thus elude diagnosis. In addition, standard therapy may be insufficient to eradicate the infection in these immunocompromised patients.[6,7]

Although syphilis is a nationally notifiable disease in the United States, ocular manifestations are not reportable to the Centers for Disease Control and Prevention (CDC). After clusters of ocular syphilis were reported in early 2015, the CDC reviewed syphilis surveillance and case investigation data from 2014, 2015, or both to ascertain syphilis cases with ocular manifestations.[8] A total of 388 suspected ocular syphilis cases were identified, 157 in 2014 and 231 in 2015. Overall the number of syphilis cases with ocular manifestations was 0.53% in 2014 and 0.65% in 2015, ranging from 0.17% to 3.9%, depending on the reporting region. Greater than 90% of the patients were men and one-half of the patients were HIV positive.

Clinical course. *T. pallidum* is a spirochete that is approximately 0.01 to 0.02 μm wide and 5 to 20 μm long. Although it cannot survive long outside of the body, it can be cultured and remains viable for several days. Syphilis is transmitted almost exclusively via sexual contact, including sexual intercourse, orogenital or anorectal contact, and occasionally kissing. The disease is most infectious in patients with untreated primary syphilis or secondary syphilis with skin lesions. Disease can also be transmitted by patients with early latent syphilis, especially if they have mucocutaneous involvement; however, disease in patients with late latent syphilis or tertiary syphilis is not infectious. Congenital syphilis occurs with transplacental spread of the spirochete. Interestingly, infection with syphilis does not confer lasting immunity, especially if treatment is received early in the course of the disease.

T. pallidum can penetrate intact mucous membranes or abraded skin. The period of incubation varies from 10 to 90 days but averages 3 weeks.[9] Before primary skin lesions appear, the spirochete spreads via the lymphatics to the bloodstream and then disseminates from there.

As with many of the spirochetal diseases, the clinical course of syphilis is divided into stages: primary, secondary, and tertiary syphilis (Box 11.1).

BOX 11.1 Syphilis: Key Features

- Caused by the spirochete *Treponema pallidum*
- Transmitted almost exclusively via sexual contact
- Congenital syphilis occurs with transplacental spread of the spirochete
- Disease is divided into stages: primary, secondary, latent, and tertiary
- Tertiary syphilis is subdivided into three subgroups: benign tertiary syphilis, cardiovascular syphilis, and neurosyphilis
- If untreated, syphilis will disseminate

Clinical manifestations

Primary syphilis. The chancre is the predominant lesion of primary syphilis. It appears about 4 weeks after infection and heals in about 1 to 2 months in untreated individuals. The lesion typically begins as a single erythematous papule at the inoculation site and later erodes to form a painless ulcer. Multiple chancres can occur, especially in patients coinfected with HIV.[10] Serous fluid from these lesions teems with spirochetes. Lesions occur on the penis, anus, and rectum in men and on the cervix, vulva, and perineum in women. Small lesions may also occur on the lips, tongue, buccal mucosa, and skin, and chancres of the eyelids and conjunctiva have also been described.[11]

Secondary syphilis. If left untreated, disease in patients with primary syphilis will progress to secondary syphilis 4 to 10 weeks after the initial manifestations of the disease. One of the unique characteristics of syphilis is that it always disseminates.[12] The skin is involved in about 90% of patients with secondary syphilis. A healing chancre may be present in patients with secondary syphilis, especially in persons with concurrent HIV infection. A generalized rash is characteristic of secondary syphilis and may be maculopapular or pustular. The rash commonly occurs on the flexor and volar surfaces of the body, typically the palms and the soles. The rash usually resolves without scarring, but some patients are left with areas of hyper- or hypopigmentation. Mucous membranes become eroded, forming erythematous patches. Condylomata lata is another characteristic dermatologic manifestation of secondary syphilis. The papules develop at the mucocutaneous junctions and in moist areas of the skin and appear as dull pink or gray hypertrophic lesions. Systemic symptoms of secondary syphilis include fever, malaise, headache, nausea, anorexia, and joint pain.[13] Generalized lymphadenopathy is found in both primary and secondary syphilis. Syphilitic infiltration of the kidneys, liver, and gastrointestinal tract also occurs in secondary syphilis, and about 10% of patients have ocular involvement. Anterior uveitis is the predominant eye finding in early secondary syphilis and may be the most common ocular lesion in syphilis.[14] Some patients may demonstrate cerebrospinal fluid (CSF) pleocytosis, and a few of these patients experience acute syphilitic meningitis with headache, neck stiffness, cranial nerve palsies, and disk edema. Similar to the clinical course of primary syphilis, the signs and symptoms of secondary disease often resolve spontaneously within 1 to 6 months.

Latent syphilis. In untreated persons, a diagnosis of latent syphilis is made with positive serologic tests for the disease in the absence of CSF abnormalities or clinical manifestations. Early latent syphilis is defined as encompassing latent syphilis during the first year after initial infection. Some of these patients may have recurrences of infectious mucocutaneous lesions. The late latent phase of syphilis occurs after 1 year of infection, and during this stage of the disease, infectious relapses are rare. Most patients who have not been treated remain in this late latent phase of the disease; however, about 30% go on to experience tertiary syphilis.

Tertiary syphilis. Tertiary syphilis is also called *late syphilis* and is often subdivided into three groups: benign tertiary syphilis, cardiovascular syphilis, and neurosyphilis, although it is important to note that syphilis can involve the central nervous system (CNS) at all stages of the disease.

Benign tertiary syphilis. Also known as *late benign syphilis,* the gumma is the typical lesion of benign tertiary syphilis and is a chronic granulomatous lesion that heals with scarring and fibrosis. It is a rare finding in the penicillin era and responds rapidly to treatment. Gummas tend to develop in the skin, mucous membranes, and skeletal system but can occur in almost any tissue and have even been found in the brain and in the choroid of the eye.[15]

Cardiovascular syphilis. The lesions of cardiovascular syphilis include aortitis and aortic aneurysms, aortic valvular insufficiency, and narrowing of the coronary ostia. The disease starts about 5 to 10 years after infection, but symptoms of cardiovascular syphilis may not be clinically evident for more than 20 years.

Neurosyphilis. This condition is said to occur in 5% to 10% of untreated patients with syphilis. Asymptomatic neurosyphilis is found in some patients who have a positive CSF–Venereal Disease Research Laboratory (VDRL) test result but no symptoms of CNS disease. In addition, invasion of the CNS by *T. pallidum* may be more common in early syphilis than once thought. Lukehart et al.[16] isolated *T. pallidum* from CSF in 12 (30%) of 40 patients with untreated primary and secondary syphilis, and an additional four patients, who did not have *T. pallidum* in the isolates but had reactive CSF on the VDRL test. Neurosyphilis can occur at any time in the course of the disease. Uveitis and hearing loss are more common in the earlier stages.[17]

One type of neurosyphilis, meningovascular syphilis, presents as aseptic meningitis, which can occur any time after primary syphilis. Unilateral or bilateral cranial nerve palsies are common, and headache, neck stiffness, dizziness, lassitude, and blurred vision occur. The classic neuro-ophthalmic finding of neurosyphilis is the Argyll Robertson (AR) pupil.[18] This is a small, irregular pupil that is unreactive to light but normally reactive to accommodation; it is commonly seen in cases of meningovascular syphilis, in which the base of the brain is involved. If the spinal cord is involved, patients may experience bulbar symptoms, muscle weakness and wasting, and slowly progressive spastic paraplegia with bladder incontinence.

T. pallidum may also invade the substance of the brain. Parenchymatous neurosyphilis is a meningoencephalitis, with progressive loss of cortical function. Patients can experience altered mental status and even syphilitic psychosis, with irritability, reduced memory, poor judgment, confusion, and delusions. Seizures may occur. On neurologic examination, patients demonstrate tremors of the mouth and tongue, hyperreflexia, and, in some cases, extensor plantar responses. Pathologically, the brain parenchyma is infiltrated with spirochetes, and the meninges are inflamed and thickened. CSF is hypercellular, and the VDRL test result is positive. Cranial nerve palsies, however, are uncommon, and optic atrophy is rare. Although pupillary abnormalities may be seen, a complete AR pupil is not characteristic. Neurosyphilis should still be considered in the differential diagnosis of advanced neurologic disease with generalized paresis, although this finding is rare in the United States.

Tabes dorsalis is a form of neurosyphilis, with involvement of the posterior columns and the posterior roots of the spinal cord, resulting in pain, ataxia, sensory changes, reduced tendon reflexes, and ocular findings. Severe stabbing pain in the lower extremities heralds this form of neurosyphilis. Unsteadiness and a wide-based gait develop later, followed by hyperesthesia and paresthesia. Incontinence and impotence are other common sequelae. Charcot arthropathy occurs in the large joints that are devoid of sensation and are prone to destructive changes. AR pupils are frequent in this form of neurosyphilis, and optic atrophy is commonly found.

Congenital syphilis. Congenital syphilis results from the transplacental transmission of *T. pallidum* from the mother to the fetus. Untreated primary or secondary syphilis is almost invariably transmitted to the fetus, whereas transmission in later stages of the disease occurs less frequently. Transmission to the fetus can occur at any time during the pregnancy, but fetal damage tends to occur after the fourth month when fetal immunologic competence starts. Congenital syphilis is preventable with proper treatment of the mother; therefore all expectant mothers should have a VDRL test at the beginning and near the end of pregnancy. In fact, serologic screening of women at the time pregnancy is first diagnosed and screening of all infants at the time of delivery is now mandatory in New York State.[5]

Signs and symptoms of early congenital syphilis may not appear until several days after birth, and Dorfman and Glaser[19] stated that the diagnosis of congenital syphilis may be missed if serologic tests are not performed for both the mother and her infant at the time of delivery. A generalized rash develops and resembles the rash of secondary syphilis, except that in the infant, the rash may be vesicular or bullous. Rhinitis (also called *snuffles*), jaundice, hepatosplenomegaly, anorexia, and pseudoparalysis may also be found. Osteochondritis and pathologic fractures are common, and radiographic changes on bone films are present in greater than 90% of patients. Chorioretinitis is often evident in the first few months of life.

Congenital syphilis may mimic other congenital infections, such as rubella, cytomegalovirus infection, and toxoplasmosis. A positive serologic test result for syphilis may be caused by passive transfer of antibody from the mother; therefore diagnosis of congenital syphilis is based on a positive FTA-ABS test result and a rising VDRL titer. Results of serologic tests performed in infants and their mothers may be negative at the time of delivery if syphilis is acquired toward the end of the pregnancy.

After 2 years, the child is described as having late congenital syphilis. Like syphilis in adults, late congenital syphilis may remain latent with few sequelae, although cardiovascular involvement does occur; and meningovascular syphilis with neurologic manifestations, including eighth cranial nerve deafness, is common. Acute syphilitic meningitis, generalized paresis, and tabes dorsalis are less common. Interstitial keratitis is the classic ophthalmic sign of congenital syphilis, occurring in 10% of patients.

Deformities of the permanent teeth occur after early syphilitic infection. The characteristic Hutchinson teeth are notched, thin, upper incisors with abnormal spacing. The term *Hutchinson triad* refers to the occurrence of Hutchinson teeth, interstitial keratitis, and deafness, but the occurrence of all three in the same patient is unusual. The bone lesions of

TABLE 11.1 Ocular Manifestations of Syphilis

Primary Syphilis
Chancres of the eyelid and conjunctiva
Secondary Syphilis
Blepharitis
Madarosis
Conjunctivitis
Dacryocystitis
Dacryoadenitis
Keratitis
Iris nodules
Iridocyclitis
Episcleritis
Scleritis
Chorioretinitis
Vitritis
Neuroretinitis
Disk edema
Exudative retinal detachment
Perivasculitis
Tertiary Syphilis
Gummas of the eyelids
Unilateral interstitial keratitis
Punctate stromal keratitis
Bilateral periostitis of the orbital bone
Episcleritis
Scleritis
Anterior and posterior uveitis
Chorioretinitis
Vasculitis
Venous and arterial occlusive disease
Exudative retinal detachment
Macular edema
Neuroretinitis
Vitritis
Pseudoretinitis pigmentosa
Chorioretinal neovascular membrane
Lens dislocation
Argyll Robertson pupil
Oculomotor palsies
Congenital Syphilis
Bilateral interstitial keratitis
Pigmentary retinitis
Glaucoma
Keratouveitis

early congenital syphilis tend to progress in late congenital syphilis, with the development of syphilitic arthritis. Finally, gummas may develop in the subcutaneous tissue and produce ulcerative skin lesions.

Ocular manifestations. Table 11.1 lists some of the more common eye manifestations of the different stages of syphilis. Ophthalmic manifestations of primary syphilis are limited to chancres of the eyelid and the conjunctiva. A primary syphilitic lesion in the lacrimal gland is extremely rare but has been reported.[20]

The eyelids are commonly involved in the rash of secondary syphilis, and blepharitis and loss of lashes and eyebrows are common. Conjunctivitis mimicking trachoma has also been seen in secondary syphilis, but dacryocystitis and dacryoadenitis are rare. Keratitis, iris nodules (Fig. 11.2), iridocyclitis, episcleritis, and scleritis have all been reported in secondary syphilis. Late in the secondary stage, vitritis and chorioretinitis may develop (Fig. 11.3A). Diffuse neuroretinitis may occur and is often localized to the peripapillary area.[21] This is followed by a pigmentary retinopathy similar in appearance to retinitis pigmentosa (see Fig. 11.3B). Disk edema, exudative retinal detachment, perivasculitis, and subretinal fibrosis can also occur (Figs. 11.4 and 11.5).[22-24]

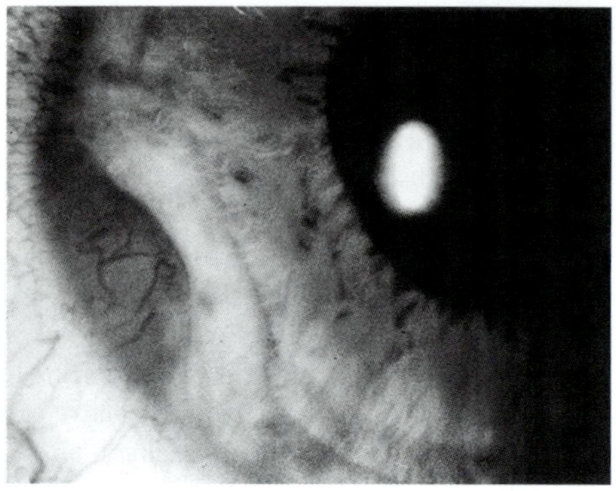

Fig. 11.2 Iris nodule caused by syphilis. (From Case records of the Massachusetts General Hospital. Weekly clinicopathological exercises. *N Engl J Med.* 1984;310:972–981.)

The gummas of tertiary syphilis can involve the eyelids and, if extensive, can cause destructive ulceration, but gummatous dacryoadenitis and infiltration of the lacrimal sac have only rarely been reported. Conjunctival vascular changes occur, but gummas of the conjunctiva almost never occur. As seen in secondary syphilis, syphilitic blepharitis with madarosis is common. Diffuse bilateral periostitis is the most common orbital finding of tertiary syphilis. Uniocular interstitial keratitis is the most common corneal finding in tertiary syphilis, but punctate stromal keratitis can occur with iritis. Episcleritis and scleritis occur, but discrete gummas of the sclera are rare. Uveitis is a common finding in late tertiary syphilis. Halperin et al.[25] stated that the main posterior segment complications of acquired syphilis include chorioretinitis, vasculitis, venous and arterial occlusive disease, retinal detachment with choroidal effusion, macular edema, neuroretinitis, optic neuritis, vitritis (see Fig. 11.3A), and pseudoretinitis pigmentosa (see Fig. 11.3B). Choroidal neovascular membranes and subretinal fibrosis (Fig. 11.6) can also occur. Posterior placoid chorioretinitis has been described in late latent syphilis.[26] Vitreous opacities are common, and lens dislocation has been reported in many patients.

The most typical manifestation of congenital syphilis is bilateral interstitial keratitis, which appears later in life. Pigmentary retinitis and glaucoma can also occur as a result of congenital syphilitic keratouveitis.

The AR pupil and disk edema are most commonly seen in meningovascular syphilis, along with oculomotor palsies and other pupillary abnormalities. Later in the course of meningovascular syphilis, optic atrophy occurs. A complete AR pupil is rare in cases of general paresis but, as with optic atrophy, is more common in cases of tabes dorsalis.

Diagnosis. The diagnosis of syphilis is based on the clinical history, physical examination, and laboratory test findings. Algorithms for testing patients suspected of having syphilis change frequently, so consultation with an infectious disease specialist can be useful in determining which tests to order, depending on the individual patient and the presumed stage of the disease. Although darkfield microscopy or immunofluorescent staining of mucocutaneous lesions can aid in the prompt diagnosis of primary, secondary, and early congenital syphilis, most physicians order serologic tests to make or confirm a

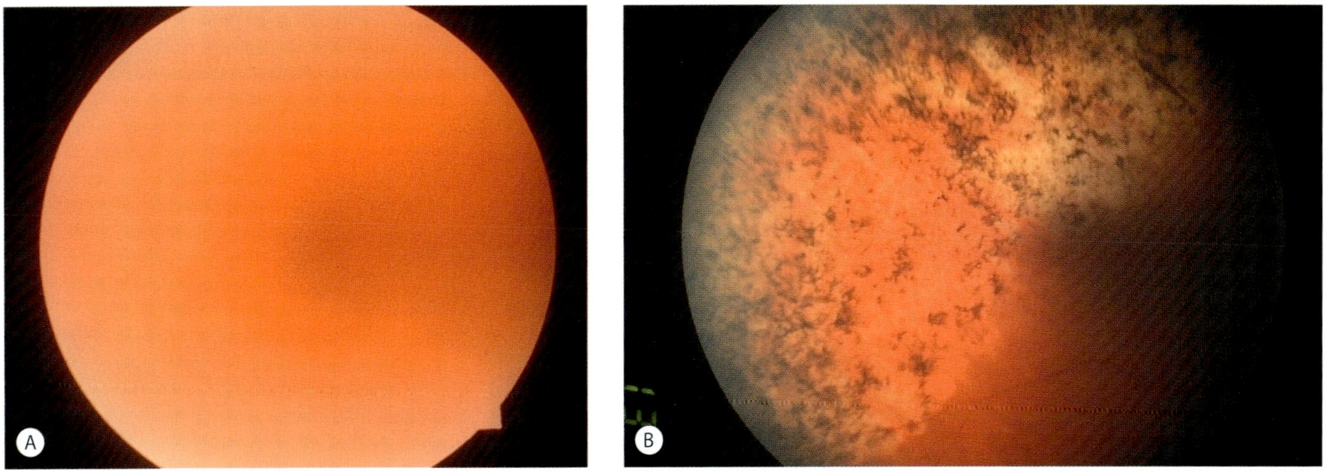

Fig. 11.3 Fundus photograph of a patient with uveitis associated with syphilis. (A) Dense vitritis obscuring the optic disc and retinal vasculature. (B) Same patient after treatment with intravenous penicillin. The vitritis and retinal infiltrates have resolved, revealing the pigmentary retinopathy characteristic of ocular syphilis.

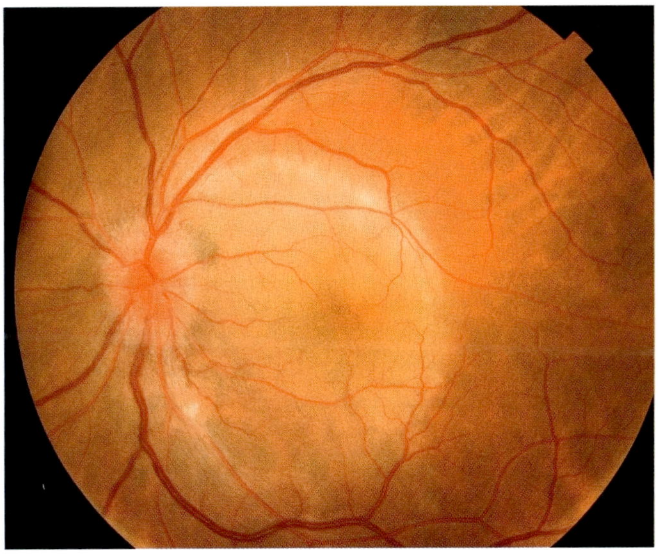

Fig. 11.4 Retinal photograph from a patient with syphilis showing disk edema and chorioretinitis involving the macula (Courtesy Rugens Belfort, Jr, MD)

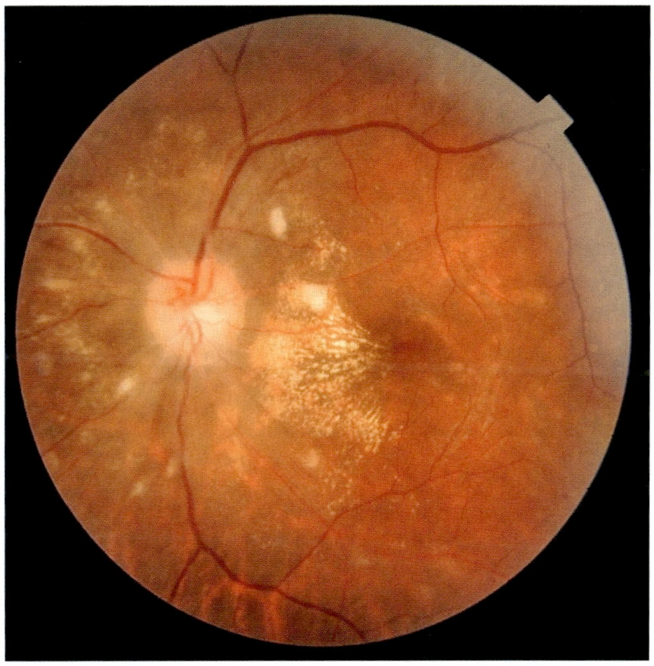

Fig. 11.5 Neuroretinitis characterized by edema of the optic disk and a macular star in a patient treated with cytotoxic agents diagnosed with syphilis (Courtesy Heloisa Nascimento, MD, PhD)

diagnosis. Darkfield microscopy can be used to identify spirochetes present in tissue fluids. *T. pallidum* is difficult to distinguish from other spirochetes, so darkfield examination requires expertise. Sensitive and specific polymerase chain reaction (PCR) tests for *T. pallidum* have been developed but are not commercially available. Serologic tests include both nontreponemal and treponemal tests. Both tests are reactive in persons with any treponemal infection, including syphilis, endemic syphilis, yaws, and pinta. Confusion often arises in determining whether a rapid plasma reagin (RPR) test or a VDRL test should be ordered, rather than an FTA-ABS test, and in the interpretation of the results. In this section, the various diagnostic tests for syphilis are explained, and a strategy for ordering tests is outlined (Box 11.2).

The two most commonly used screening tests for syphilis are the VDRL test and the RPR test. Both are nontreponemal reaginic tests. Infection with *T. pallidum* stimulates nonspecific antibodies against cardiolipin. The VDRL test quantitates these antibodies with the use of slide flocculation. The VDRL test is well standardized, and the result is reported as "reactive," "weakly reactive," "borderline," or "nonreactive." The rapid plasma reagin test is a similar assay for detecting anticardiolipin antibody. The RPR test is easier to perform than the VDRL test and is often used as a quick screening test; however, the VDRL test is more accurate for examining CSF.

The sensitivity and the specificity of the VDRL test vary, depending on the stage of disease (Table 11.2).[27,28] The VDRL test result becomes positive about 1 to 2 weeks after the appearance of the primary chancre and is positive in 99% of patients with secondary syphilis.[29] In the later stages of the disease, however, the VDRL test reactivity decreases, and only about 70% of patients with cardiovascular syphilis or neurosyphilis have a positive VDRL test result. In addition, the VDRL test often becomes nonreactive after treatment for syphilis.

Serologic tests for syphilis are not 100% specific, and false-positive results can occur, especially in patients with other spirochetal diseases

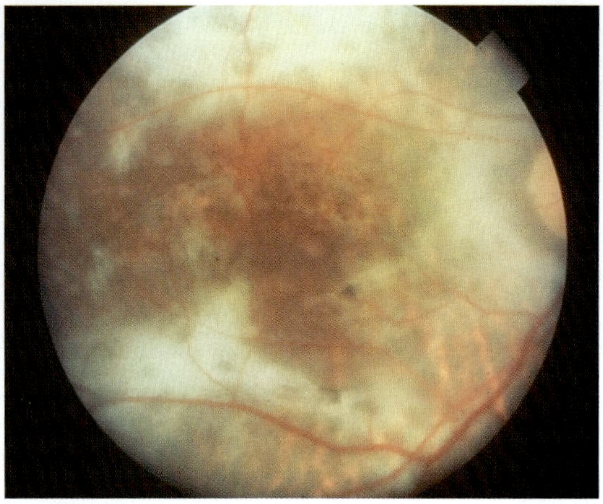

Fig. 11.6 Extensive subretinal fibrosis caused by ocular syphilis (Courtesy Rubens Belfort, Jr, MD)

BOX 11.2 Diagnosis of Syphilis: Key Points

- Diagnosis is based on clinical history, physical examination, and laboratory tests.
- There are both nontreponemal and treponemal tests for syphilis.
- Nontreponemal tests are often used to screen for syphilis. The two most common screening tests are the Venereal Disease Research Laboratory (VDRL) test and the rapid plasma reagin (RPR) test.
- Treponemal tests are more sensitive in diagnosing patients with latent or late syphilis and more specific than the VDRL test. The most commonly used treponemal test is the fluorescent treponemal antibody absorption (FTA-ABS) test.

TABLE 11.2 Sensitivity and Specificity of the VDRL and FTA-ABS tests

	SENSITIVITY BY STAGE OF SYPHILIS, % (RANGE)				
Test	**Primary**	**Secondary**	**Latent**	**Tertiary**	**Specificity of Test, % (range)**
VDRL	78 (74-87)	100	96 (88-100)	71 (37-94)	98 (96-99)
FTA-ABS	84 (70-100)	100	100	96	97 (84-100)

VDRL, Venereal Disease Research Laboratory; *FTA-ABS,* fluorescent treponemal antibody absorption.

and connective tissue diseases (Table 11.3). Any VDRL test result that is given as "weakly reactive"" or "reactive" needs to be confirmed with a more specific test. The tests used for this purpose are the treponemal tests for syphilis, such as the *T. pallidum* agglutination tests (*Treponema pallidum* hemagglutination assay [TPHA] and microhemagglutination assay with *Treponema pallidum* antigen [MHA-TP]) or the more commonly used FTA-ABS test. The *T. pallidum* immobilization test is almost completely specific for syphilis but is expensive and difficult to perform and therefore rarely used. The MHA-TP assay for antibodies to *T. pallidum* is another specific test for syphilis but is also used less frequently than the FTA-ABS test. In the FTA-ABS test, the patient's serum is absorbed with extracts of nonpathogenic treponemes to remove possible cross-reacting antitreponemal antibody that is not specific for *T. pallidum*. The absorbed serum is then made to react against *T. pallidum,* and specific antibodies are detected by the addition of fluorescein-labeled antihuman gammaglobulin. Results are

TABLE 11.3 Causes of False-Positive Serologic Test Results for Syphilis

Spirochetal Infections
Endemic syphilis (bejel)
Yaws and pinta
Leptospirosis
Lyme disease
Relapsing fever

Other Infections
Chancroid
Chickenpox
Hepatitis
Human immunodeficiency virus (HIV) infection
Infectious mononucleosis
Leprosy
Lymphogranuloma venereum
Malaria
Measles
Mycoplasma pneumonia
Pneumococcal pneumonia
Rickettsial disease
Scarlet fever
Subacute bacterial endocarditis
Tuberculosis
Trypanosomiasis

Noninfectious Causes
Blood transfusions
Chronic liver disease
Connective tissue disease
Narcotic addiction
Pregnancy
Vaccination

reported as "nonreactive" or as "1+ to 4+ positive," based on the intensity of the fluorescence.

An FTA-ABS test result reported as weakly reactive may not be reproducible. The FTA-ABS test is more sensitive than the VDRL test at all stages of syphilis, but it is more expensive and difficult to perform. The FTA-ABS test is also not entirely specific for syphilis, because false-positive results are seen in patients with systemic lupus erythematosus, biliary cirrhosis, and some connective tissue diseases, such as rheumatoid arthritis (see Table 11.3).

Because serologic tests for syphilis may take several weeks to see a reactive result, immediate diagnosis requires demonstration of treponemes in tissue fluid by darkfield microscopy. The VDRL test is an excellent screening test for patients with later primary syphilis and secondary syphilis. The sensitivity of the VDRL test is approximately 100% for patients with secondary syphilis. Because the sensitivity of the VDRL test may be only 70% in patients with tertiary syphilis, an FTA-ABS test should be ordered if a later stage of disease is suspected. From the ophthalmic standpoint, many patients with uveitis or disk edema are suspected of having late syphilis, and many uveitis specialists and neuro-ophthalmologists routinely order both VDRL and FTA-ABS tests in the evaluation of these patients. As stated earlier, in the United States, testing for syphilis has consisted of initial screening with an inexpensive nontreponemal test, with subsequent testing of reactive specimens with a treponemal test. Some clinical laboratories have started using automated treponemal tests and then retest

TABLE 11.4 Treatment of Syphilis

Primary, Secondary, and Early Latent Syphilis in Adults
Benzathine penicillin G, 2.4 million units intramuscularly (IM) in a single dose.
If penicillin allergies exist, treat with doxycycline, 100 mg orally (PO) two times daily × 2 weeks or tetracycline 500 mg PO four times daily for 2 weeks.
Latent and Tertiary Syphilis or Syphilis of Unknown Duration
Benzathine penicillin G, 7.2 million units total, administered as three doses of 2.4 million units IM each at 1-week intervals.
Neurosyphilis and Ocular Syphilis in Adults
Aqueous crystalline penicillin G 18–24 million units per day, administered as 3–4 million units intravenously (IV) every 4 hours or continuous infusion for 10–14 days.
Congenital Syphilis in Infants and Children
Early Latent Syphilis
Benzathine penicillin G, 50,000 units/kg IM, up to the adult dose of 2.4 million units in a single dose.
Late Latent Syphilis
Benzathine penicillin G, 50,000 units/kg IM, up to the adult dose of 2.4 million units, administered as three doses at 1-week intervals (total 150,000 units/kg up to the adult total dose of 7.2 million units).

reactive results with a nontreponemal test.[30] It is not clear what the recommendations are for patients who test positive with the treponemal test and then negative for the nontreponemal test. If not previously treated, these patients should probably be treated for late latent syphilis. Because the price of the FTA-ABS test has decreased and the speed of testing has improved, the FTA-ABS is being used as the initial screening test for syphilis, especially where there is a strong suspicion for the disease.[31]

In addition, all patients who may have had syphilis for more than a year should undergo lumbar puncture for CSF examination. Cell count, differential count, protein determination, and the VDRL test should be performed on CSF samples to look for evidence of neurosyphilis. As stated previously, CNS invasion by *T. pallidum* may be common in early syphilis.[16] The finding of CNS involvement is important because the recommended therapy is different from that for patients without CNS involvement. Serologic tests for neurosyphilis can also be confusing. The CSF-VDRL test is insensitive but highly specific. CSF serologic diagnosis is usually based on the production of local antitreponemal antibodies, and an intrathecal *T. pallidum* antibody index can be calculated.

Infants born with congenital syphilis have positive VDRL and FTA-ABS test results from the passive transfer of immunoglobulin G (IgG) antibodies across the placenta; therefore an immunoglobulin M (IgM) FTA-ABS test is used to diagnose congenital syphilis because IgM antibodies do not cross the placenta, and a positive test result would indicate actual infection in the infant.[32]

Patients with undiagnosed interstitial keratitis should be suspected of having late congenital syphilis. A thorough history of previous therapy should be elicited, and patients should then undergo VDRL and FTA-ABS tests and CSF examination. If the CSF-VDRL test result is positive, some experts recommend that the patient be treated as for latent syphilis (Table 11.4). Patients with a positive serum VDRL or FTA-ABS result but negative CSF findings are treated as for primary or secondary syphilis.

Although not commercially available, newer diagnostic techniques have been used to diagnose syphilis in patients with ocular manifestations of syphilis. PCR analysis may be used to detect *T. pallidum* in ocular specimens, such as aqueous humor, when available in the research setting. Finally, because individuals at the highest risk for syphilis are also at risk for HIV infection, tests for both infections should be ordered. Serologic testing after treatment is important for every patient with syphilis to ensure adequate treatment of the disease.

Prognosis. Most patients recover without long-term sequelae if syphilis is recognized and treated early. If untreated, about 25% of these patients have one or more relapses with mucocutaneous lesions. Eventually, most untreated patients remain in a latent stage of the disease; however, about one-third go on to experience tertiary syphilis. Benign tertiary syphilis occurs in about 15% of untreated patients. Cardiovascular syphilis occurs in 10% of these, and CNS involvement is seen in about 8% of untreated patients.

Treatment

General recommendations. Although there are guidelines for the treatment of syphilis, controversy persists. Before treating a patient with syphilis, one should refer to the most current recommendations for therapy, and consultation with an infectious disease specialist may be helpful. Coinfection with HIV should be ruled out because standard therapy may be insufficient to eradicate disease in these patients. Recommendations for therapy are based on the stage of disease and are presented in Table 11.4.[29] Benzathine penicillin remains the treatment of choice, except in patients with a penicillin allergy. Riedner et al. evaluated the efficacy of treating primary or latent syphilis with a single oral dose of 2 g azithromycin or a single intramuscular dose of 2.4 million units of penicillin G benzathine.[33] Cure rates were 97.7% for patients in the azithromycin group and 95% in the penicillin G benzathine group, achieving the prescribed criteria for equivalence. Parenteral penicillin G is the only therapy with documented efficacy for syphilis during pregnancy.

Unfortunately, the ideal therapy for patients with uveitic syphilis has not been studied in well-controlled clinical trials. Virulent *T. pallidum* infection has been reported to persist in the eye despite treatment with many penicillin regimens; therefore many experts suggest that patients with any ocular inflammation secondary to syphilis be treated as for neurosyphilis, even if the CSF findings are normal.[29]

In addition to treating the patient, the physician has the responsibility to report the disease to the local health department to ensure that all sexual contacts over at least the past 3 months are contacted, examined, and treated, as necessary.

Patients with syphilis should have the VDRL test repeated at 3, 6, and 12 months after treatment because titers should become nonreactive within a year after successful therapy. In addition, patients with CSF involvement should have repeated CSF examinations at 6-month intervals for at least 3 years. Patients should be treated again if clinical evidence of syphilis occurs, if a previously nonreactive VDRL test result again becomes reactive, or if an initially high-titer VDRL test result does not decrease fourfold within a year.

Finally, patients receiving therapy for syphilis, especially intravenous therapy, should be monitored for a Jarisch-Herxheimer reaction. This is a hypersensitivity response to treponemal antigens. The reaction may exacerbate preexisting ocular inflammation, such as uveitis and interstitial keratitis; prophylaxis with corticosteroids may help in some cases.

Approach to syphilis in patients with AIDS. Recognition of concurrent infection with HIV in patients with syphilis is important to the clinician because the diagnostic and therapeutic approach to syphilis may differ in these patients. Numerous reports suggest that uncharacteristic clinical manifestations of syphilis may occur in patients with concomitant HIV infection.[34,35] Unusual cases of ocular syphilis in HIV-infected patients with findings of panuveitis and retinal detachment have been reported, and some authors have stated that the incidence of ocular complications of syphilis may be increased in patients with HIV infection.[36-38] In addition, acute retinal necrosis and acute retinitis have been associated with syphilis in patients coinfected with HIV.[23,36] Despite some unique symptoms and signs, these patients usually also experience the characteristic clinical manifestations of syphilis. Patients with both HIV infection and syphilis may have an accelerated course, with a greater likelihood of uveitis and progression to neurosyphilis.[34,37,39] In the study by Berry et al.,[6] there was no difference in the detection of *T. pallidum* in CSF in patients with or without concurrent HIV infection; nevertheless, it appears that treatment failures are more common in patients with HIV.[6,40,41] In addition, serologic evidence of syphilis may be delayed. Hicks et al.[42] reported on a patient with AIDS and skin manifestations consistent with secondary syphilis in whom the VDRL and FTA-ABS results were negative on two separate occasions. A skin biopsy demonstrated spirochetes with Warthin-Starry staining of the tissue, and the patient's VDRL and FTA-ABS test results later became positive, suggesting a delayed immunologic response.

Although patients with HIV infection and syphilis have more symptoms of CNS involvement, such as acute syphilitic meningitis and hearing loss, many of them do not have positive CSF-VDRL test results, and only CSF leukocytosis or elevated CSF protein concentration, findings that are seen in patients with HIV but without syphilis, may manifest.[43] These findings have prompted some clinicians to treat all patients with concurrent HIV infection and syphilis with high-dose antibiotic therapy to cover the possibility of CNS involvement. The CDC is currently studying the question of appropriate antibiotic therapy for patients with syphilis and concurrent HIV infection. For now, recommendations include careful evaluation of all patients with syphilis for underlying HIV infection. Patients with AIDS should also be monitored for clinical signs of syphilis, and confirmation of the diagnosis should be pursued despite negative serologic results early in the course of the disease.

Patients with syphilis and HIV infection should undergo lumbar puncture to identify evidence of neurosyphilis. Because treatment failures are common, some infectious disease consultants suggest that all patients be treated with a regimen adequate for neurosyphilis. After treatment, undergoing a VDRL test is suggested every month for at least 3 months, with close observation for evidence of recurrence.[44]

Nonvenereal Treponematoses

Endemic syphilis, yaws, and pinta are three nonvenereal treponemal infections that are spread by body contact and are endemic in certain geographic areas. Like syphilis, these diseases can have severe late manifestations years after the initial infection.

Endemic Syphilis

Etiology and epidemiology. Endemic syphilis, also known as *bejel,* is caused by T. pallidum subspecies endemicum a spirochete that is morphologically and serologically indistinguishable from the *T. pallidum* that causes syphilis. Endemic syphilis is found in many arid countries, mostly in the Middle East and Africa.[45]

Clinical manifestations. The onset of endemic syphilis usually occurs in childhood and typically presents with a mucous patch on the buccal mucosa. Mucosal lesions are followed by papulosquamous and erosive papular lesions of the trunk and extremities. Latency can occur if the early stages of the disease are not treated. Periostitis of the bones of the legs and gummatous lesions of the nose and soft palate are seen in later stages. Neurologic and cardiovascular involvement and congenital transmission of endemic syphilis are uncharacteristic. Similarly, chancres, which are typical of primary syphilis, are not found as early signs of endemic syphilis.

TABLE 11.5 Ocular Manifestations of Endemic Syphilis

Anterior uveitis
Iris atrophy
Cataract
Vitreous opacity
Optic atrophy
Choroiditis
Chorioretinitis
Attenuated retinal arterioles
Patchy choroidal atrophy

Ocular manifestations. Although neurologic involvement is uncharacteristic of endemic syphilis, ocular manifestations have been reported. Tabbara et al.[46] studied 17 patients who had clinical and serologic findings that were consistent with endemic syphilis and also had ocular complaints. Ocular findings included uveitis in nine patients, optic atrophy in six, and chorioretinal scars in six. Additional findings are presented in Table 11.5.

Diagnosis. Serologic tests do not distinguish endemic syphilis from venereal syphilis. The same serologic tests that are used to diagnose venereal syphilis are used to diagnose nonvenereal treponematoses. Both the VDRL and FTA-ABS results are typically positive in endemic syphilis, and spirochetes can be isolated from skin lesions. Differentiation of venereal and nonvenereal syphilis is therefore made on clinical grounds.

Prognosis. Most patients with endemic syphilis respond well to antibiotic therapy. The prognosis of untreated endemic syphilis is unknown. Patients can experience neurologic or cardiovascular sequelae late in the course of their disease; however, symptoms are usually mild in comparison with those of tertiary syphilis.

Treatment. The current WHO-recommended therapy for patients with endemic treponematoses is either a single dose of azithromycin (30 mg/kg, up to a maximum of 2 g) or benzathine penicillin G (1.2 million units intramuscularly for adults or 600,000 units intramuscularly for children younger than 10 years of age). Treatment of all household members and other close personal contacts is recommended. After treatment, most patients become seronegative, and they should be monitored for this development.

Yaws and Pinta

Yaws, also called *frambesia,* is a nonvenereal treponematosis that is endemic in humid countries near the equator.[47] After an incubation period of 3 to 4 weeks, the first manifestation of the disease is a skin papule, often on the lower extremities. The lesion enlarges, ulcerates, and becomes encrusted, often with regional lymphadenitis. A secondary, generalized rash occurs as the initial lesion heals. Soft granulomas then erupt on the face, legs, and buttocks, often at mucocutaneous junctions. Hyperkeratotic lesions also develop and may occur on the soles of the feet. Later in the course of the disease, periostitis, exostoses of the maxillary bone, juxta-articular nodules, and gummatous skin lesions may appear.

Pinta is the third nonvenereal treponematosis and is endemic among the Native Americans of Mexico, Central America, and South America. Similar to yaws, pinta begins as a small papule at the inoculation site, with regional lymphadenitis followed by a generalized maculopapular eruption. One to several years after healing of the initial skin lesion, large blue or brown macules are found over the extremities, face, and neck. They later become depigmented and may be misdiagnosed as vitiligo. Again, as in yaws, hyperkeratotic lesions are found on the soles of the feet.

Ocular manifestations. Smith et al.[48] headed a cooperative study to determine whether neuro-ophthalmic involvement occurs in late yaws or pinta. A group of 71 patients with late yaws, 11 with late pinta, and 41 matched, positive, and negative control subjects were examined. Ocular and neurologic abnormalities were not found in patients with late pinta, although one had a bilateral interstitial keratitis. Nevertheless, several patients with late yaws had neuro-ophthalmic abnormalities, including light-near dissociation of the pupillary response, perivascular pigmentation, sheathing of the retinal vessels, and moderate optic atrophy. CNS involvement in yaws is also supported by the isolation of treponemes from the aqueous humor and by CSF abnormalities in 24.9% of 902 patients.[49]

Diagnosis. As in endemic syphilis, spirochetes may be isolated from skin lesions at the site of inoculation. Two weeks after inoculation, both the VDRL and FTA-ABS test results are positive, and the diagnosis of yaws and pinta is based on clinical findings in the setting of positive syphilis serologic findings.

Prognosis. Yaws may undergo spontaneous clinical and serologic resolution at any stage of the disease without therapy; however, antibiotic treatment improves the cure rate. Untreated patients may experience periarticular ulcers causing crippling contractures and osteomyelitis. Patients with untreated pinta experience depigmented patches of the skin, which may lead to social ostracization, which is the major consequence of pinta.

Treatment. Azithromycin or benzathine penicillin G can be used to treat yaws and pinta with the same treatment regimen recommended for endemic syphilis. The treatment recommendations are provided in the section on endemic syphilis. The WHO has undertaken a concerted effort to eradicate yaws. A longitudinal comparative cohort study showed that a single dose of azithromycin was effective in achieving serologic cure in 92% of participants with latent yaws and 94% of participants with active yaws.[50] For long-term success of disease eradication, careful follow-up is necessary to detect treatment failures and to identify individuals who did not receive treatment.[51]

Borrelia Infection

Lyme Disease

Etiology and epidemiology. In the spring and summer of 1975, a group of children living in Lyme, Connecticut, presented with an inflammatory arthropathy similar to that in juvenile rheumatoid arthritis.[52] A characteristic rash was associated with the illness, as were neurologic and cardiac abnormalities. In 1977, Steere et al.[52] labeled this illness Lyme disease. Epidemiologic studies implicated ticks as the vector for the disease, but the etiologic agent remained elusive.

Similar rashes called *erythema migrans* or *erythema chronicum migrans* had been associated with tick bites and systemic disease in Europe, and spirochete-like structures had been found in skin specimens from several patients.[53] In the United States, evidence was accumulating that patients with Lyme disease who were treated with penicillin fared better compared with untreated patients. A tick-borne organism was suspected as the causative agent, and in 1982, Burgdorfer et al.[54] found spirochetes in *Ixodes dammini* ticks while looking for the cause of Rocky Mountain spotted fever in their Montana laboratory. Spirochetes were later isolated from patients with Lyme disease in the United States and from patients in Europe with erythema migrans and Bannwarth syndrome (a chronic lymphocytic meningitis associated with erythema chronicum migrans).[55] The previously unrecognized spirochete was isolated by Burgdorfer and Barbour[56] and was named *Borrelia burgdorferi.* Today, over 20 related borrelial species are referred to as *B. burgdorferi sensu lato,* meaning "*B. burgdorferi* in the general sense."

Along with *Leptospira* and *Treponema, Borrelia* belongs to the eubacterial phylum of spirochetes.[57] These organisms are usually more

BOX 11.3 Lyme Disease: Key Features

- Caused by the spirochete *Borrelia burgdorferi*
- Transmitted by the *Ixodes dammini* tick
- Disease divided into stages: early infection divided into stage 1 (local) and stage 2 (disseminated); late infection categorized as stage 3 (persistent)
- After infection, the spirochete spreads locally in the skin in 60% to 80% of patients, causing the characteristic erythema migrans rash
- Conjunctivitis is the most common ocular finding in early Lyme disease

loosely coiled than other spirochetes, but if coiled, they have a corkscrew appearance and look exactly like *T. pallidum. Borrelia* species are easy to isolate from infected ticks but difficult to isolate from infected patients. *B. burgdorferi* is transmitted by certain *Ixodes* ticks. In the United States, the preferred host for the larval and nymphal forms of the tick is the white-footed mouse,[58] whereas the preferred host for the adult form of the tick is the white-tailed deer.[59] The ticks have now been found on at least 30 species of animals and 49 species of birds.[60] Lyme disease also occurs in domestic animals, including cats, dogs, and horses. *Ixodes* ticks are "multitalented" and transmit babesiosis and tularemia in addition to Lyme disease.

From 1980 to 1988, 13,795 cases of Lyme disease were reported in the United States.[61] During 1992–2006, a total of 248,074 cases of Lyme disease were reported in the 50 states, the District of Columbia, and U.S. territories.[62] The annual count increased 101% from 9908 cases in 1992 to 19,931 cases in 2006. Most of the cases were reported from 10 states (Connecticut, Delaware, Massachusetts, Maryland, Minnesota, New Jersey, New York, Pennsylvania, Rhode Island, and Wisconsin).[62] Lyme disease is thought to be the most common vector-borne infection in the United States, and it has been reported throughout the world, especially North America, Europe, and Asia. The rapid spread of the disease has been attributed to an increase in forested areas that house the tick-infested deer and to the migration of susceptible humans into these areas. For example, during a 7-year period, 35% of 190 residents living adjacent to a nature preserve in Ipswich, Massachusetts, acquired Lyme disease.[63] Lyme disease is currently the most common vector-borne infection in the United States and in Europe. The number of cases continues to grow as awareness of the disease by both physicians and patients increases and diagnostic tests are more commonly employed. The CDC has stated that the number of reported cases of tick-borne disease has more than doubled over the past 13 years,[64,65] and Lyme disease accounts for a majority of this.

Clinical manifestations. Lyme disease is usually described as occurring in stages (Box 11.3). Early infection is divided into stage 1 (local) and stage 2 (disseminated). Late infection is categorized as stage 3 (persistent). After infection, the spirochete spreads locally in the skin in 60% to 80% of patients and causes the characteristic rash, erythema migrans,[60,66] which is an oval or anular erythematous lesion with expanding borders that usually fades within 3 to 4 weeks in untreated patients but may recur later in the disease (Fig. 11.7). Patients recall being bitten by a tick about half of the time. Specific antibody to *B. burgdorferi* is often lacking at this stage of the disease, during which patients may have minor flu-like constitutional symptoms and regional lymphadenopathy. The most common ocular finding in early Lyme disease is conjunctivitis.[66]

Stage 2 disease occurs within days to weeks after infection, during which time the spirochete can spread to many organs via blood, causing a multitude of signs and symptoms. These systemic manifestations are mainly characterized by cardiac and neurologic involvement, although patients may experience secondary anular skin lesions. Neurologically, patients have severe headache and mild stiffness of the neck. CSF is

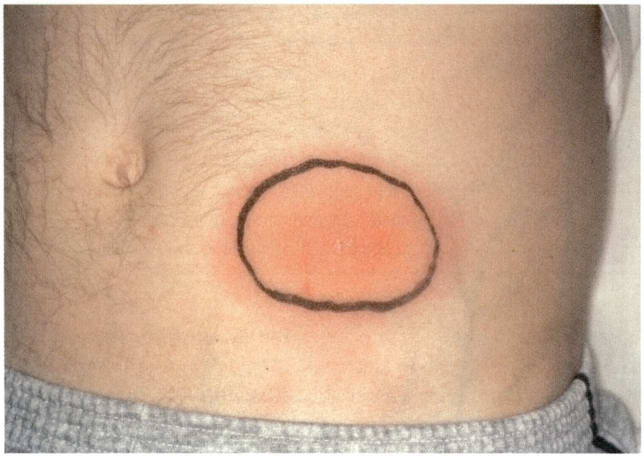

Fig. 11.7 Characteristic lesions of erythema migrans associated with Lyme disease.

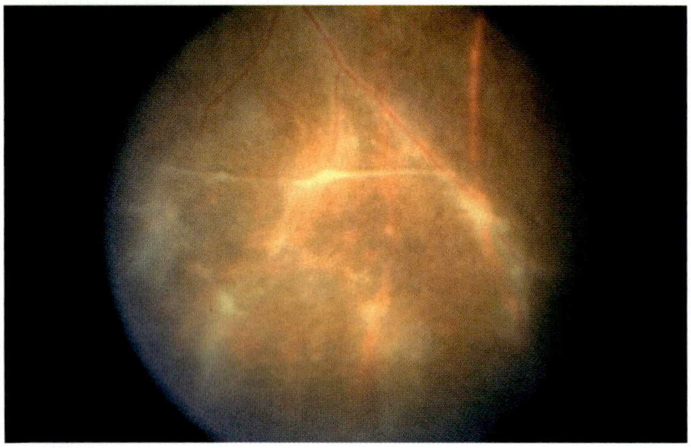

Fig. 11.8 Retinal vasculitis in a patient with ocular Lyme disease. Sheathing of peripheral retinal vessels and mild vitritis are seen in this patient on this fluorescein angiogram. The patient also had scleritis. The ocular findings resolved after treatment with intravenous ceftriaxone.

normal early on in the disease but later reveals a lymphocytic pleocytosis with a cell count in the range of 100/mm^3, elevated protein concentration, and normal glucose concentration.[67] Peripheral neuropathies, intermittent arthralgia, and musculoskeletal pain are common, and unilateral and bilateral Bell palsy is the most common cranial neuropathy.[68]

About 4% to 8% of patients have cardiac involvement, with fluctuating atrioventricular block.[69] Fewer patients have been reported with acute myopericarditis. About 6 months after infection, patients may acquire oligoarticular arthritis, with a white blood cell (WBC) count of 500 to 110,000/mm^3 in joint fluid. Other manifestations of stage 2 Lyme disease include hepatitis, nonproductive cough, microscopic hematuria or proteinuria, and orchitis.[60] The ocular findings most commonly reported in stage 2 disease are conjunctivitis and uveitis.

Stage 3 infection is characterized by prolonged episodes of arthritis. Chronic neurologic manifestations include ataxia, chronic encephalomyelitis, spastic paraparesis, and dementia. Patients often have chronic fatigue, and erythema migrans can occur late in the disease. Bilateral keratitis is described as a characteristic finding in late infection.[68-72]

Transplacental transmission of *B. burgdorferi* has been reported in two infants whose mothers had Lyme disease in the first trimester of pregnancy,[73-75] although a study of 463 infants from endemic or nonendemic areas showed no association between congenital malformations and the presence of detectable antibody to *B. burgdorferi* in cord blood.[76]

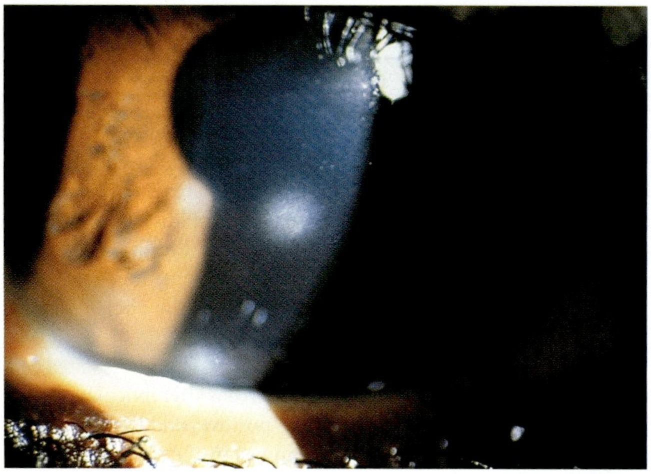

Fig. 11.9 Multiple intrastromal lesions of Lyme keratitis (Courtesy Ernest Kornmehl, MD. From Albert D, Miller J, Azar D, Blodi B, eds. *Albert & Jacobiec's Principles and Practices of Ophthalmology.* St. Louis: Elsevier. Copyright Elsevier.)

Ocular manifestations. In initial reports, the only consistently reported ocular finding in Lyme disease was transient conjunctivitis, occurring in 11% of patients with stage 1 disease.[66] Other ocular findings reported in the early stages of disease include episcleritis, iridocyclitis with posterior synechiae, and retinal vasculitis (Fig. 11.8).[77,78] Steere et al.[79] reported on a case of a 45-year-old woman who, 4 weeks after the onset of erythema migrans, experienced unilateral iritis, followed by panophthalmitis; spirochetes were found in specimens of vitreous debris obtained at surgery.

In March 1987, Bertuch et al.[70] reported on three patients with ocular findings of Lyme disease. The first patient presented with bilateral Bell palsy and late-occurring optic neuritis. The other two patients experienced patchy intrastromal infiltrates of the cornea from the Bowman layer to the Descemet membrane. These corneal infiltrates caused reduced vision but no pain, and occurred late in the course of disease. Dramatic resolution of the keratitis occurred after treatment with topical corticosteroids, suggesting an immune mechanism rather than a direct infection with the spirochete. Baum et al.[71] reported three patients who acquired bilateral keratitis long after Lyme disease was diagnosed and treated and also noted the effectiveness of topical corticosteroid therapy. Since then, several other reports have documented keratitis late in the course of Lyme disease (Fig. 11.9).[72,77,78,80-83]

Less common ocular findings associated with Lyme disease have also been reported in single case reports. Bialasiewicz et al.[84] described a patient with meningeal symptoms and diffuse choroiditis, cystoid macular edema, and exudative retinal detachments initially misdiagnosed as Vogt-Koyanagi-Harada (VKH) syndrome. Immunofluorescence results for Lyme disease were positive, and the patient improved markedly after treatment with doxycycline. Koch et al.[85] reported retinal pigment epithelial detachments in a man with neuroborreliosis. Scholes and Teske[86] tested 19 patients with intermediate uveitis for Lyme disease, and seven of 19 patients had positive antibody titers, suggesting a possible association between Lyme disease and pars planitis. Copeland et al.[87] reported on two patients with intermediate uveitis that was only partially responsive to steroids; these patients were later diagnosed with Lyme disease after positive Lyme titers were obtained. The uveitis in both patients cleared rapidly with systemic antibiotic treatment. In a report by Winward et al.,[88] patients with intermediate uveitis associated with Lyme disease demonstrated more significant anterior segment inflammation. Subsequent studies confirmed the

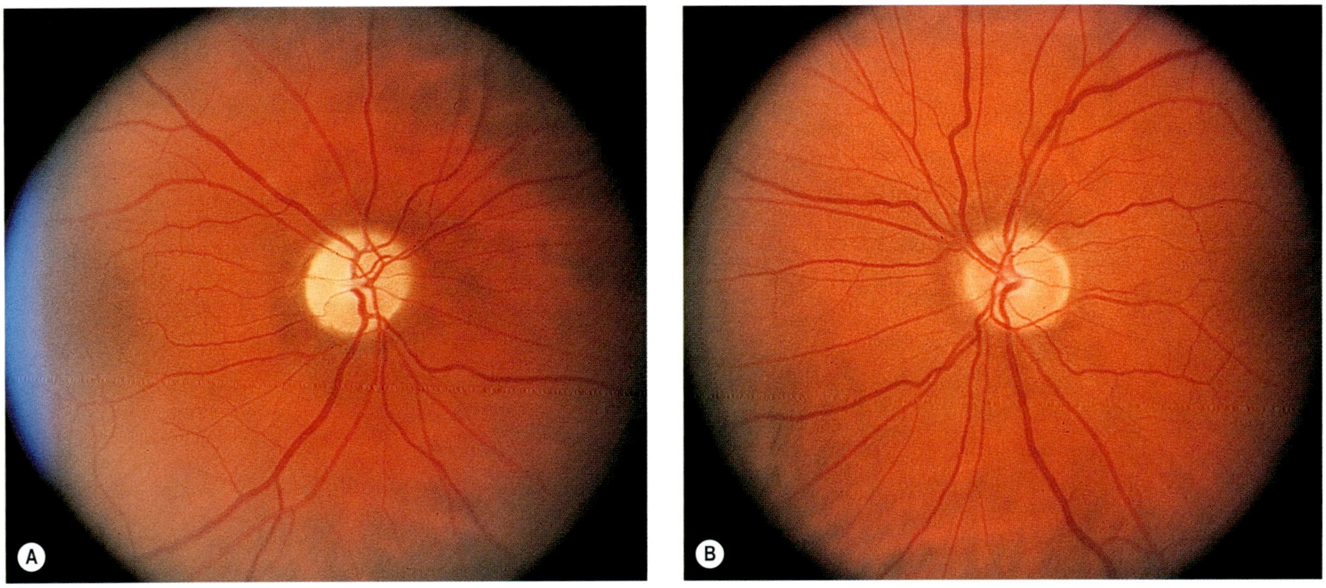

Fig. 11.10 Right (A) and left (B) optic nerves demonstrating pallor after resolution of optic neuritis associated with Lyme disease (Courtesy Ernest Kornmehl, MD. From Albert D, Miller J, Azar D, Blodi B, eds. *Albert & Jacobiec's Principles and Practices of Ophthalmology*. St. Louis: Elsevier. Copyright Elsevier.)

TABLE 11.6 **Ocular Manifestations of Lyme Disease**
Early Infection
Conjunctivitis
Episcleritis
Posterior scleritis
Iridocyclitis
Retinal vasculitis
Optic disk edema
Panophthalmitis
Choroiditis
Pars planitis
Exudative retinal detachment
Retinal pigment epithelial detachment
Exposure keratitis
Diplopia
Cortical blindness
Orbital myositis
Late Infection
Keratitis
Episcleritis

presence of significant posterior segment inflammation, especially vitritis and retinal vasculitis, in some cases of Lyme disease.[82,83,89,90]

Neuro-ophthalmic findings in Lyme disease are common.[53,91] Involvement of the CNS by Lyme disease causes cranial nerve palsies. Unilateral and bilateral Bell palsies are the most common cranial nerve palsies and often result in exposure keratitis. Diplopia caused by sixth, fourth, and third cranial nerve palsies can occur. Wu et al.[92] described a 7-year-old child who had bilateral disk edema in association with Lyme disease. A similar patient was described by Jacobson and Frens[93]; the patient was diagnosed with pseudotumor cerebri syndrome associated with Lyme disease. Optic disk edema may be the sole presenting sign of Lyme disease.[94] Other reported neuro-ophthalmic manifestations of Lyme disease include optic neuritis (Fig. 11.10), cortical blindness, and orbital myositis.[95-98] The association of some of these ocular findings with Lyme disease stems from one or two case reports, in which the diagnosis of Lyme disease was based predominantly on positive serologic findings. Because serologic results for Lyme disease may be falsely positive, some of the cases may have been wrongly diagnosed.[99] A list of the ophthalmic manifestations associated with Lyme disease is presented in Table 11.6.

Diagnosis. Techniques for the diagnosis of Lyme disease are not ideal. A patient with a history of a tick bite who later experiences erythema migrans most surely has Lyme disease; however, a tick bite is recalled in only about 50% of cases, and a pathognomonic rash may be overlooked or may not occur in a significant number of patients. Erythema migrans is the only clinical sign of clear diagnostic value; however, earlobe lymphocytoma, meningoradiculoneuritis (Garin-Bujadoux-Bannwarth syndrome), and acrodermatitis chronica atrophicans may be of some diagnostic value.[100] The spirochete can be cultured in Barbour-Stoenner-Kelly (BSK) medium, but because of the difficulty in culturing *B. burgdorferi* from patients, laboratory diagnosis is made on the basis of serologic findings. Most patients have elevated antibody titers to *B. burgdorferi* several weeks after infection. Both immunofluorescent assay and enzyme-linked immunosorbent assay (ELISA) are used in the diagnosis of Lyme disease, although ELISA is more sensitive in all stages of the disease. Unfortunately, serologic testing has not been standardized, and interlaboratory variability is significant, although the situation is improving.[101-103] The sensitivity of ELISA for Lyme disease in several laboratories approaches 90% after the first few weeks of infection. Many laboratories confirm positive ELISA results with Western blot assay. Nevertheless, the clinician must be aware of false-negative and false-positive results. False-negative results occur during the first few weeks of infection, when antibody titers may be low and may be missed by serologic tests of lower sensitivities. Early antibiotic therapy may also cause false-negative test results, and cases of seronegative Lyme disease have been reported.[104]

False-positive results may also occur as a result of cross-reaction between *B. burgdorferi* and other spirochetes, such as *T. pallidum*. Cross-reactivity between the Lyme immunofluorescence assay test and the FTA-ABS test has been reported in 11% to 54% of patients.[105-107] In a study by Hunter et al.[108]; 22% of patients with Lyme disease had

TABLE 11.7 Treatment of Lyme Disease

Early Infection
Adults
Doxycycline 100 mg orally (PO) two times daily × 10–21 days
OR Cefuroxime axetil 500 mg PO bid × 14–21 days
OR Amoxicillin 500 mg PO three times daily × 14–21 days
Children
Amoxicillin 50 mg/kg/day divided into three doses (maximum 500 mg/dose) × 14–21 days
OR Doxycycline 4 mg/kg PO two times daily × 10–21 days OR Cefuroxime 30 mg/kg PO two times daily × 14–21 days
Severe Uveitis or Neurologic Abnormalities or Arthritis
Ceftriaxone 2 g/day IV × 14–21 days

a reactive FTA-ABS test result at a dilution of 1:5, but all of these samples were negative at a dilution of 1:10. Nevertheless, the RPR test and the MHA-TP test are usually negative in patients with Lyme disease.[105] False-positive results have also been reported in many autoimmune disorders, Rocky Mountain spotted fever, infectious mononucleosis, and neurologic disorders.[107,109-111] Importantly, in most parts of the United States, the prevalence of Lyme disease is low. Even with a 90% sensitivity and specificity, the predictive value of a positive ELISA for Lyme disease is probably less than 20% in patients with a clinical picture atypical for the disease.

A fourfold increase in serial anti–*B. burgdorferi* IgM antibody levels in patients with a clinical history compatible with Lyme disease remains the most specific laboratory indicator, but this increase is not often documented by serial tests. Western blot analysis and PCR analysis[112,113] are being increasingly used for the diagnosis.

Recommendations for laboratory screening for Lyme disease include performing ELISA using both IgM-specific and IgG-specific anti-immunoglobulins or a polyvalent anti-immunoglobulin.[109] Persistence of the specific IgM response throughout infection is an unusual feature of the antibody response seen in some patients with Lyme disease and may be secondary to an impairment in the helper T-cell function needed to switch from IgM to IgG production.[114] It is suggested that positive or equivocal results on ELISA should be confirmed with Western blotting,[115,116] although new algorithms using two ELISA protocols are being developed. Because the clinical appearances of Lyme disease and syphilis are similar, RPR and FTA-ABS tests should be performed on all patients being tested for Lyme disease, and the presence of infectious mononucleosis should also be considered as a possible cause of false-positive results. Finally, the importance of pursuing a history of tick bites, residence in or travel to areas with endemic Lyme disease, rash, chronic joint complaints, or facial nerve palsy cannot be overemphasized.

The literature is now replete with articles highlighting the overdiagnosis of Lyme disease.[115-117] In cases of ocular inflammation without a clinical history of a tick bite, characteristic rash, arthritis, or neurologic complaints, the likelihood is extremely low that Lyme disease is the cause of the inflammation. In such cases, serologic testing is probably not indicated.[118,119] A cross-sectional study of patients referred to a tertiary uveitis clinic in The Netherlands showed that the prevalence of immunoblotting-confirmed *B. burgdorferi.* IgG seropositivity was slightly lower compared with that in the general population and intraocular antibody production and deoxyribonucleic acid (DNA) was absent in all tested patients, suggesting that there was no value in routine serologic screening for Lyme disease in patients with uveitis.[120] Cases of uveitis in endemic areas with suspicious nonocular symptoms should be evaluated with ELISA. As mentioned earlier, positive ELISA results should be confirmed with Western blotting, and in certain cases, ocular samples may be obtained for PCR analysis, cytologic study, or culture.[121,122] PCR analysis has been used to diagnose ocular Lyme disease[123] and is useful in detecting Lyme disease from tissue samples.

Prognosis. From 10% to 40% of patients with untreated erythema chronicum migrans progress to stage 2 Lyme disease; 3% to 10% of patients experience chronic arthritis, acrodermatitis chronica atrophicans, or neurologic disease. Once it occurs, arthritis does not always respond to antibiotic therapy. Similarly, it is not known whether neurologic involvement is prevented by oral antibiotic therapy for early Lyme disease.

Treatment. Recommendations for the treatment of Lyme disease[124] (see CDC website: https://www.cdc.gov/lyme/treatment/index.html) are listed in Table 11.7. Patients with mild ocular disease may respond well to oral antibiotics, but in cases of more severe ocular manifestations, such as posterior uveitis, intravenous antibiotic therapy with ceftriaxone is probably the treatment of choice, as recommended for cases of late Lyme neuroborreliosis.[125] Interestingly, in patients with persistent symptoms attributed to Lyme disease, longer-term antibiotic treatment did not have additional beneficial effects on health-related quality of life compared with shorter therapy.[126] Some data suggest that prior treatment with corticosteroids may predispose the patient to antibiotic failure; therefore the use of topical corticosteroids should be limited to patients who have anterior segment inflammation and are being treated with antibiotics.[88,127] Topical corticosteroids are also used to treat Lyme keratitis.[71] If the suspicion for Lyme disease is high, a therapeutic trial of antibiotics seems warranted, even in seronegative patients. Finally, chemoprophylaxis and vaccine development continue to be pursued despite early disappointments.[100]

BOX 11.4 Relapsing Fever: Key Features

- Caused by spirochetes of the genus *Borrelia*
- Two epidemiological types: epidemic (louse-borne) and endemic (tick-borne)
- Characterized by recurrent bouts of fever separated by relatively asymptomatic periods
- Eye pain, blurred vision, and photophobia are often seen with disease onset
- Diagnosis is usually based on finding *Borrelia* on thick smear of blood during a febrile episode
- Mortality reported in 2% to 5% of treated patients and up to 40% of untreated patients

Relapsing Fever

Etiology and epidemiology. Relapsing fever is an acute infectious disease caused by multiple species of the spirochetes of the genus *Borrelia* and characterized by recurrent bouts of fever separated by relatively asymptomatic periods.[128,129] Relapsing fever is divided into two epidemiologic types: epidemic, or louse-borne, and endemic, or tick-borne (Box 11.4). Epidemic relapsing fever is transmitted from person to person by the human body louse *Pediculus humanus,* which has previously ingested blood infected with *Borrelia recurrentis.*[130] Infection occurs when the hemolymph from infected body lice contaminates abraded or even normal skin, usually from scratching, when lice are crushed and come into contact with previously excoriated areas of bites. The epidemic form of relapsing fever is found in parts of Africa, South America, and China in areas where overcrowding, poor sanitation, and famine foster louse infestation.[128]

Endemic relapsing fever was first documented in the United States in 1915 after five persons contracted the disease in Bear Creek Canyon, Colorado.[131] This form of the disease is caused by at least 15 species of *Borrelia*, and the tick vectors have now been identified as several species of the genus *Ornithodoros*, with a rodent reservoir.[128,132] Transmission to humans occurs when infected saliva from the tick contaminates the site of the bite. In the United States, tick-borne relapsing fever occurs mostly in the western states, usually between May and September.[133]

Clinical manifestations. After inoculation, the spirochetes multiply in blood and invade most tissues of the body. Onset of the disease occurs 3 to 12 days after infection and is marked by fever (temperature up to 39° C to 40° C); chills; severe headache;[129] and, commonly, eye pain, blurred vision, and photophobia. Other symptoms include myalgia and joint pain; meningismus; anorexia; abdominal pain, nonproductive cough; and neurologic symptoms, including facial paralysis and altered mental status. Hepatosplenomegaly, jaundice, myocarditis, and heart failure sometimes occur late in the disease. The course of louse-borne relapsing fever tends to be more severe than that of tick-borne relapsing fever. Bleeding is common in both forms of the disease and often manifests as purpura, petechiae, or epistaxis.[134] Subconjunctival and retinal hemorrhages have been described. In more severe cases of relapsing fever, gastrointestinal or cerebral hemorrhage and disseminated intravascular coagulation may occur, resulting in death.

The initial attack of relapsing fever lasts 3 to 6 days and is followed by an afebrile period of 6 to 9 days. Defervescence may be accompanied by hypotension. Relapses tend to become shorter and less severe as the disease progresses. Mortality in relapsing fever ranges from 2% to 5% in treated cases and as high as 40% in untreated cases.[129]

Eye pain and photophobia are common, and conjunctivitis and iridocyclitis have both been reported in approximately 15% of cases of relapsing fever, usually after several relapses.[135] Cases of more severe uveitis with vitritis have been reported, but they apparently respond well to therapy.[136] Neuro-ophthalmic manifestations of relapsing fever are mostly limited to ptosis caused by paralysis of the facial nerve, but pupillary dilatation and optic neuritis have also been documented. Retinal venous occlusion with retinal hemorrhage and exudate has been documented in one case.[128]

Ocular manifestations. The ocular manifestations of relapsing fever are listed in Table 11.8.

TABLE 11.8 Ocular Manifestations of Relapsing Fever
Conjunctivitis
Subconjunctival and retinal hemorrhages
Iridocyclitis (usually after several relapses of the disease)
Vitritis
Ptosis (secondary to facial nerve paralysis)
Mydriasis
Optic neuritis
Retinal venous occlusion

Diagnosis. Despite advances in laboratory testing for many infectious diseases, definitive diagnosis of relapsing fever is still based on the presence of *Borrelia* on a thick smear of peripheral blood obtained during a febrile episode. *Borrelia* species are best seen with the Giemsa or Wright stain.[129] Repeated smears or use of an acridine orange fluorescent stain increases the sensitivity of the smears.[129,137] If direct methods of diagnosis fail, blood from the patient may be injected into mice or rats, and the blood from these animals may then be examined for spirochetes.

Immunofluorescence assays and ELISA protocols are being developed, but serologic findings are not yet useful in diagnosing relapsing fever.[131] The description of a specific antigen may facilitate the serologic detection of *Borrelia* responsible for relapsing fever, in contrast to the *B. burgdorferi* of Lyme disease.[138] PCR tests are also being developed for the disease but are not yet in common use. Nonspecific laboratory abnormalities include anemia, elevated erythrocyte sedimentation rate (ESR), platelet count less than 150,000/mm^3, and prolonged bleeding time. Serologic results for syphilis may be positive in as many as 10% of patients tested. In patients with CNS involvement, analysis of CSF usually reveals pleocytosis with an elevated protein concentration but a normal glucose level.[129]

Prognosis. Ninety-five percent of patients with relapsing fever recover with therapy, but if untreated, louse-borne relapsing fever is often fatal. Rare complications include respiratory disease, nephritis, endocarditis, neurologic disease, and bleeding diatheses. Uveitis may lead to permanent visual disability.

Treatment. The treatment for tick-borne relapsing fever in women who are not pregnant often is doxycycline, 100 mg orally two times daily for 10 days. Penicillin, erythromycin, and chloramphenicol are also effective. In louse-borne relapsing fever the treatment in women who are not pregnant can be a single dose of doxycycline 200 mg orally two times daily. A 2-week course of intravenous ceftrizone or penicillin G sodium has been recommended to treat relapsing fever accompanied by meningitis or encephalitis. Treatment for relapsing fever should be given during the early part of a febrile episode to diminish the possibility of a Jarisch-Herxheimer reaction,[139] which is caused by the release of a nonendotoxin pyrogen as *Borrelia* species are killed, and is characterized by rigors, fever, and elevated blood pressure, followed by hypotension and possible shock.

Leptospirosis

Etiology and epidemiology. Leptospirosis is a zoonosis caused by spirochetes of the genus *Leptospira*, whose natural reservoir is wild animals, mostly rodents. Weil[140] first recognized a severe form of leptospirosis as a distinct clinical entity in 1886, and the spirochetal cause of Weil disease was discovered by Inada et al. in 1915.[141] Leptospirosis can affect domestic animals, including livestock and dogs. Humans are an accidental host, acquiring the disease through contact with infected urine, tissues, or water. The spirochetes invade humans through abraded skin, mucous membranes, or the conjunctiva, although penetration through intact skin occasionally occurs. The disease is often occupational, occurring in farmers, veterinarians, and abattoir workers.[142,143] Most cases of leptospirosis in the United States are acquired during water sports and occur predominantly in young men in the late summer and early fall.[141,143] Although the exact incidence remains unknown, since 1970, physicians have reported 40 to 120 cases annually to the CDC.[144] However, these figures are probably an underestimate: active surveillance programs report a fivefold increase in the incidence of leptospirosis,[145] and outbreaks in developed countries continue to be reported.[146] Globally, there may be a million severe cases of leptospirosis annually, with substantial morbidity and mortality.

Two hundred and seven different leptospiral serovars have been identified, with pathologic leptospires belonging to the species *Leptospira interrogans*.[142] Although relatively few cases are reported annually because the signs and symptoms of the disease are not distinct, many cases go undiagnosed. Once inside the host, leptospires enter the bloodstream, can penetrate tissues, and are found in almost all organs within 24 hours. The mechanism by which leptospires cause tissue damage is not entirely clear; however, serovar-specific lipopolysaccharide has been identified in the aqueous humor of patients with leptospiral uveitis, suggesting a causative role for endotoxin in this disease.[147]

BOX 11.5 Leptospirosis: Key Features

- Caused by spirochetes of the genus *Leptospira*
- Natural reservoir is wild animals, mostly rodents
- Humans acquire disease through contact with infected urine, tissues, or water
- Disease is divided into two phases: leptospiremic and immune
- Ocular findings occur in 3% to 92% of patients; conjunctival suffusion is the characteristic finding in the leptospiremic phase; retinal findings are common in the immune phase

Clinical manifestations. The incubation period for leptospirosis ranges from 2 to 26 days, with the usual period extending from 7 to 13 days. The disease is often biphasic; the first, or leptospiremic, phase is abrupt in onset and characterized by severe frontal, bitemporal, or retro-orbital headaches; fever and chills; and severe muscle ache (Box 11.5). Conjunctival suffusion is a characteristic finding that usually appears on the third or fourth day of the disease but is frequently overlooked.[148,149] Hepatosplenomegaly and jaundice are uncommon in the first stage but occur later in the course of more severe forms of the disease. The leptospiremic phase lasts from 4 to 9 days, with recurrent fever spikes exceeding a temperature of 39° C.

For 8 to 10 days after infection, leptospires can be isolated from blood and CSF but disappear as defervescence takes place and the patient enters the second, or immune, phase of the disease. The immune phase of leptospirosis begins on day 6 to day 12 of the illness and corresponds to the time when antibodies appear in serum. The clinical course of the immune phase is variable, and some patients experience few symptoms. However, high fever and meningismus may occur in half the patients, and examination of CSF after day 7 of infection reveals pleocytosis in 50%, often with a mildly elevated protein level. Other manifestations of the disease include encephalitis; optic neuritis; cranial nerve paresis involving the sixth, seventh, and eighth cranial nerves; and peripheral neuropathies. Spontaneous abortion may result from leptospirosis acquired during pregnancy.

Ocular manifestations. The ocular manifestations of leptospirosis are listed in Table 11.9. Ocular findings have been reported in 3% to 92% of patients,[150] the most common and characteristic findings being bulbar and palpebral conjunctival hyperemia with engorged conjunctival and episcleral vessels. This hyperemia usually occurs without discomfort, lacrimation, or discharge; however, if ocular discharge is present, it can harbor leptospires and can be a source of further infection.[151] In an outbreak of leptospirosis among 74 athletes participating in triathlons, 43% reported eye pain, and 26% had red eye.[152] Uveitis is a common finding in leptospirosis. In a series of 73 patients with uveitis associated with leptospirosis, panuveitis was seen in 106 eyes (95.5%), retinal periphlebitis in 57 (51.4%), and hypopyon in 14 (12.6%).[153]

Interestingly, leptospirosis may be an important cause of recurrent uveitis in horses and is a leading cause of blindness in these animals. During a 7-year period, horses seropositive for leptospirosis were 13.2 times more likely to have uveitis compared with seronegative animals.[154] A study from India reported leptospiral antibodies in all of 15 patients with acute panuveitis and retinal vasculitis during a postmonsoon period.[155] Panuveitis with papillitis has been reported in a case of leptospirosis.[156]

Weil Disease

A severe form of leptospirosis, Weil disease, occurs with jaundice, azotemia, hemorrhages, anemia, persistent fever, and altered mental

TABLE 11.9 Ocular Manifestations of Leptospirosis

Leptospiremic Phase
Conjunctival suffusion
Immune Phase
Iridocyclitis
Optic neuritis
Facial nerve palsy
Palpebral herpes
Posterior uveitis (with retinal exudates)
Scleral icterus
Subconjunctival hemorrhages
Retinal hemorrhages

status. Renal and hepatocellular dysfunction usually occurs on day 3 to day 6 after infection. Mortality from leptospirosis occurs only in patients with jaundice and approaches 15% in younger patients and 30% in patients over 60 years of age.

In Weil disease with hepatic involvement, scleral icterus is present, and in patients with severe disease, subconjunctival and retinal hemorrhages may occur. Less commonly, during the immune phase of the disease, with CNS involvement, patients may acquire palpebral herpes, optic neuritis, and facial nerve paresis. Between 10% and 44% of patients with leptospirosis experience uveitis,[157] typically with acute, often bilateral, iridocyclitis with fine keratic precipitates, posterior synechiae, occasional vitreous opacities, and rarely retinal exudates. Patients often have blurred vision and mild ocular irritation but respond well to treatment with mydriatics and topical steroids. More severe cases of uveitis have been reported and may occur long after the disease has appeared to subside. Barkay and Garzozi[149] reported on 16 patients with predominantly anterior uveitis secondary to leptospirosis with positive serologic results. Leptospirosis should be considered as a possible cause of uveitis of unknown cause, especially in patients with occupational or recreational risk factors for the disease.

Diagnosis. The WBC count is normal to slightly elevated in most cases of leptospirosis; values greater than 15,000 cells/mm^3 suggest the presence of hepatic disease. Differential counts usually reveal greater than 70% neutrophils, a finding that may differentiate leptospirosis from viral infection. In patients with liver involvement, intravascular hemolysis may cause anemia and elevated serum bilirubin levels.

A definitive diagnosis of leptospirosis requires isolation of the spirochete from a clinical specimen, usually blood or CSF, or seroconversion (a fourfold or greater rise in antibody titer) in the presence of clinical illness. The organism is present in blood and CSF for only 8 to 10 days after infection, and the spirochete quickly disappears as antibodies appear in serum. Leptospires can be identified on darkfield microscopy, but this technique requires expertise. Leptospiruria occurs during the immune phase, although leptospires are easily confused with cellular debris in urine sediment. Tissue samples may also be examined, but tissue analysis for leptospires is predominantly limited to postmortem examination. PCR analysis can also be used to diagnose the disease, where available. Detection of leptospira DNA by using PCR in the aqueous humor of a patient with uveitis has been reported.[158]

In practice, laboratory diagnosis of leptospirosis is usually made serologically. The macroscopic slide agglutination test uses a boiled suspension of leptospires and is used mostly as a screening test. The microscopic agglutination test uses live or formalin-treated antigens, is more specific, and can be used to determine both antibody titer and serotype. Sensitive and specific complement fixation tests and ELISA

TABLE 11.10 Treatment of Leptospirosis in Women Who Are Not Pregnant

Mild Infection
Doxycycline 100 mg orally (PO) two times daily × 7 days
OR Amoxicillin 500 mg PO three times daily × 7 days
OR Ampicillin 500–750 mg PO three times daily × 7 days
Moderate to Severe Infection
Penicillin G 1.5 million units intravenously (IV) or IM every 6 hours × 7 days
OR Ceftriaxone 2g IV four times a day × 7 days
OR Cefotaxime 1g IV every 6 hours x 7 days
OR Doxycycline (loading dose of 200 mg IV; then 100 mg IV every 12 hours x 7 days)
Severe Uveltls or Neurologic Abnormalities or Arthritis
Ceftriaxone 2 g/day IV × 14–21 days

protocols for the detection of IgM antibody against leptospiral antigens have been developed. They are both inexpensive and easy to use and are playing an increasing role in the diagnosis of leptospirosis. Agglutinins appear on day 6 to day 12 of illness, and the maximum titer is reached during the third and fourth weeks. Early treatment with antibiotics may delay or suppress development of the antibody response, but if initial serologic test results are negative, the tests should be repeated 2 weeks later.

Prognosis. Patients with anicteric leptospirosis usually recover uneventfully within 2 to 6 weeks, although convalescence may extend up to 1 month. Death occurs in 5% to 30% of untreated patients and is usually attributable to acute renal failure. Uveitis occurs in 10% of patients from 2 weeks to 1 year after initial infection, but the prognosis for these patients is generally good.

Treatment. Recommendations for the treatment of leptospirosis can be found in Table 11.10. Chemotherapeutic trials were conducted during outbreaks of leptospirosis in military personnel training in Panama. Doxycycline, 200 mg orally once a week and at the end of training, prevented infection.[159] Antibiotics have been shown to reduce disease complications if they are given by the day 4 of infection; however, administration is still recommended for severe infections, even if diagnosis is made 4 days after onset of infection.

In severe cases of leptospirosis, intravenous therapy with penicillin, ceftriaxone or cefotaxime are often recommended. Less severe cases may be treated with a 7-day course of doxycycline, ampicillin, or amoxicillin.[160,161] Supportive therapy is given for renal failure, hypotension, and hemorrhage.

Prevention of leptospirosis centers on the elimination of large animal reservoirs of disease, including livestock and pets. In fact, cattle-associated leptospirosis is a problem in the British Isles, and at least 4% of all British dairy farmers are at risk for infection.[143]

The ophthalmologist must be diligent in pursuing the clinical history for evidence of previous or persistent low-grade infection that is suggestive of leptospirosis when evaluating patients with uveitis of unknown cause, especially in dairy farmers. Because many cases go unrecognized, it is not possible to state definitively how many cases of uveitis occur secondary to leptospirosis; however, one report indicated that only 17% of 483 proven cases of leptospirosis were initially diagnosed correctly.[162] In an editorial, Watt[163] suggested that a history of water or animal contact in a patient with severe myalgias and conjunctival suffusion suggests the presence of leptospirosis, particularly in someone returning from travel in Asia or Latin America. The ophthalmologist can confirm the diagnosis by sending a serum sample to a reference laboratory for the microscopic agglutination test or ELISA for leptospirosis.

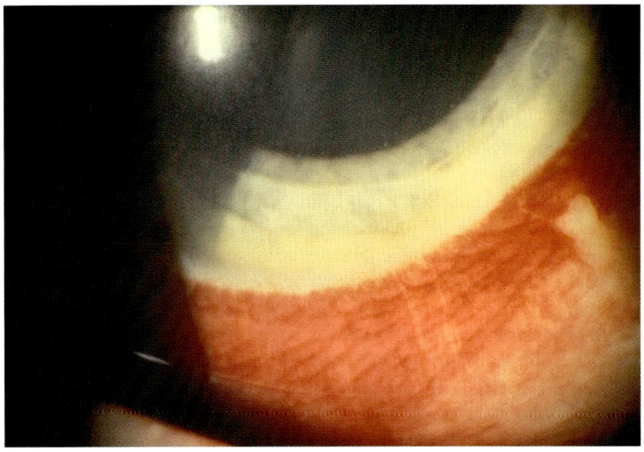

Fig. 11.11 Hypopyon uveitis in a patient with syphilis (see Case 11.1).

CASE 11.1

A 59-year-old white man who is human immunodeficiency virus (HIV)–positive experienced a sudden decrease in vision in both eyes. Visual acuity was 20/400 in the right eye (OU). Examination revealed bilateral hypopyons (Fig. 11.11), dense vitritis, and patchy areas of retinal infiltrates in both eyes (see Fig. 11.3A). The patient was referred to the National Institutes of Health (NIH) with a presumed diagnosis of cytomegalovirus retinitis. Laboratory evaluation at the NIH revealed positive results on the Venereal Disease Research Laboratory (VDRL) and fluorescent treponemal antibody absorption (FTA-ABS) tests. A diagnosis of syphilis was made, and the patient was treated with intravenous penicillin G. Within 2 weeks visual acuity improved to 20/40 OU. The retinal infiltrates also resolved, and the patient was left with a pigmentary retinopathy characteristic of resolved syphilitic retinitis (see Fig. 11.3B).

REFERENCES

1. Schaudin FR, Hoffman E. Vorlüfger Berichtüber das Vorkommen von Spirochaeten in syphilitschen Krankheitsproducten und bei Papillomen. *Arb Gesundheitsamte*. 1905;22:527.
2. Mahoney JF, Arnold RC, Harris A. Penicillin treatment of syphilis: a preliminary report. *J Vener Dis Inform*. 1943;24:355–357.
3. Continuing increase in infectious syphilis – United States. *MMWR Morb Mortal Wkly Rep*. 1988;37:35–38.
4. Congenital syphilis – New York City, 1986–1988. *MMWR Morb Mortal Wkly Rep*. 1989;38:825–829.
5. Primary and secondary syphilis – United States, 2003–2004. *MMWR Morb Mortal Wkly Rep*. 2005;55:269–273.
6. Berry CD, Hooton TM, Collier AC, et al. Neurologic relapse after benzathine penicillin therapy for secondary syphilis in a patient with HIV infection. *N Engl J Med*. 1987;316:1587–1589.
7. Johns DR, Tierney M, Felsenstein D. Alteration in the natural history of neurosyphilis by concurrent infection with the human immunodeficiency virus. *N Engl J Med*. 1987;316:1569–1572.
8. Oliver SE, Aubin M, Atwell L. Ocular syphilis—eight jurisdictions, United States, 2014–2015. *MMWR Morb Mortal Wkly Rep*. 2016;65:1185–1188.
9. Sparling PF. Natural history of syphilis. In: Holmes KK, Per-Anders M, Sparling PF, Wiesner PJ, eds. *Sexually Transmitted Diseases*. New York: McGraw-Hill; 1990:214.
10. Chapel TA. The variability of syphilitic chancres. *Sex Transm Dis*. 1978;5:68–70.
11. Pulido JS, Corbett JJ, McLeish WM. Syphilis. In: Gold DH, Weingeist TA, eds. *The Eye and Systemic Disease*. Philadelphia: JB Lippincott; 1990:234.
12. Tramont EC. Syphilis in adults: from Christopher Columbus to Sir Alexander Fleming to AIDS. *Clin Infect Dis*. 1995;21:1361–1371.

13. Chapel TA. The signs and symptoms of secondary syphilis. *Sex Transm Dis*. 1980;7:161–164.
14. Woods AC. Syphilis of the eye. *Am J Syph Gonorrhea Vener Dis*. 1943;27:133–186.
15. Wilhelmus KR. Syphilis. In: Insler MS, ed. *AIDS and Other Sexually Transmitted Diseases and the Eye*. Orlando, FL: Grune & Stratton; 1987:73–104.
16. Lukehart SA, Hook EW, Baker-Zander SA, et al. Invasion of the central nervous system by *Treponema pallidum:* implications for diagnosis and treatment. *Ann Intern Med*. 1988;109:855–862.
17. Marra CM. Update on neurosyphilis. *Curr Infect Dis Rep*. 2009;11:127–134.
18. Lowenfeld IE. The Argyll Robertson pupil, 1869–1969: A critical survey of the literature. *Surv Ophthalmol*. 1969;14:199–299.
19. Dorfman DH, Glaser JH. Congenital syphilis presenting in infants after the newborn period. *N Engl J Med*. 1990;323:1299–1302.
20. Duke-Elder S. *System of Ophthalmology. The Ocular Adnexa, Part II, Lacrimal, Orbital, and Paraorbital Diseases. Vol XIII*. St. Louis: CV Mosby; 1974:615.
21. Arruga J, Valentines J, Mauri F, et al. Neuroretinitis in acquired syphilis. *Ophthalmology*. 1985;92:262–270.
22. Morgan CM, Webb RM, O'Connor GR. Atypical syphilitic chorioretinitis and vasculitis. *Retina*. 1984;4:225–231.
23. Mendelsohn AD, Jampol LM. Syphilitic retinitis. A cause of necrotizing retinitis. *Retina*. 1985;4:221–234.
24. Jumper JM, Machemer R, Gallemore RP, et al. Exudative retinal detachment and retinitis associated with acquired syphilitic uveitis. *Retina*. 2000;20:190–194.
25. Halperin LS, Lewis H, Blumenkranz MS, et al. Choroidal neovascular membrane and other chorioretinal complications of acquired syphilis. *Am J Ophthalmol*. 1989;108:554–562.
26. Tsimpida M, Low LC, Posner E, et al. Acute syphilitic posterior placoid chorioretinitis in late latent syphilis. *Int J STD AIDS*. 2009;20:207–208.
27. Larsen SA, Seiner BM, Rudolph AH. Laboratory diagnosis and interpretation of tests for syphilis. *Clin Microbiol Rev*. 1995;8:1–21.
28. Cantor A, Nelson HD, Daeges M, Pappas M. Screening for syphilis in nonpregnant adolescents and adults. Systematic review to update the 2004 U.S. Preventive Services Task Force Recommendation [Internet]. *U.S. Preventive Services Task Force Evidence Syntheses*. 2016. No. 1367. Report No.: 14-05213-EF-1.
29. Workowski KA, Bolan GA. Sexually transmitted diseases treatment guidelines, 2015. MMWR 2015;64:34-51.
30. Syphilis testing algorithms using treponemal tests for initial screening – four laboratories, New York City, 2005–2006. *MMWR Morb Mortal Wkly Rep*. 2008;57:872–875.
31. Sena AC, White BL, Sparling PF. Novel *Treponema pallidum* serologic tests: a paradigm shift in syphilis screening for the 21st century. *Clin Infect Dis*. 2010;51:700–708.
32. Guidelines for the prevention and control of congenital syphilis. *MMWR Morb Mortal Wkly Rep*. 1988;37(Suppl 1):1–13.
33. Riedner G, Rusizoka M, Todd J, et al. Single-dose azithromycin versus penicillin G benzathine for the treatment of early syphilis. *N Engl J Med*. 2005;353:1236–1244.
34. Johns DR, Tierney M, Felsenstein D. Alterations in the natural history of neurosyphilis by concurrent infection with the human immunodeficiency virus. *N Engl J Med*. 1987;316:1569–1572.
35. Tramont EC. Syphilis in the AIDS era. *N Engl J Med*. 1987;316:1600–1601.
36. Stoumbos VD, Klein ML. Syphilitic retinitis in a patient with acquired immunodeficiency syndrome-related complex. *Am J Ophthalmol*. 1987;103:103–104.
37. Passo MS, Rosenbaum JT. Ocular syphilis in patients with human immunodeficiency virus infection. *Am J Ophthalmol*. 1988;106:1–6.
38. Levy JH, Liss RA, Maguire AM. Neurosyphilis and ocular syphilis in patients with concurrent human immunodeficiency virus infection. *Retina*. 1989;9:175–180.
39. Zaidman GW. Neurosyphilis and retrobulbar neuritis in a patient with AIDS. *Ann Ophthalmol*. 1986;18:260–261.
40. Markowitz DM, Beutner KR, Maggio RP, et al. Failure of recommended treatment for secondary syphilis. *JAMA*. 1986;255:1767–1768.
41. Richards BW, Hessburg TJ, Nussbaum JN. Recurrent syphilitic uveitis. *[Letter] N Engl J Med*. 1989;320:62.
42. Hicks CB, Benson PM, Lupton GP, et al. Seronegative secondary syphilis in a patient infected with the human immunodeficiency virus (HIV) with Kaposi sarcoma. *Ann Intern Med*. 1987;107:492–495.
43. Hollander H. Cerebrospinal fluid normalities and abnormalities in individuals infected with human immunodeficiency virus. *J Infect Dis*. 1988;158:855–858.
44. Recommendations for diagnosing and treating syphilis in HIV-infected patients. *MMWR Morb Mortal Wkly Rep*. 1988;37:600–608.
45. Pace JL, Csonka GW. Endemic non-venereal syphilis (bejel) in Saudi Arabia. *Br J Vener Dis*. 1984;60:293–297.
46. Tabbara KF, Al Kaff AS, Fadel T. Ocular manifestations of endemic syphilis (bejel). *Ophthalmology*. 1989;96:1087–1091.
47. Smith JL. Neuro-ophthalmological study of late yaws: I. An introduction to yaws. *Br J Vener Dis*. 1971;47:223–225.
48. Smith JL, David NJ, Indgin S, et al. Neuro-ophthalmological study of late yaws and pinta: II. The Caracas project. *Br J Vener Dis*. 1971;47:226–251.
49. Roman GC, Roman LN. Occurrence of congenital, cardiovascular, visceral, neurologic, and neuro-ophthalmologic complications in late yaws: a theme for future research. *Rev Infect Dis*. 1986;8:760–770.
50. Mitja O, Gonzalez-Beiras C, Godornes C, et al. Effectiveness of single-dose azithromycin to treat latent yaws: a longitudinal comparative cohort study. *Lancet Glob Health*. 2017;5:e1268–e1274.
51. Mitja O, Godornes C, Houinei W, et al. Re-emergence of yaws after single mass azithromycin treatment followed by targeted treatment: a longitudinal study. *Lancet*. 2018;391:1599–1607.
52. Steere AC, Malawista SE, Snydman DR, et al. Lyme arthritis: an epidemic of oligoarticular arthritis in children and adults in three Connecticut communities. *Arthritis Rheum*. 1977;20:7–17.
53. MacDonald AB. Lyme disease: a neuro-ophthalmologic view. *J Clin Neuroophthalmol*. 1987;7:185–190.
54. Burgdorfer W, Barbour AG, Hayes SF, et al. Lyme disease: a tick-borne spirochetosis? *Science*. 1982;216:1317–1319.
55. Berger BW, Kaplan MH, Rothenberg IR, et al. Isolation and characterization of the Lyme disease spirochete from the skin of patients with erythema chronicum migrans. *J Am Acad Dermatol*. 1985;13:444–449.
56. Barbour AG. Isolation and cultivation of Lyme disease spirochetes. *Yale J Biol Med*. 1984;57:521–525.
57. Barbour AG, Hayes SF. Biology of *Borrelia* species. *Microbiol Rev*. 1986;50:381–400.
58. Levine JF, Wilson ML, Spielman A. Mice as reservoirs of the Lyme disease spirochete. *Am J Trop Med Hyg*. 1985;34:355–360.
59. Wilson ML, Adler GH, Spielman A. Correlation between abundance of deer and that of the deer tick, *Ixodes dammini* (Acari: Ixodidae). *Ann Entomol Soc Am*. 1986;23:172–176.
60. Steere AC. Lyme disease. *N Engl J Med*. 1989;321:586–596.
61. Tsai TS, Bailey RE, Moore PS. National surveillance of Lyme disease 1987–1988. *Conn Med*. 1986;53:324–326.
62. Surveillance for Lyme Disease. United States, 1992–2006. *MMWR Morb Mortal Wkly Rep*. 2008;57(SS10):1–9.
63. Lastavica CC, Wilson ML, Berardi VP, et al. Rapid emergence of a focal epidemic of Lyme disease in coastal Massachusetts. *N Engl J Med*. 1989;320:133–137.
64. Rosenberg R, Lindsey NP, Fischer M, et al. Vital signs: trends in reported vector-borne disease cases—United States and territories, 2004-2016. *MMWR Morb Mortal Wkly Rep*. 2018;67:496–501.
65. Paules CI, Marston HD, Bloom ME, Fauci AS. Tickborne diseases – confronting a growing threat. *N Engl J Med*. 2018;379:701–703.
66. Steere AC, Bartenhagen NH, Craft JE, et al. The early clinical manifestations of Lyme disease. *Ann Intern Med*. 1983;99:76–82.
67. Pachner AR, Steere AC. The triad of neurologic manifestations of Lyme disease: meningitis, cranial neuritis, and radiculoneuritis. *Neurology*. 1985;35:47–53.
68. Clark JR, Carlson RD, Sasaki CT, et al. Facial paralysis in Lyme disease. *Laryngoscope*. 1985;95:1341–1345.
69. Steere AC, Batsford WP, Weinberg M, et al. Lyme carditis: cardiac abnormalities of Lyme disease. *Ann Intern Med*. 1980;93:8–16.

70. Bertuch AW, Rocco E, Schwartz EG. Eye findings in Lyme disease. *Conn Med*. 1987;51:151–152.
71. Baum J, Barza M, Weinstein P, et al. Bilateral keratitis as a manifestation of Lyme disease. *Am J Ophthalmol*. 1988;105:75–77.
72. Orlin SE, Lauffer JL. Lyme disease keratitis. *Am J Ophthalmol*. 1989;107:678–680.
73. Schlesinger PA, Duray PH, Burke BA, et al. Maternal–fetal transmission of the Lyme disease spirochete, *Borrelia burgdorferi*. *Ann Intern Med*. 1985;103:67–69.
74. Weber K, Bratzke HJ, Neubert U, et al. *Borrelia burgdorferi* in a newborn despite oral penicillin for Lyme borreliosis during pregnancy. *Pediatr Infect Dis J*. 1988;7:286–289.
75. Markowitz LE, Steere AC, Benach JL, et al. Lyme disease during pregnancy. *JAMA*. 1986;255:3394–3396.
76. Williams CL, Benach JL, Curran AS, et al. Lyme disease during pregnancy: a cord blood serosurvey. *Ann NY Acad Sci*. 1988;539:504–506.
77. Aaberg TM. The expanding ophthalmologic spectrum of Lyme disease. *Am J Ophthalmol*. 1989;107:77–80.
78. Flack AJ, Lavoie PE. Episcleritis, conjunctivitis, and keratitis as other manifestations of Lyme disease. *Ophthalmology*. 1990;97:973–975.
79. Steere AC, Duray PH, Kauffmann DJ, et al. Unilateral blindness caused by infection with the Lyme disease spirochete, *Borrelia burgdorferi*. *Ann Intern Med*. 1985;103:382–384.
80. Kornmehl EW, Lesser RL, Jaros P, et al. Bilateral keratitis in Lyme disease. *Ophthalmology*. 1989;96:1194–1197.
81. deLuise VP, O'Leary MJ. Peripheral ulcerative keratitis related to Lyme disease. *[Letter] Am J Ophthalmol*. 1991;111:244–245.
82. Suttorp-Schulten MSA, Kuiper H, Kijlstra A, et al. Long-term effects of ceftriaxone treatment on intraocular Lyme borreliosis. *Am J Ophthalmol*. 1993;116:571–575.
83. Karma A, Seppala I, Mikkila H, et al. Diagnosis and clinical characteristics of ocular Lyme borreliosis. *Am J Ophthalmol*. 1995;119:127–135.
84. Bialasiewicz AA, Ruprecht KW, Naumann GOH, et al. Bilateral diffuse choroiditis and exudative retinal detachments with evidence of Lyme disease. *Am J Ophthalmol*. 1988;105:419–420.
85. Koch F, Augustin AJ, Boker T. Neuroborreliosis with retinal pigment epithelium detachments. *Ger J Ophthalmol*. 1996;5:12–15.
86. Scholes GN, Teske M. Lyme disease and pars planitis. *Ophthalmology*. 1989;107(Suppl):126.
87. Copeland RA Jr, Nozik RA, Shimokaji G. Uveitis in Lyme disease. *Ophthalmology*. 1989;107(Suppl):127.
88. Winward KE, Smith JL, Culbertson WW, et al. Ocular Lyme borreliosis. *Am J Ophthalmol*. 1989;108:651–657.
89. Leys AM, Schonherr U, Lang GE, et al. Retinal vasculitis in Lyme borreliosis. *Bull Soc Belge Ophthalmol*. 1995;259:205–214.
90. Vine AK. Retinal vasculitis. *Semin Neurol*. 1994;14:354–360.
91. Logigian EL, Kaplan RF, Steere AC. Chronic neurologic manifestations of Lyme disease. *N Engl J Med*. 1990;323:1438–1444.
92. Wu G, Lincoff H, Ellsworth RM, et al. Optic disc edema and Lyme disease. *Ann Ophthalmol*. 1986;18:252–255.
93. Jacobson DM, Frens DB. Pseudotumor cerebri syndrome associated with Lyme disease. *Am J Ophthalmol*. 1989;107:81–82.
94. Federowski JJ, Hyman C. Optic disk edema as the presenting sign of Lyme disease. *Clin Infect Dis*. 1996;23:639–640.
95. Scott IU, Silva-Lepe A, Siatkowski RM. Chiasmal optic neuritis in Lyme disease. *Am J Ophthalmol*. 1997;123:136–138.
96. Schecter SL. Lyme disease associated with optic neuropathy. *Am J Med*. 1986;81:143–145.
97. Reik L Jr, Burgdorfer W, Donaldson JO. Neurologic abnormalities in Lyme disease without erythema chronicum migrans. *Am J Med*. 1986;81:73–78.
98. Seidenberg KB, Leib M. Orbital myositis with Lyme disease. *Am J Ophthalmol*. 1990;109:13–16.
99. Balcer LJ, Winterkorn JM, Galetta SL. Neuro-ophthalmic manifestations of Lyme disease. *J Neuroophthalmol*. 1997;17:108–121.
100. Stanek G, Strle F. Lyme borreliosis. *Lancet*. 2003;362:1639–1647.
101. Schwartz BS, Goldstein MD, Ribeiro JMC, et al. Antibody testing in Lyme disease: a comparison of results in four laboratories. *JAMA*. 1989;262:3431–3434.
102. Luger SW, Krauss E. Serologic tests for Lyme disease: interlaboratory variability. *Arch Intern Med*. 1990;150:761–763.
103. Barbour AG. The diagnosis of Lyme disease: rewards and perils. *Ann Intern Med*. 1989;110:501–502.
104. Dattwyler RJ, Volkman DJ, Lugt BJ, et al. Seronegative Lyme disease dissociation of specific T- and B-lymphocyte responses to *Borrelia burgdorferi*. *N Engl J Med*. 1988;319:1441–1446.
105. Russell H, Saampson JS, Schmid GP, et al. Enzyme-linked immunosorbent assay and indirect immunofluorescence assay for Lyme disease. *J Infect Dis*. 1984;149:465–470.
106. Craft JE, Grodzicki RL, Steere AC. Antibody response in Lyme disease: evaluation of diagnostic tests. *J Infect Dis*. 1984;149:789–795.
107. Magnarelli LA, Anderson JF, Johnson RC. Cross-reactivity in serological tests of Lyme disease and other spirochetal infections. *J Infect Dis*. 1987;156:183–188.
108. Hunter EF, Russell H, Farshy CE, et al. Evaluation of sera from patients with Lyme disease in the fluorescent treponemal antibody test for syphilis. *Sex Transm Dis*. 1986;13:232–236.
109. Duffy J, Mertz LE, Wobig GH, et al. Diagnosing Lyme disease: the contribution of serologic testing. *Mayo Clin Proc*. 1988;63:1116–1121.
110. Grodzicki RL, Steere AC. Comparison of immunoblotting and indirect enzyme-linked immunosorbent assay using different antigen preparations for diagnosing early Lyme disease. *J Infect Dis*. 1988;157:790–797.
111. Mandell H, Steere AC, Reinhardt BN, et al. Lack of antibodies to *Borrelia burgdorferi* in patients with amyotrophic lateral sclerosis. *N Engl J Med*. 1989;320:255–256.
112. Nocton JJ, Dressler F, Rutledge BJ, et al. Detection of *Borrelia burgdorferi* DNA by polymerase chain reaction in synovial fluid from patients with Lyme arthritis. *N Engl J Med*. 1994;330:229–234.
113. Hilton E, Sood S. Ocular Lyme borreliosis diagnosed by polymerase chain reaction on vitreous fluid. *Ann Intern Med*. 1996;125:424–425.
114. Steere AC, Grodzicki RL, Kornblatt AN, et al. The spirochetal etiology of Lyme disease. *N Engl J Med*. 1983;308:733–740.
115. Wormser GP, Nadelman RB, Dattwyler RL, et al. Practice guidelines for the treatment of Lyme disease. *Clin Infect Dis*. 2000;31(Suppl 1):S1–14.
116. Verdon ME, Sigal LH. Recognition and management of Lyme disease. *Am Fam Phys*. 1997;56:427–436.
117. Steere AC, Taylor E, McHugh GL, et al. The overdiagnosis of Lyme disease. *JAMA*. 1993;269:1812–1816.
118. Rosenbaum JT, Rahn DW. Prevalence of Lyme disease among patients with uveitis. *Am J Ophthalmol*. 1991;112:462–463.
119. Breevald J, Kuiper H, Spanjaard L, et al. Uveitis and Lyme borreliosis. *Br J Ophthalmol*. 1993;77:480–481.
120. Kazi H, De Groot-Mijnes JDF, Ten Dam-Van Loon NH, et al. No value for routine serologic screening for *Borrelia burgdorferi* in patients with uveitis in The Netherlands. *Am J Ophthalmol*. 2016;166:189–193.
121. Preac-Mursic V, Pfister HW, Spiegel H, et al. First isolation of *Borrelia burgdorferi* from an iris biopsy. *J Clin Neuroophthalmol*. 1993;13:155–161.
122. Schubert HD, Greenebaum E, Neu HC. Cytologically proven seronegative Lyme choroiditis and vitritis. *Retina*. 1994;14:39–42.
123. Hilton E, Smith C, Sood S. Ocular Lyme borreliosis diagnosed by polymerase chain reaction on vitreous fluid. *Ann Intern Med*. 1996;125:424–425.
124. Hu LT. Lyme disease. *Ann Intern Med*. 2016;165:677.
125. Rauer S, Kastenbauer S, Fingerle V, et al. Lyme neuroborreliosis. *Dtsch Arztebl Int*. 2018;115:751–756.
126. Berende A, ter Hofstede HJM, Vos FJ, et al. Randomized trial of longer-term therapy for symptoms attributed to Lyme disease. *N Engl J Med*. 2016;374:1209–1220.
127. Dattwyler RJ, Halperin JJ, Volkman DJ, et al. Treatment of late Lyme borreliosis – randomised comparison of ceftriaxone and penicillin. *Lancet*. 1988;1:1191–1194.
128. Bryceson ADM, Parry EHO, Perine PL, et al. Louse-borne relapsing fever: a clinical and laboratory study of 62 cases in Ethiopia and a reconstruction of the literature. *QJ Med*. 1970;39:129–170.
129. Southern Jr PM, Sanford JP. Relapsing fever: a clinical and microbiological review. *Medicine (Baltimore)*. 1969;48:129–149.

130. Rhee KY, Johnson Jr WD. *Borrelia* species (relapsing fever). In: Mandell GL, Bennett JE, Dolin R, eds. *Mandell, Douglas and Bennett's Principles and Practice of Infectious Diseases.* 6th ed. New York: Churchill Livingstone; 2005:2795–2796.
131. Meader CN. Five cases of relapsing fever originating in Colorado, with positive blood findings in two. *Colorado Med.* 1915;12:365–368.
132. Burgdorfer W. The enlarging spectrum of tick-borne spirochetoses: RR Parker memorial address. *Rev Infect Dis.* 1986;8:932–940.
133. Horton JM, Blaser MJ. The spectrum of relapsing fever in the Rocky Mountains. *Arch Intern Med.* 1985;145:871–875.
134. Perine PL, Parry EHO, Vukotich D, et al. Bleeding in louse-borne relapsing fever I. Clinical studies in 37 patients. *Trans Roy Soc Trop Med Hyg.* 1971;65:776–781.
135. Quin CE, Perkins ES. Tick-borne relapsing fever in East Africa. *J Trop Med.* 1946;49:30–32.
136. Hamilton JB. Ocular complications in relapsing fever. *Br J Ophthalmol.* 1943;27:68–80.
137. Sciotto CG, Lauer BA, White WL, et al. Detection of *Borrelia* in acridine orange-stained blood smears by fluorescence microscopy. *Arch Pathol Lab Med.* 1982;107:384–386.
138. Schwan TG, Schrumpf ME, Hinnebusch BJ, et al. GlpQ: an antigen for serological discrimination between relapsing fever and Lyme borreliosis. *J Clin Microbiol.* 1996;34:2483–2492.
139. Warell DA, Perine PL, Krause DW, et al. Pathophysiology and immunology of the Jarisch-Herxheimer-like reaction in louse-borne relapsing fever: comparison of tetracycline and slow-release penicillin. *J Infect Dis.* 1983;147:898–908.
140. Weil A. Über eine Eigenümliche, mit Milztumor. Ikterus and Nephritis einhergehende, akute Infektionskrankheit. *Deutsch Arch Klin Med.* 1886;39:209–232.
141. Barkay S, Garzozi H. Leptospirosis. In: Gold DH, Weingeist TA, eds. *The Eye in Systemic Disease.* Philadelphia: JB Lippincott; 1990:226–228.
142. Palmer MF. Laboratory diagnosis of leptospirosis. *Med Lab Sci.* 1988;45:174–178.
143. Waitkins SA. Update on leptospirosis. *Br Med J.* 1985;290:1502–1503.
144. Graphs and maps for selected notifiable diseases in the United States. *MMWR Morb Mortal Wkly Rep.* 1994;42:13–64.
145. Sasaki DM, Pang L, Minette HP, et al. Active surveillance and risk factors for leptospirosis in Hawaii. *Am J Trop Med Hyg.* 1993;48:35–43.
146. Guillois Y, Bourhy P, Ayral F, et al. An outbreak of leptospirosis among kayakers in Brittany, North-West France, 2016. *Euro Surveill.* 2018;23(48):1700848.
147. Priya CG, Rathinam SR, Muthukkaruppan V. Evidence for endotoxin as a causative factor for leptospiral uveitis in humans. *Invest Ophthalmol Vis Sci.* 2008;49:5419–5424.
148. Bernard N, Moshe H. Human leptospirosis associated with eye complications. *Israel Med J.* 1963;22:182.
149. Barkay S, Garzozi H. Leptospirosis and uveitis. *Ann Ophthalmol.* 1984;16:164–168.
150. Murdoch D. Leptospiral uveitis. *Trans Ophthalmol Soc NZ.* 1980;32:73–75.
151. Duke-Elder S. *System of Ophthalmology, Vol VIII: Diseases of the Outer Eye.* London: Henry Kimpton; 1965:201–203.
152. Outbreak of acute febrile illness among athletes participating in triathlons – Wisconsin and Illinois, 1998. *JAMA.* 1998;280:1473–1474.
153. Rathinam SR, Rathnam S, Slevaraj S, et al. Uveitis associated with an epidemic outbreak of leptospirosis. *Am J Ophthalmol.* 1997;124:71–79.
154. Dwyer AE, Crockett RS, Kalsow CM. Association of leptospiral seroreactivity and breed with uveitis and blindness in horses: 372 cases (1986–1993). *J Am Vet Med Assoc.* 1995;207:1327–1331.
155. Rathinamsivakumar, Ratnam S, Sureshbabu L, et al. Leptospiral antibodies in patients with recurrent ophthalmic involvement. *Indian J Med Res.* 1996;103:66–68.
156. Levin N, Nguyen-Khoa JL, Charpentier D, et al. Panuveitis with papillitis in leptospirosis. *Am J Ophthalmol.* 1994;117:118–119.
157. Duke-Elder S. *System of Ophthalmology, Vol IX: Disease of the Uveal Tract.* London: Henry Kimpton; 1966:322–325.
158. Merien F, Perolat P, Manel E, et al. Detection of leptospira DNA by polymerase chain reaction in aqueous humor of a patient with unilateral uveitis. *J Infect Dis.* 1993;168:1335–1336.
159. Takafuji ET, Kirkpatrick JW, Miller RN, et al. An efficacy trial of doxycycline chemoprophylaxis against leptospirosis. *N Engl J Med.* 1984;310:497–500.
160. Wagenaar JFP, Goris MGA. Leptospirosis. In: Jameson JL, Kasper DL, Longo DL, Fauci AS, Hauser SL, Loscalzo J, eds. *Harrison's Principles of Internal Medicines.* 20th ed. New York: McGraw Hill; 2018:1290–1295.
161. Farr RW. Leptospirosis. *Clin Infect Dis.* 1995;21:1–8.
162. Heath CW Jr, Alexander AD, Galton MM. Leptospirosis in the United States. *N Engl J Med.* 1965;273:857–922.
163. Watt GW. Leptospirosis as a cause of uveitis. *Arch Intern Med.* 1990;150:1130–1132.

12

Acquired Immunodeficiency Syndrome

Scott M. Whitcup

KEY CONCEPTS

- Despite efforts at disease prevention, in 2017, the annual number of diagnoses of human immunodeficiency virus (HIV) infection in the United States was 11.8 per 100,000 population, and HIV infection remains a global epidemic.
- Vasculopathy with cotton-wool spots and retinal hemorrhage is the most common manifestation of HIV infection.
- HIV infection can be treated with combination antiretroviral therapy (cART), also known as highly active antiretroviral therapy (HAART), or simply antiretroviral therapy (ART). Prompt initiation of ART appears to be beneficial regardless of the CD4+ T cell count.
- HIV is rarely eradicated from any individual with the currently available medications.
- Cytomegalovirus (CMV) retinitis is the most common opportunistic infection of the eye in patients with HIV infection.
- Treatment of CMV retinitis is based on the location of the disease in the eye and on the duration of ART.
- Once the immune system improves on ART and CD4+ T-cell counts increase, specific anti-CMV therapy can be stopped without causing progression of the disease.
- Immune recovery uveitis (IRU) can occur in patients receiving ART and may require therapy.
- Numerous opportunistic infections can affect the eye of the patient with HIV infection. These should be looked for and treated appropriately.

HUMAN IMMUNODEFICIENCY VIRUS

The clinical course and disease manifestations of human immunodeficiency virus (HIV) infection have dramatically changed since the widespread use of potent antiretroviral therapy (ART). The use of combinations of antiviral drugs, called *highly active antiretroviral therapy* (HAART), combination antiretroviral therapy (cART), or more simply potentent antiretroviral therapy (ART) has led to greatly improved survival and clinical outcomes. Because cART to maximally suppress HIV replication and the progression of disease is now viewed as the standard of care, many refer to HAART or cART simply as ART. However, despite the increasing use of ART, a number of treatment challenges remain. First, near-perfect adherence to complicated treatment regimens is required for sustained virologic suppression.[1] Adherence in the range of 50% to 70% is associated with poorer outcomes and development of drug resistance, and the goal should be greater than 90% adherence. Second, although patient outcomes have improved, eradication of the virus—the "cure"—has remained elusive. Third, the initial hope of a vaccine against HIV infection has also proved problematic. Finally, access to therapy is limited for many, and as a result, the incidence of HIV-1 infection continues to increase in many areas, including sub-Saharan Africa and parts of Asia.

HIV is a retrovirus and therefore has only a ribonucleic acid (RNA) copy in its genome. There are four retroviruses known to cause human disease. These include the human T-cell lymphoma viruses (HTLV)-1 and HLTV-2 and the human immunodeficiency viruses, HIV-1 and HIV-2. HIV is a member of the lentivirus subfamily of Retroviridae, and unlike HTLV, HIV-1 and HIV-2 have both genetic diversity and latency, making control and eradication difficult. The earliest evidence of HIV infection was obtained from the blood sample of a patient in the Congo. Clinical evidence of HIV-1 infection in the United States began to appear in the late 1970s, and by 1984, HIV was demonstrated to be the causative agent of acquired immunodeficiency syndrome (AIDS). Currently, HIV in humans is thought to originate from primate-to-human transmission. Most of the HIV epidemic is caused by HIV-1. HIV-2 was initially confined to West Africa but now has spread globally and accounts for a small percentage of the total number of cases.

HIV can infect many types of human cells, but much of its pathologic effect is related to infection of the helper CD4+ T cell; this occurs within hours of the virus entering the body.[2] Because this cell is crucial for the development of cell-mediated immune responses, infection of CD4+ T cells and subsequent cell death result in severe immunosuppression. The virion gp120 Env protein binds to the CD4+ T cell, and once in the cell, its RNA is translated into DNA by viral reverse transcriptase (Fig. 12.1). This DNA then enters the nucleus and incorporates into the cell genome with the assistance of integrase. The viral DNA is then capable of directing protein synthesis of new viral proteins using the infected cell's apparatus. Proteases are involved in processing HIV proteins into new viral particles, which are then shed from the cell. The infected cell eventually dies.

Epidemiology

Infection is spread mostly through sexual transmission. Until the mid-1990s, male-to-male sexual transmission dominated in the developed countries. Now, heterosexual activity is the major route of transmission globally, including many developed countries. Intravenous drug abuse is another common cause of disease transmission. Perinatal transmission from an infected mother to her offspring can occur in utero. Transmission can also occur during delivery or through breast-feeding. Finally, transmission to health care workers can occur, usually as the result of a needlestick injury. The rate of seroconversion to HIV after a needlestick injury is about 0.3%, depending on the viral load; this is about 10 to 100 times less than that with hepatitis C or B. Before the availability of a serologic test for HIV antibody, large numbers of patients, including those with hemophilia, were exposed to the virus through transfusion of infected blood products.

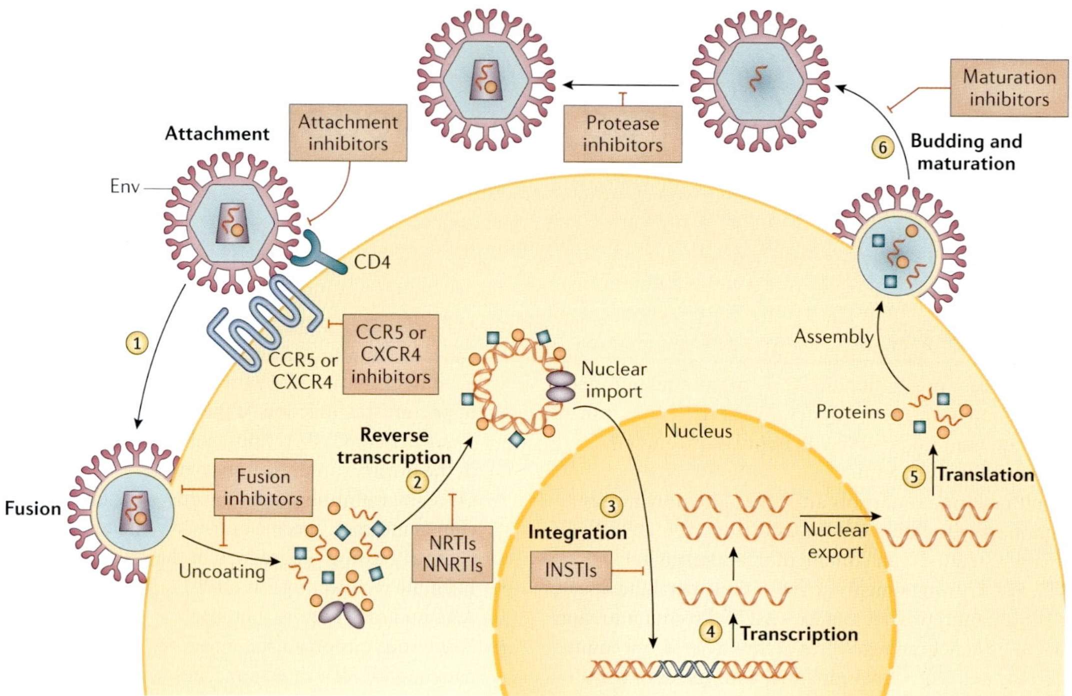

Fig. 12.1 The HIV life cycle. HIV enters its target cells via CD4 and either CC-chemokine receptor 5 (CCR5) or CXC-chemokine receptor 4 (CXCR4) through interaction with envelope (Env) glycoprotein (step 1). After fusion and uncoating, the viral RNA is then reverse transcribed into DNA (step 2). The ensuing pre-integration complex is imported into the nucleus, and the viral DNA is then integrated into the host genome (step 3). Mediated by host enzymes, HIV DNA is transcribed to viral mRNAs (step 4). These mRNAs are then exported to the cytoplasm where translation occurs (step 5) to make viral proteins and eventually mature virions (step 6). Each step — HIV entry, reverse transcription, integration and protein maturation — in the HIV life cycle is a potential target for antiretroviral drugs. INSTI, integrase strand transfer inhibitor; NNRTI, non-nucleoside reverse transcriptase inhibitor; NRTI, nucleoside reverse transcriptase inhibitor. (From Deeks SG, Overbaugh J, Phillips, et al. *HIV Infection Nature Reviews Disease Primers* 2015;1-22. Figure modified from Brenchley JM, Price DA, Douek DC. HIV disease: fallout from a mucosal catastrophe? *Nat Immunol* 2006;7:235–239.)

HIV/AIDS remains a global epidemic, with over 35 million people estimated to have the infection in 2016. Although the number of patients with newly diagnosed HIV infection appears to be declining in the United States, HIV disproportionately affects certain segments of the population, including intravenous drug users, commercial sex workers, people living in poverty, and men who have sex with men. In 2017, the number of new diagnoses of HIV infection was 11.8 per 100,000 population in the United States.[3] The annual rate of infections classified as stage 3 (AIDS) in 2017 was 5.4 per 100,000 population in the United States.

Diagnosis

HIV infection can be diagnosed on the basis of the presence of antibody to viral antigens or direct detection of HIV or one of its components. Antibodies to HIV generally occur in the circulation 3–12 weeks after infection. The antibodies do not control the infection or prevent its sequelae. Diagnosis of HIV infection is usually made by performing an immunoassay, and many experts then recommend that a positive result be confirmed with a Western blot test.[4,5] However, the Centers for Disease Control and Prevention (CDC) recommendations currently indicate that a positive result on a fourth-generation assay, confirmed with a second HIV-1 or HIV-2 specific immunoassay, is adequate for diagnosis.[6] Some strains of HIV are not detected on enzyme-linked immunosorbent assay (ELISA). Nevertheless, ELISA is almost 100% sensitive, albeit not 100% specific, so false-positive results can occur. The virus can also be cultured from blood, semen, and solid tissues, but only rarely from saliva and tears. In the eye, the virus has been found in the cornea,[7] vitreous, and retina.[8] Rapid tests for HIV are now commercially available, although testing algorithms for these tests are still being assessed.

HIV Disease

An acute retroviral syndrome occurs in approximately one-half to three-quarters of patients, usually 3 to 6 weeks after HIV infection. Typically, fever, rash, myalgias, headache, or gastrointestinal symptoms develop. The CD4+ count is reduced, and many patients have elevated liver enzyme levels. Without treatment, CD4+ counts decline by about 75 cells/μL/year. The time from initial infection to the development of a disease that meets the definition of AIDS is about 10 years. Respiratory diseases, including acute bronchitis, pneumonia, and sinusitis, are prevalent during all stages of the disease. AIDS is the most severe manifestation of HIV infection and occurs at a point at which the immune system is so impaired by the infection that opportunistic infections, such as *Pneumocystis jirovecii*, *Cryptococcus neoformans*, and cytomegalovirus (CMV) infections and oral candidiasis, and unusual malignant processes, such as Kaposi sarcoma, can emerge.[4,5] A type of encephalopathy is also caused by direct HIV infection of the brain. Fortunately, effective prophylactic regimens have significantly decreased the occurrence of many of these secondary infections, such as *Pneumocystis* pneumonia. Recommendations on the management of opportunistic infections in patients with HIV infection are evolving rapidly, and guidelines can be found online.[9]

Progression of HIV disease is related to the CD4+ lymphocyte count. The amount of HIV-1 viral RNA predicts the course of HIV disease, specifically, how rapidly the disease is likely to progress. Persons with HIV loads greater than 30,000 copies/mL have an 80% likelihood of AIDS developing within 6 years. In contrast, those with HIV loads less than 500 copies/mL have a 5.4% chance of development of AIDS.[10] CD4+ lymphocyte counts are good predictors for the development of specific clinical manifestations of the disease, particularly opportunistic infections. For example, most cases of *P. jirovecii* pneumonia occur when CD4+ counts fall to less than 200 cells/µL. Typically, CMV retinitis occurs when CD4+ counts are less than 50 cells/µL.

HIV Therapy

The discovery and widespread use of combination antiretroviral therapy (cART) has profoundly improved patient outcomes and survival in persons with HIV. Historically, there was debate on when to start ART for HIV disease. The decision regarding initiation of treatment was based on symptoms, HIV-1 RNA level, and CD4+ count. The potential benefit of ART must be based on the risks of therapy and the impact on quality of life with adherence to a strict therapeutic regimen, which is required to avoid drug resistance. Some clinicians only begin treatment when the CD4+ count drops to less than 350 cells/µL or if symptoms are present. The rapidity of the decline in CD4+ count and HIV load are other factors in the decision regarding when to start therapy. However, studies have suggested that the benefits of prompt initiation of ART outweigh the risks of treatment regardless of CD4+ T-cell count.[11,12] The benefit of prompt initiation of ART applies to both infected persons and their uninfected sexual partners.

When therapy is started, a highly active regimen consisting of a combination of antiretroviral agents should be employed to maximize efficacy and minimize resistance. The goal of therapy is to suppress plasma HIV-1 RNA to below detectable limits by using a sensitive assay. All regimens should combine drugs with synergistic antiviral activity. Four classes of anti-HIV therapy are currently available: (1) viral reverse transcriptase enzyme inhibitors (nucleoside and nucleotide reverse transcriptase inhibitors and nonnucleoside reverse transcriptase inhibitors); (2) viral protease enzyme inhibitors (protease inhibitors); (3) viral integrase enzyme inhibitors (integrase inhibitors); and (4) drugs that interfere with viral entry into the cell (fusion inhibitors and CCR5 antagonists). Box 12.1 lists the currently available antiretroviral agents. Combinations of these agents have also been approved by regulatory authorities, including the U.S. Food and Drug Administration (FDA) and the European Medicines Agency (EMA), and are available commercially.

cART regimens should be based on a number of guiding principles.[13] First, plasma HIV RNA levels indicate the extent of HIV replication and the rate of CD4+ T-cell destruction, and CD4+ T-cell counts indicate the competence of the immune system in persons with HIV infection. Regimens should be designed to provide maximal suppression of HIV infection and to minimize drug resistance. Effective strategies employ the use of combinations of anti-HIV drugs that have not been previously used in a patient and that are not cross-resistant with other drugs the patient has previously received. All drugs should be used at optimal dosages and dosing intervals. Importantly, compliance is critical for efficacy. Therefore it is critical to employ regimens that individual patients can follow. Because lack of adherence to these regimens can lead to resistance and failure of therapy, compliance must be closely monitored.

BOX 12.1 Anti–Human Immunodeficiency Virus (HIV) Medications

Multiclass Combination Drugs

- Efavirenz/emtricitabine/tenofovir disoproxil fumarate (Atripla)
- Emtricitabine/rilpivirine/tenofovir disoproxil fumarate (Complera)
- Atazanavir sulfate/cobicistat (Evotaz)
- Cobicistat/darunavir ethanolate (Prezcobix)
- Elvitegravir/cobicistat/emtricitabine/tenofovir disoproxil fumarate (Stribild)

Nucleoside Reverse Transcriptase Inhibitors

- Lamivudine/zidovudine (Combivir)
- Emtricitabine (FTC) (Emtriva)
- Lamivudine (3TC) (Epivir)
- Abacavir/lamivudine (Epzicom)
- Zalcitabine/dideoxycytidine (ddC) (Hivid)—no longer marketed
- Zidovudine (ZDV)/azidothymidine (AZT) (Retrovir)
- Abacavir/zidovudine/lamivudine (Trizivir)
- Tenofovir disoproxil fumarate/emtricitabine (Truvada)
- Didanosine/dideoxyinosine (ddI) (Videx)
- Tenofovir disoproxil fumarate (TDF) (Viread)
- Stavudine (d4T) (Zerit)
- Abacavir sulfate (ABC) (Ziagen)

Nonnucleoside Reverse Transcriptase Inhibitors

- Rilpivirine (Edurant)
- Etravirine (Intelence)
- Delavirdine (DLV) (Rescriptor)
- Efavirenz (EFV) (Sustiva)
- Nevirapine (NVP) (Viramune)

Protease Inhibitors

- Amprenavir (APV) (Agenerase)—no longer marketed
- Tipranavir (TPV) (Aptivus)
- Indinavir (IDV) (Crixivan)
- Saquinavir (Fortovase)—no longer marketed
- Saquinavir mesylate (SQV) (Invirase)
- Lopinavir (LPV)/ritonavir (RTV) (Kaletra)
- Fosamprenavir calcium (FOS-APV) (Lexiva)
- Ritonavir (RTV) (Norvir)
- Darunavir (Prezista)
- Atazanavir sulfate (ATV) (Reyataz)
- Nelfinavir mesylate (NFV) (Viracept)

Fusion Inhibitors

- Enfuvirtide (T-20) (Fuzeon)

Entry Inhibitors—CCR5 Coreceptor Antagonist

- Celsentri (Selzentry)

HIV Integrase Strand Transfer Inhibitors

- Raltegravir (Isentress)
- Dolutegravir (Tivicay)
- Elvitegravir (Vitekta)

From www.fda.gov.

Ocular Manifestations of HIV Infection

Ocular manifestations of HIV infection occur in every tissue of the eye, from the eyelids to the optic nerve (Box 12.2). The most common findings include dry eye, retinal microvasculopathy, and CMV retinitis. Although direct HIV infection in the

BOX 12.2 Ocular Manifestations of Human Immunodeficiency Virus (HIV) Infection

Eyelids
Molluscum contagiosum
Kaposi sarcoma
Herpes zoster ophthalmicus
Herpes simplex virus cutaneous vesicles
Stevens-Johnson syndrome

Conjunctiva/Sclera
Dry eye[a]
Kaposi sarcoma
Microvasculopathy
Microsporidial conjunctivitis
Herpesvirus conjunctivitis
Scleritis

Cornea
Ulcerative keratitis
Dry eye[a]
Herpes simplex keratitis
Herpes zoster ophthalmicus
Microsporidiosis
Syphilitic keratitis
Tuberculosis
Gonorrhea
Lens
Cataract

Optic Nerve
Optic neuropathy

Retina and Choroid
Microvasculopathy (cotton-wool spots, retinal hemorrhages)[a]
Cytomegalovirus (CMV) retinitis[a]
Acute retinal necrosis
Progressive outer retinal necrosis
Syphilis
Toxoplasmosis
Pneumocystis choroidopathy
Cryptococcosis
Mycobacterial infection
Intraocular lymphoma
Candidiasis
Histoplasmosis

[a] Occurs in more than 5% of patients.

brain appears to produce severe encephalopathy, there is still no definitive evidence that HIV infection of ocular tissue leads to clinically important pathologic effects. However, subclinical infection of retinal neural and endothelial cells has been reported.[8] The retinal microvasculopathy of HIV occurs in 25% to 92% of patients and includes small dot retinal hemorrhages and nerve fiber layer infarcts called cotton-wool spots (Fig. 12.2).[14-17] This retinopathy may be caused by interactions between viral antigens and antibodies that circulate in blood and then are deposited in the eye, but this has not been clearly demonstrated. The incidence of this retinal microvasculopathy increases with the degree of immunosuppression. The presence of the p24 antigen, a surface HIV antigen, in blood also increases with more advanced

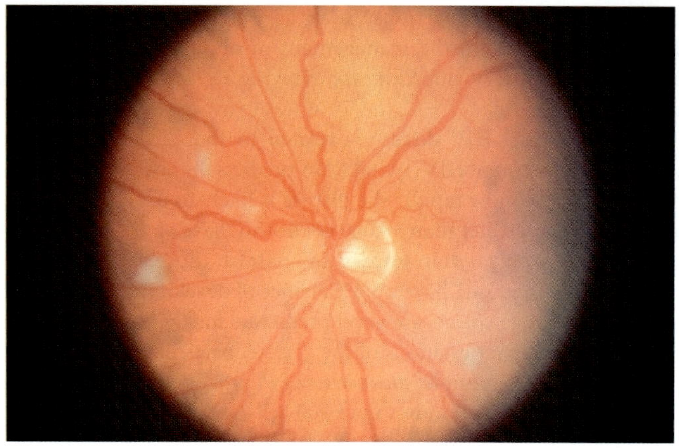

Fig. 12.2 Multiple nerve fiber layer infarcts (cotton-wool spots) in patient with acquired immunodeficiency syndrome (AIDS).

disease, and it is possible that this antigenemia may be a cause of this retinopathy, with immune complex formation in the retinal vasculature. Superficial and deep retinal hemorrhages, retinal perivasculitis, and vascular occlusions also occur. Small peripheral blot hemorrhages are frequently noted on retinal examination and appear to be more common with decreasing CD4+ counts and anemia. Electron microscopic studies of these lesions reveal swollen endothelial cells and degenerating pericytes.[18] Inflammatory cell infiltrates and infectious organisms are not seen in cotton-wool spots; however, the microvascular abnormalities are widespread throughout the retina and may provide an entrance for opportunistic viral infections of the retina.

Clinically, cotton-wool spots are seen as superficial white fluffy lesions in the retina (see Fig. 12.2). There may be small dilations of the microvasculature nearby. Visual symptoms are rarely associated with the presence of a cotton-wool spot. A cotton-wool spot cannot occur in the foveal avascular zone because there is no nerve fiber layer to become infarcted in this part of the retina. Perifoveal cotton-wool spots may cause symptoms. Patients may notice a relative, but not absolute, scotoma. This can be useful in distinguishing a cotton-wool spot from an early area of viral retinitis in which the scotoma is absolute. In patients with AIDS, these lesions can sometimes be more than 0.5 disk diameter in size. They are distinguished from infectious retinitis by the fact that they do not enlarge over time. Although individual lesions will disappear over a period of several months, new lesions often appear. The retinal hemorrhages associated with HIV infection tend to be small dot hemorrhages and rarely cause visual symptoms. Occlusive vasculopathy, such as central retinal vein occlusions, may affect vision.

Dry eye is also a common finding in patients with HIV infection and may be caused by reduced tear production associated with diminished lactoferrin and lysozyme.[19] In most patients, the condition is mild to moderately severe and can be treated with artificial tears. More severe cases of dry eye can occur. Dry eye associated with Stevens-Johnson syndrome has also been reported in patients with AIDS.[20]

Even in the era of cART, many patients with HIV infection have visual symptoms in the absence of active opportunistic infection.[21] Visual acuity, contrast sensitivity, and visual fields are worse than expected compared with a normal age-matched control group. Although the exact pathogenesis of this neuroretinopathy is unknown, causes may include HIV vasculopathy or a direct effect of HIV on the retina and optic nerve, undiagnosed coinfection, or effects from therapy.

BOX 12.3 Common Opportunistic Infections Associated with Human Immunodeficiency Virus (HIV) Infection

Cytomegalovirus (CMV)
Pneumocystis
Mycobacterium tuberculosis
Toxoplasma gondii
Mycobacterium-avium complex
Varicella-zoster virus
Cryptococcus neoformans
Coccidioides immitis
Candida

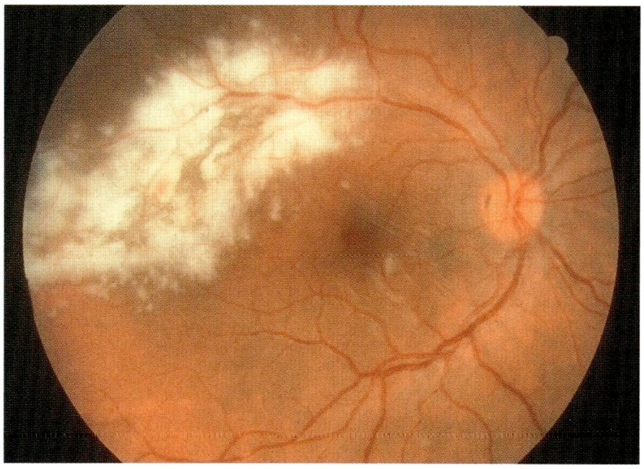

Fig. 12.3 Cytomegalovirus (CMV) retinitis in vascular distribution characterized by fluffy white retinal infiltration and small area of retinal hemorrhage.

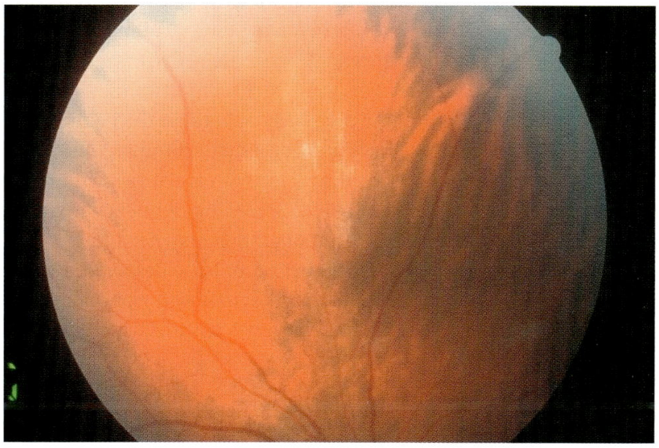

Fig. 12.4 Cytomegalovirus (CMV) retinitis may also have a granular appearance with mottling of retinal pigment epithelium (RPE) and little associated retinal hemorrhage.

Ocular Infection

Numerous other opportunistic infections are associated with HIV infection (Box 12.3). CMV retinitis is the most common ocular infection in AIDS and is discussed in the next section. Other intraocular infections that more frequently occur in patients with AIDS include syphilis, toxoplasmosis, tuberculosis, *Candida* infection, and cryptococcosis.[22-26] These have been discussed in previous chapters and must be differentiated from CMV infection. Herpesvirus infections other than CMV infection can also cause viral retinitis in patients with HIV infection. Herpes zoster ophthalmicus may be an early sign of HIV infection.[27] Herpes zoster retinitis accompanied by acute retinal necrosis (see Chapter 13) and herpes simplex retinitis have occasionally been seen in patients with AIDS.[18] These viral retinal infections are often difficult to differentiate clinically from CMV retinitis. Autopsy studies have shown that greater than 95% of viral retinitis in patients with AIDS is caused by CMV infection.[14,18] However, these studies were completed early in the history of the AIDS epidemic, and the percentages may have changed since that time.

CMV RETINITIS

CMV is a Herpesviridae class virus and contains enveloped, double-stranded DNA. Systemic CMV infection is very common in the general population and causes a heterophilic, antibody-negative mononucleosis syndrome. Therefore many adults have CMV antibodies as a result of previous infection. Approximately 50% of heterosexual men and 95% of homosexual men have evidence of a previous CMV infection. However, with the exception of a few unusual cases, CMV infection of the retina occurs as an opportunistic infection only in immunosuppressed persons or in infants with congenital CMV infection. The disease was first recognized as a congenital infection in 1947. In the past, immunosuppression associated with organ transplantation and chemotherapy was the most common cause of CMV retinitis.[28] It is interesting to note that CMV retinitis is much more frequent after renal transplantation than after bone marrow transplantation. In the current era, however, the increasing number of patients with AIDS has led to a marked increase in the incidence of CMV retinitis. CMV retinitis tends to occur in patients whose immune systems are the most significantly suppressed by HIV infection,[14,29] rarely occurring if the CD4+ count is greater than 100 cells/μL and typically occurring when CD4+ counts are less than 50 cells/μL. Before the widespread use of cART, CMV retinitis was reported in 7% to 40% of patients with AIDS in several series, and probably occurred clinically in at least 15% to 20% of these patients at some time during the course of disease.[14,15,18,22]

CMV retinitis probably reaches the eye via the bloodstream, although the possibility of reactivation of latent virus has not been ruled out. Evidence of hematogenous spread includes the fact that one eye frequently develops retinitis several months before the other and that new foci of retinitis can appear in the affected eye. It is unusual to see more than three separate areas of CMV retinitis in an eye, and most eyes contain one initial focus, which then spreads across the retina.

CMV retinitis begins as small, white retinal infiltrates which, if seen early, may resemble a large cotton-wool spot. Two types of clinical appearance may be seen. The first is a perivascular fluffy white lesion with many scattered hemorrhages (Fig. 12.3). Another manifestation is a more granular-appearing lesion that has few associated hemorrhages and often has a central area of clearing, with atrophic retina and stippled retinal pigment epithelium (Fig. 12.4). In autopsy studies, CMV has been identified in both types of lesion in patients with AIDS. However, because we do not understand what factors predispose a person to one type of lesion, we cannot exclude the possibility that some of these lesions may be other viral retinal infections. It is possible that the underlying immune status of the patient influences the clinical appearance of the lesion. However, local factors also must be important, as an occasional patient will have different-appearing lesions. Both types of lesion respond to the therapeutic approach that will be discussed later, which is consistent with herpes class viral infections of the retina.

The diagnosis of CMV retinitis is based on clinical criteria. Although it is possible to confirm the diagnosis with a polymerase chain reaction

(PCR) analysis performed on a vitreous specimen or with culture of the virus from the vitreous or the retina, this is rarely done in practice. As the number of treatment options grows and becomes more specific, accurate diagnosis will be increasingly important. Active CMV retinitis always has a faint granular border of intraretinal infiltrates, which represent the new foci of viral activity in the normal retina. In addition, the lesion grows at approximately 250 microns per week, and therefore there are usually areas that have begun to atrophy, as denoted by stippling of the retinal pigment epithelium (RPE). This is in contrast to acute retinal necrosis, in which the disease spreads rapidly, and one is less likely to find active retinitis surrounding an atrophic center. There is always low-grade mild vitreous inflammation (vitritis) with CMV retinitis, frequently less than might be expected for the degree of retinal necrosis. Usually, there are only trace vitreous cells with minimal vitreous haze. There may be fine anterior chamber keratic precipitates (KPs), although most patients have no anterior chamber reaction. Vision is normal unless the optic disk or the fovea is involved.

CMV retinitis should be classified on the basis of location and degree of activity. Therefore, determining whether the retinitis is active and the area of the retina that is involved will help guide therapy (Table 12.1 and Fig. 12.6). Active retinitis involving the macula or optic nerve will require more aggressive therapy as discussed later in this chapter.

Patients with CMV retinitis may not complain of symptoms because the lesions begin in the periphery or because the patient often does not notice an increase in floaters or a new scotoma. Therefore it may make clinical sense to screen patients who are at risk with CD4+ counts <50–100 cells/μL. A reasonable screening frequency is every 3 or 4 months for this population, although this may need to be modified as use of oral prophylactic therapies becomes widespread. Because children more rarely complain of visual symptoms, ophthalmologic screening should be performed at least every 3 months when the CD4+ count is less than 50 cells/μL.

Progression

CMV retinitis progresses in two ways. First, new lesions that are not physically near an old one may form, probably via hematogenous spread. Second, and most commonly, an old lesion spreads at its borders to involve new, previously uninfected areas of the retina. In this latter situation, the center of the old lesion eventually ceases to be white because the whiteness results from scattering of light by the edematous and necrotic retina. Once retinal cell death has occurred and only a glial scar remains, the atrophic retina is again transparent with underlying RPE stippling (see Fig. 12.4). Therefore when one assesses the progression and resolution of CMV retinitis, it is most important to pay attention to the edge of the lesions to look for advancement of the border and to not look at the center of the lesion and interpret a decrease in whiteness as an indication of improvement.

CMV infection causes vision loss in several ways. Most commonly, the infected retina is destroyed, and patients develop an absolute scotoma as a result of retinal necrosis. When the macula is involved, central vision is lost. Macular involvement can be a presenting sign of the disease but can also occur late in the course. However, until the macula is involved by active retinitis, the vision can be nearly normal unless there is secondary macular edema from a nearby area of retinitis. Patients can retain normal central vision with only a few degrees of visual field in this disease, and they can be significantly disabled by peripheral retinal destruction. The optic disk can also become involved, and the vision can be lost even when the amount of retinitis is still minimal. In some patients, paramacular CMV infection will produce macular edema, which is a reversible cause of visual loss if it can be treated before the active virus progresses through the fovea. Last, CMV retinitis can cause a rhegmatogenous retinal detachment because there is vitreous traction on the thin, atrophic retina. As you will read in more detail later in this chapter, retinal detachments with CMV retinitis are difficult to treat.

CMV Retinitis in the Era of cART

The presentation and course of CMV retinitis in patients with AIDS have dramatically changed with the use of cART: The incidence has decreased, progression is slower, the clinical manifestations have changed, and, importantly, visual prognosis has greatly improved. Before ART was available, untreated CMV retinitis progressed relentlessly, leading to retinal necrosis and blindness. Even with anti-CMV treatment, the median time to progression of CMV retinitis was approximately 2 months in patients treated with intravenous ganciclovir or foscarnet,[30,31] 2 to 4 months with intravenous cidofovir,[32,33] to 7 months with a sustained-release intravitreal ganciclovir implant.[34]

cART has led to reduced HIV replication, elevations in CD4+ cell counts, and reduced mortality.[35-37] Studying patients with HIV infection and CMV retinitis has allowed us to answer an important clinical question: whether the rejuvenated immune system that results from HAART can effectively control opportunistic infections. The progression of CMV retinitis can be accurately assessed by using the masked grading of standard retinal photographs. We know, for example, that in untreated, immunocompromised patients, CMV retinitis progresses within a median of 2 to 3 weeks.

A number of studies have suggested that ART-induced immune recovery has had a substantial impact on the course of CMV retinitis. Widespread use of cART has led to a decrease in the annual number of new cases of CMV retinitis by greater than 75%.[37,38] In a study of 1255 patients, each of whom had at least one CD4+ cell count less than 100 cells/μL, the incidence of any of three major opportunistic infections, including CMV retinitis, declined from 21.9 per 100 person-years in 1994 to 3.7 per 100 person-years in mid-1997.[37] Immune recovery has also led to improved visual outcomes in patients with CMV retinitis. In a prospective, observational cohort study, the rate of visual field loss was approximately 1% of the normal field per year in persons with immune recovery compared with approximately 7% of the normal field per year in persons without immune recovery.[39] Importantly, median survival after the diagnosis of CMV retinitis was 27 years in persons with immune recovery compared with 1.1 years in those without immune recovery.

Evidence from patients with AIDS and CMV retinitis also suggests that immune recovery with HAART can effectively control the disease in the absence of specific anti-CMV therapy. In 1997, we first reported that CMV retinitis did not progress in four patients receiving HAART despite the fact that they were not receiving anti-CMV therapy.[40] Interestingly, one of these patients never received anti-CMV therapy. Since that time, additional studies have confirmed that CMV retinitis may not be reactivated after maintenance anti-CMV therapy is stopped in patients with HAART-induced immune recovery and that active CMV retinitis may resolve in some patients who never receive specific anti-CMV treatment.[41-47] Reactivation of CMV retinitis can occur, however, especially if CD4+ counts fall to less than 50 cells/μL.[42] Furthermore, there have been some sporadic reports of CMV retinitis occurring in patients who were receiving HAART and had stable CD4+ counts of greater than 100 cells/μL. An observational study conducted in seven European HIV cohorts followed up 358 patients who were taking potent ART and in whom maintenance therapy was interrupted because of opportunistic pathogens at a CD4+ lymphocyte count greater than 50 cells/μL.[48] Of these 358 patients, 162 had CMV end-organ disease. Two relapses of CMV retinitis occurred during the study. The CD4+ counts at the time of relapse were 91 cells/μL in one patient and 247 cells/μL in the other. Nevertheless, the CD4+ count appears to be the best predictor of an effective immune response against CMV, including other laboratory

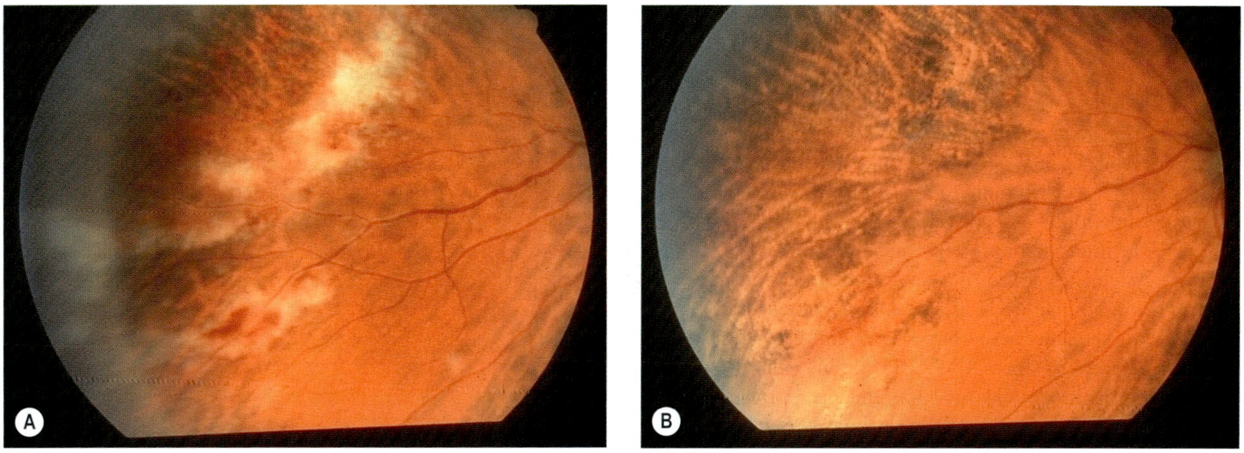

Fig. 12.5 (A) Retinal photograph of area of cytomegalovirus (CMV) retinitis in patient with acquired immunodeficiency syndrome (AIDS). (B) Same area after 6 weeks of anti-CMV therapy.

parameters, such as HIV load and CMV culture data. Researchers have investigated whether CMV load[45] or CMV-specific CD4+ cell responses quantified by flow cytometry[49] can quantify and predict an effective clinical immune response against CMV, but the incidence is currently so low that adequately powered clinical studies are difficult to conduct.

Some data have suggested that patients may need to receive cART for several months before the immune response against opportunistic infections is effectively restored.[50] Because the proportion of naïve T cells increases after about 3 months of HAART,[51] specific anti-CMV therapy should be continued for at least 3 months after CD4+ counts have increased with HAART.

Treatment

A number of medications have now been approved by the FDA for the treatment of CMV retinitis: ganciclovir and its derivatives, foscarnet, cidofovir, and fomivirsen. A sustained-release intravitreal ganciclovir implant was approved for the treatment of CMV retinitis in 1995 but was discontinued by the manufacturer in 2013 because of decreased demand. Prior to the advent of cART, patients were usually treated with induction doses of intravenous ganciclovir or foscarnet, followed by lower maintenance doses of the drug for life. Even with this therapy, recurrences were common. Use of the sustained-release ganciclovir implant more effectively treated ocular disease, but did not treat the systemic CMV infection. Now, with the use of ART and the development of orally bioavailable anti-CMV drugs, such as valganciclovir, intravenous ganciclovir and foscarnet are used less frequently.

Ganciclovir [9-(1,3-dihydroxy-2-propoxymethyl) guanine] was the first drug approved by the FDA for the treatment of CMV retinitis. Acyclovir is not sufficiently active against CMV infection, whereas ganciclovir is virostatic both in vitro and in vivo. Ganciclovir is triphosphorylated in the cell and then inhibits viral DNA polymerase. Therapy with 5 mg/kg intravenously twice daily for 14 to 21 days will halt the progression of CMV infection and the development of a less active lesion in greater than 90% of patients[52-54] (Fig. 12.5). However, because the drug is virostatic, recurrences are common unless the underlying immunosuppression can be altered. In patients with AIDS, the median time to progression of retinitis without treatment is 21 days. Intravenous administration of ganciclovir, 5 mg/kg/day, 7 days per week, prolongs the median time to relapse to 56 days, and many patients go significantly longer without a relapse.[55] After treatment visual loss caused by macular edema often improves, but visual loss caused by retinal necrosis does not. The usual therapy for CMV retinitis in immunocompromised patients includes induction therapy with intravenous ganciclovir at a dose of 5 mg/kg twice daily for 14 to 21 days, followed by maintenance therapy at a dose of 5 mg/kg once daily. The main toxicity of ganciclovir therapy is neutropenia.[55] Neutrophil counts should be maintained higher than 500/μL.

Foscarnet was the second drug approved by the FDA for the treatment of CMV retinitis. It inhibits DNA polymerase in a manner different from that of ganciclovir. In addition to being inhibitory to CMV and other herpes viruses, it inhibits reverse transcriptase and the replication of HIV. It is also administered intravenously with a 2- to 3-week induction dosage of either 60 mg/kg three times daily or 90 mg/kg twice daily, followed by maintenance therapy with 90 mg/kg or 120 mg/kg daily.[56] Foscarnet is less toxic to bone marrow compared with ganciclovir, but is nephrotoxic and leads to electrolyte abnormalities in serum calcium, phosphate, and magnesium levels.

Ganciclovir and foscarnet were compared in a multicenter trial conducted by Studies of Ocular Complications of AIDS (SOCA)[55] in which 234 patients with newly diagnosed CMV retinitis were randomly assigned to receive ganciclovir or foscarnet. Both drugs were found to be equally effective in preventing the progression of CMV retinitis, with a median time to progression of approximately 8 weeks for each drug. Although foscarnet was shown to increase survival to 12 months after diagnosis compared with 8 months with ganciclovir in patients with normal renal function, this difference in survival has not been seen in subsequent studies of the two medications. The study also showed that there was more neutropenia with ganciclovir but more infusion-related symptoms, genitourinary symptoms, nephrotoxic effects, and electrolyte abnormalities with foscarnet.[57] The combination of intravenous ganciclovir and intravenous foscarnet appears to be more effective for controlling CMV retinitis compared with monotherapy.[58,59]

Cidofovir is a cytosine-derived nucleotide analogue with a long half-life that is also FDA approved for the treatment of CMV retinitis. Cidofovir at a dose of 5 mg/kg is given intravenously once a week for 2 weeks for induction.[32] Maintenance doses of cidofovir are 3 to 5 mg/kg administered intravenously once every other week. Nephrotoxicity is the major adverse event associated with cidofovir. To reduce renal toxicity, cidofovir should be given with probenecid and adequate intravenous hydration. Because of the renal toxicity, cidofovir should not be used with foscarnet; it is less commonly used compared with other available medications.

Leflunomide is an immunosuppressive agent that inhibits virion assembly. Although not FDA approved for the treatment of CMV retinitis, systemic leflunomide has been used to treat multidrug-resistant CMV retinitis.[60]

Two anti-CMV medications have been approved for intravitreal use to treat CMV retinitis: fomivirsen and a sustained-release ganciclovir implant. The nonbioerodible ganciclovir implant releases 1 μg of drug per hour for 8 months and is surgically implanted through the pars plana. The mean time to progression with this implant is 226 days, with CMV retinitis developing in about 50% of untreated contralateral eyes during the study.[34] The efficacy of this device for treating local CMV retinitis was clearly superior to systemic therapy, but the implant does not treat systemic CMV infection or prevent occurrence in the contralateral eye. Therefore, systemic treatment is often required in addition to the ganciclovir implant. Fomivirsen is an antisense oligonucleotide that is complementary to a sequence in messenger RNA (mRNA) of the major immediate early region 2 of human CMV and inhibits replication of the virus.[61] Although intravitreous cidofovir was effective in treating CMV retinitis, its use was limited by side effects, including uveitis and macular edema.[62] However, neither the ganciclovir implant nor the intravitreous formulation of cidofovir is available from the manufacturer. Intravenous formulations of both drugs are still commercially available.

Historically, intravitreal injections of ganciclovir,[63] foscarnet,[64] or cidofovir were used for long periods to treat CMV retinitis.[65,66] Many clinicians previously used intravitreous injections of ganciclovir or foscarnet off label to treat recurrent CMV infection, especially in patients resistant to or intolerant of systemic therapy. Studies of the ganciclovir implant clearly showed that local administration with anti-CVM therapy was superior to systemic therapy in treating CMV retinitis. But patients still required systemic therapy to treat the systemic infection. Fortunately, in the era of cART, long-term CMV therapy is rarely necessary in patients with immune reconstitution.

Oral Anti-CMV Drugs

Oral formulations of ganciclovir have been developed. A randomized controlled trial (RCT) showed that once-daily oral valganciclovir was as clinically effective and well tolerated as oral ganciclovir three times daily for CMV prevention in high-risk solid organ transplant recipients.[67] Valganciclovir is an orally administered prodrug that is rapidly hydrolyzed to ganciclovir and is now the formulation most commonly used. The recommended dose for newly diagnosed CMV retinitis is 900 mg twice daily for 2 to 3 weeks, followed by 900 mg once daily. If used in combination with intravitreous ganciclovir, the dose of valganciclovir is usually 900 mg once daily. Orally administered valganciclovir appears to be as effective as intravenous ganciclovir for induction treatment and effective for long-term maintenance therapy for CMV retinitis in patients with AIDS.[68] As with intravenous ganciclovir, the major toxicity is bone marrow suppression with neutropenia and thrombocytopenia.

Current Therapeutic Approach to CMV Retinitis in the HAART Era

How has cART altered the treatment strategy for CMV retinitis? First, we now know that immune recovery after cART has reduced the incidence of opportunistic infections and can also control pre-existing infections, including CMV retinitis. As a result, lifelong anti-CMV therapy is no longer required for patients who have documented improvements in CD4+ T-cell counts after cART. In fact, most clinicians stop maintenance anti-CMV therapy in patients with stable CMV retinitis if CD4+ cell counts are stable or increasing and have been greater than 100–150 cells/μL for 6 months.[69] Freedom from anti-CMV therapy has improved the quality of life of our patients. Nevertheless, they must be closely followed up to monitor for reactivation of retinitis or the development of extraocular disease. If the CD4+ count falls to less than 50 cells/μL, the clinician should consider restarting anti-CMV therapy or, at least, plan to re-examine the patient more frequently.

TABLE 12.1 Therapeutic Approach for Cytomegalovirus (CMV) Retinitis

Zone 1 disease	Intravitreous ganciclovir or foscarnet combined with systemic anti-CMV therapy (usually oral valganciclovir)
Zone 2 or 3 disease	Systemic anti-CMV therapy (oral valganciclovir or intravenous (IV) ganciclovir or IV foscarnet)
Disease that progresses despite therapy	Intravitreous ganciclovir or foscarnet combined with systemic anti-CMV therapy (IV foscarnet should be considered if retinitis progressed on IV)

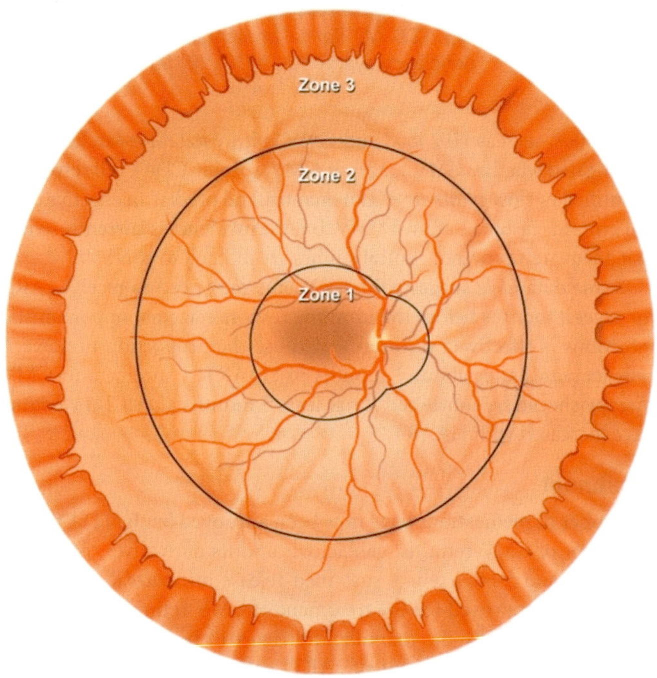

Fig. 12.6 Zones of retinal involvement developed by the Studies of Ocular Complications of AIDS (SOCA). A zone 1 lesion is present within either a circle around the fovea with a radius of 3000 μm or within 1500 μm of the edge of the optic nerve. A zone 2 lesion is present outside of zone 1 but is posterior to the ampullae of the vortex veins located at the equatorial retina. A zone 3 lesion is present between zone 2 and the ora serrata. (Reproduced with permission from Stewart MW. Optimal management of cytomegalovirus retinitis in patients with AIDS, Figure 5. *Clin Ophthalmol.* 2010;4:285–299.)

The therapeutic approach to CMV retinitis is now based on the patient's immune status in relation to cART, the location of CMV retinitis in the eye, and patient input (Table 12.1). Because we know that CMV can be effectively controlled with an improved immune status after cART, the initial goal of therapy is starting or optimizing ART to maximize efficacy in decreasing the HIV load and increasing CD4+ T-cell counts. However, if there is no significant improvement in CD4+ counts despite cART, it must be assumed that anti-CMV therapy will be required for longer than several months, and this will alter the therapeutic approach. Similarly, the approach to patients with CMV retinitis in zone 1, an area of the retina that extends 3000 μm from the center of the fovea or 1500 μm from the edge of the optic nerve (Fig. 12.6), is different from the approach to patients who have more peripheral and less immediately sight-threatening disease.

TABLE 12.2 Medications and Dosages for Cytomegalovirus Retinitis

Medication	Induction Therapy	Maintenance Therapy
Ganciclovir	Intravenous (IV) 5 mg/kg twice daily for 14–21 days	5 mg/kg daily
Foscarnet	IV 90 mg/kg twice daily for 14 days	120 mg/kg daily
Cidofovir	IV 5 mg/kg weekly for 3 weeks	5 mg/kg every 2 weeks
Valganciclovir	Oral 900 mg twice daily	900 mg daily
Ganciclovir	Intravitreal 2 mg 1–4 times to halt retinitis	2 mg weekly
Foscarnet	Intravitreal 1.2–2.4 mg 1–2 times weekly	1.2 mg weekly
Cidofovir	Intravitreal 20 μg 1–8 times	20 μg every 5–6 weeks

Again, the main treatment goal for patients who are ART naïve or who have started ART within the last several months is to limit the CMV infection until the immune system improves and controls the infection on its own. For active disease and retinitis near the macula or optic nerve (Zone 1 disease), most clinicians still recommend a combination of systemic and intravitreal injections of anti-CMV therapy.[70] This regimen provides the best ocular drug levels to control CMV retinitis and prevent potentially sight-threatening disease progression, and it also controls systemic CMV disease. Combination of systemic and intravitreal therapy is also used in patients with progressive retinitis despite systemic therapy and in patients intolerant to systemic therapy. Some patients refuse intravitreal therapy, and these patients are treated with higher induction doses of valganciclovir and watched very carefully for disease progression. Patients with peripheral, non–sight-threatening disease can be treated with systemic therapy alone. For all patients with CMV retinitis, systemic therapy is indicated to decrease the CMV viral load, improve survival, and prevent CMV retinitis in the other eye in those with uniocular retinitis.[71] A list of the medications and dosing regimens available to treat CMV retinitis is provided in Table 12.2.[70]

Oral formulations of ganciclovir can be used as maintenance therapy for CMV retinitis but may be somewhat less effective than intravenous therapy. In an open-label study, after induction therapy with intravenous ganciclovir, patients were randomly assigned to receive maintenance intravenous ganciclovir or oral ganciclovir at a dose of 1000 mg, three times a day.[72] Although the mean time to progression of retinitis was 62 days with intravenous therapy and 57 days with oral therapy, the median time to progression was 49 days with intravenous treatment and 29 days with oral treatment. Valganciclovir, the orally administered prodrug of ganciclovir, appears to be as effective as intravenous ganciclovir for induction treatment and may be effective for the long-term management of CMV retinitis in patients with AIDS.[73] The usual dose is 900 mg once daily. An effective oral preparation of foscarnet is not available. Finally, viral PCR testing of blood specimens for resistance-conferring mutations may help guide therapy in some patients.[74]

Retinal Detachment

Retinal detachment develops in approximately 20% of patients with retinitis, 50% of these patients developing detachment in the second eye if it has retinitis. Approximately 11% of patients with retinitis will experience retinal detachment 6 months after diagnosis, and 24% will have detachment over the first year after diagnosis in the first eye.[75] The greater the amount of peripheral retinal involvement, the greater is the risk of retinal detachment. Compared with eyes with 10% of the peripheral retina involved, eyes with greater than 25% involvement had a five-fold increase in the detachment rate. This risk increased 24-fold if active retinitis also was present. The use of cART did not change the outcomes of retinal detachment surgery in patients with CMV retinitis.[76]

Because the mechanism of retinal detachment in CMV retinitis is vitreous traction on the thinned, atrophic retina, multiple retinal breaks are usually present and large, relatively posterior breaks can occur. Tears can occur not only at the edge of the normal retina but also throughout the atrophic areas. The risk of retinal detachment is increased if the patient with CMV retinitis has myopia. The posterior vitreous usually adheres to the retina, and the combination of low-grade vitritis with a thinned retina allows the vitreous to pull the retina forward, causing it to become detached. The rate of growth of the detachment is variable and depends on the extent of traction and location within the eye.

The standard surgical approach for retinal detachment is not optimal for eyes with CMV retinitis. Scleral buckling is appropriate when retinal breaks are located near the vitreous base. The breaks in eyes with CMV retinitis often are more posterior and multiple. Scleral buckling may be successful in selected patients, but a more effective approach is vitrectomy, endolaser surgery, and the application of silicone oil tamponade. Head position can be more normal, although patients still cannot lie on their backs. Vision can be rehabilitated in a few days. The surgery can be performed as a local, outpatient procedure with minimal postoperative discomfort.

The use of laser surgery to demarcate areas of retinitis and thereby prevent detachment has been suggested. A similar approach is often used in acute retinal necrosis caused by herpes zoster infection. Although there is evidence in the literature to support this approach, it is not uniformly successful, and because CMV retinitis often continues to progress through a barrier of laser burns, this approach will not prevent either spread or detachment in all patients. Nevertheless, anatomic success was achieved in 14 (73.7%) of 19 eyes with CMV retinitis related retinal detachment treated with surgery.[77] Importantly, 36.8% of eyes had improvement of two or more lines in visual acuity, and 42.1% of eyes maintained visual acuity.

Prognosis

Advances in the drugs we use to treat both HIV and CMV infections have greatly improved the visual prognosis in patients with CMV retinitis. Complications, including destruction of the macula from disease progression and retinal detachment, are reduced, and this is a welcome outcome of improved treatment. Data have suggested that patients with CMV retinitis have visual impairment at a rate of 0.10 case/eye-year and blindness at a rate of 0.06 case/eye-year.[78] In a study of long-term outcomes of CMV retinitis in the era of modern ART, the rate of bilateral visual impairment was 0.9 per 100 person-years and the rate of blindness was 0.5 per 100 person-years.[79] Among patients with immune recovery, the rate of visual field loss was approximately 1% of the normal field per year compared with approximately 7% of the normal field per year in patients without immune recovery.

Immune Recovery Uveitis

Although HAART-associated improvements in immune function have improved the clinical course of CMV retinitis, immune restoration has also led to a change in the clinical manifestations of the disease. Vitritis was reported in immunocompromised patients with CMV retinitis before HAART.[80] However, more profound intraocular inflammation is occurring in patients with CMV retinitis receiving

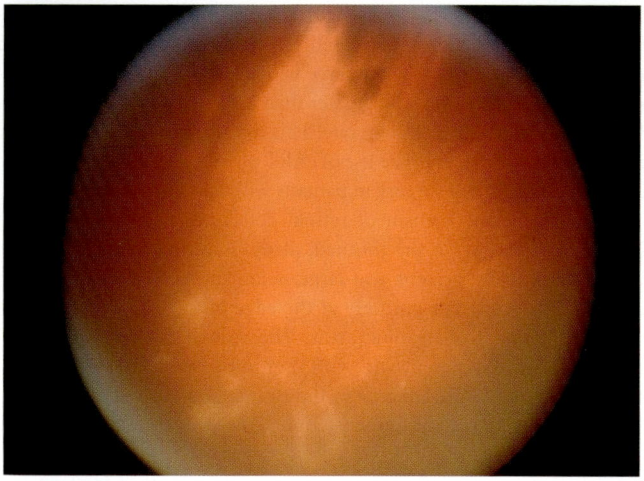

Fig. 12.7 Dense vitritis in a patient with immune-recovery uveitis in the eye with inactive cytomegalovirus (CMV) retinitis.

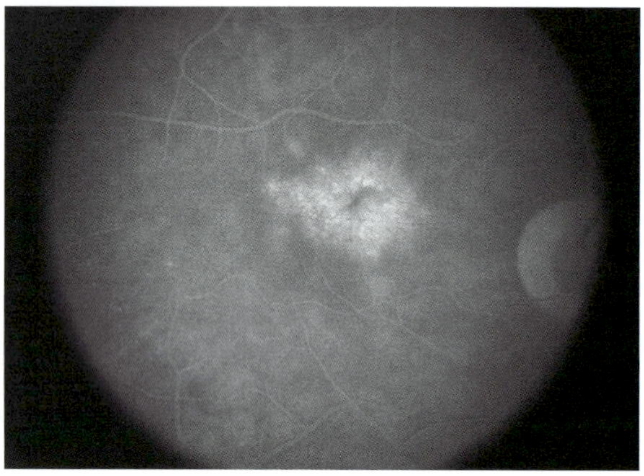

Fig. 12.8 Cystoid macular edema in a patient with immune recovery uveitis and inactive cytomegalovirus (CMV) retinitis.

HAART.[42,46,81-84] Initially, this syndrome was referred to as *immune recovery vitritis*[85]; however, because the inflammation is characterized not only by a profound vitritis (Fig. 12.7) but also by anterior uveitis, cataract, macular edema (Fig. 12.8), epiretinal membranes, and optic disk edema, we have used the term *immune recovery uveitis* (IRU).[43,86,87] In a prospective clinical trial in which specific anti-CMV therapy was discontinued in 14 patients with stable CMV retinitis and HIV infection during HAART, 12 (89.7%) of the 14 patients had IRU before their CMV therapy was stopped.[43] Three of these 12 patients had a profound increase in IRU during the course of the trial. Other investigators have reported high rates of IRU in patients with stable CMV retinitis receiving HAART;[88] however, there is large variability in the prevalence of this finding. High rates of IRU may be related to better immune responses in these patients as a result of strict compliance with aggressive HAART. The median CD4+ count at baseline in the study detailed earlier was greater than 300 cells/μL. The amount of CMV antigen in the eye may also affect the development of IRU. The incidence of IRU may be lower in patients with CMV retinitis who have not received HAART before the control of retinal disease with anti-CMV therapy.[89] With the widespread use of cART, the incidence rate of IRU is 2.2/100 person-years.[79]

Interestingly, in our prospective study of patients with CMV retinitis receiving HAART, no new retinal detachments occurred during the study.[45] This is surprising because the risk of retinal detachment in a similar population before the use of HAART was 19% at 6 months.[90] Intraocular inflammation and hypertrophy of the RPE may lead to increased adherence of the retina and a reduced risk of retinal detachment.

Immune recovery uveitis may require treatment, especially in patients with macular edema and early epiretinal membrane. Although the best therapy has yet to be established, we have treated anterior uveitis with topical prednisolone acetate. In addition, we have used periocular injections of triamcinolone or short courses of prednisone to treat vitritis and macular edema associated with decreased visual acuity. Intravitreal triamcinolone has been used to treat macular edema associated with IRU.[91] The fluocinolone implant has been used to treat macular edema in patients with AIDS and a history of CMV;[92] however, because the fluocinolone implant has been associated with the development of CMV retinitis, concurrent anti-CMV therapy should be considered, especially in patients who later develop low CD4+ T-cell counts.

The exact mechanism of immune recovery uveitis has not been elucidated. It does not occur in eyes without CMV retinitis; therefore the inflammation appears to be related to the infection, but it is unclear whether IRU is related partly to subclinical viral replication in the eye. If this were true, therapy with specific anti-CMV therapy might limit the uveitis, but this has yet to be demonstrated. In any event, the severity of IRU appears to be related to the amount of infected retina. In our experience, eyes without IRU had very small areas of retinitis. This could be related either to the amount of CMV antigen in the eye or to the degree of the breakdown in the blood–retina barrier as a result of the retinal necrosis. Finally, the type of anti-CMV therapy could also affect the amount of retinal involvement and CMV antigen in the eye. More effective treatment may reduce CMV involvement of the retina and limit the development of IRU.

Other inflammatory diseases have developed after immune recovery in patients receiving HAART. Patients with subclinical *Mycobacterium avium* complex infection develop fever, leukocytosis, and lymphadenitis after the initiation of HAART.[93] Meningitis has been reported in patients with latent cryptococcal central nervous system infection after initiation of HAART.[94] In resource-limited countries, tuberculosis is commonly noted after initiation of HAART and is one of the major opportunistic infections seen in many parts of the world.

HERPES ZOSTER

Herpes zoster ophthalmicus occurs more frequently in patients who are HIV-positive and may often be the presenting sign of the infection. Cutaneous zoster occurring in a severely immunosuppressed patient with AIDS is likely to disseminate and be difficult to treat with acyclovir, which is more effective in the immunocompetent patient. Intravenously administered acyclovir sometimes is required for cutaneous dermatomal zoster, and is certainly needed for disseminated zoster.

Varicella-zoster virus (VZV) retinitis in the patient who is HIV-positive has a somewhat more varied clinical spectrum than that seen in patients who are immunocompetent. Although the clinical picture in some patients is identical to that of acute retinal necrosis, other clinical appearances have been described. In a study by Sellitti et al., 17% of patients who are HIV-positive with herpes zoster ophthalmicus subsequently developed acute retinal necrosis.[95] A form of retinitis termed *progressive outer retinal necrosis* (PORN) appears as multifocal areas of retinitis with good preservation of the inner retina and retinal vasculature in the early clinical stages[96] (discussed in detail in Chapter 13). The areas of necrosis occasionally appear similar to those in acute retinal necrosis. In progressive outer retinal necrosis the lesions are small, often multifocal, and consist of multiple punctate white retinal

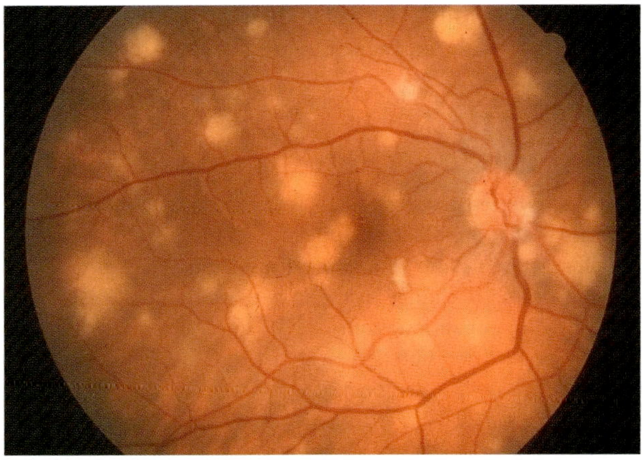

Fig. 12.9 Fundus photograph of patient with acquired immunodeficiency syndrome (AIDS) and *Pneumocystis carinii* pneumonia shows multiple yellow deep choroidal lesions. Histopathologic examination revealed not only *P. carinii* cysts but also cytomegalovirus (CMV) (see Fig. 12.10) and *Mycobacterium avium-intracellulare* (see Fig. 12.11). (From Whitcup SM, Fenton RM, Pluda JM, et al. *Pneumocystis carinii* and *Mycobacterium avium-intracellulare* infection of the choroid. *Retina.* 1992;12:331–335.)

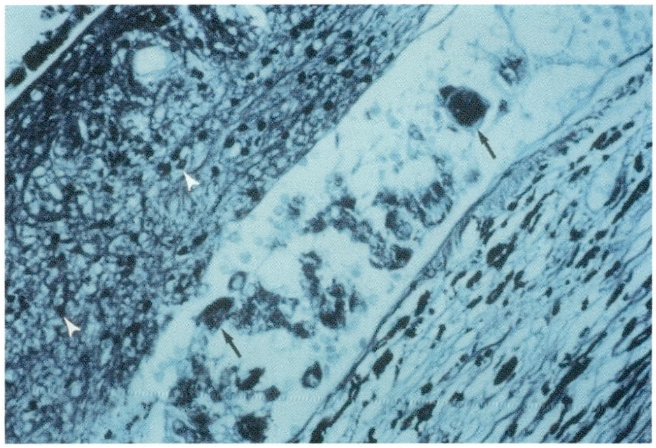

Fig. 12.10 Photomicrograph of choroidal lesion in the right eye showing numerous *Pneumocystis carinii* cysts *(white arrowheads)* and cytomegalovirus (CMV) cells in choroidal blood vessel *(arrows).* (Gomori methenamine silver stain; ×400.) (From Whitcup SM, Fenton RM, Pluda JM, et al. *Pneumocystis carinii* and *Mycobacterium avium-intracellulare* infection of the choroid. *Retina.* 1992;12:331–335.)

dots located in the outer retina (see Figs. 13.6 and 13.9). In some other patients, multiple retinal vascular occlusions with areas of retinitis may manifest initially (see Fig. 13.8).

Response to systemic acyclovir in these immunosuppressed patients is inconsistent. Approximately half have a good response to intravenous acyclovir followed by oral acyclovir, with resultant quieting of the retinitis. Some of these patients can be weaned from the oral drug, but others have recurrences without maintenance therapy.[97] In contrast, some patients experience progressive retinitis despite treatment with intravenous acyclovir. Also, because of the rapid progression of PORN and the difficulty in making a definitive diagnosis, many clinicians start therapy with acyclovir and foscarnet to treat CMV retinitis and provide "double coverage" for the PORN. A combination of intravitreal and intravenous antiviral therapy has also been used to treat the disease.[98,99] Despite therapy, the disease can be relentlessly progressive, and severe visual disability can result. The risk of retinal detachment appears to be similar in immunosuppressed and immunocompetent patients with VZV retinitis, and repair techniques are similar. With HAART, once the CD4+ T cell counts rise, antiviral therapy for zoster may be discontinued in some patients.

The major differential diagnosis in the patient who is HIV-positive is between CMV and VZV retinitis. This differentiation is important because acyclovir is considerably less toxic than either ganciclovir or foscarnet but, although effective for treating PORN, is not effective in treating CMV retinitis. Nevertheless, it is important to remember that CMV retinitis is at least 20 times more common than VZV retinitis in patients with HIV, and the differential diagnosis is based primarily on clinical criteria, taking into account the rate of progression and the multifocality.

PNEUMOCYSTIS JIROVECII CHOROIDITIS

Pneumocystis carinii was first reported by Macher et al.[100] Since that time, it has been renamed *Pneumocystis jirovecii* and classified as a fungus. The choroiditis caused by this organism is characterized by multifocal white plaques in the choroid, with little evidence of intraocular inflammation (Fig. 12.9).[101] It is an extrapulmonary form of pneumocystic disease, usually seen in patients using a prophylactic inhalant, which prevents pulmonary involvement but does not provide systemic prophylaxis. This has become a less common problem because the use of aerosolized pentamidine has decreased. Histopathologic examination in these patients shows numerous cysts in the choroid (Fig. 12.10).

The lesions rarely cause visual loss because they are located beneath the RPE and have no associated inflammation. Trimethoprim-sulfamethoxazole is usually the first-choice agent. Alternative agents include dapsone, aerosolized pentamidine, and atovaquone. Histologic examination has demonstrated large numbers of cysts with no host response. It is important to identify this disease so that the internist can be aware of the potential for extrapulmonary pneumocystic involvement. The ocular disease is associated with prophylactic aerosolized pentamidine and appears to be less common because aerosolized pentamidine use has decreased.

MYCOBACTERIUM AVIUM-INTRACELLULARE CHOROIDITIS

M. avium-intracellulare manifests as infiltrates, usually 50 to 100 μm in size and scattered throughout the fundus.[102,103] It usually causes no visual symptoms but, as in the case of pneumocystic disease, is evidence of disseminated systemic infection. *M. avium-intracellulare* is a common pathogen in patients with AIDS and often involves bone marrow and leads to marrow failure.

OTHER DISEASES

Multiple infections in a single eye may be present in patients with AIDS. Choroidal lesions, such as those caused by *Pneumocystis,* can be seen concurrently with infections by other organisms, such as CMV and *M. avium-intracellulare* (see Fig. 12.10; Fig. 12.11), but the greatest concern is a CMV infection combined with herpes zoster or herpes simplex. In this situation, the retinitis response can be atypical, and if the zoster infection is treated with acyclovir the CMV infection will continue to progress. Toxoplasmosis, which is discussed in Chapter 15, is also seen as a retinal infection with a vitritis and should be managed with an antitoxoplasmosis regimen.[103] In addition, B-cell lymphoma can occur in AIDS, manifesting as choroidal, retinal, or vitreous lesions.[104] A posterior ocular process that fails to respond to the therapy chosen on the basis of the clinical presentation may require biopsy to ascertain the

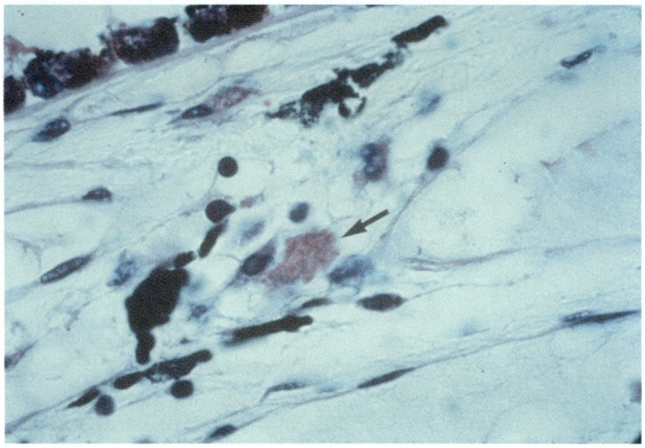

Fig. 12.11 Photomicrograph of choroid adjacent to area infiltrated with *Pneumocystis carinii* shows cluster of acid-fast bacilli *(arrow)*. (Ziehl-Neelsen stain; ×100.) (From Whitcup SM, Fenton RM, Pluda JM, et al. *Pneumocystis carinii* and *Mycobacterium avium-intracellulare* infection of the choroid. *Retina*. 1992;12:331–335.)

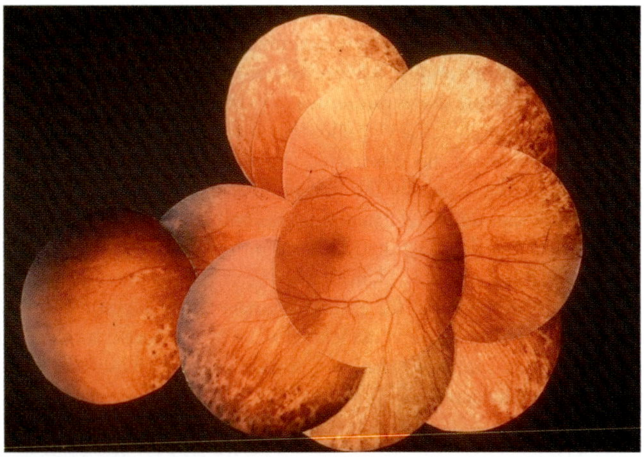

Fig. 12.12 Photographic montage of patient with didanosine-related retinal lesions. Atrophic areas of retinal pigment epithelium (RPE) hypopigmentation and hyperpigmentation are seen in the midperiphery of the fundus.

presence of lymphoma. Finally, syphilis is becoming increasingly common in HIV-infected patients and is discussed in detail in Chapter 11.[105]

DRUG-RELATED OCULAR INFLAMMATION

Several reports have identified both anterior and posterior uveitis in patients treated with rifabutin.[106] These inflammatory findings can occur months after initiation of therapy. Rifabutin is used to treat *M. avium-intracellulare* infection. Severe uveitis that is often bilateral can result. The uveitis associated with rifabutin is most commonly seen in persons also receiving fluconazole or a macrolide drug, which raises serum levels of rifabutin. The inflammation responds to appropriate steroid therapy or to a reduction in the rifabutin dosage. The mechanism of this inflammation is unclear and may be either direct drug hypersensitivity or a response to mycobacterial death, with a subsequent inflammatory response. In addition, we have described retinal lesions that appear to predominantly involve the RPE in patients treated with the antiretroviral agent didanosine (Fig. 12.12).[107] Uveitis, including intraocular inflammation and RPE changes, has been reported in about 25% of patients treated with fomivirsen, but this drug is no longer commercially available.

SUMMARY

Remarkable progress has been made in the treatment of HIV infection and the associated opportunistic infections, but, of course, we have far to go before we can claim victory over this disease. Nevertheless, there has been a dramatic change in the presentation and course of many of the ophthalmic manifestations of HIV infection, particularly CMV retinitis. Case 12.1 describes a typical case of CMV retinitis before the use of cART. Case 12.2 demonstrates the differences in the course of the disease after cART.

CASE 12.1

A 42-year-old man with a diagnosis of acquired immunodeficiency syndrome (AIDS) reported a 2-week history of reduced vision in the right eye. He had no light perception in this eye and 20/20 visual acuity in the left eye. The right eye contained 1+ vitreous cells and had a significant area of necrotic retinitis involving the optic disk. Blood cultures were positive for cytomegalovirus (CMV). The left eye had a small white infiltrate, with an associated hemorrhage near the superior vascular arcade.

Over the next few weeks, the area of involvement in the left eye increased in size. Treatment with ganciclovir was begun, resulting in a marked improvement in both eyes. Vision did not return in the right eye. Ganciclovir therapy was discontinued after 3 weeks, and the vision in the left eye remained 20/20 for 2 weeks. It then decreased to 20/300 because of macular edema. The area of necrotic retinitis was larger. A second course of ganciclovir was begun; the retinitis again resolved, and the vision returned to 20/25. Maintenance therapy was begun, but because of neutropenia, the patient could not tolerate a dose of 5 mg/kg, 5 days/week. He lost all vision in the left eye approximately 2 months later and died several weeks after that.

CASE 12.2

A 37-year-old man who had a CD4+ cell count of 5/μL was diagnosed with acquired immunodeficiency syndrome (AIDS). Routine ophthalmologic examination revealed active cytomegalovirus (CMV) retinitis in both eyes. Combination antiretroviral therapy (cART) was begun. The CMV retinitis was initially treated with intravenous ganciclovir, but the therapy was changed to intravenous foscarnet because of leukopenia.

The human immunodeficiency virus (HIV) load decreased to an undetectable level, and the CMV retinitis remained quiescent with foscarnet therapy. Upon examination, visual acuity was 20/25 in the right eye and 20/40 in the left eye. Slit-lamp biomicroscopy revealed anterior chamber cells, flare, and moderate vitritis in both eyes. Retinal examination revealed stable CMV retinitis involving the midperipheral retina bilaterally. There was slight macular edema, which was worse in the left eye. The CD4+ cell count increased, and anti-CMV therapy was stopped. The CMV retinitis remained inactive when anti-CMV therapy was stopped; however, over the next year, the vitritis and macular edema in both eyes worsened, with visual acuity dropping to 20/40 in the right eye and 20/63 in the left. The patient was offered treatment with corticosteroids as anti-inflammatory drug therapy but he refused the proposed treatment.

REFERENCES

1. Achega JB, Hislop M, Dowdy DW, et al. Adherence to nonnucleoside reverse transcriptase inhibitor-based HIV therapy and virologic outcomes. *Ann Intern Med*. 2007;146:564–573.
2. Gallo R. The AIDS virus. *Sci Am*. 1987;256:46–56.
3. Centers for Disease Control and Prevention. *HIV Surveillance Report*. Vol. 29. 2017. http://www.cdc.gov/hiv/library/reports/HIV-surveillance.html. Published November 2019. Accessed April 12, 2019.
4. Curran JW, Morgan WM, Hardy AM, et al. The epidemiology of AIDS: current status and future prospects. *Science*. 1985;229:1352–1357.
5. Layon J, Warzynski M, Idus R. Acquired immunodeficiency syndrome in the United States a selective review. *Crit Care Med*. 1986;14:819–827.
6. Centers for Disease Control and Prevention. *Quick Reference Guide: Recommended laboratory HIV testing algorithm for serum or plasma specimens*; 2018. https://stacks.cdc.gov/view/cdc/50872.
7. Salahuddin SZ, Palestine AG, Heck E, et al. Isolation of the human T-cell leukemia/lymphotropic virus type III from the cornea. *Am J Ophthalmol*. 1986;101:149–152.
8. Pomerantz RJ, Kuritzkes DR, de la Monte SM, et al. Infection of the retina by human immunodeficiency virus type I. *N Engl J Med*. 1987;317:1643–1647.
9. Panel on Opportunistic Infections in HIV-Infected Adults and Adolescents. Guidelines for the prevention and treatment of opportunistic infections in HIV-infected adults and adolescents: recommendations from the Centers for Disease Control and Prevention, the National Institutes of Health, and the HIV Medicine Association of the Infectious Diseases Society of America. http://aidsinfo.nih.gov/contentfiles/lvguidelines/adult oi.pdf. Accessed April 16, 2019.
10. Mellors JW, Munoz A, Giorgi JV, et al. Plasma viral load and CD4+ lymphocytes as prognostic markers of HIV-1 infection. *Ann Intern Med*. 1997;126:946–954.
11. Lundgren JD, Babiker AG, Gordin F, et al. The INSIGHT START Study Group. Initiation of antiretroviral therapy in early asymptomatic HIV infection. *N Engl J Med*. 2015;373:795–807.
12. Fauci AS, Marston HD. Ending the HIV-AIDS pandemic – follow the science. *N Engl J Med*. 2015;373:2197–2199.
13. Fauci AS, Folkers GK, Lane HC. Human immunodeficiency virus disease: AIDS and related disorders. In: Kasper DL, Fauci AS, Hauser SL, et al., eds. *Harrison's Principles of Internal Medicine*. 20th ed. New York: McGraw-Hill; 1393–1463.
14. Palestine AG, Rodrigues MM, Macher AM, et al. Ophthalmic involvement in the acquired immune deficiency syndrome. *Ophthalmology*. 1984;91:1092–1099.
15. Freeman WR, Lerner CW, Mines JA, et al. A prospective study of the ophthalmologic findings in the acquired immune deficiency syndrome. *Am J Ophthalmol*. 1984;97:133–142.
16. Newsome DA, Green WR, Miller ED, et al. Microvascular aspects of acquired immune deficiency syndrome retinopathy. *Am J Ophthalmol*. 1984;98:590–601.
17. Kestelyn P, Van de Perre P, Rouvroy D, et al. A prospective study of the ophthalmologic findings in the acquired immune deficiency syndrome in Africa. *Am J Ophthalmol*. 1985;100:230–238.
18. Pepose JS, Holland GN, Nestor MS, et al. Acquired immune deficiency syndrome: pathogenic mechanisms of ocular disease. *Ophthalmology*. 1985;92:474–484.
19. Meillet D, Hoang PL, Unanue F, et al. Filtration and local synthesis of lacrimal proteins in acquired immunodeficiency syndrome. *Eur J Clin Chem Clin Biochem*. 1992;30:319–323.
20. Belfort R Jr, de Smet M, Whitcup SM, et al. Ocular complications of Stevens-Johnson syndrome and toxic epidermal necrolysis in patients with AIDS. *Cornea*. 1991;10:536–538.
21. Freeman WR, Van Natta ML, Jabs D, et al. Vision function in HIV-infected individuals without retinitis: report of the Studies of Ocular Complications of AIDS Research Group. *Am J Ophthalmol*. 2008;145:453–462.
22. Schuman JS, Friedman AH. Retinal manifestations of the acquired immune deficiency syndrome. *Trans Ophthalmol Soc UK*. 1983;103:177–189.
23. Weiss A, Margo CE, Ledford DK, et al. Toxoplasmic retinochoroiditis as an initial manifestation of the acquired immune deficiency syndrome. *Am J Ophthalmol*. 1986;101:248–249.
24. Stoumbos VD, Klein ML. Syphilitic retinitis in a patient with acquired immunodeficiency syndrome-related complex. *Am J Ophthalmol*. 1987;103:103–104.
25. Croxatto JO, Mestre C, Puente S, et al. Nonreactive tuberculosis in a patient with acquired immune deficiency syndrome. *Am J Ophthalmol*. 1986;102:659–660.
26. Macher A, Rodrigues MM, Kaplan W, et al. Disseminated bilateral chorioretinitis due to *Histoplasma capsulatum* in a patient with the acquired immunodeficiency syndrome. *Ophthalmology*. 1985;92:1159–1164.
27. Sandor EV, Millman A, Croxson TS, et al. Herpes zoster ophthalmicus in patients at risk for the acquired immune deficiency syndrome (AIDS). *Am J Ophthalmol*. 1986;101:153–155.
28. Egbert PR, Pollard RB, Gallagher JG, et al. Cytomegalovirus retinitis in immunosuppressed hosts. II. Ocular manifestations. *Ann Intern Med*. 1980;93:664–670.
29. Kupperman BD, Petty JG, Richman DD, et al. Correlation between CD4+ counts and the prevalence of cytomegalovirus retinitis and human immunodeficiency virus-related noninfectious retinal vasculopathy in patients with acquired immunodeficiency syndrome. *Am J Ophthalmol*. 1993;115:575–582.
30. Studies of Ocular Complications of AIDS Research Group in collaboration with the AIDS Clinical Trials Group. Mortality in patients with the acquired immunodeficiency syndrome treated with either foscarnet or ganciclovir for cytomegalovirus retinitis. *N Engl J Med*. 1992;326:213–220.
31. Jacobson MA, O'Donnell JJ, Porteous D, et al. Retinal and gastrointestinal disease due to cytomegalovirus in patients with the acquired immune deficiency syndrome: prevalence, natural history, and response to ganciclovir therapy. *QJ Med*. 1988;67:473–486.
32. Lalezari JP, Stagg RJ, Kuppermann BD, et al. Intravenous cidofovir for peripheral cytomegalovirus retinitis in patients with AIDS: a randomized, controlled trial. *Ann Intern Med*. 1997;126:257–263.
33. Studies of Ocular Complications of AIDS Research Group in collaboration with the AIDS Clinical Trials Group. Parenteral cidofovir for cytomegalovirus retinitis in patients with AIDS: the HPMPC peripheral cytomegalovirus retinitis trial: a randomized, controlled trial. *Ann Intern Med*. 1997;126:264–274.
34. Martin DF, Parks DJ, Mellow SD, et al. Treatment of cytomegalovirus retinitis with an intraocular sustained-release ganciclovir implant. A randomized controlled clinical trial. *Arch Ophthalmol*. 1994;112:1531–1539.
35. Cavert W, Notermans DW, Staskus K, et al. Kinetics of response in lymphoid tissues to antiretroviral therapy of HIV-1 infection. *Science*. 1997;276:960–963.
36. Perelson AS, Essunger P, Cao Y, et al. Decay characteristics of HIV-1-infected compartments during combination therapy. *Nature*. 1997;387:188–191.
37. Palella FJ, Delaney KM, Moorman AC, et al. Declining morbidity and mortality among patients with advanced human immunodeficiency virus infection. *N Engl J Med*. 1998;338:853–860.
38. Holtzer CD, Jacobson MA, Hakley WK, et al. Decline in the rate of specific opportunistic infections at San Francisco General Hospital. *AIDS*. 1998;12:1931–1933.
39. Jabs DA, Ahuja A, Van Natta ML, et al. for the Studies of the Ocular Complications of AIDS Research Group. Long-term outcomes of cytomegalovirus retinitis in the era of modern antiretroviral therapy. Results from a United States cohort. *Ophthalmology*. 2015;122:1452–1463.
40. Whitcup SM, Fortin E, Nussenblatt RB, et al. Therapeutic effect of combination antiretroviral therapy on cytomegalovirus retinitis. *JAMA*. 1997;277:1519–1520.
41. Vrabec TR, Baldassano VF, Whitcup SM. Discontinuation of maintenance therapy in patients with quiescent cytomegalovirus retinitis and elevated CD4+ counts. *Ophthalmology*. 1998;105:1259–1264.
42. Whitcup SM, Cunningham ET Jr, Polis MA, et al. Spontaneous and sustained resolution of CMV retinitis in patients receiving highly active antiretroviral therapy. *Br J Ophthalmol*. 1998;82:845–846.

43. Whitcup SM, Fortin E, Lindblad AS, et al. Discontinuation of anticytomegalovirus therapy in patients with HIV infection and cytomegalovirus retinitis. *JAMA*. 1999;282:1633–1637.
44. Reed JB, Schwab IR, Gordon J, et al. Regression of cytomegalovirus retinitis associated with protease inhibitor treatment in patients with AIDS. *Am J Ophthalmol*. 1997;124:199–205.
45. Tural C, Romeu J, Siera G, et al. Long-lasting remission of cytomegalovirus retinitis without maintenance therapy in human immunodeficiency virus-infected patients. *J Infect Dis*. 1998;177:1080–1083.
46. Macdonald JC, Torriani FJ, Morse LS, et al. Lack of reactivation of cytomegalovirus (CMV) retinitis after stopping maintenance therapy in AIDS patients with sustained elevations in CD4 T cells in response to highly active antiretroviral therapy. *J Infect Dis*. 1998;177:1182–1187.
47. Jabs DA, Bolton SG, Dunn JP, et al. Discontinuing anticytomegalovirus therapy in patients with immune reconstitution after combination antiretroviral therapy. *Am J Ophthalmol*. 1998;126:817–822.
48. Kirk O, Reiss P, Uberti-Foppa C, et al. Safe interruption of maintenance therapy against previous infection with four common HIV-associated opportunistic pathogens during potent antiretroviral therapy. *Ann Intern Med*. 2002;137:239–250.
49. Komanduri KV, Viswanathan MN, Wieder ED, et al. Restoration of cytomegalovirus-specific CD4+ T-lymphocyte responses after ganciclovir and highly active antiretroviral therapy in individuals infected with HIV-1. *Nature Med*. 1998;4:953–956.
50. Connors M, Kovacs JA, Krevat S, et al. HIV induces changes in CD4+ T-cell phenotype and depletions within the CD4+ T-cell repertoire that are not immediately restored by antiviral or immune-based therapies. *Nature Med*. 1998;3:533–540.
51. Lederman MM, Connick E, Landay A, et al. Immunologic responses associated with 12 weeks of combination antiretroviral therapy consisting of zidovudine, lamivudine, and ritonavir: results of AIDS Clinical Trials Group protocol 315. *J Infect Dis*. 1998;178:70–79.
52. Palestine AG, Stevens G, Lane HC, et al. Treatment of cytomegalovirus retinitis with dihydroxy propoxymethyl guanine. *Am J Ophthalmol*. 1986;101:95–101.
53. Holland GN, Sakamoto MJ, Hardy D, et al. Treatment of cytomegalovirus retinopathy in patients with acquired immunodeficiency syndrome. *Arch Ophthalmol*. 1986;104:1794–1800.
54. D'Amico DJ, Talamo JH, Felsenstein D, et al. Ophthalmoscopic and histologic findings in cytomegalovirus retinitis treated with BW-B759U. *Arch Ophthalmol*. 1986;104:1788–1793.
55. Studies of Ocular Complications of AIDS Research Group. Mortality in patients with the acquired immunodeficiency syndrome treated with either foscarnet or ganciclovir for cytomegalovirus retinitis. *N Engl J Med*. 1992;326:213–220.
56. Palestine AG, Polis MA, De Smet MD, et al. A randomized controlled trial of foscarnet in the treatment of cytomegalovirus retinitis in patients with AIDS. *Ann Intern Med*. 1991;115:665–673.
57. Studies of Ocular Complications of AIDS Research Group, in collaboration with the AIDS Clinical Trials Group. Morbidity and toxic effects associated with ganciclovir or foscarnet therapy in a randomized cytomegalovirus retinitis trial. *Arch Intern Med*. 1995;155:65–74.
58. Combination foscarnet and ganciclovir therapy vs monotherapy for the treatment of relapsed cytomegalovirus retinitis in patients with AIDS. The Cytomegalovirus Retreatment Trial. The Studies of Ocular Complications of AIDS Research Group in Collaboration with the AIDS Clinical Trials Group. *Arch Ophthlamol*. 1996;11:23–33.
59. Walton RC, Whitcup SM, Mueller BU, et al. Combined intravenous ganciclovir and foscarnet for children with recurrent cytomegalovirus retinitis. *Ophthalmology*. 1995;102:1865–1870.
60. Levi ME, Mandava N, Chan LK, et al. Treatment of multidrug-resistant cytomegalovirus retinitis with systemically administered leflunomide. *Transpl Infect Dis*. 2006;8:38–43.
61. Perry CM, Balfour JA. Fomivirsen. *Drugs*. 1999;57:375–380.
62. Vitravene Study Group. A randomized controlled clinical trial of intravitreous fomivirsen for the treatment of newly diagnosed peripheral cytomegalovirus retinitis in patients with AIDS. *Am J Ophthalmol*. 2002;133:467–474.
63. Henry K, Cantrill H, Fletcher C, et al. Use of intravitreal ganciclovir (dihydroxy propoxymethyl guanine) for cytomegalovirus retinitis in a patient with AIDS. *Am J Ophthalmol*. 1987;103:17–23.
64. Diaz-Llopis M, Chipont E, Sanchez S, et al. Intravitreal foscarnet of cytomegalovirus in a patient with acquired immunodeficiency syndrome. *Am J Ophthalmol*. 1992;114:742–747.
65. Kirsch LS, Arevalo JF, De Clercq E, et al. Phase I/II study of intravitreal cidofovir for the treatment of cytomegalovirus retinitis in patients with the acquired immunodeficiency syndrome. *Am J Ophthalmol*. 1995;119:466–476.
66. Kirsch L, Arevalo JF, Chavez de la Pax E, et al. Intravitreal cidofovir (HPMPC) treatment of cytomegalovirus retinitis in patients with acquired immune deficiency syndrome. *Ophthalmology*. 1995;102:533–543.
67. Paya C, Humar A, Dominguez E, et al. Valganciclovir Solid Organ Transplant Study Group. Efficacy and safety of valganciclovir vs. oral ganciclovir for prevention of cytomegalovirus disease in solid organ transplant recipients. *Am J Transplant*. 2004;4:611–620.
68. Martin DF, Sierra-Madero J, Walmsley S, et al. A controlled trial of valganciclovir as induction therapy for cytomegalovirus retinitis. *N Engl J Med*. 2002;346:1119–1126.
69. Kaplan JE, Masur H, Holmes KK. USPHS, and Infectious Disease Society of America. Guidelines for preventing opportunistic infections among HIV-infected persons – 2002. Recommendations of the U.S. Public Health Service and the Infectious Diseases Society of America. *MMWR Recomm Rep*. 2009;10:1–207.
70. Port AD, Orlin A, Kiss S, et al. Cytomegalovirus retinitis: a review. *J Ocul Pharmacol Ther*. 2017;33:224–234.
71. Jabs DA, Ahuja A, Van Natta M, et al. Studies of the Ocular Complications of AIDS Research Group. Comparison of treatment regimens for cytomegalovirus retinitis in patients with AIDS in the era of highly active antiretroviral therapy. *Ophthalmology*. 2013;120:1262–1270.
72. Drew WL, Ives D, Lalezari JP, et al. Oral ganciclovir as maintenance treatment for cytomegalovirus retinitis in patients with AIDS. *N Engl J Med*. 1995;333:615–620.
73. Martin DF, Sierra-Madero J, Walmsley S, et al. A controlled trial of valganciclovir as induction therapy for cytomegalovirus retinitis. *N Engl J Med*. 2002;346:1119–1126.
74. Jabs DA, Martin BK, Ricks MO, et al. Cytomegalovirus Retinitis and Viral Resistance Study Group. Detection of ganciclovir resistance in patients with AIDS and cytomegalovirus retinitis: correlation of genotypic methods with viral phenotype and clinical outcome. *J Infect Dis*. 2006;193:1728–1737.
75. Freeman WR, Friedberg DN, Berry C, et al. Risk factors for the development of rhegmatogenous retinal detachment in patients with cytomegalovirus retinitis. *Am J Ophthalmol*. 1993;116:713–720.
76. Singh R, Bhalekar S, Parchand S, et al. Outcome of surgery in post-cytomegalovirus retinal detachment: experience before and in the era of highly active anti-retroviral therapy in Indian eyes. *Indian J Ophthalmol*. 2013;61:636–639.
77. Wong JX, Wong EP, Teoh SC. Outcomes of cytomegalovirus retinitis-related retinal detachment surgery in acquired immunodeficiency syndrome patients in an Asian population. *BMC Ophthalmol*. 2014;14:150.
78. Thorne JE, Jabs DA, Kempen JH, et al. Incidence of and risk factors for visual acuity loss among patients with AIDS and cytomegalovirus retinitis in the era of highly active antiretroviral therapy. *Ophthalmology*. 2006;113:1001–1008.
79. Jabs DA, Ahuja A, Van Natta ML, et al. Long-term outcomes of cytomegalovirus retinitis in the era of modern antiretroviral therapy; Results from a United States cohort. *Ophthalmology*. 2015;122:1452–1463.
80. Palestine AG, Rodrigues MM, Macher AM, et al. Ophthalmic involvement in acquired immunodeficiency syndrome. *Ophthalmology*. 1984;91:1092–1099.
81. Jabs DA, Bartlett JG. AIDS and ophthalmology: a period of transition. *Am J Ophthalmol*. 1997;124:227–233.
82. Zegans ME, Walton RC, Holland GN, et al. Transient vitreous inflammatory reactions associated with combination antiretroviral therapy in patients with AIDS and cytomegalovirus retinitis. *Am J Ophthalmol*. 1998;125:292–300.

83. Karavellas MP, Lowder CY, Macdonald JC, et al. Immune recovery vitritis associated with inactive cytomegalovirus retinitis: a new syndrome. *Arch Ophthalmol.* 1998;116:169–175.
84. Weinberg DV, Moorthy RS. Cystoid macular edema due to cytomegalovirus in a patient with acquired immunodeficiency virus. *Retina.* 1996;16:1443–1445.
85. Zegans ME, Walton RC, Holland GN, et al. Transient vitreous inflammatory reactions associated with combination antiretroviral therapy in patients with AIDS and cytomegalovirus retinitis. *Am J Ophthalmol.* 1998;125:292–300.
86. Whitcup SM. Cytomegalovirus retinitis in the era of highly active antiretroviral therapy. *JAMA.* 2000;283:653–657.
87. Robinson MR, Reed G, Csaky KG, et al. Immune-recovery uveitis in patients with cytomegalovirus retinitis taking highly active antiretroviral therapy. *Am J Ophthalmol.* 2000;130:49–56.
88. Karavellas MP, Plummer DJ, Macdonald JC, et al. Incidence of immune recovery vitritis in cytomegalovirus retinitis in patients following institution of successful highly active antiretroviral therapy. *J Infect Dis.* 1999;179:697–700.
89. Ortega-Larrocea G, Espinosa E, Reyes-Teran G. Lower incidence and severity of cytomegalovirus-associated immune recovery uveitis in HIV-infected patients with delayed highly active antiretroviral therapy. *Ophthalmology.* 2006;19:735–738.
90. The Studies of Ocular Complications of AIDS Research Group in collaboration with the AIDS Clinical Trials Group. Rhegmatogenous retinal detachment in patients with cytomegalovirus retinitis: the Foscarnet-Ganciclovir Cytomegalovirus Retinitis Trial. *Am J Ophthalmol.* 1997;121:61–70.
91. Morrison VL, Kozak I, LaBree LD, et al. Intravitreal triamcinolone acetonide for the treatment of immune recovery uveitis macular edema. *Ophthalmology.* 2007;114:334–339.
92. Ju J, Coassin M, Stewart JM. Fluocinolone acetonide implant (Retisert) for chronic cystoid macular edema in two patients with AIDS and a history of cytomegalovirus retinitis. *Ocul Immunol Inflamm.* 2011;19:206–209.
93. Race EM, Adelson-Mitty J, Kriegel GR, et al. Focal mycobacterial lymphadenitis following initiation of protease-inhibitor therapy in patients with advanced HIV-1 disease. *Lancet.* 1998;351:252–255.
94. Woods ML, MacGinley R, Eisen DP, et al. HIV combination therapy: partial immune restitution unmasking latent cryptococcal infection. *AIDS.* 1998;12:1491–1494.
95. Sellitti TP, Huang AJ, Schiffman J, et al. Association of herpes zoster ophthalmicus with the acquired immunodeficiency syndrome and acute retinal necrosis. *Am J Ophthalmol.* 1992;116:297–301.
96. Forster DJ, Dugel PU, Frangieh GT, et al. Rapidly progressive outer retinal necrosis in the acquired immunodeficiency syndrome. *Am J Ophthalmol.* 1990;110:341–348.
97. Johnston WH, Holland GN, Engstrom RE, et al. Recurrence of presumed varicella zoster virus retinopathy in patients with the acquired immunodeficiency syndrome. *Am J Ophthalmol.* 1993;116:42–50.
98. Yin PD, Kurup SK, Fischer SH, et al. Progressive outer retinal necrosis in the era of highly active antiretroviral therapy: successful management with intravitreal injections and monitoring with quantitative PCR. *J Clin Virol.* 2007;38:254–259.
99. Gore DM, Gore SK, Visser L. Progressive outer retinal necrosis: outcomes in the intravitreal era. *Arch Ophthalmol.* 2012;130:700–706.
100. Macher AM, Bardenstein DS, Zimmerman LE, et al. *Pneumocystis carinii* choroiditis in a male homosexual with AIDS and disseminated pulmonary and extrapulmonary *P. carinii* infection. *N Engl J Med.* 1987;316:1092.
101. Sha BE, Benson CA, Deutsch T, et al. *Pneumocystis carinii* choroiditis in patients with AIDS: clinical features, response to therapy and outcome. *J AIDS.* 1992;5:1051–1058.
102. Whitcup SM, Fenton RM, Pluda JM, et al. *Pneumocystis carinii* and *Mycobacterium avium-intracellulare* infection of the choroid. *Retina.* 1992;12:331–335.
103. Morinelli EN, Dugel PU, Riffenburgh R, et al. Infectious multifocal choroiditis in patients with acquired immune deficiency syndrome. *Ophthalmology.* 1993;100:1014–1021.
104. Stanton CA, Sloan B III, Slusher MM, et al. Acquired immunodeficiency syndrome-related primary intraocular lymphoma. *Arch Ophthalmol.* 1992;110:1614–1617.
105. Johns DR, Tierney M, Felsenstein D. Alteration in the natural history of neurosyphilis by concurrent infection with the human immunodeficiency virus. *N Engl J Med.* 1987;316:1569–1572.
106. Shafran SD, Deschenes J, Miller M, et al. Uveitis and pseudojaundice during a regimen of clarithromycin, rifabutin and ethambutol. *N Engl J Med.* 1994;330:438–439.
107. Whitcup SM, Butler KM, Caruso R, et al. Retinal toxicity in human immunodeficiency virus-infected children treated with 2′,3′-dideoxyinosine. *Am J Ophthalmol.* 1992;113:1–7.

13

Acute Retinal Necrosis and Progressive Outer Retinal Necrosis

Scott M. Whitcup

KEY CONCEPTS

- Despite effective antiviral therapies, herpes infection of the eye can lead to severe uveitis with substantial vision loss.
- Because acute retinal necrosis (ARN) can often begin as anterior uveitis, examination of the peripheral retina is important in all patients with a new onset of anterior inflammation.
- Testing of the aqueous or vitreous humor with polymerase chain reaction (PCR) testing is useful in confirming the diagnosis of ARN; however, treatment should not be delayed waiting for test results.
- Initial intravenous or oral antiviral therapy is of benefit in treating ARN; intravenous acyclovir, oral acyclovir, oral valacyclovir, and oral famciclovir have all been used.
- The adjunctive use of intravitreal foscarnet may be beneficial for some patients.
- Retinal detachment and optic nerve involvement remain important causes of vision loss in patients with ARN.
- Progressive outer retinal necrosis (PORN) is thought to be a variant of a necrotizing herpetic retinopathy in immunocompromised patients.
- Combination antiretroviral therapy in PORN may improve the prognosis.

Despite many advances in the diagnosis and treatment of ocular diseases, viral infections affecting the eye remain difficult to diagnose and to treat. Many cases of uveitis, including multifocal choroiditis, acute posterior multifocal placoid pigment epitheliopathy (APMPPE), and multiple evanescent white-dot syndrome (MEWDS), are presumed to be caused by viral infections. Nevertheless, antiviral agents rarely are used in their treatment because the evidence supporting the viral etiology is anecdotal. For example, Epstein-Barr virus (EBV) infection has been associated with multifocal choroiditis and panuveitis[1,2]; however, because EBV infection is so ubiquitous, it is difficult to prove a definite causal relationship between the virus and the choroidal disease. Many viral infections associated with uveitis are discussed in the chapter on white-dot syndromes (see Chapter 30). This chapter focuses on two disorders predominantly associated with herpes virus infections: acute retinal necrosis and progressive outer retinal necrosis. Other ophthalmic manifestations of herpes simplex virus (HSV) and herpes zoster virus (HZV) infections and other viral infections causing uveitis are discussed in Chapter 14.

ACUTE RETINAL NECROSIS

The evolution in our understanding of the etiology and pathophysiology of acute retinal necrosis (ARN) exemplifies how scientific knowledge can improve our ability to accurately diagnose and treat inflammatory eye diseases. ARN was initially described in 1971 in a report by Urayama et al.,[3] in which the authors documented the clinical findings in six patients with intraocular inflammation, retinal vascular sheathing, and large white confluent retinal infiltrates in one eye. The disease was called *Kirisawa uveitis,* and these patients, in whom rhegmatogenous retinal detachments subsequently developed, were left with poor visual acuity. No etiologic agent was identified, and no therapy appeared to affect the outcome of the disease.

Additional cases of retinitis with rhegmatogenous retinal detachment were reported in the late 1970s,[4,5] and these retinal detachments were difficult to repair because of both tractional and rhegmatogenous components. Cases of bilateral acute retinal necrosis (BARN) were also described.[6] In 1982, the finding of herpes virus in the retina of patients with ARN by Culbertson et al.[7] paved the way for specific antiviral therapy for the disease. Nevertheless, late retinal detachment remains a serious complication despite the use of prophylactic laser photocoagulation and modern vitreoretinal surgical techniques.

Was ARN a new disease or just a newly recognized one? Few, if any, similar occurrences were reported before 1971, and yet numerous reports on the topic have appeared in the literature since that time. Many investigators believe that ARN is a new disease, possibly caused by mutations in the virus or changes in host susceptibility. Others believe that improved diagnostic techniques and awareness of the disease have led to increased recognition.

Epidemiology

Initially reported in Japan, ARN has now been widely found throughout Europe and North America, with sporadic cases occurring around the world. ARN can occur in patients of either gender and at any age, although there may be a slight male preponderance. Although the disease is typically thought to affect young adults, ARN has been reported in children[8,9] and in older adults as well. Although ARN was initially described in immunocompetent patients, this disease has now been documented in patients with immunosuppression, such as those with acquired immunodeficiency syndrome (AIDS)[10,11] and in patients on immunosuppression or after bone marrow transplantation.[12] A prospective study carried out by the British Ophthalmological Surveillance Unit between September 2007 and October 2008 calculated a minimum incidence of ARN in the United Kingdom to be 0.63 cases per

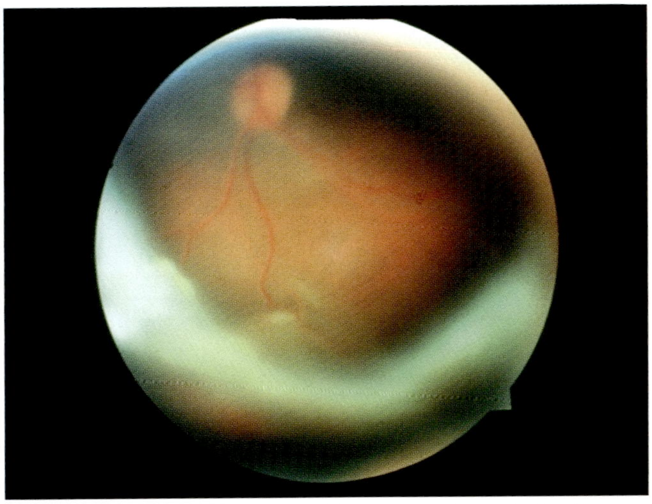

Fig. 13.1 Acute retinal necrosis with dense white retinal infiltrate in retinal periphery.

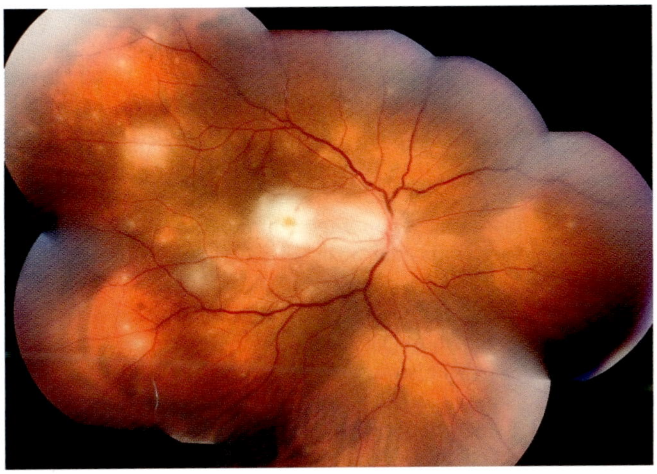

Fig. 13.2 Retina montage from a patient with acute retinal necrosis showing white infiltrative lesions predominantly involving the area around the macula and the optic nerve, although peripheral lesions are also evident. In this patient, there was no vitreous haze and minimal involvement of the retinal vessels.

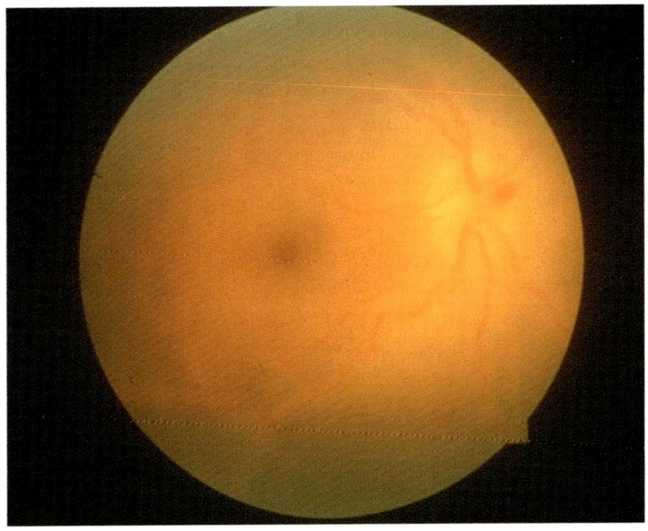

Fig. 13.3 Posterior pole of the retina 1 week after the onset of symptoms of acute retinal necrosis and after vitrectomy had been performed, demonstrating optic disk swelling and retinal perivascular sheathing.

million.[13] Patient age range was 10 to 94 years, and eight patients had a history of herpetic central nervous system (CNS) disease.

Clinical Features

The disease may affect one or both eyes; most cases begin with unilateral disease.[8] In almost one-third of cases, the second eye becomes involved, usually within 1 to 6 weeks; however, disease in the second eye has been reported to occur up to 20 years after that in the first eye.[14,15] Most patients have a history of pain, redness, floaters, and blurred vision. Anterior uveitis, with or without keratic precipitates, often occurs early in the disease, and although plasmoid aqueous has been described in these patients, hypopyon is rare. Occasionally, there is associated herpes infection at another site,[4,16] but most patients are healthy, immunocompetent, and without systemic symptoms.

With the onset of vitritis, patients report floaters and diminished visual acuity. Vitritis tends to worsen as cellular immunity to the virus occurs, and the infiltrating inflammatory cells are predominantly lymphocytes and plasma cells.[7] The earliest retinal lesions are small, patchy, white-yellow areas that tend to become enlarged, increase in number, and coalesce over time (Fig. 13.1). They usually start in the midperiphery; occasionally, they occur in the posterior pole but may not follow the architecture of the retinal vessels (Fig. 13.2). After several weeks, the lesions begin to resolve, with areas of clearing forming a "Swiss cheese" pattern. At this time, perturbation of the retinal pigment epithelium (RPE) also develops. Retinal vasculitis is another manifestation of ARN (Fig. 13.3; also see Case 13.3). Patients often have severe retinal arteritis. Capillary nonperfusion can be documented on fluorescein angiography, and periphlebitis and venous occlusions have been described less commonly. Retinal hemorrhage can occur, especially in patients with venous occlusive disease. In contrast to findings with other venous occlusive diseases, neovascularization of the iris or the retina is uncommon but has been reported.[17,18] The choroidal vasculature is also involved in this disease, and fluorescein angiography has demonstrated areas of early hypofluorescence and late staining consistent with ischemia-induced inflammatory changes.

Optic neuropathy also occurs in patients with ARN. Disk edema is a common finding early in the course of the disease,[8] and two cases of intraorbital optic nerve enlargement were reported by Sergott et al.[19] Optic nerve involvement should be suspected in patients with an afferent pupillary defect and severe visual loss, with few retinal findings. Visual field testing and color vision assessment can be informative. Visual loss may be caused by vascular occlusive disease, viral infiltration of the nerve, or optic nerve distension. Optic nerve sheath fenestration has been proposed as a possible therapeutic intervention,[20] but its effect has not been proven by well-controlled clinical trials. ARN has also been reported in patients with clinical findings of viral meningitis.[21]

The acute inflammatory disease tends to resolve over several months with or without therapy. In untreated patients, the acute phase usually resolves in 2 to 3 months. The course of the disease can also be predicted by the number of clock hours of initial retinal involvement. Unfortunately, within the next several months, tractional and rhegmatogenous retinal detachments with many large breaks develop in up to 86% of patients.[8,22] Despite control of the active viral replication in the retina, cellular infiltration into the vitreous and the formation of vitreal membranes composed of RPE and fibroblasts develop and contribute to the tearing and detachment of an already thinned retina.[23]

The Executive Committee of the American Uveitis Society published a set of standard criteria for the diagnosis of ARN syndrome,[24]

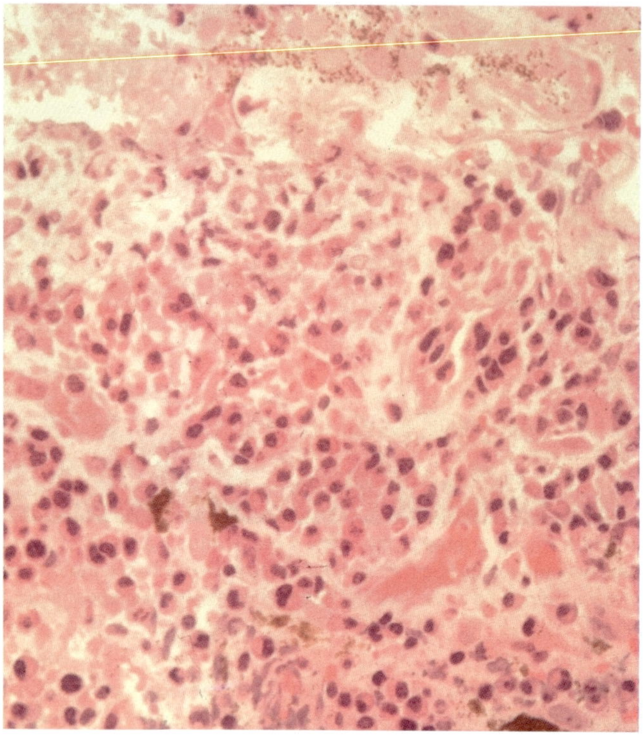

Fig. 13.4 Histologic section of chorioretinal biopsy specimen from a patient with acute retinal necrosis showing lymphocytic infiltration and areas of necrosis. (Hematoxylin & eosin stain; ×400). (Courtesy Chi-Chao Chan, MD.)

stating that the designation of ARN syndrome should be based solely on clinical appearance and the course of infection. Clinical characteristics that must be documented include (1) one or more foci of retinal necrosis with discrete borders in the peripheral retina; (2) rapid progression of disease if antiviral therapy has not been given; (3) circumferential spread of disease; (4) evidence of occlusive vasculopathy with arteriolar involvement; and (5) a prominent inflammatory reaction in the vitreous and anterior chamber. Optic nerve involvement, scleritis, and pain support the diagnosis of ARN, but are not required to make the diagnosis. Macular lesions, although less common, do not preclude a diagnosis of ARN if peripheral lesions are present.

Etiology

ARN was initially believed to be an autoimmune disease.[23] In 1982, Culbertson et al.[7] first described enucleation of an eye in a patient with ARN, in which herpesvirus particles were noted in the retina on electron microscopy. However, virus was not cultured from the eye, and serum antibodies were found to herpes simplex, herpes zoster, CMV, and EBV. Histologic examination showed prominent retinal arteritis and marked retinal necrosis, with abrupt demarcation between the normal and necrotic areas of the retina. Optic nerve inflammation was also noted. A similar histologic picture was seen in a retinal biopsy specimen we obtained from a patient with ARN in 1983, which revealed inflammatory cell infiltration and necrosis of the retina (Fig. 13.4). There was a predominance of T lymphocytes in the vitreous, but the retina contained many B lymphocytes, suggesting that antibody to the virus could be produced locally in the retina. Finally, the results of electron microscopy showed herpes class viral particles (Fig. 13.5), although virus was not cultured from the specimen. In 1986, Culbertson et al.[25] used immunohistochemical staining to reveal herpes zoster in two eyes with ARN and also succeeded in culturing the

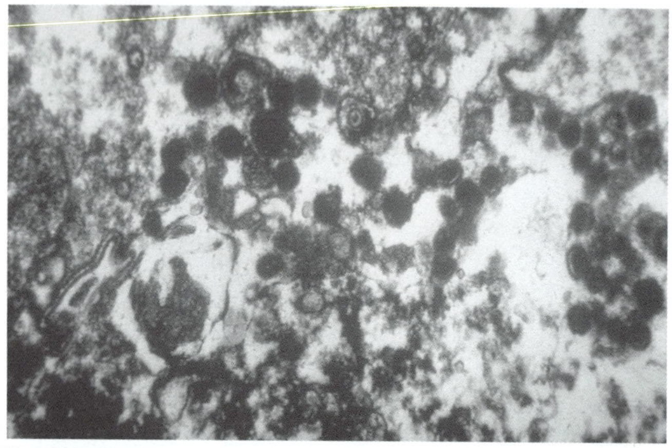

Fig. 13.5 Electron micrograph demonstrating herpes class virions in retinal biopsy specimen from a patient with acute retinal necrosis.

virus from one of the two eyes. Varicella-zoster virus (VZV) was initially thought to account for most of the typical cases of ARN; however, HSV types 1 (HSV-1) and 2 (HSV-2) and, rarely, CMV were also implicated as a cause of the disease.[26-30]

In a retrospective study of 28 patients, Ganatra et al.[31] used polymerase chain reaction (PCR) to show that VZV or HSV-1 caused ARN in patients older than 25 years of age, whereas HSV-2 caused ARN in patients younger than 25 years of age. Van Gelder et al.[32] also reported that HSV-2 is an important cause of ARN, particularly in young patients. Sugita et al. analyzed ocular fluid samples from 16 patients with ARN.[33] High copy numbers of HSV-1, HSV-2, or VZV were found in all the samples from the 16 patients, suggesting active viral replication. In a more recent study, Calvo et al. correlated visual acuity outcomes and clinical features with quantitative PCR DNA copy number in patients with ARN.[34] In this study of 14 eyes of 13 patients, quantitative DNA copy number of 5.0×10^6/mL or greater was associated with more extensive retinitis, worse visual acuity, and development of retinal detachment.

In 2017, an American Academy of Ophthalmology ophthalmic technology assessment reviewed the diagnosis and treatment of ARN.[35] In their review of the literature, PCR testing was positive for HSV or VZV DNA in 79% to 100% of cases. Studies have shown that accurate diagnosis can be made with PCR on both aqueous and vitreous samples[36]; although one epidemiologic study from the United Kingdom noted that 93% of vitreous samples, compared with 46% of aqueous samples, were positive for viral DNA.[13] Small case series have demonstrated decrease in viral DNA after antiviral therapy.[37,38]

Wherever possible, we now recommend that an aqueous or vitreous sample be obtained for PCR analysis in cases of suspected ARN. However, because the diagnosis relies heavily on the clinical picture and because prompt therapy can improve the visual outcome, we do not recommend waiting for PCR test results before starting antiviral therapy in cases of suspected ARN. Just as important, caution should be exercised in basing a diagnosis of viral infection on PCR data in the absence of any clinical signs of viral infection. Because PCR analysis is such a sensitive test, viral DNA from a previous infection years earlier may yield confusing results, especially because viral infection with HSV, CMV, and HZV are quite common.

Experimental data also support the role of herpesvirus infection in the pathogenesis of ARN. Injection of HSV-1 in BALB/c mice produces necrotizing retinitis in the contralateral eye within about 10 days.[39] This animal model is similar to ARN in humans and has yielded interesting immunologic insights into the pathophysiologic course of the

BOX 13.1 Differential Diagnosis of Acute Retinal Necrosis Syndrome

Exogenous bacterial endophthalmitis
Fungal endophthalmitis
Behçet disease
Pars planitis
Toxoplasmosis
Syphilis
Cytomegalovirus retinitis
Sarcoidosis
Intraocular lymphoma
Progressive outer retinal necrosis syndrome

disease. Necrotizing retinitis develops only in immunocompetent animals. In addition, the disease develops in the contralateral eye only if it is infected by the virus via the optic nerve. Thus, as in other inflammatory eye diseases, retinal damage, initially induced by an infectious agent, leads to a secondary immune response against previously sequestered retinal antigens. This secondary immune response can then propagate the inflammatory damage to the retina.

Other factors may play a role in the pathogenesis of ARN. Holland et al.[40] showed an association between ARN and histocompatibility lymphocyte antigen (HLA)-DQw7 and the phenotype Bw62, DR4. These data suggest that some persons may have a genetically determined predisposition to mounting an immune response against certain infectious agents that promote the development of ocular inflammatory diseases. Some data provide evidence for antigen-specific immune deviation in patients with ARN. VZV-associated ARN developed in patients in whom delayed hypersensitivity to viral antigens was absent.[41] In this study, delayed hypersensitivity responses were restored in patients who recovered from the disease. In another study, Fas and Fas ligand expression were absent in a retinal biopsy specimen from a patient with ARN.[42] Furthermore, apoptosis was noted in the specimen, suggesting a role in the disease. Finally, inflammatory cytokines may be involved in the development of ARN. Intraocular inoculation of herpesvirus was sufficient to induce vascular endothelial growth factor (VEGF), flk-1, transforming growth factor (TGF)–β_2, and interleukin (IL)-6 in the retinas of injected and contralateral eyes in experimental animals.[43]

Differential Diagnosis

Because ARN can often begin as anterior uveitis, examination of the peripheral retina is important in all patients with a new onset of anterior inflammation. The differential diagnoses of ARN are listed in Box 13.1. In general, only Behçet disease and endophthalmitis mimic the rapid progression and severity of ARN. The lesions of Behçet disease rarely present with a uniform distribution in the periphery of the retina and are often associated with systemic symptoms and signs, such as arthritis, mouth and genital ulcers, and skin lesions. Vitrectomy may be needed to rule out endophthalmitis. Toxoplasmic retinochoroiditis, syphilitic retinitis, and intraocular lymphoma more rarely mimic ARN.[44]

Therapy

Many patients appear to benefit from treatment with antiviral therapy (see Cases 13.1 and 13.2). Acyclovir has good activity against HSV and, at slightly higher concentrations, is effective against HZV. Although acyclovir is not as effective as ganciclovir or foscarnet in treating CMV infection, because CMV is rarely a cause of ARN and acyclovir is easier to administer and safer, it is the best initial therapy for the disease. Initial therapy for patients with ARN often includes intravenous acyclovir or oral valacyclovir.[35] Patients with newly diagnosed ARN can be treated with a 7- to 14-day course of intravenously administered acyclovir 500 mg/m^2, every 8 hours, followed by oral antiviral therapy.

The goal of therapy is to hasten the resolution of disease in the infected eye and to prevent contralateral spread. In a retrospective study by Palay et al.,[45] in 87.1% of patients treated with acyclovir, contralateral disease did not develop, compared with 35.1% of patients not receiving the drug. Other case series seem to show that retinal lesions resolve more quickly after initiation of acyclovir, but therapy does not appear to diminish vitritis or to prevent subsequent retinal detachment.[22,46] Patients with severe and progressive disease despite acyclovir therapy may be treated with ganciclovir or foscarnet. In addition, systemic corticosteroids, such as prednisone 0.5 to 1.0 mg/kg, can be added after the patient has received 24 to 48 hours of intravenous acyclovir. Steroids can be slowly tapered, depending on the amount of vitritis. Because of the extensive retinal arteritis and the development of retinal vascular occlusions, some have suggested aspirin therapy,[47] but again, this therapy has not been scrutinized in a clinical trial.

Although the therapeutic benefits of antiviral therapy for ARN have not been studied in well-controlled randomized clinical trials (RCTs), level II and level III data support the use of these drugs.[35] Furthermore, severe side effects with antiviral therapy are relatively rare. A reversible rise in the serum creatinine level and elevation in liver function test results may occur. The most commonly reported side effects include nausea, vomiting, and headache, but most of these occur in fewer than 5% of patients.

Both valacyclovir and famciclovir offer more convenient dosage regimens. Famciclovir at a dose of 500 mg three times daily had efficacy similar to that of acyclovir in treating patients with ophthalmic zoster.[48] Valacyclovir is rapidly converted to acyclovir, and the usual dose of valacyclovir is 1 g orally three times daily, resulting in substantial vitreous levels of acyclovir.[49] Importantly, in a 1-year prospective RCT, recurrence of any type of ocular HSV infection was 23.1% in patients receiving valacyclovir compared with 23.1% in patients receiving acyclovir.[50] The use of either oral valacyclovir or famciclovir has resulted in regression of retinitis in patients in several case series.[51-53] Finally, although there are no RCTs comparing intravenous acyclovir with oral valacyclovir for treating ARN, in a retrospective, comparative, international case series, oral valacyclovir was found to be clinically equivalent to intravenous therapy.[54] Over 5 years of follow-up, visual acuity, rates of severe vision loss, percentage of eyes maintaining good vision, and retinal detachment rates did not differ between the two therapies. Finally, intravitreal injections with antiviral agents may be useful as adjunctive therapy in patients with ARN.[55-57]

Retinal detachment and optic neuropathy remain the causes of severe visual loss in this disease. Laser photocoagulation to demarcate a zone between the involved and uninvolved areas of the retina has been tried as a prophylactic therapy to prevent retinal detachment. Sternberg et al.[58] showed that retinal detachments occurred in two of 12 eyes receiving laser therapy and in four of six eyes not receiving laser therapy. However, this retrospective analysis may be biased because the condition of patients with the most severe disease and the worst vitritis might not have been amenable to laser therapy. Others have suggested prophylactic vitrectomy, scleral buckling, and endolaser treatment for eyes at high risk for retinal detachment, but there are few data to support this therapy.[59] Additional studies are needed to better define the role of laser photocoagulation and vitrectomy in the management of ARN.

Clearly, surgery is warranted to repair retinal detachments in patients with ARN, although these detachments are difficult to repair, and proliferative vitreoretinopathy is common.[22] Vitrectomy, fluid–gas exchange, and endolaser treatment have been suggested for complicated detachments.[60] Whether this therapy is better than vitrectomy with scleral buckling is unknown. Silicone oil has also been used successfully in some patients.

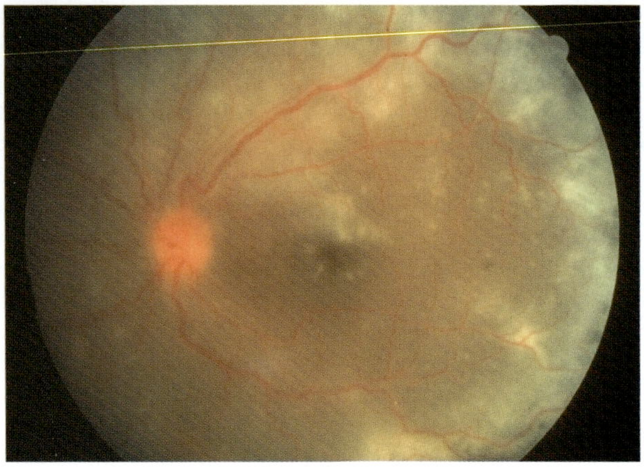

Fig. 13.6 Diffuse retinitis involving the posterior pole in a patient with progressive outer retinal necrosis. Retinitis appears to involve the outer retina with little evidence of retinal vasculitis. (Courtesy Chris Walton, MD.)

The effect of therapy on optic nerve disease is less well studied. Optic nerve fenestration and corticosteroids have been used to treat optic neuropathy in ARN, but no well-controlled study data are available to support the effectiveness of these therapeutic interventions.

With the discovery of the viral etiology of ARN, specific therapy has been employed for the treatment of this disease. Nevertheless, many questions about ARN remain. We still do not know why certain individuals are more susceptible to the disease because ARN is relatively rare but herpesvirus infection is quite common. Although acyclovir, valacyclovir, famciclovir, and corticosteroids are used to treat patients with ARN, there are still no masked RCTs to definitively show the benefits and risks of therapy.

Finally, a HZV vaccine has been developed and has been recommended by the Advisory Committee on Immunization Practices (ACIP) in immunocompetent adults age 60 years or older.[61] The vaccine was developed to prevent herpes zoster caused by reactivation of latent VZV. The effect of the vaccine of subsequent development or severity of ARN caused by VZV is unknown. However, rare cases of ARN after HZV vaccination have been reported,[62] and in one case, whole genome sequencing confirmed that the ocular virus strain was derived from the vaccine.[63]

Prognosis

Vision loss in ARN is common. Even with treatment, only about one-third of patients maintain good vision.[54] Predictors of poor visual outcome include zone 1 retinal involvement, larger areas of retinal involvement, and development of retinal detachment.[64,65]

PROGRESSIVE OUTER RETINAL NECROSIS

A syndrome characterized by rapidly progressive outer retinal necrosis (PORN) was initially described in immunocompromised patients. This syndrome seems to be different from ARN in immunocompromised patients, and the prognosis is extremely poor. Unfortunately, it is thought to be the second most frequent opportunistic retinal infection in patients with AIDS in North America.[66]

Diagnosis

PORN is thought to be a variant of a necrotizing herpetic retinopathy in immunocompromised patients. The syndrome was described by Forster et al.[67] in 1990 in two patients seropositive for human immunodeficiency virus (HIV). Margolis et al.[68] similarly described VZV retinitis in patients with AIDS, and they also noted rapidly progressive necrotizing retinitis with early patchy choroidal and deep retinal lesions, which progressed

TABLE 13.1 Diagnostic Criteria

Progressive Outer Retinal Necrosis Syndrome	Acute Retinal Necrosis Syndrome
Multifocal lesions characterized by deep retinal opacification without granular borders; there may be areas of confluent opacification	One or more foci of full-thickness retinal necrosis with discrete borders
Lesions located in the peripheral retina with or without macular involvement	Lesions located in the peripheral retina[a]
Extremely rapid progression of lesions No consistent direction of disease spread	Rapid progression of disease[b] Circumferential spread of disease around the peripheral retina
Absence of vascular inflammation	Evidence of occlusive vasculopathy, with arteriolar involvement
Minimal or Absent Intraocular Inflammation	
Characteristics that support, but are not required for, diagnosis	Prominent inflammatory reaction in the vitreous and anterior chamber
Perivenular clearing of retinal opacification	Characteristics that support, but are not required for, diagnosis
	Scleritis
	Pain

[a]Involving the area adjacent to, or outside, the major temporal vascular arcades.
[b]Progression can be successfully halted in most patients with intravenous acyclovir therapy.
From Engstrom RE, Jr, Holland GN, Margolis TP, et al. The progressive outer retinal necrosis syndrome: a variant of necrotizing herpetic retinopathy in patients with AIDS. *Ophthalmology.* 1994;101:1488–1502.

relentlessly until the patients were left with atrophic and necrotic retinas and pale optic nerves. Unlike typical ARN, there is little to no vasculitis and less vitritis, and in many patients, posterior pole involvement occurs early in the course of disease (Fig. 13.6).

Engstrom et al.[66] reviewed the cases of 38 patients with AIDS who had PORN. A definite history of cutaneous herpes zoster was documented in 22 of 33 patients (67%). The median CD4+ lymphocyte count in these patients was 21/mm^3, with a range of 0 to 130/mm^3. Most patients had a unilateral decrease in visual acuity, although about one-quarter of them had a presenting complaint of reduced peripheral vision or constriction of visual field. Asymptomatic disease was noted in seven of 65 eyes (11%). The median visual acuity at presentation was 20/30, but some patients had NLP (no light perception) vision at presentation. Inflammation of the anterior chamber and vitreous was minimal or absent in all patients. Multifocal, deep retinal lesions were typically found in the periphery; however, macular lesions were noted in 21 eyes (32%) at the time of diagnosis. Optic nerve involvement was present in 11 (17%) of 65 eyes, and an afferent pupillary defect was noted in 11 (38%) of 29 patients. The lesions, which are characteristic of this syndrome, rapidly progressed to confluence. Interestingly, although the syndrome is described as involving the outer retina, pathologic evidence suggests that the disease can cause substantial destruction of the inner retina late in its course.[67]

Differential Diagnosis

The differential diagnosis for PORN is similar to that for ARN, and a comparison of their diagnostic criteria is presented in Table 13.1. It is important to differentiate these two disorders. Retinal lesions in PORN appear to predominantly involve the deep retina, whereas lesions in ARN appear to be full-thickness ones. Posterior retinal lesions are more common in PORN, whereas anterior chamber inflammation and dense vitritis are characteristic of ARN but rare in PORN. Similarly, vascular inflammation is also rare in PORN but common in ARN. Finally, lesions progress rapidly to confluence despite therapy in PORN but are usually controlled with acyclovir therapy in ARN.

Etiology

Similar to ARN, VZV and HSV have been implicated in the cause of PORN.[69] Most patients with PORN have had impaired immune status, as a result of either an underlying disease or immunosuppressive therapy, but the disease has been reported in immunocompetent patients.[70]

Therapy

We have tried various combinations of induction doses of intravenous ganciclovir and foscarnet and intravitreal foscarnet, but visual prognosis is often poor despite therapy (see Case 13.4). High-dose intravenous acyclovir at a dosage of 10 mg/kg every 8 hours for 2 weeks has also been used with inconsistent success. Others have reported that initial intravenous antiviral therapy appeared to reduce disease activity in 17 (53%) of 32 eyes, but final visual outcome was not altered by therapy.[71] In this study, final visual acuity was NLP in 67% of eyes within 4 weeks after diagnosis. Some success has been reported with combination antiviral therapy, usually with intravenous foscarnet and either acyclovir or ganciclovir.[71] Long-term preservation of vision has been reported with the use of a combination of antiviral drugs with highly active antiretroviral therapy [HAART]).[72] Investigators in this study treated patients with a ganciclovir implant, intravenous acyclovir (10 mg/kg every 8 hours), intravitreal foscarnet (2.4 mg), and HAART. Although the ganciclovir implant is no longer commercially available, in a retrospective study of HIV-positive patients with PORN, repeated intravitreal ganciclovir injections may have resulted in better visual outcomes; however, many eyes became NLP despite therapy.[73] Complications of the disorder included retinal detachment in 70% of eyes despite prophylactic laser retinopexy in some cases.

CASE 13.1

A 22-year-old woman experienced sudden blurring of vision in the right eye, which was red and accompanied by right-sided headache. One week later, she saw an ophthalmologist, who diagnosed anterior uveitis, which was treated with topical corticosteroids. Three days later, a herpes simplex lesion developed on the lip, but the initial medical evaluation was uneventful. Two weeks after the initial symptoms, peripheral white lesions in the retina were noted. Vision in the right eye had decreased to 20/125. There were 3+ cells and 3+ flare in the anterior chamber and 4+ cells in the vitreous, and a diagnosis of acute retinal necrosis was made.

Vitrectomy was performed to aid in visualization of the retinal lesions and for obtaining specimens for viral culture. The viral culture results were negative; however, intravenous acyclovir was started after surgery. The white retinal lesions began to resolve. After 10 days, the intravenous acyclovir was discontinued, and the patient was treated with 200 mg of oral acyclovir five times daily. Laser photocoagulation was applied to the posterior edge of the white retinal lesions in an attempt to prevent retinal detachment. Two weeks later, there was increased ocular inflammation and fibrin in the vitreous and the retina. Intravenous acyclovir was restarted, and the inflammation slowly resolved. Vision 2 months later was 20/25 and remained stable without retinal detachment for longer than 1 year.

CASE 13.2

A 35-year-old African American man was referred for evaluation of enlarging chorioretinal lesions in the left eye. The patient had a 2-week history of blurred vision, photophobia, and floaters. On his visit to the referring ophthalmologist, the visual acuity was 20/25 in the left eye with vitreous cells and whitish retinal lesions. The patient was diagnosed with possible acute retinal necrosis, which was empirically treated with valganciclovir 900 mg orally two times daily. He also received topical prednisolone acetate and cyclopentolate in the left eye. On referral, his visual acuity was 20/16 in the right eye and 20/40 in the left eye. The slit-lamp biomicroscopy result was normal in the right eye and showed 2+ anterior chamber cells, 1+ anterior chamber flare, and granulomatous keratic precipitates in the left eye. Fundus examination revealed 1+ vitreous cells and white fluffy retinal infiltrates around the optic nerve and nasal periphery (Fig. 13.7A) with scattered areas of retinal vasculitis (see Fig. 13.7B). The initial laboratory workup yielded a negative result for syphilis but showed positive antibodies against cytomegalovirus (CMV) and herpes simplex virus type 2 (HSV-2). Polymerase chain reaction (PCR) analysis on the aqueous humor specimen obtained via an anterior chamber tap was positive for HSV-2 and negative for CMV, varicella zoster virus (VZV), and *Toxoplasma*. The patient was treated with five injections of intravitreal ganciclovir and foscarnet in the left eye and oral valacyclovir, 1 g three times daily, and oral prednisone, 40 mg daily. The inflammation resolved, and vision improved to 20/20, with some residual retinal scarring.

CASE 13.3

A 61-year-old woman with a history of type 2 diabetes presented with a 2-week history of pain, redness, photophobia, and decreased vision in the right eye. She was diagnosed with Behçet disease and treated with prednisone 60 mg orally four times daily. She was referred for worsening vision and pain despite corticosteroid therapy. On referral, her visual acuity was 20/125 in the right eye (OD) and 20/20 in the left eye (OS). The visual examination was notable for anterior uveitis, vitritis, and diffuse retinal vasculitis with retinal infiltrates in the right eye (Fig. 13.8). Polymerase chain reaction (PCR) analysis on the specimen obtained via an anterior chamber tap was positive for varicella zoster virus (VZV). Despite treatment with intravitreal ganciclovir and foscarnet and intravenous acyclovir, the patient's vision further deteriorated as a result of retinal ischemia.

CASE 13.4

A 32-year-old African American woman was diagnosed with human immunodeficiency virus (HIV) infection. Two years later, she developed immunoblastic B-cell non-Hodgkin lymphoma involving the lung and the nasopharynx. The patient was treated with six cycles of chemotherapy. After treatment, the patient reported a 3-day history of blurred vision in the left eye. Visual acuity was 20/16 in both eyes, and the results of slit-lamp biomicroscopy were normal. There were 1+ vitreous cells but no haze in the left eye, and funduscopic examination revealed multifocal lesions of the outer retina with no posterior pole involvement. The patient was immediately given induction doses of ganciclovir; however, the patches of retinitis continued to progress and coalesce. Induction doses of intravenous foscarnet were added to the regimen and seemed to halt the progression of retinitis. Nevertheless, 1 month later, visual acuity had decreased to 5/125, with the spread of retinitis into the posterior pole (see Fig. 13.5), and localized retinal detachment developed inferiorly. The CD4+ lymphocyte count at this time was less than 10 cells/mm^3. A diagnosis of PORN was made, and the patient was given maintenance doses of ganciclovir and foscarnet, with follow-up.

One week later, visual acuity had decreased to hand motions at a distance of 1 foot. The patient's retinitis appeared to involve the deep retina; the retinal vessels were relatively spared. The patient was again treated with induction doses of foscarnet and maintenance doses of ganciclovir. Visual acuity remained limited to light perception in the left eye, but now multifocal lesions of the outer retina in the right eye developed (Fig. 13.9) and progressed rapidly. The patient was then treated with intravenous ganciclovir and intravitreal injections of foscarnet. Disease progression appeared to be halted in the right eye for the next 2 months, but the patient lost vision in that eye. At that time, visual acuity was limited to light perception in the right eye and NLP in the left eye. Retinal examination showed a cherry-red spot in the right macula, with a diffuse area of retinitis and a large retinal detachment. The patient opted to stop therapy and died 2 years after the initial diagnosis of her ocular disease.

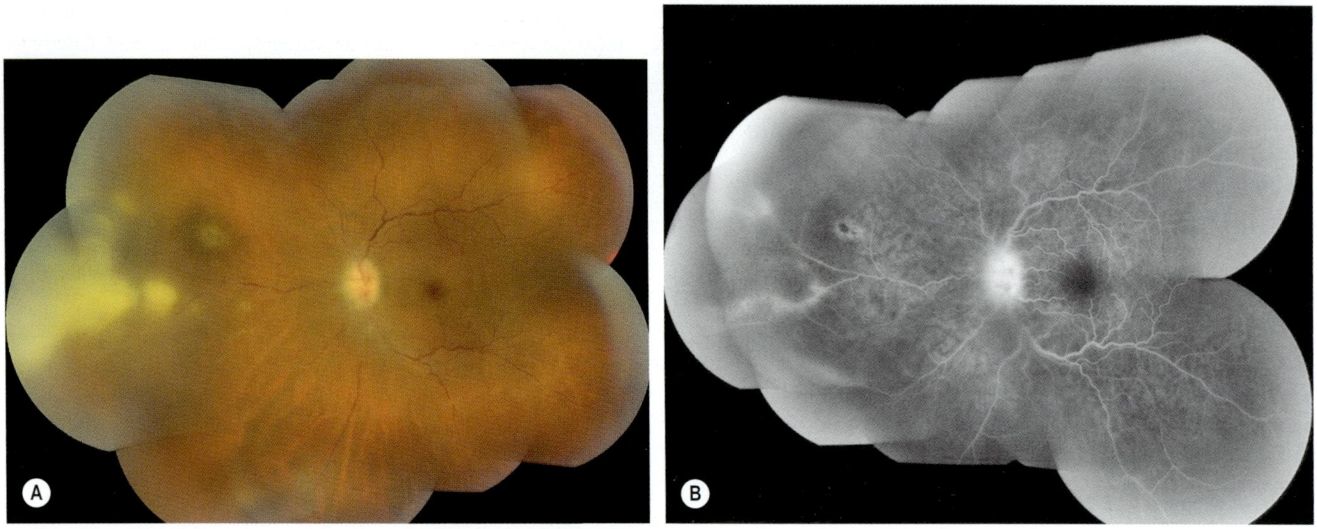

Fig. 13.7 (A) White retinal infiltrates around the optic nerve and the nasal periphery in a patient with acute retinal necrosis. (B) Fluorescein angiogram shows leakage from the optic nerve and areas of retinal vasculitis, predominantly in the nasal periphery.

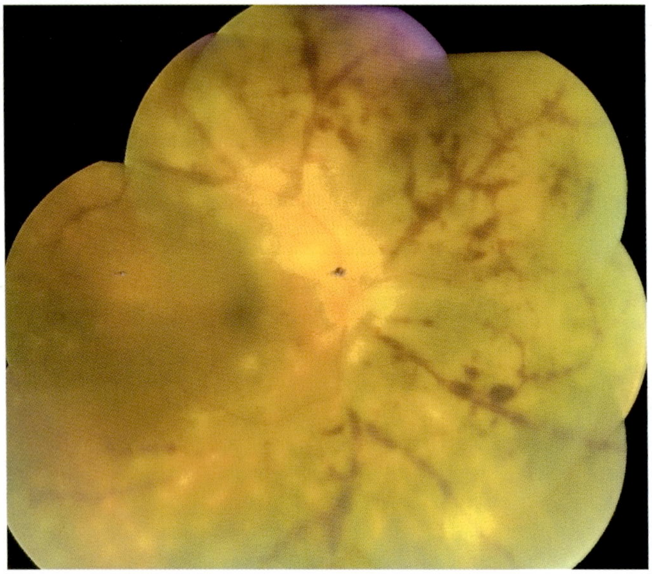

Fig. 13.8 Diffuse retinal vasculitis with retinal hemorrhage and areas of white-colored retinal infiltrates in a patient with acute retinal necrosis.

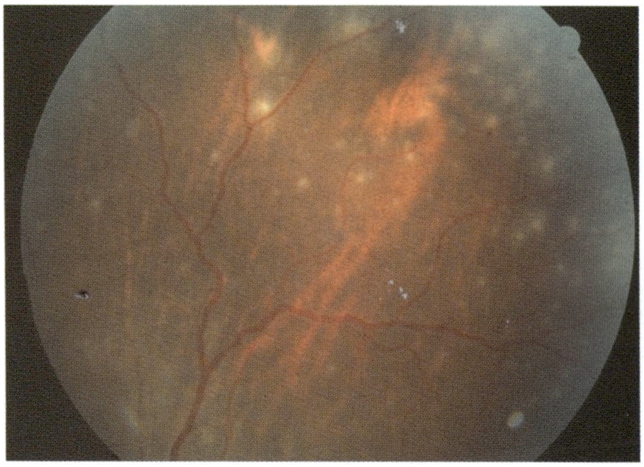

Fig. 13.9 Multifocal punctate lesions involving outer retina early in the course of progressive outer retinal necrosis. These lesions quickly spread and coalesced despite therapy. (Courtesy Chris Walton, MD.)

REFERENCES

1. Tiedeman JS. Epstein-Barr viral antibodies in multifocal choroiditis and panuveitis. *Am J Ophthalmol.* 1987;103:659–663.
2. Weber DJ, Hoffman KL, Thoft RA, et al. Endophthalmitis following intraocular lens implantation. *Rev Infect Dis.* 1986;8:12–20.
3. Urayama A, Yamada N, Sasaki T, et al. Unilateral acute uveitis with periarteritis and detachment. *Jpn J Clin Ophthalmol.* 1971;25:607–619.
4. Willerson D, Aaberg TM, Reeser FH. Necrotizing vaso-occlusive retinitis. *Am J Ophthalmol.* 1977;84:209–219.
5. Young NJA, Bird AC. Bilateral acute retinal necrosis. *Br J Ophthalmol.* 1978;62:581–590.
6. Price FW, Schlaegel TF. Bilateral acute retinal necrosis. *Am J Ophthalmol.* 1980;89:419–424.
7. Culbertson WW, Blumenkranz MS, Haines H, et al. The acute retinal necrosis syndrome. II. Histopathology and etiology. *Ophthalmology.* 1982;89:1317–1325.
8. Fisher JP, Lewis ML, Blumenkranz M, et al. The acute retinal necrosis syndrome. I. Clinical manifestations. *Ophthalmology.* 1982;89:1309–1316.
9. Tan JCH, Byles D, Stanford MR, et al. Acute retinal necrosis in children caused by herpes simplex virus. *Retina.* 2001;21:344–347.
10. Jabs DA, Schachat AP, Liss R, et al. Presumed varicella-zoster retinitis in immunocompromised patients. *Retina.* 1987;7:9–13.
11. Friberg TR, Jost BF. Acute retinal necrosis in an immunosuppressed patient. *Am J Ophthalmol.* 1984;98:515–517.
12. Kalpoe JS, van Dehn CE, Bollemeijer JG, et al. Varicella zoster virus (VZV)-related progressive outer retinal necrosis (PORN) after allogeneic stem cell transplantation. *Bone Marrow Transplant.* 2005;36:467–469.
13. Cochrane TF, Silvestri G, McDowell C, et al. Acute retinal necrosis in the United Kingdom: results of a prospective surveillance study. *Eye (Lond).* 2012;26:370–377.
14. Saari KM, Boke W, Manthey KF, et al. Bilateral acute retinal necrosis. *Am J Ophthalmol.* 1982;93:403–411.
15. Schlingemann RO, Bruinenberg M, Wertheim-van Dillen P, et al. Twenty years' delay of fellow eye involvement in herpes simplex virus type 2-associated bilateral acute retinal necrosis syndrome. *Am J Ophthalmol.* 1996;122:891–892.
16. Ludwig IH, Zegarra H, Zakov ZN. The acute retinal necrosis syndrome: possible herpes simplex retinitis. *Ophthalmology.* 1984;91:1659–1664.
17. Han DP, Abrams GW, Williams GA. Regression of disc neovascularization by photocoagulation in the acute retinal necrosis syndrome. *Retina.* 1988;8:244–246.

18. Wang CL, Kaplan HJ, Waldrep JC, et al. Retinal neovascularization associated with acute retinal necrosis. *Retina.* 1983;3:249–252.
19. Sergott RC, Belmont JB, Savino PJ, et al. Optic nerve involvement in the acute retinal necrosis syndrome. *Arch Ophthalmol.* 1985;103:1160–1162.
20. Sergott RC, Anand R, Belmont JB, et al. Acute retinal necrosis neuropathy: clinical profile and surgical therapy. *Arch Ophthalmol.* 1989;107:692–696.
21. Tada Y, Begoro K, Morimatsu M, et al. Findings in a patient with herpes simplex viral meningitis associated with acute retinal necrosis syndrome. *Am J Neuroradiol.* 2001;22:1300–1302.
22. Blumenkranz MS, Culbertson WW, Clarkson JG, et al. Treatment of the acute retinal necrosis syndrome with intravenous acyclovir. *Ophthalmology.* 1986;93:296–300.
23. Topilow HW, Nussbaum JJ, Freeman HM, et al. Bilateral acute retinal necrosis: clinical and ultrastructural study. *Arch Ophthalmol.* 1982;100:1901–1908.
24. Holland GN, Executive Committee of the American Uveitis Society. Standard diagnostic criteria for the acute retinal necrosis syndrome. *Am J Ophthalmol.* 1994;117:663–666.
25. Culbertson WW, Blumenkranz MS, Pepose JS, et al. Varicella zoster virus is a cause of the acute retinal necrosis syndrome. *Ophthalmology.* 1986;93:559–569.
26. Matsuo T, Date S, Tsuji T, et al. Immune complex containing herpes virus antigen in a patient with acute retinal necrosis. *Am J Ophthalmol.* 1986;101:368–371.
27. Sarkies M, Gregor Z, Forsey T, et al. Antibodies to herpes simplex type I in intraocular fluids of patients with acute retinal necrosis. *Br J Ophthalmol.* 1986;70:81–84.
28. Lewis ML, Culbertson WW, Post JD, et al. Herpes simplex virus type I: a cause of the acute retinal necrosis syndrome. *Ophthalmology.* 1989;93:875–878.
29. Margolis T, Irvine AR, Hoyt WF, et al. Acute retinal necrosis syndrome presenting with papillitis and arcuate neuroretinitis. *Ophthalmology.* 1988;95:937–940.
30. Rungger-Brandle E, Roux L, Leuenberger PM. Bilateral acute retinal necrosis (BARN): identification of the presumed infectious agent. *Ophthalmology.* 1984;91:1648–1658.
31. Ganatra JB, Chandler D, Santos C, et al. Viral causes of the acute retinal necrosis syndrome. *Am J Ophthalmol.* 2000;129:166–172.
32. Van Gelder RN, Willig JL, Holland GN, et al. Herpes simplex virus type 2 as a cause of acute retinal necrosis syndrome in young patients. *Ophthalmology.* 2001;108:8869–8876.
33. Sugita S, Shimizu N, Watanabe K, et al. Use of multiplex PCR and real-time PCR to detect human herpes virus genome in ocular fluids of patients with uveitis. *Br J Ophthalmol.* 2008;92:928–932.
34. Calvo CM, Khan MA, Mehta S, et al. Correlation of clinical outcomes and clinical features with quantitative polymerase chain reaction DNA copy number in patients with acute retinal necrosis. *Ocul Immunol Inflamm.* 2017;25:246–252.
35. Schoenberger SD, Kim SJ, Thorne JE, et al. Diagnosis and treatment of acute retinal necrosis. A report by the American Academy of Ophthalmology. *Ophthalmology.* 2017;124:382–392.
36. Sims JL, Yeoh J, Stawell RJ. Acute retinal necrosis: a case series with clinical features and treatment outcomes. *Clin Experiment Ophthalmol.* 2009;37:473–477.
37. Asano S, Yoshikawa T, Kimura H, et al. Monitoring herpesvirus DNA in three cases of acute retinal necrosis by real-time PCR. *J Clin Virol.* 2004;29:206–209.
38. Bernheim D, Germi R, Labetoulle M, et al. Time profile of viral DNA in aqueous humor samples of patients treated for varicella-zoster virus acute retinal necrosis by use of quantitative real-time PCR. *J Clin Microbiol.* 2013;51:2160–2166.
39. Whittum JW, McCulley JP, Niederkorn JT, et al. Ocular disease induced in mice by anterior chamber inoculation of herpes simplex virus. *Invest Ophthalmol Vis Sci.* 1984;25:1065–1073.
40. Holland GN, Cornell PJ, Park MS, et al. An association between acute retinal necrosis syndrome and HLA-DQw7 and phenotype Bw62, DR4. *Am J Ophthalmol.* 1989;108:370–374.
41. Kezuka T, Sakai J, Usui N, et al. Evidence for antigen-specific immune deviation in patients with acute retinal necrosis. *Arch Ophthalmol.* 2001;119:1044–1049.
42. Chan CC, Matteson DM, Li Q, et al. Apoptosis in patients with posterior uveitis. *Arch Ophthalmol.* 1997;115:1559–1567.
43. Vinores SA, Derevjanik NL, Shi A, et al. Vascular endothelial growth factor (VEGF), transforming growth factor-beta (TGF-beta), and interleukin-6 (IL-6) in experimental herpesvirus retinopathy: association with inflammation and viral infection. *Histol Histopathol.* 2001;16:1061–1071.
44. Balansard B, Bodaghi B, Cassoux N, et al. Necrotising retinopathies simulating acute retinal necrosis syndrome. *Br J Ophthalmol.* 2005;89:96–101.
45. Palay DA, Sternberg P, Davis J, et al. Decrease in the risk of bilateral acute retinal necrosis by acyclovir therapy. *Am J Ophthalmol.* 1991;112:250–255.
46. Matsuo T, Nakayama T, Koyama T, et al. A proposed mild type of acute retinal necrosis syndrome. *Am J Ophthalmol.* 1988;112:119–131.
47. Ando F, Kato M, Goto S, et al. Platelet function in bilateral acute retinal necrosis. *Am J Ophthalmol.* 1983;96:27–32.
48. Tyring S, Engst R, Corriveau C, et al. The Collaborative Famciclovir Ophthalmic Zoster Research Group: Famciclovir for ophthalmic zoster: a randomised aciclovir controlled study. *Br J Ophthalmol.* 2001;85:576–581.
49. Huynh TH, Johnson MW, Comer GM, et al. Vitreous penetration of orally administered valaciclovir. *Am J Ophthalmol.* 2008;145:682–686.
50. Miserocchi E, Modorati G, Galli L, et al. Efficacy of valaciclovir vs aciclovir for the prevention of recurrent herpes simplex virus eye disease: a pilot study. *Am J Ophthalmol.* 2007;144:547–551.
51. Aslanides IM, De Souza S, Wong DT, et al. Oral valaciclovir in the treatment of acute retinal necrosis syndrome. *Retina.* 2002;22:352–354.
52. Emerson GG, Smith JR, Wilson DJ, et al. Primary treatment of acute retinal necrosis with oral antiviral therapy. *Ophthalmology.* 2006;113:2259–2261.
53. Aizman A, Johnson MW, Elner SG. Treatment of acute retinal necrosis syndrome with oral antiviral medications. *Ophthalmology.* 2007;114:307–312.
54. Baltinas J, Lightman S, Tomkins-Netzer O. Comparing treatment of acute retinal necrosis with either oral valacyclovir or intravenous acyclovir. *Am J Ophthalmol.* 2018;188:173–180.
55. Luu KK, Scott IU, Chaudhry NA, et al. Intravitreal antiviral injections as adjunctive therapy in the management of immunocompetent patients with necrotizing herpetic retinopathy. *Am J Ophthalmol.* 2000;129:811–813.
56. Yeh S, Suhler EB, Smith JR, et al. Combination systemic and intravitreal antiviral therapy in the management of acute retinal necrosis syndrome. *Ophthalmic Surg Lasers Imaging Retina.* 2015;45:399–407.
57. Wong R, Pavesio CE, Laidlaw DA, et al. Acute retinal necrosis: the effects of intravitreal foscarnet and virus type on outcome. *Ophthalmology.* 2010;117:556–560.
58. Sternberg P, Han DP, Yeo JH, et al. Photocoagulation to prevent retinal detachment in acute retinal necrosis. *Ophthalmology.* 1988;95:1389–1393.
59. Blumenkranz M, Clarkson J, Culbertson WW, et al. Visual results and complications after retinal reattachment in the acute retinal necrosis syndrome: the influence of operative technique. *Retina.* 1989;9:170–174.
60. Blumenkranz MS, Clarkson J, Culbertson WW, et al. Vitrectomy for retinal detachment associated with acute retinal necrosis. *Am J Ophthalmol.* 1988;106:426–429.
61. Dooling KL, Guo A, Patel M, et al. Recommendations of the Advisory Committee on Immunization Practices for Use of Herpes Zoster Vaccines. *MMWR Morb Mortal Wkly Rep.* 2018;67:103–108.
62. Charkoudian LD, Kaiser GM, Steinmetz RL, et al. Acute retinal necrosis after herpes zoster vaccination. *Arch Ophthalmol.* 2011;129:1495–1497.
63. Heath G, Depledge DP, Brown JR, et al. Acute retinal necrosis caused by the zoster vaccine virus. *Clin Infect Dis.* 2017;65:1211–2125.
64. Kim DY, Jo J, Joe SG, et al. Clinical feature and visual prognosis of acute retinal necrosis according to the initially involved zone and extent: 10-year experience. *Eur J Ophthalmol.* 2019;29(2):244–250.
65. Meghpara B, Sulkowski G, Kessen MR, et al. Long-term follow-up of acute retinal necrosis. *Retina.* 2010;30:795–800.
66. Engstrom RE Jr, Holland GN, Margolis TP, et al. The progressive outer retinal necrosis syndrome: a variant of necrotizing herpetic retinopathy in patients with AIDS. *Ophthalmology.* 1994;101:1488–1502.

67. Forster DJ, Dugel PU, Frangieh GT, et al. Rapidly progressive outer retinal necrosis in the acquired immunodeficiency syndrome. *Am J Ophthalmol.* 1990;110:341–348.
68. Margolis TP, Iowder CY, Holland GN, et al. Varicella-zoster virus retinitis in patients with acquired immunodeficiency syndrome. *Am J Ophthalmol.* 1991;112:119–131.
69. Kashiwase M, Sata T, Yamauchi Y, et al. Progressive outer retinal necrosis caused by herpes simplex virus type 1 in a patient with acquired immunodeficiency syndrome. *Ophthalmology.* 2000;107:790–794.
70. Chawla R, Tripathy K, Gogia V, et al. Progressive outer retinal necrosis-like retinitis in immunocompetent hosts. *BMJ Case Rep.* 2016;2016:bcr2016216581.
71. Spaide RF, Martin DF, Teich SA, et al. Successful treatment of progressive outer retinal necrosis syndrome. *Retina.* 1996;16:479–487.
72. Kim SJ, Equi R, Belair ML, et al. Long-term preservation of vision in progressive outer retinal necrosis treated with combination antiviral drugs and highly active antiretroviral therapy. *Ocul Immunol Inflamm.* 2007;15:425–427.
73. Gore DM, Gore SK, Visser L. Progressive outer retinal necrosis: outcomes in the intravitreal era. *Arch Ophthalmol.* 2012;130:700–706.

14

Other Viral Diseases

Scott M. Whitcup

KEY CONCEPTS

- Herpes simplex virus (HSV) is a common cause of inflammatory eye disease. Keratitis and anterior uveitis are frequent manifestations of HSV disease; secondary glaucoma is an important cause of vision loss.
- A number of randomized controlled trials have helped guide therapy for HSV-associated ocular disease. Topical antiviral therapy is indicated for HSV keratitis. Although oral acyclovir did not improve outcomes in patients with active epithelial keratitis receiving topical antiviral therapy, it did reduce the recurrence and progression of HSV disease and appears to be beneficial for patients with HSV-associated uveitis.
- Varicella causes two distinct forms of disease: primary infection with varicella (chickenpox) and herpes zoster caused by emergence of the varicella zoster virus (VZV) from latency. Uveitis most commonly occurs with herpes zoster infection.
- Treatment with oral antiviral therapy appears to improve outcomes in patients with herpes zoster infection; however, many patients experience recurrent and chronic herpes zoster ophthalmicus.
- Viral infections associated with a transient mild uveitis during the acute stages of infection include measles (rubeola), mumps, influenza, dengue fever, Epstein-Barr virus (EBV), and human T-lymphotropic virus type 1 (HTLV-1).
- Ebola virus causes a lethal hemorrhagic disease. Acute infection can cause conjunctival hemorrhage and uveitis. Uveitis, retinal lesions, and optic nerve disease with severe vision loss are common in Ebola survivors.
- Congenital Zika virus infection has been associated with severe microcephaly. Ocular findings include chorioretinal scars in the macula, focal pigment mottling, and, more rarely, uveitis.
- Zika infection in adults has been associated with conjunctivitis, anterior and posterior uveitis, and maculopathy, but these usually resolve without visual sequelae after the viremia resolves.

Viruses are important causes of human disease and play a pathogenic role in a number of inflammatory eye diseases. Viruses were first identified in the late 1800s. Identification of the specific viral etiologies of diseases, such as foot-and-mouth disease and yellow fever, soon followed. Viruses were first classified as a distinct group based on their small size. We now know that viral genomes are composed of either RNA or DNA and that they can encode several to hundreds of proteins based on their size. Knowledge of how viruses attach, infect, and replicate in cells has allowed new therapeutic approaches to fighting viral infections. Importantly, better detection of viruses has allowed us to determine the viral causes of diseases previously thought to be idiopathic. For example, high-throughput sequencing of RNA obtained from the livers and kidneys of a cluster of patients with fatal transplant-associated diseases allowed for the identification of a new arenavirus as the cause of the outbreak.[1] Furthermore, emerging pathogens, including Zika virus and Ebola virus, have now been associated with newly described inflammatory eye diseases.

HERPES SIMPLEX VIRUS–ASSOCIATED KERATITIS AND KERATOUVEITIS

Although many viruses can induce intraocular inflammation, herpes simplex virus (HSV)–associated keratitis is probably the most common ocular disease associated with uveitis. Patients with stromal keratitis often have a concurrent anterior uveitis.[1] Although in some patients this uveitis develops during the initial onset of epithelial disease, most patients have uveitis with stromal involvement. Recurrent episodes are common and can severely damage the eye. Anterior uveitis may also occur in patients with a history of previous epithelial herpetic infection without currently active corneal disease. Herpetic keratouveitis manifests as a red, photophobic, and often very painful eye with decreased vision.[2] Secondary glaucoma frequently accompanies severe inflammatory episodes and can lead to vision loss.

Pathogenesis

It is difficult to know how much of the ocular inflammation is caused by direct viral infection, an immune response against the virus, or induced autoimmunity as a result of molecular mimicry. Each may play a role and vary among patients. A similar disease to herpes stromal keratitis can be induced in experimental animals by infecting them with HSV type 1 (HSV-1).[3,4] A herpes protein, UL6, has been identified as a viral protein resembling corneal protein. Interestingly, both tolerance and autoimmunity can be induced in the same model, depending on host susceptibility to keratitis (Fig. 14.1).[5]

Diagnosis

The diagnosis of HSV keratouveitis is most easily made in patients with a known history of HSV keratitis confirmed by typical dendritic epithelial defects (Fig. 14.2) or stromal disease confirmed on the basis of culture results (see Case 14-1). The disease should also be suspected in patients with significant corneal opacity that is accompanied by synechiae and anterior chamber cells. Keratic precipitates (KPs) in the area of corneal disease, hypopyon, and hyphema may be seen in some patients. In some patients, the corneal disease may make it difficult to examine the anterior chamber. Bacterial keratitis and possible secondary bacterial infection must be ruled out. The use of polymerase chain reaction (PCR) is starting to aid in the identification of HSV as the causative agent in patients with uveitis of unknown etiology.[6]

It remains unclear whether the uveitis associated with HSV keratitis is a secondary inflammatory response to the corneal disease or whether

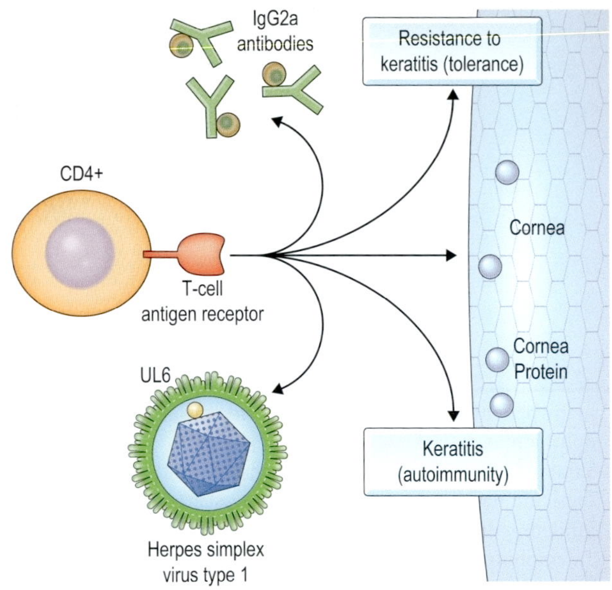

Fig. 14.1 Experimentally induced herpes keratitis. Keratitis can be induced in mice by infecting them with herpes simplex virus type 1 (HSV-1). Molecular mimicry may mediate both tolerance and autoimmunity in this animal model.[79,80] Mice that are resistant to keratitis after they have been infected with HSV-1 appear to be tolerant of the corneal protein because of similarities between a peptide sequence expressed in corneal cells and a sequence found within an immunoglobulin G $(IgG)_{2a}$-antibody variant that is unique to these animals. UL6, a protein expressed in herpes simplex virus type 1, is also similar to the corneal protein. In susceptible mice, this molecular mimicry is thought to be involved in the development of keratitis. (Albert LJ, Inman RD. Molecular mimicry and autoimmunity. *N Engl J Med.* 1999;341:2068–2074.)

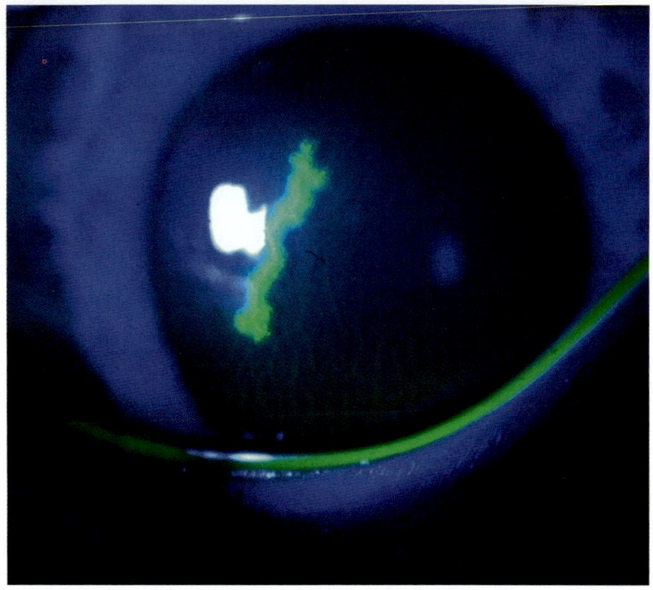

Fig. 14.2 Typical dendritic epithelial defect caused by herpes simplex virus. (Courtesy Sue Lightman, MD.)

it is induced by invasion of a virus into the anterior uvea. Nevertheless, HSV has been isolated from the aqueous humor in some patients with the disorder.[2] In experimentally induced HSV uveitis, the combination of sensitized T lymphocytes, herpes-specific antibody, and HSV antigen is required for the production of inflammation.[7] In addition, topical cyclosporin A was shown to effectively reduce stromal haze and inflammation in experimental HSV keratitis.[8] If this situation applies to human disease, therapy that inhibits the cellular arm of the immune system could control inflammation but enhance viral replication.

Experts differ on whether environmental factors could precipitate disease. Psychological stress has been cited as a potential trigger for recurrences of HSV-related ocular disease. However, with control of recall bias, a study failed to find an association between psychological stress and disease recurrence.[9]

Treatment

Findings from numerous randomized controlled trials (RCTs) have helped guide clinicians on how to best care for patients with herpetic eye disease. HSV keratitis is treated with topical antiviral therapy, such as with trifluridine solution (Viroptic) every 2 hours or vidarabine ointment (Vira A) every 3 hours. Cycloplegic agents are also employed to reduce pain and prevent synechiae. In addition, topical corticosteroids should be used in patients with associated uveitis, but their use is sometimes delayed until the corneal epithelial disease resolves. In a controlled trial of topical corticosteroids for HSV stromal keratitis, Wilhelmus et al.[10] showed that prednisolone phosphate was significantly better than placebo in reducing persistence or progression of stromal keratitis and in reducing the time to resolution of uveitis. In this study, both groups received topical trifluridine. Although some episodes may resolve without therapy, inflammation may lead to severe ocular damage.

Oral acyclovir does not appear to be beneficial for patients with HSV epithelial keratitis treated with topical antiviral agents. In an initial study, Barron et al., for the Herpetic Eye Disease Study Group,[11] reported no statistically or clinically significant beneficial effect of oral acyclovir in treating the stromal keratitis caused by HSV in patients receiving concomitant topical corticosteroids and trifluridine. The Herpetic Eye Disease Study Group also conducted a well-controlled RCT of oral acyclovir for the prevention of stromal keratitis or iritis in patients with HSV epithelial keratitis.[12] Patients with HSV epithelial keratitis of 1 week or less duration were treated with topical trifluridine and then randomly assigned to receive a 3-week course of oral acyclovir 400 mg five times a day or placebo. The study showed that stromal keratitis or iritis developed in 17 (11%) of the 153 patients treated with acyclovir and in 14 (10%) of the 134 patients treated with placebo. In a second clinical trial, the effect of oral acyclovir therapy for recurrences of HSV eye disease was investigated in 703 immunocompetent patients.[8] In this study, the cumulative probability of a recurrence of any type of ocular HSV disease was 19% in patients receiving acyclovir and 32% in patients receiving placebo. A benefit was seen for prevention of both epithelial and stromal keratitis.[9] There were only three patients with iritis; therefore the effect of treatment on uveitis could not be determined in this study. However, in another trial, the Herpetic Eye Disease Study Group assessed the benefit of adding oral acyclovir to a regimen of a topical corticosteroid and trifluridine for the treatment of HSV-associated iridocyclitis.[10] Patients with HSV iridocyclitis were randomly assigned to receive a 10-week course of either oral acyclovir 400 mg five times daily or placebo in conjunction with topical trifluridine and a topical corticosteroid. The trial was stopped early because of slow recruitment after only 50 of the planned 104 patients were enrolled. Treatment failure, defined as persistence or worsening of ocular inflammation, withdrawal of medication because of toxicity, or withdrawal for any reason occurred in 11 (50%) of 22 patients receiving acyclovir and in 19 (68%) of the 28 patients receiving placebo. Although the difference in failure rates was not statistically significant between the two groups, there was a trend toward a better outcome in the patients receiving oral acyclovir. Finally, oral acyclovir effectively prevents herpes-related recurrences after penetrating keratoplasty in herpetic eye disease, supporting the use of the drug.[13]

Valacyclovir and famciclovir are dosed less frequently than oral acyclovir and may be a useful alternative. In a small, prospective RCT of 52 immunocompetent patients, oral valacyclovir (500 mg daily) was as effective and well tolerated as acyclovir (400 mg twice daily) in reducing the rate of recurrent ocular HSV disease.[14] In another small RCT, oral valacyclovir had efficacy similar to that of topical acyclovir ointment in patients with HSV keratitis.[15] Wilhelmus[16] compared the effects of various therapeutic interventions for dendritic or geographic HSV epithelial keratitis by searching the Cochrane Central Register of Controlled Trials. The conclusion of the review was that the commercially available antiviral agents are effective and nearly equivalent. The author also noted that the combination of a nucleoside antiviral with either debridement or interferon (IFN) seemed to speed healing.

Work to develop a vaccine for HSV infection is ongoing. In a small RCT, the use of a vaccine with heat shock–inactivated HSV-1 seemed to reduce the number and duration of relapses in HSV-1–related keratitis or keratouveitis.[17]

Secondary glaucoma is associated with herpetic keratouveitis and may be difficult to control, especially in patients with rubeosis. Glaucoma in these patients often requires surgical treatment with a drainage device. Nevertheless, vision loss related to glaucoma is common in these patients.

HSV retinitis is clearly caused by direct infection of the retina by the virus. As already stated, some cases of acute retinal necrosis may be caused by HSV infection (see Chapter 13). In addition, HSV retinitis can occur in congenital HSV infection associated with herpes encephalitis.[18] This infection is usually caused by herpes simplex virus type 2 (HSV-2) and may be acquired in utero rather than during birth. Many patients with congenital HSV retinitis also have corneal and anterior chamber involvement, which obscures a clear view of the retina. When retinal lesions are seen clinically or pathologically, they appear as large, white retinal infiltrates associated with vitritis and retinal vascular sheathing. After the lesions heal, there are large areas of atrophic and scarred retina. The systemic infection by HSV is often overwhelming and fatal.

HSV retinitis has also been reported in patients who have undergone chemotherapeutic immunosuppression, and again, viral encephalitis often accompanies this ocular condition. Large areas of white retinitis with retinal necrosis result from the viral infection. The disorder may also occur in patients without immunosuppression, and in some patients, diagnosis has been made after chorioretinal biopsy.[19] In some patients, the disorder appears to respond to treatment with intravenous acyclovir.

HERPES ZOSTER OPHTHALMICUS

Varicella-zoster virus (VZV) causes two clinically distinct diseases. Primary infection causes varicella: chicken pox[20]; recurrent infection is known as *herpes zoster infection*. VZV is a DNA herpes class virus and remains latent in the ganglia after the patient has had chickenpox. Although reactivation occurs frequently in older-adult patients, reactivation may also occur in young and healthy persons with no known immunosuppression. Cutaneous herpes zoster has been associated with defects in cellular immunity, and this disorder has been frequently seen with HIV infection.

Although uveitis has been reported with varicella, most cases occur with HZV infection. In fact, uveitis associated with HZV infection often occurs with HZV ophthalmicus, defined as herpes zoster within the ophthalmic division of the fifth cranial nerve (V1). The Centers for Disease Control and Prevention (CDC) has reported that there are approximately 1 million cases of herpes zoster annually and that 32% of the United States population will experience herpes zoster in their lifetime.[21] From 1992 to 2010, the annual incidence of herpes zoster has increased by 39% to 13.9 per 1000 person-years.[22] In a retrospective medical record review of 90 patients with HZV ophthalmicus from 2010 to 2014, the overall 1-, 3-, and 5-year recurrence rates for either recurrent eye disease or rash were 8%, 17%, and 25%, respectively.[23] In this study, ocular hypertension and uveitis increased the risk of recurrent and chronic disease.

BOX 14.1 Ophthalmic Manifestations of Herpes Zoster Ophthalmicus

- Blepharoconjunctivitis
- Episcleritis
- Scleritis
- Punctate epithelial keratitis
- Dendritic keratitis
- Anterior or deep stromal keratitis
- Neurotrophic keratopathy
- Glaucoma
- Anterior uveitis, intermediate uveitis, posterior uveitis, or panuveitis
- Acute retinal necrosis
- Optic neuritis
- Oculomotor nerve palsies

Ophthalmic Manifestations

Ocular involvement is noted in two-thirds of patients with HZV ophthalmicus.[24] Involvement of the tip of the nose with skin lesions (Hutchinson sign) has been associated with a greater risk for ocular disease.[25] A list of the ophthalmic manifestations of HZV ophthalmicus are listed in Box 14.1. Anterior uveitis can accompany herpes zoster ophthalmicus and may result from vascular occlusion and secondary ischemia or an immune response against virus in the eye. Intraocular inflammation occurs in one-third to one-half of patients.[24,26] Severe glaucoma often arises in patients with severe inflammatory disease, and corneal disease manifested by dendritic keratitis, stromal keratitis, or exposure keratitis is a common finding. Large KPs and posterior synechiae accompany anterior uveitis. Although anterior uveitis may appear with the initial cutaneous lesions, it often develops 1 to 2 weeks after the onset of dermatologic disease. In a small number of patients, scleritis may be seen. The iris should be closely examined because it may be the key to correct diagnosis. Sector and patchy iris atrophy consistent with ischemic damage is characteristic of the disorder. Hyphema may occur, and some eyes develop phthisis because of severe ischemic destruction of the iris and the ciliary body. Histologic study in severe disease reveals vascular inflammation and a granulomatous cellular infiltrate in the uvea.[27] Occasionally, retinal vascular occlusive disease or severe choroiditis with associated vitreal inflammation may be seen.

Treatment

Treatment with oral acyclovir early in the course of HZV infection, when the cutaneous lesions are still active, appears to reduce viral proliferation and the complications of the infection, including anterior uveitis.[28-30] In immunocompetent patients, the usual dose of acyclovir is 800 mg five times daily for 7 to 10 days. Famciclovir at a dose of 500 mg three times daily had efficacy similar to that of acyclovir for treating patients with ophthalmic zoster,[31] and valacyclovir, usually dosed 1 g three times daily for 7 days, has also been used effectively to treat the severity and duration of HZV infection. In contrast, acyclovir appears to have little effect on the development of postherpetic neuralgia. A Cochrane review was unable to discern the relative benefits and harms of valacyclovir versus acyclovir in the treatment of HZV ophthalmicus in immunocompetent patients,[32] and the authors suggested that additional well-controlled RCTs are needed. Another review of 1515 articles and abstracts concluded that oral famciclovir and valacyclovir are reasonable alternatives to oral acyclovir in the treatment of active HZV ophthalmicus in immunocompetent individuals.[33]

The value of antiviral therapy for uveitis later in the course of the disease is unclear. It appears that weeks into the course of the disease, anterior uveitis may not be caused by active viral replication but by ischemia. Therefore antiviral therapy appears to be no longer useful. Anterior uveitis and glaucoma may persist for weeks to months and must be treated with topical corticosteroids, cycloplegics, and appropriate glaucoma therapy. It is not clear whether the prolonged inflammatory course is solely caused by residual ischemia or whether an immunologic response against retained viral antigen in the ocular tissue also promotes persistent inflammation.

Although oral corticosteroids are sometimes necessary to treat postherpetic neuralgia, they should be used cautiously in the acute phase of ophthalmic zoster infection because of reports of associated ipsilateral cerebrovascular occlusion with contralateral hemiparesis.[24] Systemic corticosteroids should also be used cautiously in patients with HZV infection associated with acquired immunodeficiency syndrome (AIDS) because these agents may cause increased immunosuppression. Local corticosteroid therapy should be used with caution in these patients, especially early in the course of disease if no antiviral therapy has been started. Local corticosteroids, including intravitreous corticosteroids, have been reported to decrease inflammation and improve vision without reactivation of infectious ocular disease.[34] Topical therapy for skin lesions, including treatment for postherpetic neuralgia, should also be considered.

Therapy requires a commitment to long-term management because even after the acute inflammation resolves, residual damage that limits acuity may be surgically repaired. Many patients are left with severe visual loss. A combination of dry eye, corneal disease, cataract, and posterior synechiae contributes to visual loss and often precludes a thorough evaluation of the posterior segment of the eye. Because the optic nerve and the retina may also be involved in the disease process, it is often difficult to determine the exact cause of visual loss in any given patient. Nevertheless, it is important to try to ensure that the retina and optic nerve are not severely damaged before surgery for cataract, corneal disease, or glaucoma is performed.

In 2006, the U.S. Food and Drug Administration (FDA) approved a live attenuated vaccine for the prevention of herpes zoster and its sequelae. In a large, placebo-controlled clinical trial, the zoster vaccine reduced the overall incidence of zoster by 51.3%.[35] The Advisory Committee on Immunization Practices (ACIP) recommends routine vaccination of persons 60 years of age and older. The labeled indication was expanded to patients age 50 years and older. In 2017, a recombinant zoster vaccine was approved for adults 50 years of age and older. This vaccination requires a two-dose series of injections. Zoster vaccine should not be administered to persons with primary or acquired immunodeficiency.

In 2018, the American Academy of Ophthalmology (AAO) published a policy statement with recommendations for a herpes zoster vaccine for patients age 50 years and older.[36] It is noted that people with a history of herpes zoster ophthalmicus may be at risk for recurrent eye disease after vaccination with either of the approved vaccines.[37,38] The CDC recommends the recombinant zoster vaccine based on efficacy, but the live vaccine is an option where compliance with two doses is an issue, especially in immunocompetent adults 50 to 59 years of age, in whom efficacy was good and fewer systemic reactions were noted. The AAO Policy Statement states, "Ophthalmologists should recommend strongly that patients 50 years of age and older without contraindications obtain vaccination with the recombinant zoster vaccine and should work with primary care physicians, internists, dermatologists, other medical doctors, and health care professionals to recommend vaccination strongly against herpes zoster starting at 50 years of age."

WEST NILE VIRUS

West Nile virus (WNV) is now the leading cause of mosquito-borne disease and arboviral encephalitis in the continental United States. The virus was initially reported as being transmitted among birds by *Culex* mosquitoes in Africa, Asia, the Middle East, and parts of Europe. It is most commonly spread to humans via the bite of an infected mosquito. Originally identified in Africa in 1937, it was first detected in the western hemisphere in New York City in 1999 and has now spread across the United States.[39] WNV is an enveloped single-stranded RNA virus of the Flaviviridae family. Other flaviviruses cause yellow fever, dengue fever, Japanese encephalitis, St. Louis encephalitis, and tick-borne encephalitis.

Epidemiology

Because WNV is transmitted to humans by mosquitoes, in the United States, disease outbreaks occur during the summer season. In 2007, from January 1 through November 13, 43 states reported 3304 cases of human WNV illness to the CDC.[40] A total of 93 cases were fatal. The CDC stated that as of January 8, 2019, a total of 49 states and the District of Columbia reported WNV infections in humans, birds, or mosquitoes. In total, 2544 cases of WNV disease in people were reported; 1594 (63%) were cases of neuroinvasive disease. The incidence of neuroinvasive WNV disease reported in the United States in 2018 is shown in Fig. 14.3.[41]

Diagnosis

A definitive diagnosis of WNV infection is based on findings from laboratory testing. An enzyme-linked immunosorbent assay (ELISA) can be used to detect WNV-specific immunoglobulin M (IgM). However, clinicians must understand the presentations of the disease to know when to order the test and that both false-positive and false-negative results are possible. It is therefore recommended that all positive results be confirmed with neutralizing antibody testing of acute-phase and convalescent-phase serum specimens at a state public health laboratory or at the CDC.

Clinical Description

Although about 80% of WNV infections are asymptomatic, the virus can produce a flu-like illness, with fever and chills, headache, arthralgia, myalgia, and retro-orbital pain.[42] A rash can be seen, and, occasionally, neurologic disease, including optic neuritis, has been reported. The incubation period for WNV disease is about 2 to 6 days but can be up to 14 days longer in immunocompromised patients. WNV disease should be considered in any person with a febrile or an acute neurologic illness who has had recent exposure to mosquitoes, blood transfusions, or organ transplantation.

The differential diagnosis of WNV disease includes other causes of encephalitis and aseptic meningitis, including HSV and enteroviruses. Other arboviral infections, such as St. Louis encephalitis and Eastern equine encephalitis, should also be considered.

Ophthalmic Manifestations

Intraocular involvement with WNV infection was first reported in 2003.[43] Multifocal choroiditis is the most common ocular finding in the disease. Other ophthalmic manifestations are listed in Box 14.2 and include chorioretinitis and optic neuritis.[44-47]

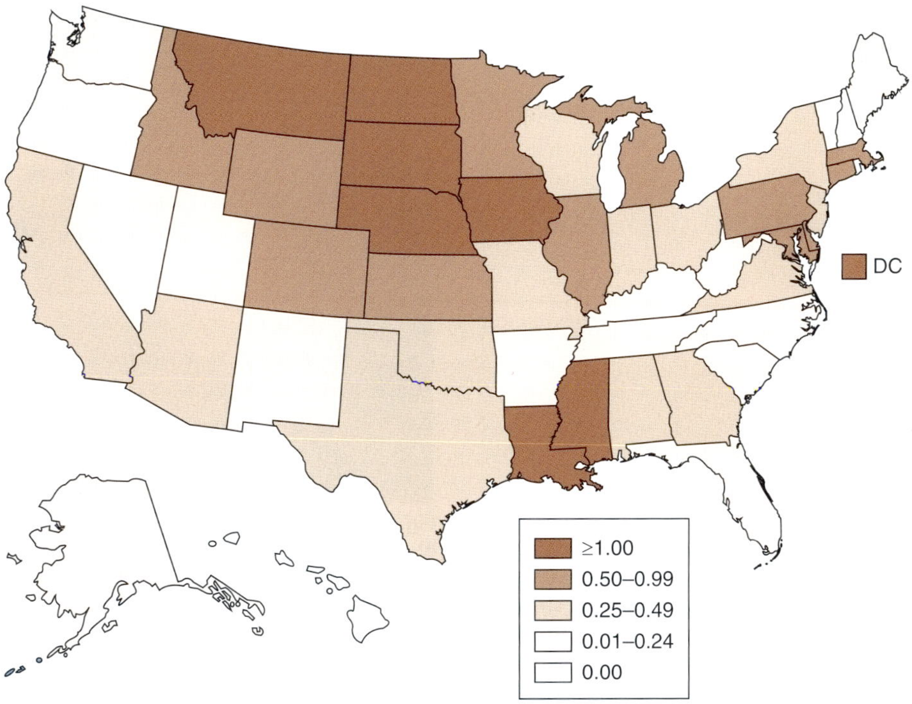

Fig. 14.3 Incidence* of reported cases of West Nile virus neuroinvasive disease—United States, 2018. *Cases per 100,000 population. *DC,* District of Columbia. (From McDonald E, Martin SW, Landry K, et al. West Nile virus and other domestic nationally notifiable arboviral diseases - United States, 2018. *MMWR Morb Mortal Wkly Rep.* 2019;68:673–678.)

BOX 14.2 Ocular Manifestations of West Nile Virus Infection

Multifocal chorioretinitis
Retinal hemorrhages
Vitritis
Chorioretinal linear streaks
Occlusive vasculitis
Optic neuritis
Optic atrophy
Sixth-nerve palsy

Inflammation can be caused by direct infection, an immune response against the virus, or autoimmunity induced by molecular mimicry.

Treatment

There is no proven treatment for WNV infection; no vaccine or specific antiviral treatments are available. Over-the-counter pain relievers can be used to alleviate fever and pain. Supportive care should be provided to patients with severe manifestations of the disease, including neurologic complications. Fatalities occur mainly in older and compromised patients with underlying disease, such as diabetes. Although nonspecific antiviral agents have shown some activity against WNV in vitro, these agents have not been effective against the virus clinically.[48] A number of researchers are working on vaccines for WNV and other flaviviruses.[49] As with other mosquito-transmitted diseases, control of mosquito populations and the use of insect repellents are important in limiting the disease.

Prognosis

The symptoms and signs of WNV infection can persist for months after disease presentation. In a longitudinal cohort study of 156 patients with WNV infection, physical and mental functions, mood, and fatigability mostly returned to normal within 1 year of symptom onset.[50] Recovery was slightly longer in patients with neuroinvasive disease. Lack of comorbid conditions was associated with faster recovery of physical function.

ZIKA VIRUS

Zika virus was first isolated from the blood of a sentinel rhesus macaque that had been placed in the Zika Forest of Uganda in 1947.[51] Human illness caused by Zika virus was first reported in 1954[52] and sporadically until 2007, when an outbreak occurred in 5000 of 6700 inhabitants on several islands in the Federated States of Micronesia.[53] Zika virus infection in humans was reported on Easter Island in Chile in 2014, in Brazil in 2015, and globally in 85 countries by 2017.

Zika virus is an arthropod-borne virus that is transmitted by infected *Aedes* mosquitoes, and there is substantial evidence that the virus can be transmitted from mother to fetus during pregnancy.[54] Human infections are usually asymptomatic or present with mild symptoms and are misdiagnosed as influenza or dengue. Zika virus disease is characterized by low-grade fever, headache, malaise, a macular or papular rash, and vomiting. A relationship between Guillain-Barré syndrome and Zika virus outbreaks has been reported.[55]

Ophthalmic Manifestations

Conjunctivitis and retro-orbital pain are common ophthalmic manifestations. A list of the ophthalmic signs of Zika virus infection is provided in Box 14.3. In adults, Zika virus infection can present as nonpurulent conjunctivitis. Iridocyclitis with KPs, posterior uveitis, and retinal pigment epithelium (RPE) lesions have also been described.[46,56-58] Congenitally acquired Zika virus infection causes birth defects in newborns, including microcephaly, impaired brain development, seizures, hearing loss, facial deformities, and a number of ophthalmic manifestations leading to vision loss.[59] The ocular findings were characterized in a

BOX 14.3 Ocular Manifestations of Zika Virus Infection

Adult Infection
Nonpurulent conjunctivitis
Anterior uveitis
Keratic precipitates
Disruption of retinal pigment epithelium (RPE)

Congenital Infection
Mottling of RPE in the macula
Loss of foveal reflex
Chorioretinal atrophy
Optic neuritis
Optic nerve hyperplasia
Retinal hemorrhage
Iris coloboma
Lens subluxation
Congenital glaucoma

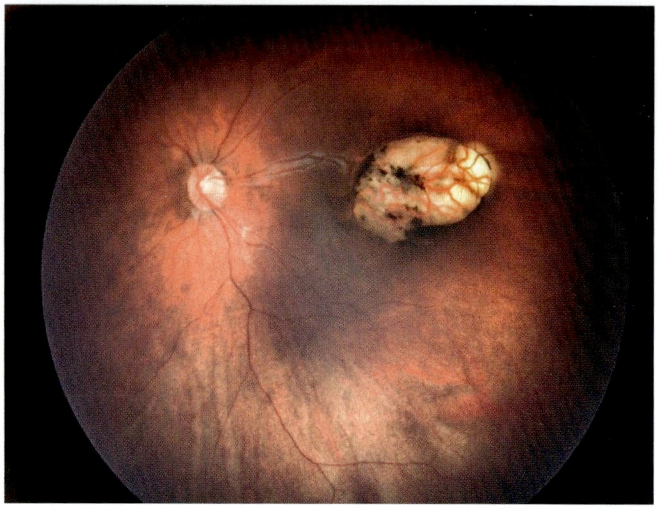

Fig. 14.4 A large chorioretinal lesion in the macula and diffuse stippling of the retinal pigment epithelium in the eye of a child with congenital Zika virus infection. (Courtesy Rubens Belfort, Jr, MD.)

series of 29 infants with microcephaly examined at a tertiary hospital in Salvador, Brazil.[60] Of the 58 eyes examined, ocular abnormalities were present in 17 eyes (29.3%) of 10 children (34.5%). Bilateral findings were found in 70% of the infants. The most common lesions were focal pigment mottling of the retina and chorioretinal atrophy in 11 eyes (Fig. 14.4), followed by optic nerve abnormalities in eight eyes, bilateral iris coloboma in two eyes, and lens subluxation in one eye.

Treatment

There are no antiviral treatments or licensed vaccines against Zika virus infection. Anterior segment inflammatory disease has been treated with topical corticosteroids.[57] Supportive care is warranted for more symptomatic adult infections, and infants with birth defects and ophthalmic involvement often have severe vision loss.

EBOLA VIRUS

Ebola virus is one of the three genera of the family Filoviridae; Cueva virus and Marburg virus are the other two. Filoviruses have linear, nonsegmented, single-stranded, negative sense RNA genomes approximately 19 kb in length. The current outbreak of Ebola virus disease (EVD) began in 2013.[61] Ebola virus infection usually occurs through direct exposure of skin lesions or mucosal surfaces to contaminated body fluids, tissues, or materials. The virus suppresses both the intrinsic and innate immune responses and also inhibits the clotting system. After an incubation period of 3 to 25 days, patients develop an initial influenza-like syndrome, with fever, chills, headaches, myalgias, and a maculopapular rash, followed by more severe manifestations, including vomiting, diarrhea, cough, chest pain, hypotension, confusion, coma, and hemorrhagic findings of conjunctival injection, epistaxis, hematemesis, hematuria, and melena. Most patients succumb to the disease within a couple of weeks; however, with aggressive supportive care, including intravenous fluid hydration, correction of electrolyte abnormalities, nutritional support, and management of respiratory and renal diseases, survival rates greater than 80% have been reported.[62]

Ophthalmic Manifestations

Conjunctival injection and hemorrhagic conjunctivitis are initial ocular findings in EVD.[63] In patients who survive the acute infection, uveitis is the most common ophthalmic finding, including anterior uveitis, posterior uveitis, and panuveitis.[64] Other complications include cataract, optic neuropathy, hypotony, retinal scarring, and phthisis bulbi. The uveitis in EVD has been successfully treated with corticosteroids and topical cycloplegia. Persistent presence of Ebola virus in the eye has been documented,[65] and the uveitis may represent an immune response against the virus as the patient's immunity is restored during convalescence. Interestingly, a unilateral uveitis was similarly described in a patient recovering from Marburg virus infection, and Marburg virus was cultured from the anterior chamber of the involved eye.[66]

SEVERE ACUTE RESPIRATORY SYNDROME CORONAVIRUS 2 (SARS-COV-2)

The severe acute respiratory syndrome coronavirus 2 (SARS-CoV-2) is an enveloped RNA betacoronavirus, which has been identified as the causative pathogen of coronavirus disease 2019 (COVID-19).[67] The disease was first recognized as pneumonia of unknown origin in Wuhan, China, and quickly progressed to a global pandemic.[68] Transmission occurs primarily through close contact with an infected person, mainly via respiratory droplets and after touching contaminated surfaces. Symptoms of COVID-19 appear approximately 2 to 14 days after exposure and include cough, shortness of breath, and difficulty breathing. Other findings associated with the disease include fever, chills, headache, myalgias, sore throat, and loss of taste or smell.

The eye can be involved in COVID-19 in a number of ways. Importantly, it has been implicated as a route of infection, and SARS-CoV-2 has been found in tears. A number of ocular findings have been associated with COVID-19; conjunctivitis appears to be the most common. In a case series of 38 patients with clinically confirmed COVID-19 from a hospital center in the Hubei province in China, 12 (31.6%) had ocular manifestations: conjunctivitis with conjunctival hyperemia, chemosis, and epiphora.[69] Eleven of the 12 patients with ocular abnormalities and positive results for SARS-CoV-2 on reverse transcription–polymerase chain reaction (RT-PCR) from nasopharyngeal swabs, and two of these patients had positive results from both conjunctival and nasopharyngeal swabs. Conjunctivitis rarely can be the only presenting finding of COVID-19.[70]

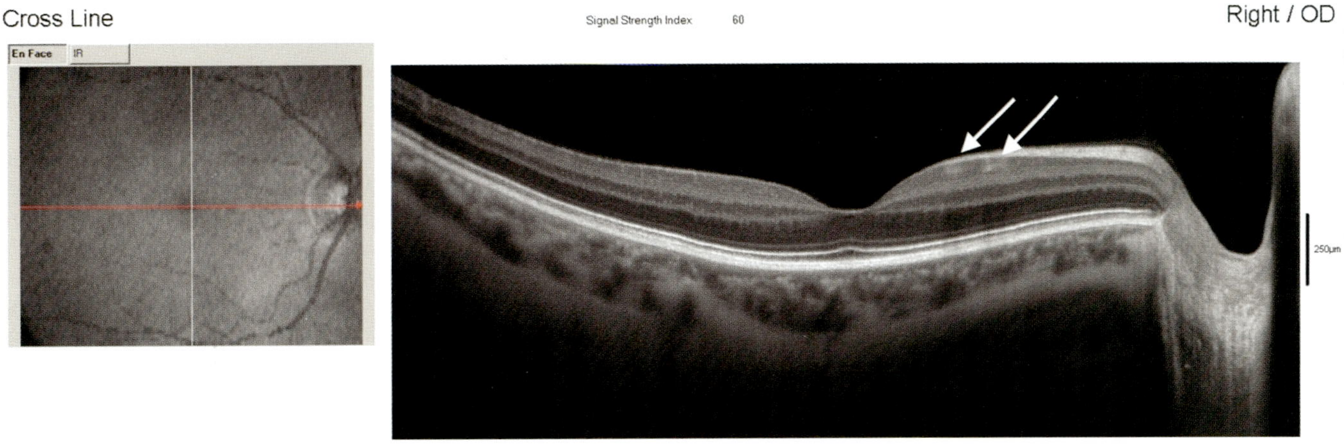

Fig. 14.5 Optical coherence tomography (OCT) scan of the right eye of a 35-year-old woman with coronavirus disease 2019 (COVID-19). The patient presented with fever, dyspnea, anosmia, and mesenteric adenitis, but no visual complaints. The OCT scan of the right eye shows two hyperreflective lesions at the level of the inner plexiform and ganglion cell layers *(arrows)*. (Courtesy Paula Marinho, MD.)

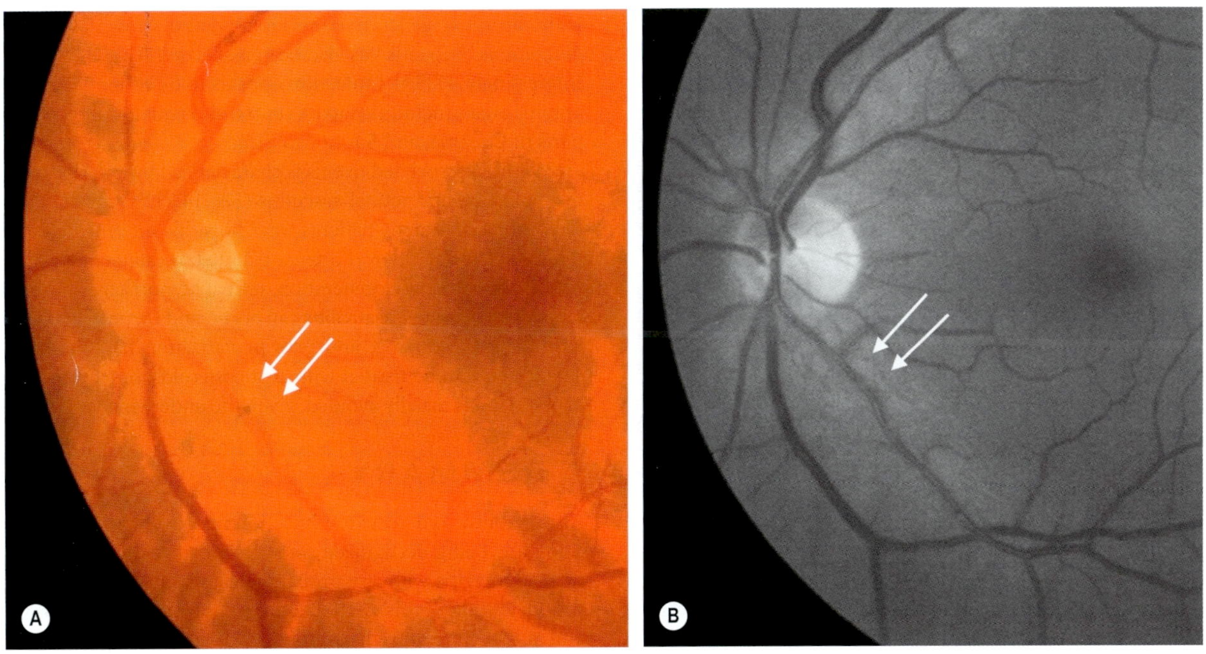

Fig. 14.6 Retinal lesions in patients with SARS-CoV-2 infection. (A) Retinal photograph showing two focal dot hemorrhages *(arrows)*. (B) Red-free photograph showing the same two retinal hemorrhages in the patient with coronavirus disease 2019 (COVID-19). (Courtesy Paula Marinho, MD.)

Retinal findings have now been reported in patients with COVID-19.[71] Retinal and optical coherence tomography (OCT) changes were reported in 12 adults. All patients showed hyperreflective lesions at the level of the ganglion cell and inner plexiform layers, more prominently at the papillomacular bundle (Fig. 14.5). Cotton-wool spots and microhemorrhages of the retina were also noted in four patients (Fig. 14.6). Visual acuity and pupillary reflexes were normal in all eyes, and no signs of ocular inflammation, such as vitreous cells or anterior chamber cells, were seen. Interestingly, 11 of the 12 patients presented with anosmia. One case of acute anterior uveitis was reported in a 30-year old woman with COVID-19.[72] The patient had bilaterial conjunctivitis and uniocular anterior segment inflammation in the right eye with miosis and slightly decreased visual acuity. The patient was treated with topical administration of a fixed antibiotic-steroid medication and tropicamide with resolution of the inflammation and improvement in visual acuity.

It is not unexpected that SARS-CoV-2 would be associated with ocular findings. A number of coronaviruses infect animals and cause ocular diseases, including uveitis. Feline infectious peritonitis is a common disease in cats and is caused by feline coronavirus (FCoV).[73] Ocular signs of the disease include anterior uveitis, retinal hemorrhage, and retinal detachment.[74]

Numerous antiviral agents for COVID-19 are being tested. Remdesivir has been shown to have a beneficial clinical effect in patients with more advanced disease,[76] and has been approved by the US FDA to treat COVID-19 for use in adults and pediatric patients 12 years of age and older and weighing at least 40 kg requiring hospitalization.In a clinical trial of patients with COVID-19, two monoclonal antibodies

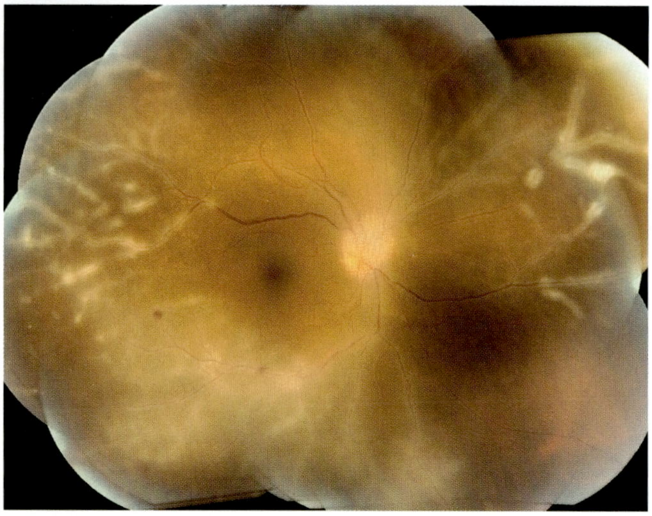

Fig. 14.7 Retinal vasculitis with retinal infiltrates and extensive vasculitis in the retinal periphery in a patient with human T-lymphotropic virus type 1 (HTLV-1)–associated uveitis.

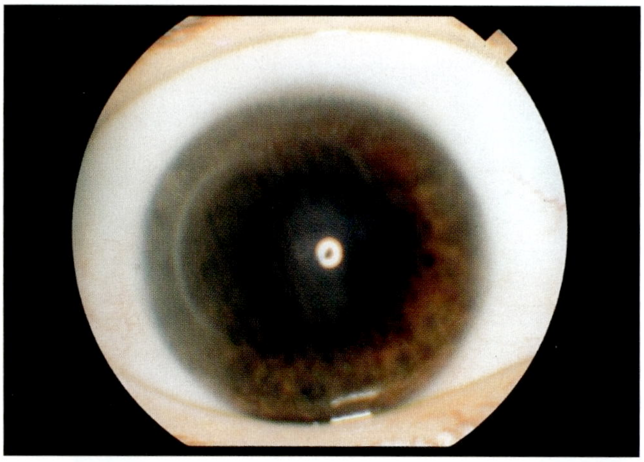

Fig. 14.8 A 12-year-old girl with herpes simplex virus infection–associated keratitis complicated by anterior uveitis, disciform stromal keratitis, and formation of a Wessely immune ring. (Courtesy Roger George, MD.)

administered together, casirivimab and imdevimab, were shown to reduce COVID-19-related hosptitalization or emergency room visits in patients at high risk for disease progression within 28 days after treatment when compared to placebo. These data led the FDA to issue an emergency use authorization for these monoclonal antibodies for treatment of OCVID-19.[77] A number of antiviral agents and antibodies against SARS-CoV-2 are currently in clinical trials. Finally, in record time, vaccines against COVID-19 have been developed and are being distributed globally in the effort to end the pandemic.

OTHER VIRAL INFECTIONS

A number of other viral infections are associated with transient mild anterior uveitis during the acute stages. These include measles (rubeola), mumps, influenza, dengue fever, Epstein-Barr virus (EBV), and human T-lymphotropic virus type I (HTLV-1). HTLV-1 uveitis is described in more detail in a later section. Anterior uveitis rarely is accompanied by symptoms and often goes undiagnosed because these patients do not undergo an ophthalmologic examination in the first week or two after onset of disease. Retinitis and choroiditis caused by German measles (rubella) is rarely seen in the active stages of disease because rubella is a congenital infection. One other manifestation of measles virus infection is the rare, late presentation of subacute sclerosing panencephalitis. In addition to the progressive, fatal central nervous system disease characterized by dementia, ataxia, and myoclonus, associated necrotizing retinitis involving the macula has developed in some patients.[78] Lesions have occasionally been mistaken for Vogt-Koyanagi-Harada (VKH) syndrome, toxoplasmosis, or juvenile macular degeneration. Uveitis of varying severity has been associated with EBV infection.[79,80] One study reported positive antibody titers to early antigen (viral capsid antigen IgM) in 10 patients with multifocal choroiditis[81]; however, subsequent studies have not confirmed this association.[82]

Finally, Rift Valley fever is an emerging, mosquito-borne disease caused by the family Bunyaviridae, genus Phlebovirus. The virus causes an acute, febrile disease and can be acquired through mosquito bites, contact with viremic blood and body fluids, inhalation of virus aerosols, or possibly ingestion of infected unpasteurized milk. Complications include jaundice and hemorrhagic meningoencephalitis. Ophthalmic manifestations include conjunctivitis and retinal lesions.[83]

Human T-lymphotropic Virus Type I

HTLV-1 is the first human retrovirus to be associated with malignancy, an adult T-cell leukemia/lymphoma.[84] HTLV-1 was initially associated with chronic degenerative myelopathy, also known as *tropical spastic paraparesis*.[85] Uveitis has also been associated with HTLV-1 infection. Interestingly, HTLV-I infection appears to be endemic to specific geographic areas, including Japan, central and equatorial regions of Africa, parts of Oceania, and South America.

HTLV-I–associated uveitis is characterized by anterior uveitis, vitreous opacities, and retinal vasculitis (Fig. 14.7).[86,87] In the past, the initial diagnosis in many patients was idiopathic intermediate uveitis, and reduced visual acuity was often attributed to cataract and cystoid macular edema. Retinal degeneration, retinal hemorrhage, epiretinal membrane, and optic nerve atrophy can occur, and corneal involvement with corneal haze, scarring, and neovascularization have been reported.[88] The uveitis can be treated with corticosteroids, but systemic immunosuppression is usually avoided, given the underlying viral infection.

SUMMARY

As our ability to detect viral infection improves and as new viral infections are being recognized and described, a number of idiopathic forms of uveitis will very probably be attributed to viral etiologies. In the 4th edition of this textbook, the section on WNV uveitis was added, and at that time, I predicted that additional new viral causes of uveitis would be identified. WNV-associated uveitis is now more commonly recognized and inflammatory eye disease associated with Zika virus and Ebola virus have been added to this edition. Again, the list of virus-specific causes of uveitis will undoubtedly grow over time. The hope is that more specific antiviral therapies will be developed to improve the outcomes of patients with these infections.

CASE 14.1

Herpes simplex virus (HSV) infection–associated keratitis was diagnosed in a 12-year-old girl with dendritic keratitis. She was treated with topical trifluridine, resulting in resolution of the keratitis. Over the course of the subsequent year, the patient had several recurrences of dendritic keratitis but later developed disciform stromal keratitis with associated anterior uveitis. She was then treated with topical trifluridine and topical corticosteroids. When an attempt was made to taper the topical corticosteroids, there was exacerbation of the stromal keratitis and anterior uveitis and the formation of a Wessely immune ring (Fig. 14.8). The patient's clinical course was complicated by cataract and glaucoma, and she required long-term therapy with topical trifluridine, corticosteroids, and a topical beta-blocker.

REFERENCES

1. Palacios G, Druce J, Tran T, et al. A new arenavirus in a cluster of fatal transplant-associated diseases. *N Engl J Med*. 2008;358:991–998.
2. O'Connor GR. Recurrent herpes simplex uveitis in humans. *Surv Ophthalmol*. 1976;21:165–170.
3. Streilein JW, Dana MR, Ksander BR. Immunity causing blindness: five different paths to herpes stromal keratitis. *Immunol Today*. 1997;18:443–449.
4. Zhao Z-S, Granucci F, Yeh L, et al. Molecular mimicry by herpes simplex virus type 1: autoimmune disease after viral infection. *Science*. 1998;279:1344–1347.
5. Albert LJ, Inman RD. Molecular mimicry and autoimmunity. *N Engl J Med*. 1999;341:2068–2074.
6. Sugita S, Shimizu N, Watanabe K, et al. Use of multiplex PCR and real-time PCR to detect human herpes virus genome in ocular fluids of patients with uveitis. *Br J Ophthalmol*. 2008;92(7):928–932.
7. Oh JO, Minasi P. Role of lymphocyte and antibody in the pathogenesis of immune-mediated herpetic uveitis. *Curr Eye Res*. 1985;4:685–691.
8. Yoon KC, Heo H, Is K, et al. Effect of topical cyclosporin A on herpetic stromal keratitis in a mouse model. *Cornea*. 2008;27:454–460.
9. Herpetic Eye Disease Study Group. Psychological stress and other potential triggers for recurrences of herpes simplex virus eye infections. *Arch Ophthalmol*. 2000;118:1617–1625.
10. Wilhelmus KR, Gee L, Hauck WW, et al. Herpetic eye disease study: a controlled trial of topical corticosteroids for herpes simplex stromal keratitis. *Ophthalmology*. 1994;101:1883–1896.
11. Barron BA, Gee L, Hauck WW, et al. Herpetic eye disease study: a controlled trial of oral acyclovir for herpes simplex stromal keratitis. *Ophthalmology*. 1994;101:1871–1882.
12. The Herpetic Eye Disease Study Group. A controlled trial of oral acyclovir for the prevention of stromal keratitis or iritis in patients with herpes simplex virus epithelial keratitis: the Epithelial Keratitis Trial. *Arch Ophthalmol*. 1997;115:703–712.
13. van Rooij J, Rijneveld WJ, Remeijer L, et al. Effect of oral aciclovir after penetrating keratoplasty for herpetic keratitis: a placebo-controlled multicenter trial. *Ophthalmology*. 2003;110:1916–1919.
14. Miserocchi E, Modorati G, Galli L, et al. Efficacy of valaciclovir vs aciclovir for the prevention of recurrent herpes simplex virus eye disease: a pilot study. *Am J Ophthalmol*. 2007;144:547–551.
15. Sozen E, Avunduk AM, Akyol N. Comparison of efficacy of oral valaciclovir and topical aciclovir in the treatment of herpes simplex keratitis: a randomized clinical trial. *Chemotherapy*. 2006;52:29–31.
16. Wilhelmus KR. Therapeutic interventions for herpes simplex virus epithelial keratitis. *Cochrane Database Syst Rev*. 2008;1:CD002898.
17. Pivetti-Pezzi P, Accoriniti M, Colabelli-Gisoldi RA, et al. Herpes simplex virus vaccine in recurrent herpetic ocular infection. *Cornea*. 1999;18:47–51.
18. Reynolds JD, Griebel M, Mallory S, et al. Congenital herpes simplex retinitis. *Am J Ophthalmol*. 1986;102:3336.
19. Grutzmacher RD, Henderson D, McDonald PJ, et al. Herpes simplex chorioretinitis in a healthy adult. *Am J Ophthalmol*. 1983;96:788–796.
20. Strachman J. Uveitis associated with chicken pox. *J Pediatr*. 1955;46:327–328.
21. Harpaz R, Ortega-Sanchez IR, Seward JF. Advisory Committee on Immunization Practices (ACIP). Prevention of herpes zoster: recommendations of the Advisory Committee on Immunization Practices (ACIP). *MMWR Recomm Rep*. 2008;57:1–30. Quiz CE2–CE4.
22. Hales CM, Harpaz R, Joesoef MR, et al. Examination of links between herpes zoster incidence and childhood varicella vaccination. *Ann Intern Med*. 2013;159:739–745.
23. Tran KD, Falcone MM, Choi DS, et al. Epidemiology of herpes zoster ophthalmicus. *Ophthalmology*. 2016;123:1469–1475.
24. Womack LW, Liesegang TJ. Complications of herpes zoster ophthalmicus. *Arch Ophthalmol*. 1983;101:42–45.
25. Harding SP, Lipton JR, Wells JC. Natural history of herpes zoster ophthalmicus: predictors of postherpetic neuralgia and ocular involvement. *Br J Ophthalmol*. 1987;71:353–358.
26. Cobo M, Foulks GN, Liesegang T, et al. Observations on the natural history of herpes zoster ophthalmicus. *Curr Eye Res*. 1987;6:195–199.
27. Hedges TR, Albert DM. The progression of the ocular abnormalities of herpes zoster: histopathologic observations of nine cases. *Ophthalmology*. 1982;89:165–177.
28. Balfour HH Jr. Acyclovir therapy for herpes zoster: advantages and adverse effects. *JAMA*. 1986;255:387–388.
29. Balfour HH Jr, Bean B, Laskin OL, et al. Acyclovir halts progression of herpes zoster in immunocompromised patients. *N Engl J Med*. 1983;308:1448–1452.
30. Cobo LM, Foulks GN, Liesegang TJ, et al. Oral acyclovir in the treatment of acute herpes zoster ophthalmicus. *Ophthalmology*. 1986;93:763–770.
31. Tyring S, Engst R, Corriveau C, et al. Famciclovir for ophthalmic zoster: a randomised aciclovir controlled study. *Br J Ophthalmol*. 2001;85:576–581.
32. Schuster AK, Harder BC, Schlichtenbrede FC, et al. Valacyclovir versus acyclovir for the treatment of herpes zoster ophthalmicus in immunocompetent patients. *Cochrane Database Syst Rev*. 2016;11:CD011503.
33. Fan S, Stojanovic D, Malvankar-Mehta MS, et al. Treatment of herpes zoster ophthalmicus: a systematic review and Canadian cost-comparison. *Can J Ophthalmol*. 2018;53:117–123.
34. Fonollosa A, Llorenc V, Artaraz J, et al. Safety and efficacy of intravitreal dexamethasone implants in the management of macular edema secondary to infectious uveitis. *Retina*. 2016;36:1778–1785.
35. Oxman MN, Levin MJ, Johnson GR, et al. A vaccine to prevent herpes zoster and postherpetic neuralgia in older adults. *N Engl J Med*. 2005;352:2271–2284.
36. American Academy of Ophthalmology Policy Statement. Recommendations for herpes zoster vaccine for patients 50 years and older. *Ophthalmology*. 2018;125:1813–1816.
37. Hwang CW Jr, Steigleman WA, Saucedo-Sanchez E, et al. Reactivation of herpes zoster keratitis in an adult after varicella zoster vaccination. *Cornea*. 2013;32:508–509.
38. Jastrzebski A, Brownstein S, Ziai S, et al. Reactivation of herpes zoster keratitis with corneal perforation after zoster vaccination. *Cornea*. 2017;36:740–742.
39. Hayes EB, Gubler DJ. West Nile virus: epidemiology and clinical features of an emerging epidemic in the United States. *Annu Rev Med*. 2006;57:181–194.
40. Centers for Diseases Control and Prevention (CDC). West Nile virus update—United States, January 1–November 13, 2007. *MMWR Morb Mortal Wkly Rep*. 2007;16:1191–1192.
41. McDonald E, Martin SW, Landry K, et al. West Nile Virus and Other Domestic Nationally Notifiable Arboviral Diseases—United States, 2018. *MMWR Morb Mortal Wkly Rep*. 2019;68:673–678.
42. Campbell GL, Marfin AA, Lanciotti RS, et al. West Nile virus. *Lancet Infect Dis*. 2002;9:519–529.
43. Bains HS, Jampol LM, Caughron MC, et al. Vitritis and chorioretinitis in a patient with West Nile virus infection. *Arch Ophthalmol*. 2003;121:205–207.
44. Chan CK, Limstrom SA, Tarasewicz DG, et al. Ocular features of West Nile virus infection in North America: a study of 14 eyes. *Ophthalmology*. 2006;113:1539–1546.
45. Garg S, Jampol LM. Systemic and intraocular manifestations of West Nile virus infection. *Surv Ophthalmol*. 2005;50:3–13.
46. Singh S, Kumar A. Ocular manifestations of emerging flaviviruses and the blood-retinal barrier. *Viruses*. 2018;10(10):E530.
47. Chan CK, Limstrom SA, Tarasewicz DG, et al. Ocular features of West Nile virus infection in North America: a study of 14 eyes. *Ophthalmology*. 2006;113:1539–1546.
48. Anderson JF, Rahal JJ. Efficacy of interferon alpha-2b and ribavirin against West Nile virus in vitro. *Emerg Infect Dis*. 2002;8:107–108.
49. Chang DC, Liu WJ, Anraku I, et al. Single-round infectious particles enhance immunogenicity of a DNA vaccine against West Nile virus. *Nat Biotechnol*. 2008;26:571–577.
50. Loeb M, Hanna S, Nicole L, et al. Prognosis after West Nile virus infection. *Ann Intern Med*. 2008;149:232–241.
51. Dick GW, Kitchen SF, Haddow AJ. Zika virus. I. Isolations and serological specificity. *Trans R Soc Trop Med Hyg*. 1952;46:509–520.
52. MacNamara FN. Zika virus: a report on three cases of human infection during an epidemic of jaundice in Nigeria. *Trans R Soc Trop Med Hyg*. 1954;48:139–145.

53. Duffy MR, Chen T-H, Hancock WT, et al. Zika virus outbreak on Ypa Island, Federated States of Micronesia. *N Engl J Med*. 2009;360:2536–2543.
54. Petersen LR, Jamieson DJ, Powers AM, et al. Zika virus. *N Engl J Med*. 2016;374:1552–1563.
55. Oehler E, Watrin L, Larre P, et al. Zika virus infection complicated by Guillain-Barre syndrome—case report, French Polynesia, December 2013. *Euro Surveill*. 2014;19(9):20720.
56. Kodati S, Palmore TN, Spellman FA, et al. Bilateral posterior uveitis associated with Zika virus infection. *Lancet*. 2017;389:125–126.
57. Furtado JM, Esposito DL, da Fonesca BA, et al. Uveitis associated with Zika virus infection. *N Engl J Med*. 2016;375:394–395.
58. Jampol LM, Goldstein DA. Zika virus infection and the eye. *JAMA Ophthalmol*. 2016;134(5):535–536.
59. Schuler Faccini L, Ribeiro EM, Feitosa IM, et al. Possible association between Zika virus infection and microcephaly – Brazil, 2015. *MMWR Mortal Wkly Rep*. 2016;65:59–62.
60. de Paula Freitas B, de Oliveira Dias JR, Prazeres J, et al. Ocular findings in infants with microcephaly associated with presumed Zika virus congenital infection in Salvador, Brazil. *JAMA Ophthalmol*. 2016;134(5):529–535.
61. *Global alert and response: Ebola virus disease*. Geneva: World Health Organization; 2014. http://www.who.int/csr/don/archive/disease/ebola/en.
62. Uyeki TM, Mehta AK, Davey RT Jr, et al. Clinical management of Ebola virus disease in the United States and Europe. *N Engl J Med*. 2016;374:636–646.
63. Moshifar M, Fenzi CR, Zhan L. What we know about ocular manifestations of Ebola. *Clin Ophthalmol*. 2014;8:2355–2357.
64. Shantha JG, Crozier I, Yeh S. An update on ocular complications of Ebola virus disease. *Curr Opin Ophthalmol*. 2017;28:600–606.
65. Varkey JB, Shantha JG, Crozier I, et al. Persistence of Ebola virus in ocular fluid during convalescence. *N Engl J Med*. 2015;372:2423–2427.
66. Gear JS, Cassel GA, Gear AJ, et al. Outbreak of Marburg virus disease in Johannesburg. *Br Med J*. 1975;29:489–493.
67. Lu R, Zhao X, Li J, et al. Genomic characterisation and epidemiology of 2019 novel coronavirus: implications for virus origins and receptor binding. *Lancet*. 2020;395:565–574.
68. Castagnoli R, Votto M, Licari A, et al. Severe acute respiratory syndrome coronavirus 2 (SARS-CoV-2) infection in children and adolescents. A systematic review. *JAMA Pediatr*. 2020 Apr 22. https://doi.org/10.1001/jamapediatrics.2020.1467. Online ahead of print.
69. Wu P, Duan F, Luo C, et al. Characteristics of ocular findings of patients with coronavirus disease 2019 (COVID-19) in Hubei Province, China. *JAMA Ophthalmol*. 2020;138(5):575–578.
70. Scalinci SZ, Trovato Battagliola E. Conjunctivitis can be the only presenting sign and symptom of COVID-19. *IDCases*. 2020;20:e00774.
71. Marinho PM, Marcos AAA, Romano AC, et al. Retinal findings in patients with COVID-19. *Lancet*. 2020;395(10237):1610.
72. Mazzotta C, Giancipoli E, Anterior acute uveitis report in a SARS-CoV-2 patient managed with adjunctive topical antiseptic prophylaxis preventing 2019-nCoV spread through the ocular surface route. *International Medical Case Reports Journal*. 2020;13:513–520.
73. Viner RM, Whittaker E. Kawasaki-like disease: emerging complication during the COVID-19 pandemic. *Lancet*. 2020;395(10239):1741–1743.
74. Andrew SE. Feline infectious peritonitis. *Vet Clin North Am Small Anim Pract*. 2000;30:987–1000.
75. Doherty MJ. Ocular manifestations of feline infectious peritonitis. *J Am Vet Med Assoc*. 1971;159:417–424.
76. Grein J, Ohmagari N, Shin D, et al. Compassionate use of remdesivir for patients with severe COVID-19. *N Engl J Med*. 2020;382(24):2327–2336.
77. FDA News Release. Coronavirus (COVID-19) Update: November 9, 2020.
78. Otradovec J. Chorioretinitis centralis bei leuco-encephalitis subacuta sclerotisans. *Van Bogaert Ophthalmol*. 1963;146:65–73.
79. Wilhelmus KR. Ocular involvement in infectious mononucleosis. *Am J Ophthalmol*. 1981;91:117–118.
80. Wong KW, D'Amico DJ, Hedges TR III, et al. Ocular involvement associated with chronic Epstein-Barr virus infection. *Br J Ophthalmol*. 1989;73:1002–1003.
81. Tiedman JS. Epstein-Barr viral antibodies in multifocal choroiditis and panuveitis. *Am J Ophthalmol*. 1987;103:659–663.
82. Spaide RF, Sugin S, Yanuzzi LA, et al. Epstein-Barr virus antibodies in multifocal choroiditis and panuveitis. *Am J Ophthalmol*. 1991;112:410–413.
83. El-Bahnasawy M, Megahed LA, Abdella Saleh HA, et al. The Rift Valley fever: could re-emerge in Egypt again? *J Egypt Soc Parasitol*. 2013;43:41–56.
84. Manns A, Hisada M, La Grenade L. Human T-lymphotropic virus type I infection. *Lancet*. 1999;353:1951–1958.
85. Osame M, Usuku K, Izumo S, et al. HTLV-I associated myelopathy, a new clinical entity. *Lancet*. 1986;1:1031–1032.
86. Mochizuki M, Watanabe T, Yamaguchi K, et al. HTLV-I uveitis: a distinct clinical entity caused by HTLV-I. *Jpn J Cancer Res*. 1992;83:236–239.
87. Nakao K, Ohba N, Nakagawa M, et al. Clinical course of HTLF-I associated uveitis. *Jpn J Ophthalmol*. 1999;43:404–409.
88. Buggage RR, Levy-Clarke GA, Smith JA. New corneal findings in human T-cell lymphotrophic virus type 1 infection. *Am J Ophthalmol*. 2001;132:950–951.

Ocular Toxoplasmosis

H. Nida Sen

KEY CONCEPTS

- Ocular disease can occur with both congenital and acquired diseases.
- Disease is often unilateral, and the majority of recurrences are seen as satellite lesions.
- Immunodeficient patients are at risk for acquired disease, reactivation of old disease, and bilateral and multifocal disease.
- Pregnancy and cataract surgery may be associated with increased risk for recurrence.

Toxoplasmosis is a common disease in both mammals and birds. The disease is caused by the obligate intracellular protozoan *Toxoplasma gondii.* It is thought that this organism infects at least 500 million persons worldwide.[1] According to the Centers for Disease Control and Prevention (CDC), 11% of the population age 6 years and older in the United States have been infected by *Toxoplasma.*[2] Age-adjusted serologic prevalence in the United States is estimated at 22.5%.[3] In the United Kingdom, the estimated lifetime risk for ocular toxoplasmosis has been calculated to be 18 in 100,000.[4] In the developing world, its prevalence is probably underestimated. In some parts of the world, greater than 60% of the population has been infected with *Toxoplasma,* especially in hot, humid climates and lower altitudes because the oocysts survive better in these climates.[2]

The disease can cause a passing flu-like condition that has little consequence, but it can also cause lymphadenopathy, serious and sometimes fatal disease in immunocompromised hosts, spontaneous abortions, and congenital disease. For the ophthalmologist, it is one of the most frequently encountered posterior uveitides, classically producing necrotic retinitis. It is also one of the few uveitides which can be definitively diagnosed. In the past few years, our understanding of the organism and the interrelationship between it and its host has brought into question several concepts that had been previously accepted in ophthalmology practice.

ORGANISM AND TRANSMISSION

In 1908, *T. gondii* was first found in the brain of a rodent, the gondi, in North Africa by Nicolle and Manceaux[5] and then by Splendore[6] in a rabbit in Brazil. Janku[7] first described postmortem findings in a child who had died of disseminated toxoplasmosis. He noted what were probably *Toxoplasma* organisms in the eye, but inoculation of animals with infected tissue did not induce disease. Transmission of the organism to animals via inoculation of infected human tissue was accomplished by Wolf et al.[8] Helenor Campbell Wilder identified the presence of the organism in the human eye in 1952, confirming that it was the cause of uveitis.[9]

T. gondii is a "cosmopolitan" parasite, being found all over the world. Members of the cat family are the definitive hosts. Oocysts of *Toxoplasma* are 10 to 12 μm in length and oval in shape. They are found uniquely in the intestinal mucosa of cats. Once they are released, they can be spread to humans or to other animals through a variety of vectors. Although invariably thought to be ingested, the organism may also enter the host through other mucosal surfaces.[10]

Common routes of transmission to humans are accidental ingestion of oocysts through cat litter or contaminated soil or water and transplacental transmission, resulting in primary infection during pregnancy. Humans can also be infected secondarily by ingesting meat (pork, lamb, venison, shellfish, and chicken in endemic areas, but probably not beef) contaminated by *Toxoplasma* cysts or by eating food contaminated by knives and utensils, and drinking unpasteurized goat's milk (tachyzoites). *Toxoplasma* can be acquired rarely through blood transfusion or organ transplantation.[2]

The two forms of the organism that can be found in humans are cysts and tachyzoites (Fig. 15.1). The cysts are up to 200 μm in diameter, contain hundreds to thousands of organisms, and have a propensity for infecting cardiac tissue, muscle, and neural tissue, including that of the retina. The cyst structure is complex and can include elements from the host. Cysts can remain intact outside of a host in soil for at least 1 year. It is not entirely clear what factors cause ultimate rupture of the cyst and release of tachyzoites. The tachyzoite is oval or arc shaped and about 6 to 7 mm in length. It is an obligate intracellular organism that actively proliferates and is the cause of the acute disease. The organism's entry into and residence within the host cell are clearly complex and dynamic events, and much is still not known. Joiner[11] found that the organism forms a parasitophorous vacuole that surrounds the parasite and that lacks plasma membrane markers from the host. It will not fuse with other compartments in the cell and is sheltered from all cellular traffic.

Many of the antigens of the organism have been identified (Table 15.1 and Fig. 15.2), with SAG 1 or p30 being the most studied. This major surface antigen has a molecular mass between 27 and 30 kDa. It is useful in the serologic diagnosis of infection[12] and may play a role in the parasite's ability to invade a cell.[13] In animal models, immunization with this antigen or adoptive transfer of immune cells recognizing this antigen will confer a degree of protection against active infection. The *p30* gene sequence has been deduced,[14] and its messenger ribonucleic acid (mRNA) appears to be 1500 nucleotides in length.

A second antigen that has been characterized is SAG 2, or p22. This cell surface antigen (molecular mass 22 kDa) can participate in antibody-dependent, complement-mediated lysis of the tachyzoite.[15] It appears to be part of a complex phagosomal reticular network.[16] A third antigen that has been studied is known as the *F3G3 antigen.*

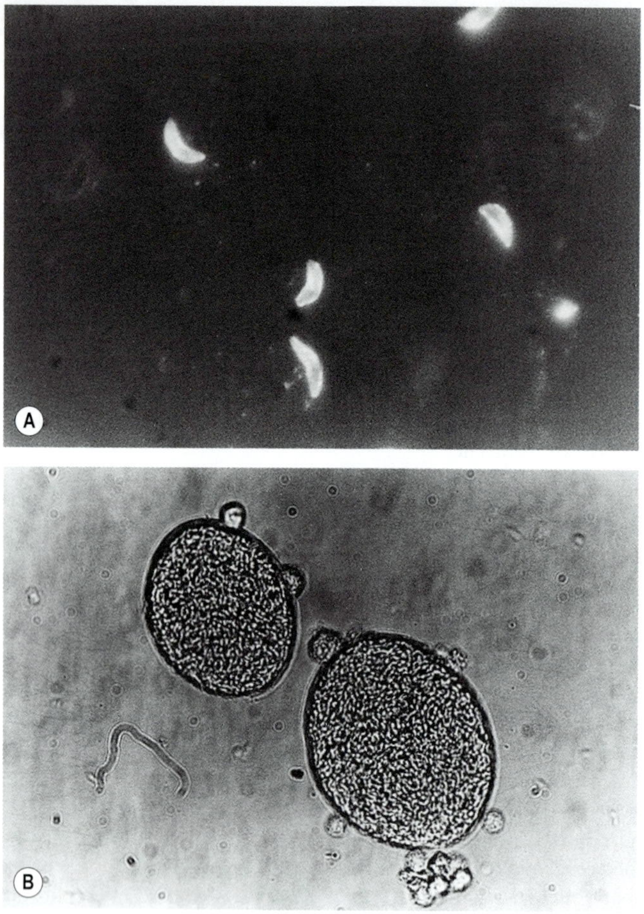

Fig. 15.1 (A) Tachyzoites in culture stained with immunofluorescent dye. (B) *Toxoplasma* cysts containing large numbers of tachyzoites. (Courtesy Leon Jacobs, MD.)

This 58-kDa antigen is cytoplasmic and not expressed on the cell surface. Passive transfer of antibody that reacts to this antigen has been successful in protecting animals from a lethal challenge by the *Toxoplasma* organism.[17] The study of excreted/secreted antigens of toxoplasmosis continues[18] because it has been demonstrated that 90% of the circulating antigens detected during active infection are those that are actively excreted.[19] These antigens could be used as a basis for vaccine development in that immunization against these antigens might abrogate rapid entry of the tachyzoite into the cell. Attempts to classify the specific clonal lineages that may cause human toxoplasmosis have been of interest. Howe and Sibley[20] determined the population genetic structure of *T. gondii* by using multiple restriction fragment length polymorphism analysis. They studied six loci in 106 independent *Toxoplasma* isolates from humans and animals. Although not separate strains, three distinct lineages were found, with only four of the isolates showing an extensively mixed genotype. In this study, human isolates were found in all three lineages, although the majority of those had a type III genotype. However, one study performed in Europe reported that the cases evaluated were of the type I genotype.[21] This was also the type reported from Brazil.[22] However, the story is most probably more complicated than that. Grigg et al.[23] reported an abundance of atypical strains (i.e., lineages) that were associated with disease.

Howe et al.[24] genotyped 68 of 72 samples isolated from human disease by using the p22 (SAG2) antigen. They found that the vast majority of these 68 isolates (81%) were classified as type II, whereas only 10% were type I, and 9% were type III. Genotypes I, II, and III and recombinant atypical genotypes can be distinguished serologically. Most human infections in North America and Europe have been attributed to type II parasites, which are less virulent than type I parasites and the atypical recombinant genotypes in animal models.

TABLE 15.1 *Toxoplasma gondii* Antigens

Bradyzoite	Surface antigen (S-Ag) 2C, 2D, and 4
	Bradyzoite specific recombinant (BSR) 4
	Matrix antigen (MAG) 1
	Lactate dehydrogenase (LDH) 2
	Enolase (ENO) 1
	Bradyzoite antigens (BAG) 1
	Phosphatidylinositol (PtdIns)
	p-ATPase
Tachyzoite	SAG 1 (p30)
	SAG 2A and 2B (p22)
	LDH 1
	ENO 2
	PtdIns t
	SAG-related sequences (SRS) 1–3

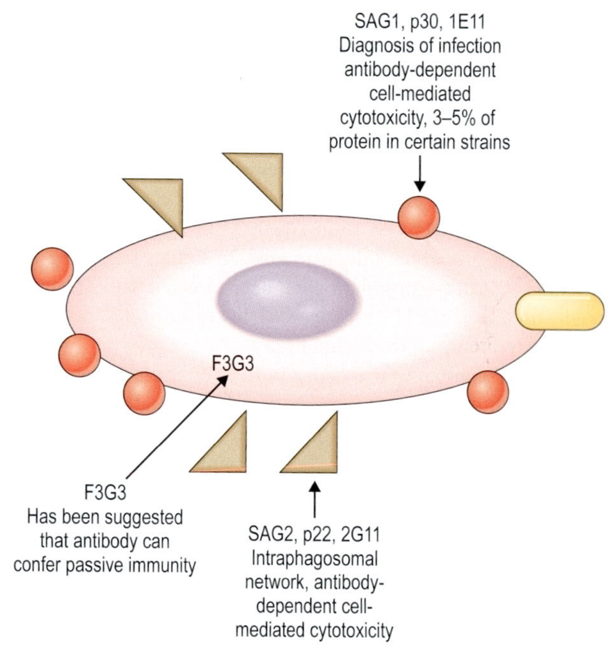

Fig. 15.2 Diagram showing anatomic areas from which purified *Toxoplasma* antigens have been isolated.

CLINICAL MANIFESTATIONS

Systemic

Acquired disease in immune competent adults leads to lymphadenopathy in 90% of patients, with fever, malaise, and sore throat in some cases. More severe disease can occur, affecting muscle, skin, brain, heart, kidney, and other organs. Death resulting from toxoplasmosis rarely occurs in the immunocompetent individual. However, in the immunocompromised patient, toxoplasmosis can be a fulminant central nervous system (CNS) disease that rapidly leads to death.

Ocular

Ocular toxoplasmosis can occur with both the congenital and acquired forms of the disease. Acquisition of the disease causes most concern when it occurs during pregnancy. An older article suggests that in the United States, up to six in 1000 women acquire the infection while pregnant,[1] with an approximately 40% risk of transmission of the infection to the fetus. In a report describing the national neonatal screening program for congenital toxoplasmosis in Denmark, 2.1 congenital toxoplasmosis cases were identified per 10,000 newborns.[25] The congenital form of the disease can lead to a wide range of symptoms, but most important to this discussion is that most cases of ocular toxoplasmosis are conjectured to be acquired congenitally, with activation occurring later in life. In the Danish study, 9.6% of those with congenital toxoplasmosis were born with retinal or macular lesions, with 15.6% manifesting these changes at age 3 years.[25] In a European study reported by Koppe and Kloosterman in 1982,[26] 5% of the infants infected would either die or become severely affected by the disease. Furthermore, about 70% of infants with congenital infections will show chorioretinal scars compatible with toxoplasmosis after a follow-up of 16 years, with 1% to 2% suffering severe visual impairment because of this infection. However, evidence suggests that acquired infection may be responsible for the majority of the cases with ocular disease (Case 15.1).[27] In following up the results of an outbreak of systemic toxoplasmosis that occurred in October 1977 in Atlanta, Georgia, in the United States, Wilson and Teutsch[28] reported that one patient in the original group of patients who became ill or had serologic evidence of acute infection showed evidence of ocular disease.

A large atrophic scar, frequently in the macula—a result of congenital toxoplasmosis—is usually seen (Fig. 15.3). Although such lesions help in diagnosing an old problem, they do not present the ophthalmologist with a therapeutic problem. Rather, it is the reactivation or the recent acquisition of toxoplasmosis that poses the problem (Case 15.2). In these instances, ocular toxoplasmosis manifests as focal retinitis. The active lesion can vary greatly in size but is usually oval or circular in shape and rarely bullous. Frequently, reactivation sites will be "satellite" lesions next to old atrophic lesions, indicative of previous toxoplasmic infections. During the acute stage of infection, the retina appears thickened, rather than transparent, and is cream colored (Fig. 15.4). Cells are found in the vitreous, particularly overlying the active lesion. Some eyes may have one or two small, old lesions, whereas others may have many, with some lesions being very large and involving several clock-hours of peripheral retina. In some large and particularly recalcitrant lesions, the vitreous haze and cellular reaction can be so profound as to cause decreased vision. In the area surrounding active retinitis, hemorrhage and sheathing of the retinal blood vessels may be seen. Fluorescein angiography

CASE 15.1

A 20-year-old woman from Ghana presented with blurry vision in the right eye. Her visual acuity was 20/100 in the right eye and 20/20 in the left eye. Best corrected visual acuity (BVCA) in the right eye was 20/40. The left eye examination was normal, whereas the right eye showed +3 anterior chamber cells, +2 vitreous cells, and trace vitreous haze with a large inferotemporal yellowish chorioretinal lesion, papillitis, and arteriolar sheathing and plaques, also known as *Kyrieleis plaques* (see Fig. 15.14A). Fluorescein angiography showed extensive vascular leakage, both arteriolar and venular (see Fig. 15.14B). The patient received 4 weeks of triple therapy (pyrimethamine, sulfadiazine, and oral prednisone), which was started 48 hours after antimicrobial therapy. Even though the lesion was smaller and more consolidated on follow-up, more vascular plaques and increased haze were noted (see Fig 15.14C); therefore the triple therapy was continued for another 6 weeks. Four months after the initial presentation, the lesion was completely atrophic, with the Kyrieleis plaques, vitreous haze, papillitis, and vascular leakage all resolved, as shown by fluorescein angiography (see Figs. 15.14D and E). The patient's visual acuity improved to 20/25 in the right eye.

CASE 15.2

A 43-year-old white man presented with congenital toxoplasmosis. He had never had good vision in the left eye because of a large atrophic scar in the macula. The right eye had multiple lesions, all compatible with the diagnosis of ocular toxoplasmosis. In the right eye, there was a lesion that encroached on the temporal side of the fovea, but visual acuity was 20/25 in that eye when the patient was first seen at the National Eye Institute. Two years later, he complained of "haziness" in his vision in the right eye. Examination of the parafoveal lesion could not detect an area of activity. Despite this, therapy with clindamycin, sulfadiazine, pyrimethamine (Daraprim), folinic acid, and prednisone was begun.

The haziness disappeared over the course of the 3-week therapy period. During the ensuing years, the patient's vision in the right eye varied from 20/25 to 20/32. He had a recurrence of inflammation every 12 to 18 months. Examination of serial retinal photographs shows greater pigmentation around the atrophic scars but rarely any clinical evidence of activity.

The lack of observable activity on the edge of the old lesion abutting the fovea did not dissuade us from treating the patient each time he complained of a change in his vision. A small nidus of infection, enough to alter his vision but not enough for the observer to note, could very well be there. This patient always maintained a supply of his medication and started on the antimicrobial therapy (sulfadiazine and clindamycin) immediately whenever symptoms appeared. He was always seen within 24 hours, and therapy with pyrimethamine (after a baseline platelet count), folinic acid, and steroids were started.

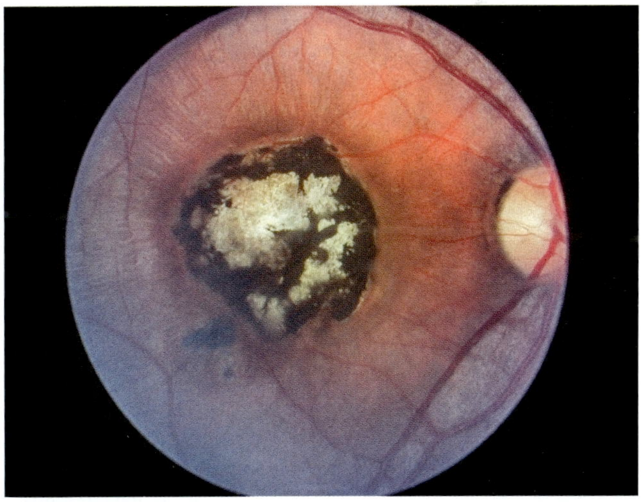

Fig. 15.3 Large macular atrophic scar caused by congenital toxoplasmosis.

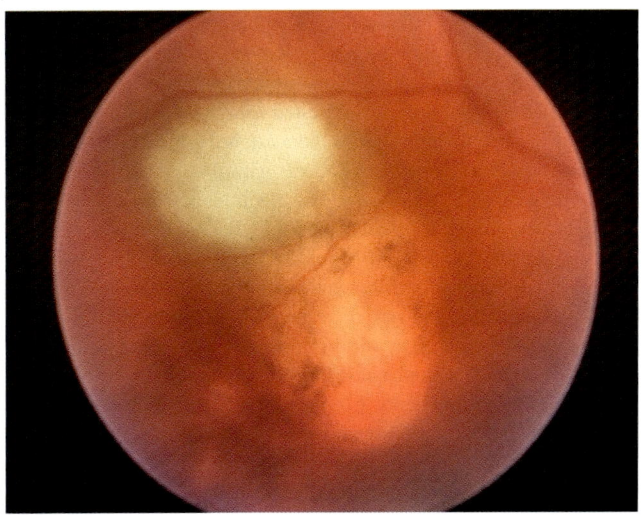

Fig. 15.4 Large active toxoplasmic infection in retina; seen as "satellite" to old healed atrophic lesion.

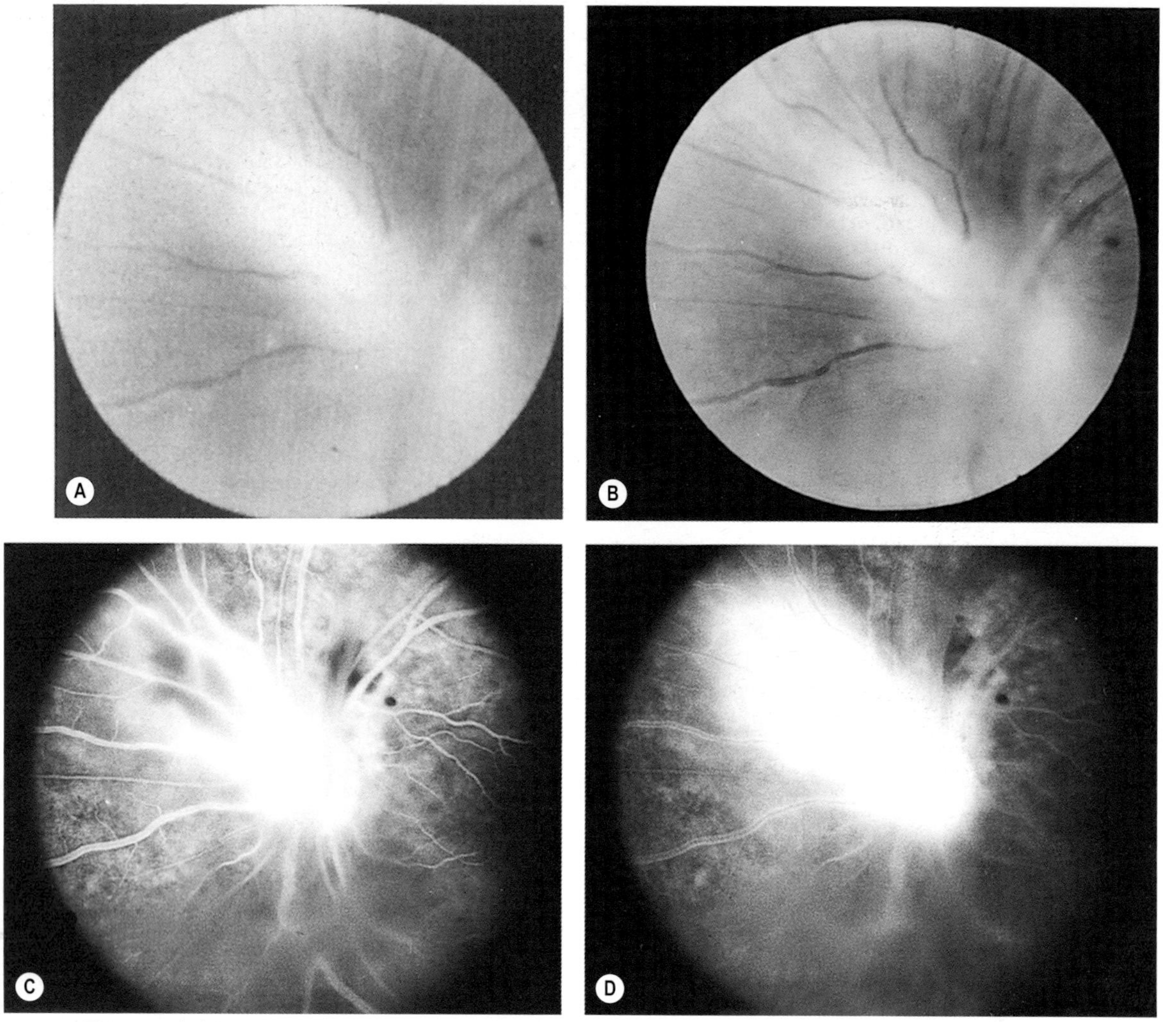

Fig. 15.5 (A) Fluorescein angiogram showing leakage around borders of macular lesion of toxoplasmosis. Note staining of retinal vein below lesion. (B) Large toxoplasmosis lesion encroaching on optic disk. (C and D) Fluorescein angiogram of lesion showing hyperfluorescence peripherally with later photograph showing leakage of dye from both lesion and disk. (A, Courtesy J.D.M. Gass, MD.)

of the active lesion demonstrates early blockage with subsequent leakage of the lesion (Fig. 15.5). Indocyanine green (ICG) angiography can show hypofluorescence of both active and inactive lesions.[29] It can also show other areas of choroidal hypofluorescence that do not correspond to the defects seen on fluorescein angiography[30] (Fig. 15.6). Spectralis optical coherence tomography (OCT) has shown that the retinal layers are abnormally hyperreflective at sites of active lesions, with thickening of the posterior hyaloids, which is often focally detached.[31] When the lesions are close to the optic nerve, there can be considerable field loss[32]; one study reported that 94% of patients with toxoplasmosis had visual field loss as a result of the disease.[33] As mentioned, there is a real risk of disease recurrence, hence the finding of "satellite" lesions. It has been suggested that *Toxoplasma* cysts would be found in greater numbers near the site of a previous infection, which would seem reasonable. Holland et al.[34] reported that the risk of recurrence was greatest immediately after an episode, particularly within the first few years and that younger patients with ocular toxoplasmosis have a greater chance of recurrence compared with older patients.[34,35] The longer interval from the first episode was strongly associated with decreased risk of recurrence.[34]

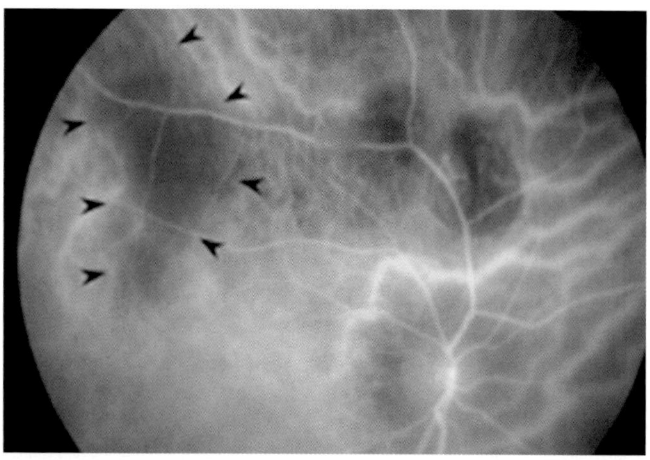

Fig. 15.6 The indocyanine green (ICG) angiogram in the early phase can show hypofluorescent areas that do not correlate with that seen on fluorescein angiography *(arrowheads)*. (Reproduced with permission from: Khairallah M, Yahia SB, Zaouali S, et al. Acute choroidal ischemia associated with toxoplasmic retinochoroiditis. *Retina*. 2007;27(7):947–951. Copyright 2007 Wolters Kluwer.)

Because the *Toxoplasma* organism has a propensity for neural tissue, it is important to bear in mind that the lesion classically begins in the retina, and only with ongoing inflammation will it involve not only

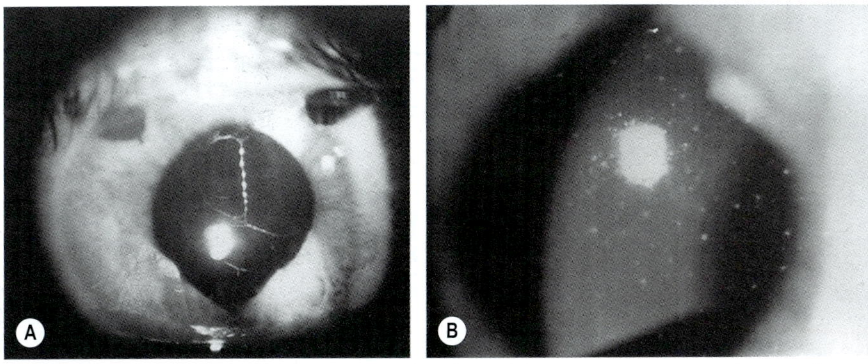

Fig. 15.7 **(A)** "Scaffolding" seen in the vitreous of patient with severe recurrent ocular toxoplasmosis. **(B)** Keratic precipitates on cornea of same eye during inflammatory episode.

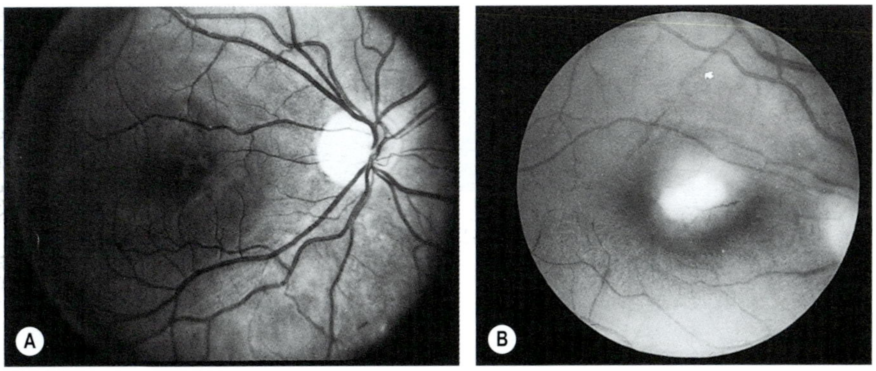

Fig. 15.8 Punctate inner retinal layer toxoplasmosis. **(A)** Lesion begins as subtle alteration in normal macular pattern. **(B)** In a follow-up photograph, lesion takes on appearance of more classic type of toxoplasmic infection. (Courtesy J.D.M. Gass, MD.)

multiple layers of the retina but also the choroid. Cells in the anterior chamber may also be noted and may appear to be either a granulomatous or nongranulomatous uveitis. In the immunocompetent host, although evidence of old toxoplasmic activity may be present, the disease activates in only one eye at a time in the majority (up to 90%) of patients.[34] With continuing inflammatory disease, the lesion and overlying vitreous will undergo several changes. The vitreous may contract, and posterior vitreal detachment is not uncommon. Further vitreal condensation leads to "scaffolding" of vitreal strands (Fig. 15.7). Roizenblatt et al.[36] described the development of vitreous cylinders in toxoplasmosis as a result of condensation of the collagen fibers. As the lesion becomes less acute, the area of retinal involvement takes on a less bright-yellow appearance, ultimately becoming atrophic, often with pigment heaping around its edges. Pigment clumping, however, does not surround all old lesions and should not be considered a diagnostic cue. The associated retinal disturbance will also begin to resolve. All patients will have visual field defects that correspond to the interruption of the retinal nerve fiber layer.[37] Although unusual, unilateral toxoplasmic anterior optic neuropathy, presenting with sudden painless loss of vision, has been reported.[38]

Decreased vision. Vision decreases in the patient with toxoplasmosis for several reasons. The disease has a propensity to occur in the posterior pole and can cause macular scars, more in the congenital form (46%) than in the acquired form (16%).[39,40] Lesions in the posterior pole can lead to macular edema and probable inflammatory by-products of the reactions affecting central vision, even if the fovea is relatively far from the center of the retinitis. Another cause of decreased vision is infection directly involving the macula. Once the fovea is involved in the actual infection itself, the chances of return of good vision are poor, and all efforts must be made to prevent this from occurring. Schlaegel and Weber[41] noted that in 60 attacks of ocular toxoplasmosis, seven patients (12%) had active retinitis within 5 degrees of the umbo, and another seven (12%) demonstrated some evidence of mild macular edema. Additionally, the vitreal inflammation, by itself, may be so great as to significantly reduce vision. The observer should not forget that patients with ocular toxoplasmosis often have elevated intraocular pressure (IOP). These patients need to be monitored closely because loss of vision could be caused by glaucoma.[42]

Ocular toxoplasmosis has been noted to present in a variety of ways besides the classic manifestation already described. Friedmann and Knox[43] and Doft and Gass[44] observed a subset of cases of ocular toxoplasmosis characterized by gray-white fine punctate lesions of the deep retina and retinal pigment epithelium (RPE), initially with little or no overlying vitreal activity (Fig. 15.8). The resolution of these lesions may leave a typical toxoplasmosis scar. Another important presentation is papillitis. These patients may have severe papillitis even with central retinal artery occlusion,[45] white-centered retinal hemorrhages,[46] vitreal inflammation, and sector nerve, fiber-bundle defects, with no apparent retinal foci, as described by Folk and Lobes.[47] Other presentations that we are aware of are bullous-like inflammatory lesions in the midperiphery of the retina (Fig. 15.9), a wide ring-like lesion near the extreme periphery of the retina that resembles a severe uniocular pars planitis, and scleritis resulting from the severe retinal inflammation caused by the *Toxoplasma* infection. The acute inflammation may be so severe that choroidal ischemia manifests as retinal whitening.[30] Numerous anecdotal reports of various presentations can be found in the literature. Although some may be without foundation, these reports emphasize the need to suspect this disorder in a variety of clinical situations. Toxoplasmosis lesions can, on occasion, be confused with other infectious disorders (see Case 15.3). In a patient who received an allogeneic bone marrow transplant for leukemia, ocular toxoplasmosis presented as bilateral cytomegalovirus (CMV) retinitis, with the patient also found to have CNS lesions[48] (see Fig. 15.5). Friedmann and Knox[28] noted that of the 63 cases they reviewed, each had, on average, 2.7 episodes.

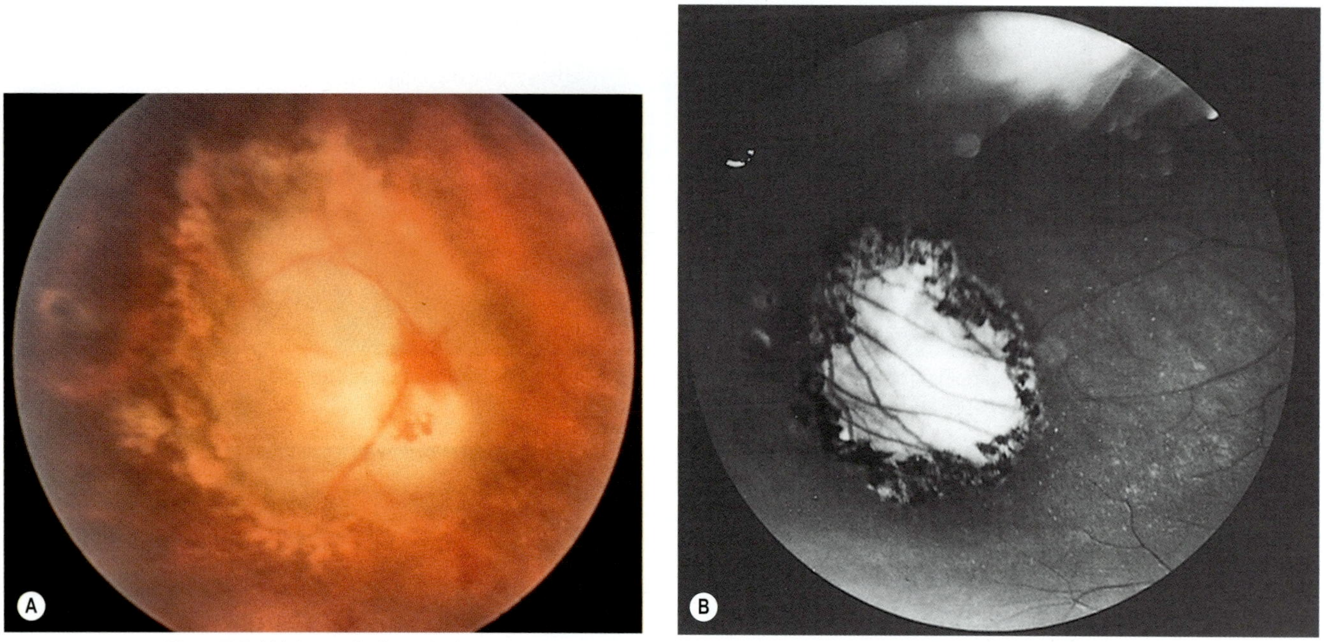

Fig. 15.9 (A) Large bullous lesion caused by toxoplasmosis, with titer of 1:125. (B) Lesion involuted only after antitoxoplasmosis medication.

CASE 15.3

A 36-year-old white man with acquired immunodeficiency syndrome (AIDS)–related complex had chronic granulomatous skin disease, chronic hepatitis, thrombocytopenia, and evidence of exposure to both human immunodeficiency virus (HIV) and human T-cell leukemia/lymphoma-1 virus (HTLV-1). When he was first seen, he had had uveitis in the right eye for several months. He had active toxoplasmic retinitis in the right eye and an old pigmented lesion in the left eye, also compatible with ocular toxoplasmosis. The left eye also had a dense cataract. He was treated with clindamycin and sulfadiazine, with resolution of his inflammation after a 6-week course of sulfadiazine. The clindamycin was stopped after 3 weeks because of severe gastrointestinal problems, and pyrimethamine with folinic acid was begun for the next 3 weeks. Computed tomography (CT) of the head showed no evidence of cerebral toxoplasmosis. Under this therapeutic regimen, the patient underwent cataract surgery, which resulted in a good visual outcome.

The patient continued to have recurrences of his ocular toxoplasmosis as soon as the specific antimicrobial therapy was discontinued. It was therefore decided to maintain long-term sulfadiazine therapy, but this needed to be stopped because of hives. Pyrimethamine was then used. In August 1985, the cataract in the patient's right eye significantly reduced his vision and made it difficult to maintain close monitoring of his retinitis. There were now cotton-wool spots in both eyes and cells in the left, but the lesion in the right eye seemed to be stable. The patient therefore underwent lensectomy and vitrectomy in the right eye. Vitreous specimen demonstrated HIV; his Witmer quotient was markedly elevated for Toxoplasma, supporting the preoperative diagnosis; and after surgery, his right eye revealed 4+ cells and 3+ haze. These conditions responded only to the addition of sulfadiazine.

This patient's course of ocular disease emphasized the rapidity of the changes and the difficulty treating them because of his immunosuppressed state. The presence of HIV in the vitreous, in addition to the patient's history of chronic hepatitis, emphasized the great care needed in handling these samples. Furthermore, without intact cell-mediated immunity, the disease simply recurred once therapy was discontinued. Fortunately effective antiretroviral therapy has significantly improved management of such cases.

The involvement of the retinal vasculature needs to be emphasized. In one review of 64 patients,[49] 59 had vascular changes in the quadrant of the active lesion. Five eyes had changes in all quadrants. Three of these patients also had retinal vascular occlusions. Frosted branch angiitis has been reported in eyes with ocular toxoplasmosis even years after the acute event.[50]

In patients with ocular toxoplasmosis who are undergoing eye surgery, there is a risk of reactivation of disease. Bosch-Driessen et al.[51] reported that in patients with toxoplasmosis undergoing cataract extraction, five of 15 eyes had reactivation of disease. These authors suggested that perioperative prophylactic anti-*Toxoplasma* therapy may be warranted.

The most important sequela of ocular toxoplasmosis is loss of vision resulting from direct involvement of the fovea by the infection. However, choroidal neovascularization (CNV) can also occur as a late complication of the disease.[52,53] Skorska et al.[53] found that subretinal neovascular lesions were present in seven of 36 patients studied. The new vessels were located either directly on the border of the scar or at a distance, with feeder vessels arising from the scar (Fig. 15.10). Retinochoroidal anastomoses have also been observed to occur in toxoplasmosis, with one study reporting an incidence of 2.7%[54] (Fig. 15.11). Other vascular complications have been reported. Rose[55] reported the case of a patient with ocular toxoplasmosis with retinal vein occlusion, papillitis, and florid disk neovascularization. Pakalin and Arnaud[56] observed an occurrence that manifested as arteriolar branch occlusion at a site passing through an area of necrosis. They emphasized the need to include toxoplasmosis in the differential diagnosis of even arterial inflammatory phenomena, something not usually done. Bosch-Driessen et al.[57] reported that nine (6%) of 150 patients with ocular toxoplasmosis had retinal detachments, and another seven (5%) had retinal breaks. Retinal detachment was seen more commonly in those with myopia, and the visual prognosis is guarded: five of nine eyes with retinal detachment were left with 20/200 visual acuity or worse. As with any disorder that disrupts the Bruch membrane, CNV, usually at the rim of an old lesion, needs to be looked for. One report described multiple CNV lesions in one eye with punctate outer retinal *Toxoplasma* lesions.[58]

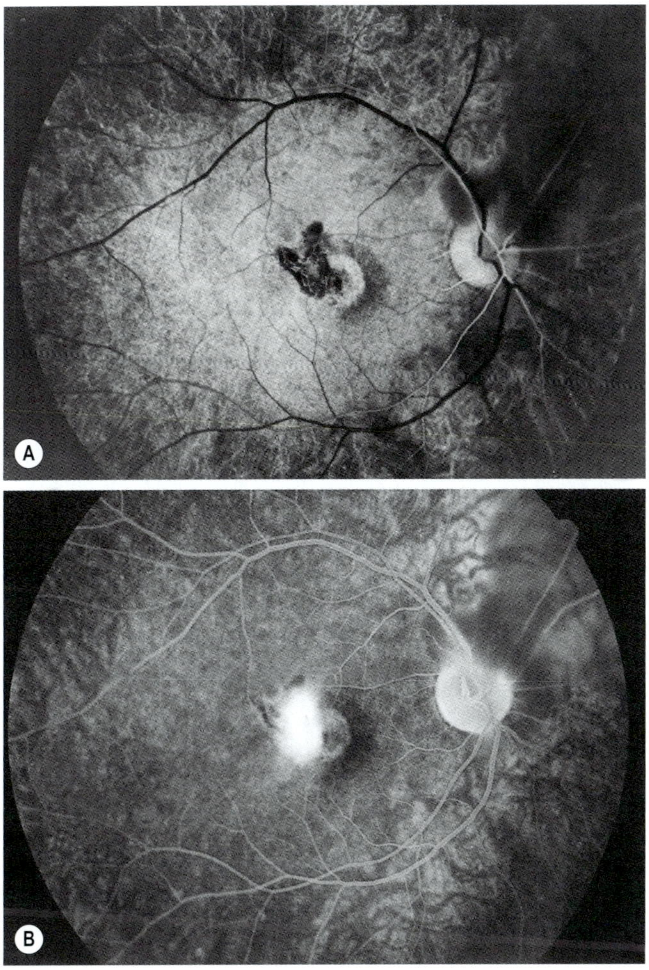

Fig. 15.10 Subretinal neovascularization 8 months after acute attack of ocular toxoplasmosis. **(A)** Nasal portion of lesion that stains corresponds to area of old scarred lesion. **(B)** In the late-stage angiogram, nasal hyperfluorescence has not increased in size; however, temporal subretinal neovascular lesion can be seen. (Courtesy Prof. G. Coscas. Reproduced with permission from Skorska I, Soubrane G, Coscas G. Toxoplasmic choroiditis and subretinal neovessels. *J Fr Ophtalmol.* 1984;7(3):211–218 [in French], © Masson.)

A curious association between Fuchs heterochromia and ocular toxoplasmosis was initially made by Toledo de Abreu et al.[59] They studied 13 patients with Fuchs syndrome who had focal necrotizing chorioretinal toxoplasmic lesions; none of these patients had ciliary injection or posterior synechiae, but most had keratic precipitates, anterior chamber reactions, and cataracts. Six of the 13 had iris transillumination. La Hey et al.[60] evaluated this possible association in a series of 88 patients with Fuchs heterochromia, comparing them with control subjects and other patients with uveitis. Although nine (10.2%) of these patients with Fuchs heterochromia had scars compatible with toxoplasmosis, the authors were unable to establish a special relationship between the two entities. Others have confirmed these observations.[61] Schwab,[62] in an interesting review, also looked for a relationship between toxoplasmosis and Fuchs heterochromic iridocyclitis. In his review, he found that 13 (52%) of 25 patients with Fuchs heterochromic iridocyclitis had scars typical of toxoplasmosis and serologic evidence of the organism compared with only 4% of patients in a general retina clinic. Sabhapandit et al. could not find any association between toxoplasma and Fuchs heterochromic uveitis by using aqueous polymerase chain reaction (PCR) testing in 25 patients.[63]

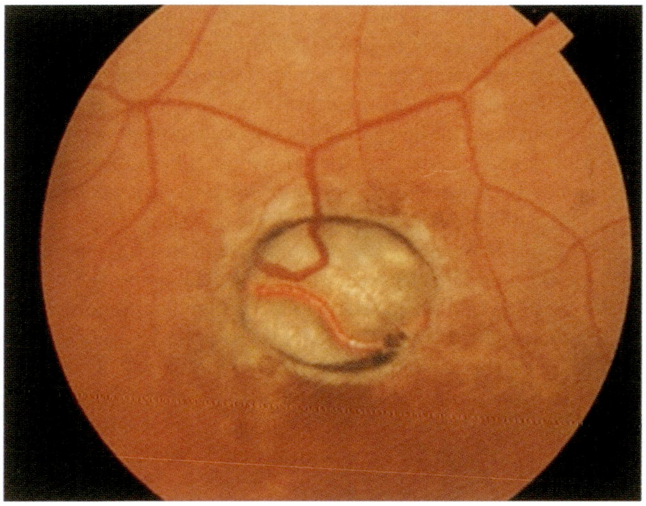

Fig. 15.11 Fundus photograph of eye with congenital toxoplasmosis, with retinochoroidal shunt. (Courtesy J. Melamed, MD, Porto Alegre, Brazil.)

Although there may be a relationship between the two entities, at least in a subgroup of patients, this is not entirely clear at this time.

Effects in the Immunocompromised Host

Special mention of ocular toxoplasmosis in the immunocompromised host seems appropriate, particularly the patient with acquired immunodeficiency syndrome (AIDS) not being treated with highly active antiretroviral therapy (HAART) (see Chapter 12). In these patients, the development of ocular toxoplasmosis does not meet the diagnostic criteria for an opportunistic infection but can indicate to the clinician that a change in the patient's immune state has occurred. Indeed, we have seen active ocular toxoplasmosis in a patient with the AIDS-related complex in whom the full-blown picture of AIDS soon developed. In the patient with AIDS, the degree of inflammatory disease associated with toxoplasmic retinitis is usually far greater than that seen with CMV retinitis, perhaps indicating that reactivation (or acquisition) of the disease occurs earlier in the course of AIDS than in CMV retinitis, when the immune system is still capable of mustering a significant inflammatory response. In the United States, toxoplasmic retinitis is still a relatively uncommon disorder in patients with AIDS. Often, in toxoplasmic retinitis, numerous lesions will appear to be active at the same time, which is a unusual finding in the immunocompetent patient.

The diagnosis of ocular toxoplasmosis in a patient with AIDS should initiate evaluation for possible CNS disease as well. CNS toxoplasmosis has become a problem frequently seen in this patient population. The reason for the disparity between the incidences of the CNS and eye diseases is not known. Therapeutic management of these ocular lesions can be difficult. Despite therapy, disease can progress. Moorthy et al.[64] reported on two cases of severe necrotizing retinitis, with one developing panophthalmitis and orbital cellulitis despite therapy with sulfadiazine, pyrimethamine, and folinic acid. It is not known whether the ocular manifestations of this disease represent reactivation or acquired disease. One could conjecture that both routes are possible. Gagliuso et al.[65] observed that most ocular lesions in patients with AIDS are not associated with a pre-existing retinochoroidal scar and that this would therefore suggest acquired disease. This may be true, but it is possible that cysts in the retina may remain dormant and become activated only in the immunosuppressed state. It is also possible that small lesions indicative of previous disease are simply engulfed in the large retinal necrotic lesion present in the patient with AIDS.

The patient who has undergone iatrogenic immunosuppression has a high risk of reactivation of ocular toxoplasmosis. As with patients with AIDS, if the immunosuppression cannot be reversed, serious consequences may ensue, as reported by Yeo et al.[66] Singer et al.[67] and Blanc-Jouvan et al.[68] have reported cases of ocular toxoplasmic retinochoroiditis occurring after liver transplantation. In one of the patients in the study by Singer et al., because of the difficulty in diagnosing the disorder, the eye had to be ultimately enucleated. These authors emphasize the fulminant nature of the disease, which is far more suggestive of the type of ocular disease seen in patients with AIDS.

We conclude with the interesting observation that immune recovery uveitis may be driven by *Toxoplasma* antigens and not only by CMV, as it is generally thought. Sendi et al.[69] reported the case of a 34-year-old man with human immunodeficiency virus (HIV) with a CD4 count of 11; after the patient was placed on HAART therapy, uveitis developed after an increase in his CD4 count. Aqueous PCR for CMV was negative but positive for *Toxoplasma,* and the patient's disease abated only after periocular steroid injections.

In summary, the diagnosis of ocular toxoplasmosis is primarily a clinical diagnosis. The typical lesions, as described, constitute the most important factor in the decision making. The one additional supportive test we believe to be important is a positive toxoplasmosis titer at any dilution. When the presentation is highly unusual, the diagnosis rests on a combination of multiple factors. In young children, infection with Lymphocytic choriomeningitis (LCM) virus, found in rodent feces, urine, and saliva, has been reported to mimic the ocular lesions associated with toxoplasmosis.[70] In these patients, toxoplasmosis could be confused with ocular histoplasmosis syndrome, although vitreal cells are not present in the latter entity and the peripapillary changes are rarely evident in toxoplasmosis. The deep retinal presentation of toxoplasmosis may be confused with white-dot syndromes, such as an unusual case of acute posterior multifocal placoid pigment epitheliopathy (see Chapter 30). In the immunocompromised host, a single toxoplasmosis lesion early on in the course of the disease may be confused with CMV retinitis. One possible way to discriminate between the two entities is the use of fluorescein angiography. In an active toxoplasmosis lesion, the central area will block fluorescein early and stain late because the central part is where the greatest inflammatory response is taking place. This is in contrast to CMV retinitis, in which the central area will be atrophic and more readily hyperfluorescent early in the angiography (Phuc LeHoang, MD, personal communication, 1989). ICG angiography will show that the lesion extends beyond the visible area, with hypofluorescent foci at all phases.[71] A very good review of ocular disease can be found in Dr. Gary Holland's Jackson Memorial lecture.[72,73]

HISTOPATHOLOGY AND IMMUNE FACTORS

In ocular toxoplasmosis, cysts and tachyzoites can be found in the retina (Fig. 15.12). The *Toxoplasma* organism most frequently is seen in the superficial portions of the retina. The lesion induced is necrotic, destroying the architecture of the retina. In many cases, the underlying structures are destroyed as well, so the disease at this point can certainly be classified as chorioretinitis. Clinically, this destruction will permit the examiner to see the underlying sclera quite clearly. Dutton et al.[74,75] were able to study these alterations more carefully by using a murine model of congenital toxoplasmic retinochoroiditis. They noted that the inflammation ranged from a low-grade mononuclear infiltrate to total destruction of the outer retina, the RPE, and the choroid. Of great interest was the fact that photoreceptor outer segments were phagocytosed by macrophages, whereas the *Toxoplasma* cysts did not appear to be the center of the inflammatory attack. Roberts et al.[76] histologically characterized the eyes from 10 fetuses and two infants with congenital toxoplasmosis. Retinitis was present in 10 of 18 eyes, necrosis in four of 18, RPE changes in 12 of 18, choroidal inflammation in 15 of 18, and optic neuritis in five of eight fetal eyes. Parasites were found on immunohistologic examination in 10 of 18 eyes. It appeared to the authors that the inflammatory response mounted by the host accounted for part of the damage observed.

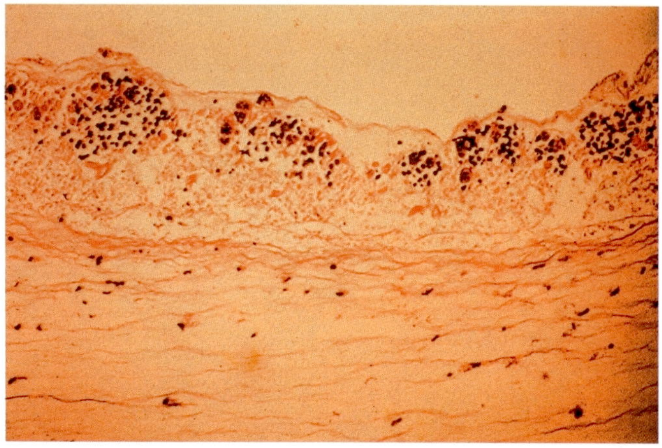

Fig. 15.12 Photomicrograph showing toxoplasmic cysts in retina. Cysts are larger circular structures, located mainly in or close to the nerve fiber layer. (Courtesy D. Cogan, MD.)

Because of the selective photoreceptor destruction, one can speculate that autoimmune mechanisms may be important in the tissue destruction seen (see discussion of autoimmunity in Chapter 1). Indeed, when we had the opportunity to evaluate this issue, we found that in 16 (40%) of 40 patients with ocular toxoplasmosis, an in vitro proliferative response to the retinal S-antigen (S-Ag) was seen.[77] This finding could indicate that an autoimmune component to the inflammatory disease is initiated, with destruction of the retina by a parasite and subsequent sensitization to the uveitogenic antigen. We also found that proliferative responses to the p22 antigen approached antigens to crude toxoplasmosis antigen, whereas the response to the p30 membrane antigen was considerably less striking. Others have shown that the *Toxoplasma* antigen stimulates CD25+ helper cells.[78]

Immune Response

The host's immune response is exceptionally important in the ultimate expression of toxoplasmosis. In animal models, resistance, as measured by survival after challenge with the organism, has been reported to be regulated by at least five genes,[79] one of which is within the region of the H-2 antigen (the equivalent of the major histocompatibility complex [MHC] in humans).[80] Brown and McLeod[81] found that class I MHC genes and the CD8+ fraction of T cells determine the cyst number in *Toxoplasma* infection. Jamieson et al.[82] reported polymorphism associations at the COL2A1 encoding type II collagen only in those who had ocular disease. Others have looked at the effect of cytokines on the multiplication of the *Toxoplasma* organism. Interferon (IFN)-γ, tumor necrosis factor (TNF)-α, and transforming growth factor-β all appear to play a role in inhibiting multiplication.[83,84] Gazzinelli et al.[85] reported that reactivation of *T. gondii,* at least in the experimental mouse model, results from downregulation of IFN-γ and TNF-α, which leads to reduced macrophage (with a decrease in inducible nitric oxide synthase and macrophage activation gene 1) and glial activation, a release of parasite growth, and tissue damage. Shen et al.[86] found IFN in the eyes of *Toxoplasma*-infected mice but that inflammation-induced apoptosis was caused by several factors, not only Fas/FasL interactions. Beamon et al.[87] reported that interleukin (IL)-6 enhanced intracellular reproduction of *T. gondii* and actually reversed the effect of IFN-γ–mediated killing, which contradicts the finding of Lyons et al.[88] who stated that IL-6 knockout mice in a chronic toxoplasmosis model had more severe disease and an increased parasite burden. This finding is particularly important in light of the fact that the RPE produces large amounts of IL-6. An analysis of ocular fluids from uveitic eyes (including those from patients with toxoplasmosis) demonstrated the presence of various cytokines, including IL-6, IFN, and IL-10. Furtado et al. showed in ex vivo assays that tachyzoites preferentially infect glial cells over neuronal cells. The same group also showed that migration of human dendritic cells across the RPE is increased after infection and that although neutrophils may not be infected by *T. gondii* or may not assist in the transport of tachyzoites across the retina, they appear to participate actively in the inflammatory reaction against *T. gondii*.[89-91] Zamora et al. showed that the *Toxoplasma* organism invades human retinal endothelial cells more efficiently than they do human dermal endothelial cells.[92] In another study, Feron et al.[93] characterized 10 T-cell specimens from the vitreous of patients with toxoplasmosis. Although the cell lines were initially generated by mitogenic stimulation, they were all CD4+ and appeared reactive to *Toxoplasma* antigens and not to any retinal antigens. The majority had a helper T cell type 2 (Th2) profile. It has also been suggested that CD8+ T cells directed against the *Toxoplasma* organism appear during the acute phase of the disease, whereas CD4+ parasite-specific T cells appear with chronicity of the disease.[94] Denkers et al.[95] reported that the *Toxoplasma* organism possesses a superantigen that expands murine Vβ5-expressing cells, most of which were CD8+. It may be that this superantigen-driven expansion of predominantly IFN-γ-secreting CD8+ cells is partly why the early immune response is seen. Curiel et al.[96] reported the cloning of human CD3+, CD4+ T cells that lysed autologous target cells that had been pulsed with *Toxoplasma* antigen or infected with live tachyzoites. These results suggest that specific immunotherapy with a vaccine may be possible. Patients with acute toxoplasmosis have increased serum levels of CXCL8, part of the chemokines that control leukocyte infiltration and can even modulate angiogenesis.[97]

Although antibodies are usually readily made, it is the intactness of the cellular component of the immune system that is important for resolution of the disease process. However, antibody production may play an important role in establishing a state of premunition (immunity from infection) in *Toxoplasma* infection.[98] In an attempt to evaluate why newborns seem to have difficulty fighting the *Toxoplasma* infection, Wilson and Haas[99] evaluated the cellular defenses against *T. gondii* in newborns. They noted that newborn and adult macrophages killed the organism equally well, but supernatants from cord blood–derived, concanavalin A-stimulated mononuclear cells activated macrophages less effectively compared with the supernatants produced from adult blood cells. This difference appeared to lie in the CD4+ fraction of T cells. Cord blood appeared to produce fewer lymphokines capable of activating macrophages, including IFN-γ. The authors did not believe that enhanced generation of reactive oxygen intermediates was important in explaining the differences between the responses in adults and newborns. Roberts et al.[100] demonstrated in a murine model that inhibition of nitric oxide by administration of Lω-*nitro*-L-arginine methyl ester made the disease worse. Of interest is the fact that the organism replicates in macrophages, and this reduced killing in the newborn may then lead to greater susceptibility.

Inflammatory Response

What then is the cause of the focal retinal inflammatory response? So far, data still support the notion that it is the release of actively proliferating tachyzoites, often from a long-dormant cyst. We know now of many immune components that can stimulate this tachyzoite–bradyzoite interconversion (Fig. 15.13). However, immune studies with patients with ocular toxoplasmosis suggested that other factors are involved. Wyler et al.[101] noted that lymphocytes from patients with ocular toxoplasmosis demonstrated in vitro responses not only to *Toxoplasma* antigens but also to a crude retinal preparation. As mentioned earlier, our patients with toxoplasmosis have demonstrated in vitro cellular responses to the retinal S-Ag, a purified antigen from the photoreceptor region and the site of the most intense inflammatory response in Dutton et al.'s murine model for toxoplasmosis.[75] Abrahams and Gregerson[102] detected circulating antibodies to various retinal antigens in patients with toxoplasmosis. Whittle et al.,[103] using indirect immunofluorescent techniques over normal human cadaver retina, determined the presence of human antiretinal antibodies in patients with ocular toxoplasmosis. Of the sera from 36 patients with toxoplasmosis, 94% demonstrated photoreceptor layer reactivity. However, only 27 of these patients had anti–S-Ag antibodies, as determined with enzyme-linked immunosorbent assay (ELISA). The authors concluded that antiretinal activity can be accounted for by antibodies directed not only against S-Ag but also against other antigens. These observations raise the provocative argument that the inflammatory disease we see is, at least partly or occasionally, autoimmune driven. However, Vallochi et al.[104] reported that peripheral blood from patients with ocular toxoplasmosis also recognized retinal antigens. But their data suggest that such autoimmune responses are associated with less severe disease. We know that the *Toxoplasma* cyst may include tissue from the host and that S-Ag may be sequestered there until the cyst breaks open. Alternatively, the initial destruction caused by the proliferating organism releases immunogenic antigens to the general circulation, thereby causing sensitization. This then results in a secondary autoimmune response, which can prolong the initial response or become the center of a recurrent inflammatory episode sometime in the future.

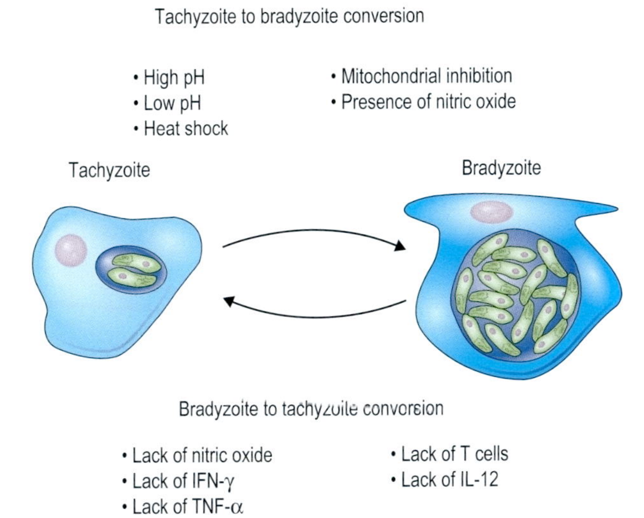

Fig. 15.13 Factors that affect conversion from tachyzoite to bradyzoite. (From Lyons RE, McLeod R, Roberts CW. *Toxoplasma gondii* tachyzoite–bradyzoite interconversion. *Trends Parasitol.* 2002;18:198, with permission.)

The mechanism of the anterior uveitis and the Fuchs-like syndrome seen in conjunction with the retinitis of ocular toxoplasmosis still is a subject of conjecture. In a rabbit model of experimental ocular toxoplasmosis, toxoplasmic antigen was found in the vitreous.[105] In a feline model of ocular toxoplasmosis, chorioretinal lesions formed

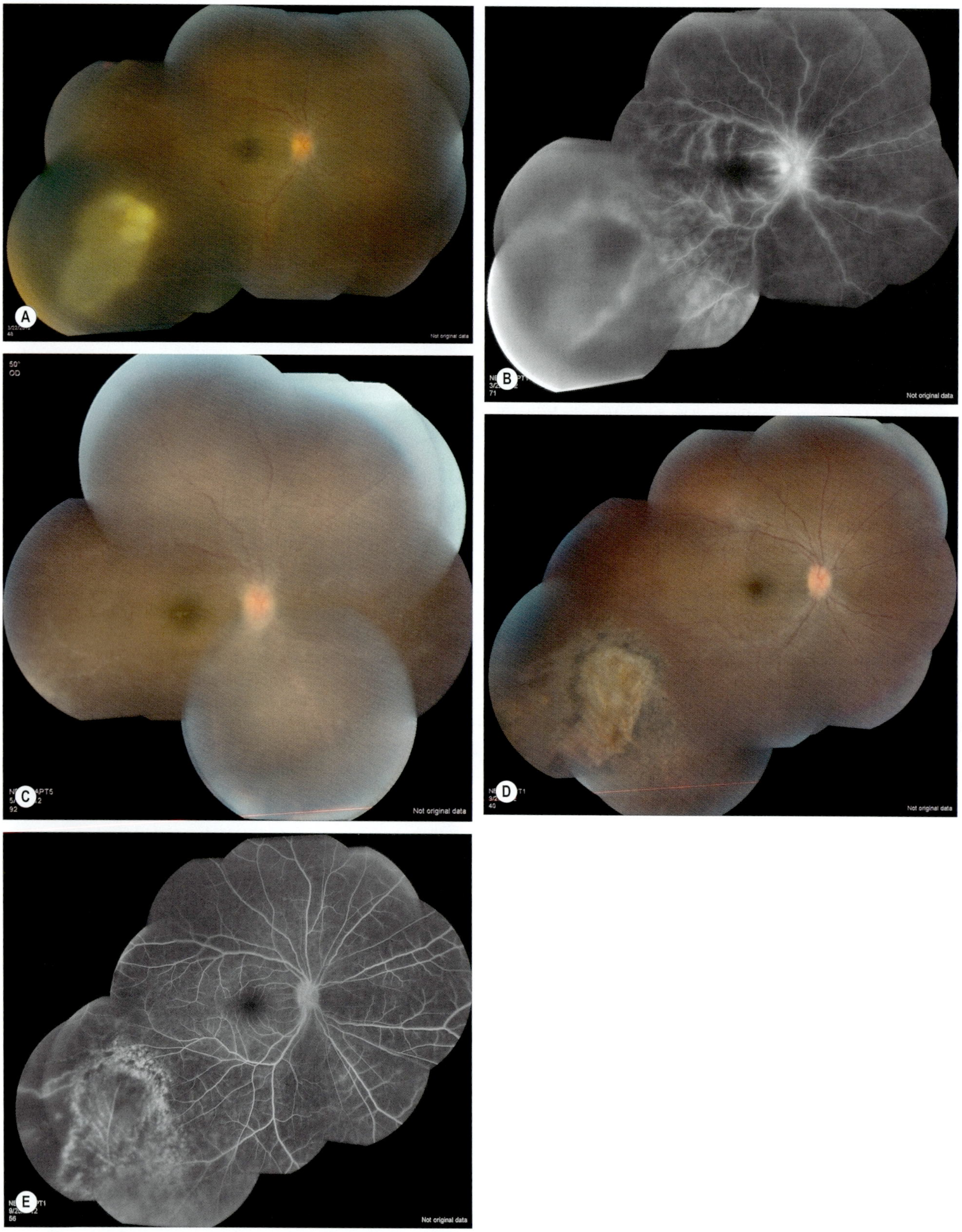

Fig. 15.14 Patient with ocular toxoplasmosis with typical inferotemporal yellowish chorioretinal lesion, papillitis, and arteriolar sheathing and plaques, also known as *Kyrieleis plaques* (A). The fluorescein angiogram shows extensive vascular leakage (B). Because of persistent inflammation and vascular plaques (C), the patient received a long course of antibiotic therapy, resulting in resolution of inflammation and visual acuity improvement (D, E) (see Case 15.1).

after injection of organisms into the carotid, and anterior uveitis could be seen in some of the animals.[106] It may be that in human cases, the antigen is also found in the anterior chamber, producing an inflammatory response there; alternatively, immune complexes formed more posteriorly in the eye may become fixed to the tissue in the anterior chamber, including the iris, giving the clinical findings described. However, an intact *Toxoplasma* organism has been found in only one case of an immunocompromised person with AIDS.[107] Greven and Teot[108] reported recovering encysted bradyzoites from the cytospin of a vitrectomy specimen obtained in the course of a retinal detachment repair, helping confirm the clinical impression and leading to initiation of therapy.

Methods of Diagnosis

Serologic evidence of the *Toxoplasma* organism is of immense importance in making the diagnosis. Research has suggested that there is selective activation of a subset of B cells locally in nonlymphoid tissue, such as the eye.[109] Indeed, research evaluating serum and intraocular antibody responses has shown differences.[110] Antibody from the aqueous of patients with chronic toxoplasmosis stained more intensely to a 28-kDa antigen, believed to be the GRA-2 antigen, which is expressed in both tachyzoites and bradyzoites. The presence of immunoglobulin M (IgM) titers to the organism suggests a recently acquired infection. Diagnostic tests for toxoplasmosis include the dye test (DT); indirect fluorescent antibody test (IFA); enzyme immunoassays (ELISA, immunoblots); agglutination test; and AVIDITY test.[111] If acute infection is suspected, serum should be tested for IgG and IgM specific antibodies. The presence of IgM is considered to be suggestive of acute infection and, in most cases, disappears within several months; however, in some patients, IgM can persist for years. Serologic testing can also be unreliable in immunocompromised patients. Confirmatory testing through a *Toxoplasma* reference laboratory (i.e., Palo Alto Medical Foundation Toxoplasma Serology Laboratory) should be sought if acute infection is suspected.

Weiss et al.[112] reported their experience comparing the immunofluorescence antibody test, the Sabin-Feldman dye test, and ELISA. They found that for three patients, the immunofluorescence test result was negative (titer < 1:16), whereas the Sabin-Feldman test result was positive for these three patients, as was the ELISA result in the one patient tested. These data suggest that the Sabin-Feldman test or the ELISA antibody test should be performed before the diagnosis of ocular toxoplasmosis is excluded on the basis of a negative antibody test result.[112]

PCR testing is being used increasingly for diagnostic purposes and has become one of the mainstays of diagnosis, but it does have its drawbacks.[113] Questions regarding initial problems in this methodology have been raised. In one early study comparing antibody determinations with the detection of *T. gondii* DNA,[114] intraocular IgG was more commonly found in recurrent ocular toxoplasmosis than in recently acquired disease (81% versus 41% of patients). However, DNA from *T. gondii* was found intraocularly in recently acquired disease compared with recurrent ocular toxoplasmosis (37% versus 4% of patients).[115]

The diagnosis of ocular disease by using serologic means alone may not always be reliable.[116] Rothova et al. noted that even though IgG antibody positivity was seen in 100% of their patients with clinically apparent ocular toxoplasmosis, 58% of the control subjects also showed positive results. Although seven (28%) of 25 patients with toxoplasmosis had detectable circulating immune complexes with IgG and *Toxoplasma* antigen, 2 (16%) of 12 control subjects did as well. In reviewing findings from normal control subjects and patients with suspected ocular toxoplasmosis, Phaik et al.[117] estimated that at least 77% of those with ocular toxoplasmosis had serotiters 1:256 or greater, somewhat higher than those found in control subjects. Nonetheless, we believe that the diagnosis is very much a clinical one, with serologic findings being supportive but not definitive.

The serologic examination of the aqueous is a technique reported by Desmonts.[118] In a classic article, Desmonts postulated that in patients with a purely ocular recurrence of toxoplasmosis, local antibody formation against the organism will occur and that the local titer will therefore be greater than that found in the circulation. His impressive demonstration of this phenomenon and the calculation of the C value is a result that the ophthalmologist should be aware of (see Chapter 5). This technique is not as widely used in the United States but is used in Europe.[119] Although the clinical appearance of the disease is straightforward in most patients we have seen, this added technique can be helpful in the evaluation of those whose disease presents real diagnostic dilemmas. Turunen et al.[120] emphasized the reliability of this test and found that in both patients with toxoplasmosis and control subjects, intraocular antimumps antibody formation was within the normal range, suggesting that the response may be specific.

When comparing PCR and antibody levels in the eye, Westeneng et al.[121] found that antibody levels helped diagnose toxoplasmosis in immunocompromised patients more often compared with PCR, which often becomes negative in disease present for an extended period. Alternatively, PCR seemed better for the diagnosis of viral retinitis. This was the finding in the study by Rothova et al. when comparing all patients regardless of their immune status.[115] In their report, they calculated that in 26 (87%) of 30 patients with toxoplasmosis, the diagnosis would not have been made by using PCR testing alone. This is in contrast to the Goldmann-Witmer quotient; if this were the only test performed, only two of the 30 patients with toxoplasmosis would not have been diagnosed. In contrast, Mahalakshmi et al.[122] compared local antibody production with a nested PCR method and found no difference in sensitivity between the tests. They preferred using the PCR method because of the amount of specimen needed, the rapidity of the test, and the cost.

Histologic diagnosis can be helpful in rare and specific circumstances. Palkovacs et al.[123] used fine-needle aspiration biopsy to diagnose acquired toxoplasmosis in a 34-year-old woman who received bone marrow transplantation for leukemia. The biopsy showed crescent-shaped intraretinal organisms and cysts.

Pregnancy. Testing for toxoplasmosis is routinely performed in pregnant women. It is generally believed that if the mother has anti-*Toxoplasma* antibodies before the beginning of the pregnancy, then the fetus is protected. Most of the children born with symptoms of *Toxoplasma* infection are infected during the third trimester of the pregnancy. It is believed that if one child is born with signs of ocular toxoplasmosis, then succeeding siblings will be protected. There are some anecdotal reports that may disprove this concept, but in most instances, the presence of extenuating circumstances could explain the unusual findings without disproving the concept. Rarely, disease may be transmitted from a toxoplasmosis-positive mother. Pregnancy is a period of relative immunodepression: The body does not wish to reject the immunologically foreign object (the fetus) that is maturing in the uterus. For some autoimmune diseases, this immune state may reduce the possibility of disease. However, with an infectious disorder, the risk of disease may increase. There have been several reported cases of reactivation of ocular toxoplasmosis during pregnancy and improvement of disease in some with delivery.[124,125] Although this supports the notion mentioned earlier, it is still a fairly unusual event, suggesting that immune surveillance still works in most cases. However, it does need to be considered when monitoring a patient with ocular toxoplasmosis who becomes pregnant. What should be done when there is reactivation of ocular disease during pregnancy? Many clinicians will try to monitor the lesion if it appears not to be sight threatening. Martinez et al.[126] reported successful management of ocular toxoplasmosis during pregnancy with intraocular injections of clindamycin and dexamethasone combined with systemic sulfadiazine.

Other Methods

Other methods for diagnosis of toxoplasmosis have been developed. Western blot analysis[127] has been used to identify cytoplasmic and membrane antigens of *T. gondii.* Immunoblotting has also been shown to be useful.[128] Using identified genes that are specific to this organism as a template and by means of the PCR method, one can search for toxoplasmic DNA, even when it is present in minute quantities. PCR analysis will permit adequate amplification of these DNA fragments to allow detection with standard laboratory techniques, such as Southern blot analysis. To date, two genes have been used. The gene for the p30 antigen encodes one of the major surface proteins of the organism.[12-14] The *B1* gene,[129] which contains an intron but does not encode for a known protein, has been shown to be in the genome of many *Toxoplasma* strains, but not in the mammalian genome. In one study, the PCR technique was applied to deparaffinized ocular sections from two patients. Although cysts could be identified by use of standard microscopic examination in one eye, PCR analysis permitted the identification of the parasite in both patients.[113] This study demonstrated the feasibility of the PCR method even when paraffin slides are used. By means of this method, toxoplasmic DNA was identified in the aqueous of three patients with ocular toxoplasmosis.[130] The positive PCR response in these three patients was not related to the C coefficient, which is the analysis used to determine local production of a specific antibody. Finally, tissue culturing with the use of ocular tissue has been used to diagnose toxoplasmosis in HIV-positive patients.[131]

Another approach to diagnosis has been offered by the development of in vivo tests. One method shown to work in rabbits is the use of in vivo immunofluorescence. Scheiffarth et al.[132] tagged specific anti-*Toxoplasma* antibodies with fluorescein, injected them intravenously, and found that samples from experimentally induced chorioretinitis would stain with this technique. Much work is still needed before this technique can be used for the diagnosis of the human form of the disease.

Congenital versus Acquired Disease

As discussed earlier, it was formerly an established "given" in ophthalmology that most, if not all, of the ocular lesions ascribed to toxoplasmosis were caused by a congenitally acquired infection. As mentioned earlier, Perkins,[133] in reviewing the literature, found that uveitis was described in 52 (3.1%) of 1669 cases of acquired toxoplasmosis and was most commonly seen with toxoplasmic encephalitis.[133] In his treatise *Uveitis and Toxoplasmosis,*[134] Perkins stated: "It is probable that the vast majority of cases of toxoplasmic uveitis in adults and children are recurrences of a congenital infection." It has therefore been assumed that acquired disease rarely manifests as purely ocular disease.

These ophthalmic "givens" have been seriously questioned by the seminal observations of a family of ophthalmologists, the Silveiras of Erechim, a small city located in the southernmost state (Rio Grande do Sul) of Brazil. These physicians had noted a very high rate of toxoplasmosis in the population of this region. In a survey of 100 healthy children, they found that 98% of those between ages 10 and 15 years had antibodies to toxoplasmosis. On the basis of their observations, the frequency of retinal scars in the population of this area was calculated to be 40 in 200, compared with 1 in 200 in the United States and 6 in 200 in São Paulo, Brazil. In a search for an explanation of this very high rate, it was noted that the residents of this region prepared sausages from raw or poorly cooked pork. The preparation of sausages is a family endeavor requiring much tasting, which could partly explain the high incidence of the disease. Additionally, toxoplasmic cysts in the eye, which provided a definitive diagnosis of this disorder after enucleation, suggest that the disease was an acquired one, rather than a congenital one.[135]

To corroborate these earlier observations, a household survey was undertaken in the Erechim region. Of the 1042 persons examined, 184 (17.7%) were found to have ocular toxoplasmosis. On the basis of these observations, the prevalence of ocular toxoplasmosis was calculated to be 30 times higher than estimates for this disease in other parts of the world.[136] Also of interest was the finding that only 0.9% of young children tested had antibodies to *T. gondii,* further suggesting that the ocular disease seen was caused by postnatal infection rather than congenital infection.

A prospective study investigating the incidence of congenital toxoplasmosis in this region was then undertaken.[137] During a 5-month period, serum was obtained from 283 of 599 newborns and 190 infants younger than 1 year of age. The study showed that 2.1% of the newborns and 0.5% of the infants had evidence of circulating antibodies to the *Toxoplasma* organism. For 21% of adults in this region of Brazil to have ocular toxoplasmosis caused by a congenital infection, greater than 20% of the mothers would have to be infected during pregnancy. Indeed, only 0.5% to 0.6% of the cord blood tested revealed anti-*Toxoplasma* antibodies. A questionnaire given to patients in the Erechim region newly diagnosed with ocular toxoplasmosis showed that eating undercooked or raw meat, having a garden, and eating frozen lamb meat were associated with acquiring the disease.[138]

These studies clearly demonstrated that acquired disease is a major mode of transmission of this parasite that leads to the ocular form of the disease.[139,140] In a study detailing results from the French program against congenital toxoplasmosis, Delair et al.[141] reported that there were more cases of acquired disease than congenital cases. Only 4% of the acquired cases were bilateral, whereas 43.5% of the congenital cases were bilateral. In addition to the difference in seroprevalence of toxoplasma between Erechim and Rio Grande do Sul[142] the role of the environment was further emphasized in a report finding that residents of the United Kingdom born in West Africa had a 100 times higher incidence of ocular symptoms compared with those born in the United Kingdom.[4] An outbreak of toxoplasmosis in British Columbia, Canada, which lasted from October 1994 to March 1995 and appeared to be caused by contaminated drinking water, resulted in 100 patients with the acquired form of the disease and 12 with the congenital form.[143] Of the 100 patients with acquired disease, 20 presented with retinal findings; seven of these lesions were in the macular region. The concept that acquired disease can lead to ocular lesions has now become accepted.

The notion that an unborn child may be "protected" by the mother's seropositivity at the time of pregnancy has been questioned for years. The group in Brazil[144] has reported the case of a woman who had been diagnosed with toxoplasmosis 20 years earlier and who then delivered a child with toxoplasmosis. Both reactivated and newly acquired disease with genetically different strains or lineages of *T. gondii* are possible explanations.[145]

THERAPY

An initial decision must be made with regard to the need to treat the *Toxoplasma*-induced lesion. We know that in the immunocompetent person, the disease is ultimately self-limiting. The decision to treat is based on the following criteria:

- A lesion within the temporal arcade
- A lesion abutting the optic nerve or threatening a large retinal vessel

- A lesion that has induced a large degree of hemorrhage
- A lesion that has induced significant vitritis
- A relative indication being multiple recurrences resulting in marked vitreal condensation

Results of a nonrandomized study comparing three therapeutic regimens in 149 patients—pyrimethamine, sulfadiazine, and steroid; clindamycin, sulfadiazine, and steroid; and trimethoprim and sufa- methoxazole—did not show a difference in the duration of the inflammation or in the rate of recurrence.[146] However, 52% of the patients in the group receiving pyrimethamine experienced reduction in the size of the retinal inflammatory focus versus 25% of the untreated group (peripheral lesions). Stanford et al.,[147] after performing an evidence-based systematic review of antibiotic therapy for toxoplasmosis, felt that there was lack of evidence to support routine antibiotic treatment for acute ocular disease. A single-masked randomized study of 59 patients in Iran compared trimethoprim/sulfamethoxazole versus pyrimethamine/sulfadiazine (both groups received oral steroids) and found no difference in the two groups in terms of retinal lesion resolution and visual acuity.[148] A survey by Holland and Lewis[149,150] found that of the 79 respondents, 15% of experts in uveitis treated ocular toxoplasmosis regardless of clinical features, whereas 85% to 94% treated all cases with zone 1 involvement. Decline in visual acuity was a significant consideration in the treatment decision. The participants reported using a total of nine drugs in 25 different regimens, with the most common regimen being the classic triple therapy followed by trimethoprim/sulfamethoxazole therapy. In contrast, a survey of Brazilian ophthalmologists showed that 67.9% treated all active cases regardless of clinical features. The majority used classic therapy for zone 1 lesions.[150] Triple therapy includes sulfadiazine (1 g orally four times daily) and pyrimethamine (a 50-mg loading dose, followed by 25 mg orally twice daily)—always given concomitantly with folinic acid 3 to 5 mg three times per week— and systemic prednisone. A baseline platelet count and weekly counts are obtained for the duration of the pyrimethamine therapy. Typical treatment duration is 3 to 6 weeks with this regimen,[149] and prednisone is added 24 hours after initiation of antimicrobial therapy. If the macula or the optic nerve is threatened, the patient is monitored more frequently to try to taper the prednisone in such a way that it is stopped before the anti-*Toxoplasma* therapy is discontinued. It is important to stress that immunosuppressive therapy (prednisone) should never be used alone, but only under the therapeutic cover of the specific antimicrobial therapy; we do not give prednisone at higher doses for any prolonged period. Periocular injections of corticosteroids are generally avoided. Sabates et al.[151] reported on seven patients with particularly destructive and disseminated disease, and all were initially treated with corticosteroids alone. We do not use intravitreal steroid injections to treat this disease, our concern being that such high levels in the eye will overcome the antimicrobial effect and lead to reactivation, echoing concerns raised by others.[152] Cytotoxic agents do not have a role in the treatment of this infection.

Clindamycin (150–300 mg orally three or four times daily) combined with sulfadiazine has also been shown to be effective in treating this disorder[153,154] and, as mentioned earlier, has been used intravitreally in pregnant patients[126] and in those unable to tolerate systemic medication.[155] Because the two agents affect unrelated pathways, it may be that the combination could have synergistic effects, although not perhaps as effective as the combination of pyrimethamine and sulfadiazine.[156] Although it is a useful approach, the potential for diarrhea and the serious complication of pseudomembranous colitis, at worst, is problematic. Clindamycin has also been given as 50-mg subconjunctival injections, with positive clinical results observed.[157] Kishore et al.[158] reported treating four patients with 1 mg of clindamycin (in 0.1 mL injection) and 1 mg of dexamethasone (in 0.1 mL injection) given intravitreally. In three of the patients systemic medications were continued. A favorable response was seen within 2 weeks. All patients needed three to four injections. In a randomized controlled trial (RCT), 68 patients with ocular toxoplasmosis involving or threatening the macula or the optic nerve, being located adjacent to a large vessel, and/or being associated with severe vitritis were randomized to receive intravitreal clindamycin (1 mg) and dexamethasone (400 mg) or the classic triple therapy. The results of the RCT showed that mean reduction in lesion size, increase in visual acuity, and decrease in vitreous inflammation were not significantly different between the groups.[159] One of the caveats is that the use of lower-than-standard dosing of pyrimethamine and sulfadiazine may have resulted in underestimation of the effectiveness of systemic therapy. Systemic therapy appeared superior in patients with positive *T. gondii* IgM. In the injection arm, 47% required two to three injections, which were given at 2-week intervals. Local treatment is preferable in patients who cannot tolerate systemic therapy or in pregnant patients. It should not be the treatment of choice in immunocompromised patients (Case 15.3). Although depot corticosteroids are avoided, short-acting dexamethasone injections can be used cautiously in combination with intravitreal clindamycin.

Evidence suggests that treating congenitally acquired disease does have a positive therapeutic effect. In a cohort of 25 children diagnosed with congenital toxoplasmosis, who were not treated during their first year of life and who had an average follow-up of 5.7 years, 18 (72%) had at least one new lesion, with 13 of them having lesions in their macula.[160] Indeed, new lesions were noted after the first decade of life in some. This is in contrast to 132 children with congenital toxoplasmosis who were treated with anti-*Toxoplasma* medication (pyrimethamine, sulfadiazine, and leucovorin) during the first year: 34 (31%) developed new eye lesions, with 15 (14%) being in the macula.[161] McLeod et al.[162] reported the overall neurologic long-term effects of therapy for 1 year (with sulfadiazine and pyrimethamine) in children with congenital toxoplasmosis. Those with no substantial neurologic damage all had normal cognitive, neurologic, and auditory outcomes. For those with significant neurologic damage early in their life, the results are not as positive.

A trimethoprim/sulfamethoxazole combination (160–800 mg twice daily orally) has become an attractive alternative, given its low cost, wide availability, and favorable side-effect profile. In principle, this combination would inhibit the synthesis of tetrahydrofolic acid, as does pyrimethamine. The combination of trimethoprim/sulfamethoxazole was evaluated in the treatment of toxoplasmosis by Opremcak et al.,[163] who found that in all 16 patients studied, active retinochoroiditis resolved and vision improved. This observation was further supported by the results of an RCT comparing classic therapy with trimethoprim/sulfamethoxazole combination therapy, which showed comparable results. An RCT performed in Brazil[164] of 124 patients with a history of ocular toxoplasmosis showed that intermittent trimethoprim/sulfamethoxazole (Bactrim) therapy was associated with a significant reduction in ocular recurrences compared with the observation group (6.6% versus 23.8%).

Another drug that has shown positive results in the treatment of toxoplasmosis is atovaquone (Mepron). Of great potential interest is its ability to kill *Toxoplasma* cysts in vitro,[165] and other studies have shown that atovaquone reduced the number of cerebral cysts in a Syrian gold hamster model.[166] If this action held true for humans, it would be conceivable that one therapeutic course with this agent could prevent recurrences, assuming that adequate levels of the drug were available to resolve the infection completely. Atovaquone is a quinolone derivative first developed for its antimalarial properties. It has been used most extensively in the treatment of CNS toxoplasmosis, with reasonably good results.[167] It was used successfully in a patient with AIDS who was unable to continue more standard therapy.[168] Anecdotal reports do not seem to support the notion that recurrences can be eliminated with atovaquone.[169] In a study of 17 immunocompetent patients, therapy with atovaquone 750 mg four times daily for 3 months combined with 40 mg of prednisone resulted in a positive therapeutic outcome.[170] In another cohort of 41 patients,[171] similar results were reported. However, in both studies, recurrences were reported in 12% to 44% of patients, although the time to recurrence appeared to be prolonged.

Azithromycin (250 mg daily orally) has also been used for the treatment of ocular toxoplasmosis. Rothova et al. showed clinical resolution of disease in 11 patients within 4 weeks of azithromycin used as single therapy, but 27% experienced recurrence within the first year.[172] In a separate clinical trial of 46 patients, the same group found no significant difference between the classic therapy and the pyrimethamine/azithromycin regimen, although the latter was better tolerated.[173]

Empiric observations in the immunocompromised host (e.g., patients with AIDS) have shown that the disease will be arrested only with therapy and will be reactivated once therapy has been stopped as long as the immunocompromised state persists. Because cellular response is very important for host defense, before the availability of HAART, long-term anti-*Toxoplasma* therapy was needed. Systemic corticosteroids are typically not added to the antimicrobial regimen in immunocompromised patients.

Additional Therapeutic Approaches

Cryotherapy of peripheral lesions has been suggested as an alternative therapeutic approach. However, excessive cryotherapy applied to these "hot" eyes could potentially induce unwanted and excessive vitreous condensation and membrane formation, ultimately pulling on the retina and causing retinal detachment. Photocoagulation has also been advocated by some as a means to treat toxoplasmosis. Ghartey and Brockhurst[174] described their experience in treating five eyes with toxoplasmic lesions unresponsive to antimicrobial therapy and corticosteroids. Photocoagulation treatment was thought to benefit four eyes, with healing of lesions after a few weeks. Others have suggested that such treatment could reactivate dormant cysts, leading to renewal of ocular disease.

CNV is a rare complication (2%) of ocular toxoplasmosis.[175] Therapies for CNV have been evaluated in the treatment of this complication secondary to ocular toxoplasmosis. Photodynamic therapy (PDT)[176,177] and anti–vascular endothelial growth factor (VEGF) injections[178,179] have been used by several, with results (albeit in a small number of patients) showing that CNV may be amenable to these therapies.

Vitrectomy and lensectomy can be performed to remove vitreous and lens opacities that affect vision.[180] Significant vitreous condensations can form in eyes having a history of multiple episodes of inflammation caused by toxoplasmosis. In patients with toxoplasmosis undergoing vitrectomy, we usually begin antimicrobial therapy before surgery and continue it postoperatively. Prophylaxis is also suggested for cataract extraction.[51] The rationale for this approach is the concern that the nonspecific inflammation induced by vitrectomy might initiate an inflammatory episode of toxoplasmosis. We would not use periocular steroid injection after the procedure but will give oral steroids (in the setting of antimicrobial therapy), if indicated.

REFERENCES

1. Krick J, Remington J. Current concepts in parasitology. Toxoplasmosis in the adult – an overview. *N Engl J Med.* 1978;298:550–553.
2. Centers for Disease Control and Prevention (CDC). https://www.cdc.gov/parasites/toxoplasmosis/epi.html.
3. Jones JL, Kruszon-Moran D, Wilson M, et al. *Toxoplasma gondii* infection in the United States: seroprevalence and risk factors. *Am J Epidemiol.* 2001;154:357–365.
4. Gilbert RE, Dunn DT, Lightman S, et al. Incidence of symptomatic toxoplasma eye disease: aetiology and public health implications. *Epidemiol Infect.* 1999;123:283–289.
5. Nicolle C, Manceaux L. Sur une infection a corps de Leishman (ou organismes voisins) du gondi. *Compt Rend Acad Sci.* 1908;147:763–766.
6. Splendore A. Un nouvo protozoa parassita dei conigli: incontrato nell lesoni anatomiche d'une malattia che ricorda in molti punti il Kala-azar dell'uomo. *Rev Soc Sci São Paulo.* 1908;3:109–112.
7. Janku J. Pathogenesis and pathologic anatomy of coloboma of macula lutea in eye of normal dimensions, and in microphthalmic eye, with parasites in retina. *Cas Lek Cesk.* 1923;62:1021–1027. 154–1059, 1111–1115, 1138–1143.
8. Wolf A, Cowen D, Paige B. Human toxoplasmosis: occurrence in infants as an encephalomyelitis: verification by transmission to animals. *Science.* 1939;89:226–227.
9. Holland GN, Lewis KG, O'Connor GR. Ocular toxoplasmosis: a 50th anniversary tribute to the contribution of Helenor Campbell Wilder Foerster. *Arch Ophthalmol.* 2002;120:1081–1084.
10. O'Connor G. The mucosae as possible sites of entrance for *Toxoplasma gondii*. In: O'Connor G, ed. *Immunologic Diseases of the Mucous Membranes.* New York: Masson Publishing USA Inc.; 1989:71–78.
11. Joiner K. Cell entry by *Toxoplasma gondii*: all paths do not lead to success. *Res Immunol.* 1993;144(1):34–38.
12. Santoro F, Afchain D, Pierce R, et al. Serodiagnosis of *Toxoplasma* infection using a purified parasite protein. *Clin Exp Immunol.* 1985;62:262–269.
13. Kasper L, Khan I. Role of p30 in host immunity and pathogenesis of *T. gondii* infection. *Res Immunol.* 1993;144(1):45–48.
14. Burg J, Perelman D, Kasper LH, et al. Molecular analysis of the gene coding the major surface antigen of *Toxoplasmosis gondii. J Immunol.* 1988;141:3584–3591.
15. Kasper L, Crabb J, Pfefferkor E. Isolation and characterization of a monoclonal antibody-resistant antigenic mutant of *Toxoplasma gondii. J Immunol.* 1982;129:1694–1699.
16. Sibley L, Krahenbuhl JL, Adams GM, et al. *Toxoplasma* modifies macrophage phagosomes by secretion of a vesicular network rich in surface proteins. *J Cell Biol.* 1986;103:867–874.
17. Sharma S, Araujo F, Remington J. Toxoplasma antigen isolated by affinity chromatography with monoclonal antibody protects mice against lethal infection with *Toxoplasma gondii. J Immunol.* 1984;133:2818–2820.
18. Cesbron-Delauw M, Capron A. Excreted/secreted antigens of *Toxoplasmosis gondii* – their origin and role in the host – parasite interaction. *Res Immunol.* 1993;144(1):41–44.
19. Hughes H, Van Knapen F. Characterization of a secretory antigen from *Toxoplasma gondii* and its role in circulating antigen production. *Int J Parasit.* 1982;12:433–437.
20. Howe DK, Sibley LD. *Toxoplasma gondii* comprises three clonal lineages: correlation of parasite genotype with human disease. *J Infect Dis.* 1995;172:1561–1566.
21. Switaj K, Master A, Borkowski PK, et al. Association of ocular toxoplasmosis with type I *Toxoplasma gondii* strains: direct genotyping from peripheral blood samples. *J Clin Microbiol.* 2006;44(11):4262–4264.
22. Vallochi AL, Muccioli C, Martins MC, et al. The genotype of *Toxoplasma gondii* strains causing ocular toxoplasmosis in humans in Brazil. *Am J Ophthalmol.* 2005;139(2):350–351.
23. Grigg ME, Ganatra J, Boothroyd JC, et al. Unusual abundance of atypical strains associated with human ocular toxoplasmosis. *J Infect Dis.* 2001;184:633–639.

24. Howe DK, Honore S, Derouin F, et al. Determination of genotypes of *Toxoplasma gondii* strains isolated from patients with toxoplasmosis. *J Clin Microbiol.* 1997;35:1411–1414.
25. Schmidt DR, Hogh B, Andersen O, et al. The national neonatal screening programme for congenital toxoplasmosis in Denmark: results from the initial four years, 1999–2002. *Arch Dis Child.* 2006;91(8):661–665.
26. Koppe J, Kloosterman G. Congenital toxoplasmosis: long term follow-up. *Paediatr Padol.* 1982;17:171–179.
27. Arantes TE, Silveira C, Holland GN, et al. Belfort ocular involvement following postnatally acquired *Toxoplasma gondii* infection in Southern Brazil: a 28-year experience. *Am J Ophthalmol.* 2015;159:1002–1012.
28. Wilson L, Teutsch S. Acquired toxoplasmosis. *Ophthalmology.* 1982;89:1299–1302.
29. Atmaca LS, Simsek T, Atmaca SP, et al. Fluorescein and indocyanine green angiography in ocular toxoplasmosis. *Graefes Arch Clin Exp Ophthalmol.* 2006;244(12):1688–1691.
30. Khairallah M, Yahia SB, Zaouali S, et al. Acute choroidal ischemia associated with toxoplasmic retinochoroiditis. *Retina.* 2007;27(7):947–951.
31. Orefice JL, Costa RA, Campos W, et al. Third-generation optical coherence tomography findings in punctate retinal toxoplasmosis. *Am J Ophthalmol.* 2006;142(3):503–505.
32. Stanford MR, Tomlin EA, Comyn O, et al. The visual field in toxoplasmic retinochoroiditis. *Br J Ophthalmol.* 2005;89(7):812–814.
33. Scherrer J, Iliev ME, Halberstadt M, et al. Visual function in human ocular toxoplasmosis. *Br J Ophthalmol.* 2007;91(2):233–236.
34. Holland GN, Crespi CM, ten Dam-van Loon N, et al. Analysis of recurrence patterns associated with toxoplasmic retinochoroiditis. *Am J Ophthalmol.* 2008;145(6):1007–1013.
35. Garweg JG, Scherrer JN, Halberstadt M. Recurrence characteristics in European patients with ocular toxoplasmosis. *Br J Ophthalmol.* 2008;92(9):1253–1256.
36. Roizenblatt J, Grant S, Foos R. Vitreous cylinders. *Arch Ophthalmol.* 1980;98:734–739.
37. Benson W. Ocular toxoplasmosis and visual field defects. *Am J Ophthalmol.* 1980;90:25–29.
38. Song A, Scott IU, Davis JL, et al. Atypical anterior optic neuropathy caused by toxoplasmosis. *Am J Ophthalmol.* 2002;133:162–164.
39. Holland GN. Ocular toxoplasmosis: a global reassessment. Part II: disease manifestations and management. *Am J Ophthalmol.* 2004;137:1–17.
40. Bosch-Driessen LE, Berendschot TT, Ongkosuwito JV, Rothova A. Ocular toxoplasmosis: clinical features and prognosis of 154 patients. *Ophthalmology.* 2002;109(5):869–878.
41. Schlaegel TJ, Weber J. The macula in ocular toxoplasmosis. *Arch Ophthalmol.* 1984;102:697–698.
42. Westfall AC, Lauer AK, Suhler EB, et al. Toxoplasmosis retinochoroiditis and elevated intraocular pressure: a retrospective study. *J Glaucoma.* 2005;14(1):3–10.
43. Friedmann C, Knox D. Variations in recurrent active toxoplasmic retinochoroiditis. *Arch Ophthalmol.* 1969;81:481–493.
44. Doft B, Gass J. Outer retinal layer toxoplasmosis. *Graefes Arch Clin Exp Ophthalmol.* 1986;224:78–82.
45. Tandon R, Menon V, Das GK, et al. Toxoplasmic papillitis with central retinal artery occlusion. *Can J Ophthalmol.* 1995;30(7):374–376.
46. Hayashi S, Kim MK, Belfort RJ. White-centered retinal hemorrhages in ocular toxoplasmosis. *Retina.* 1997;17(4):351–352.
47. Folk J, Lobes L. Presumed toxoplasmic papillitis. *Ophthalmology.* 1984;91:64–67.
48. Chung H, Kim JG, Choi SH, et al. Bilateral toxoplasma retinochoroiditis simulating cytomegalovirus retinitis in an allogeneic bone marrow transplant patient. *Korean J Ophthalmol.* 2008;22(3):197–200.
49. Theodossiadis P, Kokolakis S, Ladas I, et al. Retinal vascular involvement in acute toxoplasmic retinochoroiditis. *Int Ophthalmol.* 1995;19:19–24.
50. Oh J, Huh K, Kim SW. Recurrent secondary frosted branch angiitis after toxoplasmosis vasculitis. *Acta Ophthalmol Scand.* 2005;83(1):115–117.
51. Bosch-Driessen LH, Plaisier MB, Stilma JS, et al. Reactivations of ocular toxoplasmosis after cataract extraction. *Ophthalmology.* 2002;109:41–45.
52. Fine S, Owens S, Haller J. Choroidal neovascularization as a late complication of ocular toxoplasmosis. *Am J Ophthalmol.* 1981;91:318–322.
53. Skorska I, Soubrane G, Coscas G. Toxoplasmic choroiditis and subretinal neovessels. *J Fr Ophthalmol.* 1984;7:211–218.
54. Potter J. Vascular anastomoses in ocular toxoplasmosis. *J Am Optom Assoc.* 1982;53:549–552.
55. Rose G. Papillitis, retinal neovascularization and recurrent retinal vein occlusion in *Toxoplasma* retinochoroiditis: a case report with uncommon clinical signs. *Aust NZ J Ophthamol.* 1991;19:155–157.
56. Pakalin S, Arnaud B. Arterial occlusion associated with toxoplasmic chorioretinitis. *J Fr Ophthamol.* 1990;13:554–556.
57. Bosch-Driessen LH, Karimi S, Stilma JS, et al. Retinal detachment in ocular toxoplasmosis. *Ophthalmology.* 2000;107:36–40.
58. Fujiwara T, Machida S, Hasegawa Y, et al. Punctate outer retinal toxoplasmosis with multiple choroidal neovascularizations. *Retina.* 2006;26(3):360–362.
59. Toledo de Abreu M, Belfort RJ, Hirata P. Fuch's heterochromic cyclitis and ocular toxoplasmosis. *Am J Ophthamol.* 1982;93:739–744.
60. La Hey E, et al. Fuch's heterochromia iridocyclitis is not associated with ocular toxoplasmosis. *Arch Ophthamol.* 1992;110:806–811.
61. Saraux H, Laroche L, Le Hoang P. Secondary Fuch's heterochromic cyclitis: a new approach to an old disease. *Ophthalmologica.* 1985;190:193–198.
62. Schwab I. The epidemiologic association of Fuch's heterochromic iridocyclitis and ocular toxoplasmosis. *Am J Ophthalmol.* 1991;1:356–362.
63. Sabhapandit S, Murthy SI, Balne PK, Sangwan VS, Sumanth V, Reddy AK. Clinical spectrum, diagnostic criteria, and polymerase chain reaction of aqueous humor in viral and toxoplasma detection in Fuchs' uveitis syndrome. *Indian J Ophthalmol.* 2016;64(8):555–558.
64. Moorthy R, Smith R, Rao N. Progressive ocular toxoplasmosis in patients with acquired immunodeficiency syndrome. *Am J Ophthalmol.* 1993;115:742–747.
65. Gagliuso D, Teich SA, Friedman AH, et al. Ocular toxoplasmosis in AIDS patients. *Trans Am Ophthalmol Soc.* 1990;88:63–86.
66. Yeo J, Jakobiec F, Iwamoto T. Opportunistic toxoplasmic retinochoroiditis following chemotherapy for systemic lymphoma. A light and electron microscopic study. *Ophthalmology.* 1983;90:885–898.
67. Singer M, Hagler W, Grossniklaus H. *Toxoplasma gondii* retinochoroiditis after liver transplantation. *Retina.* 1993;13:40–45.
68. Blanc-Jouvan M, Boibieux A, Fleury J, et al. Chorioretinitis following liver transplantation: detection of *Toxoplasma gondii* in aqueous humor. *Clin Infect Dis.* 1996;22(1):184–185.
69. Sendi P, Sachers F, Drechsler H, et al. Immune recovery vitritis in an HIV patient with isolated toxoplasmic retinochoroiditis. *AIDS.* 2006;20(17):2237–2238.
70. Brezin AP, Thulliez P, Cisneros B, et al. Lymphocytic choriomeningitis virus chorioretinitis mimicking ocular toxoplasmosis in two otherwise normal children. *Am J Ophthalmol.* 2000;130:245–247.
71. Auer C, Bornasconi O, Herbort CP. Indocyanine green angiography features in toxoplasmic retinochoroiditis. *Retina.* 1999;19(1):22–29.
72. Holland GN. Ocular toxoplasmosis: a global reassessment. Part I: Epidemiology and course of disease. *Am J Ophthalmol.* 2003;136(6):973–988.
73. Holland GN. Ocular toxoplasmosis: a global reassessment. Part II: Disease manifestations and management. *Am J Ophthalmol.* 2004;137(1):1–17.
74. Dutton G, Hay J, Hair DM, et al. Clinicopathological features of a congenital murine model of ocular toxoplasmosis. *Graefes Arch Clin Exp Ophthalmol.* 1986;224:256–264.
75. Dutton G, McMenamin PG, Hay J, et al. The ultrastructural pathology of congenital murine toxoplasmic retinochoroiditis. Part II: The morphology of the inflammatory changes. *Exp Eye Res.* 1986;43:545–560.
76. Roberts F, Mets MB, Ferguson DJ, et al. Histopathological features of ocular toxoplasmosis in the fetus and infant. *Arch Ophthalmol.* 2001;119(1):51–58.
77. Nussenblatt R, Mittal KK, Fuhrman S, et al. Lymphocyte proliferative responses of patients with ocular toxoplasmosis to parasite and retinal antigens. *Am J Ophthamol.* 1989;107:632–641.

78. Fatoohi F, Cozon GJ, Wallon M, et al. Systemic T cell response to *Toxoplasma gondii* antigen in patients with ocular toxoplasmosis. *Jpn J Ophthalmol.* 2006;50(2):103–110.
79. McLeod R, Skamene E, Brown C, et al. Genetic regulation of early survival and cyst number after peroral *Toxoplasma gondii* infection of AXB/BXA recombinant inbred and B10 congenic mice. *J Immunol.* 1989;142:3247–3255.
80. McLeod R, Brown C, Mack D. Immunogenetics influence outcome of *Toxoplasma gondii* infection. *Res Immunol.* 1993;144(1):61–65.
81. Brown C, McLeod R. Class I MHC genes and CD8+ T cells determine cyst number in toxoplasma infection. *J Immunol.* 1990;145:3438–3441.
82. Jamieson SE, de Roubaix LA, Cortina-Borja M, et al. Genetic and epigenetic factors at COL2A1 and ABCA4 influence clinical outcome in congenital toxoplasmosis. *PLoS One.* 2008;3(6):e2285.
83. Chan C, Hu S, Gekker G, et al. Effects of cytokines on multiplication of *Toxoplasma gondii* in microglial cells. *J Immunol.* 1993;150:3404–3410.
84. Nagineni CN, Pardhasaradhi K, Martins MC, et al. Mechanisms of interferon-induced inhibition of *Toxoplasma gondii* replication in human retinal pigment epithelial cells. *Infect Immun.* 1996;64(10):4188–4196.
85. Gazzinelli R, Eltoum I, Wynn TA, et al. Acute cerebral toxoplasmosis is induced by in vivo neutralization of TNF-alpha and correlates with the down-regulated expression of inducible nitric oxide synthase and other markers of macrophage activation. *J Immunol.* 1993;(151):3672–3681.
86. Shen DF, Matteson DM, Tuaillon N, et al. Involvement of apoptosis and interferon-gamma in murine toxoplasmosis. *Invest Ophthalmol Vis Sci.* 2001;42:2031–2036.
87. Beamon M, Hunter C, Remington J. Enhancement of intracellular replication of *Toxoplasma gondii* by IL-6. *J Immunol.* 1994;153:4583–4587.
88. Lyons RE, Anthony JP, Ferguson DJ, et al. Immunological studies of chronic ocular toxoplasmosis: up-regulation of major histocompatibility complex class I and transforming growth factor β and a protective role for interleukin-6. *Infect Immun.* 2001;69(4):2589–2595.
89. Ashander LM, Lie S, Ma Y, et al. Neutrophil activities in human ocular toxoplasmosis: an in vitro study with human cells. *Invest Ophthalmol Vis Sci.* 2019;60(14):4652–4660.
90. Furtado JM, Ashander LM, Mohs K, Chipps TJ, Appukuttan B, Smith JR. *Toxoplasma gondii* migration within and infection of human retina. *PLoS One.* 2013;8(2):e54358.
91. Furtado JM, Bharadwaj AS, Ashander LM, Olivas A, Smith JR. Migration of *Toxoplasma gondii*-infected dendritic cells across human retinal vascular endothelium. *Invest Ophthalmol Vis Sci.* 2012;53(11):6856–6862.
92. Zamora DO, Rosenbaum JT, Smith JR. Invasion of human retinal vascular endothelial cells by *Toxoplasma gondii* tachyzoites. *Br J Ophthalmol.* 2008;92(6):852–855.
93. Feron EJ, Klaren VNA, Wierenga EA, et al. Characterization of *Toxoplasma gondii*-specific T cells recovered from vitreous fluid of patients with ocular toxoplasmosis. *Invest Ophthalmol Vis Sci.* 2001;42:3228–3232.
94. Herion P, Saavedra R. Human T-cell clones as tools for the characterization of the cell-mediated immune response to *Toxoplasma gondii*. *Res Immunol.* 1993;144(1):48–51.
95. Denkers E, Caspar P, Sher A. *Toxoplasma gondii* possesses a superantigen activity that selectively expands murine T cell receptors Vβ5-bearing CD8+ lymphocytes. *J Exp Med.* 1994;180:985–994.
96. Curiel T, Krug ED, Purner MB, et al. Cloned human CD4+ cytotoxic T lymphocytes specific for *Toxoplasma gondii* lysetachyzoite-infected target cells. *J Immunol.* 1993;151:2024–2031.
97. Goncalves RM, Rodrigues DH, Camargos da Costa AM, et al. Increased serum levels of CXCL8 chemokine in acute toxoplasmic retinochoroiditis. *Acta Ophthalmol Scand.* 2007;85(8):871–876.
98. Hafizi A, Modabber F. Effect of cyclophosphamide on *Toxoplasma gondii* infection: reversal of the effect by passive immunization. *Clin Exp Immunol.* 1978;33:389–394.
99. Wilson C, Haas J. Cellular defense against *Toxoplasma gondii* in newborns. *J Clin Invest.* 1984;73:1606–1616.
100. Roberts F, Roberts CW, Ferguson DJ, et al. Inhibition of nitric oxide production exacerbates chronic ocular toxoplasmosis. *Parasite Immunol.* 2000;22:1–5.
101. Wyler D, Blackman J, Lunde M. Cellular hypersensitivity to toxoplasmal and retinal antigens in patients with toxoplasmal retinochoroiditis. *Am J Trop Med Hyg.* 1980;29:1181–1186.
102. Abrahams IW, Gregerson DS. Longitudinal study of serum antibody responses to retinal antigens in acute ocular toxoplasmosis. *Am J Ophthalmol.* 1982;93(2):224–231.
103. Whittle RM, Roberts CW, Ferguson DJ, et al. Human antiretinal antibodies in toxoplasma retinochoroiditis. *Br J Ophthalmol.* 1998;82:1017–1021.
104. Vallochi AL, da Silva Rios L, Nakamura MV, et al. The involvement of autoimmunity against retinal antigens in determining disease severity in toxoplasmosis. *J Autoimmun.* 2005;24(1):25–32.
105. Rollins D, Tabbara K, O'Connor G. Detection of toxoplasmal antigen and antibody in ocular fluids in experimental ocular toxoplasmosis. *Arch Ophthalmol.* 1983;101:455.
106. Davidson MG, Lappin MR, English KV, et al. A feline model of ocular toxoplasmosis. *Invest Ophthalmol Vis Sci.* 1993;34:3653–3660.
107. Rehder JR, Burnier MB Jr, Pavesio CE, et al. Acute unilateral toxoplasmic iridocyclitis in an AIDS patient. *Am J Ophthalmol.* 1988;106(6):740–741.
108. Greven C, Teot L. Cytologic identification of *Toxoplasma gondii* from vitreous fluid. *Arch Ophthalmol.* 1994;112:1086–1088.
109. Klaren VNA, van Doornik CE, Ongkosuwito JV, et al. Differences between intraocular and serum antibody responses in patients with ocular toxoplasmosis. *Am J Ophthalmol.* 1998;126:698–706.
110. Klaren VNA, Peek R. Evidence for a compartmentalized B cell response as characterized by IgG epitope specificity in human ocular toxoplasmosis. *J Immunol.* 2001;167:6263–6269.
111. Centers for Disease Control and Prevention (CDC). https://www.cdc.gov/parasites/toxoplasmosis/health_professionals/index.html. Accessed November, 2019.
112. Weiss M, Velazquez N, Hofeldt A. Serologic tests in the diagnosis of presumed toxoplasmic retinochoroiditis. *Am J Ophthalmol.* 1990;109:407–411.
113. Brezin A, Egwuagu CE, Burnier Jr M, et al. Identification of *Toxoplasma gondii* in paraffin-embedded sections by the polymerase chain reaction. *Am J Ophthalmol.* 1990;110:599–604.
114. Ongkosuwito JV, Bosch-Driessen EH, Kijlstra A, et al. Serologic evaluation of patients with primary and recurrent ocular toxoplasmosis for evidence of recent infection. *Am J Ophthalmol.* 1999;128:407–412.
115. Rothova A, van Knapen F, Baarsma GS, et al. Usefulness of aqueous humor analysis for the diagnosis of posterior uveitis. *Ophthalmology.* 2008;115(2):306–311.
116. Rothova A, van Knapen F, Baarsma G. Serology in ocular toxoplasmosis. *Br J Ophthalmol.* 1986;70:615–622.
117. Phaik C, Seah S, Guan OS, et al. Anti-toxoplasma serotitres in ocular toxoplasmosis. *Eye.* 1991;5(5):636–639.
118. Desmonts G. Definitive serological diagnosis of ocular toxoplasmosis. *Arch Ophthalmol.* 1966;76:839–853.
119. Goichot E, Bloch-Michel E. Interet de l'etude detaillee de la serologie quantitative de l'humeur aqueuse pour le diagnostic de la toxoplasmose oculaire. A propos de 180 cas. *J Fr Ophthalmol.* 1980;3:21–26.
120. Turunen H, Leinikki P, Saari K. Demonstration of intraocular synthesis of immunoglobulin G toxoplasma antibodies for specific diagnosis of toxoplasmic chorioretinitis by enzyme immunoassay. *J Clin Microbiol.* 1983;17:988–992.
121. Westeneng AC, Rothova A, de Boer JH, et al. Infectious uveitis in immunocompromised patients and the diagnostic value of polymerase chain reaction and Goldmann-Witmer coefficient in aqueous analysis. *Am J Ophthalmol.* 2007;144(5):781–785.
122. Mahalakshmi B, Therese KL, Madhavan HN, et al. Diagnostic value of specific local antibody production and nucleic acid amplification technique-nested polymerase chain reaction (nPCR) in clinically suspected ocular toxoplasmosis. *Ocul Immunol Inflamm.* 2006;14(2):105–112.
123. Palkovacs EM, Correa Z, Augsburger JJ, et al. Acquired toxoplasmic retinitis in an immunosuppressed patient: diagnosis by transvitreal fine-needle aspiration biopsy. *Graefes Arch Clin Exp Ophthalmol.* 2008;246(10):1495–1497.

124. Kump LI, Androudi SN, Foster CS. Ocular toxoplasmosis in pregnancy. *Clin Exp Ophthalmol.* 2005;33(5):455–460.
125. Garweg JG, Scherrer J, Wallon M, et al. Reactivation of ocular toxoplasmosis during pregnancy. *Br J Obstet Gynaecol.* 2005;112(2):241–242.
126. Martinez CE, Zhang D, Conway MD, et al. Successful management of ocular toxoplasmosis during pregnancy using combined intraocular clindamycin and dexamethasone with systemic sulfadiazine. *Int Ophthalmol.* 1999;22:85–88.
127. Ware P, Kasper L. Strain-specific antigens of *Toxoplasma gondii. Infect Immun.* 1987;55:778–783.
128. Ho-Yen DO, Ashburn D. Immunoblotting can help the diagnosis of ocular toxoplasmosis. *J Clin Pathol.* 2000;53:155–158.
129. Boothroyd J, Burg JL, Nagel S, et al. Antigen and tubulin genes *Toxoplasma gondii.* In: Nogueria N, ed. *Molecular Strategies of Parasitic Invasion.* New York: A R Liss; 1987:237–250.
130. Brezin A, Egwuagu CE, Silveira C, et al. Analysis of aqueous humor in ocular toxoplasmosis. *N Engl J Med.* 1991;324:699.
131. Miller D, Davis J, Rosa R, et al. Utility of tissue culture for detection of *Toxoplasma gondii* in vitreous humor of patients diagnosed with toxoplasmic retinochoroiditis. *J Clin Microbiol.* 2000;38:3840–3842.
132. Scheiffarth O, Zrenner E, Disko R, et al. Intraocular in vivo immunofluorescence. *Invest Ophthalmol Vis Sci.* 1990;31:272–276.
133. Perkins E. Ocular toxoplasmosis. *Br J Ophthalmol.* 1973;57:7–17.
134. Perkins ES. *Uveitis and Toxoplasmosis.* Boston, MA: Little, Brown; 1961.
135. Silveira C, Belfort R Jr, Burnier M, et al. Acquired toxoplasmosis infection as the cause of toxoplasmic retinochoroiditis in families. *Am J Ophthalmol.* 1988;106:362–364.
136. Glasner P, Silveria C, Kruszon-Moran D, et al. An unusually high prevalence of ocular toxoplasmosis in southern Brazil. *Am J Ophthalmol.* 1992;114:136–144.
137. Glasner P, Silveria CN, Carmargo MG, et al. Low frequency of congenital *Toxoplasmosis gondii* (TG) infection in the Erechim region of Rio Grande do Sul, Brazil. *Ophthalmology.* 1992;(Suppl 99):150.
138. Jones JL, Muccioli C, Belfort R Jr, et al. Recently acquired *Toxoplasma gondii* infection, Brazil. *Emerg Infect Dis.* 2006;12(4):582–587.
139. Nussenblatt R, Belfort R Jr. Ocular toxoplasmosis, an old disease revisited. *JAMA.* 1994;271:304–307.
140. Abreu MT, Boni D, Belfort R Jr. Toxoplasmose ocular em Venda Nova do Imagrante, ES, Brasil. *Arq Bras Oftalmol.* 1998;61:541–545.
141. Delair E, Monnet D, Grabar S, et al. Respective roles of acquired and congenital infections in presumed ocular toxoplasmosis. *Am J Ophthalmol.* 2008;146(6):851–855.
142. Melamed J, Sebben JC, Maestri M, et al. Epidemiology of ocular toxoplasmosis in Rio Grande do Sul, Brazil. In: Dernouchamps JP, ed. *Recent Advances in Uveitis: Proceedings of the Third International Symposium on Uveitis, Brussels, Belgium.* Amsterdam: Tassignon Kugler Publications; 1993:211–214.
143. Burnett AJ, Shortt SG, Isaac-Renton J, et al. Multiple cases of acquired toxoplasmosis retinitis presenting in an outbreak. *Ophthalmology.* 1998;105(6):1032–1037.
144. Silveira C, Ferreira R, Muccioli C, et al. Toxoplasmosis transmitted to a newborn from the mother infected 20 years earlier. *Am J Ophthalmol.* 2003;136(2):370–371.
145. Silveira C. *Toxoplasmose Duvidas e Controversias. Erechim.* RS, Brazil: Edifapes; 2002.
146. Rothova A, Buitenhuis HJ, Meenken C, et al. Therapy of ocular toxoplasmosis. *Int Ophthalmol.* 1989;13:415–419.
147. Stanford MR, See SE, Jones LV, et al. Antibiotics for toxoplasmic retinochoroiditis: an evidence-based systematic review. *Ophthalmology.* 2003;110(5):926–931. Quiz 931–932.
148. Soheilian M, Sadoughi MM, Ghajarnia M, et al. Prospective randomized trial of trimethoprim/sulfamethoxazole versus pyrimethamine and sulfadiazine in the treatment of ocular toxoplasmosis. *Ophthalmology.* 2005;112:1876–1882.
149. Holland GN, Lewis KG. An update on current practices in the management of ocular toxoplasmosis. *Am J Ophthalmol.* 2002;134(1):102–114.
150. Morais FB, Arantes TEFE, Muccioli C. Current practices in ocular toxoplasmosis: a survey of Brazilian uveitis specialists. *Ocul Immunol Inflamm.* 2018;26(2):317–323.
151. Sabates R, Pruett R, Brockhurst R. Fulminary ocular toxoplasmosis. *Am J Ophthalmol.* 1981;92:497–503.
152. Aggio FB, Muccioli C, Belfort R Jr. Intravitreal triamcinolone acetonide as an adjunct in the treatment of severe ocular toxoplasmosis. *Eye.* 2008;22(9):1200–1201.
153. Tabbara K, O'Connor G. Treatment of ocular toxoplasmosis with clindamycin and sulfadiazine. *Ophthalmology.* 1980;87:129–134.
154. Lakhanpal V, Schocket S, Nirankari V. Clindamycin in the treatment of toxoplasmic retinochoroiditis. *Am J Ophthalmol.* 1983;95:605–613.
155. Sobrin L, Kump LI, Foster CS. Intravitreal clindamycin for toxoplasmic retinochoroiditis. *Retina.* 2007;27(7):952–957.
156. Thiermann E, Apt W, Atias A. Comparative study of some combined treatment regimens in acute toxoplasmosis in mice. *Am J Trop Med Hyg.* 1978;27:747–750.
157. Ferguson JJ. Clindamycin therapy for toxoplasmosis. *Ann Ophthalmol.* 1981;13:95–100.
158. Kishore K, Conway MD, Peyman GA. Intravitreal clindamycin and dexamethasone for toxoplasmic retinochoroiditis. *Ophthalmic Surg Lasers.* 2001;32(3):183–192.
159. Soheilian M, Ramezani A, Azimzadeh A, et al. Randomized trial of intravitreal clindamycin and dexamethasone versus pyrimethamine, sulfadiazine, and prednisolone in treatment of ocular toxoplasmosis. *Ophthalmology.* 2011;118:134–141.
160. Phan L, Kasza K, Jalbrzikowski J, et al. Longitudinal study of new eye lesions in children with toxoplasmosis who were not treated during the first year of life. *Am J Ophthalmol.* 2008;146(3):375–384.
161. Phan L, Kasza K, Jalbrzikowski J, et al. Longitudinal study of new eye lesions in treated congenital toxoplasmosis. *Ophthalmology.* 2008;115(3):553–559. e8.
162. McLeod R, Boyer K, Karrison T, et al. Outcome of treatment for congenital toxoplasmosis, 1981–2004: the National Collaborative Chicago-Based, Congenital Toxoplasmosis Study. *Clin Infect Dis.* 2006;42(10):1383–1394.
163. Opremcak EM, Scales DK, Sharpe MR. Trimethoprim-sulfamethoxazole therapy for ocular toxoplasmosis. *Ophthalmology.* 1992;99:920–925.
164. Silveira C, Belfort R Jr, Muccioli C, et al. The effect of long-term, intermittent trimethoprim/sulfamethoxazole treatment on recurrences of toxoplasmic retinochoroiditis. *Am J Ophthalmol.* 2002;134:41–46.
165. Araujo F, Huskinson J, Remington J. Remarkable in vitro and in vivo activities of the hydroxynaphthoquinone 566C80 against tachyzoites and tissue cysts of *Toxoplasma gondii. Antimicrob Agents Chemother.* 1991;35:293–299.
166. Gormley PD, Pavesio CE, Minnasian D, et al. Effects of drug therapy on Toxoplasma cysts in an animal model of acute and chronic disease. *Invest Ophthalmol Vis Sci.* 1998;39:1171–1175.
167. Lane H, Laughon BE, Falloon J, et al. NIH Conference: recent advances in the management of AIDS-related opportunistic infections. *Ann Intern Med.* 1994;120:945–955.
168. Lopez J, de Smet MD, Masur H, et al. Orally administered 566C80 for treatment of ocular toxoplasmosis in a patient with the acquired immunodeficiency syndrome. *Am J Ophthalmol.* 1992;113:331–333.
169. Baatz H, Mirshahi A, Puchta J, et al. Reactivation of toxoplasma retinochoroiditis under atovaquone therapy in an immunocompetent patient. *Ocul Immunol Inflamm.* 2006;14(3):185–187.
170. Pearson PA, Piracha AR, Sen HA, et al. Atovaquone for the treatment of toxoplasma retinochoroiditis in immunocompetent patients. *Ophthalmology.* 1999;106:148–153.
171. Winterhalter S, Severing K, Stammen J, Maier AK, Godehardt E, Joussen AM. Does atovaquone prolong the disease-free interval of toxoplasmic retinochoroiditis? *Graefes Arch Clin Exp Ophthalmol.* 2010;248:1187–1192.
172. Rothova A, Bosch-Driessen LE, van Loon NH, Treffers WF. Azithromycin for ocular toxoplasmosis. *Br J Ophthalmol.* 1998;82:1306–1308.

173. Bosch-Driessen LH, Verbraak FD, Suttorp-Schulten MS, et al. A prospective, randomized trial of pyrimethamine and azithromycin vs pyrimethamine and sulfadiazine for the treatment of ocular toxoplasmosis. *Am J Ophthalmol*. 2002;134:34–40.
174. Ghartey K, Brockhurst R. Photocoagulation of active toxoplasmic retinochoroiditis. *Am J Ophthalmol*. 1980;89:858–864.
175. Atmaca LS, Simsek T, Batioglu F. Clinical features and prognosis in ocular toxoplasmosis. *Jpn J Ophthalmol*. 2004;48(4):386–391.
176. Wirthlin R, Song A, Song J, et al. Verteporfin photodynamic therapy of choroidal neovascularization secondary to ocular toxoplasmosis. *Arch Ophthalmol*. 2006;124(5):741–743.
177. Mauget-Faysse M, Mimoun G, Ruiz-Moreno JM, et al. Verteporfin photodynamic therapy for choroidal neovascularization associated with toxoplasmic retinochoroiditis. *Retina*. 2006;26(4):396–403.
178. Benevento JD, Jager RD, Noble AG, et al. Toxoplasmosis-associated neovascular lesions treated successfully with ranibizumab and antiparasitic therapy. *Arch Ophthalmol*. 2008;126(8):1152–1156.
179. Ben Yahia S, Herbort CP, Jenzeri S, et al. Intravitreal bevacizumab (Avastin) as primary and rescue treatment for choroidal neovascularization secondary to ocular toxoplasmosis. *Int Ophthalmol*. 2008;28(4):311–316.
180. Fitzgerald C. Pars plana vitrectomy for vitreous opacity secondary to presumed toxoplasmosis. *Arch Ophthalmol*. 1980;98:321–323.

16

Ocular Histoplasmosis

H. Nida Sen

KEY CONCEPTS

- Presumed ocular histoplasmosis syndrome (POHS) is characterized by a triad of peripapillary pigment changes, white round chorioretinal macular and midperipheral scars, and absence of vitritis.
- Amphotericin therapy does not help.
- Lesions have a high possibility of choroidal neovascularization.
- Laser therapy and anti–vascular endothelial growth factor (VEGF) therapies have been used to treat neovascularization.
- Subretinal surgical removal of neovascular lesions is of minimal value.

In the spectrum of ocular inflammation, ocular histoplasmosis is the only syndrome with the word *presumed* being part of its name. Epidemiologic evidence supports the concept that an invading organism is the cause of this ocular disease. However, there is accruing evidence to support the notion that there is a complex interaction between the exogenous pathogen and the immune response. Also, advances in submacular surgery have offered patients with this disease a possible, but yet-to-be-fully-proven, alternative therapeutic approach to consider besides medical and laser therapy or simply observation.

SYSTEMIC FINDINGS

Histoplasma capsulatum, a fungus found worldwide in valleys with rivers, is endemic to the midwestern United States. Found in the soil, it is readily inhaled and phagocytosed. Although histoplasmosis may start in the lungs, it can spread to the liver and the spleen, leaving small calcified lesions that can be seen on x-ray examination. The disease can take three major forms: a nonfatal acute pneumonitis with fever; an acute progressive form that can be fatal in 1 to 2 months; and a chronic form similar to tuberculosis.[1] These disease presentations rarely have ocular manifestations. Ocular histoplasmosis syndrome is a rather distinct entity found almost exclusively in the United States, and it usually occurs in symptom-free persons living in endemic regions. However, a similar clinical entity has been seen in nonendemic regions both in the United States and in other countries.

OCULAR APPEARANCE

It was probably Reid et al.[2] who described the first ocular case that we now recognize as ocular histoplasmosis syndrome, but Woods and Wahlen[3] were the first to describe this ocular syndrome in full detail. They believed that *H. capsulatum* might be the cause of both the typical atrophic spots in the retinal periphery and the disciform changes in the macula. Although the disorder is found most commonly in the midwestern United States, particularly in the Ohio–Mississippi River valleys, it also appears in the Middle Atlantic states, such as Maryland. In these areas, skin tests for histoplasmosis show positive results in a high percentage of the population, indicating systemic sensitization by the immune system. Ocular histoplasmosis syndrome is a rare disease in other parts of the world, even in areas endemic for histoplasmosis.[4] From countries other than the United States, there are reports of patients with symptoms that meet the criteria for the diagnosis; however, test results are negative for evidence of histoplasmosis infection and sensitization.[5,6]

Studies in the United States have suggested that typical findings of ocular histoplasmosis will be found in 1.6%[1] to 12.9%[7] of the population in an endemic area. Furthermore, Smith and Ganley[8] determined from the study in Walkersville, Maryland, that maculopathy caused by ocular histoplasmosis will develop in 1 of 1000 adults in an endemic area. The disease appears most commonly in the third to fourth decades of life, with men more likely to have involvement of both maculae.[4] It appears that the disease is considerably less common in African Americans[9] (Box 16.1). *H. capsulatum* causes four major clinical manifestations of the ocular disease: "histo" spots, maculopathy, peripapillary pigment changes, and clear vitreous.

"Histo" Spots

A disseminated choroiditis produces the typical histo spots. Numbering, on average, four to eight per eye, these choroidal scars are circular, depigmented, and atrophic; they have a disk diameter of 0.2 to 0.7 and may have a pigment clump centrally[10] (Fig. 16.1). The peripheral lesions are not thought to be significant in terms of prognosis with regard to good visual acuity. In a small number of patients, these lesions occur in the equatorial ocular region as streaks running parallel to the ora serrata. They can become larger or smaller, and they may disappear.

Maculopathy

Maculopathy results in a macular lesion that is sight threatening, causing a sudden, abrupt change in vision. During the initial stage, the choroid may take on a ground-glass appearance and push the retina upward. In the macula, detachment of the retinal pigment epithelium (RPE) can occur, and in 7% of patients, central serous choroidopathy is seen.[11] In a large number of patients (63%), the lesion is hemorrhagic[11] and, in rare instances, causes vitreous hemorrhage.[12] Intervals between macular attacks may vary from 1 month to years, leading to a disciform scar (Fig. 16.2). Schlaegel[4] stated that he informed his patients that if there were histo scars in the macula, then there was a one-in-four chance of recurrence in the macula over the ensuing 3 years. However, if no scars are noted, then the chances for ocular problems are about 1 in 50. About 60% of the time, this process leads to severe visual impairment, and only 10% to 15% of patients will maintain 20/20 vision in the affected eye after a 2-year period. The development of a disciform lesion in the second eye depends on the presence of old atrophic histo scars in the macular region because new lesions appear to arise at the edges of old ones.[9] These membranes can sometimes be difficult to diagnose because of the absence of hemorrhage or pigmentation.[13] Rarely, subretinal neovascularization leading to a disciform scar can appear in the absence of previous pigmentary changes, usually denoting a nidus of activity,[14] supporting the concept that there are invisible foci of choroidal inflammation in this disorder.[15] Indocyanine green (ICG) angiography has shown areas of hypofluorescence in areas that can be mapped to points where patients were reporting visual disturbances.[16]

In a longitudinal study of 28 eyes of 20 patients with POHS, Adhi et al. found that in all eyes with maculopathy, choroidal neovascularization (CNV) developed; ellipsoid zone, RPE, and the Bruch disruption in 100% and pigment epithelial detachment (PED) in 75% of eyes.[17] Unique patterns of choroidal hypoperfusion were identified by Wang et al. using optical coherence tomography angiography (OCTA). Areas of choroidal hypoperfusion correlated well with clinically visible lesions in POHS.[18] A point of great interest is the natural history of disciform lesions caused by ocular histoplasmosis, particularly in light of new surgical techniques (see later discussion). In ocular histoplasmosis, spontaneous improvement of visual acuity is possible in patients with disciform changes caused by this disorder. Jost et al.[19] found that 10 of 700 patients with ocular histoplasmosis experienced spontaneous improvement. In a study by Kleiner et al.,[20] visual outcomes were evaluated in 74 eyes with ocular histoplasmosis and active subretinal neovascular membranes. Over a follow-up period that ranged from 12 to 109 months (median, 36.5 months), the authors found that 14% of eyes retained a visual acuity of 20/40 or better.

Some of the factors associated with the retention of good vision were the patient's age (< 30 years), the small size of the membrane, and an absence of visual loss caused by ocular histoplasmosis in the other eye. Campochiaro et al.[21] reported on five patients who maintained or spontaneously regained good visual acuity in the presence of a subfoveal neovascular membrane. These authors believed that a typical pattern emerged in all of these patients when sequential photographs and angiograms were studied. A pigmented ring forms around the membrane, and the membrane begins to change character, as seen on the angiogram, going from one that leaks fluorescein to one that stains but does not leak. With time, there is resorption of subretinal fluid, with limitation of the hemorrhage and fibrosis (Fig. 16.3).

BOX 16.1 Characteristics of Ocular Histoplasmosis Syndrome

- Resident of histoplasmosis belt of the United States
- White, 20 to 50 years of age
- Multiple choroidal spots ("histo" spots)
- Peripapillary pigmentary changes
- Disciform scar
- No vitreous inflammation
- HLA-B7 positivity (macular disease)

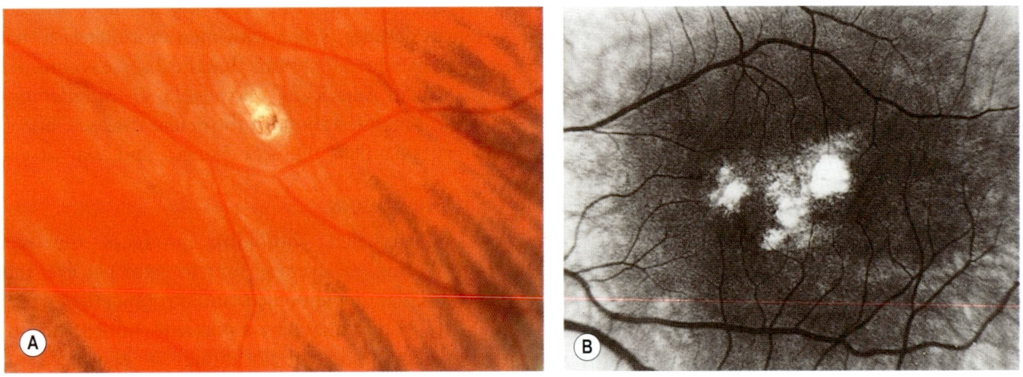

Fig. 16.1 (A) Peripheral "histo" lesion. These lesions are round and deep to the retina. The medium has no cells. (B) Similar lesions in the macula.

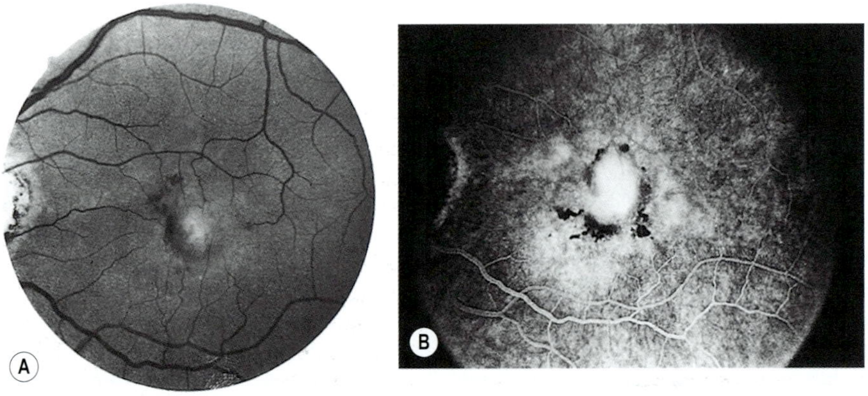

Fig. 16.2 (A) Patient with macular disciform lesion caused by multiple recurrences of presumed ocular histoplasmosis. (B) Late-stage fluorescein angiogram showing subretinal alterations.

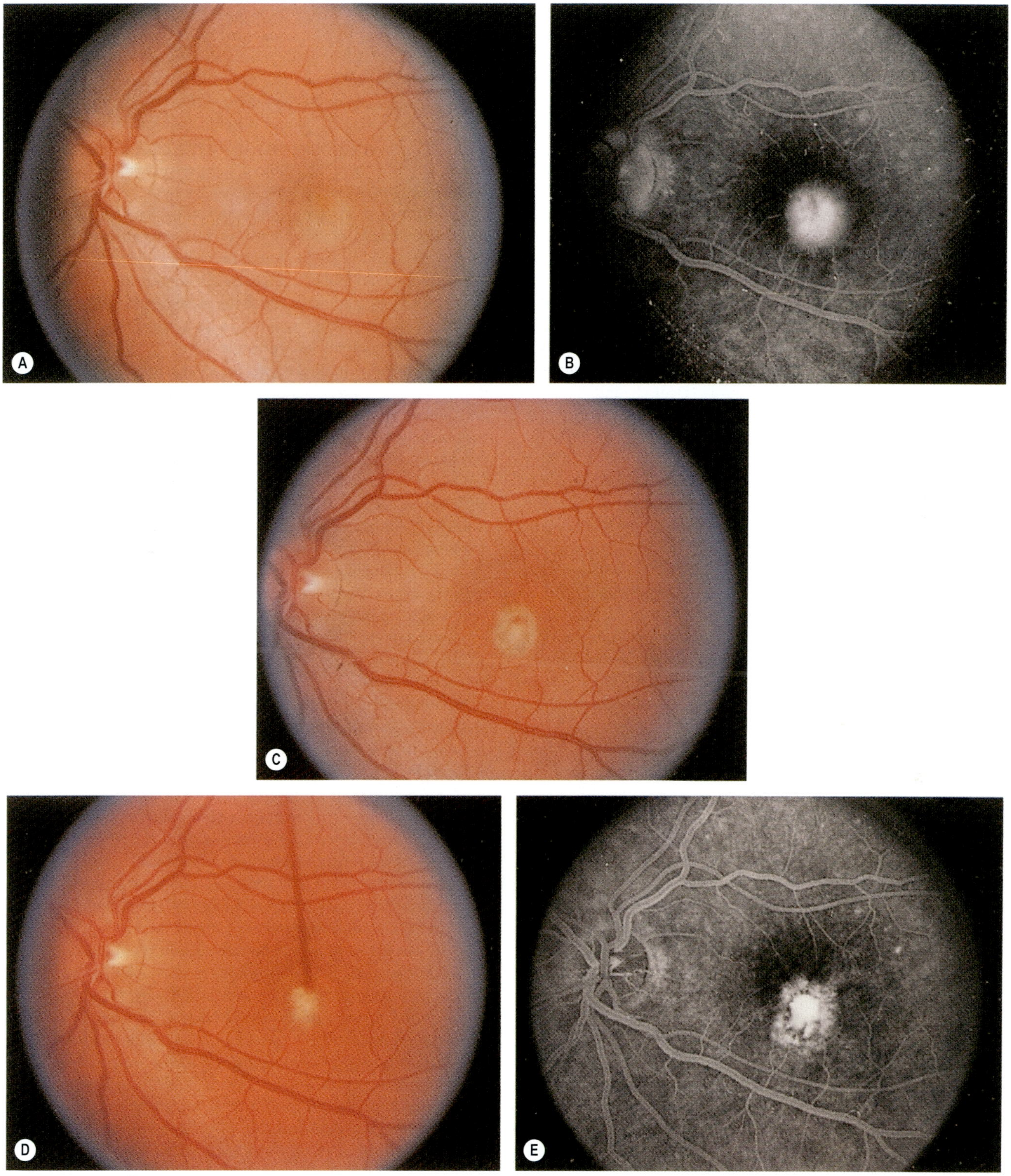

Fig. 16.3 Fundus photographs and angiograms of a 30-year-old patient who reported metamorphopsia for several weeks in the left eye. Visual acuity was 20/40, with 20/20 vision in the right eye. (A) Raised macular lesion. (B) Angiogram shows hyperfluorescence compatible with subfoveal neovascularization. Vision in the left eye decreased to 20/100 at 3 months and was 20/80 at 6 months. However, a pigmented ring around the lesion (C) was noted. By 24 months, vision had returned to 20/20, with an atrophic lesion in the macula (D), with staining but no leakage noted on angiography (E). (Courtesy Peter A. Campochiaro, MD.)

Peripapillary Pigment Changes

Peripapillary pigment changes occur, presumably as a result of underlying choroiditis. These changes are important because they can help the ophthalmologist diagnose the disease. A line of pigment is seen bordering the disk inside a depigmented area. These lesions sometimes appear to be nodular and can harbor subretinal nets, with resultant hemorrhagic episodes. In a patient with documented disseminated histoplasmosis,[22] optic neuropathy and gaze palsy were also reported.

Clear Vitreous

Clear vitreous is an important part of the clinical appearance of ocular histoplasmosis. The presence of cells must make the observer reconsider the diagnosis.

The differential diagnosis of this condition includes many diseases, including tuberculosis, coccidioidomycosis, cryptococcosis, multifocal choroiditis,[23] and sarcoidosis, in which granulomatous lesions appear deep to the retina. In pseudohistoplasmosis, an entity reported by Nozik and Dorsch,[24] lesions are present in the posterior segment, highly suggestive of ocular histoplasmosis. Deutsch and Tessler[25] found that sarcoidosis could be identified as the underlying cause of the histoplasmosis-like profile in many of the patients they observed. In the report by Parnell et al.,[23] experienced observers felt (and showed) that they were able to differentiate between histoplasmosis syndrome and multifocal choroiditis. In multifocal choroiditis, symptoms wax and wane, and patients (mostly women) will have an enlarged blind spot or other changes on visual field testing not explained by the clinical examination. Usually, patients with ocular histoplasmosis are asymptomatic unless the lesion affects their central vision. Most importantly, unlike ocular histoplasmosis syndrome, all of these entities should have obvious inflammatory activity in the vitreous. Some noninflammatory conditions that simulate this condition include myopic degeneration, drusen of the optic disk, and angioid streaks. Again, it is important to keep in mind the fact that if vitreal cells are present, then the diagnosis of ocular histoplasmosis must be reconsidered.

Several reports describing ocular disease compatible with this diagnosis have appeared but in areas where *H. capsulatum* is not found.[26,27] In one study from The Netherlands, 51 patients were identified with the classic findings of the disease and an incomplete form in another 31.[28] No evidence of *Histoplasma* could be found. Three patients with ocular disease suggestive of ocular histoplasmosis have been reported from India[29]; five cases of patients with classic findings but no antibodies to *Histoplasma* have been reported from Brazil.[30] These studies do not negate the reality of this syndrome but, rather, emphasize the fact that various insults to the eye may result in the same or similar clinical entities.

ETIOLOGY AND IMMUNOLOGY

Few clinically relevant tests are required to corroborate the clinical impression of ocular histoplasmosis. A skin test using histoplasmin antigen is most helpful, with reactivity usually appearing early after exposure and persisting throughout the patient's life. However, there is a risk that ocular lesions may be reactivated with the use of this test, so it is best not undertaken in patients with macular disease. One can argue that because "invisible" lesions may be present in the macula, the test may pose a risk to all patients. The test is therefore not often performed. The complement fixation test for circulating antibodies is not a particularly effective way to evaluate exposure; Schlaegel[4] found seropositivity in only one-third of typical cases. Chest x-ray to detect any calcification can help establish whether the patient had been previously exposed to this pathogen.

The exact role that *H. capsulatum* plays in ocular histoplasmosis remains to be elucidated. *Histoplasma* organisms have been found in the eyes of patients who have been immunosuppressed.[31] Indeed, in one report of a patient with a 12-year history of relapsing disseminated histoplasmosis, the ocular lesion manifested was endophthalmitis, rather than the typical findings of ocular histoplasmosis syndrome.[32] Specht et al.[33] reported ocular findings in a patient with acquired immunodeficiency syndrome (AIDS) and disseminated histoplasmosis. Creamy white intraretinal and subretinal lesions were noted, and postmortem examination of the globe showed the presence of *Histoplasma* yeast cells in the area of the retinitis and in the optic nerve. Pulido et al.[34] reported a case of exogenous postoperative *Histoplasma* endophthalmitis. The enucleated specimen (obtained after intraocular lens surgery) from the 60-year-old patient showed *Histoplasma* organisms but seronegativity and absence of systemic infection. However, other histopathologic correlations in which the presence of *Histoplasma* antigen has been suspected have occurred in cases thought to be compatible with ocular histoplasmosis syndrome.[35-37]

Histoplasmosis has been seen to occur naturally in both cats and dogs, inducing choroiditis and retinitis, respectively.[38] Intracarotid inoculation of nonhuman primates with live *H. capsulatum* showed that acute lesions took on several clinical features seen in humans, including chorioretinal scarring, RPE defects, and "disappearing" lesions. However, organisms were not demonstrated, on culture or with special staining techniques, in lesions present for longer than 6 weeks.[39] Subretinal neovascularization was observed in one eye of a nonhuman primate 1 year after injection with the organism.[40] Of interest was the failure of fluorescein angiography to demonstrate the presence of this abnormality, presumably because of the presence of tight junctions and therefore no leakage.

Anderson et al.[41] have characterized the lesions of histoplasmic choroiditis in the nonhuman primate with the use of antihuman monoclonal antibodies. They found variability in the cellular components of typical histo spots, even in the same eye. Of interest was a chronic lesion with a B-cell focus having high numbers of mature B cells and helper/inducer T cells.

Immunologic monitoring has not been very helpful in understanding the basic mechanisms of this disease. Check et al.[42] believed that in vitro lymphocyte proliferation assays with *Histoplasma* organisms seemed to correlate with the severity of disease. Brahmi et al.[43] found similar lymphocyte transformation responses in patients with both presumed ocular disease and acute histoplasmosis syndrome, whereas other parameters, such as natural killer (NK) cell activity and helper/suppressor cell ratios, were different among these groups.

With the use of human leukocyte antigen (HLA) typing, a potential immunogenetic predisposition to the development of the macular lesions appears to have been identified. Godfrey et al.[44] and Braley et al.[45] found an association between HLA-B7 and the macular lesions of this syndrome, giving a calculated relative risk of 11.8. This association has not been noted in those patients with manifestation of only peripheral retinal lesions. Spaide et al.[46] noted the absence of HLA-DR2 in 17 patients with multifocal choroiditis and panuveitis, whereas this antigen was found in 17 patients with subretinal neovascularization associated with ocular histoplasmosis syndrome. These authors believed, as the data suggested, that despite the ocular fundus similarities of these two entities, the disorders appear to have differing genetic dispositions. Ongkosuwito et al.,[47] analyzing DR sequencing, suggested that isoleucine at amino acid 67 was most strongly associated with ocular histoplasmosis syndrome.

Chheda et al. investigated risk factors for POHS and CNV development in a large case control study.[48] They found that smoking was associated with a threefold higher risk of CNV. Additionally, they

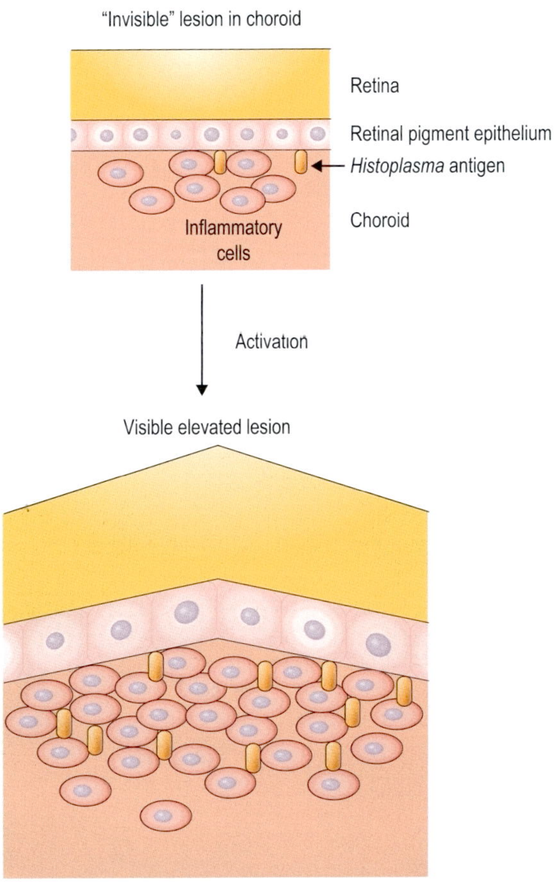

Fig. 16.4 Diagram showing the presence of "invisible" lesions in the choroid. *Histoplasma* antigen may be present, inducing a minimal inflammatory response, and therefore is not seen. If more antigen is released from distant site and lodges in the same area, or if *Histoplasma* antigen already there acts as adjuvant, more pronounced inflammatory response will occur, which now can be visualized as "active" lesion.

found that younger age and higher education were associated with a lower likelihood of CNV as well.

Many questions remain concerning the underlying mechanism of this entity. Many years ago, Richard O'Connor, who at that time was at the University of California, San Francisco, studied patients in whom typical lesions of ocular histoplasmosis developed several decades after they left an endemic area. There are several explanations for this. It may be that genetically prone persons are unable to clear the organism and that they continuously "shed" antigen from a site, such as the spleen. Once the organism has lodged in the eye, the low-grade inflammatory response in the choroid occurs again. Another possibility is that molecular mimicry may be the reason for repeated attacks (see Chapter 1). A third possibility is that in genetically prone persons, the fungal antigen acts as an adjuvant to induce an inflammatory response wherever it lodges, for example, in the choroid (Fig. 16.4). Ongkosuwito et al.,[49] in The Netherlands, studied 23 patients with peripapillary atrophy, punched-out retinal lesions, and macular disciform scars but no cells in the vitreous. None had antibodies to *H. capsulatum*, and no other risk factors could be identified.

The subretinal membranes resulting from ocular histoplasmosis syndrome have been studied. In a study by Grossniklaus et al.,[50] 17 ocular histoplasmosis membranes were evaluated. All were fibrovascular, and some showed hemorrhage. The most common cellular elements were vascular endothelium and RPE. It should be added that Mann et al.[51] reported a case of granulomatous inflammation, where the membranes were thinner and smaller in diameter, and photoreceptors were less likely to be found than in membranes removed from eyes with age-related macular degeneration (AMD).[50]

NONSURGICAL THERAPIES

Amphotericin B has no role in the treatment of ocular histoplasmosis. Not only is it ineffective, but it also exposes the patient to a medication with serious secondary effects.

Corticosteroids can be given for the acute macular lesion that causes a sudden drop in visual acuity or in preparation for laser therapy. Patients with macular lesions, particularly those with one eye already visually handicapped because of the disease, may consider carrying prednisone with them and checking daily for any changes in vision or distortions that occur, as noted on an Amsler grid. Short-term corticosteroid therapy should be given in high doses (60 mg daily, 50–120 mg every other day) to achieve an effect. The chronicity of the disorder (at least 2 years) suggests that a long-term therapeutic commitment must be made by both patient and physician. The final visual outcome when subretinal neovascular nets encroach on the foveal and juxtafoveal region is not affected by corticosteroid therapy[52]; with a follow-up of 39 months on average, 81% of eyes had visual acuities worse than 6/12, and almost 70% of these were 6/60 or worse with the use of this form of therapy.

Steroids, given locally and systemically, have been used as antiangiogenic agents. In one study, 18 patients with ocular histoplasmosis were treated with either oral prednisone for 4 to 6 weeks (n = 10) or a single sub-Tenon injection of triamcinolone (n = 8).[53] Oral prednisone resulted in short-term improvement in visual acuity and stabilization of the lesion. Intraocular steroid has also been used. Rechtman et al.[54] reported the use of intraocular triamcinolone injections in 10 patients with ocular histoplasmosis with subfoveal or juxtafoveal choroidal neovascular lesions. They reported that three experienced improvement in visual acuity, two had loss of visual acuity, and five had no change in visual acuity. This was with an average follow-up of 17 months (6–41 months). Increased intraocular pressure and "mild" cataract development were noted as adverse effects. Continued intraocular injections of steroid would theoretically be necessary to achieve a long-term result.

Holekamp et al.[55] reported the use of either a 2-mg or a 6-mg fluocinolone acetonide implant in 14 eyes with CNV not caused by AMD, seven of them being caused by ocular histoplasmosis. In 10 of the 14 eyes, involution of the CNV occurred, but, interestingly, four patients, all of whom received the 2-mg implant, had recurrence of their lesions. The authors reported "significant" complications with the device.

Antiangiogenic therapies, particularly the intravitreal injection of anti-VEGF agents, have provided the practitioner with a new approach to ocular neovascular lesions. Adan et al.[56] reported a case of juxtafoveal CNV responding well in the short term to an injection of bevacizumab. Schadlu et al.[57] performed a retrospective chart review of 28 eyes in 28 patients who received intravitreal injections of bevacizumab for CNV secondary to ocular histoplasmosis. The mean follow-up period was 22 weeks, and the patients received an average of almost two injections. Twenty of the eyes monitored experienced improvement in central visual acuity; in four eyes, visual acuity stayed unchanged, and in four, a decrease in vision occurred. The real question is the long-term stability of these visual outcomes or whether continued injections of an anti-VEGF agent are needed (Fig. 16.5). To date, bevacizumab, ranibizumab, and aflibercept have all been used for the treatment of CNV associated with POHS, resulting in improvement in vision, and anti-VEGF injections have become the standard of care.[58-60] One large retrospective comparative case series of 150 eyes (of 140 patients) showed

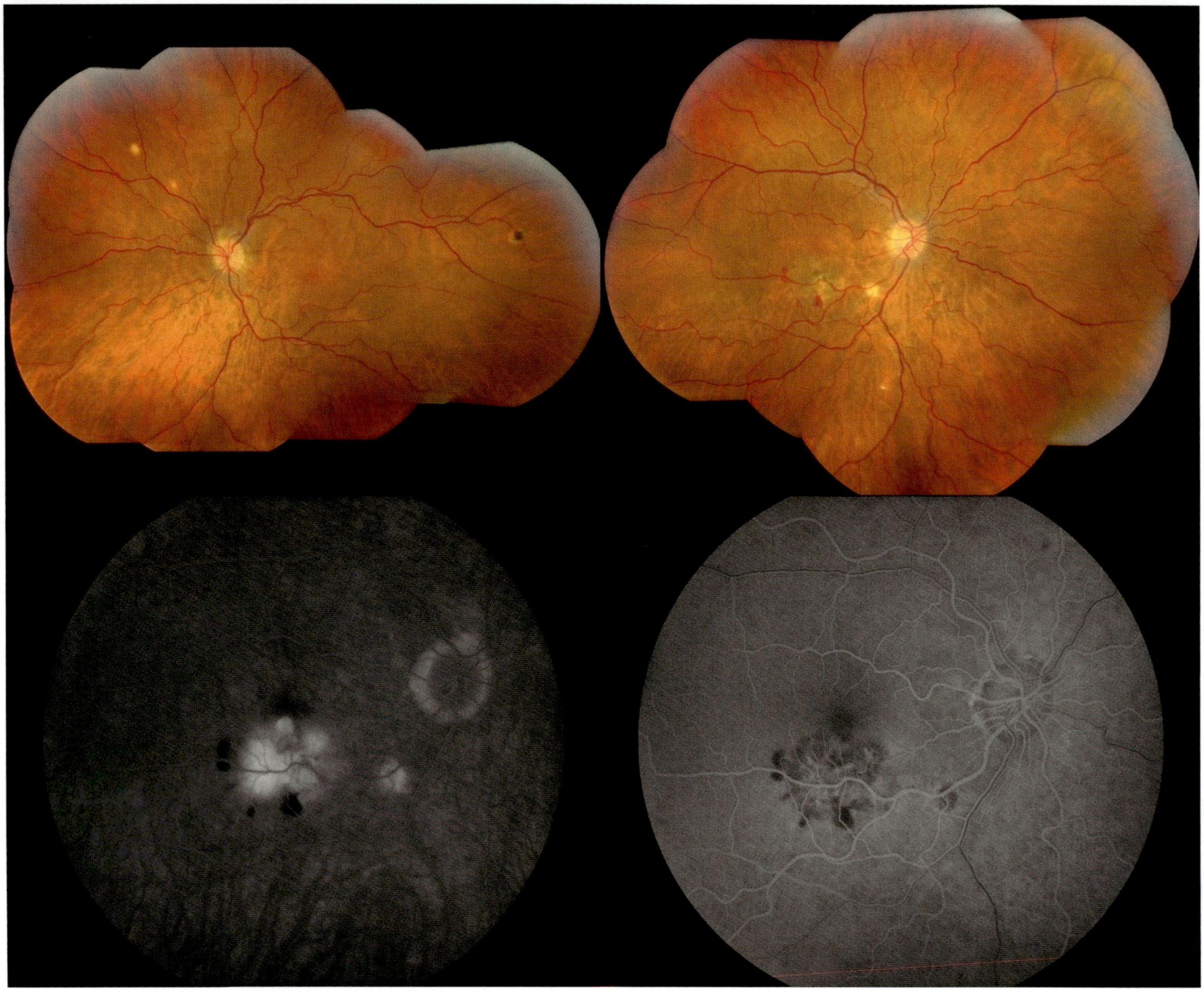

Fig. 16.5 This white man had granulomatous nodules in the lung that upon workup (lavage) were positive for histoplasmosis. He developed an active choroidal neovascularization (CNV) in the right eye requiring intravitreal bevacizumab injections.

no difference in visual outcomes between intravitreal bevacizumab monotherapy compared with combined intravitreal bevacizumab and photodynamic therapy (PDT). Visual acuity improved by three lines or more in 38%; in 82%, visual acuity was maintained or improved.[58]

Laser Therapy

Maumenee[37] first suggested the use of laser photocoagulation to treat ocular histoplasmosis syndrome. The results of a randomized controlled trial (RCT) evaluating the effectiveness of argon laser photocoagulation for choroidal neovascular membranes have shown this approach to be the treatment of choice until the advent of vascular endothelial growth factor (VEGF) inhibitors.[61] After an 18-month follow-up, 34% (39 of 114) of untreated eyes versus 9.4% (11 of 117) of treated eyes lost visual acuity of six lines or more from baseline. In 1991, the Macular Photocoagulation Study Group[62] published their 5-year results of three RCTs using argon laser photocoagulation in the treatment of extrafoveal CNV caused by various disorders, including ocular histoplasmosis. In these studies, untreated eyes with extrafoveal CNV caused by ocular histoplasmosis had a 3.6 times greater risk of losing visual acuity of six or more lines compared with laser-treated eyes. However, recurrent CNV was noted in 26% of the treated eyes. In a multicenter RCT, the Canadian Ophthalmology Study Group[63] found that krypton red laser photocoagulation was no better for well-defined extrafoveal nets compared with argon green laser photocoagulation.

A study by Fine et al. reported the use of laser therapy to treat subfoveal neovascular nets.[64] Only 25 patients were enrolled, and the follow-up period was fairly short. The observers could not conclude whether the approach was useful or not, but a marked decrease in vision did not appear to occur in the group treated with laser photocoagulation, nor was there a striking increase. One interesting aspect of this report was the difficulty in recruiting patients; the authors hypothesized that in most patients, the nets begin outside the fovea and therefore are treated before reaching the more advanced stage. Recurrence of subretinal neovascular nets is problematic. Green[65] reported a clinicopathologic study of treated choroidal neovascular membranes and noted that recurrences of CNV, some contiguous and some not contiguous to treated areas, occurred in nine of 12 lesions in the 10 eyes he studied. It is interesting to note that the scar induced by laser photocoagulation resembled that of the naturally occurring scar, portions of which consisted of hyperplastic RPE (Fig. 16.6).

PDT can be considered a therapeutic approach for macular subretinal neovascular lesions associated with this disease.[66] Saperstein et al.[67] reported the results of a small (26-patient), open-label, three-center,

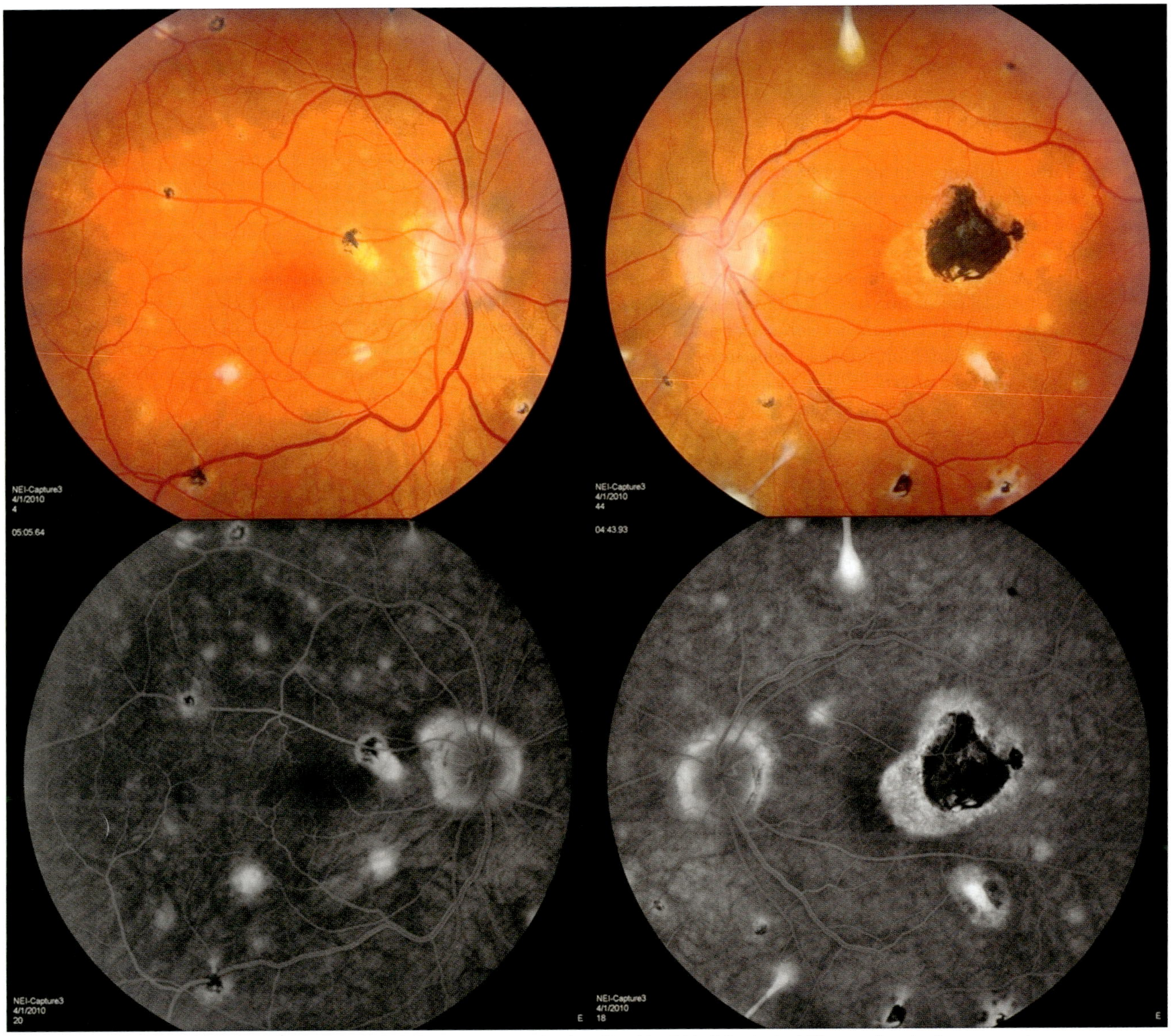

Fig. 16.6 This 40-year-old Caucasian woman, who has lived in Ohio-Mississippi River valley, had presumed ocular histoplasmosis in both eyes complicated by choroidal neovascularization (CNV) in the left eye which was treated with laser in early 1990s, with resultant large macular hyperpigmented scar.

noncomparative case series using PDT in the treatment of subfoveal neovascular lesions related to ocular histoplasmosis. By month 12, patients received, on average, 2.9 treatments, and there was a median improvement of seven letters from baseline in 14 patients, whereas four patients lost eight or more letters, and two lost 15 or more. No serious systemic side effects or ocular adverse events were reported. Leslie et al.[68] retrospectively reviewed the cases of six patients with predominantly classic CNV secondary to inflammatory disease and whose lesions apparently did not regress with immunosuppressive therapy. According to the report, two of the six patients had ocular histoplasmosis. With a median follow-up of 10 months, an improvement in vision (median improvement of 18 letters) occurred in all cases. Thus the authors felt that PDT was a useful consideration in such patients. Lim et al.[69] came to a different conclusion in their study, stating that PDT may stabilize, but not improve, visual acuity in eyes with CNV secondary to inflammatory disease. A systematic literature review of CNV associated with rare diseases such as POHS, uveitis and CSCR treatment showed that both intravitreal ranibizumab and PDT showed significant improvement from baseline best corrected visual acuity (BCVA) over a 12-month period; however, all patients in the PDT group required rescue ranibizumab therapy.[70] With the introduction of anti-VEGF agents, laser therapy and PDT are seldom used.

SUBRETINAL SURGERY

The removal of choroidal neovascular nets by means of subretinal surgery has especially thought-provoking implications. Although reports of subretinal surgery appeared in the 1980s,[71,72] this type of surgery did not really develop until the 1990s, with the advent of new instruments and indications. CNV caused by ocular histoplasmosis has been one disease in which this approach has been explored in some depth. An initial article by Thomas and Kaplan[73] reported two cases of subfoveal neovascularization caused by ocular histoplasmosis syndrome whose visual acuities were 20/400. After surgery and a short follow-up time, visual acuity was found to have returned to 20/20 in one patient and to 20/40 in the other. Subsequent reports have put the technique in perspective, albeit not definitively. Berger and Kaplan[74] reported that eight of 15 patients with subfoveal CNV caused by ocular histoplasmosis experienced improvement in visual acuity of two lines or better after subretinal surgery and removal of the membrane. They noted an improvement in vision even after 6 months of reduced vision. Recurrent CNV occurred in two of the 15 eyes. Thomas et al.[75] performed two types of procedures on patients with histoplasmosis who had subfoveal nets. After performing vitrectomy, the authors either disconnected the choroidal circulation or extracted the net through the retinotomy site. Of 16 eyes that had membranes removed, six improved by at least two Snellen lines, whereas none of the eyes in the four cases where the membranes' choroidal circulation was disconnected showed such improvement. A large study of 117 patients with ocular histoplasmosis and subretinal neovascularization provided some insight into the long-term effects of subretinal surgery.[76,77] In a median 13-month follow-up, recurrence of disease was noted in 51 eyes (44%), the median time to recurrence being 3 months. Recurrences were extrafoveal (16%), juxtafoveal (18%), or subfoveal (66%). In this group of eyes with recurrent disease, 16 were treated with laser, 17 had repeat surgery, and 18 were only under observation. Visual outcome was better in the eyes treated with laser. During this median 13-month follow-up, approximately 35% of eyes experienced 20/40 or better visual acuity, and 40% had improvement of three lines or better than before surgery. In those patients followed up for at least 1 year, vision appeared to be stable or better compared with the 3-month postoperative visual acuity measurements. Almony et al.[78] reported their findings from a retrospective review of patients with extensive peripapillary CNV, which is a type of lesion different from the ones discussed earlier. These authors found that this approach yielded positive results, with stabilization or improvement of visual acuity.

There was certainly enough information to support an RCT to evaluate the use of surgery for foveal or perifoveal choroidal neovascular lesions secondary to ocular histoplasmosis or those that appear to be idiopathic. The results of this study were published in a series of reports and are important reading for those interested in the subject. The Submacular Surgery Trials (SST) Research Group randomized 225 patients to either observation (n = 113) or subretinal surgery (n = 112): 46% of the observation arm and 55% of those in the surgery arm had a successful outcome.[79] Five in the surgery arm had rhegmatogenous detachments. The conclusion overall was that there was no or a smaller benefit to surgery than the trial was designed to detect. One subgroup that may have benefited more from surgery was a group with a visual acuity of 20/100 or worse and had other criteria mentioned in the report. To be fair, another report[80] of this study measured vision-targeted quality of life measures in these patients, and the surgical arm did show a larger improvement in the measure of this parameter than did the observation arm. The authors called it a "possible small overall benefit."

REFERENCES

1. Asbury T. The status of presumed ocular histoplasmosis: including a report of a survey. *Trans Am Ophthalmol Soc.* 1966;64:371–400.
2. Reid JD, Scherer JH, Herbut PA, et al. Systemic histoplasmosis diagnosed before death and produced experimentally in guinea pigs. *J Lab Clin Med.* 1942;27:419–434.
3. Woods AC, Wahlen HE. The probable role of benign histoplasmosis in the etiology of granulomatous uveitis. *Am J Ophthalmol.* 1960;49:205–220.
4. Schlaegel TFJ. *Ocular Histoplasmosis.* New York: Grune & Stratton; 1977.
5. Saraux H, Pelosse B, Guigui A. Multifocal inner choroiditis: pseudohistoplasmosis—the European form of the presumed American histoplasmosis. *J Fr Ophtalmol.* 1986;9:645–651.
6. Braunstein RA, Rosen DA, Bird AC. Ocular histoplasmosis syndrome in the United Kingdom. *Br J Ophthalmol.* 1974;58:893–898.
7. Davidorff FH, Anderson JD. Ocular lesions in the Earth Day 1970 histoplasmosis epidemic. *Int Ophthalmol Clin.* 1975;15:51–60.
8. Smith RE, Ganley JP. An epidemiologic study of presumed ocular histoplasmosis. *Trans Am Acad Ophthalmol Otolaryngol.* 1971;1971:994–1005.
9. Gass JDM, Wilkinson CP. Follow-up study of presumed ocular histoplasmosis. *Trans Am Acad Ophthalmol Otolaryngol.* 1972;76:672–694.
10. Smith RE, Ganley JP, Knox DL. Presumed ocular histoplasmosis. II. Patterns of peripheral scarring in persons with nonmacular disease. *Arch Ophthalmol.* 1972;87:251–257.
11. Walma D, Schlaegel TFJ. Presumed ocular histoplasmosis. *Am J Ophthalmol.* 1964;57:107–110.
12. Kranias G. Vitreous hemorrhage secondary to presumed ocular histoplasmosis syndrome. *Ann Ophthalmol.* 1985;17:295–298.
13. Rivers MB, Pulido JS, Folk JC. Ill-defined choroidal neovascularization within ocular histoplasmosis scars. *Retina.* 1992;12:90–95.
14. Ryan SJJ. De novo subretinal neovascularization in the histoplasmosis syndrome. *Arch Ophthalmol.* 1976;94:321–327.
15. Schlaegel TFJ. The concept of invisible choroiditis in the ocular histoplasmosis syndrome. *Int Ophthalmol Clin.* 1983;23:55–63.
16. Weinberger AWA, Kube T, Wolf S. Dark spots in late-phase indocyanine green angiographic studies in a patient with presumed histoplasmosis syndrome. *Graefes Arch Clin Exp Ophthalmol.* 1999;237:524–526.
17. Adhi M, Jusufbegovic D, Schaal S. Sequential chorioretinal changes in presumed ocular histoplasmosis syndrome analyzed using spectral domain optical coherence tomography. *Ocul Immunol Inflamm.* 2017;25(4):545–553.
18. Wang JC, Laíns I, Sobrin L, Miller JB. Distinguishing white dot syndromes with patterns of choroidal hypoperfusion on optical coherence tomography angiography. *Ophthalmic Surg Lasers Imaging Retina.* 2017;48(8):638–646.
19. Jost BF, Olk RJ, Burgess DB. Factors related to spontaneous visual recovery in the ocular histoplasmosis syndrome. *Retina.* 1987;7:1–8.
20. Kleiner RC, Ratner CM, Enger C, et al. Subfoveal neovascularization in the ocular histoplasmosis syndrome: a natural history study. *Retina.* 1988;8:225–227.
21. Campochiaro PA, Morgan KM, Conway BP, et al. Spontaneous involution of subfoveal neovascularization. *Am J Ophthalmol.* 1990;109:668–675.
22. Perry JD, Girkin CA, Miller NR, et al. Disseminated histoplasmosis causing reversible gaze palsy and optic neuropathy. *J Neuro-Ophthalmol.* 1999;19:140–143.
23. Parnell JR, Jampol LM, Yannuzzi LA, et al. Differentiation between presumed ocular histoplasmosis syndrome and multifocal choroiditis with panuveitis based on morphology of photographed fundus lesions and fluorescein angiography. *Arch Ophthalmol.* 2001;119:208–212.
24. Nozik RA, Dorsch W. A new chorioretinopathy associated with anterior uveitis. *Am J Ophthalmol.* 1973;76:758–762.
25. Deutsch TA, Tessler HH. Inflammatory pseudohistoplasmosis. *Ann Ophthalmol.* 1985;17:461–465.
26. Suttorp-Schulten MSA. The etiology of the presumed ocular histoplasmosis syndrome. *Ocul Immunol Inflamm.* 1997;5:71–72.
27. Watzke RC, Klein ML, Weiner MH. Histoplasmosis-like choroiditis in a nonendemic area. The Northwest United States. *Retina.* 1998;18:204–212.
28. Suttorp-Schulten MSA, Bollemeijer JG, Bos PJ, et al. Presumed ocular histoplasmosis in the Netherlands—an area without histoplasmosis. *Br J Ophthalmol.* 1997;81:7–11.
29. Sinha R, Raju S, Garg SP, et al. Presumed ocular histoplasmosis syndrome in India. *Ocul Immunol Inflamm.* 2007;15(4):315–317.
30. Amaro MH, Muccioli C, Abreu MT. Ocular histoplasmosis-like syndrome: a report from a nonendemic area. *Arq Bras Oftalmol.* 2007;70(4):577–580.
31. Scholz R, Green WR, Kutys R, et al. Histoplasma capsulatum in the eye. *Ophthalmology.* 1984;91:1100–1104.
32. Goldstein BG, Buettner H. Histoplasmic endophthalmitis: a clinicopathologic correlation. *Arch Ophthalmol.* 1983;101:774–777.
33. Specht CS, Mitchell KT, Bauman AE, et al. Ocular histoplasmosis with retinitis in a patient with acquired immune deficiency syndrome. *Ophthalmology.* 1991;98:1356–1359.
34. Pulido JS, Folberg R, Carter KD, et al. Histoplasma capsulatum endophthalmitis after cataract extraction. *Ophthalmology.* 1990;97:217–220.

35. Khalil MK. Histopathology of presumed ocular histoplasmosis. *Am J Ophthalmol.* 1982;94:369–376.
36. Ryan SJJ. Histopathological correlates of presumed ocular histoplasmosis. *Int Ophthalmol Clin.* 1975;15:125–137.
37. Maumenee AE. Clinical entities in 'uveitis': an approach to the study of intraocular inflammation. *Am J Ophthalmol.* 1970;69:1–27.
38. Gwin RM, Makley TA Jr, Wyman M, et al. Multifocal ocular histoplasmosis in a dog and a cat. *J Am Vet Med Assoc.* 1980;176:638–642.
39. Smith RE, Dunn S, Jester JV. Natural history of experimental histoplasmic choroiditis in the primate. *Invest Ophthalmol Vis Sci.* 1984;25:810–819.
40. Jester JV, Smith RE. Subretinal neovascularization after experimental ocular histoplasmosis in a subhuman primate. *Am J Ophthalmol.* 1985;100:252–258.
41. Anderson A, Clifford W, Palvolgyi I, et al. Immunopathology of chronic experimental histoplasmic choroiditis in the primate. *Invest Ophthalmol Vis Sci.* 1992;33:1637–1641.
42. Check IJ, Diddie KR, Jay WM, et al. Lymphocyte stimulation by yeast phase Histoplasma capsulatum in presumed ocular histoplasmosis syndrome. *Am J Ophthalmol.* 1979;87:311–316.
43. Brahmi Z, Wheat J, Rubin RH, et al. Humoral and cellular immune response in ocular histoplasmosis. *Ann Ophthalmol.* 1985;17:440–444.
44. Godfrey WA, Sabates R, Cross DE. Association of presumed ocular histoplasmosis with HLA-B7. *Am J Ophthalmol.* 1978;85:854–858.
45. Braley RE, Meredith TA, Aaberg TM, et al. The prevalence of HLA-B7 in presumed ocular histoplasmosis. *Am J Ophthalmol.* 1978;85:859–861.
46. Spaide RF, Skerry JE, Yannuzzi LA, et al. Lack of HLA-DR2 specificity in multifocal choroiditis and panuveitis. *Br J Ophthalmol.* 1990;74:536–537.
47. Ongkosuwito JV, Tilanus MG, Van der Lelij A, et al. Amino acid residue 67 (isoleucine) of HLA-DRB is associated with POHS. *Invest Ophthalmol Vis Sci.* 2002;43:1725–1729.
48. Chheda LV, Ferketich AK, Carroll CP, Moyer PD, Kurz DE, Kurz PA. Smoking as a risk factor for choroidal neovascularization secondary to presumed ocular histoplasmosis syndrome. *Ophthalmology.* 2012;119(2):333–338.
49. Ongkosuwito JV, Kortbeek LM, Van der Lelij A, et al. Aetiological study of the presumed ocular histoplasmosis syndrome in The Netherlands. *Br J Ophthalmol.* 1999;83:535–539.
50. Grossniklaus HE, Green WR, the Submacular Surgery Trials Research Group. Histopathologic and ultrastructural findings of surgically excised choroidal neovascularization. *Arch Ophthalmol.* 1998;116:745–749.
51. Mann ES, Forgary SJ, Kincaid MC. Choroidal neovascularization with granulomatous inflammation in ocular histoplasmosis syndrome. *Am J Ophthalmol.* 2000;130:247–250.
52. Olk RJ, Burgess DB, McCormick PA. Subfoveal and juxtafoveal subretinal neovascularization in the presumed ocular histoplasmosis syndrome. *Ophthalmology.* 1984;91:1592–1602.
53. Martidis A, Miller DG, Ciulla TA, et al. Corticosteroids as an antiangiogenic agent for histoplasmosis-related subfoveal choroidal neovascularization. *J Ocul Pharmacol Ther.* 1999;15:425–428.
54. Rechtman E, Allen VD, Danis RP, et al. Intravitreal triamcinolone for choroidal neovascularization in ocular histoplasmosis syndrome. *Am J Ophthalmol.* 2003;136(4):739–741.
55. Holekamp NM, Thomas MA, Pearson A. The safety profile of long-term, high-dose intraocular corticosteroid delivery. *Am J Ophthalmol.* 2005;139(3):421–428.
56. Adan A, Navarro M, Casaroli-Marano RP, et al. Intravitreal bevacizumab as initial treatment for choroidal neovascularization associated with presumed ocular histoplasmosis syndrome. *Graefes Arch Clin Exp Ophthalmol.* 2007;245(12):1873–1875.
57. Schadlu R, Blinder KJ, Shah GK, et al. Intravitreal bevacizumab for choroidal neovascularization in ocular histoplasmosis. *Am J Ophthalmol.* 2008;145(5):875–878.
58. Cionni DA, Lewis SA, Petersen MR, Foster RE, Riemann CD, Sisk RA, et al. Analysis of outcomes for intravitreal bevacizumab in the treatment of choroidal neovascularization secondary to ocular histoplasmosis. *Ophthalmology.* 2012;119(2):327–332.
59. Walia HS, Shah GK, Blinder KJ. Treatment of CNV secondary to presumed ocular histoplasmosis with intravitreal aflibercept 2.0 mg injection. *Can J Ophthalmol.* 2016;51(2):91–96.
60. Yılmaz T, Dikci S, Genç O, Mutlu K. Multiple intravitreal ranibizumab injections for persistent choroidal neovascularization associated with presumed ocular histoplasmosis syndrome. *Turk J Ophthalmol.* 2017;47(2):115–118.
61. Ocular Histoplasmosis Study. Argon laser photocoagulation for ocular histoplasmosis: results of a randomized clinical trial. *Arch Ophthalmol.* 1983;101:1347–1357.
62. Macular Photocoagulation Study Group. Argon laser photocoagulation for neovascular maculopathy: five year results from randomized clinical trials. *Arch Ophthalmol.* 1991;109:1109–1114.
63. Canadian Ophthalmology Study Group. Argon green vs krypton red laser photocoagulation for extrafoveal choroidal neovascularization. *Arch Ophthalmol.* 1994;112:1166–1173.
64. Fine SL, Wood WJ, Isernhagen RD, et al. Laser treatment for subfoveal neovascular membranes in ocular histoplasmosis syndrome: results of a pilot randomized clinical trial. *Arch Ophthalmol.* 1993;111:19–20.
65. Green WR. Clinicopathologic studies of treated choroidal neovascular membranes: a review and report of two cases. *Retina.* 1991;11:328–356.
66. Sickenberg M, Schmidt-Erfurth U, Miller JW, et al. A preliminary study of photodynamic therapy using verteporfin for choroidal neovascularization in pathologic myopia, ocular histoplasmosis syndrome, angioid streaks, and idiopathic causes. *Arch Ophthalmol.* 2000;117:327–336.
67. Saperstein DA, Rosenfeld PJ, Bressler NM, et al. Photodynamic therapy of subfoveal choroidal neovascularization with verteporfin in the ocular histoplasmosis syndrome. One-year results of an uncontrolled, prospective case series. *Ophthalmology.* 2002;109:1499–1505.
68. Leslie T, Lois N, Christopoulou D, et al. Photodynamic therapy for inflammatory choroidal neovascularisation unresponsive to immunosuppression. *Br J Ophthalmol.* 2005;89(2):147–150.
69. Lim JI, Flaxel CJ, LaBree L. Photodynamic therapy for choroidal neovascularisation secondary to inflammatory chorioretinal disease. *Ann Acad Med Singapore.* 2006;35(3):198–202.
70. Bennett N, John L, Likhar N, Agrawal R, Amoaku WM. Clinical efficacy and safety of current interventions for choroidal neovascularization associated with rare diseases: a systematic literature review. *Adv Ther.* 2018;35(5):591–603.
71. Machemer R. Surgical approaches to subretinal strands. *Am J Ophthalmol.* 1980;90:81–85.
72. de Juan EJ, Machemer R. Vitreous surgery for hemorrhage and fibrous complications of age-related macular degeneration. *Am J Ophthalmol.* 1988;105:25–29.
73. Thomas MA, Kaplan HJ. Surgical removal of subfoveal neovascularization in the presumed ocular histoplasmosis syndrome. *Am J Ophthalmol.* 1991;111:1–7.
74. Berger AS, Kaplan HJ. Clinical experience with the surgical removal of subfoveal neovascular membranes: short term postoperative results. *Ophthalmology.* 1992;99:969–975.
75. Thomas MA, Grand MG, Williams DF, et al. Surgical management of subfoveal choroidal neovascularization. *Ophthalmology.* 1992;99:952–968.
76. Melberg NS, Thomas MA, Dickinson JD, et al. Managing recurrent neovascularization after subfoveal surgery in presumed ocular histoplasmosis syndrome. *Ophthalmology.* 1996;103:1064–1069.
77. Holekamp NM, Thomas MA, Dickinson JD, et al. Surgical removal of subfoveal choroidal neovascularization in presumed ocular histoplasmosis. *Ophthalmology.* 1997;104:22–26.
78. Almony A, Thomas MA, Atebara NH, et al. Long-term follow-up of surgical removal of extensive peripapillary choroidal neovascularization in presumed ocular histoplasmosis syndrome. *Ophthalmology.* 2008;115(3):540–545. e5.
79. Hawkins BS, Bressler NM, Bressler SB, et al. Surgical removal vs observation for subfoveal choroidal neovascularization, either associated with the ocular histoplasmosis syndrome or idiopathic: I. Ophthalmic findings from a randomized clinical trial: Submacular Surgery Trials (SST) Group H Trial: SST Report No. 9. *Arch Ophthalmol.* 2004;122(11):1597–1611.
80. Hawkins BS, Miskala PH, Bass EB, et al. Surgical removal vs observation for subfoveal choroidal neovascularization, either associated with the ocular histoplasmosis syndrome or idiopathic: II. Quality-of-life findings from a randomized clinical trial: SST Group H Trial: SST Report No. 10. *Arch Ophthalmol.* 2004;122(11):1616–1628.

17

Ocular Toxocariasis

Scott M. Whitcup

KEY CONCEPTS

- Toxocariasis is a zoonotic infection caused by the roundworms *Toxocara canis* and *Toxocara cati.*
- Although ocular toxocariasis is relatively uncommon, it mostly affects young children and frequently causes permanent vision loss, including blindness.
- The diagnosis is predominantly based on clinical findings and exposure to puppies or kittens.
- Enzyme-linked immunosorbent assay (ELISA) is the most reliable and readily available test for the evaluation of antibodies directed against this organism and may be helpful in the diagnosis of the disease.
- Most *Toxocara* infections are self-limiting and resolve without therapy.
- Corticosteroids may be useful to control inflammation in infected tissues, including the eye, lungs, heart, and central nervous system (CNS).
- Although the use of available anthelmintic drugs, including albendazole and mebendazole, have not been conclusively shown to alter the course of the disease, the combination of anthelmintics and corticosteroids appears useful in some cases of ocular toxocariasis.
- Surgery may be useful in treating ophthalmic complications of infection, including retinal detachment.
- Prevention is the best approach. Routine deworming of pets and avoidance of contaminated areas are warranted.

Ocular toxocariasis is a zoonotic infection that is caused by the roundworms *Toxocara canis* and *Toxocara cati.* Humans become infected with *Toxocara* by ingesting embryonated eggs that can be shed in the feces of infected dogs and cats. The roundworms can cause damage as they migrate through the tissues in the body, and the resultant disease has been termed *larva migrans syndrome.* Other parasitic worms that can cause larva migrans syndrome include *Ascaris suum. T. canis, T. cati,* and *A. suum.* These are all large intestinal roundworms that belong to the family Ascarididae. In addition to causing similar clinical diseases in humans, they share biological features that cause similar risk factors for infection.

LIFE CYCLE

T. canis is an ascarid that can only complete its life cycle in the dog. Fig. 17.1 shows the life cycle of *Toxocara* species. *Toxocara* can follow a direct (single host) or indirect (multiple host) life cycle. An adult dog can acquire the infection by ingesting eggs with stage I encapsulated larvae that are found in the soil; by ingesting second-stage larvae from infected meat from animals, such as mice or rabbits; or by ingesting advanced-stage larvae from the feces of prenatally infected pups.[1] In some parts of the United States, toxocariasis is found in 100% of puppies less than 6 months of age.[2] Eggs in the intestine will ultimately hatch, and the larvae will migrate out of the intestine to all parts of the body. Most of the eggs will encyst as stage II larvae and not develop further. However, pregnancy can reactivate some of these dormant larvae, allowing them to re-enter the bloodstream and pass through the placenta to infest the growing pups. At birth, the larvae will migrate to the lungs and reach stage III. These can be coughed up and then swallowed, whereupon these larvae develop into stage IV eggs that then develop into the adult worm. These adult worms lay massive numbers of eggs that pass out of the host in feces.

Humans can then be infected when they ingest soil, food, or other materials contaminated by the eggs. Once in the human intestine, the stage II larva will enter the bloodstream, migrating throughout the body until the vascular lumen becomes small enough to block its progress. At this point, the larva bores into the tissue and encysts. In addition to the eye, *Toxocara* cysts are frequently found in the brain, liver, and lungs. Because the larvae cannot migrate out of the tissue, the life cycle ends at the stage II larval state, and *Toxocara* eggs are not found in the feces of infected persons.

The encysted larvae may stay dormant without causing any clinically overt symptoms, even when present in large numbers. However, two clinical syndromes have been well described: visceral larva migrans and ocular toxocariasis.

T. cati has a life cycle similar to that of *T. canis* (see Fig. 17.1). Humans usually become infected either by contact with eggs in contaminated litter boxes or by petting the infected animals and then touching the mouth because the eggs can adhere to the animal's fur. Clinical signs of *T. cati* in the cat include vomiting, decreased appetite, and stunted growth; however, mild infections with small numbers of worms may have no obvious signs or symptoms. Ocular disease caused by *T. cati* is similar to that caused by *T. canis.*[3]

EPIDEMIOLOGY

Toxocara infection is one of the most common zoonotic infections worldwide, but because most infections are asymptomatic, it remains relatively unknown to the public and is often overlooked by clinicians. The first nematode infection of the eye was reported by Calhoun,[4] in 1937, who observed a larva in the anterior chamber of an 8-year-old boy; and that the larva was ultimately was resorbed. The description of the organism led to its being considered an ascarid. In 1950, Wilder described endophthalmitis caused by nematodes,[5] and Nichols subsequently identified *T. canis* as the etiologic factor.[6]

Toxocara spp. can be found across the globe. Seropositivity varies widely by study and geographic area. In one study, seropositivity to *Toxocara* in adults on the island of Réunion was reported to be 92.8%.[7]

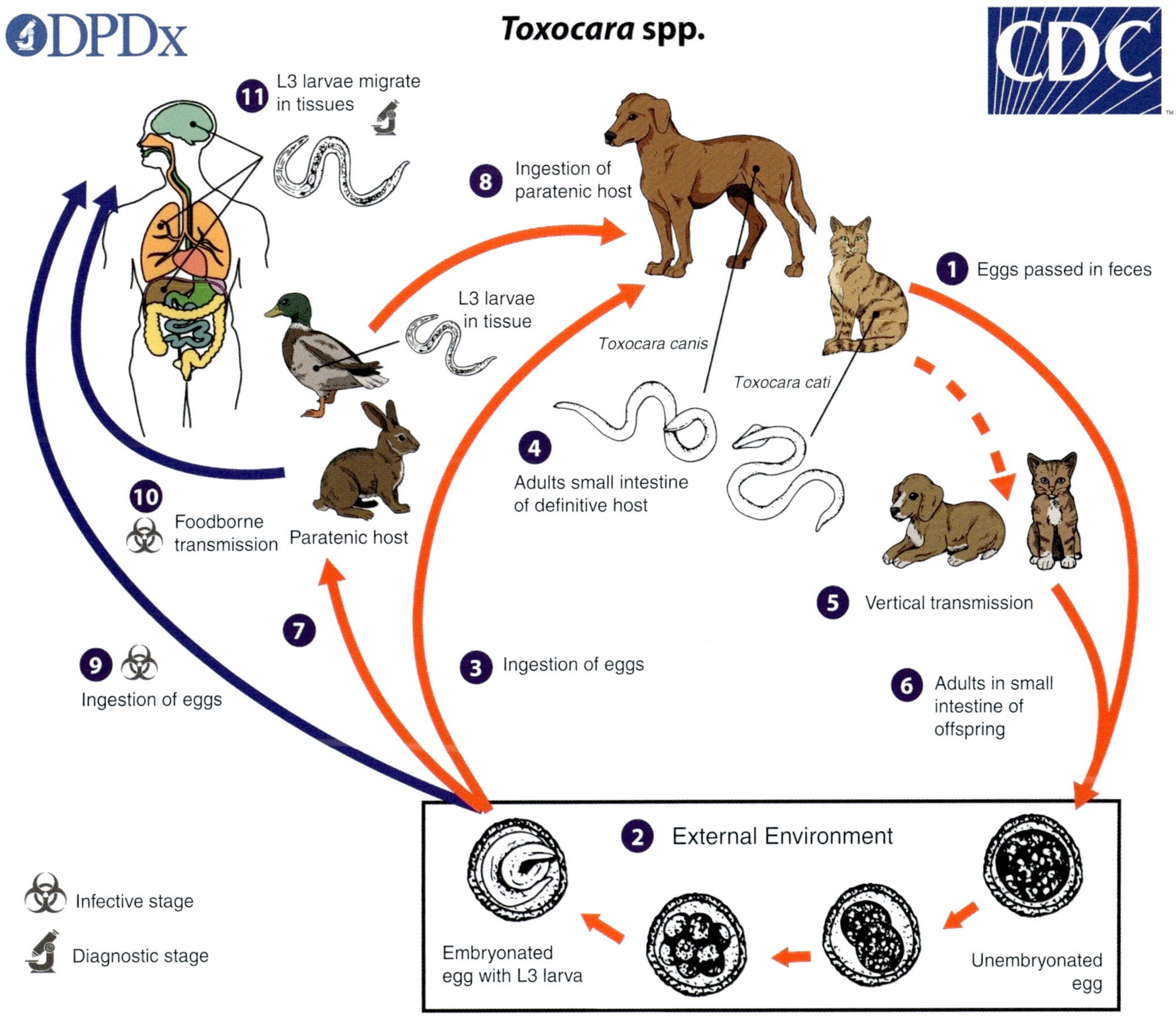

Fig. 17.1 Life cycle of *Toxocara*. *Toxocara* spp. can have a direct (one host) or indirect (multiple host) life cycle. Unembryonated eggs are shed in the feces of the definitive host (canids: *T. canis;* felids: *T. cati*). Eggs embryonate over a period of 1 to 4 weeks in the environment and become infective, containing third-stage (L3) larvae. After ingestion by a definitive host, the infective eggs hatch, and larvae penetrate the gut wall. In younger dogs *(T. canis)* and in cats *(T. cati)*, the larvae migrate through the lungs, bronchial tree, and esophagus, where they are coughed up and swallowed into the gastrointestinal tract; adult worms develop and oviposit in the small intestine. In older dogs, patent (egg-producing) infections can also occur, but larvae more commonly become arrested in tissues. Arrested larvae are reactivated in female dogs during late gestation and may infect pups by the transplacental (major) and transmammary (minor) routes; in the small intestine of the pup, adult worms become established. In cats, *T. cati* larvae can be transmitted via the transmammary route to kittens if the dam is infected during gestation, but somatic larval arrest and reactivation do not appear to be important as in *T. canis*. *Toxocara* spp. can also be transmitted indirectly through ingestion of paratenic hosts. Eggs ingested by suitable paratenic hosts hatch, and larvae penetrate the gut wall and migrate into various tissues, where they encyst. The life cycle is completed when definitive hosts consume the larvae within the paratenic host tissue, and the larvae develop into adult worms in the small intestine. Humans are accidental hosts and become infected by ingesting infective eggs or undercooked meat/viscera of infected paratenic hosts. After ingestion, the eggs hatch, and larvae penetrate the intestinal wall and are carried by the circulation to a variety of tissues (liver, heart, lungs, brain, muscle, eyes). Although the larvae do not undergo any further development in these sites, they can cause local reactions and mechanical damage that causes clinical toxocariasis. (From https://www.cdc.gov/dpdx/toxocariasis/index.html)

Human disease caused by *Toxocara* has been reported in countries worldwide, with most cases occurring in France, Austria, India, Japan, Korea, China, the United States, and Brazil.[8] In this review, the authors stated that 823 cases of ocular toxocariasis had been reported. Over a 20-year period, at the Francis I. Proctor Foundation at the University of California, San Francisco, of the 22,185 cases encountered, 22 were diagnosed with ocular toxocariasis (Table 17.1).[9] In a study of school children, the prevalence of consultant-diagnosed ocular toxocariasis was 6.6 cases per 100,000 persons. It should be mentioned here that another member of the Ascarididae family, *T. cati,* also needs to be considered in the differential diagnosis.[3]

T. canis and *T. cati* are very common parasites of most domestic and peridomestic dogs and cats, with even higher rates of infection found in puppies and kittens. The incidence of infected puppies has been estimated to vary: 33% in London; 98% in Columbus, Ohio; and 100% in Brisbane, Australia.[10] In one case-control study comparing patients with visceral larvae migrans (VLM) with age- and sex-matched control subjects, 23 of the 24 patients had dogs in their homes some time before their illness, and there was a significant association between puppies in the household within 1 year of symptoms and VLM.[11] Having a litter of puppies in the home was identified as a significant risk factor for toxocariasis.[12] In a study by Good et al., dog ownership in the past 2 years, convulsion, and geophagia were identified as risk factors for toxocariasis (Table 17.2).[13]

Parks, playgrounds, and yards frequented by dogs and cats are common sources for *Toxocara* infection. In addition, increasing populations of semiwild cats and dogs are contributing to high levels of *Toxocara* eggs in the environment.[14] Preventing dog and cat feces being deposited in play areas appears to be the best way to control infection. Routine deworming of pets and nonferal cats and dogs are also important health measures to limit human exposure.

CLINICAL SYNDROMES

As stated previously, VLM and ocular toxocariasis are the two common clinical presentations of the disease. VLM occurs mainly in young children and usually presents with fever, hepatomegaly, splenomegaly, and pulmonary symptoms often resembling asthma. Myocarditis, nephritis, and central nervous system (CNS) involvement causing

TABLE 17.1 Demographics and Other Information on *Toxocara* Patients Seen at the Proctor Foundation, University of California, San Francisco

Variable	Finding
Sex (%)	
Male	10 (45.5)
Female	12 (54.5)
Ethnicity (%)	
Non-Hispanic, white	15 (68.1)
Hispanic	3 (13.6)
Asian	4 (18.1)
Residence (%)	
United States	20 (90.9)
California	18 (81.8)
International	2 (9.1)
Ophthalmologist Referral (%)	22 (100)
Puppy/kitten Exposure (%)	18 (81.8)
Mean/median age at presentation in years (range)	
All patients	16.5/14 (1–37)
Male	15.3/11.5 (3–34)
Female	17.4/17.5 (1–37)
Mean/median time from onset to presentation in months (range)	
All patients	18.8/5.5 (< 1–212)
Male	7.9/6.3 (< 1–22)
Female	28/5.5 (< 1–212)

From Stewart JM, Cubillan LD, Cunningham ET, Jr. Prevalence, clinical features, and causes of vision loss among patients with ocular toxocariasis. *Retina.* 2005;25:1005–1013, with permission.

TABLE 17.2 Risk Factors for Toxocariasis in a European Population

Factor	Patients, n/N (%)[a]	Controls n/N (%)[a]	OR (95% CI)	*P*
Dog ownership ever	10/11 (90.9)	24/44 (54.5)	7.6 (0.97–394.4)	0.0552
Cat ownership ever	4/9 (44.4)	22/44 (50)	0.55 (0.05–4.2)	0.8214
Bird ownership ever	3/9 (33.3)	8/44 (18.2)	2.2 (0.31–12.7)	0.5248
Dog ownership in the past 2 years	9/11 (81.8)	18/44 (40.9)	5.5 (1.04–56.1)	0.0422
Cat ownership in the past 2 years	4/8 (50)	20/44 (45.5)	0.82 (0.08–6.7)	1
Bird ownership in the past 2 years	3/8 (37.5)	4/44 (9.1)	4.1 (0.54–28.1)	0.1884
Wheezing in the past 12 months	4/11 (36.4)	8/44 (18.2)	2.5 (0.43–13.3)	0.3687
Asthma	3/11 (27.3)	3/44 (6.8)	8.9 (0.62–498.4)	0.1312
Eczema	1/11 (9.1)	4/44 (9.1)	1 (0.02–14.1)	1
Hay fever	3/11 (27.3)	7/44 (15.9)	2.3 (0.25–20.0)	0.6149
Convulsion	4/10 (40)	1/44 (2.3)	16 (1.58–788)	0.0134
Geophagia	5/9 (55.6)	4.44 (9.1)	8.2 (1.4–62.2)	0.0183

Additional matching factors were age, sex, and urban/rural residence (patients, n = 11; controls n = 44).
[a]Number positive for the factor/replying to the question.
From Good B, Holland CV, Taylor MR, et al. Ocular toxocariasis in schoolchildren. *Clin Infect Dis.* 2004;39(2):173–178, with permission.

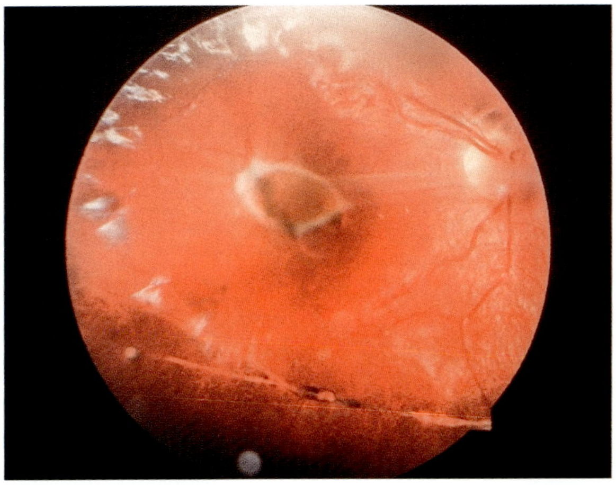

Fig. 17.2 *Toxocara* lesion in the macula of a 6-year-old girl. The choroidal lesion is raised, pushing the overlying retina upward; note the epiretinal changes.

seizures, neuropsychiatric symptoms, or encephalopathy can occur. Eosinophilia can occur with VLM. In this chapter, we will focus predominantly on ocular toxocariasis.

OCULAR MANIFESTATIONS

Toxocariasis is typically found in children. In one study, the average age of diagnosis was estimated to be 7.5 years (age range 2–31 years)[15]; and most patients are younger than 16 years of age.[16] In a study published by the U.S. Centers for Disease Control and Prevention (CDC) on ocular toxocariasis between 2009 and 2010, the median patient age was 8.5 years (age range 1–60 years).[17] Importantly, however, ocular toxocariasis also occurs in adults[18,19] and can be a cause of severe vision loss in these patients.[20] The disease is almost always uniocular; however, bilateral cases of *T. canis* infection have been reported.[21]

Several presentations of ocular toxocariasis have been described. Probably the most common presenting sign is a granuloma either in the posterior pole or in the retinal periphery. This is presumed to develop after a stage II larva has been lodged in a choroidal vessel and becomes encysted.[22] The lesion is often raised; is whitish in color; has a width of 0.75 to 2 or 3 disk diameters; and may have an associated fibrous band (Fig. 17.2). Ocular toxocariasis can also present as chronic endophthalmitis. *Toxocara* infection in the eye can cause leukocoria and may be misdiagnosed as retinoblastoma. In a review of 22 cases of ocular toxocariasis, 50% presented with a peripheral retinal granuloma, 25% with macular lesions, and 25% with moderate to severe vitreous inflammation mimicking endophthalmitis.[9] Severe vitritis may occur, representing an immune response against highly immunogenic antigens from a dead worm.

A plethora of less common ocular findings may be present. Live larvae have been observed in the retinal vessels.[23] Fuchs heterochromia has been reported as being associated with this entity, just as it has been noted in cases of ocular toxoplasmosis[24] (Fig. 17.3). Optic nerve disease[25,26] and occlusion of a branch retinal artery have been reported.[24] Karel et al.[27] reported a patient case of *Toxocara*, in which the larva had migrated into the lens through the posterior capsule. Unilateral pars planitis and diffuse unilateral subacute neuroretinitis are other rare presentations of the disease.

Because the disease often occurs in young children and because it typically involves only one eye, patients may be asymptomatic. When symptoms occur, vision loss is the most frequent complaint. As noted earlier, leukocoria may precipitate a visit to the doctor. In addition to vision loss, adult patients may complain of floaters.

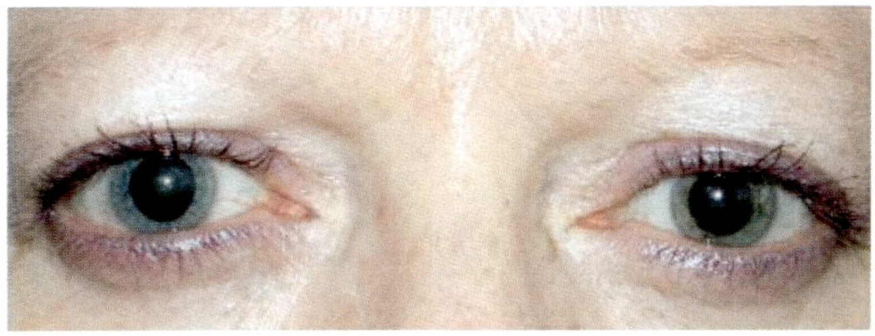

Fig. 17.3 Right eye with heterochromia in a 20-year-old woman. The right eye has a peripheral retinal lesion compatible with *Toxocara*. (Reproduced with permission from Teyssot N, Cassoux N, Lehoang P, et al. Fuchs heterochromic cyclitis and ocular toxocariasis. *Am J Ophthalmol*. 2005;139:915–916.)

BOX 17.1 Differential Diagnosis of Ocular Toxocariasis

- Retinoblastoma
- Idiopathic uveitis
- Infectious endophthalmitis
- Noninfectious endophthalmitis
- Sarcoidosis
- Pars planitis
- Other helminthic disease
- Ocular toxoplasmosis
- Diffuse unilateral subacute neuroretinitis
- Coats disease
- Retinopathy of prematurity
- Combined hamartoma of the retina and retinal pigment epithelium
- Familial exudative vitreoretinopathy
- Persistent fetal vasculature

The clinical features of ocular toxocariasis in adults are relatively similar to those in children.[28] In a review of 14 adult patients with ocular toxocariasis, the mean age at diagnosis was 45.6 years and the mean duration between the first symptoms and diagnosis was 15.1 months.[29] The disease was unilateral in all cases, and the main baseline findings were a peripheral granuloma in 57%, vasculitis in 57%, vitreoretinal traction in 57%, and chronic macular edema in 71%. Toxocariasis can occur in older adults as well. A *Toxocara* lesion presenting as a vasoproliferative tumor was reported in a 64-year-old man.[30]

In children, the most important alternative diagnosis to consider is retinoblastoma.[31] Shields[32] has stated that *T. canis* endophthalmitis is most commonly confused with retinoblastoma. Furthermore, presumed ocular toxocariasis accounted for 26% of the pseudoretinoblastomas seen at the Oncology Service of Wills Eye Hospital in Philadelphia. Children with retinoblastoma are typically younger than those with ocular toxocariasis, the vitreous in retinoblastoma is usually clear, and there may be a familial history of retinoblastoma. Ultrasonography,[33] radiography, or other imaging methods will usually help distinguish toxocariasis from retinoblastoma because calcification is frequently found in retinoblastoma and is only rarely reported in patients with toxocariasis.[34] A list of diseases to be considered in the differential diagnosis of ocular toxocariasis is provided in Box 17.1. In addition to retinoblastoma, infectious endophthalmitis should be considered in these patients. Other forms of uveitis, including pars planitis and sarcoidosis, can occur in these patients as well. Other infectious causes to consider are ocular toxoplasmosis and other

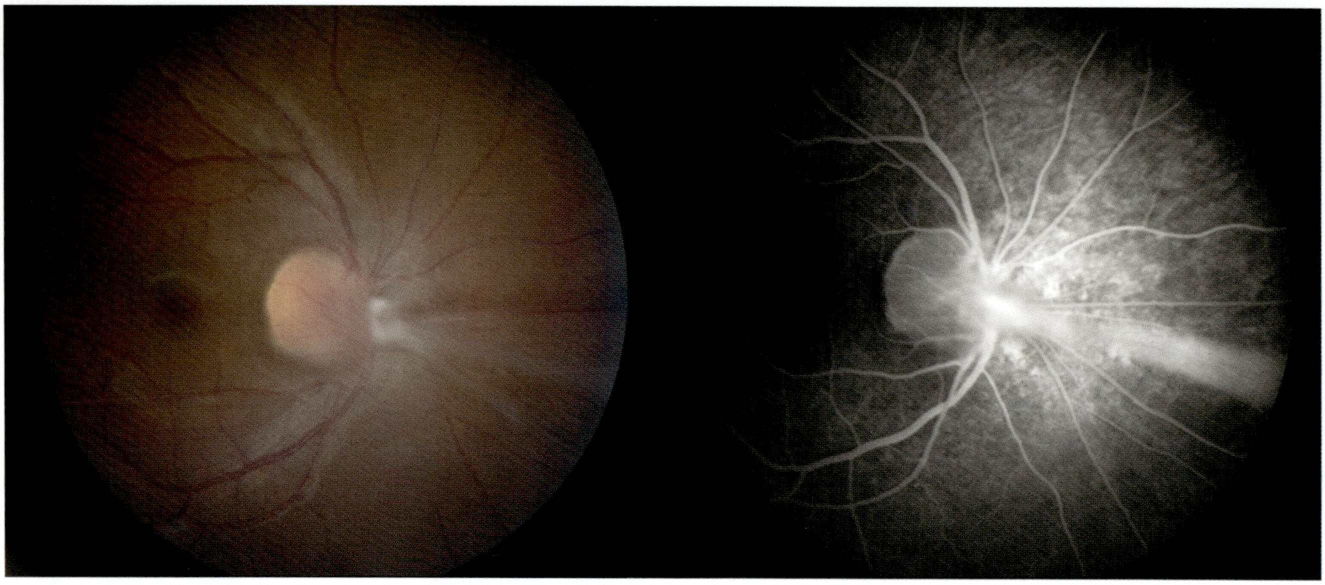

Fig. 17.4 Fundus photograph and fluorescein of an adult patient with ocular toxocariasis seen at the National Eye Institute (NEI). Note the lesion adjacent to the disk with fibrotic stalk extending toward the periphery *(left)*. This is also noted on fluorescein angiogram *(right)*. (Reproduced with permission from the NEI.)

helminthic diseases. Retinal disorders, such as Coats disease, familial exudative vitreoretinopathy, retinopathy of prematurity, and a combination hamartoma of the retina and the RPE are also included in the list of disorders that can appear similar to ocular toxocariasis.

DIAGNOSIS

The diagnosis of ocular toxocariasis is based primarily on clinical findings and a history of exposure to puppies and kittens or a history of pica or geophagia. In addition to clinical examination, imaging may be helpful in differentiating ocular toxoplasmosis from other disorders in the differential diagnosis. In cases where it is difficult to visualize the retina, echography can be useful. Using standard echography, Wan et al.[35] identified the characteristic findings of ocular toxocariasis (Fig. 17.4): a solid, highly reflective mass; vitreous bands or membranes that extended from the mass to the posterior pole; and a traction retinal detachment or fold from the mass to the posterior pole. The migration of the *Toxocara* larva in the retina has been documented with the use of optical coherence tomography (OCT) and fluorescein angiography.[36,37] Larvae moving through the nerve fiber layer of the retina produce a highly reflective signature (Fig. 17.5).

Laboratory Testing

Enzyme-linked immunosorbent assay (ELISA) is the most reliable and readily available test for the evaluation of antibodies directed against *Toxocara*. This test uses at least two *Toxocara*-derived antigens: one from embryonated eggs and one from the excretory–secretory antigens or exoantigen. One report[38] suggested that the exoantigen may give more consistent findings, and the CDC has suggested that the excretory–secretory antigens are preferable to larval extracts because they are convenient to produce and an absorption–purification step is not required for obtaining maximum specificity. Gillespie et al.[39] found that a two-site antigen-capture ELISA that detects a carbohydrate epitope on the excretory–secretory antigens of *Toxocara* was reasonably efficient (in 50% of patients) in detecting antibodies in patients with acute toxocariasis, but not in those with inactive or ocular disease. One ELISA kit evaluated[40] had a calculated diagnostic sensitivity of 91%, but 14% of serum samples showed false-positive results because of cross-reactions with other protozoan or helminthic infections. This is why some authors suggest that a negative serum test warrants testing of ocular fluids if the clinical suspicion is high enough. De Visser et al.[41] paired fluid samples with serum samples. In their study, two children with ocular disease had low serum titers but significantly high antibody titers in their ocular fluids, supporting a diagnosis of ocular toxocariasis.

There is some debate as to what endpoint titer should be considered positive for this ELISA. Sensitivity and specificity of the test will vary, depending on the titer selected as positive (Table 17.3). As with most diagnostic tests, the toxocariasis ELISA is not 100% sensitive and 100% specific for the disease. At the CDC, a titer greater than 1:32 is considered positive.[42] Evaluation of their ELISA in patients with presumptive diagnoses of either VLM or ocular larvae migrans indicated sensitivity of 78% and 92% and specificity of 73% and 91%, respectively. Another report showed that at a cut-off value of 0.258, the sensitivity and specificity of a serum immunoglobulin G (IgG) ELISA were 93% and 100%, respectively, for ocular toxocariasis in patients with uveitis.[43] Confirmation of ELISA results can be obtained by testing aqueous or vitreous samples or when serum samples are negative but clinical suspicion is high. Albert and Marcus[44] reported the case of a 4-year-old boy with a serum ELISA titer of 1:4; examination of the enucleated eye revealed a second-stage larva of *Toxocara*. Kieler[45] reported the case of a 5-year-old with an ELISA titer of 1:2, where the *Toxocara* parasite was present in an eosinophilic granuloma in the vitreous cavity, and Sharkey and McKay[46] reported the case of a patient who had repeatedly negative ELISA test results. In a review of 383 Japanese patients with uveitis,[47] 55 had serum antibodies to *T. canis*, whereas 11 of 22 vitreous samples obtained from these patients showed positive results. Interestingly, samples from eight patients had antibodies to *T. canis* in both serum and the vitreous, but three had antibodies only in the vitreous. In another case reported by Schneider et al.,[48] results of serum analysis were negative, but results from polymerase chain reaction (PCR) analysis performed on the aqueous were positive. A possible confounding factor is a cross-reactivity with *T. cati*. Sakai et al.[49] reported the case of a patient who was presumed to have *T. canis* infestation and observed that the titer for ELISA directed against the second larval stage of *T. canis* was minimal. ELISA using

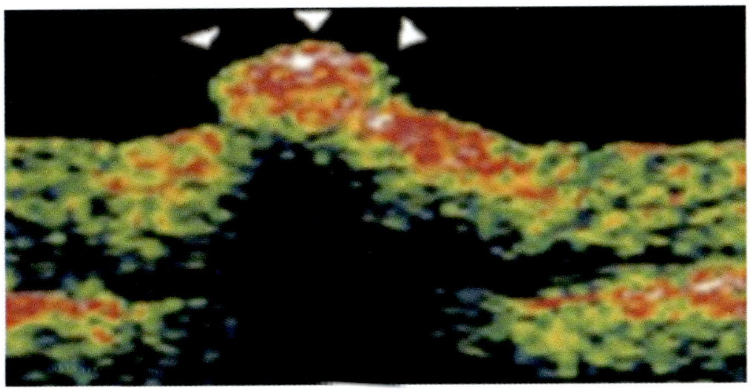

Fig. 17.5 Optical coherence tomography (OCT) scan of a *Toxocara* mass protruding into the vitreous. (Reproduced with permission and reprinted in part from Suzuki T, Joko T, Akao N, et al. Following the migration of a *Toxocara* larva in the retina by optical coherence tomography and fluorescein angiography. *Jpn J Ophthalmol.* 2005;49:159–161.)

antigens from adult *T. canis* and *T. cati* showed very high antibody levels to *T. cati.*

Magnaval et al.[50] tested the value of Western blotting techniques against that of the standard ELISA. Using the same excretory–secretory antigens for both, results from the Western blotting technique correlated well with those from the ELISA technique. Although potentially more specific with less cross-reactivity against other helminths, Western blotting is not widely available.

Other laboratory tests can be important in the diagnosis of *T. canis* infection. Children with VLM often have an eosinophilia and hyperglobulinemia.[32] No eggs are found in the stool because the life cycle of *T. canis* in humans does not reach this stage. Because there is no acute systemic illness, elevated immune parameters in serum are rarely evident.

Histopathology and Immune Factors

The immune reaction to the *Toxocara* organism is similar to that seen for other parasites of this type. Initially, there is a profound eosinophilic response, followed by infiltration of macrophages, lymphocytes, and epithelioid cells. A large granulomatous response to the organism is not unusual (see Fig. 17.2). Scarring may occur late in the immune response. The inflammatory response may be quite profound and cause more destruction than that caused by the offending organism. In severe inflammatory reactions, *Toxocara* may be destroyed, and therefore the diagnosis can only be suspected on the basis of the massive inflammatory response. In vitro work by Del Prete et al.[51] isolated clones of T cells from patients by using the *T. canis* excretory–secretory antigen. They found that these clones secreted interleukin (IL)-4 and IL-5 but no or only minimal amounts of IL-2 and interferon-γ, the reverse of what was seen from clones that were specific to the purified protein derivative of *Mycobacterium tuberculosis.*

An eosinophilic amorphous material, called the *Splendore-Hoeppli phenomenon,* can be seen in the organs of children with VLM. Werner et al.[52] showed eosinophilic amorphous material resembling the Splendore-Hoeppli phenomenon on histopathologic examination of subretinal material removed from an eye with *T. canis* infection. This reaction is not specific to *Toxocara* and occurs with other parasitic diseases as well. Experimentally induced disease will produce a marked eosinophilic response and a histologic picture not unlike that seen in humans.[53] Furthermore, Rockey et al.[54] have noted that eosinophils adhere firmly to the larval sheath. Interestingly, the parasite is able to evade eosinophils in culture by shedding its sheath. This in vitro observation supports the notion that the larval sheath could act as an antigenic stimulus without the presence of the parasite itself. In addition

TABLE 17.3 Sensitivity and Specificity of ELISA for Diagnosis of Ocular Toxocariasis

Cut-off Titer of Positive Test	Sensitivity (%)	Specificity (%)
1:2	95	72
1:4	93	86
1:8	90	91
1:16	85	94
1:32	73	95
1:64	51	97
1:128	24	99
1:256	15	100
1:512	5	100

ELISA, enzyme-linked immunosorbent assay. From Hagler WS, Pollard ZF, Jarrett WH, et al. Results of surgery for ocular *Toxocara canis. Ophthalmology.* 1981;88:1081–1086, with permission.

to eosinophils, T cells appear to be important in the host's immune response to this parasite.[55]

Researchers have also studied the extent of infection by quantifying the number of organisms in various tissues. Carter[56] used 35S-labelled *T. canis* to determine larval numbers in various tissues. It was found that although initially the larvae congregated in the liver, by day 14 after infection, the majority of the isotope was found in the brain. Cuellar et al.[57] reported that measuring the levels of immune complexes may be a good technique for monitoring treatment efficiency because these levels fell quickly and remained low with therapy. Various animal models have been used to study this disease.[58] Hamsters and gerbils seem most susceptible to *Toxocara.* Gerbils may develop ocular lesions 55% of the time. Ollero et al.[59] studied the prevalence of eye disease in a mouse model of *Toxocara.* Eye disease occurred after the larva reached the brain but was not dependent on the inoculating dose.[58] Another animal model using Swiss mice[60] tested the use of cyclosporin. Of interest was the fact that the medication increased the susceptibility of the mice to the *Toxocara* larvae, but the antiparasitic effect of the medication was significant, leading to a diminution in the number of living larvae.

TREATMENT AND PROGNOSIS

Most *Toxocara* infections are self-limiting and resolve without therapy. Certain systemic infections, however, may warrant treatment. Glucocorticoids are frequently used in patients with severe myocardial, pulmonary, or CNS involvement to reduce the inflammatory response. The use of available anthelmintic drugs, including albendazole and mebendazole, has not been conclusively shown to alter the course of disease. Nevertheless, some data suggest that the combination of the anthelmintic drugs with corticosteroids may be useful in treating ocular toxocariasis. Rubin et al.[23] reported the use of systemic prednisone (40 mg/day) with thiabendazole (2 g daily for 5 days), which caused disappearance of active larvae 24 hours after the initiation of therapy but no change in pre- and posttreatment visual acuity. However, some reports have described this approach as ineffective in altering the course of disease. Wilkinson and Welch[61] reported that thiabendazole and prednisone given to different groups of patients were not found to be successful in treating the disorder.

Evidence suggests that live larvae do not induce a substantial inflammatory response but that considerable inflammation occurs after the death of the organism. This may explain the variable response to anthelmintic drugs. As noted earlier, most published reports of

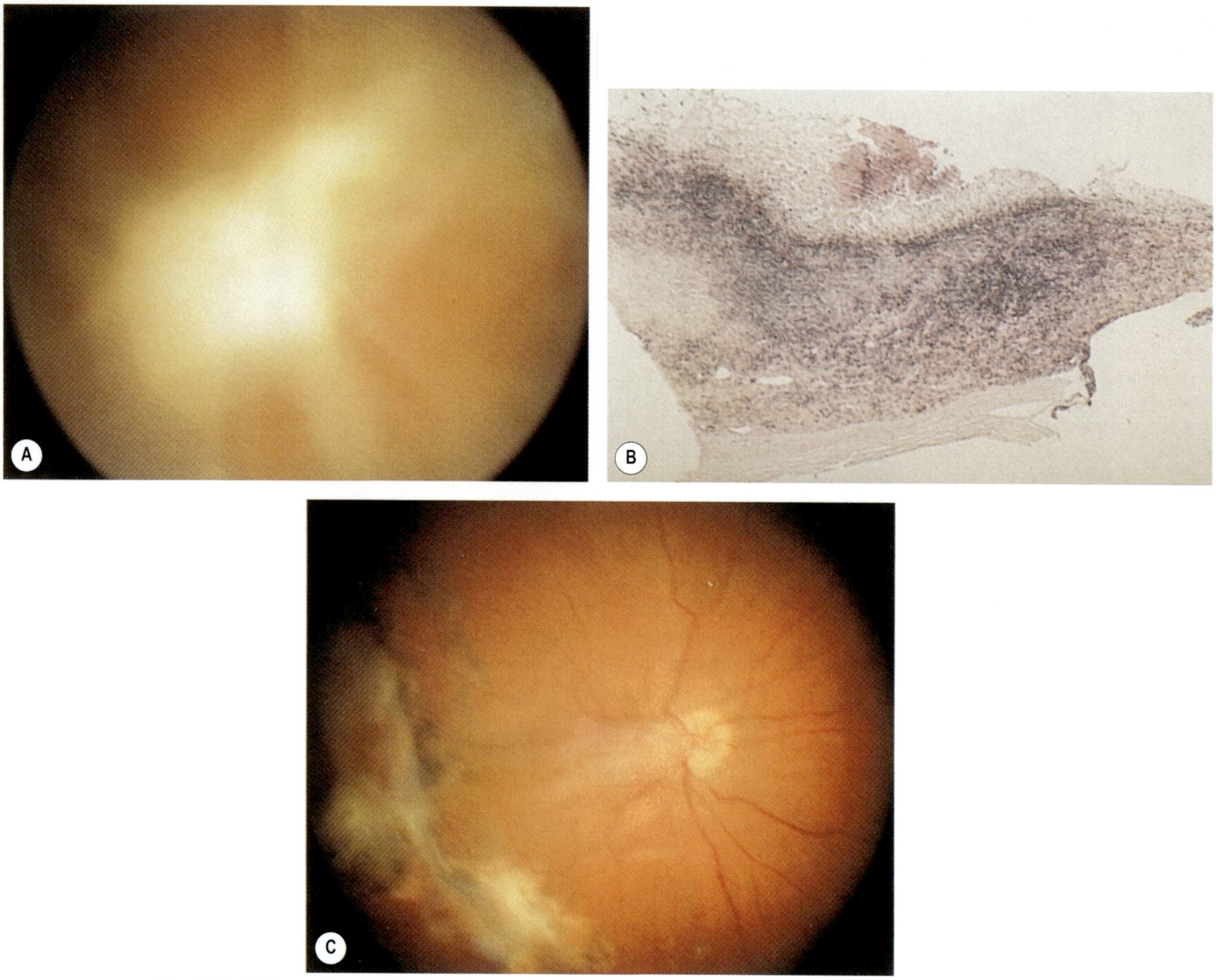

Fig. 17.6 (A) Posterior traction detachment caused by a large granuloma. After pars plana vitrectomy, the lesion was removed in toto through the retinotomy site. (B) The histologic findings of the lesion were characteristic of toxocariasis. Result of enzyme-linked immunosorbent assay (ELISA) for *Toxocara canis* showed the vitreous sample as markedly positive. (C) Posterior pole after surgery. Vision improved from hand motion to 15/200. (Courtesy Prof. M. Gonvers, Lausanne, Switzerland.)

successful treatment described the simultaneous use of corticosteroids with anthelmintic agents, and most experts agree that corticosteroids should be considered part of any treatment regimen for ocular toxocariasis. Furthermore, evidence suggests that the mere movement of the larva through the retina induces an inflammatory response and justifies the combined use of anthelmintics and corticosteroids.[36]

Many experts suggest combining albendazole with a corticosteroid in the treatment for ocular toxocariasis, although the dose and duration of therapy vary. Some recommend a dose of albendazole is 800 mg twice daily for adults and 400 mg twice daily for children for a period of 5 to 20 days, where others suggest 400 mg twice daily for 5 days in both adults and children.[62]

Surgery may also have a beneficial role in the management of ocular toxocariasis.[63,64] Vitrectomy has been used to treat vitreomacular traction and there is one report of the organism being recovered via vitrectomy.[64] Hagler et al.[65] operated on 17 patients with retinal complications of ocular toxocariasis; three of them had active infection at the time of surgery. The authors were able to reattach the retina in 12 of these patients, and in 15, a stabilization or improvement of visual acuity was obtained. Belmont et al.[66] also reported favorable outcomes in patients with ocular toxocariasis who underwent pars plana vitrectomy for retinal complications of disease. Gonvers et al.[67] reported the case of a 30-year-old patient with traction detachment as a result of an inflammatory granuloma (Fig. 17.6). The granuloma was removed in toto, and examination revealed a typical toxocariasis retinal lesion. Results of ELISA performed on the vitreous sample were strongly positive. Maguire et al.[68] performed vitrectomy for vitreopapillary traction and extracted an intact *T. canis* organism. If the larva is visible and is at least 3 mm from the foveola, photocoagulation can be attempted to kill it.[69] This may induce inflammation that will require prednisone therapy. Amin et al.[70] reported improvement in visual acuity in five of 10 eyes with *Toxocara* lesions having a traction retinal detachment needing repair, membrane removal, scleral buckle, and fluid–gas exchange or silicone oil. Monshizadeh et al.[71] reported choroidal neovascular membrane as a complication of an inactive *Toxocara* lesion in a 17-year-old woman. The lesion was treated with laser therapy, and vision improved from 20/40 to 20/20. Cryopexy was used to treat a patient with a vasoproliferative lesion secondary to the organism.[30]

Vision outcomes vary widely in patients with ocular toxocariasis, depending on the extent and location of the parasite and the resulting tissue damage. Nevertheless, vision loss is reported in most patients. In a review of 159 patients with ocular toxocariasis, 85% had vision loss; vision loss was permanent in 71% of patients.[72] Of the patients with permanent vision loss, 94% had a subretinal granulomatous mass or scar, a peripheral granuloma with traction bands, or a posterior pole granuloma (see Case 17.1). Unfortunately, as stated earlier, there are no RCTs showing that treatment with anthelmintics and corticosteroids improve the prognosis. There are, however, data suggesting that treatment can help some patients. Clearly, surgery can improve vision in patients with a number of ophthalmic complications of the disease. Most importantly, prevention of infection is the best approach. Deworming of pets and avoiding exposure to contaminated areas are clearly warranted.

CASE 17.1

A 5-year-old boy was referred to an ophthalmologist after failing a routine eye-screening examination in his pediatrician's office. According to his parents, the boy had no visual complaints, and assessment of his behavior, physical examination performed by the pediatrician, and a complete blood cell count with a differential all showed normal results. Although the family had no pets, several neighbors owned dogs. The boy's visual acuity was 20/400 in the left eye and 20/20 in the right eye. There was small-angle exotropia. The anterior segment was quiet. Intraocular pressure was normal. The lens was clear. The vitreous in the right eye had 1+ cells, with trace haze. The vitreous of the left eye was normal. A gray-white subretinal granuloma was present in the left macula, with preretinal gliosis extending from the disk to the macula and associated with retinal wrinkling. The left retina was normal. Results of ELISA for *T. canis* were positive, with a titer of 1:64, and the diagnosis of ocular toxocariasis was made. A course of systemic corticosteroids was started, but there was no improvement in visual acuity in the left eye, and the therapy was stopped. The posterior segment has remained unchanged for more than 3 years.

REFERENCES

1. Molk R. Ocular toxocariasis: a review of the literature. *Ann Ophthalmol.* 1983;15:216–231.
2. Kazacos KR. Visceral and ocular larva migrans. *Semin Vet Med Surg (Small Animal).* 1991;6:227–235.
3. Sakai R, Kawashima H, Shibui H, et al. *Toxocara cati*-induced ocular toxocariasis. *Arch Ophthalmol.* 1998;116:1686–1687.
4. Calhoun FP. Intraocular lesion by the larva of ascaris. *Arch Ophthalmol.* 1937;18:963–970.
5. Wilder HC. Nematode endophthalmitis. *Trans Am Acad Ophthalmol Otolaryngol.* 1950;55:99–109.
6. Nichols RL. The etiology of visceral larva migrans. I. Diagnostic morphology of infective second stage *Toxocara* larvae. *J Parasitol.* 1956;42:349–362.
7. Magnaval JF, Michault A, Calon N, et al. Epidemiology of human toxocariasis in La Reunion. *Trans Roy Soc Trop Med Hyg.* 1994;88:531–533.
8. Chen J, Liu Q, Liu G-H, et al. Toxocariasis: a silent threat with a progressive public health impact. *Infect Dis Poverty.* 2018;7:59.
9. Stewart JM, Cubillan LD, Cunningham ET Jr. Prevalence, clinical features, and causes of vision loss among patients with ocular toxocariasis. *Retina.* 2005;25(8):1005–1013.
10. Mok CH. Visceral larva migrans. *Clin Pediatr.* 1968;7:565–573.
11. Schantz PM, Weis PE, Pollard ZF, et al. Risk factors for toxocaral ocular larva migrans: a case-control study. *Am J Public Health.* 1980;12:1269–1272.
12. Marmor M, Glickman L, Shofer F. *Toxocara canis* infection of children: epidemiologic and neuropsychological findings. *Am J Public Health.* 1987;77:554–559.
13. Good B, Holland CV, Taylor MR, et al. Ocular toxocariasis in schoolchildren. *Clin Infect Dis.* 2004;39(2):173–178.
14. Ruiz de Ybanez MR, Garijo M, Goyena M, et al. Improved methods for recovering eggs of *Toxocara canis* from soil. *J Helminthol.* 2000;74:349–353.
15. Brown DH. Ocular *Toxocara canis.* II. Clinical review. *J Pediatr Ophthalmol.* 1970;7:182–191.
16. Syndromes de Larva Migrans. In: Diallo JS, ed. *Manifestations Ophtalmologiques des Parasitoses.* Paris: Masson; 1985:155–161.
17. Ocular toxocariasis. United States, 2009–2010. *MMWR Morbid Mortal Wkly Rep.* 2011;60:734–746.
18. Beerlandt N, Dralands L, Vanginderdeuren R, et al. Ocular toxocariasis in a 36 year old patient: a case report. *Bull Soc Belge Ophtalmol.* 1995;259:177–181.
19. Yokoi K, Goto H, Sakai J, et al. Clinical features of ocular toxocariasis in Japan. *Ocul Immunol Inflamm.* 2003;11(4):269–275.
20. Taylor MR. The epidemiology of ocular toxocariasis. *J Helminthol.* 2001;75:109–118.
21. Benitez del Castillo JM, Herreros G, Guillen JL, et al. Bilateral ocular toxocariasis demonstrated by aqueous humor enzyme-linked immunosorbent assay. *Am J Ophthalmol.* 1995;119:514–516.
22. Upadhyay M, Rai NC. *Toxocara* granuloma of the retina. *Jpn J Ophthalmol.* 1980;24:278–281.
23. Rubin ML, Kaufman HE, Tierney JP, et al. An intraretinal nematode. *Trans Am Acad Ophthalmol Otolaryngol.* 1968;72:855–866.
24. Teyssot N, Cassoux N, Lehoang P, et al. Fuchs heterochromic cyclitis and ocular toxocariasis. *Am J Ophthalmol.* 2005;139(5):915–916.
25. Bird AC, Smith JL, Curtin VT. Nematode optic neuritis. *Am J Ophthalmol.* 1964;69:72–77.
26. Cox TA, Haskins GE, Gangitano JL, et al. Bilateral *Toxocara* optic neuropathy. *J Clin Neurol Ophthalmol.* 1983;3:267–274.
27. Karel I, Peleska M, Uhlíková M, et al. Larval migrans lentis. *Ophthalmologia.* 1977;174:14–19.
28. Steahly LP, Mader T. Acute ocular toxocariasis in adults. *J Ocul Ther Surg.* 1985;4:93–99.
29. Despreaux R, Fardeau C, Touhami S, et al. Ocular toxocariasis: clinical features and long-term visual outcomes in adult patients. *Am J Ophthalmol.* 2016;166:162–168.
30. Mori K, Ohta K, Murata T. Vasoproliferative tumors of the retina secondary to ocular toxocariasis. *Can J Ophthalmol.* 2007;42(5):758–759.
31. Shields CL, Honavar S, Shields JA, et al. Vitrectomy in eyes with unsuspected retinoblastoma. *Ophthalmology.* 2000;107:2250–2255.
32. Shields JA. Ocular toxocariasis: a review. *Surv Ophthalmol.* 1984;28:361–381.
33. Kennedy JJ, Defeo E. Ocular toxocariasis demonstrated by ultrasound. *Ann Ophthalmol.* 1981;13:1357–1358.
34. Howard GM, Ellsworth RM. Differential diagnosis of retinoblastoma. *Am J Ophthalmol.* 1965;60:610–616.
35. Wan WL, Cano MR, Pince KJ, et al. Echographic characteristics of ocular toxocariasis. *Ophthalmology.* 1991;98:28–31.
36. Suzuki T, Joko T, Akao N, et al. Following the migration of a *Toxocara* larva in the retina by optical coherence tomography and fluorescein angiography. *Jpn J Ophthalmol.* 2005;49(2):159–161.
37. Hashida N, Nakai K, Nishida K. Diagnostic evaluation of ocular toxocariasis using high-penetration optical coherence tomography. *Case Rep Ophthalmol.* 2014;5:16–21.
38. Glickman LT, Grieve RB, Lauria SS, et al. Serodiagnosis of ocular toxocariasis: a comparison of two antigens. *J Clin Pathol.* 1985;38:103–107.
39. Gillespie SH, Bidwell D, Voller A, et al. Diagnosis of human toxocariasis by antigen capture enzyme linked immunosorbent assay. *J Clin Pathol.* 1993;46:551–554.
40. Jacquier P, Gottstein B, Stingelin Y, et al. Immunodiagnosis of toxocariasis in humans: evaluation of a new enzyme-linked immunosorbent assay kit. *J Clin Microbiol.* 1991;29:1831–1835.
41. de Visser L, Rothova A, de Boer JH, et al. Diagnosis of ocular toxocariasis by establishing intraocular antibody production. *Am J Ophthalmol.* 2008;145(2):369–374.
42. Centers for Disease Control and Prevention (CDC). https://www.cdc.gov/dpdx/toxocariasis/index.html.
43. Abd El-Aal NF, Basha MAA, Eid AM. New insight into the diagnostic cut-off value of serum anti-*Toxocara* IgG for ocular toxocariasis in uveitis patients. *J Helminthol.* 2018;94:e12.

44. Albert DM, Marcus L. Ocular toxocariasis presenting as leukocoria in a patient with low ELISA titer to *Toxocara canis*. *Ophthalmology*. 1981;88:1302–1306.
45. Kieler RA. *Toxocara canis* endophthalmitis with low ELISA titer. *Ann Ophthalmol*. 1983;15:447–449.
46. Sharkey JA, McKay PS. Ocular toxocariasis in a patient with repeatedly negative ELISA titre to *Toxocara canis*. *Br J Ophthalmol*. 1993;77:253–254.
47. Yoshida M, Shirao Y, Asai H, et al. A retrospective study of ocular toxocariasis in Japan: correlation with antibody prevalence and ophthalmological findings of patients with uveitis. *J Helminthol*. 1999;73:357–361.
48. Schneider C, Arnaud B, Schmitt-Bernard CF. Toxocarose oculaire. Interet de l'immunodiagnostic local. *J Fr Ophthalmol*. 2000;23:1016–1019.
49. Sakai R, Kawashima H, Shibui H, et al. *Toxocara cati*-induced ocular toxocariasis. *Arch Ophthalmol*. 1998;116:1686–1687.
50. Magnaval JF, Fabre R, Maurières P, et al. Application of the Western blotting procedure for the immunodiagnosis of human toxocariasis. *Parasitol Res*. 1991;77:697–702.
51. Del Prete GF, De Carli M, Mastromauro C, et al. Purified protein derivative of *Mycobacterium tuberculosis* and excretory-secretory antigen(s) of *Toxocara canis* expand in vitro human T cells with stable and opposite (type 1 T helper or type 2 T helper) profile of cytokine production. *J Clin Invest*. 1991;88:346–350.
52. Werner JC, Ross RD, Green WR, et al. Pars plana vitrectomy and subretinal surgery for ocular toxocariasis. *Arch Ophthalmol*. 1999;117:532–534.
53. Rockey JH, Donnelly JJ, Stromberg BE, et al. Immunopathology of *Toxocara canis* and *Ascaris suum* infections of the eye: the role of the eosinophil. *Invest Ophthalmol Vis Sci*. 1979;18:1172–1184.
54. Rockey JH, John T, Donnelly JJ, et al. In vitro interaction of eosinophils from ascarid-infected eyes with *Ascaris suum* and *Toxocara canis* larvae. *Invest Ophthalmol Vis Sci*. 1983;24:1346–1357.
55. Kayes SG. Human toxocariasis and the visceral larva migrans syndrome: correlative immunopathology. *Chem Immunol*. 1997;66:99–124.
56. Carter KC. The use of 35S-labelled *Toxocara canis* to determine larval numbers in tissues. *J Helminthol*. 1992;66:279–287.
57. Cuellar C, Fenoy S, Aguila C, et al. Evaluation of chemotherapy in experimental toxocariasis by determination of specific immune complexes. *J Helminthol*. 1990;64:279–289.
58. Fenoy S, Ollero MD, Guillén JL, et al. Animal models in ocular toxocariasis. *J Helminthol*. 2001;75:119–124.
59. Ollero MD, Fenoy S, Cuéllar C, et al. Experimental toxocariosis in BALB/c mice: effect of the inoculation dose on brain and eye involvement. *Acta Trop*. 2008;105(2):124–130.
60. el-Ganayni GA, Handousa AE. The effect of cyclosporin A (CSA) on murine visceral toxocariasis canis. *J Egypt Soc Parasitol*. 1992;22:487–494.
61. Wilkinson CP, Welch RB. Intraocular *Toxocara*. *Am J Ophthalmol*. 1971;71:921–930.
62. Barisani-Asenbauer T, Maca SM, Hauff W, et al. Treatment of ocular toxocariasis with albendazole. *J Ocul Pharmacol Ther*. 2001;17:287–294.
63. Dinning WJ, Gillespie SH, Cooling RJ, et al. Toxocariasis: a practical approach to management of ocular disease. *Eye*. 1988;2:580–582.
64. Acar N, Kapran Z, Utine CA, et al. Pars plana vitrectomy revealed *Toxocara canis* organism. *Int Ophthalmol*. 2007;27(4):277–280.
65. Hagler WS, Pollard ZF, Jarrett WH, et al. Results of surgery for ocular *Toxocara canis*. *Ophthalmology*. 1981;88:1081–1086.
66. Belmont JB, Irvine A, Benson W, et al. Vitrectomy in ocular toxocariasis. *Arch Ophthalmol*. 1982;100:1912–1915.
67. Gonvers M, Mermoud A, Uffer S, et al. Ocular *Toxocara canis* in a 30-year-old adult. *Klin Monatsbl Augenheilkd*. 1992;200:522–524.
68. Maguire AM, Green WR, Michels RG, et al. Recovery of intraocular *Toxocara canis* by pars plana vitrectomy. *Ophthalmology*. 1990;97:675–680.
69. Brown GC, Tasman WS. Retinal arterial obstruction in association with presumed *Toxocara canis* neuroretinitis. *Ann Ophthalmol*. 1981;13:1385–1387.
70. Amin HI, McDonald HR, Han DP, et al. Vitrectomy update for macular traction in ocular toxocariasis. *Retina*. 2000;20:80–85.
71. Monshizadeh R, Ashrafzadeh MT, Rumelt S. Choroidal neovascular membrane: a late complication of inactive *Toxocara* chorioretinitis. *Retina*. 2000;20:219–220.
72. Woodhall D, Starr MC, Montgomery SP, et al. Ocular toxocariasis: epidemiologic, anatomic, and therapeutic variations based on a survey of ophthalmic subspecialists. *Ophthalmology*. 2012;119:1211–1217.

18

Onchocerciasis and Other Parasitic Diseases

Alan G. Palestine

KEY CONCEPTS

- Onchocerciasis, or river blindness, is a disease that affects 17.7 million people worldwide, and some 123 million people live in regions where onchocerciasis is endemic; ivermectin is usually the drug of choice, but use of it has not eradicated the disease.
- Worms of two sizes have been described in eyes with diffuse unilateral subacute neuroretinitis (DUSN).
- The number of parasitic disorders affecting the eye is very large.

ONCHOCERCIASIS

Clinical Appearance

Onchocerciasis, or river blindness, is a disease that affects 17.7 million people worldwide, with more than 123 million people living in its endemic regions.[1] It is estimated that some 270,000 persons are blinded and a half million are severely visually handicapped because of this disease. In developing countries, blindness occurs at 10 times the rate reported in the developed world.[2,3] Ocular onchocerciasis has been declared by the World Health Organization (WHO) as one of the five major preventable causes of blindness (the others are cataract, trachoma, glaucoma, and xerophthalmia). The disease is caused by a tissue-dwelling parasite, the nematode *Onchocerca volvulus.* It is spread by the blackflies of the Simulium species and is found in a broad belt across western and central Africa, in Central America, and in small pockets in northern South America and the Arabian peninsula. Zoonotic infections have been reported in many countries, including Hungary.[4] The blackfly needs rapid running water to propagate, and therefore the endemic areas are usually the most fertile, which makes this disease of extraordinary importance for the affected Third World countries.

The infected blackfly bites humans, thereby introducing the infection. Polymerase chain reaction (PCR)–mediated amplification methods and immunoblotting of the silk proteins permit identification of sibling species of biting adult females.[5] Adult worms will ultimately develop and form the nodules found throughout the body, often subcutaneously. These adults will produce microfilariae that are released in extraordinary numbers. The diagnosis of the disease and the determination of the infestation rate are made by counting the number of microfilariae found in skin snips (Fig. 18.1) The microfilariae are the major cause of most of the ocular disease. Table 18.1 lists other ocular manifestations involved in parasitic infections of the eye.

A major complication of *Onchocerca* infestation is corneal disease. Microfilarial infestation in the cornea is related to visual loss over time,[6] and the presence of a large number of microfilariae in the anterior segment is related to irreversible visual loss.[7] In the cornea, there is punctate keratitis; the presence of "snowflake" opacities in the cornea is associated with a fairly mild infestation. With more intense infestation and over time, sclerosing keratitis and loss of vision are seen (Figs. 18.2 and 18.3).

Iridocyclitis can be seen in conjunction with other aspects of onchocerciasis, although the intensity of reaction can vary considerably.[8] In addition to atrophy of the iris, more serious complications, such as glaucoma and cataract, can occur. Glaucoma has been recognized as a possibly important cause of irreversible visual loss in these patients.[9] In addition, even without the presence of the inflammatory response, microfilariae can be seen in the anterior chamber. However, the patient needs to be placed in a darkened room with the head held down between the knees for a few minutes. With the use of a slit lamp, the observer will note the presence of the swirling microfilariae in the anterior chamber.

Alterations of the posterior pole have been seen as well, and the degree of visual impairment caused by these changes has probably been underestimated in the past. Large areas of chorioretinitis and optic nerve disease leading to atrophy can be seen (Fig. 18.4). Newland et al.[10] examined 800 patients in a hyperendemic region of the rainforest in Liberia, West Africa. They found chorioretinal changes in 75% of those examined, which strongly suggested that visual impairment in those living in this region was largely caused by chorioretinal disease and not by anterior segment changes. In a report describing recent Ethiopian immigrants to Israel, Enk et al.[11] examined 1200 patients and found that 83 had cutaneous signs of onchocerciasis, with 48% having positive skin snip results for the presence of microfilaria. Of the 65 patients who underwent ocular examination, four eyes had evidence of active anterior segment inflammation, and 11 had retinal or choroidal changes.

Relatively few eyes with this condition have been studied histologically. It is thought that the microfilariae may enter through the long and short ciliary vessels.[12,13] Another possibility is the passage of microfilariae through cerebrospinal fluid (CSF) into the optic nerve sheath[14] or direct invasion through the sclera by the parasite's release of digestive enzymes.[15]

It should be noted that the ocular disease in most patients is thought to be a result of slow, chronic, and relatively insidious changes. However, acute episodes of glaucoma, uveitis, and optic nerve disease may be important components of the disease in some patients. Egbert et al.[16] examined patients in Ghana and found that 10.6% of those with glaucoma had concomitant onchocerciasis compared with 2.6% of those needing cataract extraction.

Laboratory studies have been attempted to better deduce the mechanism of systemic infestation, and, to a lesser degree, work has concentrated on ocular disease. The only known natural animal host besides the human is the gorilla,[17] although the disease has been induced in the chimpanzee[18] and the cynomolgus monkey, in which *Onchocerca lienalis* was used.[19] Using a rabbit model, Duke and Garner[20] placed *O. volvulus* into the vitreous or subretinally and observed chorioretinal alterations. The injection of *O. lienalis* subconjunctivally in guinea pigs produced a lesion resembling that seen in human onchocercal punctate keratitis.[21] In a monkey model for this disease, disease was induced with the injection of 10,000 live *O. volvulus* microfilariae into the vitreous and this produced posterior segment lesions similar to those seen in the human disease.[22]

Immune Characteristics

Laboratory studies have suggested that the parasite induces a complex immune response, perhaps partly autoimmune. Immunoglobulin E (IgE) production is a prominent feature of *Onchocerca* infestation, and

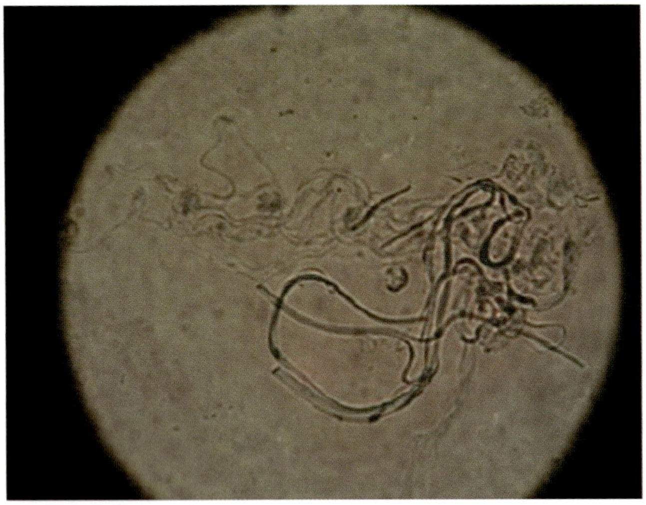

Fig. 18.1 Microfilariae seen after immersion of skin snips in saline for 30 minutes. (From Terranova M. Padovese V, Klaus S, Morrone A. Onchocerciasis in Tigray. *Int J Dermatol.* 2007;46(Suppl 2):39–41.)

circulating immune complexes that presumably contain parasite antigen can be detected.[23] Cell-mediated responsivity is reduced,[24] a phenomenon also noted in other helminth infections. Indeed, it appears that in addition to a predominantly B-cell (i.e., antibody) response, the immune system tries to minimize bystander tissue damage after the death of microfilariae by producing blocking antibodies and down-regulating cytokines.[25] Chan et al.[26] examined the ocular fluid and serum from patients with onchocerciasis for the presence of antiretinal autoantibodies and found that these patients had antibodies directed toward the inner retina (nerve fiber, ganglion cell, and Müller cell) that could not be absorbed with the use of either S-antigen (S-Ag) or the interphotoreceptor-binding protein. These observations suggested that autoimmune mechanisms may play a role in the retinal degeneration and optic nerve disease seen so frequently in these patients. Van der Lelij et al.[27] found high titers of anti-*Onchocerca* antibodies in the aqueous of patients with onchocerciasis and ocular disease and believed that retinal autoimmunity was an improbable factor in the pathogenesis of onchocercal chorioretinopathy.

However, immunologic cross-reactivity between an antigen of *O. volvulus* and that found in the retinal pigment epithelium (RPE) has been identified. Antisera from patients with onchocerciasis identified a 22-kDa antigen from *Onchocerca*, whereas a 44-kDa antigen from cultured human RPE was immunoprecipitated with the same antiserum.[28] Klager et al.[29] used Western blotting to show that antibody reactions to this antigen were seen in all patients with onchocerciasis and posterior pole disease but were not seen in controls. These interesting results suggest that molecular mimicry plays a role in the development of at least certain aspects of the ocular complications noted in this disorder. It also strengthens the notion that, as with ocular toxoplasmosis, inflammatory systems can no longer be restricted to only one mechanism and that in some ways, contradictory routes may be stimulated. Autoantibody responses are not restricted to the eye. Such cross-reactivity has been reported against five major autoantigens, anticalreticulin activity, and the 65-kDa arthritis-associated mycobacterial heat shock protein.[30]

TABLE 18.1 Parasitic Infections of the Eye

Ocular Manifestation	Disease
Anterior Chamber	
Hyphema	Loiasis (Central and West Africa),[157–159] gnathostomiasis (Asia)[160–162]
Hypopyon	Amebiasis (worldwide),[163] cysticercosis (Latin America, India), gnathostomiasis, onchocerciasis (Africa, Latin America), toxocariasis
Anterior uveitis	Amebiasis, angiostrongyliasis (Pacific),[162] hookworm, ascariasis, schistosomiasis (tropics),[164] caterpillar setae, cestodes (sparganosis),[165] cysticercosis, giardiasis, gnathostomiasis,[166] leishmania (Asia, Latin America), loiasis, myiasis, onchocerciasis, tapeworm trichinosis, toxocariasis, trypanosomiasis (Africa, Latin America), kala-azar (with HIV+),[167] Bancroft filariasis (tropics)[168]
Vitreous	
Hemorrhage	Ascariasis, schistosomiasis, loiasis, trichinosis
Vitritis	Schistosomiasis,[169] caterpillar setae, cysticercosis, gnathostomiasis, onchocerciasis, toxocariasis, trichinosis
Choroid/Retina	
Degeneration, exudates, nodules, detachment	Angiostrongyliasis, amebiasis, babesiosis, caterpillar setae, cysticercosis, *Echinococcus* (hydatid cyst),[170] leishmania, loiasis, myiasis, onchocerciasis, trichinosis,[171] toxocariasis
Hemorrhage	Amebiasis, hookworm, ascariasis, schistosomiasis, cysticercosis giardiasis, gnathostomiasis, leishmania, linguatulosis, loiasis, myiasis, malaria,[152] toxocariasis, trichinosis, trypanosomiasis
Arteriolar and venule occlusion	Toxocariasis, schistosomiasis, loiasis
Inflammation of retinal pigment epithelium and retinal vasculitis	Filariasis (*Wuchereria bancrofti*),[172] onchocerciasis, kala-azar (with HIV+)[173]

HIV+, human immunodeficiency virus–positive.

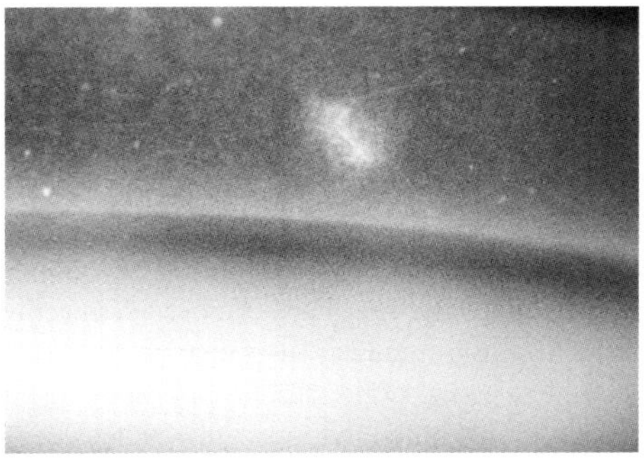

Fig. 18.2 Dead microfilaria of *Onchocerca* in cornea inducing localized inflammatory response recognized clinically as snowflake opacity. (Courtesy Hugh Taylor, MD.)

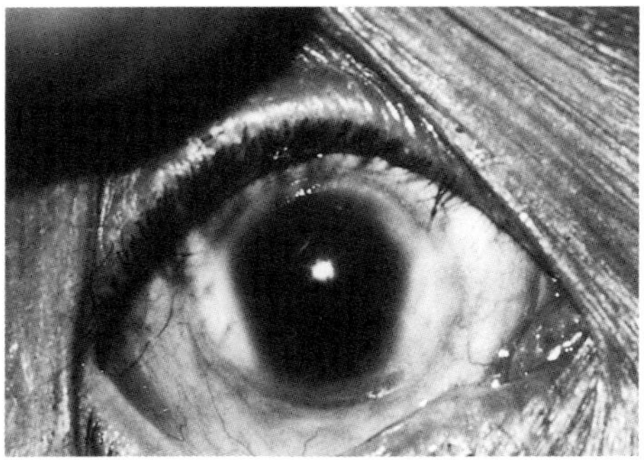

Fig. 18.3 Sclerosing keratitis in a patient with onchocerciasis. (Courtesy Hugh Taylor, MD.)

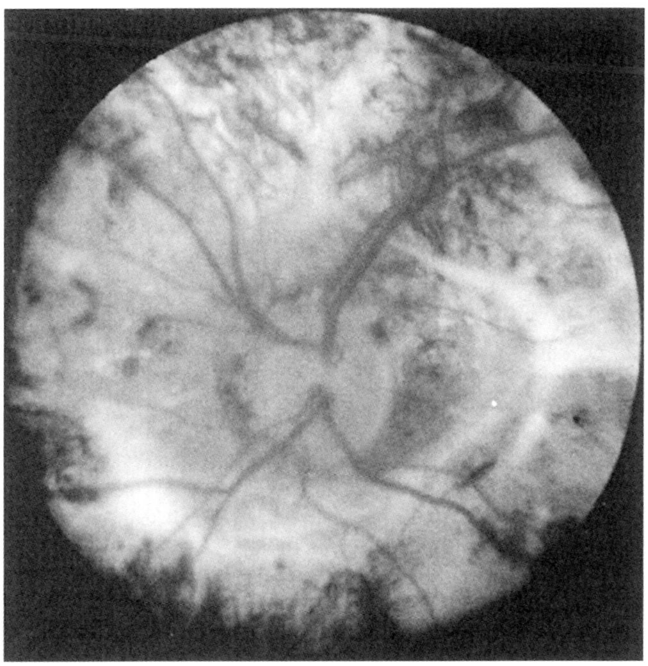

Fig. 18.4 Montage of retina from a patient with ocular manifestations of onchocerciasis. Extensive chorioretinal alterations can be seen. This change is underrecognized as a cause of visual handicap in this disorder. (Courtesy David Cogan, MD.)

The corneal lesions of onchocerciasis have been studied using animal models. There is infiltration of granulocytes and eosinophils into the clear structures. Kaifi et al.[31] found that vascular adhesion molecules are important in this process. These authors demonstrated a regulatory role for platelet endothelial cell adhesion molecule 1 and intercell adhesion molecule in that they recruit neutrophils and eosinophils to the cornea, as does P-selectin.[32] Because there are antibodies that are directed against these molecules, it raises the possibility of their use in immune therapy for the cornea. Other studies by the same group[33,34] demonstrated the importance of CD4+ T cells in the development of corneal opacification, but not in the early stages of the disease. Saint Andre et al.[35] proposed that the predominant inflammatory response seen in the cornea of *Onchocerca*-infected animals is, in fact, directed against the endosymbiont of *Onchocerca and Wolbachia.* Indeed, it may be the essential player in the pathogenesis of river blindness.[36] This endosymbiont is so essential to the nematode that embryogenesis of *Onchocerca* is completely dependent on the presence of *Wolbachia.* The *O. volvulus–Wolbachia* combination initiates activation of many immune indicators[37] (Table 18.2). Indeed, this may open a new avenue for therapy (see below).

TABLE 18.2 Filarial and Endobacterial Molecules Capable of Inducing an Inflammatory Response*

Response	Mechanisms Operative in Immunopathogenesis of Onchocerciasis	
	Proinflammatory	Anti-inflammatory
Regulatory cells	Th2, Th1 Macrophage Mast cell	Th3 Alternatively activated macrophage
Regulatory molecules	IL-5, IL-4, IL-13 IFN-γ TNF-α, IL-8, IL-12	IL-10, TGF-β IL-4
Effector cells	B cell Eosinophil, neutrophil Macrophage, mast cell	B cell Alternatively activated macrophage
Effector molecules	IgG1, IgG3, IgE MBP, EDN, ECP Peroxidases (EPO, MPO) Defensins Oxygen, nitrogen radicals Proteases	IgG4, polyclonal IgE

*Pathogenesis and host responses in human onchocerciasis: impact of *Onchocerca filariae* and *Wolbachia endobacteria*.
IFN, interferon.; *IG,* immunoglobulin; *IL,* interleukin; *TGF,* transforming growth factor; *Th,* T helper; *TNF,* tumor necrosis factor.
Reproduced with permission from: Brattig NW. Pathogenesis and host responses in human onchocerciasis: impact of *Onchocerca filariae* and *Wolbachia endobacteria. Microbes Infect.* 2004;6(1):113–128.

With studies of the specialized mechanisms of the parasite, an interesting concept has emerged.[38] Lipid-binding proteins in the nematode, with no known counterpart in mammalian systems, exist. One of these, Ov-FAR-1, has a high affinity for retinal and fatty acids and is present in all life stages of the parasite.[39] Retinol is believed to be important for the growth and differentiation of the organism and for its embryogenesis and glycoprotein synthesis.[40] The concentration of retinol is eight times higher in the *Onchocerca* nodule than in the surrounding tissue.[41] It is possible that Ov-FAR-1 causes a relatively local or systemic depletion of vitamin A in patients with onchocerciasis and may also be a trigger for the production of collagen, which is found in large quantities in

Onchocerca nodules. These could explain why ivermectin therapy may not be effective for the retinal disease in this disorder because microfilaria already present in the retina would continue to produce this lipid-binding protein (see later discussion on ivermectin).

The regulation of interleukin (IL)-5 production in onchocerciasis has been evaluated. It has been suggested that in some helminthic infections, the production of IL-5 may be associated with an immune or a resistant state. It appears that in patients who are "immune" to the effects of *Onchocerca,* both IL-2 and IL-5 are produced in significantly higher levels than in those with acute infection. IL-2 production is required to induce IL-5.[42] Toll-like receptor 2 (TLR2) appears to regulate chemokine production and neutrophil recruitment to the cornea in experimentally induced *Onchocerca/Wolbachia* keratitis.[43] Interferon (IFN)-γ responses from TLR2 knockout mice are also deficient.[44]

Therapy

Varied therapeutic strategies have been employed. A long-term approach has attempted to eliminate the vector, the blackfly, in endemic regions. This approach has been moderately successful in a large area of West Africa, but it has been expensive, needs constant monitoring to prevent encroachment of blackflies from non–insecticide-treated regions, and is officially coming to an end. Three modalities were traditionally available to treat the patient. The first was nodulectomy, that is, removing the adult worms that produce the microfilariae. Nodulectomy was reported by Rodolfo Robles in Central America in 1915 to treat the ophthalmic disease, and this approach has been practiced in Guatemala since 1935. Indeed, although hard evidence concerning its effectiveness is lacking, the rate of blindness in endemic regions has decreased from 1935 to 1979, during which time 1.5 million people have been examined and 257,883 nodules excised.[45] Nodulectomy has not significantly altered the number of microfilariae found in skin snips from patients in West Africa.

Other modalities available are specific therapies against the *Onchocerca* organism. For many years, these were limited to diethylcarbamazine citrate (DEC-C) and suramin. DEC-C is microfilaricidal, and with the massive killing of these organisms, a severe systemic reaction occurs (Mazzotti reaction). Aggravation of the ocular condition can also occur, with limbitis, an increase in corneal opacities, and advancement of sclerosing keratitis. Furthermore, Bird et al.[46] observed that DEC-C administration induced transient RPE lesions, optic disk leakage, and visual field loss. The side effects of DEC-C sometimes necessitate corticosteroid treatment. Although suramin is more toxic to adult worms than to microfilariae, killing of the microfilariae still leads to secondary reactions. Furthermore, suramin has intrinsic toxicity, which may be fatal. For these reasons, suramin is best given in progressive doses over 6 to 8 weeks until a total dosage of 60 to 67 mg/kg is reached. Both these drugs were used in the past with great care, and patients needed to be followed up closely by physicians with experience in their use. They are not used often today.

Other drugs that have been evaluated include the benzimidazoles, and quantification of ocular reactions as a result of the therapy has been published.[47] These compounds have an effect on the embryogenesis of various *Onchocerca* species, thereby sterilizing the adult worms. Testing of these compounds has suggested that embryogenesis is interrupted in adult worms in the nodules of patients with onchocerciasis 2 months after therapy.[48] However, these drugs are poorly absorbed orally, and standard dosages may not be particularly effective.

In 1982, the agent ivermectin was shown to be successful in the treatment of onchocerciasis.[49] The belief was that given as a single oral dose of 150 μg/kg, it would control or curtail the disease when administered on a wide scale in endemic areas.[2,50] Ivermectin is not thought to kill adult worms, nor does it affect embryogenesis or spermatogenesis; rather, it prevents the release of the microfilariae from the adult female worm, resulting in their in utero degeneration. Ivermectin was compared with DEC-C in a randomized, double-masked study in the treatment of ocular changes caused by onchocerciasis.[51] It was found that although DEC-C caused a marked increase in both living and dead microfilariae in the cornea by inducing limbitis and punctate keratitis, ivermectin did not. Furthermore, ivermectin resulted in long-term reduction in intraocular microfilariae when given as a single oral dose of 200 μg/kg. Other studies have demonstrated similar results.[52,53] Diallo et al.[52] noted that microfilarial densities reached 4% of pretherapy levels 1 year after a single 12-mg dose of ivermectin, but one of 10 ivermectin-treated patients needed systemic steroid therapy to treat adverse systemic reactions. In this study, adult worms taken from patients treated with ivermectin were examined; they contained deformed and degenerated intrauterine forms of the microfilariae. In one report outlining the preliminary findings regarding the distribution of ivermectin to 118,925 persons in Nigeria, Ogunba and Gemade[54] found that the drug was extremely well tolerated: only 0.7% of recipients reported adverse reactions within 3 days of treatment. Whitworth et al.[55] reported the results of a randomized, double-masked study performed in Sierra Leone comparing the effects of ivermectin with those of placebo on ocular disease. They found that the 296 persons who received ivermectin had less anterior segment disease, a lower prevalence of microfilariae in the anterior chamber and cornea, and less punctate keratitis and iritis compared with the 272 patients who received placebo. No difference was found between the two groups with regard to optic atrophy or chorioretinitis, and the visual acuities in the two groups were not statistically significantly different, although the results for the ivermectin group were more favorable. Dadzie et al.[56] found very low ocular microfilariae loads in 334 patients in Ghana who were treated twice with the medication. Blindness did occur in three patients in the ivermectin group; these patients were thought to have advanced disease. Because of these and other reports, between March 1992 and February 1993, an estimated 1.5 million people were treated in the Onchocerciasis Control Programme (OCP) area.[57] The OCP has covered 11 countries in West Africa, and by 2002, 10 million people had received ivermectin[50]; by 2006, nongovernmental development organizations had helped treat 62 million people[58] (Fig. 18.5). Will this therapeutic program eradicate this disease? In some smaller endemic regions, such as Ecuador, it has the potential to do so.[59] However, in the vast area of West Africa, the challenge is enormous. Because of the characteristics of ivermectin, it has been estimated that 90 million at-risk individuals would need to be treated for 25 years, a daunting task.[60] Some reports, such as those by Semba et al.[61] and Njoo et al.,[62] have not shown encouraging results. The study reported by Njoo et al. included a fairly small number of patients with onchocerciasis from an hyperendemic area with no vector control, and 44% of 25 patients who received three doses of ivermectin still had positive results on skin snip analyses, but the number of adverse reactions did decrease with repeated administration. In one long-term follow-up study performed in Sierra Leone and reported by Mabey et al.,[63] ivermectin-treated patients had full ocular examinations in 1989 and again in 1994. These authors concluded that annual treatment with ivermectin controlled all aspects of ocular disease except chorioretinal lesions. Changing the dosing interval to every 6 months did not seem to help either. Chippaux et al.[64] found that repeated ivermectin doses failed to prevent the initial occurrence of retinal lesions or the worsening of preexisting ones. Awadzi et al.[65] treated patients with doses of ivermectin varying from 150 μg/kg to 1600 μg/kg of body weight. Their findings suggested that administration of larger doses of the medication was probably no better than giving repeated lower doses. It appears that ivermectin therapy needs to be

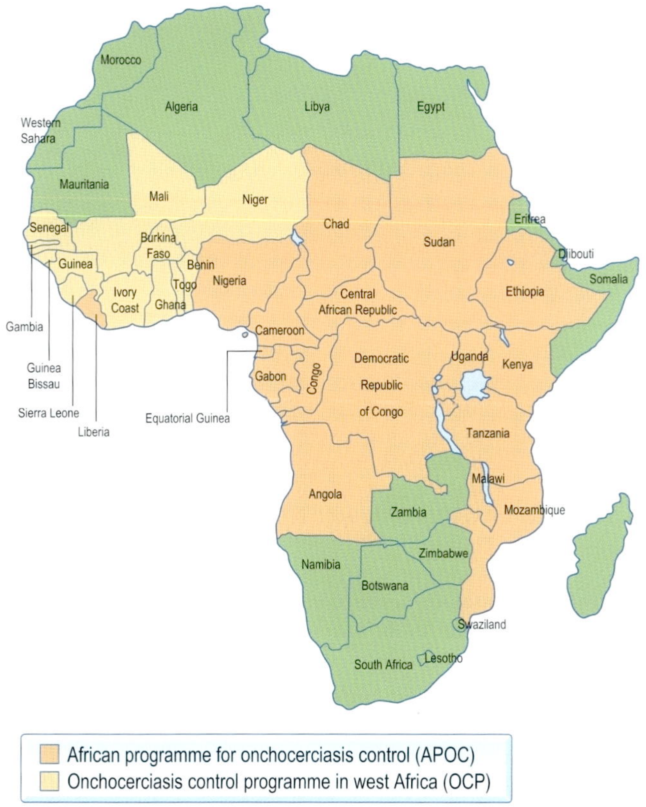

Fig. 18.5 The geographic distribution of African programs for onchocerciasis control. (Reproduced with permission from: Hopkins AD. Onchocerciasis—is it all solved? *Eye*. 2005;19:1057–1066.)

given regularly to produce any long-term benefit.[66] A controlled study on administration of ivermectin every 3 months showed that this regimen greatly reduced the number of female worms and acute itching and skin lesions.[67] Studies in the past with at least 1 year of follow-up did not show a statistically significant difference in visual outcome between ivermectin and placebo.[68] Awadzi et al.[69] reported that over a 30-month period, they were able to confirm the existence of a population of female *O. volvulus* that responded poorly to ivermectin. A randomized study[70] giving patients high doses (800 μg/kg) annually or the normal dose at 3-month intervals did show a greater effect compared with the standard dose (150 μg/kg) annually. However, in this particular study, transitory ocular complaints were noted, suggesting that the higher-dose approach should be considered with caution. Other studies have suggested that therapy alone, without vector control, may not control the disease in endemic areas, and models of this approach[71,72] have suggested that therapy alone (without vector control) will not control disease in the next quarter-century. These projections once again point to the need to find new drugs to treat this disorder.

As mentioned earlier, *Wolbachia* appears to be one of the major sources of antigenic stimulation for the corneal disease, and in its symbiotic relationship with *Onchocerca*, it appears to be essential for the fertility of *O. volvulus*. Treatment with doxycycline, 100 mg/day for 6 weeks, will deplete *Wolbachia* in *Onchocerca* after several months and inhibit embryogenesis.[3] However, a Cochrane review of ivermectin with or without doxycycline was inconclusive in proving that the addition of doxycycline was useful for treatment.[73] Furthermore, even if a medication that safely kills adult organisms becomes available, there is interest in other medications, such as moxidectin, that inhibits embryogenesis and may last longer than ivermectin.[3]

GIARDIASIS

Giardia lamblia is a flagellated binucleate protozoan about 12 to 14 μm in length. It can be in a motile form (trophozoite) or in a cystic state. The organism was first seen microscopically by van Leeuwenhoeck in 1681.[74] Ingestion of contaminated food or drinking water is the usual mode of spread. In humans, *Giardia* has a propensity to inhabit the jejunum, where it will multiply and cause swelling of the microvilli of the intestinal epithelial cells. Gastrointestinal symptoms include epigastric burning, cramps, diarrhea, constipation, and weight loss. Although extraintestinal spread of the organism has not been documented, to date, there have been reports of patients with extraintestinal manifestations attributed to *Giardia*.[75,76] These include nervousness, headache, and emotional instability. To our knowledge, Barraquer[77] was the first to make the association between giardiasis and ocular inflammatory disease, noting choroiditis, hemorrhagic retinopathy, and iridocyclitis. Knox and King[78] reported finding *Giardia* in the stools of three patients with retinal arteritis, which was associated with iridocyclitis in two of them. These authors thought that antiparasitic therapy improved the ocular state in these patients. Pettoello Mantovani et al.[79] examined 90 children with intestinal *Giardia* for ocular disease. They noted that eight of them (9%) had "salt-and-pepper" alterations at the level of the RPE in all quadrants of the midperiphery. Some of these patients also had atrophic regions and hard exudates associated with the lesions. In addition, one other patient was noted to have temporal "discoloration" of the optic disk, and another had chorioretinitis, which resolved with steroid therapy. These patients were treated, and after 1 year of follow-up, no alterations in the salt-and-pepper changes were noted. In two control groups, one of 200 children with gastrointestinal symptoms not caused by *Giardia* and 200 healthy children did not have salt-and-pepper changes. In a similar study reported by Corsi et al.,[80] 141 children with *Giardia* were examined, and 28 (19.9%) were noted to have salt-and-pepper changes in their fundus.

The underlying cause of the ocular inflammatory disease is unknown, although the most plausible explanation at this point is that the inflammation results from a hypersensitivity reaction. The organism has never been isolated from lesions (besides the gut) associated with the parasite (e.g., urticarial lesions). Immune complexes have been reported in patients with *Giardia*,[81] and it has been suggested that the ocular lesions are a hypersensitivity reaction. Human leukocyte antigen studies have been performed, with a higher expected frequency seen for HLA-A1 (46.7% versus 32%) and HLA-B12 (47.8% versus 25.3%).[82]

Diagnosis is based on finding the organism in the stool, and this is not always easy to do. Multiple examinations or even biopsy of jejunal tissue may be needed. In the past, the disease was treated with quinacrine hydrochloride (Atabrine) (100 mg) given three times a day for 10 days, but a single dose of tinidazole (50 mg/kg) has been used more recently.[80] In one study, oral corticosteroids and metronidazole (250 mg three times daily) were used.[83]

OPHTHALMOMYIASIS

The term *ophthalmomyiasis* refers to infestation of the eye by the larval forms of flies (maggots) of the order Diptera. *Ophthalmomyiasis externa* is infestation of the conjunctiva, whereas *ophthalmomyiasis interna* (posterior or anterior) is infestation inside the globe.[84] Usually, these larval forms are obligate tissue parasites that require the host's tissue to complete their developmental cycle. In addition to humans, the usual hosts for these larvae include cattle, deer, sheep, horses, and reindeer. The larvae may get to the eye via a vector, such as an adult fly that carries the larvae or eggs to the region, or through touching of the

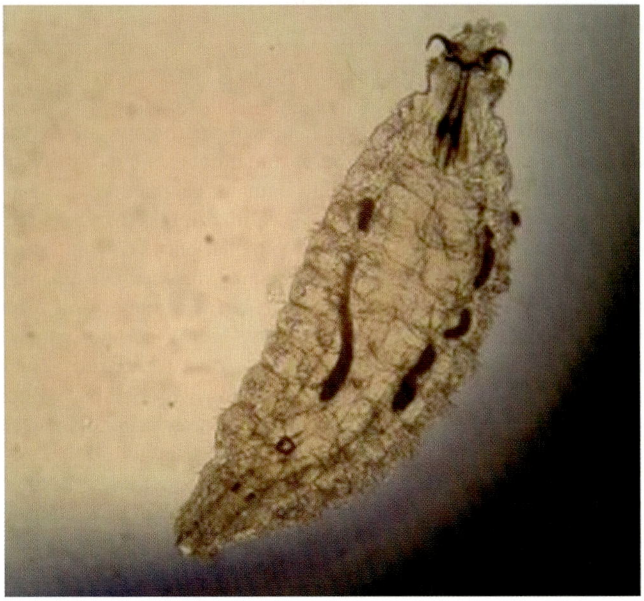

Fig. 18.6 First instar larva from *Oestrus ova*. Note the oral hooks. Removed from the conjunctiva of a patient. (Reproduced with permission from: James Dunbar et al. An outbreak of human external ophthalmomyiasis due to *Oestrus ovis* in Southern Afghanistan. *Clin Infect Dis.* 2008;46:e124–e126. University of Chicago Press.)

ocular region with hands contaminated by the larvae. Most patients do not report being "bitten." The larva is thought to bore through the coats of the eye until they come to rest within. However, an early report by DeBoe[85] described the emergence of the larva from the optic nerve head into the vitreous. A few cases have been described in the literature.

Seventeen patients with ophthalmomyiasis externa were seen by Amr et al.[86] in northern Jordan. These occurrences were caused by the sheep nasal botfly *Oestrus ovis;* the symptoms were mild to severe conjunctivitis, cellulitis, and lacrimation. Four cases of *O. ovis* infection in Kuwait, both before and after Operations Desert Shield and Desert Storm, were reported.[87] Another species involved is *Cochliomyia hominivorax,*[88] whose larvae can lie over the conjunctiva and can be removed with a cotton swab[89] (Fig. 18.6).

With ophthalmomyiasis interna, the invading larva may initially cause little or no pain, but discomfort and an intraocular inflammatory reaction can certainly occur,[90] particularly after its death.[91] The characteristic features of ophthalmomyiasis interna include the presence of subretinal tracks,[92,93] along with the finding of an encysted larva either subretinally or even free floating in the vitreous. Without finding the maggot in the eye, a definitive diagnosis cannot be made; the maggot is white or semitranslucent, segmented, and tapered at both ends.[92] Vision may be lost because of macular hemorrhage, optic nerve invasion by the maggot, or retinal detachment. Jakobs et al.[94] reported the case of a patient with a larva that appeared to have entered the eye via the optic nerve, migrated subretinally yielding tracts, and then apparently entered the optic nerve again. Billi et al.[95] reported such a case after cataract extraction, conjecturing that the site of entry into the eye was the surgical wound. The organism, which was removed from the eye with vitrectomy, was thought to be of the Sarcophagidae family of flies. Interestingly, no RPE tracking was noted. Campbell et al.[96] reported that an interesting retinopathy that resembled ophthalmomyiasis interna was seen in 10% of a sample Chamorro population examined on the island of Guam. In addition, this retinopathy was found in 50% of a population with the amyotrophic lateral sclerosis

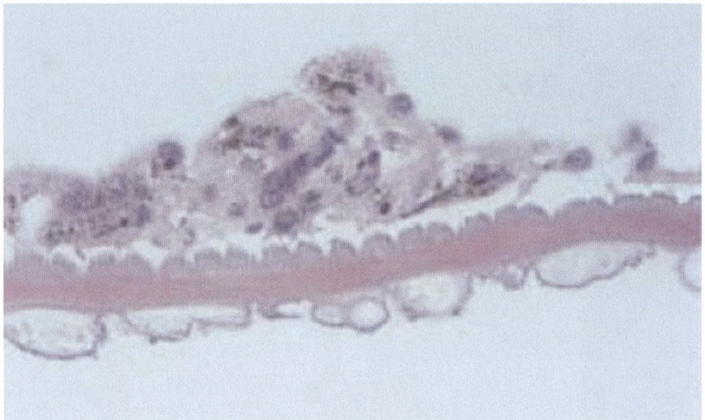

Fig. 18.7 Macrophages and foreign body giant cells on the surface (cuticle) of the larva (hematoxylin and eosin [H&E]; original magnification ×600). (Reproduced with permission from: Saraiva VS, Amaro MH, Belfort R, Jr., Burnier MN, Jr. A case of anterior internal ophthalmomyiasis: case report. *Arq Bras Ofthalmol.* 2006;69 (5):741–743.)

(ALS)–parkinsonism–dementia complex. Although the retinopathy appeared to be similar to the changes seen with parasitic infestation, Campbell et al. were not able to establish a definitive diagnosis despite obtaining eyes for histologic study.

The treatment of ophthalmomyiasis must be based on the ocular findings. If the worm is found in the anterior chamber, it should be removed as quickly as possible because it may migrate to other areas of the eye.[97] Heterochromic iridocyclitis has been described after a case of ophthalmomyiasis interna posterior.[98] Saraiva et al.[99] reported a case where a worm was removed from the anterior segment, with histology showing the larva to be covered with macrophages and foreign body giant cells (Fig. 18.7). The granulomatous reaction cleared with removal of the worm. In the case of an immobile subretinal worm, with no inflammatory disease and good vision, the ophthalmologist may elect to only observe the patient. However, if there is a severe inflammatory reaction, anti-inflammatory therapy should be initiated. Hemorrhage may require vitrectomy because it may indicate that the larva is alive and migrating. If the larva can be visualized in the subretinal space and if the decision is made to treat it, Gass and Lewis[92] have recommended the use of photocoagulation versus removal of the organism with sclerotomy. Others have suggested either laser or vitrectomy.[100] Forman et al.[101] described the case of a 16-year-old patient with a subretinal fly larva, which was killed with argon laser therapy. The patient's visual acuity improved from 20/200 to 20/20. Syrdalen et al.[102] reported that removal of a reindeer warble fly larva through a pars plana opening after vitrectomy freed the surrounding vitreous attachments. There is also a report of a caribou botfly infecting an eye and the patient retaining good vision.[100] However, the visual result varies, depending on whether the macula and the optic nerve were involved in the process.[94]

CYSTICERCOSIS

Cysticercosis is more common in areas with poor hygiene conditions. It is usually seen in the first four decades of life; it is rare in the United States but is frequently seen in Central and South America and is the most common parasitic infection affecting the nervous system.[103] This disease is caused by ingestion of the eggs of *Taenia solium,* the pork tape worm. The larva migrates to the eye, where it encysts (Fig. 18.8). The cyst can be located in any part of the eye. In the anterior chamber, it can induce anterior uveitis with fibrous changes and secondary glaucoma. Excision of the cyst containing the worm has been reported

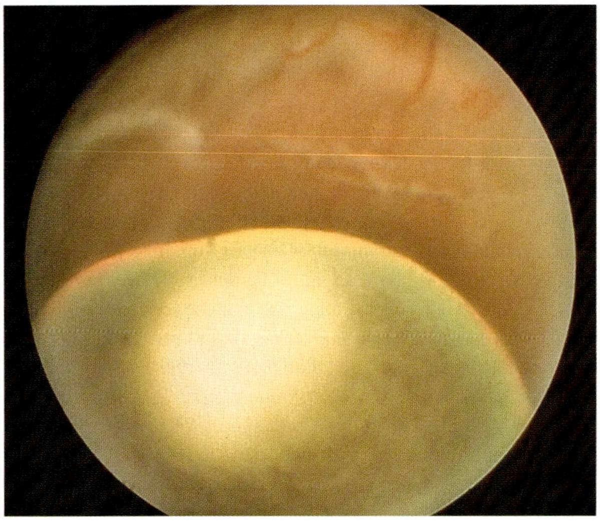

Fig. 18.8 *Cysticerca* organism seen through cystic retina. (Courtesy Miguel Burnier, Jr., MD.)

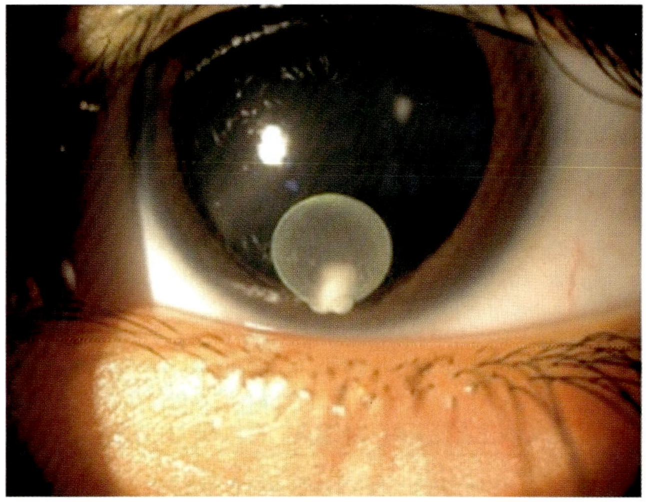

Fig. 18.9 A 6-year-old girl with discomfort and drop in vision in one eye. Scolex exiting the cyst. (From Cortez MA, Giuliari GP, Escaf L, et al. Ocular cysticercosis of the anterior segment. *J AAPOS*. 2007;11:628–662, with permission.)

to be therapeutic[104,105] (Fig. 18.9). Often, the scolex of the larva can be seen moving slowly in the vitreous.[106] An anterior chamber tap will reveal a large number of eosinophils. The presence of the parasite could be disastrous for the eye, particularly if the parasite is located in the subretinal space. Vitrectomy can be used to remove the larva if it is in the vitreous[107] and offers the potential for good vision postoperatively. However, the removal of subretinal lesions may not lead to a good visual outcome.[108] The larva can be removed via a sclerotomy site, and repair of the detachment caused by the presence of the parasite with a scleral buckling procedure can be tried.[107] Some authors have reported removing the organism through retinotomy at the apex of the induced serous retinal detachment by using a soft silicone-tipped extrusion cannula.[109] There are usually no overt systemic findings in this disorder. However, cysticercosis has been identified as the cause of severe medial rectus muscle myositis.[110] Menon et al. reported finding an optic nerve lesion (no confirmatory biopsy could be obtained) identified by using high-resolution computed tomography (CT).[111] Albendazole has been used to treat neurocysticercosis, with regression of the cyst in some patients.[112]

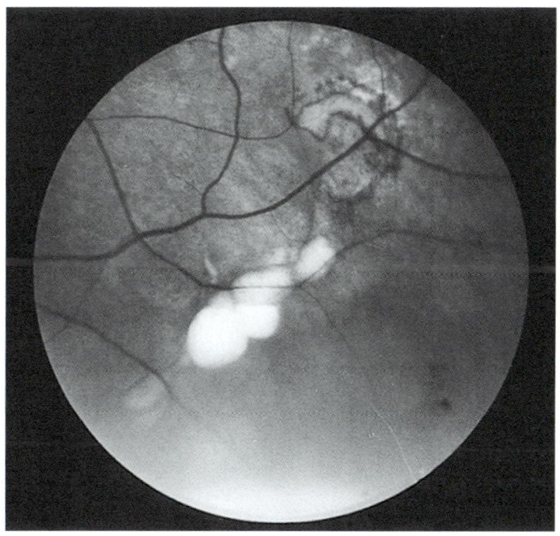

Fig. 18.10 Presumed caterpillar setae causing track anteroposteriorly in temporal retina.

CATERPILLAR SETAE

Caterpillar setae have been known since ancient times to be toxic to humans. Ocular disease was first associated with the caterpillar when it was reported by Schon in 1861. Several species of caterpillar have setae forming a row on their dorsal surface and containing histamine-liberating substances,[113] which are released only if the setae break off. It is theorized that these setae reach the eye by being airborne or when a person prunes a tree or bush containing these caterpillars. Once a hair reaches the eye, the movement of the globe and lids may force the hair into the eye itself and cause the disease described here. If it stays on the surface of the globe, then a small granulomatous reaction in the conjunctiva will ensue. Caterpillar setae keratitis has also been reported.[114] A seasonal epidemic was reported in the Kangra district of India, with over 136 individuals being affected.[115]

The initial entry of the caterpillar hair into the eye may cause an immediate inflammatory reaction, with pain, photophobia, and anterior uveitis. Later findings include chorioretinal lesions. According to Raspiller et al.,[116] this may occur anywhere from 6 months to 16 years after the initial insult. These authors highlighted two characteristics of these chorioretinal lesions. The first is the presence of one or more tracks that align in the anteroposterior direction and reflect the setae migration from the anterior portion of the globe to the posterior portion. The second aspect is the formation of white nodules or outpouchings along the track (Fig. 18.10).

The best management is avoidance of situations in which caterpillar setae can be released. Certainly, if a caterpillar hair can be seen sticking out of the ocular surface, an attempt should be made to remove it under light from the slit lamp. It has been suggested that setae can be asymptomatic subconjunctivally and intracorneally.[115] If the hair is noted in the anterior chamber or the vitreous, then surgical removal may be considered. Only about 10% of cases have vitreoretinal involvement. Fraser et al.[117] reported performing vitrectomy to remove the setae. Raspiller et al.[116] suggested placing a barrier of laser photocoagulation in front of the progressing track to prevent it from extending into the macular region. The use of anti-inflammatory agents is certainly indicated to reduce the inflammatory response and to make the patient more comfortable.

AMEBIASIS

It is estimated that 10% of the world population is infested by amebae, and at least half the populations of Central and South America and Asia. Most of the symptoms are gastrointestinal. However, intraocular inflammatory disease has, on occasion, been associated with the parasite. Rodger et al.[118] reported that intermediate uveitis was common in patients with amebic dysentery. Several researchers have reported that various entamoebae[119] and *Acanthamoeba*[120] species cause chorioretinal lesions. The disease is characterized by a subretinal whitish exudative lesion, most commonly in the macular region. Hemorrhage and disturbances of the RPE are associated with this lesion. In patients with dysentery, the ameba can be found in stool samples, but this is not always the case in hepatic amebiasis.

DIFFUSE UNILATERAL SUBACUTE NEURORETINITIS

Although *Toxocara canis* involvement of the eye has long been recognized, there is certainly a possibility that other nematodes not recognized so far may also cause ocular disease. An example of this is diffuse unilateral subacute neuroretinitis (DUSN). A description of this ocular disorder was first published in 1978 by Gass and Scelfo[121] with features that included insidious, usually severe loss of peripheral and central vision; vitritis; diffuse and focal pigment epithelial derangement with relative sparing of the macula; narrowing of the retinal vessels; optic atrophy; increased retinal circulation time; and subnormal electroretinographic findings. For the previous eleven years they had categorized these patients as the "unilateral wipeout syndrome". Interestingly, they initially thought that the disease may be a viral inflammation affecting primarily the retina, pigment epithelium, and optic nerve head. Gass later published an article in which he reported observing a motile subretinal nematode in two patients with DUSN.[122] On further searching of the literature, Gass was able to identify previously reports appearing as early as 1952 of cases of similar nematodes producing the same clinical picture. Hence a syndrome of initially unknown cause that was classified only by clinical description was later found to be related to a nematode in the subretinal space. The understanding of the cause suggested possible therapies that had not been considered when the disease was thought to be idiopathic.[123]

DUSN begins as scattered, recurrent, deep gray-white retinal lesions, accompanied by marked loss of central acuity. There is often moderate vitreal inflammation, but in some patients, there may be no observable inflammation. Optic disk swelling may be present. As the disease advances, there is progressive optic atrophy, narrowing of the retinal vessels, RPE stippling, and further visual field loss. Electroretinography shows significantly reduced response. Careful examination with a contact lens may disclose a motile worm moving in the subretinal space. The details of the worm's size will be discussed later. Occasionally, the worm may be seen in the vitreous. In some patients, subretinal tracks that correspond to previous movements of the worm can be seen. The examination light may cause the worm to move. Granulomatous masses, such as those seen in classic *T. canis* infestation, are not observed in DUSN. There have been reports of unusual presentations of the disease, including a worm that appeared to be below the RPE[124] and a large worm that produced a macular cyst.[125] Fluorescein angiography has demonstrated no fluorescence of the gray-white lesions in the early stages, with late staining of these lesions.[84] Perivascular staining and mottled RPE window defects are also seen. Indocyanine green (ICG) staining has demonstrated choroidal areas of hypofluorescence, suggesting the involvement of the choroid in addition to that of the subretinal space.[126] Before the worm is identified, several disorders can be considered in the differential diagnosis. These include acute multifocal posterior placoid epitheliopathy, toxoplasmosis, optic neuritis, and posttraumatic retinal and choroidal ischemia.

Because the movement of the worm is thought to cause destruction of the retinal outer segments, visual loss is rarely reversible. Visual acuity of less than 20/200 is seen in about one-half of patients.[122] Occasional patients have retained good vision without treatment. An associated creeping skin eruption that is suggestive of systemic nematode infection is seen in some patients.

Worms of two sizes have been described in eyes with DUSN. A smaller worm 400 to 700 μm in length was seen in most patients who lived in southeastern United States and was reported in the Caribbean and South America (Brazil).[127] A larger worm (1500–2000 μm) has been seen in patients residing in the northern and midwestern United

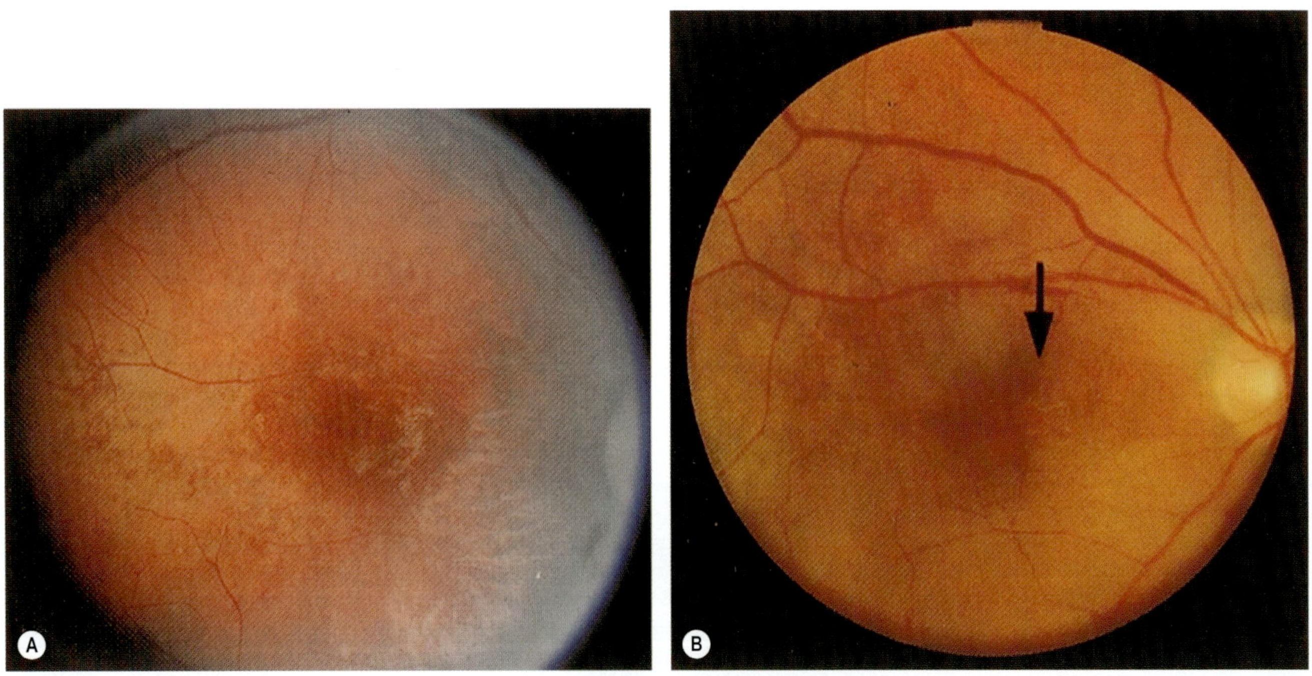

Fig. 18.11 Fundus photographs of worms causing diffuse unilateral subacute neuroretinitis (DUSN) from (A) the southern part of the United States and (B) the northern part of United States. (Courtesy J. Donald Gass, MD.)

States (Fig. 18.11) and in Germany,[128,129] China,[130] and Brazil.[131] However, this geographic relationship does not always hold up to careful scrutiny. The worms have been described as being about 1/20th their length in diameter (Fig. 18.12).

The method of identification of the type of nematode that causes DUSN is still being debated. *Toxocara* organisms rarely exceed 400 μm in length. Titers for *T. canis* have been looked for in patients with DUSN, and the results are invariably negative.[132] Eosinophilia is occasionally seen. In 1984, it was suggested that the larger worms in patients living in more northern climates were *Baylisascaris procyonis*, a nematode found in raccoons.[133] Experimental infection of subhuman primates and other laboratory animals with oral administration of *B. procyonis* eggs has produced a clinical picture similar to that of DUSN.[134] Goldberg et al.[135] reported the case of a patient from the western United States with unilateral DUSN whose evaluation implicated *Baylisascaris* as the causative agent. However, no patient with DUSN has had the neurologic complications that have been associated with infection by this nematode. It is likely that the clinical picture of DUSN can be produced by a variety of nematodes that, by chance, find their way to the eye and destroy the retina. These may include *Toxocara* in some patients despite the very low levels of *Toxocara* antibodies that are found because the smaller worms seen in DUSN are of the correct size for *Toxocara*. Indeed, in one report in which the organism was removed from the eye transvitreally, the larva was thought to be a third-stage *Toxocara*.[136]

Therapy with thiabendazole, an anthelmintic agent, or corticosteroids had not been successful in the treatment of DUSN. However, Souza et al.[137] treated 12 patients with DUSN in Brazil with albendazole, 400 mg/day for 30 days, and observed improvement in visual acuity and reduction in inflammation. The worm has also been successfully destroyed with photocoagulation.[123,138] The need to treat with laser as rapidly as possible is emphasized by several authors. Venkatesh et al.[139] reported from India a case where the worm was photographed but not initially treated with laser therapy, and although laser therapy was applied later, it resulted in only partial improvement in visual acuity. In a series of two reports, Garcia et al.[140,141] emphasized the need to treat with laser as early as possible. Their results suggested that early therapy resulted in improvement in vision, whereas late therapy helped few. It has been shown that the thickness of the nerve fiber layer is decreased in DUSN; thus it would make sense that early treatment would minimize this.[142] In this disease, the death of the worm is usually not associated with an increased inflammatory response. However, as reported by Muccioli and Belfort,[143] a patient with DUSN did develop acute iridocyclitis and hypopyon uveitis, presumably related to the death of the organism. Therefore most practitioners add oral steroids

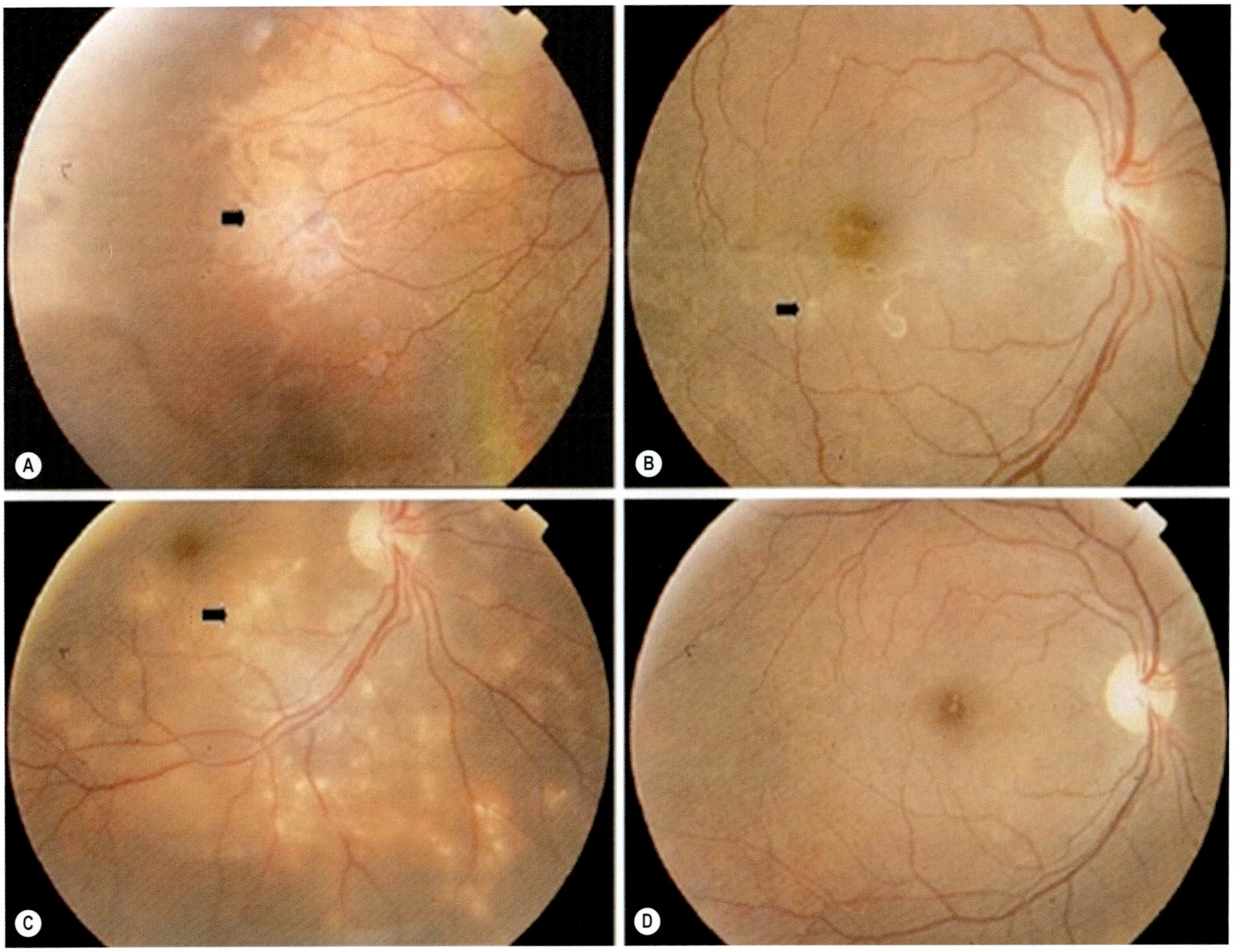

Fig. 18.12 Migratory worm in diffuse unilateral subacute neuroretinitis (DUSN). (A) Motile worm surrounded by tracts. (B) Worm (1500–2000 mm) migrating below the macula after laser had been applied *(arrow)*. (C) Dead worm with multiple white dots. (D) Resolution 3 weeks after laser therapy. (Reproduced from: Myint K, Sahay R, Mon S, Saravanan VR, Narendran V, Dhillon B. "Worm in the eye": the rationale treatment of DUSN in South India. *Br J Ophthalmol.* 2006;90:1125–1127. Copyright 2006, with permission of the BMJ Publishing Group.)

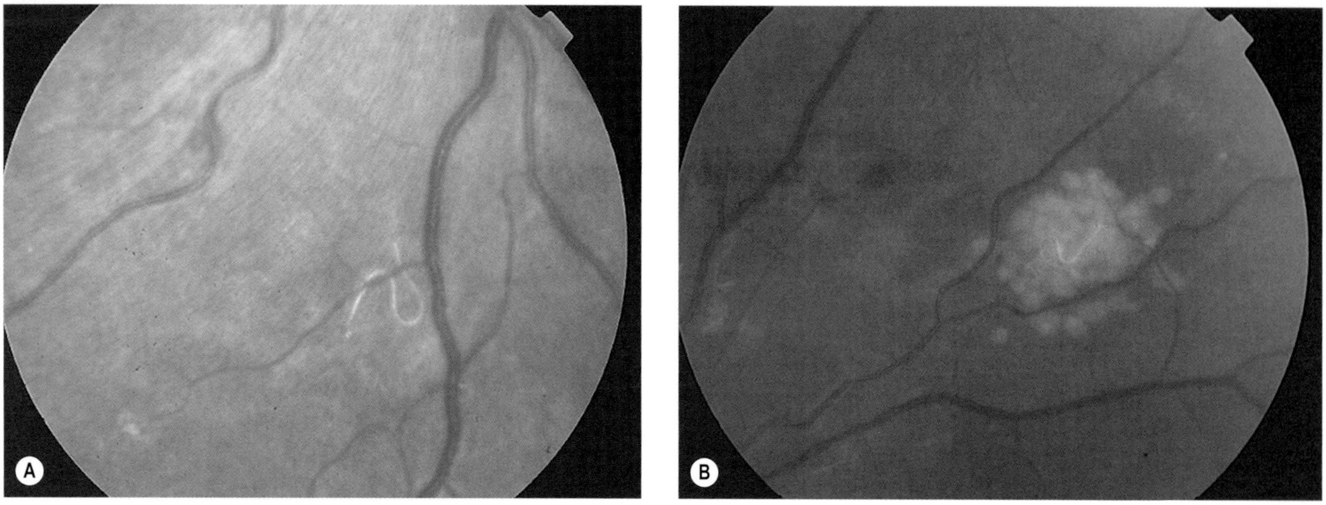

Fig. 18.13 Fundus photo of a subretinal worm (A), which was successfully photocoagulated (B). (Courtesy Rubens Belfort, MD and Marcelo Casela, MD.)

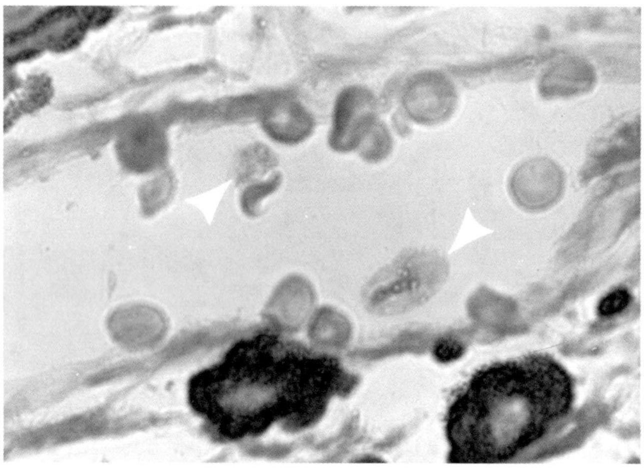

Fig. 18.14 Photomicrograph showing schizonts of *Plasmodium vivax* in the choroid. (Hematoxylin & eosin [H&E]; original magnification ×1000.) (Courtesy Professor Jyotirmay Biswas. Reproduced from Biswas J, Fogla R, Srinivasan P, Narayan S, Haranath K, Badrinath V. Ocular malaria. A clinical and histopathologic study. *Ophthalmology.* 1996;103:1471–1475, with permission.)

to the therapeutic regimen after laser therapy is initiated.[144] In addition, if the worm can be localized in the periphery of the retina, it can be surrounded by photocoagulation and then excised. Destruction of the worm by using photocoagulation appears to halt the progression of DUSN (Fig. 18.13). Although the risk factors for the development of this type of ocular larval migrans are uncertain and the exact type of nematode in each case is still not specified, the recognition of the cause of this disease has led to the beginnings of a logical therapeutic approach. An epiretinal membrane may result, needing surgical removal, which could cause a persistent traction detachment even after adequate photocoagulation has been administered.[145]

Although nematodes in the eye have been reported, there are few reports of trematodes. McDonald et al.[146] reported finding *Alaria mesocercaria,* a trematode, in the eyes of two unrelated Asian men who presumably were exposed to the organism when they consumed poorly cooked frogs' legs. They both presented with unilateral disease, choroidal tracks, and other findings similar to those of DUSN. In one patient, the organism was killed with laser therapy, and in the other, the trematode was removed surgically from the vitreous.

Finally, it is fitting to finish this section with a footnote from Gass et al. In a report from Brazil, Cunha de Souza et al.[147] described the first patient with the documented presence of nematodes in both eyes. That report's discussion ends with the proposal, based on the bilaterality of this disease entity, that the more appropriate term is *diffuse subacute neuroretinitis.*

MALARIA

Malaria is caused by a protozoon, most commonly *Plasmodium falciparum* and *Plasmodium vivax.* It is estimated that approximately 300 million people in the world harbor the parasite, and it has been suggested that malaria was the underlying cause of the chronic ocular problems experienced by Jefferson Davis (President of the Confederacy during the American Civil War).[148] Of patients with malaria, 10% to 20% have been reported to have ocular manifestations,[149] which range from subconjunctival hemorrhages to optic neuritis and retinal hemorrhages. In a report generated from the Blantyre (Malawi) Malaria Project,[150] 1000 children with cerebral malaria underwent ophthalmologic examination. The age range of these children was 2 to 14 years; 5% of them had cotton-wool spots. There were retinal vessel abnormalities and retinal hemorrhages with white centers, resembling Roth spots. Retinal whitening, perhaps caused by retinal edema, was seen very frequently. Although papilledema was not seen often, it was a poor prognostic sign. Biswas et al.[151] reported a clinical and histopathologic study of three patients, one with multiple, blotchy retinal hemorrhages; a second with bilateral panuveitis, perivasculitis, retinal hemorrhages, and glaucoma; and a third with cerebral malaria and retinal hemorrhages as well.[151] Histopathologic examination showed cytoadherence of the parasitized erythrocytes, schizonts, and gametocytes of *P. vivax* in the retinal and choroidal blood vessels (Fig. 18.14).

SEASONAL HYPERACUTE PANUVEITIS

A curious entity that has been reported by Malla[152] and by Upadhyay et al.[153] in Nepal may be a parasite-related ocular disease. This severe and usually unilateral disease has been noted to occur principally in children, with sporadic cases in adults. The oldest reported patient was 44 years of age. About one-third to one-half of patients revealed a history of contact with a moth in the few days preceding the onset of ocular symptoms. In 249 patients with newly diagnosed uveitis seen at the

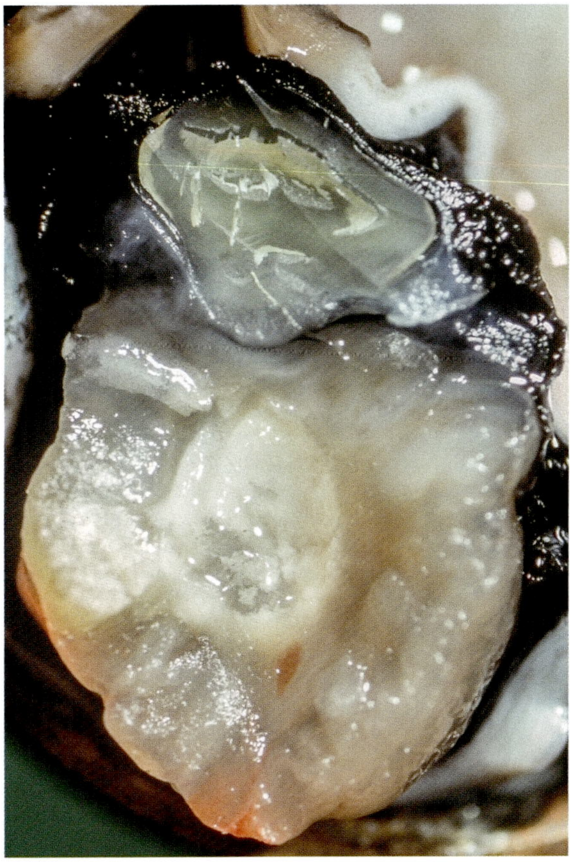

Fig. 18.15 Sectioned eye with seasonal hyperacute panuveitis. The eye has intraocular hemorrhage and cataract. The dense white structure in the center of the vitreous is a totally detached retina.

Eye Department of Tribhuvan University's Teaching Hospital, from October 1997 to September 1999, 13 patients with seasonal hyperacute panuveitis (SHAPU) were seen. All racial groups in Nepal seem to be affected (Dr. Dev Shah, personal communication).

SHAPU has occurred in 2-year cycles, the first having been recognized soon after the monsoon season of 1975. The disease begins very acutely with a red eye and leukocoria with little pain. There may be a fibrinoid reaction in the anterior chamber, and often there is also a hypopyon. This is followed by hypotony and a very sudden decrease in vision, and it may be referred to as *malignant hypotension*. Examination of the posterior segment is obscured by the leukocoria. The anterior chamber ultimately becomes flat and the eye becomes phthisical (Fig. 18.15). Ultrasonography may show remarkable choroidal thickening. So far, therapy has not been able to reverse the course of the disease.

In a study by Upadhyay et al.,[154] examination of children with SHAPU revealed no systemic abnormalities. The erythrocyte sedimentation rate was normal or minimally elevated, and the results of tests for rheumatoid factor and antinuclear antibodies were negative. The levels of circulating immune complexes were not elevated. Anti-*Toxoplasma* antibodies were not present in the majority of patients, and anti-*Toxocara* antibodies were found only in a few. Evidence of S-Ag sensitization could not be demonstrated.[154] In another study, several children were noted to have been exposed to moths, but laboratory experiments attempting to define whether antigens from the moth-induced uveitis were not successful.[86] Histologic examination revealed a severe inflammatory response, with lymphocytes and plasma cells noted and the retina drawn up into the retrolenticular mass. Eosinophils did not contain a significant proportion of the cell population. Scanning electron microscopy showed prominent Russel bodies and plasma cells. Neither worms nor virus particles could be identified. The underlying cause of this disorder remains unknown, and therapy has been problematic. In a study performed in Pokhara, Nepal, 14 patients underwent vitrectomy, and half of them had a final visual acuity of 6/60, which appears to be an improvement over the phthisis that is frequently seen as the end result.[155]

REFERENCES

1. World Health Organization (WHO). Onchocerciasis and its control. *WHO Tech Rep Ser*. 1995;852:1–103.
2. Narita AS, Taylor HR. Blindness in the tropics. *Med J Aust*. 1993;159:416–420.
3. Boatin BA, Richards FO Jr. Control of onchocerciasis. *Adv Parasitol*. 2006;61:349–394.
4. Sallo F, Eberhard ML, Fok E, et al. Zoonotic intravitreal Onchocerca in Hungary. *Ophthalmology*. 2005;112(3):502–504.
5. Brockhouse CL, Vajime CG, Marin R, et al. Molecular identification of onchocerciasis vector sibling species in black flies (Diptera: Simuliidae). *Biochem Biophys Res Commun*. 1993;194:628–634.
6. Anderson J, Fuglsang H, Marshall TF. Effects of diethylcarbamazine on ocular onchocerciasis. *Tropenmed Parasit*. 1976;(27):263–275.
7. Thylefors B, Brinkman UK. The microfilarial load in the anterior segment of the eye. A parameter of intensity of onchocerciasis. *Bull Org Mond Santé*. 1977;5:731–737.
8. Maertens K. Tonography in onchocerciasis. *Bull Soc Panafr Ophthalmol*. 1982;5:23–27.
9. Thylefors B, Duppenthaler JL. Epidemiological aspects of intra-ocular pressure in an onchocerciasis endemic area. *Bull Org Mond Santé*. 1979;57:963–969.
10. Newland HS, White AT, Greene BM, et al. Ocular manifestations of onchocerciasis in a rain forest area of West Africa. *Br J Ophthalmol*. 1991;(75):163–169.
11. Enk CD, Anteby I, Abramson N, et al. Onchocerciasis among Ethiopian immigrants in Israel. *Isr Med Assoc J*. 2003;5(7):485–488.
12. Neumann E, Gunders AE. Pathogenesis of the posterior segments lesion of ocular onchocerciasis. *Am J Ophthalmol*. 1973;75:82.
13. Budden FH. The natural history of ocular onchocerciasis over a period of 14–15 years and the effect on this of a single course of suramin. *Trans Roy Soc Med Hyg*. 1976;70:484–491.
14. Duke BOL, Vincelette J, Moore PJ. Microfilariae in the cerebrospinal fluid, and neurological complications during treatment of onchocerciasis with diethylcarbamazine. *Tropenmed Parasit*. 1976;(27):123–132.
15. Tonjum AM, Thylefors B. Aspects of corneal changes in onchocerciasis. *Br J Ophthalmol*. 1978;(62):458–461.
16. Egbert PR, Jacobson DW, Fiadoyor S, et al. Onchocerciasis: a potential risk factor for glaucoma. *Br J Ophthalmol*. 2005;89(7):796–798.
17. Van den Berghe L, Chardome M, Peel E. The filarial parasites of the eastern gorilla in the Congo. *J Helminthol*. 1964;38:349–368.
18. Duke BOL. Experimental transmission of *Onchocerca volvulus* from man to chimpanzee. *Trans Roy Soc Trop Med Hyg*. 1962;56:271.
19. Donnelly JJ, Taylor HR, Young E, et al. Experimental ocular onchocerciasis in cynomolgus monkeys. *Invest Ophthalmol Vis Sci*. 1986;27:492–499.
20. Duke BOL, Garner A. Fundus lesions in the rabbit eye following inoculation of *Onchocerca volvulus* microfilariae into the posterior segment. II. Pathology. *Tropenmed Parasitol*. 1976;(27):19–29.
21. Sakla AA, Donnelly JJ, Lok JB, et al. Punctate keratitis induced by subconjunctivally injected microfilariae of *Onchocerca lienalis*. *Arch Ophthalmol*. 1986;104:894–898.
22. Semba RD, Donnelly JJ, Young E, et al. Experimental ocular onchocerciasis in cynomolgus monkeys. IV. Chorioretinitis elicited by *Onchocerca volvulus* microfilariae. *Invest Ophthalmol Vis Sci*. 1991;32:1499–1507.
23. Somorin AO, Hewer DC, Ajugwo RE. Immunoglobulin in Nigerian onchocerciasis. *Ann J Trop Med Hyg*. 1977;(26):872–876.
24. Ngu JL, Blackett K. Immunological studies in onchocerciasis in Cameroon. *Trop Geog Med*. 1976;28:111–120.

25. Ottesen EA. Immune responsiveness and the pathogenesis of human onchocerciasis. *J Infect Dis.* 1995;171:659–671.
26. Chan CC, Nussenblatt RB, Kim MK, et al. Immunopathology of ocular onchocerciasis. 2. Anti-retinal autoantibodies in serum and ocular fluids. *Ophthalmology.* 1987;(94):439–443.
27. Van der Lelij A, Rothova A, De Vries JP, et al. Analysis of aqueous humour in ocular onchocerciasis. *Curr Eye Res.* 1991;10:169–176.
28. Braun G, McKechnie NM, Connor V, et al. Immunological crossreactivity between a cloned antigen of *Onchocerca volvulus* and a component of the retinal pigment epithelium. *J Exp Med.* 1991;174:169–177.
29. Klager S, McKechnie NM, Braun G, et al. Immunologic crossreactivity in the pathogenesis of ocular onchocerciasis. *Invest Ophthalmol Vis Sci.* 1993;34:2888–2902.
30. Meilof JF, Van der Lelij A, Rokeach LA, et al. Autoimmunity and filariasis: autoantibodies against cytoplasmic cellular proteins in sera of patients with onchocerciasis. *J Immunol.* 1993;151:5800–5809.
31. Kaifi JT, Diaconu E, Pearlman E. Distinct roles for PECAM-1, ICAM-1, and VCAM-1 in recruitment of neutrophils and eosinophils to the cornea in ocular onchocerciasis (river blindness). *J Immunol.* 2001;166:6795–6801.
32. Kaifi JT, Hall LR, Diaz C, et al. Impaired eosinophil recruitment to the cornea in P-selectin-deficient mice in *Onchocerca volvulus* keratitis (river blindness). *Invest Ophthalmol Vis Sci.* 2000;41(12):3856–3861.
33. Hall LR, Pearlman E. Pathogenesis of onchocercal keratitis (river blindness). *Clin Microbiol Rev.* 1999;12:445–453.
34. Hall LR, Kaifi JT, Diaconu E, et al. CD4+ depletion selectively inhibits eosinophil recruitment to the cornea and abrogates *Onchocerca volvulus* keratitis (river blindness). *Infect Immun.* 2000;68(9):5459–5461.
35. Saint Andre AV, Blackwell NM, Hall LR, et al. The role of endosymbiotic *Wolbachia* bacteria in the pathogenesis of river blindness. *Science.* 2002;295:1892–1895.
36. Gillette-Ferguson I, Hise AG, Sun Y, et al. *Wolbachia*- and *Onchocerca volvulus*-induced keratitis (river blindness) is dependent on myeloid differentiation factor 88. *Infect Immun.* 2006;74(4):2442–2445.
37. Brattig NW. Pathogenesis and host responses in human onchocerciasis: impact of *Onchocerca filariae* and *Wolbachia* endobacteria. *Microbes Infect.* 2004;6(1):113–128.
38. Bradley JE, Nirmalan N, Kläger SL, et al. River blindness: a role for parasite retinoid-binding proteins in the generation of pathology? *Trends Parasitol.* 2001;17(10):471–475.
39. Tree TI, Gillespie AJ, Shepley KJ, et al. Characterization of an immunodominant glycoprotein antigen of *Onchocerca volvulus* with homologues in other filarial nematodes and *Caenorhabditis elegans. Mol Biochem Parasitol.* 1995;69:185–195.
40. Gudes LJ, Sporn MB. Roberts AB. Cellular biology and biochemistry of retinoids. In: Sporn MB, et al., eds. The Retinoids. New York: Raven Press; 1994; 443–520.
41. Sturcheler D, Wyss F, Hanck A, et al. Retinol, onchocerciasis, and *Onchocerca volvulus. Trans Roy Soc Trop Med Hyg.* 1981;75:617.
42. Steel C, Nutman TB. Regulation of IL-5 in onchocerciasis. A critical role for IL-2. *J Immunol.* 1993;(150):5511–5518.
43. Gillette-Ferguson I, Daehnel K, Hise AG, et al. Toll-like receptor 2 regulates CXC chemokine production and neutrophil recruitment to the cornea in *Onchocerca volvulus/Wolbachia*-induced keratitis. *Infect Immun.* 2007;75(12):5908–5915.
44. Daehnel K, Gillette-Ferguson I, Hise AG, et al. *Filaria/Wolbachia* activation of dendritic cells and development of Th1-associated responses is dependent on toll-like receptor 2 in a mouse model of ocular onchocerciasis (river blindness). *Parasite Immunol.* 2007;29(9):455–465.
45. United Nations Development Program (UNDP), World Bank, and World Health Organization (WHO). Report of the eighth meeting on the Scientific Working Group On Filariasis in collaboration with the Programme For The Prevention Of Blindness. In: *Special Programme for Research and Training in Tropical Disease: The Pathogenesis and Treatment of Ocular Onchocerciasis.* Geneva, Switzerland: WHO; 1982.
46. Bird AC, el-Sheikh H, Anderson J, et al. Changes in visual function and in the posterior segment of the eye during treatment of onchocerciasis with diethylcarbamazine citrate. *Br J Ophthalmol.* 1980;64:191–200.
47. Hero M, Bird AC, Awadzi K. Quantification of the ocular reactions to microfilaricides in the chemotherapy of onchocerciasis. *Eye.* 1992;6:93–96. [Pt 1].
48. Rivas-Alcala AR, Greene BM, Taylor HR, et al. Chemotherapy of onchocerciasis: a controlled comparison of mebendazole, levamisole, and diethylcarbamazine. *Lancet.* 1981:485–492. ii.
49. Aziz MA, Diallo S, Diop IM, et al. Efficacy and tolerance of ivermectin in human onchocerciasis. *Lancet.* 1982;2:171–173.
50. Boatin B. The Onchocerciasis Control Programme in West Africa (OCP). *Ann Trop Med Parasitol.* 2008;102(Suppl 1):13–17.
51. Taylor HR, Murphy RP, Newland HS, et al. Treatment of onchocerciasis. The ocular effects of ivermectin and diethylcarbamazine. *Arch Ophthalmol.* 1986;104:863–870.
52. Diallo S, Aziz MA, Lariviere M, et al. A double-blind comparison of the efficacy and safety of ivermectin and diethylcarbamazine in a placebo controlled study of Senegalese patients with onchocerciasis. *Trans Roy Soc Trop Med Hyg.* 1986;80:927–934.
53. Dadzie KY, Bird AC, Awadzi K, et al. Ocular findings in a double-blind study of ivermectin versus diethylcarbazine versus placebo in the treatment of onchocerciasis. *Br J Ophthalmol.* 1987;71:78–85.
54. Ogunba EO, Gemade EL. Preliminary observations on the distribution of ivermectin in Nigeria for control of river blindness. *Ann Trop Med Parasitol.* 1992;(86):649–655.
55. Whitworth JA, Gilbert CE, Mabey DM, et al. Effects of repeated doses of ivermectin on ocular onchocerciasis: community-based trial in Sierra Leone. *Lancet.* 1991;338:1100–1103.
56. Dadzie KY, Remme J, De Sole G. Changes in ocular onchocerciasis after two rounds of community-based invermectin treatment in a holo-endemic onchocerciasis. *Doc Ophthalmol.* 1991;79:261–267.
57. WHO. Onchocerciasis and its control. Report of a WHO Expert Committee on Onchocerciasis Control. In: In Tech Rep Ser No 852, vol. 852. pp. 1–104. Geneva: World Health Organization; 1995. p. 1–104.
58. Haddad D. The NGDO Co-ordination Group for Onchocerciasis Control. *Ann Trop Med Parasitol.* 2008;102(Suppl 1):35–38.
59. Vieira JC, Cooper PJ, Lovato R, et al. Impact of long-term treatment of onchocerciasis with ivermectin in Ecuador: potential for elimination of infection. *BMC Med.* 2007;5:9.
60. Hopkins AD. Ivermectin and onchocerciasis: is it all solved? *Eye.* 2005;19(10):1057–1066.
61. Semba RD, Murphy RP, Newland HS, et al. Longitudinal study of lesions of the posterior segment in onchocerciasis. *Ophthalmology.* 1990;97:1334–1341.
62. Njoo FL, Stilma JS, van der Lelij A. Effects of repeated ivermectin treatment in onchocerciasis. *Doc Ophthalmol.* 1992;79:261–267.
63. Mabey D, Whitworth JA, Eckstein M, et al. The effects of multiple doses of ivermectin on ocular onchocerciasis. *Ophthalmology.* 1996;103:1001–1008.
64. Chippaux JP, Boussinesq M, Fobi G, et al. Effect of repeated ivermectin treatments on ocular onchocerciasis: evaluation after six to eight dosings. *Ophthalmic Epidemiol.* 1999;6(4):229–246.
65. Awadzi K, Attah SK, Addy ET, et al. The effects of high-dose ivermectin regimens on *Onchocerca volvulus* in onchocerciasis patients. *Trans Roy Soc Trop Med Hyg.* 1999;93:189–194.
66. Gardon J, Boussinesq M, Kamgno J, et al. Effects of standard and high doses of ivermectin on adult worms on *Onchocerca volvulus*: a randomised controlled trial. *Lancet.* 2002;360:203–210.
67. Klager SL, Whitworth JA, Downham M. Viability and fertility of adult *Onchocerca volvulus* after 6 years of treatment with ivermectin. *Trop Med Int Health.* 1996;1(5):581–589.
68. Ejere H, Schwartz E, Wormald R. Ivermectin for onchocercal eye disease (river blindness). *Cochrane Database Syst Rev.* 2001;1:CD002219.
69. Awadzi K, Attah SK, Addy ET, et al. Thirty-month follow-up of sub-optimal responders to multiple treatments with ivermectin, in two onchocerciasis-endemic foci in Ghana. *Ann Trop Med Parasitol.* 2004;98(4):359–370.
70. Fobi G, Gardon J, Kamgno J, et al. A randomized, double-blind, controlled trial of the effects of ivermectin at normal and high doses, given annually or three-monthly, against *Onchocerca volvulus:* ophthalmological results. *Trans Roy Soc Trop Med Hyg.* 2005;99(4):279–289.

71. Plaisier AP, van Oortmarssen GJ, Remme J, et al. The risk and dynamics of onchocerciasis recrudescence after cessation of vector control. *Bull WHO*. 1991;69:169–178.
72. Davies JB. Description of a computer model of forest onchocerciasis transmission and its application to field scenarios of vector control and chemotherapy. *Ann Trop Med Parasitol*. 1993;87:41–63.
73. Abegunde AT, Ahuja RM, Okafor NJ. Doxycycline plus ivermectin versus ivermectin alone for treatment of patients with onchocerciasis. *Cochrane Database Syst Rev*. 2016;15(1):CD011146.
74. Sucs FE, Zanen A. Ocular manifestations secondary to giardiasis. *Bull Soc Belge Ophtalmol*. 1986;219:63–69.
75. Welch PB. Giardiasis with unusual clinical findings. *Am J Digest Dis*. 1943;1943:10.
76. Webster BH. Human infection with *Giardia lamblia*. *Am J Dig Dis (New Series)*. 1958;(3):64–71.
77. Barraquer I. Sur la coincidence de la lambliase et de certaines lesions du fond de l'oeil. *Bull Soc Pathol Exot (Paris)*. 1938;(31):55–58.
78. Knox DL, King JJ. Retinal arteritis, iridocyclitis, and giardiasis. *Ophthalmology*. 1982;89:1303–1308.
79. Pettoello Mantovani M, Giardino I, Magli A, et al. Intestinal giardiasis associated with ophthalmologic changes. *J Pediatr Gastroenterol*. 1990;11:196–200.
80. Corsi A, Nucci C, Knafelz D, et al. Ocular changes associated with *Giardia lamblia* infection in children. *Br J Ophthalmol*. 1998;(82):59–62.
81. De Ocampo Lecture Wania J. The eye and intestinal parasitic diseases. In: Shimizu K, ed. *Current Aspects of Ophthalmology*. Amsterdam: Elsevier Science; 1992:1–7.
82. Roberts-Thornson IC, Mitchel GI. Genetic studies in human and murine giardiasis. *Gut*. 1980;21:397–401.
83. Anderson ML, Griffith DG. Intestinal giardiasis associated with ocular inflammation. *J Clin Gastroenterol*. 1985;7(2):169–172.
84. Behr C. Ophthalmomyiasis interna and externa. *Klin Mbl Augenheilkd*. 1920;64:161–180.
85. DeBoe MP. Dipterous larva passing from the optic nerve into the vitreous chamber. *Arch Ophthalmol*. 1933;(10):824–825.
86. Amr ZS, Amr BS, Abo-Shehada MN. Ophthalmomyiasis externa caused by *Oestrus ovis* L. in the Ajloun area of northern Jordan. *Ann Trop Med Parasitol*. 1993;(87):259–262.
87. Hira PR, Hajj B, al-Ali F, et al. Ophthalmomyiasis in Kuwait: first report of *Oestrus ovis* before and after the Gulf conflict. *J Trop Med Hyg*. 1993;96:241–244.
88. Chodosh J, Ophthalmomyiasis Clarridge J. A review with special reference to *Cochliomyia hominivorax*. *Clin Infect Dis*. 1992;14:444–449.
89. Dunbar J, Cooper B, Hodgetts T, et al. An outbreak of human external ophthalmomyiasis due to *Oestrus ovis* in southern Afghanistan. *Clin Infect Dis*. 2008;46(11):e124–e126.
90. Dixon JM, Winkler CH, Nelson JH. Ophthalmomyiasis interna caused by *Cuterebra* larva. *Trans Am Ophthalmol Soc*. 1969;67:110–115.
91. Godde-Jolly D, Brumpt ML, Stofft P. Un cas d'ophthalmomyase "hypoderma boris" de la chambre anterieure. *Bull Soc Ophthal Fr*. 1966;(2):48–56.
92. Gass JDM, Lewis RA. Subretinal tracks in ophthalmomyiasis. *Arch Ophthalmol*. 1976;94:1500–1505.
93. Slusher MM, Holland WD, Weaver RG, et al. Ophthalmomyiasis interna posterior. Subretinal tracks and intraocular larvae. *Arch Ophthalmol*. 1979;97:885–887.
94. Jakobs EM, Adelberg DA, Lewis JM, et al. Ophthalmomyiasis interna posterior. Report of a case with optic atrophy. *Retina*. 1997;17:310–317.
95. Billi B, Lesnoni G, Audisio P, et al. Pars plana vitrectomy for retinal detachment due to internal posterior ophthalmomyiasis after cataract extraction. *Graefes Arch Clin Exp Ophthalmol*. 1997;235:255–258.
96. Campbell RJ, Steele JC, Cox TA, et al. Pathologic findings in the retinal pigment epitheliopathy associated with the amyotrophic lateral sclerosis/Parkinsonism-dementia complex of Guam. *Ophthalmology*. 1993;100:37–42.
97. Sharifipour F, Feghhi M. Anterior ophthalmomyiasis interna: an ophthalmic emergency. *Arch Ophthalmol*. 2008;126(10):1466–1467.
98. Spirn MJ, Hubbard GB, Bergstrom C, et al. Ophthalmomyiasis associated with Fuchs heterochromic iridocyclitis. *Retina*. 2006;26(8):973–974.
99. Saraiva V da S, Amaro MH, Belfort R, et al. A case of anterior internal ophthalmomyiasis: case report. *Arq Bras Oftalmol*. 2006;69(5):741–743.
100. Lagace-Wiens PR, Dookeran R, Skinner S, et al. Human ophthalmomyiasis interna caused by *Hypoderma tarandi*, Northern Canada. *Emerg Infect Dis*. 2008;14(1):64–66.
101. Forman AR, Cruess AF, Benson WE. Ophthalmomyiasis treated by argon-laser photocoagulation. *Retina*. 1984;(4):163–165.
102. Syrdalen P, Nitter T, Mehl R. Opthalmomyiasis interna posterior: report of case caused by reindeer warble fly larva and review of previous reported cases. *Br J Ophthalmol*. 1982;66:589–593.
103. Barry M, Kaldiian LC. *Neurocysticercosis. Semin Neurol*. 1993;13:131–143.
104. Cortez MA, Giuliari GP, Escaf L, et al. Ocular cysticercosis of the anterior segment. *J Am Assoc Pediatr Ophthalmol Strabismus*. 2007;11(6):628–629.
105. Mahendradas P, Biswas J, Khetan V. Fibrinous anterior uveitis due to cysticercus cellulosae. *Ocul Immunol Inflamm*. 2007;15(6):451–454.
106. Meyerson L, Pienaar BT. Intraocular cysticercus. *Br J Ophthalmol*. 1961;(45):148–153.
107. Topilow HW, Yimoyines DJ, Freeman HM, et al. Bilateral multifocal intraocular cysticercosis. *Ophthalmology*. 1981;88:1166–1172.
108. Segal P, Mrzyglod S, Dudarewiex JS. Subretinal cysticercosis in the macular region. *Am J Ophthalmol*. 1964;57:655–664.
109. Chuck RS, Olk RJ, Weil GJ, et al. Surgical removal of a subretinal proliferating cysticercus of *Taeniaeformis crassiceps*. *Arch Ophthalmol*. 1997;115(4):562–563.
110. Stewart CR, Salmon JF, Murray AD, et al. Cysticercosis as a cause of severe medical rectus muscle myositis. *Am J Ophthalmol*. 1993;116:510–511.
111. Menon V, Tandon R, Khanna S, et al. Cysticercosis of the optic nerve. *J Neuro-Ophthalmol*. 2000;20(1):59–60.
112. Takayanagui OM, Jardim E. Therapy for neurocysticercosis: comparison between albendazole and praziquantel. *Arch Neurol*. 1992;49:290–294.
113. Diallo JS. *Manifestations Ophtalmologiques des Parasitoses*. Paris, France: Masson; 1985.
114. Teske SA, Hirst LW, Gibson BH, et al. Caterpillar induced keratitis. *Cornea*. 1991;10:317–321.
115. Sood P, Tuli R, Puri R, et al. Seasonal epidemic of ocular caterpillar hair injuries in the Kangra District of India. *Ophthalmic Epidemiol*. 2004;11(1):3–8.
116. Raspiller A, Lepori JC, George JL. Chorioretinopathie par migration de poils de chenilles. *Bull Mem Soc Fr Ophtalmol*. 1984;95:153–156.
117. Fraser SG, Dowd TC, Bosanquet RC. Intraocular caterpillar hairs (setae): clinical course and management. *Eye*. 1994;8(Pt 5):596–598.
118. Rodger FC, Chir PK, Hosain ATMM. Night blindness in the tropics. *Arch Ophthalmol*. 1960;(63):927–935.
119. Braley AE, Hamilton HE. Central serous choroiditis associated with amebiasis. *Arch Ophthalmol*. 1957;(58):1–14.
120. Schlaegel TFJ, Culbertson C. Experimental *Hartmanella* optic neuritis and uveitis. *Ann Ophthalmol*. 1972;(4):103–112.
121. Gass JDM, Scelfo R. Diffuse unilateral subacute neuroretinitis. *J Roy Soc Med*. 1978;71:95–111.
122. Gass JDM, Braunstein RA. Further observations concerning the diffuse unilateral subacute neuroretinitis syndrome. *Arch Ophthalmol*. 1983;101:1689–1697.
123. Parson HE. Nematode chorioretinitis: report of a case with photographs of a viable worm. *Arch Ophthalmol*. 1952;(47):799–800.
124. Anshu A, Chee SP. Diffuse unilateral subacute neuroretinitis. *Int Ophthalmol*. 2008;28(2):127–129.
125. Vedantham V, Vats MM, Kakade SJ, et al. Diffuse unilateral subacute neuroretinitis with unusual findings. *Am J Ophthalmol*. 2006;142(5):880–883.
126. Vianna RN, Onofre G, Ecard V, et al. Indocyanine green angiography in diffuse unilateral subacute neuroretinitis. *Eye*. 2006;20(9):1113–1116.
127. Küchle M, Knorr HL, Medenblik-Frysch S, et al. Diffuse unilateral subacute neuroretinitis syndrome in a German most likely caused by the raccoon roundworm, *Baylisascaris procyonis*. *Graefes Arch Clin Exp Ophthalmol*. 1993;231:48–51.
128. Naumann GOH, Knorr HLJ. DUSN occurs in Europe. Letter to the Editor. *Ophthalmology*. 1994;101(6):971–972.

129. Cunha de Souza E, Lustosa da Cunha S, Gass JDM. Diffuse unilateral subacute neuroretinitis in South America. *Arch Ophthalmol.* 1992;110:1261 1263.
130. Cai J, Wei R, Zhu L, et al. Diffuse unilateral subacute neuroretinitis in China. *Arch Ophthalmol.* 2000;118:721–722.
131. Cialdini AP, Cunha de Souza E, Avila MP. The first South American case of diffuse unilateral subacute neuroretinitis caused by a large nematode. *Arch Ophthalmol.* 1999;117:1431–1432.
132. Garcia CA, Sabrosa NA, Gomes AB, et al. Diffuse unilateral subacute neuroretinitis—DUSN. *Int Ophthalmol Clin.* 2008;48(3):119–129.
133. Kazacos KR, Vestre WA, Kazacos EA, et al. Diffuse unilateral subacute neuroretinitis syndrome: a probable cause. *Arch Ophthalmol.* 1984;102:967–968.
134. Kazacos KR, Raymond LA, Kazacos EA, et al. The raccoon ascarid: a probable cause of human ocular larva migrans. *Ophthalmology.* 1985;(92):1735–1744.
135. Goldberg MA, Kazacos KR, Boyce WM, et al. Diffuse unilateral subacute neuroretinitis. Morphologic, serologic, and epidemiologic support for *Baylisascaris* as a causative agent. *Ophthalmology.* 1993;100:1695–1701.
136. Cunha de Souza E, Nakashima Y. Diffuse unilateral subacute neuroretinitis. Report of transvitreal surgical removal of a subretinal nematode. *Ophthalmology.* 1995;102:1183–1186.
137. Souza EC, Casella AM, Nakashima Y, et al. Clinical features and outcomes of patients with diffuse unilateral subacute neuroretinitis treated with oral albendazole. *Am J Ophthalmol.* 2005;140(3):437–445.
138. Raymond LA, Gutierrez Y, Strong LE, et al. Living retinal nematode destroyed by photocoagulation. *Ophthalmology.* 1978;85:944–949.
139. Venkatesh P, Sarkar S, Garg S. Diffuse unilateral subacute neuroretinitis: report of a case from the Indian subcontinent and the importance of immediate photocoagulation. *Int Ophthalmol.* 2005;26(6):251–254.
140. Garcia CA, Gomes AH, Garcia Filho CA, et al. Early-stage diffuse unilateral subacute neuroretinitis: improvement of vision after photocoagulation of the worm. *Eye.* 2004;18(6):624–627.
141. Garcia CA, Gomes AH, Vianna RN, et al. Late-stage diffuse unilateral subacute neuroretinitis: photocoagulation of the worm does not improve the visual acuity of affected patients. *Int Ophthalmol.* 2005;26(1–2):39–42.
142. Garcia CA, de Oliveira AG, de Lima CE, et al. Retinal nerve fiber layer analysis using GDx in 49 patients with chronic phase DUSN. *Arq Bras Oftalmol.* 2006;69(5):631–635.
143. Muccioli C, Belfort RJ. Hypopyon in a patient with presumptive diffuse unilateral subacute neuroretinitis. *Ocul Immunol Inflamm.* 2000;8(2):119–121.
144. Myint K, Sahay R, Mon S, et al. "Worm in the eye": the rationale for treatment of DUSN in south India. *Br J Ophthalmol.* 2006;90(9):1125–1127.
145. Matsumoto BT, Adelberg DA, Del Priore LV. Transretinal membrane formation in diffuse unilateral subacute neuroretinitis. *Retina.* 1995;15:146–149.
146. McDonald HR, Kazacos KR, Schatz H, et al. Two cases of intraocular infection with *Alaria mesocercaria* (Trematoda). *Am J Ophthalmol.* 1994;177(4):447–455.
147. Cunha de Souza E, Abujamra, Nakashima S, Gass Y. JDM Diffuse bilateral subacute neuroretinitis. *Arch Ophthalmol.* 1999;117:1349–1351.
148. Hertle RW, Spellman R. The eye disease of Jefferson Davis (1808–1889). *Surv Ophthalmol.* 2006;51(6):596–600.
149. Hidayet AA, Nalbandian RM, Sammons DW, et al. The diagnostic histopathologic features of ocular malaria. *Ophthalmology.* 1993;100:1183–1186.
150. Hirneiss C, Klauss V, Wilke M, et al. Ocular changes in tropical malaria with cerebral involvement—results from the Blantyre Malaria Project. *Klin Monatsbl Augenheilkd.* 2005;222(9):704–708. [in German].
151. Biswas J, Fogla R, Srinivasan P, et al. Ocular malaria. A clinical and histopathologic study. *Ophthalmology.* 1996;103:1471–1475.
152. Malla OK. *Endophthalmitis probably caused by Tussock moth. Report of the Proceedings of the First National Seminar on Prevention of Blindness. Kathmandu.* ; 1978:44.
153. Upadhyay MP, Rai NC, Ogg JE, et al. Seasonal hyperacute panuveitits of unknown etiology. *Ann Ophthalmol.* 1984;16:38–44.
154. Upadhyay MP, Rai NC, Ogg JE, et al. Seasonal hyperacute panuveitits. In: Saari K, ed. *Uveitis Update.* Amsterdam: Excerpta Medica; 1984: 257–262.
155. Byanju RN, Pradhan E, Rai SC, et al. Visual outcome of vitrectomy in seasonal hyperacute panuveitis. *Kathmandu Univ Med J.* 2003;1(2):121–123.
156. Botero D, Aguledo LM, Uribe FJ, et al. Intraocular filaria, a *Loaina* species, from a man in Columbia. *Am J Trop Med Hyg.* 1984;33:578–582.
157. Lee BY, McMillian R. *Loa loa:* ocular filariasis in an African student in Missouri. *Ann Ophthalmol.* 1984;16:456–458.
158. Padgett JJ, Jacobsen KH. Loiasis: African eye worm. *Trans Roy Soc Trop Med Hyg.* 2008;102(10):983–989.
159. Tuder RC, Blair E. *Gnathostoma spinigerum:* an unusual cause of ocular nematodiasis in the western hemisphere. *Am J Ophthalmol.* 1971;(72):185–190.
160. Bathrick ME, Mango CA, Mueller JF. Intraocular gnathostomiasis. *Ophthalmology.* 1981;88:1293–1295.
161. Singalavanija A, Wangspa S, Teschareon S. Intravitreal angostrongyliasis. *Aust NZ J Ophthalmol.* 1986;14:381–384.
162. Matsuo T, Notohara K, Shiraga F, et al. Endogenous amoebic endophthalmitis. *Arch Ophthalmol.* 2001;119:125–128.
163. Newton JC, Kanchanaranya C, Previte LR. Intraocular *Schistosoma mansoni. Am J Ophthalmol.* 1968;65:774–778.
164. Mougeot G, Cambon M, Menerath JM, et al. Human eye anterior chamber sparganosis. *Parasite.* 1999;6:365–366.
165. Kannan KA, Vasantha K, Venugopal M. Intraocular gnathostomiasis. *Indian J Ophthalmol.* 1999;47(4):252–253.
166. Blanche P, Gombert B, Rivoal O, et al. Uveitis due to *Leishmania major* as part of HAART-induced immune restitution syndrome in a patient with AIDS. *Clin Infect Dis.* 2002;34(9):1279–1280.
167. Mathai E, David S. Intraocular filariasis due to *Wuchereria bancrofti. Trans Roy Soc Trop Med Hyg.* 2000;94:317–318.
168. Vedy J, Carrica A, Rivaud C, et al. A propos d'un cas de retinite chez un bilharzien. *Med Trop.* 1979;39:603–609.
169. Behrens-Baumann W, Freissler G. Retinochoroidopathy in a patient with seropositive trichinosis. *Klin Monatsbl Augenheilkd.* 1991;119:114–117.
170. Muftuoglu G, Cicik E, Ozdamar A, et al. Vitreoretinal surgery for a subretinal hydatid cyst. *Am J Ophthalmol.* 2001;132:435–437.
171. Gupta A, Agarwal A, Dogra MR. Retinal involvement in *Wucheria bancrofti* filariasis. *Acta Ophthalmol Copenh.* 1992;(70):832–835.
172. Ramos A, Cruz I, Muñez E, et al. Post-kala-azar dermal leishmaniasis and uveitis in an HIV-positive patient. *Infection.* 2008;36(2):184–186.

19

Postsurgical Uveitis

Alan G. Palestine

KEY CONCEPTS

- The causes of postoperative inflammation are divided into those occurring acutely and those occurring after 6 weeks.
- Bacterial infections are the most common, but fungal endophthalmitis may also occur sometime after surgery.
- Lens-induced uveitis may occur spontaneously in an eye with a hypermature lens or after ocular trauma or cataract surgery.
- Postoperative noninfectious inflammation that persists longer than 3 months occurs in a small subset of postsurgical patients.

Intraocular inflammation can occur after any ocular surgical procedure. It is especially important in the postoperative patient to differentiate infectious causes of uveitis from other causes of intraocular inflammation because bacterial and fungal endophthalmitis require prompt treatment with specific antimicrobial therapy. The major causes of postsurgical uveitis are listed in Box 19.1.

Patients with a pre-existing uveitis often experience exacerbation of intraocular inflammation after surgery. The flare-up usually occurs 3 days to a week postoperatively in patients who receive subconjunctival corticosteroids at the end of the surgical procedure. In patients who do not receive steroids, the inflammation may occur earlier. Patients with a history of uveitis undergoing retinal detachment repair develop more proliferative vitreoretinopathy (PVR) compared with other patients but have an overall similar prognosis.[1] Occasionally, uveitis occurring after cataract surgery can be severe enough to be confused with infectious endophthalmitis, although hypopyon and severe pain are rare in patients with noninfectious postsurgical uveitis. In contrast, low-grade intraocular inflammation is common after many ocular procedures, especially after cataract extraction. This inflammation appears to be mediated by prostaglandins and can be inhibited by prostaglandin inhibitors.[2] In contrast, a rat model of bacterial endophthalmitis showed that a wide range of proinflammatory cytokines are released, including tumor necrosis factor (TNF)-α, interleukin (IL)-1β, and the rat equivalent of IL-8.[3] A better idea that is emerging is that of host/pathogen interactions during these severe infections[4]; the eye upregulates αB crystallin in an attempt to prevent apoptosis of the retinal cells.[5] However, some infectious agents, such as *Propionibacterium acnes,* may produce low-grade postsurgical endophthalmitis, which may take months to develop.

There are many options for the management of patients with uveitis undergoing ocular surgery. A common paradigm is for the eye to be quiet for 3 months before surgery. However, the perioperative corticosteroid regimen varies among surgeons, with preoperative topical, periocular, and systemic drugs being used from a few days to 2 weeks before surgery. After surgery, tapering can be tailored to the inflammatory response. It is unclear whether patients with a distant history of uveitis require prophylactic preoperative corticosteroids, and there are no clear guidelines as to the risk of uveitis recurrence in patients whose condition has been controlled with long-term systemic immunosuppressive therapy. Likewise, we do not have strong data regarding the risk of posterior uveitic recurrence after ocular surgery, although patients with anterior or intermediate uveitis appear to be at the highest risk for postsurgical complications. A patient with active uveitis with a dense cataract and iris bombé, similar to the one shown in Fig. 19.1, would need several months of therapy before cataract surgery. However, if urgent surgery for glaucoma or retinal detachment is needed, an intensive course of oral, periocular, intraocular, and systemic corticosteroid therapy would be needed and surgery cannot be delayed for the customary 3 months of quiescence.

ACUTE BACTERIAL ENDOPHTHALMITIS

Most cases of bacterial endophthalmitis occur after intraocular surgery and are considered surgical emergencies. Fortunately, postoperative endophthalmitis is a rare condition. Allen and Mangiaracine[6] reported 22 occurrences (0.11%) of endophthalmitis in a series of 20,000 ocular operations and 9 occurrences (0.056%) in a second series of 16,000 operations.[7] The overall prevalence has been estimated to be 0.07%.[8] Postkeratoplasty endophthalmitis is associated with grafts obtained from those who die in hospital as a result of cancer.[9] The rate of endophthalmitis after pars plana vitrectomy is low, reported at 0.039%,[10] with the incidence of infection after 20- and 25-gauge vitrectomies being similar (0.03%).[11] However, visual outcome in these cases is usually not good. For cataract extraction, older studies have suggested a rate between 0.07% and 0.12%[12,13]; 75% of patients present within 11 days of cataract surgery or a secondary implant.[14] West et al.[15] have suggested that the rate has been increasing over the years, from 0.1% in the 1990s to 0.2% for the period 2000–2003. Ng et al.[16] reported that in their series, 48% of cases with endophthalmitis secondary to cataract surgery occurred after phacoemulsification and 39% after planned extracapsular extraction. In Sweden, the rate was calculated to be 0.048%, with a higher rate seen with the clear cornea approach (0.053%) versus the sclerocorneal approach (0.036%); the difference was statistically significantly different.[17] Thoms et al.[18] reviewed 815 cases of cataract extraction with the clear cornea approach, almost equally divided into sutured and unsutured groups, and found that there were five cases of culture-positive endophthalmitis in the unsutured group and none in the sutured group ($P = 0.022$). In addition, those who did not receive topical antibiotics until the day after surgery and those who did not receive 5% povidone-iodine drops immediately after wound closure were found to be at greater risk. In a survey sent to 4000 members of the American Society of Cataract and Refractive Surgery (ASCRS), of the 1312 who responded, 30% reported that they used intracameral antibiotics either via injection or in the irrigating solution.[19] Wound problems appear to be an important contributing factor in about 25% of occurrences of endophthalmitis,[20] and infectious endophthalmitis may be a more common problem after glaucoma surgery, with late-onset endophthalmitis after trabeculectomy and antimetabolites seen

BOX 19.1 Causes of Postoperative Intraocular Inflammation

Day 1 to Day 30 Post Operation

Acute aerobic bacterial endophthalmitis
Sterile endophthalmitis
Increased activity of previous uveitis
Phacogenic (lens-related) uveitis
Toxic reaction to intraocular lens

Day 15 to 2 Years Post Operation

Fungal endophthalmitis
Endophthalmitis caused by *Propionibacterium acnes* or other anaerobic organisms
Endophthalmitis caused by low-virulence aerobic bacteria
Phacogenic (lens-related) uveitis
Sympathetic ophthalmia
Toxic reaction to intraocular lens
Iris–ciliary body irritation related to physical contact with intraocular lens
Glaucoma drainage device
Persistent anterior uveitis after ocular surgery
New onset of idiopathic uveitis

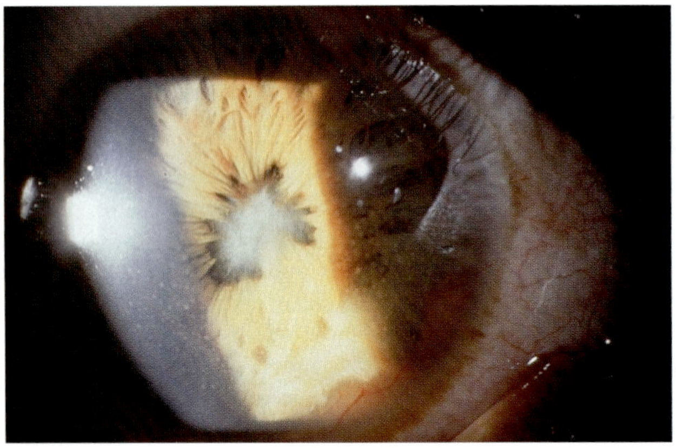

Fig. 19.1 Active granulomatous uveitis with keratic precipitates, posterior synechia, iris bombé, and a dense cataract.

in 2.7% to 8% of patients.[21-23] Other authors[24] have reported endophthalmitis associated with glaucoma drainage implants, usually as a result of exposure of the drainage tube. Kuang et al.[25] evaluated 988 trabeculectomy procedures performed over a 5-year period. In their experience, there was one case of early endophthalmitis, but there were six cases (0.6%) that had a late onset. Mitomycin use increased the risk of late-onset infection. It has been reported after Ahmad valve placement. Endophthalmitis was noted in one study in nine (1.7%) of 542 eyes, and the rate was five times higher in children.[26]

The interval between surgery and the onset of inflammation is sometimes helpful in distinguishing bacterial endophthalmitis from other causes of postoperative inflammation. Most bacterial infections occur within 11 days after surgery, but the vast majority of these occur within 2 to 5 days. Pain and diminished vision are accompanied by conjunctival hyperemia, chemosis, and lid edema. Anterior uveitis, with fibrin, hypopyon, and vitritis, is also characteristic of bacterial endophthalmitis. These symptoms and signs should prompt a diagnostic evaluation that includes culture of intraocular fluids, usually obtained via vitreous aspiration. Even in patients with endophthalmitis after anterior segment surgery, cultures of the vitreous yield positive results more frequently than those of the aqueous.[27] The most common organisms are the gram-positive ones, particularly coagulase-negative *Staphylococcus*.[28] Methicillin-resistant *Staphylococcus aureus* (MRSA) needs to be considered in the diagnosis. Deramo et al.[29] reported that in 64 cases of acute endophthalmitis secondary to cataract extraction, 33 of the 64 were culture positive, and 6 (18.2%) of the 33 showed MRSA. All were sensitive to gentamicin and vancomycin.

The management of bacterial endophthalmitis in the past included vitrectomy; intravitreal, systemic, subconjunctival, and topical antibiotics; and corticosteroids.[20,30] The approach to postoperative endophthalmitis was clarified by the results of the Endophthalmitis Vitrectomy Study,[31] in which all patients received intravitreal amikacin and vancomycin. One group was randomized to pars plana vitrectomy, and the other group received a vitreous tap. Each of these larger groups was further subdivided into those who received systemic antibiotics and those who did not. In general, patients did reasonably well in terms of visual results. It was noted that vitrectomy was helpful in patients presenting with poor vision. Systemic antibiotics did not seem to improve the outcome. Therefore the current approach is usually vitrectomy and the use of broad-spectrum antibiotics, such as vancomycin and ceftazidime or vancomycin and amikacin, given intravitreally.[32] Increasing numbers of surgeons have begun to deviate from the EVS guidelines, which initially suggested vitrectomy only if vision was restricted to hand motions only.[33] It is important to recognize that the EVS study made recommendations only for post–cataract surgery infections, and guidelines for the management of infections occurring after other types of surgery have often been extrapolated from these results without direct evidence.[34]

Only 50% to 75% of eyes with a clinical picture consistent with bacterial endophthalmitis will show positive bacterial culture results.[19] Polymerase chain reaction (PCR) analysis can be more specific in these situations, often with pan-bacterial 16S ribosomal deoxyribonucleic acid (rDNA) gene primers or cytochrome P-450L primers for fungi.[35] PCR techniques have developed rapidly and have real clinical importance. Chiquet et al.[36] used eubacterial PCR primers for bacterial detection in 100 acute post–cataract surgery endophthalmitis cases. When they evaluated the detection rate of culture versus PCR, when using aqueous specimens, there was little difference from when a vitreous tap was used (38.2% versus 34.6%). However, with vitrectomy, the positivity rate was 70% for PCR versus 9% for culture. When PCR and culture were combined, the detection rate was 68% with a vitreous tap specimen, 72% with a vitrectomy specimen, and 47% from an aqueous specimen. Culture-negative infections have been presumed to be caused by bacteria that grow poorly in culture. However, a study by Lee in 2015 showed good agreement between bacterial cultures and the presence of 16S DNA detected on PCR analysis in culture-positive endophthalmitis, but they found no cases of culture-negative endophthalmitis, which were 16S PCR positive.[37] Furthermore, this study detected torque teno virus sequences in 57% of bacterial culture-positive specimens and 100% of culture-negative specimens but none in the control specimens. This raises the concern that acute bacterial endophthalmitis may be more complex than a simple postoperative bacterial infection.

These patients should, however, initially be treated as though they have bacterial endophthalmitis until their condition has improved or until other clinical information suggests an alternative diagnosis. Although sterile endophthalmitis can occur in the early postoperative period and may mimic a bacterial infection, the consequences of untreated bacterial endophthalmitis are so severe that culture and antibiotic therapy should not be delayed.

Patients with infections occurring after intraocular foreign bodies present a more complex problem. In a retrospective study of 589 cases of eyes with an intraocular foreign body, encountered over a 12-year period at the King Khaled Eye Hospital (Riyadh, Saudi Arabia),[38] 44 (7.5%) showed clinical evidence of endophthalmitis. A positive culture result, however, was obtained on 17 eyes. The question regarding prophylactic use of antibiotics to diminish the risk of infection in cases of intraocular foreign bodies was addressed by Soheilian et al.,[39] who performed a randomized study on 346 eyes with intraocular foreign bodies. In addition to receiving surgical treatment (repair of the globe and removal of the object), the eyes were randomized to receiving either 40 μg of gentamicin sulfate and 45 μg of clindamycin intravitreally or balanced salt solution (BSS) injected intravitreally; endophthalmitis developed in 8 of the 167 eyes receiving BSS compared with 1 of the 179 eyes in the antibiotic group. Some have questioned the specifics of the study,[40] but the larger issue regarding the value of antibiotics in these circumstances is supported.

Intravitreal injections are frequently used to treat many ocular diseases. Contamination from the ocular surface with secondary infection is thought to be the mechanism of postinjection acute infection. De Caro et al.[41] performed cultures on specimens from sites and needles used in patients undergoing intravitreal injections and found that 2% (2 of 114) of the needles were contaminated by bacteria. Injection site prophylaxis does make a big difference, with positive culture results found in 43% of the sites without betadine prophylaxis and 13% in sites that received prophylaxis. Although endophthalmitis has been reported after bevacizumab intravitreal injections,[42] in one study of 5233 consecutive injections, only one case of acute endophthalmitis was found.[43] Other studies have reported rates between 0.039%[44] and 0.09%.[45] It has been suggested that not talking during administration of the injection decreases the risk of infection, but complete agreement on the best practices to prevent this type of infection is lacking.[46] There is no role for preinjection antibiotics. Postinjection infections present similarly to postsurgical infections, but usually within a few days of injection. The current management approach is vitreous aspiration for culture combined with intravitreal injection of vancomycin and ceftazidime.

CHRONIC BACTERIAL ENDOPHTHALMITIS

Although most patients with postoperative bacterial endophthalmitis present with acute onset of severe inflammation, loss of vision, and pain, some bacteria can cause chronic indolent intraocular infection. These organisms are more difficult to culture and grow more slowly.

Propionibacterium acnes (now renamed *Cutibacterium acnes*) has been recognized as an organism that can cause chronic postoperative uveitis, especially after cataract extraction with intraocular lens placement.[47-49] It has also been reported after cataract extraction and Molteno placement in a 7-year-old with congenital glaucoma.[50] The typical patient with *P. acnes* endophthalmitis presents with chronic low-grade anterior segment inflammation, which starts from 2 months to 2 years after cataract surgery. Topical corticosteroids often suppress the inflammation early in the course of the disease but do not prevent the protracted low-grade inflammatory response. Hence the inflammation resembles chronic intermediate uveitis. White plaques composed of bacteria are often seen between the intraocular lens and the posterior capsule or on the intraocular lens haptics (Fig. 19.2). The clinical course of *P. acnes* endophthalmitis may resemble that of pseudophakic phacoanaphylaxis,[51,52] and it is not clear whether some of these patients actually had undiagnosed *P. acnes* infections.

In addition to the predominance of polymorphonuclear cells, the inflammatory infiltrate in eyes with *P. acnes* endophthalmitis includes a large number of macrophages (10%–15%).[53] The presence of residual lens material in some patients suggests that lens-induced uveitis may be contributing to the inflammation.[48,52] Others have suggested

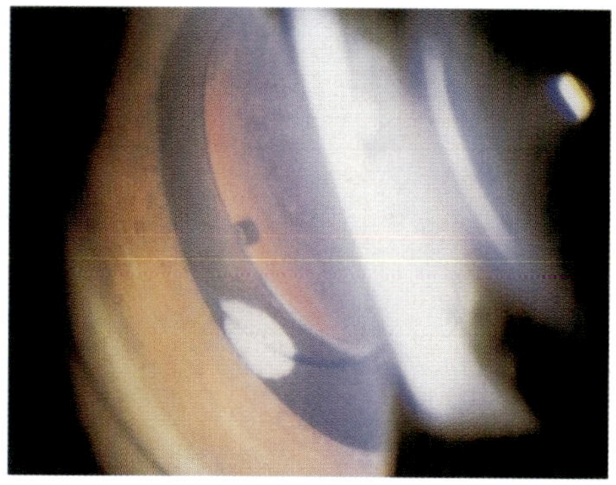

Fig. 19.2 Infiltrate on lens haptic in patient with late-onset postoperative endophthalmitis caused by *Propionibacterium acnes.* (From Murase KH, Goto H, Kezuka T, et al. A case of lens induced uveitis following metastatic endophthalmitis. *Jpn J Ophthalmol.* 2007;51(4):304–306, with permission.)

CASE 19.1

A 66-year-old woman underwent bilateral extracapsular cataract surgery, followed by posterior chamber intraocular lens implantation. The two surgical procedures were performed 6 weeks apart. After surgery, the patient's visual acuity was 20/20 in each eye. Two months after surgery, anterior uveitis developed in the right eye, and white material was noted on the polypropylene lens haptic (see Fig. 19.2).

The anterior uveitis initially resolved with administration of topical and periocular corticosteroids. However, the patient had recurrent episodes of uveitis, and eventually a hypopyon and vitritis developed. The intraocular lens was removed and replaced with a new one. Bacterial and fungal culture results were reported as negative. The intraocular inflammation persisted despite therapy with oral corticosteroids. Repeat aqueous and vitreous cultures were performed, and both results were positive for *Propionibacterium acnes* 5 days after inoculation. Cytologic examination of the specimens showed macrophages and neutrophils, with few lymphocytes. The patient received intravitreal cefazolin and intravenous cephalexin. Two weeks later, there was a moderate amount of persistent inflammation and a second intravitreal injection of cefazolin was given. The inflammation resolved, and the patient's vision improved to 20/20.

that *P. acnes* immunopotentiation may be the result of inhibition of suppressor T cells caused by stimulated macrophages.[54]

Diagnosis of *P. acnes* endophthalmitis is based on culture results. It is important to instruct the microbiology laboratory not to discard the cultures after the usual 3 to 4 days because the organism is slow growing, and cultures should be maintained by the laboratory for 14 days before they are read as negative. Therapy for *P. acnes* endophthalmitis usually involves a combination of vitrectomy, posterior capsulectomy, intravitreal vancomycin, and sometimes systemic cephalosporins. Although the intraocular lens does not need to be removed at the time of initial therapy, recurrent disease is managed with repeat courses of intravitreal antibiotics and removal of the residual posterior capsule and the intraocular lens. Clark et al.[55] reported the following results in their study of eyes with *P. acnes:* 100% of eyes treated with intraocular antibiotics only had persistent disease; 50% of eyes treated with pars plana vitrectomy and antibiotics had persistent disease; and 14% of eyes treated with pars plana vitrectomy, antibiotics, and subtotal capsulotomy had persistent disease. None of the eyes receiving total capsulotomy and removal of the intraocular lens had recurrent disease.

Despite the delay in diagnosis and therapy for this chronic endophthalmitis, the visual prognosis is usually good. *P. acnes* infection has been reported after Ahmed valve placement (Case 19.1).[56] Other

TABLE 19.1 **Characteristics of Fungal Infections (Postsurgical and Endogenous)**

Organism	Risk Factors	Ocular Characteristics
Candida sp.	Intravenous (IV) drug use, chronic IV therapy, surgery	Yellow-white chorioretinal lesions, vitreous fluff balls
Aspergillus sp.	IV drug use, immunosuppression, surgery	Yellow-white chorioretinal lesions, vitreous fluff balls
Coccidioides immitis	Residence in southwestern United States	Multiple yellow-white chorioretinal lesions, punched-out choroidal lesions; often associated with pulmonary *C. immitis* infection
Cryptococcus neoformans	Immunosuppression, lymphoma	Small or large yellow-white chorioretinal lesions; often associated with meningitis
Histoplasma capsulatum	Immunosuppression	Panuveitis with iris involvement
Sporotrichum schenckii	Horticulturists	Panuveitis
Blastomyces dermatitidis	Systemic North American blastomycosis	Panuveitis or multiple small chorioretinal lesions

organisms, including *Propionibacterium granulosum, Achromobacter, Pseudomonas oryzihabitans,*[57] *Mycobacterium,*[58] and *Staphylococcus epidermidis* may also cause chronic bacterial endophthalmitis.[59] However, in addition to these bacteria, fungal endophthalmitis may also cause chronic smoldering postoperative intraocular inflammation.

FUNGAL ENDOPHTHALMITIS

Fungal endophthalmitis is a relatively rare condition; however, as diagnostic abilities improve, the incidence of this condition appears to be increasing. Studies show that fungi account for 8% to 13% of culture-positive isolates; in some reports, the *Candida* species predominate[20,27] and *Aspergillus* in others.[60] Fungal infections may not become symptomatic until months after surgery. They often start with low-grade iridocyclitis or vitritis, and some may have corneal involvement.[60] Symptoms of blurred vision, redness, and pain gradually increase. Corticosteroid therapy can temporarily alleviate the symptoms, giving the impression that this condition is not infectious. With time, the infection progresses, and "fluff balls" may form in the vitreous in addition to the occurrence of anterior uveitis and vitritis. A discrete fungal mass may be present in the vitreous or in the anterior chamber in some eyes.[61] There may be a "string of pearls" in the posterior segment, a mass in the iris, corneal infiltrate, or necrotizing scleritis.[62] The risk factors for and the ocular characteristics of postoperative and endogenous fungal infections are listed in Table 19.1.

Untreated fungal endophthalmitis leads to blindness. Even after the correct diagnosis is made, treatment initiated late in the course of the disease may not successfully restore vision. In one study only 42% of eyes had a visual acuity of 20/400 or better after treatment for fungal endophthalmitis.[61] Patients who present early with good visual acuity (better than 20/60) have a more favorable visual prognosis.[61] Infections by *Acremonium* or *Fusarium* are associated with a poorer prognosis. Some fungal infections are difficult to eliminate from the eye even with vitrectomy and removal of the intraocular lens and the lens capsule.

Fungal endophthalmitis should be suspected in all patients with postoperative inflammation that occurs weeks to months after surgery. Rarely, fungal infection may occur within 1 week after the surgical procedure. If fungal infection is suspected, it is helpful to pass part of the vitreous specimen through a Millipore filter and to culture the filter as a method of concentrating the organisms. Fungal organisms do not stain well on Gram staining. One needs to search for these organisms by using either the Giemsa stain or the Gomori methenamine silver stain. It can take several weeks for the cultures to grow, and *Candida, Fusarium,* and *Aspergillus* are the most common causes of the disorder. The use of Cellufluor or Calcofluor white staining techniques on vitreous samples allows for rapid identification of fungal elements and has improved diagnostic speed and accuracy.[63] As with bacterial conditions, PCR analysis is being employed more and more often, with as much usefulness as has been shown in bacterial disease. In one study of 50 cases of nonbacterial endophthalmitis, six cases were detected by using panfungal primers (ITS1 and ITS4).[64]

Antifungal therapy combined with vitrectomy and removal of an intraocular lens offers the best chances of a favorable outcome. Some patients have been successfully managed without intraocular lens removal, especially those with *Candida* endophthalmitis.[61,65] Intravitreal and intravenous amphotericin B, intravitreal and oral voriconazole, oral fluconazole, and oral flucytosine are used to treat the infection. Because of its lower toxicity, voriconazole, 100 μg intravitreally, is preferred over amphotericin. Five to 10 μg of amphotericin B can be used as well; this dose can be repeated once, if needed. Intraocular miconazole (25–50 μg) can be used in patients not responding to treatment with amphotericin B. Topical and subconjunctival antifungal agents may be used in infections that involve the cornea. Oral flucytosine is useful in candidal infections that are not resistant to this drug.

ENDOGENOUS ENDOPHTHALMITIS

The majority of these cases occur in patients with intravenous drug use or chronic intravenous catheters, but this disorder increasingly needs to be considered because more patients with altered immune states are being seen. At present, they account for a small number, 5% to 7%, of documented cases.[66] Most series have shown that the majority of these cases are fungal infections, but a large minority of cases are bacterial in origin.[67-70] Vitreous aspirates usually yield negative results, and even vitrectomy cultures can show negative results. The diagnosis is most often made when vitritis and vitreous fluff balls are seen in a patient with fungemia. A change in vision in any patient with sepsis should raise concerns regarding endogenous endophthalmitis. Routine screening of patients with fungemia has a low yield for discovery of endogenous fungal endophthalmitis.[71] Schiedler et al.[69] reviewed 21 eyes with culture-proven endogenous endophthalmitis, and fungal isolates were found in 13 of them. Six of these patients died within 2 months of the diagnosis. Perhaps as a harbinger of the future, Agarwal et al.[72] reported the case of a 65-year-old woman who experienced gradual loss of vision in the right eye during treatment with infliximab (3 mg/kg). Gram-positive cocci were cultured from the eye. Some of the factors predisposing to endogenous endophthalmitis include immunosuppressive therapy, acquired immunodeficiency syndrome

(AIDS), systemic autoimmune disease, intravenous hyperalimentation, malignancy, diabetes, intravenous drug use, and hematologic disorders[67] (Box 19.2). Because the infection in these cases originates in the choroid and spreads to the vitreous and the majority of cases are of fungal origin, systemic antifungal therapy is often sufficient.[73] Intravitreal drugs and vitrectomy may be helpful in treating bacterial infections and the more severe or nonresponsive ones.[73]

LENS-INDUCED UVEITIS

Phacoanaphylactic (phacoantigenic) uveitis is a granulomatous inflammatory response that is thought to represent an immunologic reaction against lens proteins released after surgical or traumatic disruption of the lens capsule. The term *phacoanaphylactic uveitis* is somewhat of a misnomer because the reaction is not an anaphylactoid or type I hypersensitivity reaction. This form of lens-induced uveitis is differentiated from nongranulomatous phacogenic (phacotoxic) uveitis, although there is no evidence to support the theory that lens degradation products are directly toxic to the eye.[74,75] It now appears that all these entities may represent varying severities of the same immunologic process that is better termed *lens-induced uveitis*.

BOX 19.2 Factors Putting Patients at Higher Risk for Endogenous Endophthalmitis

- Acquired immunodeficiency syndrome (AIDS)
- Intravenous drug use
- Intravenous hyperalimentation
- Indwelling catheters
- Diabetes mellitus
- Cancer
- Hemodialysis
- Immunosuppression for autoimmune disease and transplantation
- Bone marrow suppression
- Hepatic disease
- Postpartum status
- Underlying systemic autoimmune disease

Lens-induced uveitis may occur spontaneously in an eye with a hypermature lens or after ocular trauma or cataract surgery. It may occur under rather unusual circumstances. One such example is a case of lens-induced uveitis occurring after metastatic endophthalmitis secondary to septic pneumonia. Six months after the event, the patient experienced pain and decreasing vision; this led to enucleation, which demonstrated changes compatible with this disease[76] (Fig. 19.3). A number of researchers have reported a high incidence of lens-induced uveitis after sympathetic ophthalmia.[74,75] However, isolated lens-induced uveitis is usually uniocular, occurring after recent surgery; sympathetic ophthalmia is a bilateral disease.[77] The inflammation may occur hours or months after disruption of the lens capsule. Granulomatous keratic precipitates, anterior chamber cells and flare, and occasionally a hypopyon may be seen.

The inflammation can be severe and associated with both anterior uveitis and vitritis. Removal of all residual lens material is usually curative. Response to the administration of corticosteroids is poor. If some lens material is found to be mixed with the vitreous, vitrectomy may be indicated. Lens-induced uveitis was rare in the 1960s when intracapsular cataract surgery was performed but became more common with extracapsular cataract extraction. Improved surgical techniques in which all lens material is removed have significantly decreased the incidence of this condition. Lens-induced uveitis may be difficult to distinguish clinically from chronic endophthalmitis, such as that caused by *P. acnes* infection[47,48]; therefore culture specimens should be obtained from most eyes with chronic postoperative intraocular inflammation. Some authors have proposed the use of modified Papanicolaou or May-Grunwald-Giemsa staining of the aqueous cytospin or thin prep to guide the diagnosis.[78]

TOXIC ANTERIOR SEGMENT SYNDROME

Toxic anterior segment syndrome (TASS) is a sterile postoperative inflammatory response to noninfectious agents entering the anterior chamber.[79] It is usually seen early—2 days or less—after anterior segment surgery. Initially, the entity was seen with early intraocular lenses. These lenses were associated with a variety of toxic reactions caused by problems with lens material. Some causes of intraocular lens–related uveitis included reactions against metal haptics,[52] impurities on the

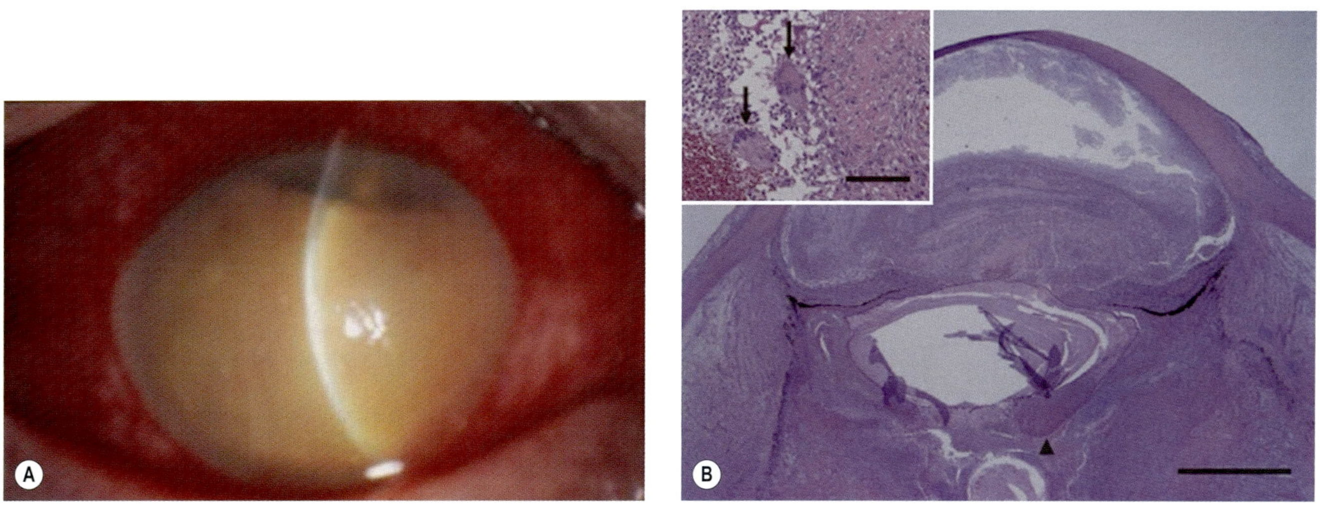

Fig. 19.3 (A) Eye of patient who developed a severe anterior chamber immune response 6 months after suffering from metastatic endophthalmitis secondary to septic pneumonia. The eye was enucleated. (B) Histopathology of eye showing phacoanaphylaxis. (From Murase KH, Goto H, Kezuka T, et al. A case of lens-induced uveitis following metastatic endophthalmitis. *Jpn J Ophthalmol.* 2007;51(4):304–306, with permission.)

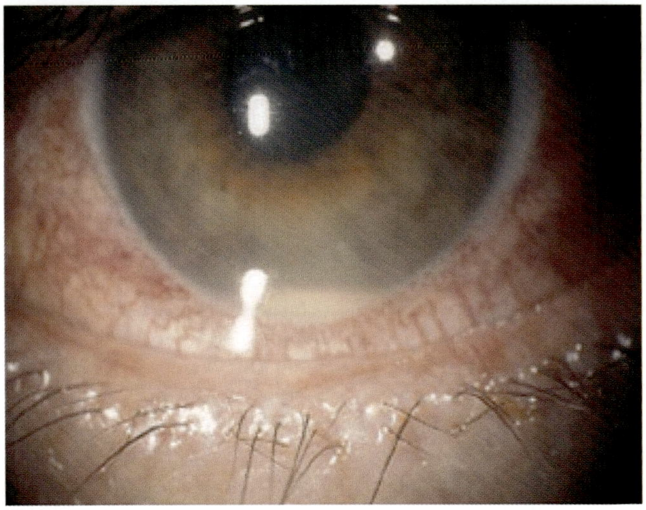

Fig. 19.4 Example of toxic anterior segment syndrome. (From Mamalis N, Edelhauser HF, Dawson DG, et al. Toxic anterior segment syndrome. *J Cataract Refract Surg.* 2006;32(2):324–333, with permission.)

lens by the manufacturer,[68] certain methods of sterilization,[80] and degradation of lens haptics.[81] Although these reactions are usually not immunologically driven, the resultant tissue damage can then lead to prostaglandin and cytokine release and the recruitment of lymphocytes and other inflammatory cells into the eye. This secondary immune-mediated inflammation can often be more damaging than the initial toxic reaction to the intraocular lens.

Some old models of anterior chamber intraocular lenses were associated with the development of a syndrome characterized by uveitis, glaucoma, and hyphema (UGH syndrome).[82] Fortunately, UGH syndrome is uncommon with current anterior chamber intraocular lenses with flexible haptics, but a posterior intraocular lens that is not within the capsular bag can rub on the posterior iris or ciliary body causing mechanically induced inflammation. This is best detected by using ultrasonic biomicroscopy and with the presence of iris transillumination defects.

Intraocular lenses sometimes cause mild inflammation that leads to the accumulation of cellular deposits on the anterior surface of the lens.[10,14,83] These deposits are often composed of macrophages and giant cells but may be acellular,[58] and membranes are often associated with them. Clearly, most eyes tolerate a posterior chamber intraocular lens with little inflammation.[84] However, some patients have mild iridocyclitis, which can be seen histologically, even if the lens was clinically well tolerated.[85] Indeed, over the years, many causes of TASS have been recognized. These include the irrigating solutions or viscosurgical devices not at the correct pH or osmolality; incorrect chemical composition or residual preventatives; instrument contaminants; and intraocular lens contaminants, such as polishing, cleaning, and sterilizing materials (Fig. 19.4).

PERSISTENT POSTOPERATIVE ANTERIOR UVEITIS

Inflammation is commonly seen after ocular surgery and usually resolves within a month after surgery, aided by postoperative topical steroids and topical nonsteroidal drops. However, in some patients, this inflammation can persist for greater than 3 months after surgery and is termed *persistent anterior uveitis (PAU)*. In a 2018 study of endoscopic ciliary body photocoagulation for glaucoma, Edmiston noted that 22% of patients had PAU and that this was more common in blacks.[86] There was no difference in final visual acuity or intraocular pressure. Similarly, Reddy noted, in 2019, that 2% of eyes with uncomplicated phacoemulsification and intraocular lens insertion developed PAU and that black patients were 11-fold more likely to experience this complication.[87] There do not appear to be any other definable risk factors for the development of PAU except for intraoperative complications, such as a broken posterior capsule, vitreous loss, or lysis of synechia. Final visual acuity was not worse for patients with PAU, but 30% did develop postoperative cystoid macular edema.

LASER-INDUCED UVEITIS

Yttrium–aluminum–garnet (YAG) laser capsulotomy has been associated with low-grade inflammation.[88] The shock wave created by the laser is capable of causing a physical alteration in the blood–eye barrier. We have observed several patients with a history of ongoing intraocular inflammation in which YAG laser capsulotomy caused a significant increase in inflammation. In some patients, increased amounts of topical, periocular, or even systemic corticosteroids may be required at the time of the laser procedure. We encountered an unusual case of endophthalmitis that appeared to be induced by YAG laser iridectomy. The iridectomy was performed in this patient who had closed-angle glaucoma with minimal bleeding from an iris vessel. Two days after the procedure, the patient developed a hypopyon. Sepsis was diagnosed, and the same organism was grown in cultures of specimens from both the eye and blood.

In summary, there are many possible causes of postsurgical inflammatory eye disease, and it is important to distinguish among mechanical, immunologic, and infectious etiologies because each mechanism requires a specific treatment approach. Going forward, our understanding of infectious endophthalmitis will evolve as surgical techniques change and alter the risk factors for specific types of infections, leading to different treatment paradigms.[89]

REFERENCE

1. Slingsby TJ, Pecen PE, Palestine AG. Outcomes and complications associated with noninfectious uveitis in patients presenting with rhegmatogenous retinal detachment. *Ophthalmol Retina.* 2020;4(8): 823–828.
2. Huang K, Peyman GA, McGetrick J, et al. Indomethacin inhibition of prostaglandin mediated inflammation following intraocular surgery. *Invest Ophthalmol Vis Sci.* 1977;16:1760–1762.
3. Giese MJ, Sumner HL, Berliner JA, et al. Cytokine expression in a rat model of *Staphylococcus aureus* endophthalmitis. *Invest Ophthalmol Vis Sci.* 1998;39(13):2785–2790.
4. Callegan MC, Gilmore MS, Gregory M, et al. Bacterial endophthalmitis: therapeutic challenges and host-pathogen interactions. *Prog Retin Eye Res.* 2007;26(2):189–203.
5. Whiston EA, Sugi N, Kamradt MC, et al. αB-crystallin protects retinal tissue during *Staphylococcus aureus*-induced endophthalmitis. *Infect Immun.* 2008;76(4):1781–1790.
6. Allen HF, Mangiaracine AB. A study of 22 infections in 20,000 operations. *Arch Ophthalmol.* 1964;72:454–462.
7. Allen HF, Mangiaracine AB. Bacterial endophthalmitis after cataract extraction. II. Incidence in 36,000 consecutive operations with special reference to preoperative topical antibiotics. *Arch Ophthalmol.* 1974;91:3–7.
8. Kattan HM, Flynn HW Jr, Pflugfelder SC, et al. Nosocomial endophthalmitis survey. *Ophthalmology.* 1991;98:227–238.
9. Hassan SS, Wilhelmus KR, Dahl P, et al. Infectious disease risk factors of corneal graft donors. *Arch Ophthalmol.* 2008;126(2):235–239.
10. Eifrig DE. Deposits on the surface of intraocular lenses. *South Med J.* 1980;73:6–8.
11. Shimada H, Nakashizuka H, Hattori T, et al. Incidence of endophthalmitis after 20- and 25-gauge vitrectomy: causes and prevention. *Ophthalmology.* 2008;115(12):2215–2220.

12. Results of the Endophthalmitis Vitrectomy Study. A randomized trial of immediate vitrectomy and of intravenous antibiotics for the treatment of postoperative bacterial endophthalmitis. Endophthalmitis Vitrectomy Study Group. *Arch Ophthalmol.* 1995;113(12):1479–1496.
13. Javitt JC, Vitale S, Canner JK, et al. National outcome of cataract extraction. *Arch Ophthalmol.* 1991;109:1085–1089.
14. Berrocal AM, Davis JL. Uveitis following intraocular surgery. *Opthalmol Clin North Am.* 2002;15:357–364.
15. West ES, Behrens A, McDonnell PJ, et al. The incidence of endophthalmitis after cataract surgery among the U.S. Medicare population increased between 1994 and 2001. *Ophthalmology.* 2005;112(8):1388–1394.
16. Ng JQ, Morlet N, Pearman JW, et al. Management and outcomes of postoperative endophthalmitis since the Endophthalmitis Vitrectomy Study: the Endophthalmitis Population Study of Western Australia (EPSWA)'s fifth report. *Ophthalmology.* 2005;112(7):1199–1206.
17. Lundstrom M, Wejde G, Stenevi U, et al. Endophthalmitis after cataract surgery: a nationwide prospective study evaluating incidence in relation to incision type and location. *Ophthalmology.* 2007;114(5):866–870.
18. Thoms SS, Musch DC, Soong HK. Postoperative endophthalmitis associated with sutured versus unsutured clear corneal cataract incisions. *Br J Ophthalmol.* 2007;91(6):728–730.
19. Chang DF, Braga-Mele R, Mamalis N, et al. Prophylaxis of postoperative endophthalmitis after cataract surgery: results of the 2007 ASCRS member survey. *J Cataract Refract Surg.* 2007;33(10):1801–1805.
20. Driebe WT, Mandelbaum S, Forster RK, et al. Pseudophakic endophthalmitis: diagnosis and management. *Ophthalmology.* 1986;93:442–448.
21. Higgenbotham EJ, Stevens RK, Musch DC. Bleb-related endophthalmitis after trabeculectomy with mitomycin C. *Ophthalmology.* 1996;103:650–656.
22. Wolner B, Liebmann JM, Sassani JW, et al. Late bleb-related endophthalmitis after trabeculectomy with adjunctive 5-fluorouracil. *Ophthalmology.* 1991;98:1053–1060.
23. Katz IJ, Cantor LB, Spaeth GL. Complications of surgery in glaucoma: early and late bacterial endophthalmitis following glaucoma filtering surgery. *Ophthalmology.* 1985;92:959–963.
24. Gedde SJ, Scott IU, Tabandeh H, et al. Late endophthalmitis associated with glaucoma drainage implants. *Ophthalmology.* 2001;108:1323–1327.
25. Kuang TM, Lin YC, Liu CJ, et al. Early and late endophthalmitis following trabeculectomy in a Chinese population. *Eur J Ophthalmol.* 2008;18(1):66–70.
26. Al-Torbak AA, Al-Shahwan S, Al-Jadaan I, et al. Endophthalmitis associated with the Ahmed glaucoma valve implant. *Br J Ophthalmol.* 2005;89(4):454–458.
27. Forster RK, Zachary IG, Cottingham AJ Jr, et al. Further observation on the diagnosis, cause, and treatment of endophthalmitis. *Am J Ophthalmol.* 1976;81:52–56.
28. Han DP, Wisniewski SR, Kelsey SF, et al. Microbiologic yields and complication rates of vitreous needle aspiration versus mechanized vitreous biopsy in the Endophthalmitis Vitrectomy Study. *Retina.* 1999;19:98–102.
29. Deramo VA, Lai JC, Winokur J, et al. Visual outcome and bacterial sensitivity after methicillin-resistant *Staphylococcus aureus*-associated acute endophthalmitis. *Am J Ophthalmol.* 2008;145(3):413–417.
30. Weber DJ, Hoffman KL, Thoft RA, et al. Endophthalmitis following intraocular lens implantation. *Rev Infect Dis.* 1986;8:12–20.
31. Doft BH. Treatment of postcataract extraction endophthalmitis: a summary of the results from the Endophthalmitis Vitrectomy Study. *Arch Ophthalmol.* 2008;126(4):554–556.
32. Bron A. Le traitment curatif des endophtalmies aigues post chirurgicales. *J Fr Ophtalmol.* 1999;22:1076–1083.
33. Fliney GD, Pecen PE, Cathcart JN, Palestine AG. Trends in treatment strategies for suspected bacterial endophthalmitis. *Graefes Arch Clin Exp Ophthalmol.* 2018;256(4):833–838.
34. Palestine AG, Pecen PE. Infectious endophthalmitis in the current era. *Ophthalmol Retina.* 2020;4(6):553–554.
35. Okhravi N, Adamson P, Lightman S. Use of PCR in endophthalmitis. *Ocul Immunol Inflamm.* 2000;8:189–200.
36. Chiquet C, Cornut PL, Benito Y, et al. Eubacterial PCR for bacterial detection and identification in 100 acute postcataract surgery endophthalmitis. *Invest Ophthalmol Vis Sci.* 2008;49(5):1971–1978.
37. Lee AY, Akileswaran L, Tibbetts MD, Garg SJ, Van Gelder RN. Identification of torque teno virus in culture-negative endophthalmitis by representational deep DNA sequencing. *Ophthalmology.* 2015;122(3):524–530.
38. Chaudhry IA, Shamsi FA, Al-Harthi E, et al. Incidence and visual outcome of endophthalmitis associated with intraocular foreign bodies. *Graefes Arch Clin Exp Ophthalmol.* 2008;246(2):181–186.
39. Soheilian M, Rafati N, Mohebbi MR, et al. Prophylaxis of acute posttraumatic bacterial endophthalmitis: a multicenter, randomized clinical trial of intraocular antibiotic injection, report 2. *Arch Ophthalmol.* 2007;125(4):460–465.
40. Essex RW, Lamoureux E, Charles PG, et al. Prophylaxis for posttraumatic endophthalmitis. *Arch Ophthalmol.* 2008;126(5):742–743. Author reply 743–744.
41. de Caro JJ, Ta CN, Ho HK, et al. Bacterial contamination of ocular surface and needles in patients undergoing intravitreal injections. *Retina.* 2008;28(6):877–883.
42. Yenerel NM, Dinc UA, Gorgun E. A case of sterile endophthalmitis after repeated intravitreal bevacizumab injection. *J Ocul Pharmacol Ther.* 2008;24(3):362–363.
43. Mason JO 3rd, White MF, Feist RM, et al. Incidence of acute onset endophthalmitis following intravitreal bevacizumab (Avastin) injection. *Retina.* 2008;28(4):564–567.
44. Torres-Costa S, Ramos D, Brandão E, Carneiro Â, Rosas V, Rocha-Sousa A, Falcão-Reis F, Falcão M. Incidence of endophthalmitis after intravitreal injection with and without topical antibiotic prophylaxis. *Eur J Ophthalmol.* 2020 Feb 4. 1120672120902028. doi: 10.1177/1120672120902028. [Epub ahead of print].
45. Levinson JD, Garfinkel RA, Berinstein DM, Flory M, Spellman FA. Timing of povidone-iodine application to reduce the risk of endophthalmitis after intravitreal injections. *Ophthalmol Retina.* 2018;2(7):654–658.
46. Patel SN, Gangaputra S, Sternberg P Jr, Kim SJ. Prophylaxis measures for postinjection endophthalmitis. *Surv Ophthalmol.* 2020;65(4):408–420.
47. Meisler DM, Palestine AG, Vastine DW, et al. Chronic *Propionibacterium* endophthalmitis after extracapsular cataract and intraocular lens implantation. *Am J Ophthalmol.* 1986;102:733–739.
48. Roussel TJ, Culbertson WW, Jaffe NS. Chronic postoperative endophthalmitis associated with *Propionibacterium acnes. Arch Ophthalmol.* 1987;105(9):1199–1201.
49. Jaffe NS. *Propionibacterium acnes* and endophthalmitis seven months after extracapsular cataract extraction and intraocular lens implantation. *Ophthalmic Surg.* 1986;17:791–793.
50. Hollander DA, Dodds EM, Rossetti SB, et al. *Propionibacterium acnes* endophthalmitis with bacterial sequestration in a Molteno's implant after cataract extraction. *Am J Ophthalmol.* 2004;138(5):878–879.
51. Apple DJ, Mamalis N, Steinmetz RL, et al. Phacoanaphylactic endophthalmitis associated with extracapsular cataract extraction and posterior chamber intraocular lens. *Arch Ophthalmol.* 1984;102:1528–1532.
52. McMahon MS, Weiss JS, Riedel KG, et al. Clinically unsuspected phacoanaphylaxis after extracapsular cataract extraction with intraocular lens. *Br J Ophthalmol.* 1985;69:836–840.
53. Whitcup SM, Belfort R Jr, de Smet MD, et al. Immunohistochemistry of the inflammatory response in *Propionibacterium acnes* endophthalmitis. *Arch Ophthalmol.* 1991;109:978.
54. Maguire HCJ, Cipriano D. Immunopotentiation of cell-mediated hypersensitivity by *Corynebacterium parvum (Propionibacterium acnes). Int Arch Allergy Appl Immun.* 1983;70:34–39.
55. Clark WL, Kaiser PK, Flynn HW Jr, et al. Treatment strategies and visual acuity outcomes in chronic postoperative *Propionibacterium acnes* endophthalmitis. *Ophthalmology.* 1999;106:1665–1670.
56. Gutierrez-Diaz E, Montero-Rodríguez M, Mencía-Gutiérrez E, et al. *Propionibacterium acnes* endophthalmitis in Ahmed glaucoma valve. *Eur J Ophthalmol.* 2001;11:383–385.
57. Yu EN, Foster CS. Chronic postoperative endophthalmitis due to *Pseudomonas oryzihabitans. Am J Ophthalmol.* 2002;134:613–614.
58. Abu El-Asrar A, Tabbara K. Chronic endophthalmitis after extracapsular cataract extraction caused by *Mycobacterium chelonae* subspecies abscessus. *Eye.* 1995;9(6):798–801.
59. Flicker L, Meredith TA, Wilson LA, et al. Chronic bacterial endophthalmitis. *Am J Ophthalmol.* 1987;103:745–748.

60. Narang S, Gupta A, Gupta V, et al. Fungal endophthalmitis following cataract surgery: clinical presentation, microbiological spectrum, and outcome. *Am J Ophthalmol.* 2001;132(5):609–617.
61. Pflugfelder SC, Flynn HW Jr, Zwickey TA, et al. Exogenous fungal endophthalmitis. *Ophthalmology.* 1988;95:19–30.
62. Samson CM, Foster CS. Chronic postoperative endophthalmitis. *Int Ophthalmol Clin.* 2000;40:57–67.
63. Sutphin JE, Robinson NM, Wilhelmus KR, et al. Improved detection of oculomycoses using induced fluorescence with Cellufluor. *Ophthalmology.* 1986;93:416–417.
64. Tarai B, Gupta A, Ray P, et al. Polymerase chain reaction for early diagnosis of post-operative fungal endophthalmitis. *Indian J Med Res.* 2006;123(5):671–678.
65. Gilbert CM, Novak MA. Successful treatment of postoperative *Candida* endophthalmitis in an eye with an intraocular lens implant. *Am J Ophthalmol.* 1984;97:593–595.
66. Smith SR, Kroll AJ, Lou PL, et al. Endogenous bacterial and fungal endophthalmitis. *Int Ophthalmol Clin.* 2007;47(2):173–183.
67. Jackson TL, Eykyn SJ, Graham EM, et al. Endogenous bacterial endophthalmitis: a 17-year prospective series and review of 267 reported cases. *Surv Ophthalmol.* 2003;48(4):403–423.
68. Romero CF, Rai MK, Lowder CY, et al. Endogenous endophthalmitis: case report and brief review. *Am Fam Phys.* 1999;60(2):510–514.
69. Schiedler V, Scott IU, Flynn HW Jr, et al. Culture-proven endogenous endophthalmitis: clinical features and visual acuity outcomes. *Am J Ophthalmol.* 2004;137(4):725–731.
70. Zhang YQ, Wang WJ. Treatment outcomes after pars plana vitrectomy for endogenous endophthalmitis. *Retina.* 2005;25(6):746–750.
71. Wang K, Krishnan G, Pershing S. Ophthalmology consultation to detect endogenous endophthalmitis: clinical characteristics in consulted versus diagnosed cases among at-risk inpatients. *Ophthalmic Surg Lasers Imaging Retina.* 2020;51(3): 159-A3.
72. Agarwal PK, Gallaghar M, Murphy E, et al. Endogenous endophthalmitis in a rheumatoid patient on tumor necrosis factor alpha blocker. *Indian J Ophthalmol.* 2007;55(3):230–232.
73. Chhablani J. Fungal endophthalmitis. *Expert Rev Anti Infect Ther.* 2011;9(12):1191–1201.
74. Blodi FC. Sympathetic uveitis as an allergic phenomenon. *Trans Am Acad Ophthalmol Otolaryngol.* 1959;63:642–656.
75. Easom HA, Zimmerman LE. Sympathetic ophthalmia and bilateral phacoanaphylaxis. *Arch Ophthalmol.* 1964;72:9–15.
76. Murase KH, Goto H, Kezuka T, et al. A case of lens-induced uveitis following metastatic endophthalmitis. *Jpn J Ophthalmol.* 2007;51(4):304–306.
77. Meltzer DW. Sterile hypopyon following intraocular lens surgery. *Arch Ophthalmol.* 1980;98:100–104.
78. Kalogeropoulos CD, Malamou-Mitsi VD, Asproudis I, et al. The contribution of aqueous humor cytology in the differential diagnosis of anterior uvea inflammations. *Ocul Immunol Inflamm.* 2004;12(3):215–225.
79. Mamalis N, Edelhauser HF, Dawson DG, et al. Toxic anterior segment syndrome. *J Cataract Refract Surg.* 2006;32(2):324–333.
80. Stark WJ, Rosenblum P, Maumenee AE, et al. Postoperative inflammatory reactions to intraocular lens sterilized with ethylene oxide. *Ophthalmology.* 1980;87:385–389.
81. Krause U, Alanko HI. Dislocated intraocular lens after biodegradation of fixation loops. *Acta Ophthalmol.* 1986;64:338–343.
82. Ellington FT. The uveitis–glaucoma–hyphema syndrome associated with the Mark VIII anterior-chamber lens implant. *J Am Intraocul Implant Soc.* 1978;4:50–53.
83. Wolter JR, Sugar A, Meyer RF. Reactive membranes on posterior chamber lens implants. *Ophthalmic Surg.* 1985;16:699–702.
84. Crawford JB. A histopathologic study of the position of the Shearing intraocular lens in the posterior chamber. *Am J Ophthalmol.* 1981;91:458–461.
85. McDonnell PJ, Green WR, Maumenee AE, et al. Pathology of intraocular lenses in 33 eyes examined postmortem. *Ophthalmology.* 1983;90:386–403.
86. Edmiston AM, SooHoo JR, Seibold LK, Kahook MY, Palestine AG, Pantcheva MB. Postoperative inflammation after endoscopic cyclophotocoagulation: racial distribution and effect on outcomes. *J Glaucoma.* 2018;27:266–268.
87. Reddy AK, Patnaik JL, Miller DC, Lynch AM, Palestine AG, Pantcheva MB. Risk factors associated with persistent anterior uveitis after cataract surgery. *Am J Ophthalmol.* 2019;206:82–86.
88. Flohr MJ, Robin A, Kelley JS. Early complications following Q-switched neodymium YAG laser posterior capsulotomy. *Ophthalmology.* 1985;92:360–363.
89. Palestine AG, Pecen PE. Infectious endophthalmitis in the current era. *Ophthalmol Retina.* 2020;4:553–554.

20

Anterior Uveitis

Scott M. Whitcup

KEY CONCEPTS

- Anterior uveitis is the most common form of uveitis, with an annual incidence of 8:100,000 population, and is the least likely to be referred to a uveitis specialist.
- Although anterior uveitis is usually the most easily managed form, associated complications, such as glaucoma, may result in severe visual loss.
- Many disorders that can cause panuveitis, such as sarcoidosis, Behçet disease, bacterial endophthalmitis, and ocular malignancies, start as anterior uveitis. As with all cases of uveitis, it is important to diagnose infection and malignancy so that prompt and appropriate therapy can be started.
- Diagnostic evaluation should be based on the medical history and clinical examination findings and used to narrow the differential diagnosis.
- Anterior uveitis is associated with systemic disease in about half the patients. Diagnosis of the underlying condition is important to ensure proper treatment of both uveitis and the systemic disease.

Anterior uveitis is the most common form of uveitis and the least likely to be referred to a uveitis specialist. The diagnosis of anterior uveitis is based on inflammation limited to the anterior chamber. Because many patients have only a single episode of disease without recurrence or complications, there is debate as to the right approach to evaluate and treat patients with newly diagnosed anterior uveitis. Although anterior uveitis is usually the most easily managed form, associated complications, such as glaucoma, may result in severe visual loss. In addition, many disorders that can cause a sight-threatening panuveitis, such as sarcoidosis, Behçet disease, and bacterial endophthalmitis, can start as anterior uveitis. Furthermore, ocular malignancies, such as leukemia, can masquerade as anterior uveitis. Therefore the approach to patients with anterior uveitis requires careful thought and planning.

As we learn more about the pathophysiology of uveitis, it is becoming increasingly clear that many forms of uveitis may be triggered by microbial agents. There are numerous conditions in which the line between infectious and noninfectious causes becomes blurred. Therefore this chapter is included in the section on noninfectious uveitic conditions. Infectious causes of anterior uveitis are reviewed in other relevant chapters in this text.

EPIDEMIOLOGY

Anterior uveitis accounts for approximately three-quarters of cases of uveitis, with an annual incidence rate of about eight per 100,000 population.[1-3] Most cases have no identifiable cause and are classified as idiopathic; however, in some series, human leukocyte antigen (HLA)-B27 is associated with the disease in one-third to almost two-thirds of patients.[4,5] Furthermore, in a single center series of patients with spondyloarthritis, the prevalence of uveitis at the time of diagnosis was 11.5%, and 20 years after diagnosis, it reached nearly 40%.[6]

CLINICAL DESCRIPTION

Anterior uveitis includes diseases previously categorized as both iritis (inflammation of the iris) and iridocyclitis (inflammation of the iris and ciliary body). Patients with anterior uveitis often complain of redness, pain, and photophobia; some are relatively asymptomatic. Tearing may occur, but ocular discharge is rare. Some patients with severe anterior uveitis may also complain of blurred vision. Conjunctival injection is frequently noted on examination. *Ciliary flush,* that is, conjunctival injection in the perilimbal area, is characteristic of many forms of the disease. Pupillary miosis, posterior synechiae, and dilated iris vessels are common findings in all forms of anterior uveitis. However, sector abnormalities of the iris may suggest herpes zoster ophthalmicus as an underlying cause. The iris may also adhere to the trabecular meshwork, forming peripheral anterior synechiae (PAS). These PAS should be looked for on gonioscopic examination because patients with severe PAS are at increased risk for secondary glaucoma. In addition, patients with severe posterior synechiae, that is, iris adhesions to the lens, can develop pupillary block and may require prophylactic iridectomy.

The major indicators of anterior uveitis are the presence of cells and flare in the anterior chamber. Anterior chamber inflammation is assessed on slit-lamp biomicroscopic examination and is discussed in detail in Chapter 3. These cells and flare represent extravasated inflammatory cells and protein as a result of a breakdown of the blood–aqueous barrier. The clinical examination remains the gold standard in assessing anterior segment uveitis. A commercial device using laser photometry to objectively assess anterior chamber flare is available, although it is not routinely used

TABLE 20.1 **Syndromes of Anterior Uveitis**

Disease	Age (years)	Sex	Ocular Redness	HLA-B27	Systemic Findings	Steroid Response
Idiopathic	Any	Either	Yes	No	None	Yes
HLA-B27, ocular only	15–40	M > F	Yes	Yes	None	Yes
Ankylosing spondylitis	15–40	M > F	Yes	Yes	Spondylitis, sacroiliitis	Yes
Reactive arthritis	15–40	M > F	Yes	Yes	Arthritis, urethritis, mucocutaneous lesions	Yes
Juvenile rheumatoid arthritis	3–16	F > M	No	No	Pauciarticular arthritis, ANA-positive, RF-negative	Yes
Fuchs iridocyclitis	Any	Either	No	No	None	Yes/no
Posner-Schlossman syndrome	Adult	Either	No	No	None	Yes
Schwartz syndrome	Adult	Either	No	No	None	No
Ocular ischemia	>50	Either	Yes	No	Carotid insufficiency	No
Kawasaki disease	1–18	Either	Yes	No	Skin rash, lymphadenopathy fever, cardiac lesions	Yes

ANA, antinuclear antibody; *RF*, rheumatoid factor.

in clinical practice. Guex-Crosier et al.[7] used laser flare-cell photometry to demonstrate that disruption of the blood–aqueous barrier was very pronounced in idiopathic anterior uveitis and acute retinal necrosis but minimal in patients with toxoplasmosis or Fuchs heterochromic cyclitis. These authors have suggested that laser flare-cell photometry provides quantitative and sensitive assessment of anterior segment inflammation and may be useful in the management of patients with uveitis.

Fibrin may accumulate in the anterior chamber and may cause the once-mobile cells that circulate in the aqueous to become frozen. This plasmoid aqueous is a sign of severe anterior uveitis, which requires aggressive therapy. Another sign of severe anterior uveitis is a hypopyon composed of layered leukocytes. A hypopyon can be seen in a number of forms of anterior uveitis, but it is frequently associated with Behçet disease or infectious endophthalmitis. Anterior uveitis, including some cases with hypopyons, has been described in patients with acquired immunodeficiency syndrome (AIDS) receiving the drug rifabutin as treatment or prophylaxis for mycobacterial infection.[8-10] Also, hyphema may occur in patients with anterior uveitis, but it usually resolves without permanent damage.[11]

Inflammatory cells may also collect and adhere to the corneal endothelium and form keratic precipitates (KPs). The mechanism appears to involve the expression of cell adhesion molecules that are upregulated in the presence of inflammatory cytokines, such as interleukin-1 (IL-1).[12-14] Large, greasy-appearing KPs are suggestive of a granulomatous inflammation and may help in determining the cause of the uveitis (see Chapter 4). In vivo confocal microscopy of keratic precipitates showed heterogeneous features of KPs and may have diagnostic relevance.[15] Furthermore, anterior segment inflammation can damage the corneal endothelium and may lead to long-term damage, particularly with intraocular surgery.[16]

During the acute inflammatory episode, intraocular pressure (IOP) is often reduced because of ciliary body shutdown and reduced aqueous fluid production. As the inflammation subsides, however, IOP may rapidly increase, especially in patients with severe PAS. In some patients, it is difficult to determine whether the increased IOP is a result of underlying inflammation or a response to the corticosteroids used to control the disease. In secondary glaucoma caused by active inflammatory disease, increased corticosteroid therapy leads to a reduction in IOP.

Although some of the clinical symptoms and signs of anterior uveitis are specific for certain diseases, most disorders are differentiated by their associated systemic findings. The clinical findings of the common disorders that cause anterior uveitis are summarized in Table 20.1. Some disorders, such as postsurgical inflammation, infectious uveitis, Behçet disease, sarcoidosis, and masquerade syndromes, are discussed in separate chapters.

Finally, there is now interest in exploring the use of artificial intelligence to improve the diagnosis and treatment of many disorders, including anterior uveitis. For example, machine learning has been employed in the selection of intraocular lenses and the analysis of photographic and optical coherence tomography (OCT) images in the diagnosis of retinal diseases.[17] Algorithms and networks to aid in differential diagnoses and treatment approaches help with the application of artificial intelligence to diagnoses of specific disease entities and are specifically being developed for anterior uveitis.[18] It is hoped that these tools will help clinicians improve outcomes in patients with anterior uveitis.

IDIOPATHIC ANTERIOR UVEITIS

After a thorough medical history and ocular and general physical examinations, almost 50% of patients are found to have anterior segment inflammation that is not associated with other defined clinical syndromes. This form of anterior uveitis is referred to as *idiopathic anterior uveitis.* To diagnose idiopathic anterior uveitis, patients must not only lack systemic disease associations but also cannot have the HLA-B27 haplotype, which is associated with anterior segment inflammatory disease. In one study, 47% of patients with anterior uveitis had HLA-B27-associated anterior uveitis[1]; however, about one-quarter of these patients also had underlying systemic disorders, including ankylosing spondylitis and Reiter syndrome. Nevertheless, the diagnosis of idiopathic anterior uveitis depends greatly on the extent of the evaluation for an underlying condition. Many patients initially diagnosed with idiopathic anterior uveitis are later found to have a specific disorder causing their ocular inflammatory disease.

Importantly, one should rule out masquerade syndromes that present with anterior uveitis (see Chapter 31). Some conditions, including the presence of intraocular foreign bodies; malignancies, including leukemia and lymphoma; ocular infections, such as postsurgical infections; and pigment dispersion syndrome, can all be misdiagnosed as idiopathic anterior uveitis. Medications, including rifabutin, sulfonamides, topical prostaglandin analogues for glaucoma and ocular hypertension, and vaccines, have been associated with anterior uveitis.[19,20] Nevertheless, even after a thorough evaluation, a specific etiology cannot be determined in many patients. It has been hypothesized that these patients may have an immune responsiveness that may explain the development of anterior segment inflammation. In a study, patients with a history of acute anterior uveitis but no signs of ocular inflammation at the time of recruitment showed a high innate immune responsiveness compared with control subjects.[21] In a whole blood culture assay, levels of tumor necrosis factor-α and cross-reactive protein (CRP) were significantly higher in patients with a history of anterior uveitis than in control subjects.[21]

Diagnostic Workup

How should you evaluate a patient with a first episode of anterior uveitis? This is a controversial topic among uveitis specialists. Some have suggested that no evaluation is needed. Others have stated that a long list of laboratory tests and diagnostic procedures should be ordered on every patient. The prudent approach probably lies somewhere in the middle, and, as discussed in Chapter 5, a complete medical history and a thorough examination can help focus the workup. For example, if the patient complains of lower back pain, a diagnosis of ankylosing spondylitis is suggested and the evaluation might consist solely of sacroiliac joint radiography and HLA-B27 testing. Similarly, for a child with anterior uveitis with band keratopathy and a history of arthritis, a diagnosis of juvenile rheumatoid arthritis is suggested, and a targeted evaluation consisting of tests for antinuclear antibody (ANA) and rheumatoid factor with a referral to a pediatric rheumatologist may be appropriate.

However, when thorough history taking and physical examination fail to suggest specific diagnoses, what tests should be ordered? Many uveitis specialists will do a limited workup of all patients with anterior uveitis even if it is their first episode. If the uveitis is nongranulomatous, I request testing for syphilis serology because syphilis is a frequently missed diagnosis, and early treatment can prevent long-term complications. Similarly, I request a complete blood cell count and urinalysis to rule out an underlying systemic disorder, such as connective tissue disease, because the associated renal disease or anemia may be asymptomatic and yet warrant therapy. If the inflammation is granulomatous, a number of other disorders are suggested (see Chapter 4). For granulomatous anterior uveitis, I will also request a purified protein derivative test, chest x-ray, serum and urine calcium test, and serum angiotensin-converting enzyme level measurement to rule out asymptomatic tuberculosis or sarcoidosis. Although it is important to rule out infection as a cause of idiopathic anterior uveitis, anterior chamber paracentesis with polymerase chain reaction (PCR) has a relatively low diagnostic utility.[22] Importantly, most of my evaluation is based on using the tests to discern among the diseases in my differential diagnosis based on medical history and clinical examination. Without knowing the pretest probability of a disease, even relatively sensitive and specific diagnostic test results can mislead the clinician (see Chapters 4 and 5 on Differential Diagnosis and Diagnostic Testing).

Treatment

The breakthrough in the treatment of ocular inflammation came with the discovery of corticosteroids. In 1949, Hench et al.[23] reported the beneficial effects of 17-hydroxy-11-dehydrocorticosterone and pituitary adrenocorticotropic hormone in patients with rheumatoid arthritis. During the subsequent year, two reports were published in the *Journal of the American Medical Association (JAMA)* on their effects on ocular inflammatory disease.[24,25] A vast improvement was seen compared with the outcomes of previous therapies. Earlier in the twentieth century, patients with ocular inflammation were treated by inducing hyperpyrexia. Early on, patients were placed in steam baths in which their temperature was raised to 40–41° C for 4 to 6 hours. In some patients, the inflammation subsided, but many patients experienced severe complications. Later, patients were injected with milk protein or typhoid toxin to induce fever. Despite complications with their use, corticosteroids were a welcome advancement in the treatment of inflammation.

Patients with idiopathic anterior uveitis tend to have nongranulomatous inflammation that responds well to topical corticosteroid therapy. Acetate preparations of topical corticosteroids tend to penetrate the cornea better compared with other preparations, especially if the epithelium is intact, and many clinicians tend to use prednisolone acetate 1%. Prednisolone acetate can be used hourly to treat severe anterior segment inflammation. Difluprednate 0.05% has been approved by the U.S. Food and Drug Administration (FDA) to treat endogenous anterior uveitis. In a phase III, multicenter, randomized controlled trial (RCT), difluprednate 0.05% four times daily was shown to be not inferior to prednisolone acetate 1% given eight times daily with decreasing anterior chamber cells at 14 days in patients with anterior uveitis.[26] The study also showed that complete clearing of anterior chamber cells was greater in difluprednate-treated patients and that increased IOP was also more common with difluprednate treatment.

To prevent the development of posterior synechiae and to reduce pain and photophobia caused by inflammation of the ciliary muscle, mydriasis and cycloplegia are indicated. Scopolamine 0.25% given twice daily is usually sufficient. For resistant disease, periocular injections of corticosteroids may be useful. Systemic corticosteroids or other systemic anti-inflammatory drugs are rarely needed to treat anterior uveitis. However, patients with anterior uveitis may develop posterior segment disease. These patients frequently require more aggressive anti-inflammatory therapy, including periocular or systemic corticosteroids, or other immunosuppressive therapy. Local corticosteroid therapy, such as periocular injections, may also be warranted for severe or recalcitrant anterior uveitis with inadequate response to topical therapy. In some patients, topical nonsteroidal anti-inflammatory drugs are used to taper topical corticosteroids. Systemic anti-inflammatory drugs, including the biologics, are more frequently used when there is an underlying systemic disease requiring therapy.

HLA-B27–ASSOCIATED ANTERIOR UVEITIS

HLA-B27–associated anterior uveitis appears to be a distinct clinical disorder. This form of the disease has frequent associations with systemic diseases, including ankylosing spondylitis, Reiter syndrome, inflammatory bowel disease, Whipple disease, and psoriatic arthritis.[27] Nevertheless, as stated earlier, many patients with the HLA-B27 haplotype and anterior uveitis have no associated systemic illness, and not all patients with the HLA-B27 haplotype have uveitis; the prevalence of HLA-B27 is about 7% in North American whites.

Epidemiology

Some studies suggest that as many as 50% of patients with acute anterior uveitis are HLA-B27 positive, and half of these have spondyloarthropathies.[28] In a systematic review of 126 articles describing 29,877 patients with spondyloarthropathy, Zeboulon et al.[29] reported a uveitis prevalence rate of 32.7%. This prevalence rate increased with the duration of disease. As noted earlier, in a series of 798 patients with anterior uveitis, 60% were HLA-B27 positive, and a total of 50% had axial spondyloarthritis.[5]

Demographics and Clinical Findings

Patients with HLA-B27–associated anterior uveitis are more often males and tend to develop uveitis at a younger age compared with those who are HLA-B27 negative.[3] Although some studies have indicated that the long-term visual prognosis is similar for both groups,[3] data suggest that spondyloarthritis is more common in patients who are HLA-B27 positive.[5]

In a retrospective cohort study of 177 patients with HLA-B27–associated uveitis, the average age at onset of acute anterior uveitis was 36 years, with no difference between males and females.[30] HLA-B27–associated systemic disease developed earlier in males, and bilateral uveitis developed more frequently in females.

Should HLA typing be performed in all patients with anterior uveitis? We obtain HLA typing for male patients presenting with their first episode of acute anterior uveitis and in all patients if they have back pain or other systemic symptoms or signs. In addition, if patients have severe chronic anterior uveitis, we request HLA typing for the patient because the finding of the HLA-B27 haplotype often obviates the need for an extensive laboratory evaluation to rule out infectious or other treatable causes of the disease.

Etiology

The finding of the HLA-B27 haplotype is also of interest as a clue to the possible pathogenesis of both the spondyloarthropathies and anterior uveitis. We know that major histocompatibility complex (MHC) class I molecules, such as HLA-B27, are involved in antigen presentation and the initiation of an immune response. Some hypothesize that HLA-B27 interacts with certain endogenous antigens, leading to the development of inflammatory disease. HLA-B27 also has a tendency to misfold and may lead to a number of outcomes, including dimer formation with unique binding properties or activation of the IL-23–IL-17 axis, predisposing to inflammatory disease (Fig. 20.1).[31-33]

A number of studies have examined the associations among HLA-B27, infections, and the development of inflammatory disease. The role of gram-negative bacteria and their interaction with MHC class I antigens in triggering anterior uveitis has been of particular interest.[27,34] *Helicobacter pylori* has also been associated with anterior uveitis.[28] Unfortunately, this possible link among microbial antigens, HLA-B27, and anterior uveitis remains speculative because antimicrobial agents have not been proven to affect the course of disease. This may be attributed to lack of efficacy of antimicrobial agents or the dearth of trials investigating this therapeutic approach. A possible explanation for the lack of efficacy of antimicrobial agents is that the infection induces inflammation through Toll-like receptors (TLRs), and the process becomes separate from the active infection.[35]

Other immunologic studies have been performed in an attempt to determine the pathogenesis of anterior uveitis. Increased levels of complement and immunoglobulin G (IgG) compatible with breakdown of the blood–aqueous barrier can be detected in the aqueous of patients with anterior uveitis.[36] There is also evidence of complement activation in the aqueous of patients with anterior uveitis, indicated by the presence of C3a, C4a, and C5a.[37] Evidence of increased serum fibrin degradation products has suggested a pathogenic role of the clotting pathways.[38] Increased expression of cell adhesion molecules has been associated with the development of intraocular inflammation. Increased expression of intercellular adhesion molecule-1 (ICAM-1) in the irides of patients with uveitis has been reported,[39] and expression of cell adhesion molecules in the anterior uvea has been shown to precede infiltration of inflammatory cells in animal models of acute anterior uveitis.[12,13] Polymorphisms within the tumor necrosis factor (TNF)-α promoter region have been identified, and individuals with these single-nucleotide polymorphisms (SNPs) show higher susceptibility to the development of uveitis.[40]

HLA-B27–ASSOCIATED ANTERIOR UVEITIS WITH SYSTEMIC DISEASE

Ankylosing Spondylitis

Ankylosing spondylitis is chronic, inflammatory arthritis that primarily affects the spine and the sacroiliac joints. The disease was previously known as Bechterew disease and Marie-Strumpell disease and is now classified as a spondyloarthropathy. Without treatment, the disease can progress and result in fusion and rigidity of the spine, known as *bamboo spine.* Diagnosis of ankylosing spondylitis is usually based on imaging, with characteristic active inflammation seen on magnetic resonance imaging (MRI) or definite sacroiliitis on radiography, with at least one other clinical feature of the disease. Clinical features of ankylosing spondylitis include anterior uveitis, arthritis, inflammatory back pain, psoriasis, dactylitis, inflammatory bowel disease, heel enthesitis, a family history of spondyloarthropathies, presence of HLA-B27, elevated CRP, and good response to nonsteroidal anti-inflammatory drugs (NSAIDs).

Ocular involvement occurs in 25% of patients with ankylosing spondylitis.[41] In 80% of patients, both eyes are involved but are rarely inflamed simultaneously. Although the ocular findings associated with ankylosing spondylitis include both iritis and conjunctivitis, iritis is the more significant manifestation. The disease course is quite variable. Recurrence of the ocular inflammation may occur as frequently as every 2 to 3 weeks. Some patients have fewer than one exacerbation per year. Interestingly, recurrence may be seasonal, although this variation appears to be more frequent in patients with idiopathic anterior uveitis.[42]

The anterior uveitis associated with ankylosing spondylitis usually has a presentation similar to that of idiopathic disease, occurring as unilateral acute iritis with pain, photophobia, and redness (Fig. 20.2A). Patients often report onset of an attack 1 to 2 days before anterior chamber cell and flare are evident on slit-lamp biomicroscopy. The use of laser photometry may help determine when the initial breakdown of the blood–aqueous barrier occurs in relation to the development of symptoms and clinical signs of inflammation. Vision may decrease transiently during an acute episode as a result of anterior chamber inflammation or, less often, because of associated cystoid macular edema. A fibrin clot may form in the anterior chamber (see Fig. 20.2B). Posterior synechiae commonly develop unless the attacks are treated promptly with corticosteroids and cycloplegic agents (Fig. 20.3).

Ankylosing spondylitis has been reported to affect men 2.5 to three times more frequently in comparison with women. Women may have a milder disease that may present with more peripheral joint manifestations. It is a common disorder that affects 0.1% of white adults.[43] Because the HLA-B27 antigen is dominantly inherited and expressed, 50% of offspring will carry the gene, but the disease will be manifest in only 10% of them. Approximately 96% of patients with ankylosing spondylitis have the HLA-B27 antigen compared with 6% to 14% of a control white population without ankylosing spondylitis. HLA-B27 is found in 0% to 4% of African Americans. Thus the relative risk for ankylosing spondylitis in patients with the HLA-B27 antigen is as high as 100. Nevertheless, only 1.3% of all HLA-B27–positive patients will have the disease.

Sacroiliitis may be asymptomatic early in the course of disease but may be associated with severe lower back pain and debilitating stiffness and decreased range of motion. X-rays of the sacroiliac joints show blurring of the joints, followed by sclerotic changes and eventually obliteration as the disease progresses (see Fig. 20.2C). A common

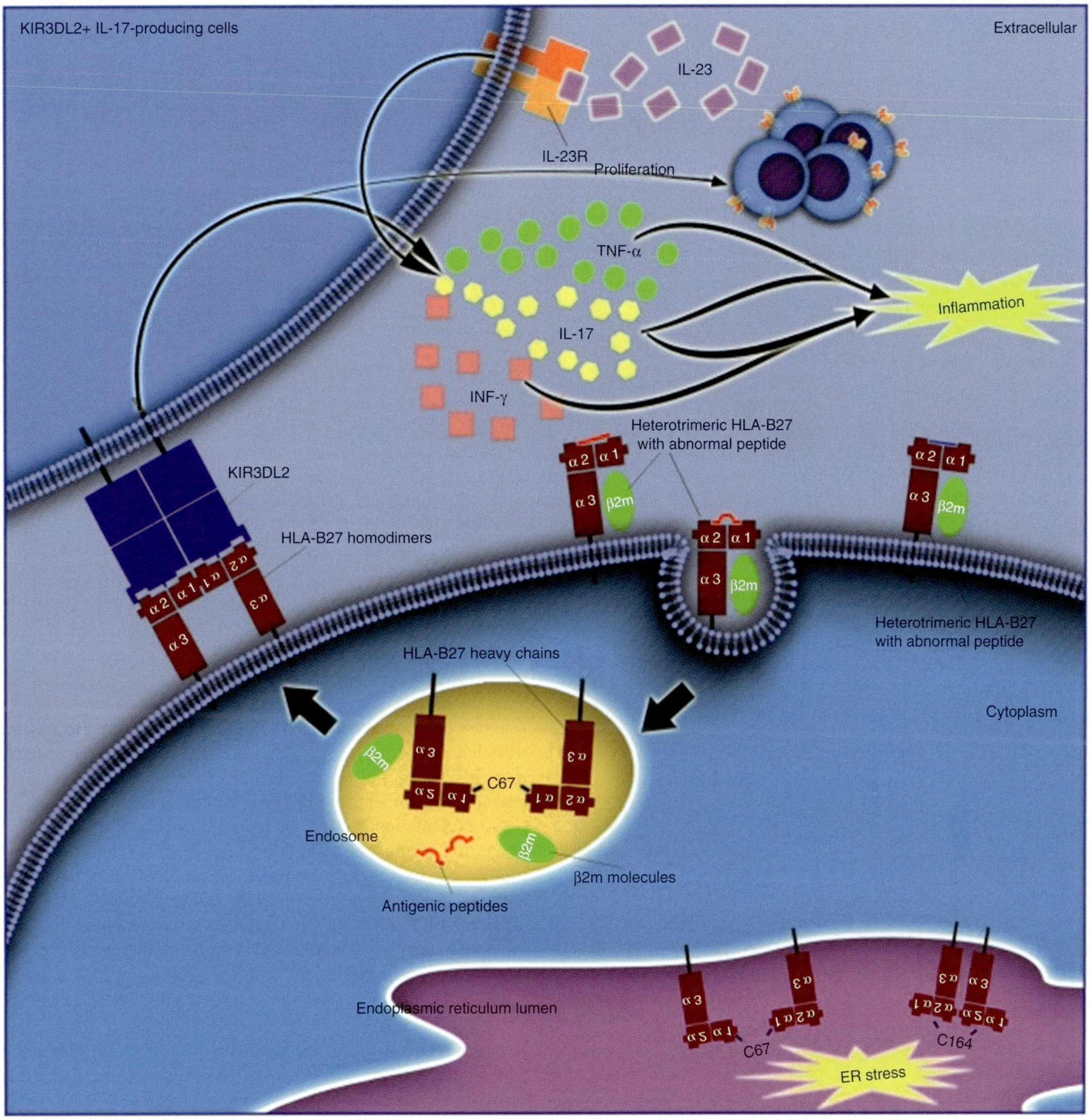

Fig. 20.1 Different pathogenic roles of ER-resident and cell surface HLA-B27 dimers. ER-resident dimers may result in ER stress as a cellular response and lead to activation of the unfolded protein response. Cell surface dimers are reported to form after the recycling of fully folded HLA-B27 cell surface molecules via the endocytic pathway, and re-express as dimers for presentation to immunoreceptors, including KIR and LILR. Enhanced proliferation and survival of KIR3DL2+ CD4+ T cells and increased IL-17 production in patients with ankylosing spondylitis after stimulation with antigen-presenting cells expressing HLA-B27 homodimers has been previously demonstrated. The majority of these cells have been reported to produce TNF-α and IFN-γ. IL-17 has been demonstrated to synergize with TNF-α or IFN-γ to promote the release of inflammatory mediators and influence bone metabolism, thus demonstrating its important role in the pathogenesis of ankylosing spondylitis. *ER*, endoplasmic reticulum; *HLA*, human leukocyte antigen; IFN-γ, interferon-gamma, *IL-17*, interleukin-17; *KIR*, killer cell immunoglobulin-like receptor; *KIR3DL2*, killer cell immunoglobulin-like receptor three domains long cytoplasmic tail 2; *LILR*, leukocyte immunoglobulin-like receptor; *TNF-α*, tumor necrosis factor-alpha. (From Chen R, Li J, He C, et al. Role of HLA-B27 in the pathogenesis of ankylosing spondylitis. *Mol Med Rep*. 2017;15:1943–1951.)

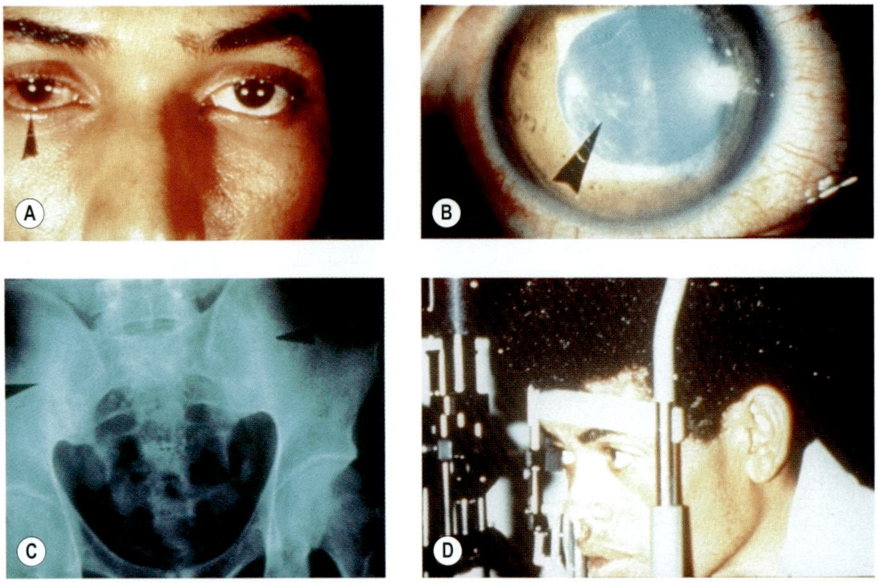

Fig. 20.2 (A) Unilateral redness caused by iritis associated with ankylosing spondylitis. (B) Fibrin clot in the anterior chamber in iritis associated with ankylosing spondylitis. (C) X-ray of the sacroiliac joints demonstrating increased radiodensity caused by ankylosing spondylitis. (D) Flexed neck caused by ankylosis of the cervical spine in ankylosing spondylitis. (Courtesy Fernando Orefice, MD, and Rubens Belfort, Jr., MD.)

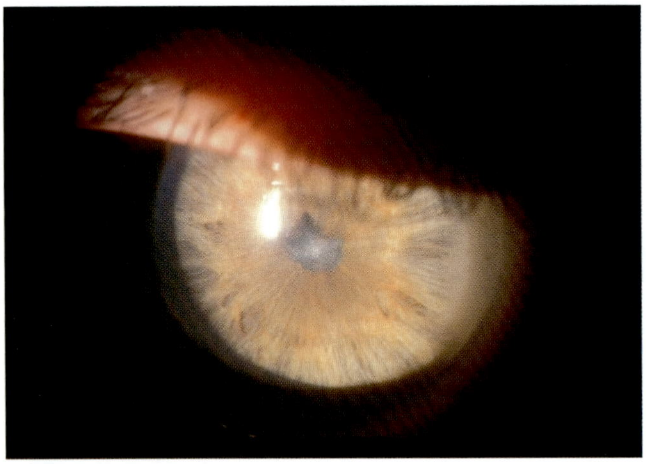

Fig. 20.3 Occluded pupil in a patient with ankylosing spondylitis and recurrent iritis.

mistake in the initial evaluation of patients with possible ankylosing spondylitis is to order lumbosacral spine films instead of imaging of the sacroiliac joints. MRI of the sacroiliac joints often provides definitive evidence of active sacroiliitis and is useful in the diagnosis of ankylosing spondylitis.

As noted earlier, early diagnosis and treatment is imperative because of the risk of fusion of the spine, which begins in the lumbar region but can involve all parts of the spine. This leads to back pain and stiffness and, in severe disease, may cause pulmonary restriction and a stiff, flexed neck, making positioning for slit-lamp biomicroscopic examination difficult (see Fig. 20.2D). Interestingly, the associated uveitis does not appear to correlate with the severity of the underlying spondylitis. Aortic insufficiency, cardiomegaly, and conduction defects are also associated with this disease.

Etiology

The reason for the association between HLA-B27 and ankylosing spondylitis remains unknown. As mentioned earlier, some data suggest that environmental triggers, such as infections by gram-negative bacteria, are an important factor in the development of the disease. This information has led to several theories. One hypothesis suggests that HLA-B27 is a receptor for the infectious agent. A second suggests that HLA-B27 may cross-react with foreign antigens and induce tolerance. Others have suggested that HLA-B27 is a marker for an immune response gene that determines susceptibility to an environmental stimulus, or that microbial agents activate TLRs and induce inflammation. Polymorphisms of ERAP1, which encode an endoplasmic reticulum aminopeptidase involved in peptide trimming before MHC class I presentation, suggest that HLA-B27 operates through aberrant processing of antigenic peptides.[44] Additional genetic studies further support the hypothesis that disease susceptibility may be caused by aminopeptidases involved in peptide processing before MHC class I presentation.[45] Finally, the IL-23–IL-17 pathway has been shown to be involved in the pathogenesis of ankylosing spondylitis, and this has led to new therapeutic options for the disease.[46]

Treatment

It is important to make the diagnosis of ankylosing spondylitis in patients with uveitis because, if the disease is recognized and treated early, spinal deformity can be prevented. Treatment usually involves physical therapy and anti-inflammatory drugs, including NSAIDs. Sulfasalazine has been used in patients who fail to respond to NSAIDs or who have contraindications to NSAID therapy. Cytotoxic agents, such as methotrexate, are reserved for severe cases but can reduce rates of recurrence.[47] More recently, biologics, including anti-TNF drugs and anti–IL-17A antibody, have been used to treat ankylosing spondylitis.[48]

Anterior uveitis associated with ankylosing spondylitis is usually managed with topical corticosteroids and mydriatic agents. NSAIDs may have some role in treating the uveitis associated with this disorder; however, data from large RCTs are lacking. A meta-analysis of four placebo-controlled studies in ankylosing spondylitis treated with anti-TNF agents reviewed their effect on anterior uveitis. The frequency of flares of anterior uveitis was significantly less in patients receiving anti-TNF therapy than in patients receiving placebo (6.8

anterior uveitis flares per 100 patient-years versus 15.6 uveitis flares per 100 patient-years),[49] although there are some reports of paradoxical development or exacerbation of uveitis after therapy with anti-TNF drugs.[50] Interestingly, a paradoxical effect of blocking TNF-α was demonstrated in an experimental model of anterior uveitis.[51-53] Some clinical trials have demonstrated the efficacy of anti–IL-17A treatment for noninfectious uveitis, but intravenous dosing may be required for better efficacy.[54]

Reactive Arthritis (Reiter Syndrome)

Reactive arthritis is a systemic disorder characterized by arthritis, conjunctivitis, and urethritis. It was first described in 1818, but it was named after Reiter, who described the entity in 1916.[55] Reiter syndrome is now more commonly referred to as reactive arthritis, a form of seronegative spondyloarthropathy that includes ankylosing spondylitis, psoriatic arthritis, juvenile chronic arthritis, and the arthropathy associated with inflammatory bowel disease.[56] This change has resulted, in part, from the desire to use names that are more clinically descriptive and because of Reiter's involvement with the Nazis during World War II. Reactive arthritis is the most common cause of inflammatory oligoarthropathy in young males and, like ankylosing spondylitis, is related to both HLA-B27 and a specific infection that may trigger the disease. The disease develops in at least 1% of patients with nonspecific urethritis and occurs in about 2% of patients after dysentery caused by *Shigella* spp.

In many patients, the classic triad of arthritis, conjunctivitis, and urethritis does not manifest. In addition, many of the findings of reactive arthritis are easily missed. For example, urethritis may be mild and missed. Other systemic associations include scaling skin eruption, called *keratoderma blennorrhagicum;* balanitis; and aphthous stomatitis. Rheumatologic features of the disease include arthralgias, plantar fasciitis, and tenosynovitis. In about 20% of patients with reactive arthritis, sacroiliitis and ascending spinal disease similar to ankylosing spondylitis develop. Hyperkeratotic skin lesions occur and may be indistinguishable from psoriasis. A number of classification systems have been proposed for reactive arthritis (Box 20.1),[57] but none has been used uniformly in clinical practice.

In one review, arthritis was the presenting symptom in 25% of patients and genitourinary symptoms in 19%.[57] As the syndrome progresses, 94% of patients developed arthritis at some point, mostly in the joints of the hands, wrists, feet, and knees. Sacroiliitis occurred in 19% of patients, and almost any joint can be involved. Urethritis occurs in 75% of patients, with cystitis, orchitis, vaginitis, and epididymitis occurring in occasional patients. Oral ulcers occur in 19% of patients and external genital lesions in 39%. Skin lesions are common in reactive arthritis: they are seen in about 20% of patients but occur rarely in patients with ankylosing spondylitis.

Conjunctivitis is the most common ocular finding in patients with reactive arthritis and occurs in 30% to 60% of patients. Some patients experience a mucoid discharge, but the conjunctivitis is usually not chronic. Iritis and keratitis are less common. Iritis occurs in 3% to 12% of patients and is nongranulomatous and mild. The keratitis is characterized by multifocal punctate subepithelial and anterior stroma infiltrates. A small pannus may also develop.

As stated previously, reactive arthritis may occur after dysentery caused by gram-negative bacteria or after nongonococcal urethritis caused by *Chlamydia trachomatis* and *Ureaplasma urealyticum*.[58] Nevertheless, treatment of the dysentery does not appear to alter the development or course of the syndrome. Most patients have signs of this syndrome 2 to 4 weeks after the onset of dysentery, but the full syndrome may take years to develop.[57]

BOX 20.1 Reactive Arthritis

Major Criteria
Polyarthritis
Conjunctivitis, iridocyclitis
Urethritis
Keratoderma blennorrhagica, balanitis circinata

Minor Criteria
Fasciitis, tendonitis, sacroiliitis, spondylitis
Keratitis
Cystitis, prostatitis
Oral mucosal lesions, psoriasis-like rash, nail changes
Diarrhea, leukocytosis, increased serum globulins, inflammation in the synovial fluid
Reactive arthritis is:
Definite if three major criteria or two major and three minor
Probable if two major and two minor

Modified from Lee DA, Barker SM, Su WPD, et al. The clinical diagnosis of Reiter's syndrome. *Ophthalmology.* 1986;93:350–356.

The diagnosis of reactive arthritis is based on clinical findings in association with the HLA-B27 haplotype. Rheumatoid factor and autoantibodies are usually absent. The ocular disease associated with reactive arthritis is usually mild and can be treated with topical corticosteroids and mydriatic agents. However, the joint involvement may lead to significant long-term dysfunction and require treatment with NSAIDs. Prompt antibiotic therapy is required for underlying infections, such as acute chlamydial urethritis or enteric infection. Immunosuppressive therapy with azathioprine or methotrexate may be required for systemic sequelae. Anti-TNF agents have also been used to treat the disease.

Juvenile Idiopathic Arthritis

Juvenile idiopathic arthritis (JIA) is chronic arthritis that was previously called *juvenile rheumatoid arthritis* (JRA). The term *juvenile rheumatoid arthritis* was previously used to describe all forms of childhood arthritis. As in adults, arthritis in children may be associated with infections, such as Lyme disease, psoriasis, inflammatory bowel disease, and other systemic diseases. The diagnosis is based on the presence of arthritis in a child younger than 16 years of age and usually with a negative rheumatoid factor test result and no other known cause for the joint disease.[59] Incidence/prevalence in North American populations ranges from 16 to 150 cases per 100,000.[60] The joint inflammation may be polyarticular or pauciarticular, and most patients have negative rheumatoid factor test results. A systemic form of JIA is characterized by a symmetric polyarthritis, with associated fever, rash, hepatosplenomegaly, and leukocytosis.

Diagnosis

Identifying the subclassification of JIA is important to determine the risk for uveitis. There is no perfect classification system; however, a system developed by the International League of Associations for Rheumatology (ILAR) lists seven disease categories (Box 20.2).[61,62] JIA is a diagnosis of exclusion, and there are numerous infectious diseases, such as septicemia, brucellosis, and viral infections, that can mimic JIA. Malignancies such as leukemia and lymphoma; connective tissue diseases, such as systemic lupus erythematosus and Kawasaki disease; and sarcoidosis can all cause clinical pictures similar to that of JIA. Radiographs of the joints are usually obtained to evaluate joint disease, although MRI can also be beneficial to assess bone and synovial diseases.

BOX 20.2 International League of Associations for Rheumatology (ILAR) Disease Classification for Juvenile Idiopathic Uveitis

Systemic arthritis
Oligoarthritis
Polyarthritis rheumatoid factor negative
Polyarthritis rheumatoid factor positive
Psoriatic arthritis
Enthesitis-related arthritis
Undifferentiated arthritis

Children with juvenile idiopathic arthritis and uveitis are often asymptomatic and rarely complain of ocular symptoms, especially if the disease is uniocular. Uveitis is rare in children with systemic JIA.[63,64] Uveitis develops only occasionally in patients with polyarticular arthritis. In contrast, patients with the pauciarticular form of JIA (≤ 4 joints involved) have a much higher risk for the development of ocular inflammation. Girls with pauciarticular arthritis and a positive ANA test result have the highest risk for chronic iridocyclitis.[59] A higher risk of uveitis is also associated with arthritis sparing the wrists but involving a lower-extremity joint: chronic anterior uveitis will develop in 14% of girls in this high-risk group.

A group of boys with pauciarticular arthritis also have an increased risk for anterior uveitis[65]: 75% of boys with pauciarticular arthritis are HLA-B27 positive, and the ocular inflammation they experience is similar in appearance to that of ankylosing spondylitis. The uveitis is characterized by acute, episodic, nongranulomatous anterior uveitis, and some of these boys have ankylosing spondylitis later in life.[65] It may be that many of these boys have HLA-B27–related spondyloarthropathy and not JIA.

Unlike boys with JIA who have uveitis, girls with JIA tend to have chronic indolent disease, which can cause permanent ocular damage before it is recognized. In fact, the inflammation is clinically silent in greater than 50% of patients. Therefore girls with pauciarticular arthritis with test results that are positive for ANA and negative for rheumatoid factor should be screened every 3 to 4 months for the development of chronic smoldering uveitis. Parents should be told that a red eye should not be dismissed as conjunctivitis. Frequently, the first sign of uveitis in these girls is an irregular pupil as a result of posterior synechiae.

The chronic uveitis in JIA is characterized by anterior chamber cells and flare. Usually, patients only have 1 to 2+ cells, and once the uveitis has developed, chronic flare is typical. Anterior chamber cells and not flare should be used to determine the severity of disease and the need for therapy. The number of cells will fluctuate with the severity of inflammation and diminish with corticosteroid therapy. Similar to the uveitis associated with other arthropathies, the severity of the uveitis is unrelated to the severity of the underlying joint disease. Although the joint disease often diminishes with age, ocular disease frequently persists into adulthood. Chronic inflammation may lead to band keratopathy, posterior synechiae, cataract, hypotony, and glaucoma. Glaucoma has been reported in up to 20% of eyes and may be caused by pupillary block or chronic inflammatory disease, with presumed damage to the trabecular meshwork.[66] Band keratopathy occurs in more than half the patients and can cause significant visual disturbance (Fig. 20.4).[65] Cataract occurs in at least 60% of eyes and, in young patients, may lead to amblyopia. Chronic inflammation in the presence of posterior synechiae and a small pupil can lead to the development of a fibrin membrane over the pupil. Finally, although the ocular inflammatory disease associated with JIA primarily involves the anterior segment, vitritis, macular edema, and macular folds may occur. Therefore visual loss may be caused by multiple factors in patients with JIA, and a thorough evaluation is necessary to determine the appropriate therapeutic approach.

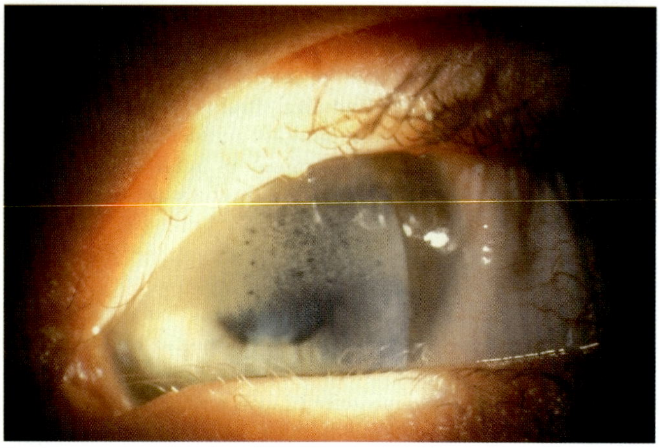

Fig. 20.4 Band keratopathy in a patient with long-standing pauciarticular juvenile rheumatoid arthritis and chronic iritis.

The average age of onset of joint disease in patients who have acute uveitis is 7.5 to 9 years.[59,65] In contrast, joint symptoms develop earlier in life in patients with chronic uveitis, with an average age of onset of 4 to 6.3 years. In one study, half the patients had chronic uveitis by age 6 years.[66] Joint inflammation usually precedes ocular disease by several years, but iritis can precede the joint symptoms by months to years.[65]

Pathology

Histopathologic studies have been performed only on a few eyes of patients with JIA.[67,68] Histologic findings show that the inflammation predominantly involves the iris and the ciliary body. Plasma cells and lymphocytes are the most common inflammatory cells, and scattered giant cells have been noted. A similar histologic picture is seen in the involved joints of these patients. In view of the association between ANAs and other autoantibodies with JIA, some have hypothesized that infiltrating plasma cells are responsible for local synthesis of autoantibodies against ocular antigens.[68] However, these proposed autoantibodies or ocular antigens have not been identified.

Differential Diagnosis

Ocular sarcoidosis in children is the disease that most closely mimics JIA. Children with sarcoidosis develop arthritis and skin lesions, and often radiographic evidence of pulmonary disease is lacking. JIA can be distinguished from sarcoidosis by the presence of a positive ANA test result, the characteristic distribution of involved joints, the nongranulomatous inflammation limited primarily to the anterior segment of the eye, and the absence of systemic symptoms and signs. Nevertheless, early in the course of JIA, the affected children may have no history of joint disease and present only with chronic uveitis and band keratopathy. Other diseases to consider include Lyme disease, psoriatic arthritis, juvenile Reiter syndrome, ankylosing spondylitis, inflammatory bowel disease–associated anterior uveitis, Kawasaki disease, trauma, and keratouveitis caused by herpes simplex or herpes zoster infection.

Treatment and Prognosis

Children who are at high risk for uveitis should have ophthalmic screening every 3 months. Patients with chronic anterior uveitis associated with JIA also need to be seen regularly—usually every 3 months or more frequently if the disease is very active. Topical corticosteroids remain the mainstay of therapy.[69,70] Corticosteroid therapy should be used to reduce the number of anterior chamber cells, but chronic flare in the absence of cells should not be treated. Glaucoma and cataract are frequent side effects of topical steroid therapy in children with JIA. Especially in young patients, cataracts may lead to the development of amblyopia and require prompt surgical removal. Guidelines for the screening, monitoring, and treatment of uveitis associated with JIA have been published by the American College of Rheumatology and the Arthritis Foundation.[71]

Chylack[70] studied 210 patients with JIA and found that in 39% of patients, the uveitis responded to short courses of topical corticosteroids. However, in 61% of patients, JIA did not respond to corticosteroids or required prolonged treatment. Repeated periocular injections of depot preparations of corticosteroids are needed to manage some occurrences of chronic active inflammation that cannot be controlled with topical corticosteroids alone. In most children, this requires general anesthesia for each injection. Short courses of oral corticosteroids can be tried, but we do not favor the long-term use of oral corticosteroids in children because of the overwhelming side effects on growth and bone formation. Alternate-day therapy may reduce the side effects and may be tried for unusually severe ocular disease requiring prolonged therapy.

The use of NSAIDs may allow for a reduction in the dosage of corticosteroids required to treat chronic uveitis.[72] Tolmetin and naproxen are the NSAIDs most commonly used in children. A number of other immunosuppressive agents, including azathioprine, chlorambucil, cyclophosphamide, and methotrexate, have been used to treat severe uveitis associated with JIA. Methotrexate remains the most widely used conventional disease-modifying antirheumatic drug (DMARD) because of its efficacy and safety profile.[62] A double-masked trial of methotrexate versus placebo in the treatment of resistant JIA showed that joint disease improved with methotrexate therapy; however, the study did not address the response of the uveitis.[73] At the National Eye Institute (NEI), we have found cyclosporin to be useful for the treatment of many forms of childhood uveitis but have rarely treated children with JIA using this agent.

More recently, anti-TNF agents have been used to treat JIA. In a retrospective case series, the use of the anti-TNF agents led to a prompt reduction in intraocular inflammation.[74] In children and adolescents with JIA and uveitis on a stable dose of methotrexate, addition of adalimumab therapy controlled inflammation, with a lower rate of treatment failure compared with placebo, although side effects were also much higher with adalimumab.[75] However, not all patients respond to anti-TNF therapy, and children need to be monitored closely for therapeutic response and potential relapse.[76]

Surgery is often needed in the management of JIA-associated uveitis. Cataracts are common in children with JIA and require surgical removal, but only in eyes that have been "quiet" for at least 3 months. Cataract extraction may be performed by either phacoemulsification or as pars plana lensectomy.[77,78] The need for a secondary surgical procedure appears to be reduced in patients undergoing pars plana lensectomy with vitrectomy.[78] Many uveitis specialists also recommend removal of the posterior capsule at the time of surgery because a secondary laser posterior capsulotomy may be difficult to perform in children. Foster and Barrett[79] reported their surgical experience in patients with JIA. Cataracts were common in their patients and developed in 13 (18%) of 72 patients during follow-up. These authors performed phacoemulsification extracapsular cataract extraction, followed by pars plana vitrectomy, and emphasized the need for aggressive anti-inflammatory therapy both before and after surgery. The average postoperative visual acuity in this study was 20/40.

Medical management of glaucoma in patients with JIA is problematic. Aggressive use of topical IOP-lowering agents is warranted. Surgery is required for a number of patients in whom medical management has failed. Laser iridectomy is indicated for glaucoma caused by pupillary block with iris bombé. In patients with secondary glaucoma caused by chronic intraocular inflammation, the success rate of traditional surgery with trabeculectomy is poor.[80] Filtering devices, such as Molteno implants, may improve the prognosis. Cyclocryotherapy should only be used when other surgical procedures have failed to control IOP.

Band keratopathy is seen in 77% of patients with severe JIA-associated iridocyclitis.[64] This band keratopathy can be treated with chemical chelation and topical application of 0.37 M ethylenediaminetetraacetic acid (EDTA) solution after debridement of the epithelium with 70% isopropyl alcohol and scraping. The excimer laser may have a role in the management of this complication in the future. Keratoconjunctivitis sicca can also occur in JIA. In a study of 64 patients with JIA, 12.5% complained of dry eye with poorer Schirmer test results and tear breakup times compared with age- and sex-matched controls.[81]

Prognosis is related to early diagnosis and meticulous treatment of ocular inflammation and management of secondary complications. Because ocular inflammation does not always mirror joint disease, routine ophthalmologic examinations at least every 3 months are recommended.[82] This makes sense because complications and vision loss are common. In a retrospective cohort study of 75 patients with JIA, the incidence of any ocular complication was 0.33 per eye-year.[83] Rates of vision loss to 20/50 or worse and 20/200 or worse were 0.10 per eye-year and 0.08 per eye-year, respectively. Risk factors included anterior chamber flare 1+ or greater and elevated IOP. Immunosuppressive drug therapy reduced the rates of complications, including hypotony and blindness. Additional use of biologic agents to control inflammatory disease may further improve the long-term visual prognosis and even delay the onset of uveitis. In a study of 3512 patients with JIA, the use of DMARDs significantly reduced the risk for uveitis onset.[84] Early methotrexate use within the first year of disease and the combination of methotrexate with a TNF inhibitor were shown to have the highest protective effect in this study.

Psoriatic Arthritis

Psoriasis is a skin disease caused by hyperproliferation of the epidermis with resultant scaling. Uveitis occurs predominantly in patients who develop arthropathy. About 20% of patients with psoriasis develop psoriatic arthropathy, and about 20% of these patients develop uveitis, sacroiliitis, and ascending spinal disease.[85] The arthropathy usually involves the distal joints of the hands and feet and the sacroiliac joints. The uveitis predominantly involves the anterior segment of the eye and is similar to HLA-B27–associated disease. One small case series has suggested that the uveitis associated with psoriatic arthritis is more likely to be insidious and bilateral, with posterior segment involvement compared with uveitis in spondyloarthropathy.[86] Because psoriasis is a common disorder, not all anterior uveitis that occurs in patients with psoriasis will be causally related, especially if the patient does not have arthritis. In these patients, psoriasis and arthropathy are treated separately. Anti-TNF agents have also been used to treat both components of the disease.[87] The uveitis in these patients tends to respond well to standard therapy with topical corticosteroids and a drop to induce cycloplegia and mydriasis.

Inflammatory Bowel Disease

Uveitis may develop in patients with both ulcerative colitis and Crohn disease.[88,89] About 5% of patients (range 0.3%–13%) with

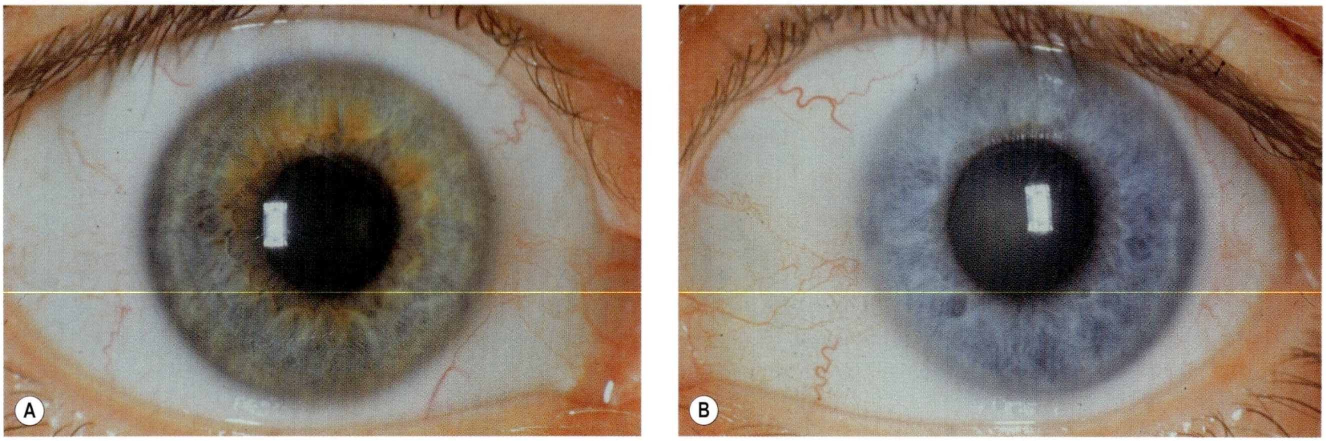

Fig. 20.5 Photograph of irides of a patient with Fuchs heterochromic iridocyclitis demonstrating heterochromia. (A) The unaffected right eye. (B) The affected left eye has the lighter colored iris.

inflammatory bowel disease will have ocular disease.[90] Conjunctivitis, episcleritis, and anterior uveitis are most commonly described; however, posterior uveitis may also occur.[91] The ophthalmologist should ask the patient with anterior uveitis about recurrent diarrhea, bloody diarrhea, or abdominal cramping. Although the uveitis often responds to therapy with topical corticosteroids, early diagnosis of inflammatory bowel disease will lead to prompt treatment for the gastrointestinal complications that frequently occur. Similar to other spondyloarthropathies, anti-TNF agents are now used in the management of the disease. The effect on uveitis is less well documented in clinical trials.

Whipple Disease

Whipple disease is a chronic infectious disease caused by *Tropheryma whipplei* and has been associated with uveitis.[92] Because the causative organism has been identified, the description of this disease has been moved to the chapter on bacterial and fungal diseases (Chapter 10).

DISEASE ASSOCIATIONS

Fuchs Heterochromic Iridocyclitis

The association of iris heterochromia and cataract was initially described by Lawrence in 1843.[93] In 1906, Fuchs[94] described seven patients with heterochromic iridocyclitis and later described 38 patients with the disease and reported on the pathologic features of six eyes. The classic hallmark of Fuchs heterochromic iridocyclitis is, as the name suggests, iris heterochromia (Fig. 20.5A and B). However, this classic finding may be difficult to perceive. It is easiest to see in blue-eyed patients, in whom the affected eye appears more intensely blue.[95] In addition, 7% to 15% of patients have bilateral involvement and no obvious heterochromia. A more consistent finding appears to be blurring of the iris stroma and loss of detail and density of the iris surface that can only be seen on careful slit-lamp biomicroscopic examination.[95,96] Fuchs observed that most patients with this disorder had cataracts.

The typical patient is young and presents with iris heterochromia and a mild disturbance of vision. In one series from Italy, 18% of patients were 16 years of age or younger.[97] Pain and redness are rare. Slit-lamp examination shows small stellate KPs, with fine filaments that are uniformly scattered over the endothelium, unlike most other occurrences of anterior uveitis where the KPs occur predominantly on the lower half of the cornea. Anterior chamber inflammation is mild, and low-grade vitritis may be seen. The posterior segment of the eye is usually unaffected, although cystoid macular edema has been reported in a few patients. Abnormal vessels bridging the anterior chamber angle are frequently described, but iris neovascularization and neovascular glaucoma are rare.[98] It is well documented that hyphema is likely to occur after intraocular surgery. Amsler[99] first noted the occurrence of hyphema after paracentesis. Anterior chamber paracentesis was initially proposed as a diagnostic test for Fuchs heterochromic iridocyclitis but appears unwarranted for this purpose.[98]

Many patients with Fuchs heterochromic iridocyclitis are unaware of their disease until their vision decreases because of cataract or progressive glaucoma. Rarely, vitreous inflammation is severe enough to cause floaters. The presence of fine, evenly distributed KPs in a white eye with mild anterior chamber cells and flare, cataract, and increased IOP should suggest the diagnosis. Patients often note that one iris has been lighter in color for many years. Brown eyes become less brown and blue eyes appear bluer with this disorder because the heterochromia is caused by loss of anterior iris pigment. Gray eyes may appear green.

The differential diagnosis of Fuchs heterochromic iridocyclitis includes disorders that produce iris heterochromia. Malignant melanoma of the iris, Horner syndrome, and chronic anterior uveitis with iris atrophy caused by infections, such as herpes zoster, should all be considered. In addition, Posner-Schlossman syndrome and neovascular glaucoma may cause ocular disease that looks like Fuchs heterochromic iridocyclitis.

Etiology

A number of researchers have hypothesized an infectious cause for Fuchs heterochromic iridocyclitis. Fuchs described peripheral chorioretinal scars in some patients with this disease. Several authors have associated Fuchs heterochromic iridocyclitis with toxoplasmosis (Fig. 20.6). Ocular toxoplasmosis may cause fine KPs and anterior uveitis and mimic Fuchs heterochromic iridocyclitis. This would explain why many patients with Fuchs heterochromic iridocyclitis lack findings of toxoplasmosis. Others suggest that infection with *Toxoplasma* may be causally related to the disorder. Chorioretinal scars consistent with ocular histoplasmosis have also been noted, but a causal relationship between infectious agents and Fuchs heterochromic iridocyclitis remains unproven. Others have proposed that lack of normal sympathetic innervation and neurogenic factors cause the findings associated with the disease, but again these associations are unproven.[98]

Investigators have suggested an association between rubella virus and Fuchs heterochromic iridocyclitis. In one study, rubella virus, but not herpes simplex virus, varicella zoster virus, or toxoplasmosis, was associated with the disease.[100] Antibody against rubella was identified in the aqueous humor of 13 of 14 patients studied; antibody against the other infectious agents was not found. In another study, using nested PCR, antibody against rubella virus was found in all 52 eyes with Fuchs heterochromic cyclitis.[101]

The finding of infiltrating plasma cells and lymphocytes on pathologic examination of ocular specimens from patients with Fuchs iridocyclitis confirms an inflammatory cause for the disease.[102] Electron microscopic examination of iris biopsy specimens has shown both a reduction in the number of stromal melanocytes and a decrease in melanosome size.[103] In that study, plasma cells, mast cells, and lymphocytes were found to be present in the tissue, but no infectious organisms were seen. Although Fuchs heterochromic iridocyclitis may be a single pathologic entity with a single cause, much of the evidence suggests that many occurrences represent a common ocular response that can develop from a variety of etiologic insults.

Treatment and Prognosis

Fuchs heterochromic iridocyclitis is generally chronic. Although therapy with topical corticosteroids can reduce the clinical signs of inflammation, long-term topical therapy is often unnecessary and may serve only to hasten cataract formation and induce glaucoma in responders to steroid therapy. Cataracts can be safely removed in patients with Fuchs heterochromic iridocyclitis; however, the glaucoma associated with the disease may not be easily controlled and can result in significant and permanent visual loss. Uveitis in these patients must be controlled. Although medications can control the glaucoma, surgery is often required but is fraught with the complications and difficulties associated with glaucoma surgery in other patients with uveitis.[96,98]

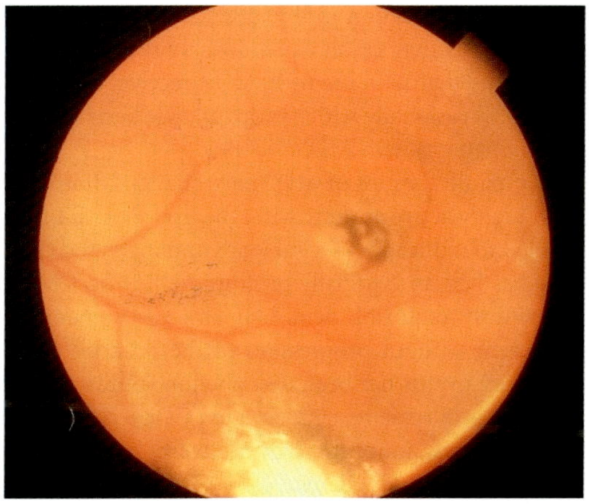

Fig. 20.6 Chorioretinal scar consistent with toxoplasmosis observed in the patient shown in Fig. 20-5. (Courtesy Rubens Belfort, Jr., MD.)

Kawasaki Disease

Kawasaki disease, also called *mucocutaneous lymph node syndrome,* is a disease of children and young adults characterized by an erythematous and desquamative exanthem (Fig. 20.7A), oral mucosal erythema (see Fig. 20.7B), conjunctivitis, fever, and an asymmetric cervical adenopathy.[104] Anterior uveitis has also been noted in many patients with this disorder and may lead to earlier diagnosis. In a study of 111 patients with incomplete Kawasaki disease, 37% had uveitis and received an earlier diagnosis and treatment than patients without uveitis.[105] Although the cause is unknown, patients with active Kawasaki disease have an antibody to interferon-α–activated endothelial cells from the umbilical vein that express MHC class II antigens.[106] In one study, 66% of patients had evidence of anterior uveitis that occurred most commonly during the first week of illness.[107] The uveitis does not appear to be severe or chronic and usually resolves without therapy. Optic disk edema and dilated retinal veins may also be seen (see Figs. 20.7C and D).

Most patients with Kawasaki disease have a good prognosis for recovery, although fatal complications develop in approximately 3%. Treatment for the systemic disease usually involves high-dose intravenous gamma globulin and aspirin. The anterior uveitis associated with Kawasaki disease is usually managed with topical corticosteroids.

Tubulointerstitial Nephritis and Uveitis Syndrome

Anterior uveitis has been associated with acute interstitial nephritis. In 1975, two publications reported two patients with interstitial nephritis

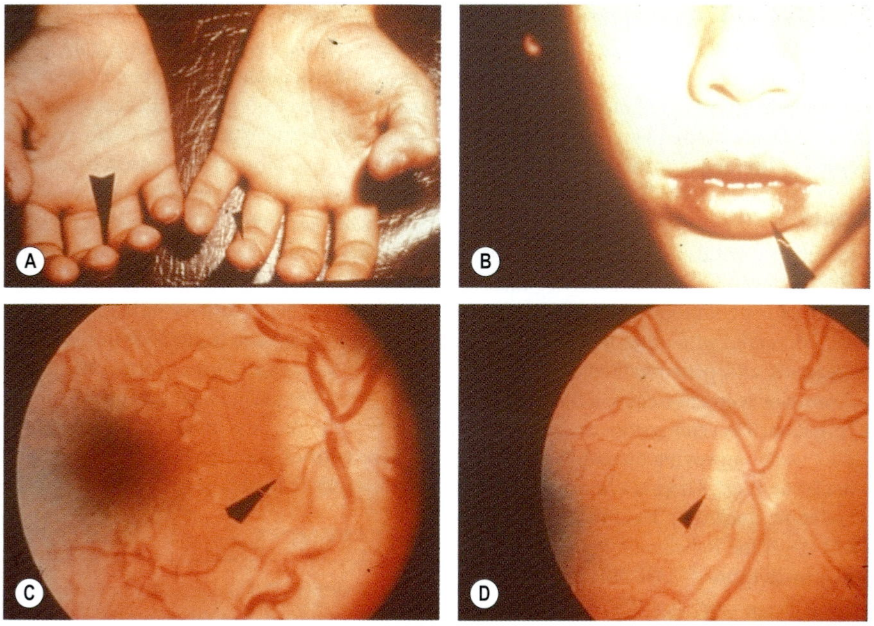

Fig. 20.7 (A) Distal cutaneous erythematous lesions seen in patient with Kawasaki disease. (B) Oral mucocutaneous lesions in a patient with the disease. (C) Papilledema and dilated retinal veins in a patient with Kawasaki disease that (D) resolved after the acute phase. (Courtesy Fernando Orefice, MD, and Rubens Belfort, Jr., MD.)

and anterior uveitis.[108,109] This syndrome is now called *tubulointerstitial nephritis and uveitis syndrome* (TINU).[110] The clinical and laboratory features of the disease were reviewed in a series of 111 patients.[111] Patients usually present with acute uveitis and later show manifestations of acute interstitial nephritis with cellular casts in urine.[112] Renal biopsy results show infiltration with eosinophils and mononuclear cells. The nephritis usually responds to corticosteroid therapy. Anterior uveitis has also been reported in patients with IgA nephropathy.[113] This disease often occurs in children and is associated with an upper respiratory tract infection. The uveitis appears to occur with the pulmonary disease and responds to standard therapy with topical corticosteroids and mydriatic and cycloplegic drops.

Pathogenesis

The pathogenesis of TINU appears to involve an immune response mediated by a number of possible environmental insults, including infection and certain medications. There appears to be a genetic component, and the disease has been described in monozygotic twins.[114] Seroreactivity against renal and retinal antigens has been reported.[115]

Glaucomatous Cyclitic Crisis

Glaucomatous cyclitic crisis, also known as *Posner-Schlossman syndrome,* is inflammatory glaucoma manifesting as unilateral fine KPs, mydriasis, and elevated IOP.[116] Conglomerates of inflammatory cells are occasionally noted in the anterior chamber angle, and accompanying reduction in aqueous outflow has been documented. Infectious agents, including cytomegalovirus (CMV), have been associated with Posner-Schlossman syndrome, as demonstrated by quantitative PCR.[117] Episodes are treated with topical corticosteroids and drugs to manage the increased IOP.[118] Surgical treatment of glaucoma is sometimes required, and successful outcomes have been reported.[119]

Schwartz Syndrome

Rhegmatogenous retinal detachment is frequently associated with a mild reduction in IOP. In some patients, IOP is elevated and associated with anterior uveitis. This syndrome of increased IOP, an open anterior chamber angle, and anterior segment inflammation is termed *Schwartz syndrome.*[120] It remains unclear whether the increased IOP is secondary to the anterior uveitis, concomitant damage to the trabecular meshwork, or blockage of the trabecular meshwork from retinal pigment epithelium (RPE) or components of the photoreceptors.[121] It should also be noted that anterior uveitis is a frequent finding in blunt ocular trauma and usually resolves with topical corticosteroid therapy.

Anterior Segment Ischemia

Anterior segment ischemia caused by carotid artery insufficiency may, in older patients, simulate anterior uveitis with the presence of cells and flare. The amount of flare is often out of proportion to the number of cells in the anterior chamber compared with other types of anterior uveitis. The pupil is poorly reactive, and patients often complain of dull, deep, and chronic pain. Anterior segment ischemia is often associated with other signs of ischemia, such as venous stasis and neovascularization.[122] Therapy should focus on improving the ischemia, rather than treating the secondary ocular findings. There is a long list of other causes of anterior segment ischemia, including local insults, such as surgery. Again, therapy should target the ischemia, although intraocular anti–vascular endothelial growth factor (VEGF) therapy has been used in cases with rubeosis iridis.[123]

Lens-Induced Uveitis

Anterior uveitis occurs in association with several forms of lens-induced glaucoma. Phacolytic glaucoma occurs when a hypermature cataract leaks liquefied cortical material into the anterior chamber. Macrophages are found in the aqueous humor, although KPs are rare.[124] Treatment involves suppressing the inflammation with topical corticosteroids and removing the cataract. Phacoantigenic glaucoma occurs after rupture of the lens capsule and is characterized by conjunctival chemosis and anterior segment inflammation, which develop within days to weeks after the capsular disruption. Phacotoxic glaucoma may also occur after recent cataract extraction or traumatic rupture of the lens capsule.[125] In these patients, inflammation is treated with topical, periocular, or systemic corticosteroids, in addition to antiglaucoma medications. These conditions must be distinguished from endophthalmitis, especially in the context of recent trauma or ocular surgery.

Anterior Uveitis Associated With AIDS

Anterior uveitis is found in a number of patients with AIDS and is also reviewed in the chapter on human immunodeficiency virus (HIV) infection (Chapter 12).[126] The anterior uveitis is often associated with other infectious diseases, such as syphilis, CMV retinitis, toxoplasmosis, herpes simplex, or herpes zoster.[127] A mild anterior uveitis may be associated with HIV infection in the absence of coinfection. In addition, anterior uveitis may result as an adverse reaction to one of the many medications that patients with AIDS receive. As stated earlier, anterior uveitis, occasionally with hypopyon, has been associated with rifabutin use in patients with AIDS.[8-10,128]

The ocular manifestations of AIDS have changed dramatically with the advent of highly active antiretroviral therapy (HAART). The use of HAART has led to reduced HIV viral loads and increased CD4+ T-cell counts. This has had an especially profound effect on CMV retinitis. Patients previously requiring persistent anti-CMV therapy are able to stop treatment without progression of the retinitis. However, an immune recovery uveitis has been described in some eyes with quiescent CMV retinitis in patients with elevated CD4+ counts.[129] In addition to anterior uveitis, immune recovery uveitis can include cataract, vitritis, and cystoid macular edema.

Other Disease Associations

In addition to the disorders described here, anterior uveitis can occur in many forms of uveitis. Infectious causes of uveitis, such as syphilis, herpes simplex virus keratitis, herpes zoster infection, and toxoplasmosis, are frequently accompanied by anterior uveitis. Noninfectious causes of uveitis, such as Behçet disease, sarcoidosis, and multiple sclerosis, are also associated with anterior segment inflammation. Anterior uveitis may be caused by postoperative infection as well. Acute bacterial endophthalmitis may present with a hypopyon. *Propionibacterium acnes* infection after cataract surgery has been associated with indolent smoldering anterior uveitis. Anterior uveitis may also be a sign of corneal allograft rejection, especially when seen in conjunction with corneal inflammation, such as a Khodadoust line. Anterior uveitis can occur after immunization or vaccination and may develop as a toxic effect of certain medications.[8,128,130] Finally, a number of malignancies, such as leukemia, retinoblastoma, and intraocular lymphoma, may masquerade as idiopathic anterior uveitis.[131,132] These entities are discussed in detail in the chapter on masquerade syndromes (Chapter 31).

REFERENCES

1. Wakefield D, Dunlop I, McClusky PJ, et al. Uveitis: aetiology and disease associations in an Australian population. *Aust NZ J Ophthalmol.* 1986;14:181–187.
2. Vedot E, Barth E, Billet P. Epidemiology of uveitis: preliminary results of a prospective study in Savoy. In: Sarri KM, ed. *Uveitis Update.* Amsterdam: Elsevier; 1984:13–16.

3. Rothova A, Veenedaal WG, Linssen A, et al. Clinical features of acute anterior uveitis. *Am J Ophthalmol.* 1987;103:137–145.
4. Wakefield D, Montanaro A, McCluskey P. Acute anterior uveitis and HLA-B27. *Surv Ophthalmol.* 1991;36:223–232.
5. Juanola X, Loza Santamaria E, Cordero-Coma M. for the SENTINEL Working Group. Description and prevalence of spondyloarthritis in patients with anterior uveitis. *Ophthalmology.* 2016;123:1632–1636.
6. Frantz C, Portier A, Etcheto A, et al. Acute anterior uveitis in spondyloarthritis: a monocentric study of 301 patients. *Clin Exp Rheumatol.* 2019;37:26–31.
7. Guex-Crosier Y, Pittet N, Herbort CP. Evaluation of laser flare-cell photometry in the appraisal and management of intraocular inflammation in uveitis. *Ophthalmology.* 1994;101:728–735.
8. Frank MO, Graham MB, Wispelway B. Rifabutin and uveitis [letter]. *N Engl J Med.* 1994;330:868.
9. Jacobs DS, Piliero PJ, Kuperwaser MG, et al. Acute uveitis associated with rifabutin use in patients with human immunodeficiency virus infection. *Am J Ophthalmol.* 1994;118:716–722.
10. Saran BR, Maguire AM, Nichols C, et al. Hypopyon uveitis in patients with acquired immunodeficiency syndrome treated for systemic *Mycobacterium avium* complex infection with rifabutin. *Am J Ophthalmol.* 1994;112:1159–1165.
11. Fong DS, Raizman MB. Spontaneous hyphema associated with anterior uveitis. *Br J Ophthalmol.* 1993;77:635–638.
12. Whitcup SM, Wakefield D, Li Q, et al. Endothelial leukocyte adhesion molecule-1 in endotoxin-induced uveitis. *Invest Ophthalmol Vis Sci.* 1992;33:2626–2630.
13. Whitcup SM, DeBarge LR, Rosen H, et al. Monoclonal antibody against CD11b/CD18 inhibits endotoxin-induced uveitis. *Invest Ophthalmol Vis Sci.* 1993;34:673–681.
14. Elner VM, Elner SG, Pavilack MA, et al. Intercellular adhesion molecule-1 in human corneal endothelium: modulation and function. *Am J Pathol.* 1991;138:525–536.
15. Wertheim MS, Mathers WD, Planck SJ, et al. In vivo confocal microscopy of keratic precipitates. *Arch Ophthalmol.* 2004;122:1773–1781.
16. Alfawaz AM, Holland GN, Yu F, et al. Corneal endothelium in patients with anterior uveitis. *Ophthalmology.* 2016;123:1637–1645.
17. Lee A, Taylor P, Kalpathy-Cramer J, et al. Machine learning has arrived! *Ophthalmology.* 2017;1234:1726–1728.
18. Gonzalez-Lopez JJ, Garcia-Aparico AM, Sanchez-Ponce D, et al. Development and validation of a Bayesian network for the differential diagnosis of anterior uveitis. *Eye.* 2016;30:865–872.
19. Moorthy RS, Valluri S, Jampol LM. Drug-induced uveitis. *Surv Ophthalmol.* 1998;42:557–570.
20. Fraunfelder FW, Rosenbaum JT. Drug-induced uveitis. Incidence, prevention and treatment. *Drug Safety.* 1997;17:197–207.
21. Huhtinen M, Repo H, Laasila K, et al. Systemic inflammation and innate immune response in patients with previous anterior uveitis. *Br J Ophthalmol.* 2002;86:412–417.
22. Anwar Z, Galor A, Albini TA, et al. The diagnostic utility of anterior chamber paracentesis with polymerase chain reaction in anterior uveitis. *Am J Ophthalmol.* 2013;155:781–786.
23. Hench PS, Kendall EC, Slocumb CH, et al. The effect of a hormone of the adrenal cortex (17-hydroxy-11-dehydrocorticosterone: compound E) and of pituitary adrenocorticotropic hormone on rheumatoid arthritis. *Proc Staff Meet Mayo Clin.* 1949;24:181–197.
24. Gordon DM, McLean JM. Effects of pituitary adrenocorticotropic hormone (ACTH) therapy in ophthalmologic conditions. *JAMA.* 1950;142:1271–1276.
25. Olson JA, Steffensen EH, Margulis RR, et al. Effect of ACTH on certain inflammatory diseases of the eye. *JAMA.* 1950;142:1276–1278.
26. Sheppard JD, Toyos MM, Kempen JH, et al. Difluprednate 0.05% versus prednisolone acetate 1% for endogenous anterior uveitis: a phase III, multicenter, randomized study. *Invest Ophthalmol Vis Sci.* 2014;55:2993–3002.
27. Wakefield D, Montanaro A, McCluskey P. Acute anterior uveitis and HLA-B27. *Surv Ophthalmol.* 1991;36(3):223–232.
28. Otasevic L, Zlatanovic G, Stanojevic-Paovic A, et al. *Helicobacter pylori:* an underestimated factor in acute anterior uveitis and spondyloarthropathies? *Ophthalmologica.* 2007;221:6–13.
29. Zeboulon N, Dougados M, Gossec L. Prevalence and characteristics of uveitis in the spondyloarthropathies: a systematic literature review. *Ann Rheum Dis.* 2008;67:955–959.
30. Braakenburg AM, de Valk HW, de Boer J, et al. Human leukocyte antigen-B27-associated uveitis: long-term follow-up and gender differences. *Am J Ophthalmol.* 2008;145:472–479.
31. Colbert RA, Tran TM, Layh-Schmitt G. HLA-B27 misfolding and ankylosing spondylitis. *Mol Immunol.* 2014;57:44–51.
32. Colbert RA, Navid F, Till T. The role of HLA-B*27 in spondyloarthritis. *Best Pract Res Clin Rheumatol.* 2017;31:797–815.
33. Chen B, Li J, He C, et al. Role of HLA-B27 in the pathogenesis of ankylosing spondylitis (review). *Molecular Med Rep.* 2017;15:1943–1951.
34. Wakefield D, Abi-Hanna D. HLA antigens and their significance in the pathogenesis of anterior uveitis: a mini review. *Curr Eye Res.* 1986;5:465–473.
35. Chang JH, McCluskey PJ, Wakefield D. Toll-like receptors in ocular immunity and the immunopathogenesis of inflammatory eye disease. *Br J Ophthalmol.* 2006;90:103–108.
36. Mondino BJ, Rao H. Hemolytic complement activity in aqueous humor. *Arch Ophthalmol.* 1983;101:465–468.
37. Mondino BJ, Sumner H. Anaphylatoxin levels in human aqueous humor. *Invest Ophthalmol Vis Sci.* 1986;27:1288–1292.
38. Sen DK, Sarin GS, Mathur MD. Serum fibrin degradation products in acute idiopathic anterior uveitis. *Acta Ophthalmol.* 1986;64:632–636.
39. Wakefield D, McCluskey P, Palladinetti P. Distribution of lymphocytes and cell adhesion molecules in iris biopsy specimens from patients with uveitis. *Arch Ophthalmol.* 1992;110:121–125.
40. El-Shabrawi Y, Wegscheider BJ, Weger M, et al. Polymorphisms within the tumor necrosis factor-alpha promoter region in patients with HLA-B27-associated uveitis: association with susceptibility and clinical manifestations. *Ophthalmology.* 2006;113:695–700.
41. Brewerton DA, Caffrey M, Hart FD, et al. Ankylosing spondylitis and HLA-B27. *Lancet.* 1973;1:904–907.
42. Ebringer R, White L, McCoy R, et al. Seasonal variation in acute anterior uveitis: differences between HLA-B27 positive and HLA-B27 negative disease. *Br J Ophthalmol.* 1985;69:202–204.
43. Masi AT. Epidemiology of B27 associated disease. *Ann Rheum Dis.* 1979;38:131–134.
44. Evans DM, Spencer CC, Pointon JJ, et al. Interaction between ERAP1 and HLA-B27 in ankylosing spondylitis implicates peptide handling in the mechanism for HLA-B27 in disease susceptibility. *Nat Genet.* 2011;43:761–767.
45. International Genetics of Ankylosing Spondylitis Consortium (IGAS), Cortes A, Hadler J, Pointon JP, et al. Identification of multiple risk variants for ankylosing spondylitis through high-density genotyping of immune-related loci. *Nat Genet.* 2013;45:730–738.
46. Jethwa H, Bowness P. The interleukin (IL)-23/IL-17 axis in ankylosing spondylitis: new advances and potentials for treatment. *Clin Exp Immunol.* 2016;183:30–36.
47. Munoz-Fernandez S, Garcia-Aparicio AM, Hidalgo MV, et al. Methotrexate: an option for preventing the recurrence of acute anterior uveitis. *Eye.* 2009;23:1130–1133.
48. Jones A, Ciurtin C, Ismajli M, et al. Biologics for treating axial spondyloarthritis. *Expert Opin Biol Ther.* 2018;18:641–652.
49. Braun J, Baraliakos X, Listing J, et al. Decreased incidence of anterior uveitis in patients with ankylosing spondylitis treated with the anti-tumor necrosis factor agents infliximab and etanercept. *Arthritis Rheum.* 2005;52:2447–2451.
50. Sfikakis PP. The first decade of biologic TNF antagonists in clinical practice: lessons learned, unresolved issues and future directions. *Curr Dir Autoimmun.* 2010;11:180–210.
51. Lie E, Lindstrom U, Zverkova-Sandstrom T, et al. Tumour necrosis factor inhibitor treatment and occurrence of anterior uveitis in ankylosing spondylitis: results from the Swedish biologics register. *Ann Rheum Dis.* 2017;76(9):1515–1521.

52. Reddy AR, Backhouse OC. Does etanercept include uveitis? *Br J Ophthalmol.* 2003;87:925.
53. Kasner L, Chan CC, Whitcup SM, et al. This increase in anterior uveitis with anti-TNF therapy may be more associated with etanercept than with other anti-TNF agents. The paradoxical effect of tumor necrosis factor alpha (TNF-α) in endotoxin-induced uveitis. *Invest Ophthalmol Vis Sci.* 1993;34:2911–2917.
54. Letko E, Yeh S, Foster CS, et al. AIN457A2208 Study Group. Efficacy and safety of intravenous secukinumab in non-infectious uveitis requiring steroid-sparing immunosuppressive therapy. *Ophthalmology.* 2015;122:939–948.
55. Reiter H. Uber eine bisher unerkannte Spirochateninfektion. *Dtsch Med Wochenschr.* 1916;42:1535–1536.
56. Garcia-Kutzbach A, Chacon-Suchite J, Garcia-Ferrer H, et al. Reactive arthritis: update 2018. *Clin Rheumatol.* 2018;37:869–874.
57. Lee DA, Barker SM, Su WPD, et al. The clinical diagnosis of Reiter's syndrome. *Ophthalmology.* 1986;93:350–356.
58. Keat A. Reiter's syndrome and reactive arthritis in perspective. *N Engl J Med.* 1983;39:1606–1615.
59. Cassidy JT, Levinson JE, Bass JC, et al. A study of classification criteria for a diagnosis of juvenile rheumatoid arthritis. *Arthritis Rheum.* 1986;29:274–281.
60. Ravelli A, Martini A. Juvenile idiopathic arthritis. *Lancet.* 2007;369:767–768.
61. Petty RF, Southwood TR, Manners P, et al. International League of Associations for Rheumatology Classification of Juvenile Idiopathic Arthritis: second revision, Edmonton, 2001. *J Rheumatol.* 2004;31:390–392.
62. Giancane G, Consolaro A, Lanni S, et al. Juvenile idiopathic arthritis: diagnosis and treatment. *Rheumatol Ther.* 2016;3:187–207.
63. Rosenberg AM. Uveitis associated with juvenile rheumatoid arthritis. *Semin Arthritis Rheum.* 1987;16:158–173.
64. Wolf MD, Lichter PR, Ragsdale CG. Prognostic factors in the uveitis of juvenile rheumatoid arthritis. *Ophthalmology.* 1987;94:1242–1247.
65. Smiley WK. The eye in juvenile rheumatoid arthritis. *Trans Ophthalmol Soc UK.* 1974;94:817–829.
66. Key SW III, Kimura SJ. Iridocyclitis associated with juvenile rheumatoid arthritis. *Am J Ophthalmol.* 1975;80:425–429.
67. Merriam JC, Chylack LT, Albert DM. Early onset pauciarticular juvenile rheumatoid arthritis: a histopathologic study. *Arch Ophthalmol.* 1983;101:1085–1092.
68. Sabates R, Smith T, Apple D. Ocular histopathology in juvenile rheumatoid arthritis. *Ann Ophthalmol.* 1979;1979:733–737.
69. Kanski JJ. Anterior uveitis in juvenile rheumatoid arthritis. *Arch Ophthalmol.* 1977;95:1794–1797.
70. Chylack LT. The ocular manifestations of juvenile rheumatoid arthritis. *Arthritis Rheum.* 1977;20:217–223.
71. Angeles-Han ST, Ringold S, Beukelman T, et al. American College of Rheumatology/Arthritis Foundation guideline for the screening, monitoring, and treatment of juvenile idiopathic arthritis-associated uveitis. *Arthritis Rheumatol.* 2019;71:864–877.
72. Olson NY, Lindsley CB, Godfrey WA. Nonsteroidal antiinflammatory drug therapy in chronic childhood iridocyclitis. *Am J Dis Child.* 1988;142:1289–1292.
73. Giannini EH, Brower EJ, Kuzmind N, et al. Methotrexate in resistant juvenile rheumatoid arthritis. Results of the USA–USSR double-blind, placebo-controlled trial. *N Engl J Med.* 1992;326:1043–1049.
74. Kahn P, Weiss M, Imundo LF, et al. Favorable response to high-dose infliximab for refractory childhood uveitis. *Ophthalmology.* 2006;113:860–864.
75. Ramanan AV, Dick AD, Jones AP, et al. for the SYCAMORE Study Group. Adalimumab plus methotrexate for uveitis in juvenile idiopathic arthritis. *N Engl J Med.* 2017;376:1637–1646.
76. Sauremann RK, Levin AV, Rose JB, et al. Tumour necrosis factor alpha inhibitors in the treatment of childhood uveitis. *Rheumatology (Oxford).* 2006;45:92–99.
77. Diamond JG, Kaplan HG. Lensectomy and vitrectomy for complicated cataract secondary to uveitis. *Arch Ophthalmol.* 1978;96:1798–1804.
78. Praeger DL, Schneider HA, Sakowski AD, et al. Kelman procedure in the treatment of complicated cataract of the uveitis of Still's disease. *Trans Ophthalmol Soc UK.* 1976;96:168–171.
79. Foster CS, Barrett F. Cataract development and cataract surgery in patients with juvenile rheumatoid arthritis-associated iridocyclitis. *Ophthalmology.* 1993;100:809–817.
80. O'Brien JM, Albert DM. Therapeutic approaches for ophthalmic problems in juvenile rheumatoid arthritis. *Rheum Dis Clin North Am.* 1989;15:413–437.
81. Akinci A, Cakar N, Uncu N, et al. Keratoconjunctivitis sicca in juvenile rheumatoid arthritis. *Cornea.* 2007;26:941–944.
82. Reininga JK, Los LI, Wulffraat NM, et al. The evaluation of uveitis in juvenile idiopathic arthritis (JIA) patients: are current ophthalmologic screening guidelines adequate? *Clin Exp Rheumatol.* 2008;26:367–372.
83. Thorne JE, Woreta F, Kedhar SR, et al. Juvenile idiopathic arthritis-associated uveitis: incidence of ocular complications and visual acuity loss. *Am J Ophthalmol.* 2007;143:840–846.
84. Tappeiner C, Schenck S, Nieweth M, et al. Impact of anti-inflammatory treatment on the onset of uveitis in juvenile idiopathic arthritis: longitudinal analysis from a nationwide pediatric rheumatology database. *Arthritis Care Res.* 2016;68:46–54.
85. Calin A. The spondyloarthropathies. In: Wyngaarden JB, Smith LH Jr, Bennett JC, eds. *Cecil Textbook of Medicine.* 19th. Philadelphia: WB Saunders; 1992:1515–1521.
86. Paiva E, Macaluso D, Edwards A, et al. Characterisation of uveitis in patients with psoriatic arthritis. *Ann Rjeum Dis.* 2000;59:67–70.
87. Tobin AM, Kirby B. TNF alpha inhibitors in the treatment of psoriasis and psoriatic arthritis. *BioDrugs.* 2005;19:47–57.
88. Ellis PP, Gentry JH. Ocular complications of ulcerative colitis. *Am J Ophthalmol.* 1964;58:779–784.
89. Duker JS, Brown GC, Brooks L. Retinovasculitis in Crohn's disease. *Am J Ophthalmol.* 1987;103:654–668.
90. Lopes Troncoso LL, Biandardi AL, Veira de Moraes HV Jr, et al. Ophthalmic manifestations in patients with inflammatory bowel disease: a review. *World J Gatroenterol.* 2017;23:5836–5848.
91. Karmiris K, Avgerinos A, Tavernaraki A, et al. Prevalence and characteristics of extra-intestinal manifestations in a large cohort of Greek patients with inflammatory bowel disease. *J Crohns Colitis.* 2016;10:429–436.
92. Selsky EJ, Knox DL, Maumanee AE, et al. Ocular involvement in Whipple's disease. *Retina.* 1984;4:103–106.
93. Lawrence W. Changes in colour in the iris. In: Hays I, ed. *A Treatise on Diseases of the Eye.* Philadelphia: Lea & Blanchard; 1843:411–416.
94. Fuchs E. Über Komplicaationen der Heterochromie. *Z Augenheilkd.* 1906;15:191–212.
95. Kimura SJ, Hogan MJ, Thygeson P. Fuchs' syndrome of heterochromic cyclitis. *Arch Ophthalmol.* 1955;54:179–186.
96. Liesegang TJ. Clinical features and prognosis in Fuchs' uveitis syndrome. *Arch Ophthalmol.* 1982;100:1622–1626.
97. Accorinti M, Spinucci G, Pia Pirraglia M, et al. Fuchs' heterochromic iridocyclitis in an Italian tertiary referral centre: Epidemiology, clinical features, and prognosis. *J Ophthalmol.* 2016;2016:1458624.
98. Jones NP. Fuchs' heterochromic uveitis: an update. *Surv Ophthalmol.* 1993;37:253–272.
99. Amsler M. New clinical aspects of the vegetative eye. *Trans Ophthalmol Soc UK.* 1948;68:45–74.
100. de Groot-Mijnes JD, de Visser L, Rothova A, et al. Rubella virus is associated with Fuchs' heterochromic iridocyclitis. *Am J Ophthalmol.* 2006;141:212–214.
101. Quentin CD, Reiber H. Fuchs' heterochromic cyclitis: rubella virus antibodies and genome in aqueous humor. *Am J Ophthalmol.* 2004;138:46–54.
102. Goldberg MF, Erozan YS, Duke JR, et al. Cytopathologic and histopathologic aspects of Fuchs' heterochromic iridocyclitis. *Arch Ophthalmol.* 1965;74:604–609.
103. McCartney AC, Bull TB, Spalton DJ. Fuchs' heterochromic cyclitis: an electron microscopy study. *Trans Ophthalmol Soc UK.* 1986;105:324–329.
104. Bligard CA. Kawasaki disease and its diagnosis. *Pediatr Dermatol.* 1987;4:75–84.

105. Lee KJ, Kim HJ, Kim MJ, et al. Usefulness of anterior uveitis as an additional tool for diagnosing incomplete Kawasaki disease. *Korean J Pediatr.* 2016;59:174077.
106. Leung DY, Collins T, Lapierre LA, et al. Immunoglobulin M antibodies present in the acute phase of Kawasaki syndrome lyse cultured vascular endothelial cells stimulated by gamma interferon. *J Clin Invest.* 1986;77:1428–1435.
107. Burns JC, Joffe L, Sargent RA, et al. Anterior uveitis associated with Kawasaki syndrome. *Pediatr Infect Dis.* 1985;4:258–261.
108. Kikkawa Y, Sakurai M, Mano T, et al. Interstitial nephritis with concomitant uveitis. Report of two cases. *Contrib Nephrol.* 1975;4:1–11.
109. Dobrin RS, Venier RL, Fish AL. Acute eosinophilic interstitial nephritis and renal failure with bone marrow-lymph node granulomas and anterior uveitis: a new syndrome. *Am J Med.* 1975;59:325–333.
110. Vanhaesebrouck P, Carton D, De Bel C, et al. Acute tubulo-interstitial nephritis and uveitis syndrome (TINU syndrome). *Nephron.* 1985;40:418–422.
111. Mandeville JT, Levinson RD, Holland GN. The tubulointerstitial nephritis and uveitis syndrome. *Surv Ophthalmol.* 2001;46:195–208.
112. Gafter U, Ben-Basat M, Zevin D, et al. Anterior uveitis, a presenting symptom in acute interstitial nephritis. *Nephron.* 1986;42:249–251.
113. Moller-Jensen J, Marthinsen L, Linne T. Anterior uveitis in IgA nephropathy. *Am J Ophthalmol.* 1989;108:604–605.
114. Howarth L, Gilbert RD, Bass P, et al. Tubulointerstitial nephritis and uveitis in monozygotic twin boys. *Pediatr Nephrol.* 2004;19:917–919.
115. Shimazaki K, Jirawuthiworavong GV, Nguyen EV, et al. Tubulointerstitial nephritis and uveitis syndrome: a case with an autoimmune reactivity against retinal and renal antigens. *Ocul Immunol Inflamm.* 2008;16:51–53.
116. Posner A, Schlossman A. Syndrome of unilateral recurrent attacks of glaucoma with cyclitic symptoms. *Arch Ophthalmol.* 1948;39:517–528.
117. Teoh SB, Thean L, Koay E. Cytomegalovirus in aetiology of Posner-Schlossman syndrome: evidence from quantitative polymerase chain reaction. *Eye (Lond).* 2005;19:1338–1340.
118. Megaw R, Agarwal PK. Posner-Schlossman syndrome. *Surv Ophthalmol.* 2017;62:277–285.
119. Artini W, Bani AP. The effectiveness of trabeculectomy with mitomucin C and releasable suture in Posner-Schlossman syndrome with secondary glaucoma: a case series. *Niger J Clin Pract.* 2019;22:138–143.
120. Schwartz A. Chronic open-angle glaucoma secondary to rhegmatogenous retinal detachment. *Am J Ophthalmol.* 1973;75:205–211.
121. Matsuo N, Takabatake M, Ueno H, et al. Photoreceptor outer segments in the aqueous humor in rhegmatogenous retinal detachment. *Am J Ophthalmol.* 1986;101:673–679.
122. Jacobs NA, Ridgway AE. Syndrome of ischaemic ocular inflammation: six cases and a review. *Br J Ophthalmol.* 1985;69:682–687.
123. Janssens K, Zeyen T, Van Calster J. Anterior segment ischemia with rubeosis iridis after a circular buckling operation treated successfully with an intravitreal bevacizumab injection: a case report and review of the literature. *Bull Soc Belge Ophthalmol.* 2012;319:5–9.
124. Epstein DL, Jedziniak JA, Grant WM. Identification of heavy molecular weight protein in aqueous humor in human phacolytic glaucoma. *Invest Ophthalmol.* 1978;17:398–402.
125. Irvine SR, Irvine AR Jr. Lens-induced uveitis and glaucoma. II. The "phacotoxic" reaction. *Am J Ophthalmol.* 1952;35:370–375.
126. Shuler JD, Engstrom RE, Holland GN. External ocular disease and anterior segment disorders associated with AIDS. *Int Ophthalmol Clin.* 1989;29:98–104.
127. Verma S, Hughes JD, Mabey D, et al. Symptomatic anterior uveitis in HIV-positive patients. *Int J STD AIDS.* 1999;10:268–274.
128. Fuller JD, Stanfield LE, Craven DE. Rifabutin prophylaxis and uveitis [letter, comment]. *N Engl J Med.* 1994;330:1315–1316.
129. Robinson MR, Reed G, Csaky KG, et al. Immune-recovery uveitis in patients with cytomegalovirus retinitis taking highly active antiretroviral therapy. *Am J Ophthalmol.* 2000;130:49–56.
130. Yeomans SM, Knox DL, Green WR, et al. Ocular inflammatory pseudotumor associated with propranolol therapy. *Ophthalmology.* 1983;90:1422–1425.
131. Woog JJ, Chess J, Albert DM, et al. Metastatic carcinoma of the iris simulating iridocyclitis. *Br J Ophthalmol.* 1984;68:167–173.
132. Hertler AA, Rosenwasser GO, Gluck WL. Isolated anterior chamber relapse in acute monoblastic leukemia. *Am J Hematol.* 1986;23:401–403.

21

Scleritis

Scott M. Whitcup

KEY CONCEPTS

- Scleritis is a painful and potentially sight-threatening inflammation of the sclera and is associated with immune or infectious causes. Treatment often requires systemic anti-inflammatory therapy, including corticosteroids and immunosuppressive drugs.
- Biologic agents, including the anti–tumor necrosis factor (TNF)-α medications, may be useful in treating scleritis.
- Episcleritis is an inflammatory disorder of the episclera and is often mild in severity, rarely impairs vision, and frequently resolves with topical anti-inflammatory agents or with no therapy.
- Antimicrobial therapy and surgical treatment are often required for treating bacterial or fungal scleritis.

Scleritis is a painful and potentially sight-threatening disorder. From a strict anatomic viewpoint, scleritis is not a form of uveitis but, rather, an inflammatory disorder that is similar in pathogenesis to many forms of uveitis. When severe, scleritis is often associated with inflammation in the underlying uveal tissue. Entire books have been written on scleritis, so only some of its key features are discussed in this chapter. Like uveitis, scleritis is often associated with underlying systemic disease. Additionally, the therapeutic approaches to scleritis and uveitis share many similarities. In contrast to scleritis, episcleritis is a disorder involving the more superficial episclera and tends to be more acute and less severe than scleritis. Importantly, episcleritis is rarely, if ever, vision threatening and may resolve without therapy. Episcleritis is also discussed in this chapter.

EPISCLERITIS

Episcleritis is an inflammatory disorder involving the episcleral tissue that lies superficial to the sclera, just beneath the Tenon capsule. Although it occurs in both sexes and at all ages, it is seen more frequently in young to middle-aged women. Episcleritis is usually mild and is characterized by slight conjunctival injection and the presence of a foreign body sensation. The episodes often resolve without treatment, but episcleritis can recur. Occasionally, patients may experience more severe redness and pain. Inflamed episcleral blood vessels tend to have a salmon color in natural light, radiate from the limbus, and can be moved over the sclera with a cotton-tipped applicator. In addition, these more superficial vessels will blanch after administration of topical phenylephrine. Nodular episcleritis has also been described.

In 50% or greater of cases, episcleritis is idiopathic; however, many of the diseases associated with scleritis have also been associated with episcleritis. In a review of 100 patients with episcleritis, an associated systemic disease was found in 36 (36%).[1] Although often self-limiting, episcleritis can be associated with corneal involvement, uveitis, and glaucoma.

Extensive evaluation for underlying disease may not be warranted for mild forms of the disease, especially if it is not recurrent. When treatment is required, the disease often responds to topical or oral nonsteroidal anti-inflammatory drugs (NSAIDs) or to topical corticosteroids. Although topical vasoconstrictors can reduce the redness, they should be used sparingly. In patients with episcleritis that fails to respond to initial therapy, one should suspect the possibility of a masquerade syndrome, such as a conjunctival malignancy or an underlying systemic disease.

The differential diagnosis of episcleritis includes conjunctivitis; a conjunctival malignancy, such as lymphoma; medications; and scleritis. Conjunctivitis, whether allergic or infectious, can frequently be distinguished from episcleritis on the basis of symptoms and examination findings. Infectious conjunctivitis is usually associated with a discharge and allergic conjunctivitis with itching and chemosis. Scleritis is anatomically deeper and has a distinct appearance. Malignant conjunctival lesions also tend to have a specific appearance and are rarely mistaken for episcleritis. A number of medications associated with both episcleritis and scleritis are listed in Box 21.1.

The visual prognosis for patients with episcleritis is usually good.[2] Some patients have a single episode, and in those with recurrent disease, the frequency of episodes tends to diminish over time. Because up to one-third of patients can have an associated systemic disease and because episcleritis can be associated with ocular complications, such as uveitis and glaucoma, patients with more severe or recurrent episcleritis should be carefully assessed and treated. Table 21.1 compares the features of episcleritis and scleritis.

SCLERITIS

The severity of scleritis varies greatly, but the disease can result in loss of vision and be difficult to treat. Scleritis is characterized by eye pain and redness of the sclera and episclera. The pain is usually gradual in onset but can become excruciating, with the feeling of something boring into the eye, and can wake the patient from sleep. The pain may radiate to the forehead or to other parts of the face and may be associated with photophobia and tearing. Corneal involvement, anterior uveitis, and exudative retinal detachments can occur and cause decreased vision. The inflamed sclera is deep to the episclera, typically with a violaceous hue, and the inflamed vessels cannot be moved with a cotton-tipped applicator (Fig. 21.1). The disease is most common in the fourth to sixth decades of life and more common in women. Scleritis is bilateral in greater than 50% of patients, but it frequently starts in one eye. It can be divided into anterior and posterior diseases (see Table

21.1). Anterior scleritis has been classified into four additional categories (Table 21.2): diffuse, nodular, necrotizing with inflammation, and necrotizing without inflammation.[3] Necrotizing scleritis without inflammation is also called *scleromalacia perforans*. A standardized grading system for scleritis has been published and may be useful for clinical assessment and research purposes (Fig. 21.2).[4]

Necrotizing scleritis is a severe form of the disorder, frequently associated with both blinding ocular disease and life-threatening systemic disease. An underlying systemic disease was found in approximately one-half of patients with necrotizing scleritis.[3] Necrotizing scleritis with inflammation is almost always painful. The sclera is edematous, and inflammation leads to scleral thinning, which allows the underlying choroid to become visible. Intraocular inflammation is often seen in severe cases of scleritis. Fluorescein angiography shows hypoperfusion or nonperfusion of the scleral vessels. Other complications of scleritis include cataract and glaucoma. In one review, an increase in intraocular pressure was noted in about one-fifth of patients.[5]

BOX 21.1 Medications Associated with Episcleritis and Scleritis

Bisphosphonates
Erlotinib
Procainamide

TABLE 21.1 Characteristics of Episcleritis and Scleritis

Feature	Episcleritis	Scleritis
Anatomy	Episclera (deep to Tenon capsule)	Sclera
Age (years)	20s–40s	20s–60s
Sex	Predominantly women	Predominantly women
Clinical features	Mild pain, transient	Painful
Underlying systemic disease	Occasional	Common
Complications	Rare	Frequent
Treatment	May not be needed Topical anti-inflammatory drugs, when needed	Needed Systemic corticosteroids, immunosuppressive medications, or biologic agents frequently required
Prognosis	Excellent; rarely vision threatening	Variable; frequently vision impairing

Posterior scleritis is defined as inflammation of the sclera posterior to the ora serrata. Symptoms of posterior scleritis can be subtle, and the disease is frequently misdiagnosed. As with other forms of scleritis, pain is the most common symptom; however, vision is affected more frequently. Unlike other forms of scleritis, redness can be subtle and missed on examination. Other findings include retinal and/or choroidal folds, exudative retinal detachments, or choroidal masses. As with anterior scleritis, masquerade syndromes should be suspected in atypical cases of posterior scleritis, especially when the disease does not respond to treatment. Some of the malignant diseases masquerading as posterior scleritis include lymphoma, metastatic carcinoma, and choroidal melanoma. We have also seen occurrences of benign lymphoid hyperplasia involving the choroid and juvenile xanthogranuloma misdiagnosed as posterior scleritis. Nonmalignant disorders, including retinal detachments and central serous retinopathy, can also masquerade as posterior scleritis.

Scleritis occurs in children, although the characteristics of the disease can differ from those in adults. Episcleritis appears to occur less frequently in children but usually has a similar mild course as in adults. In a series of 24 eyes from 20 children with scleritis, the mean age at presentation was 12 years with equal sex distribution.[6] The disease was unilateral in 80% of patients. Most eyes had posterior scleritis, and tuberculosis was the only associated systemic disease found in three (15%) patients. In a study of posterior scleritis in children, underlying systemic disease was also uncommon.[7] Scleritis in children can occur after surgery, including strabismus surgery.

Disease Associations

An underlying systemic disease is diagnosed in about one-half of patients with scleritis. Box 21.2 lists some of the diseases associated with scleritis. Rheumatoid arthritis is probably the most common of these. Scleritis has been associated with several forms of systemic

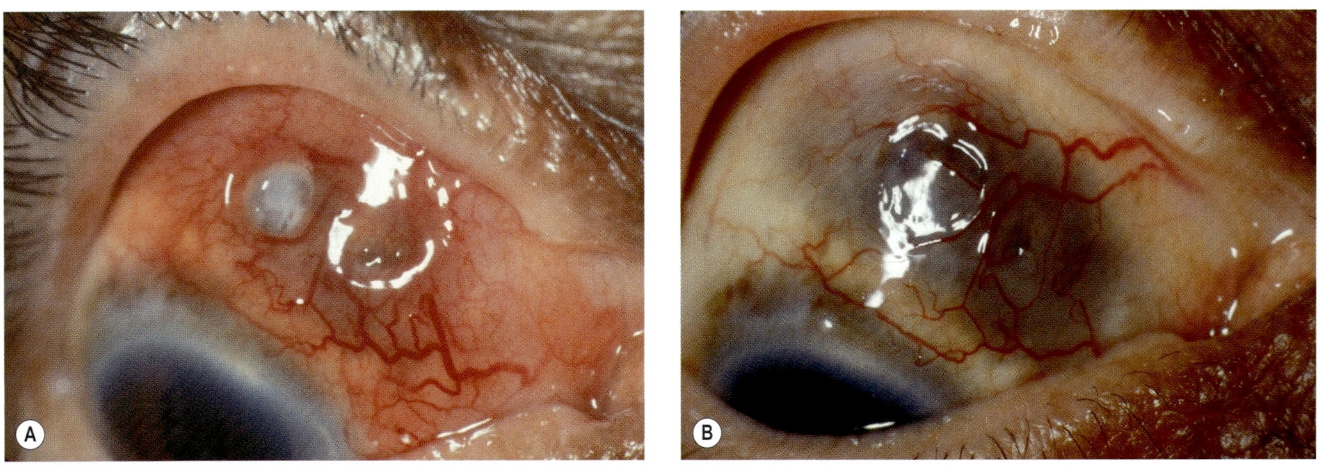

Fig. 21.1 (A) Nodular anterior scleritis in patient with rheumatoid arthritis. Inflammation of the deep scleral vessels is characterized by violaceous hue. (B) After 2 months of systemic corticosteroids, the scleral vessels are less inflamed; however, signs of scleral thinning can be noted.

vasculitis, including Wegener granulomatosis (Fig. 21.3), polyarteritis nodosa, and relapsing polychondritis. The presence of necrotizing scleritis is thought to be associated with increased severity of disease in patients with rheumatoid arthritis[8] and is an indication for systemic immunosuppression; however, this association may not hold true for other autoimmune diseases. Wegener granulomatosis is a multiorgan disease characterized by necrotizing granulomatous vasculitis. The disease frequently involves the kidneys and the respiratory tract; the eye is involved in more than half these patients. Polyarteritis nodosa is another systemic vasculitis that affects multiple organs. It involves small- and medium-sized arteries and is associated with abdominal pain, myalgia, peripheral neuritis, and renal disease. Eye involvement can also occur. Cogan syndrome is a form of systemic vasculitis associated with interstitial keratitis and hearing loss. Arthritis, aortitis, and vasculitis resembling polyarteritis nodosa have also been described.

A number of infectious diseases have been associated with scleritis. Historically, tuberculosis and syphilis were common causes. Scleritis has also been described in patients with Lyme disease and other infections, such as bartonellosis.

TABLE 21.2 Classification of Scleritis with Approximate Disease Prevalence

Classification	Prevalence (%)
Anterior scleritis	90–99
Diffuse scleritis	30–45
Nodular scleritis	30–45
Necrotizing scleritis with inflammation	10
Necrotizing scleritis without inflammation (scleromalacia perforans)	1–5
Posterior scleritis	1–10

Other Causes of Scleritis

Scleritis has been associated with a number of surgical procedures, including cyclodestructive procedures, pterygium surgery, vitreoretinal surgery, and other corneal and anterior segment operations. These cases of scleritis can be severe and require prolonged therapy.[9] Medications, including the bisphosphonates, have been associated with both episcleritis and scleritis (see Box 21.1).[10,11]

Diagnostic Testing

Although the diagnosis of scleritis is based on medical history and clinical examination, diagnostic testing is often indicated because many patients have an associated systemic disease. Posterior scleritis is more difficult to diagnose on the basis of clinical signs and symptoms, and B-scan ultrasonography can be useful in demonstrating thickening of the posterior sclera. Optical coherence tomography (OCT) may also be useful in the diagnosis and management of some patients with scleritis. In one study, patients with active anterior scleritis showed increased thickness of the sclera, with intrascleral hyporeflective areas consistent with edema compared with patients

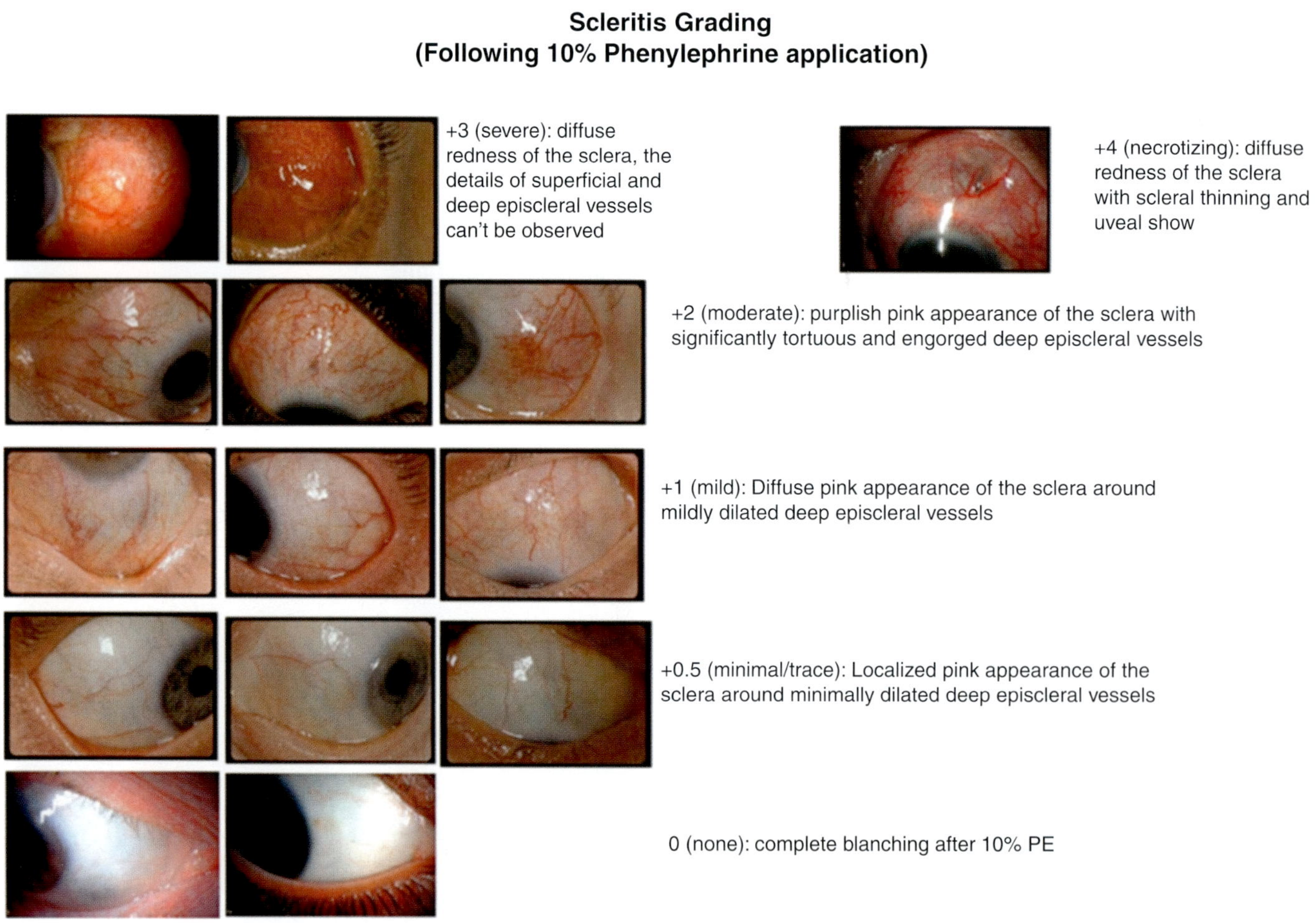

Fig. 21.2 Scleritis grading system. Standardized digital photographs of scleritis of varying severity. (From Sen HN, Sangave AA, Goldstein DA, et al. A standardized grading system for scleritis. Ophthalmology. 2011;118:768–771.)

BOX 21.2 Diseases Associated with Scleritis

Rheumatoid arthritis
Juvenile rheumatoid arthritis
Reiter syndrome
Crohn disease
Ankylosing spondylitis
Ulcerative colitis
Polymyositis
Relapsing polychondritis
Systemic lupus erythematosus
Wegener disease
Polyarteritis nodosa
Cogan syndrome
Sarcoidosis
Lyme disease
Bartonellosis
Syphilis
Tuberculosis
Herpes zoster infection
Acanthamoeba keratitis

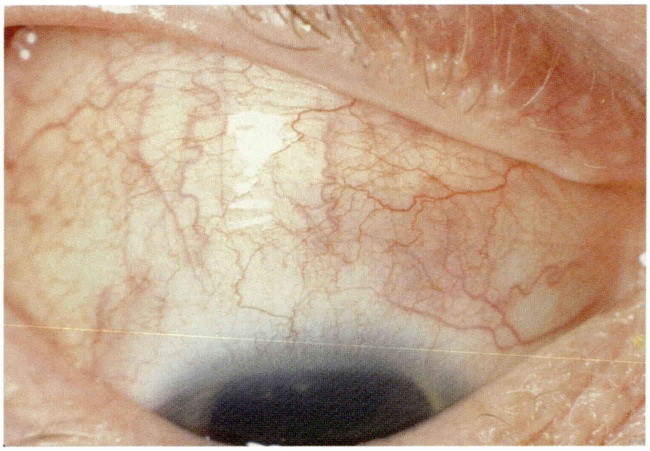

Fig. 21.3 Diffuse anterior scleritis in a patient with Wegener granulomatosis.

with episcleritis and normal eyes.[12] In complicated cases, computed tomography (CT) may be useful in identifying associated orbital disease. If an underlying rheumatologic disease is suspected, laboratory assessment should be based on the history and physical examination of the patient. A fluorescent treponemal antibody absorption (FTA-ABS) test should be performed to rule out any treatable cause of scleritis. The antineutrophil cytoplasmic antibody (ANCA) test may be useful in predicting the presence of an underlying systemic disease in patients with scleritis.[13] ANCA-positive patients with scleritis are also more likely to have ocular complications and thus warrant more aggressive anti-inflammatory therapy.

Pathogenesis

Most of the pathologic data suggest that scleritis is an immune-mediated disease.[14] Pathologic examination shows both granulomatous and nongranulomatous inflammation and associated vasculitis.[15] Histologic examination reveals diffuse infiltration with inflammatory cells that eventually replaces collagen, leading to scleral thinning (Fig. 21.4).

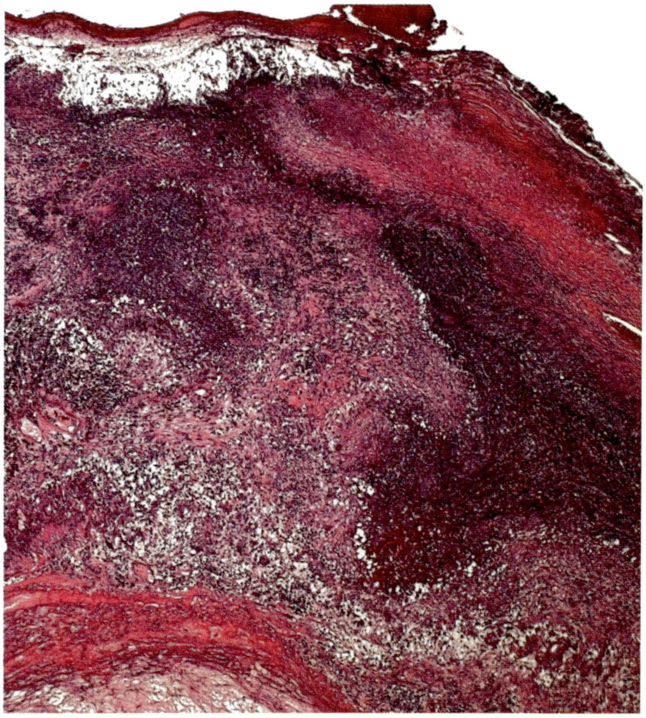

Fig. 21.4 Photomicrograph showing diffuse replacement of the collagen fibers of the sclera with inflammatory infiltrates. The inflammation consists of focal granulomas, vasculitis, hemorrhage, and necrosis. (Hematoxylin & eosin; original magnification ×50.) (Courtesy Chi-Chao Chan, MD.)

Deposition of circulating immune complexes has been thought to be the cause of the disorder; however, the disease may also be caused by a T-cell–mediated response to antigens in the sclera, such as type II collagen, or to antigens in the scleral blood vessels. Increased expression of cell adhesion molecules, such as intercellular adhesion molecule 1 (ICAM-1) on the sclera may play a role in the pathogenesis of the disease.[16] Sporadic case reports have discussed possible infectious causes of scleritis.[17]

Differential Diagnosis

Episcleritis is the most challenging condition to differentiate from scleritis, and because the severity and treatment of episcleritis differ greatly from those of scleritis, it is important to distinguish the two diseases. Severe uveitis can be associated with overlying scleral inflammation, but the diagnosis of underlying uveitis is obvious on ophthalmic examination. Malignancies, such as melanoma or metastatic disease, can mimic scleritis and should be considered. It is also important to diagnose underlying immunologic diseases because systemic therapy is often required for both scleritis and the underlying condition.

Treatment

Use of topical corticosteroids or oral NSAIDs usually controls inflammation in patients with mild scleritis. For more severe forms of the disease, treatment with oral corticosteroids or other systemic immunosuppressive agents is often required.[18-20] Methotrexate is commonly used to treat moderately severe scleritis, and mycophenolate mofetil was shown to have efficacy in treating patients with scleritis, some of whom had failed or were intolerant to other therapies.[21,22]

The scleritis associated with necrotizing systemic vasculitis may be diffuse, nodular, or necrotizing. Necrotizing scleritis in these diseases is especially difficult to treat and almost always requires systemic immunosuppressive therapy.[23–26] Importantly, immunosuppression is required to control the underlying necrotizing systemic vasculitis because, in untreated patients, mortality is high. Treatment recommendations are therefore based, to a large degree, on findings from trials examining the effect of immunosuppression on mortality and disease severity in patients with Wegener granulomatosis and polyarteritis nodosa. Treatment with cyclophosphamide was shown to produce complete remission in 93% of patients.[27] Deaths occurred in only 7% of patients over a mean follow-up period of 51 months. Similarly, cyclophosphamide reduced the 5-year mortality in patients with polyarteritis nodosa from 53% to 20%.[28]

Although there have been no randomized controlled trials (RCTs), several studies have evaluated the treatment of scleritis associated with necrotizing systemic vasculitis. Cyclophosphamide was the only effective immunosuppressive drug used in three patients with necrotizing scleritis associated with relapsing polychondritis; in these patients, treatment with high-dose systemic corticosteroids, penicillamine, methotrexate, and azathioprine had failed.[23] Treatment of scleritis in patients with necrotizing systemic vasculitis should be guided both by the ophthalmic response and by control of the underlying disease. The ANCA test, for example, is a useful laboratory measure of the therapeutic response in patients with Wegener granulomatosis. Cyclophosphamide, starting at a dose of 2 mg/kg/day, may be the drug of choice for scleritis associated with necrotizing systemic vasculitis. Concomitant administration of prednisone at a dose of 1 mg/kg/day may be needed for disease uncontrolled by a maximally tolerated dose of cyclophosphamide. Oral corticosteroids can usually be tapered and often discontinued over the first 6 to 12 weeks of cytotoxic therapy.

Other immunosuppressive agents, including methotrexate, azathioprine, cyclosporin, and chlorambucil, have been successfully used for the treatment of necrotizing systemic vasculitis, but the reports in the literature are of small case series. Because of its widespread use in the treatment of rheumatologic disease, methotrexate is probably more commonly used to treat scleritis compared with some of the other agents. Inflammation control was achieved in 11 of 18 patients with chronic, noninfectious, nonnecrotizing scleritis treated with methotrexate at a dose of 7.5 to 35 mg weekly.[29] Complete corticosteroid sparing was achieved in 10 of these 11 patients.

Periocular injections of corticosteroids have not been widely used for the treatment of scleritis, mainly for fear of exacerbating scleral thinning or precipitating scleral perforation. Subconjunctival corticosteroid injections for nonnecrotizing anterior scleritis resistant to topical or systemic therapy was evaluated in 38 eyes of 35 patients.[30] Thirty-six of the 38 eyes had complete resolution of signs and symptoms within 6 weeks of therapy. However, 15 had perforation, and other adverse events included cataract and glaucoma. No scleral necrosis or scleral melting was observed over a median follow-up period of 29 months. Use of intravitreal sustained-release implants have also been used to treat refractory scleritis.[31] Although preliminary, these data suggest that there may be a role for local corticosteroid therapy in some patients with anterior scleritis; however, additional data are needed to fully assess the safety and efficacy of this therapeutic approach. Other therapeutic approaches have included the use of rituximab[32] and topical cyclosporin A.[33]

Bacterial and fungal causes of scleritis require specific antimicrobial therapy.[34] In addition to local and systemic antimicrobial treatment, surgical intervention may also be needed to control progressive suppuration. With appropriate therapy, vision outcomes in these patients can be good.

Although there has been success in treating rheumatologic diseases, such as rheumatoid arthritis with inhibitors of tumor necrosis factor (TNF), the initial clinical experience in treating scleritis was more variable. A case series reported nine patients with uveitis and seven with scleritis treated with etanercept or infliximab.[35] Only six of the 16 patients experienced improvement, and five developed inflammatory eye disease for the first time while taking a TNF inhibitor. More recently, there have been a number of other reports of patients successfully treated with anti-inflammatory biologic agents, including TNF inhibitors, rituximab, tofacitinib, and gevokizumab.[36–42] However, it is important to note that there are no findings from large, well-controlled RCTs to guide therapy for patients with scleritis. Nevertheless, these biologic agents offer additional therapeutic options for patients with scleritis. As with all immunotherapy, it is critical to rule out underlying infections, such as tuberculosis, before these agents are used.

Prognosis

Patients with episcleritis have a good prognosis. The disease rarely impairs vision and often resolves with topical nonsteroidal anti-inflammatory agents or, in many cases, without therapy. In contrast, scleritis can cause profound vision loss and often requires systemic immunosuppressive therapy. Scleral perforation and severe glaucoma are two of the more devastating complications of scleritis. Surgical treatment of scleral perforation can be successfully performed, but it is critical that inflammation be well controlled with systemic immunosuppressive medications. Glaucoma can also lead to blindness in patients with scleritis. The glaucoma can usually be controlled with topical medications; however, surgical treatment may be warranted in rare cases where intraocular pressure cannot be controlled with eye drops. In a study of 104 patients with scleritis, a loss of more than two lines of Snellen acuity was observed in 23 patients, three of whom had a final visual acuity of no light perception.[43] Importantly, with appropriate diagnosis and therapy of scleritis and the underlying systemic disease, when present, visual and patient outcomes can be good.

CASE 21.1

A 64-year-old Asian woman with a history of diabetes and hypertension presented with pain and redness in her left eye. She was initially diagnosed with an inflamed pinguecula and treated with topical corticosteroids, without improvement. The patient reported occasional pain in her hands and knees, and she had been previously diagnosed with osteoarthritis and treated with nonsteroidal anti-inflammatory drugs. On examination, she was found to have nodular scleritis of the left eye (Fig. 21.5A). Laboratory evaluation revealed a positive result for rheumatoid factor, and a positive result for anticyclic citrullinated peptide (anti-CCP), consistent with a diagnosis of rheumatoid arthritis. The patient was initially treated with oral prednisone, resulting in improvement in the scleritis within a week (see Fig. 21.5B). Low-dose methotrexate and infliximab were started as the prednisone was tapered. The scleritis resolved, and the patient's arthritis remained quiet; her medications were slowly tapered and discontinued. After 2 years, the scleritis (see Fig. 21.5C) and joint disease recurred, and the patient was treated with a similar regimen.

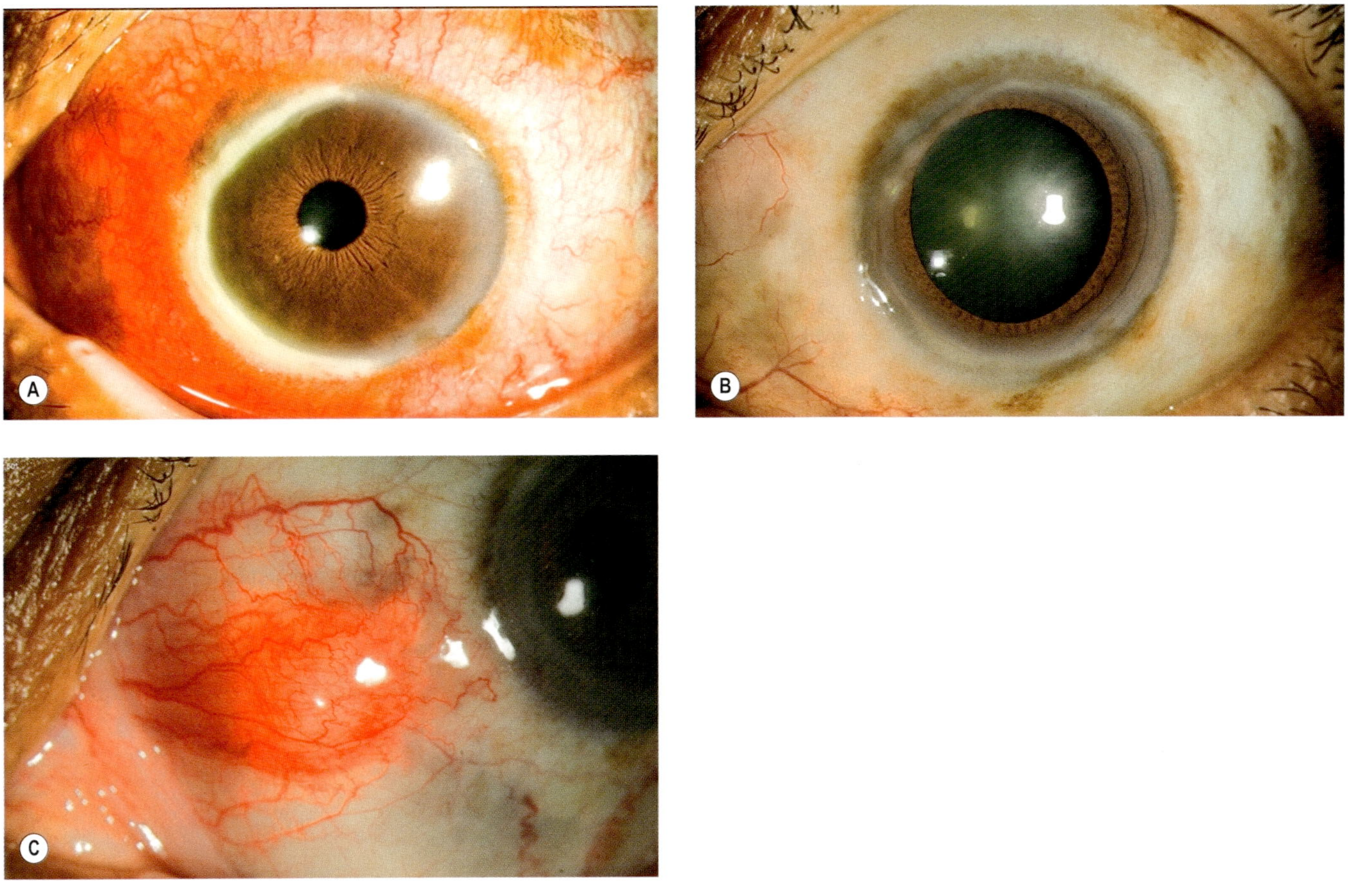

Fig. 21.5 (A) Nodular scleritis in a patient with rheumatoid arthritis. (B) Improvement of the scleritis within 1 week of starting oral prednisone. (C) Recurrent nodular scleritis 2 years after the patient's systemic anti-inflammatory medications had been tapered.

REFERENCES

1. Akpek EK, Uy HS, Christen W, et al. Severity of episcleritis and systemic disease association. *Ophthalmology*. 1999;106:729–731.
2. Heron E, Gutzwiller-Fontaine M, Bourcier T. Scleritis and episcleritis: diagnosis and treatment. *Rev Med Intern*. 2014;35:577–585.
3. Watson PG, Hayreh SS. Scleritis and episcleritis. *Br J Ophthalmol*. 1976;60:163–191.
4. Sen HN, Sangave AA, Goldstein DA, et al. A standardized grading system for scleritis. *Ophthalmology*. 2011;118:768–771.
5. Heinz C, Bograd N, Koch J, et al. Ocular hypertension and glaucoma incidence in patients with scleritis. *Graefes Arch Clin Exp Ophthalmol*. 2013;251:139–142.
6. Majumder PD, Ali S, George A, et al. Clinical profile of scleritis in children. *Ocul Immunol Inflamm*. 2019;27(4):535–539.
7. Cheung CM, Chee SP. Posterior scleritis in children: clinical features and treatment. *Ophthalmology*. 2012;119:59–65.
8. Foster CS, Forstot L, Wilson LA. Mortality rate in rheumatoid arthritis patients with destructive ocular lesions: effect of systemic immunosuppression. *Ophthalmology*. 1984;91:1253–1263.
9. Galanopoulos A, Snibson G, O'Day J. Necrotising anterior scleritis after pterygium surgery. *Aust N Z J Ophthalmol*. 1994;22:167–173.
10. Fraunfelder FW. Ocular side effects associated with bisphosphonates. *Drugs Today (Barc)*. 2003;39:829–835.
11. Turgeon PW, Slamovits TL. Scleritis as the presenting manifestation of procainamide-induced lupus. *Ophthalmology*. 1989;96:68–71.
12. Shoughy SS, Jaroudi MO, Kozak I, et al. Optical coherence tomography in the diagnosis of scleritis and episcleritis. *Am J Ophthlamol*. 2015;159:1045–1049.
13. Hoang LT, Lim LL, Vaillant B, et al. Antineutrophil cytoplasmic antibody-associated active scleritis. *Arch Ophthalmol*. 2008;126:651–655.
14. Watson PG. Doyne Memorial Lecture, 1982. The nature and the treatment of scleral inflammation. *Trans Ophthalmol Soc UK*. 1986;102:257–281.
15. Sevel D. Necrogranulomatous scleritis. Clinical and histologic features. *Am J Ophthalmol*. 1967;64:1125–1134.
16. Sangwan VS, Merchant A, Sainz de la Maza M, et al. Leukocyte adhesion molecule expression in scleritis. *Arch Ophthalmol*. 1998;116:1476–1480.
17. Krist D, Wenkel H. Posterior scleritis associated with *Borrelia burgdorferi* (Lyme disease) infection. *Ophthalmology*. 2002;109:143–145.
18. Foster CS, Sainz de la Maza M. *The Sclera*. New York: Springer-Verlag; 1994.
19. Jabs DA, Mudun A, Dunn JP, et al. Episcleritis and scleritis: clinical features and treatment results. *Am J Ophthalmol*. 2000;130:469–476.
20. Okhravi N, Odufuwa B, McCluskey P, et al. *Scleritis. Surv Ophthalmol*. 2006;51:351–363.
21. Thorne JE, Jabs DA, Qazi FA, et al. Mycophenolate mofetil therapy for inflammatory eye disease. *Ophthalmology*. 2005;112:1472–1477.
22. Sobrin L, Christen W, Foster CS. Mycophenolate mofetil after methotrexate failure or intolerance in the treatment of scleritis and uveitis. *Ophthalmology*. 2008;115:1416–1421.
23. Hoang Xuan T, Foster CS, Rice BA. Scleritis in relapsing polychondritis. *Ophthalmology*. 1990;97:892–898.
24. Sainz de la Maza M, Molina N, Gonzalez-Gonzalez LA, et al. Scleritis therapy. *Ophthalmology*. 2012;119:51–58.
25. Daniel Diaz J, Sobol EK, Gritz DC. Treatment and management of scleral disorders. *Surv Ophthalmol*. 2016;61:702–717.
26. Beardsley RM, Suhler EB, Rosenbaum JT, et al. Pharmacotherapy of scleritis: current paradigms and future directions. *Expert Opin Pharmacother*. 2013;14:422–424.

27. Fauci AS, Haynes BF, Katz P, et al. Wegener's granulomatosis: prospective clinical and therapeutic experience with 85 patients for 21 years. *Ann Intern Med.* 1983;98:76–85.
28. Leib ES, Restivo C, Paulus HE. Immunosuppression and corticosteroid therapy of polyarteritis nodosa. *Am J Med.* 1979;67:941–947.
29. Jachens AW, Chu DS. Retrospective review of methotrexate therapy in the treatment of chronic, noninfectious, nonnecrotizing scleritis. *Am J Ophthalmol.* 2008;145:487–492.
30. Albini TA, Zamir E, Read RW, et al. Evaluation of subconjunctival triamcinolone for nonnecrotizing anterior scleritis. *Ophthalmology.* 2005;112:1814–1820.
31. Ahn SJ, Hwant SJ, Lee BR. Intravitreal dexamethasone implants for the treatment of refractory scleritis combined with uveitis in adult-onset Still's disease: a case report. *BMC Ophthlmol.* 2016;16:196.
32. Ahmadi-Simab K, Lamprecht P, Nolle B, et al. Successful treatment of refractory anterior scleritis in primary Sjogren's syndrome with rituximab. *Ann Rheum Dis.* 2005;64:1087–1088.
33. Shimura M, Yasuda K, Fuse N, et al. Effective treatment with topical cyclosporin A of a patient with Cogan syndrome. *Ophthalmologica.* 2000;214:429–432.
34. Cunningham MA, Alexander JK, Matoba AY, et al. Management and outcome of microbial anterior scleritis. *Cornea.* 2011;30: 1020–1023.
35. Smith JR, Levinson RD, Holland GN, et al. Differential efficacy of tumor necrosis factor inhibition in the management of inflammatory eye disease and associated rheumatic disease. *Arthritis Rheum.* 2001;45:252–257.
36. Murphy CC, Ayliffe WH, Booth A, et al. Tumor necrosis factor alpha blockage with infliximab for refractory uveitis and scleritis. *Ophthalmology.* 2004;111:352–356.
37. Sobrin L, Kim EC, Christen W, et al. Infliximab therapy for the treatment of refractory ocular inflammatory disease. *Arch Ophthalmol.* 2007;125:895–900.
38. Beardsley RM et al. *Expert Opin Pharmacother.* (see above)
39. Cao JH, Orgy M, Cocho L, et al. Rituximab in the treatment of refractory noninfectious scleritis. *Am J Ophthalmol.* 2016;164:22–28.
40. Suhler EB, Lim LL, Beardsley RM, et al. Rituximab therapy for refractory scleritis: results of a phase I/II dose-ranging, randomized, clinical trial. *Ophthalmology.* 2014;121:1885–1891.
41. Paley MA, Karacal H, Rao PK, et al. Tofacitinib for refractory uveitis and scleritis. *Am J Ophthalmol Case Rep.* 2018;13:53–55.
42. Knickelbein JE, Tucker WR, Bhatt N, et al. Gevokizumab in the treatment of autoimmune non-necrotizing anterior scleritis: results of a phase I/II clinical trial. *Am J Ophthalmol.* 2016;172:104–110.
43. Wieringa WG, Wieringa JE, ten Dam-van Loon NH, et al. Visual outcome, treatment results, and prognostic factors in patients with scleritis. *Ophthalmology.* 2013;120:379–386.

22

Intermediate Uveitis

Scott M. Whitcup

KEY CONCEPTS

- Diagnosis is based on the anatomic location of ocular inflammation: vitreous and peripheral retina with macular edema.
- Intermediate uveitis is frequently associated with a systemic or infectious disease.
- Pars planitis is a subtype of intermediate uveitis.
- Complications include macular edema, epiretinal membrane, vitreous hemorrhage, retinal detachment, and glaucoma.
- Uveitis in patients with multiple sclerosis may be associated with a shorter time to first disease recurrence and a higher annualized relapse rate.
- Treatment involves corticosteroids and immunosuppressive agents, including biologic agents.
- Cryoretinopexy and vitrectomy may be beneficial for some patients.

The diagnosis of intermediate uveitis is based on the anatomic location of ocular inflammation; it is not a distinct clinicopathologic condition. The diagnosis is made when ocular inflammation primarily involves the vitreous and the peripheral retina. Intermediate uveitis was first described as chronic cyclitis by Fuchs in 1908.[1] The clinical description of intermediate uveitis was further elucidated in 1950 by Schepens,[2] who described patients with a peripheral uveitis characterized by inflammation centered on the vasculature and exudative changes in the retinal periphery. In 1960, Brockhurst et al.[3] described additional patients with peripheral vascular abnormalities and exudate along the ora serrata and pars plana, and Welch et al.[4] used the term *pars planitis* to describe inflammation characterized by the white accumulation on the pars plana. Other terms used in the literature to describe patients with intermediate uveitis include *vitritis, peripheral exudative retinitis, cyclochorioretinitis, chronic posterior cyclitis,* and *peripheral uveoretinitis.* Unfortunately, there is still confusion and controversy, even among uveitis specialists, regarding how to classify patients with this anatomic distribution of intraocular inflammation. Grouping conditions with the anatomic features of intermediate uveitis does provide value because it helps with developing a differential diagnosis and in determining response to therapy and long-term prognosis. The Standardization of Uveitis Nomenclature (SUN) Working Group has defined intermediate uveitis as disease where the vitreous is the major site of inflammation.[5]

We use the term *intermediate uveitis,* as suggested by the International Uveitis Study Group, to classify patients with intraocular inflammation predominantly involving the vitreous and the peripheral retina. Some specialists use this term only if a more specific diagnosis cannot be made. Specific diseases, such as sarcoidosis and multiple sclerosis, are known to cause intermediate uveitis, and we often classify patients as having intermediate uveitis associated with sarcoidosis or associated with multiple sclerosis, when an underlying disease can be identified. The reason for this is that some diseases, such as sarcoidosis, can also present with other manifestations, such as predominant retinitis, and these patients will respond differently to therapy. We also use the term *pars planitis* to describe a subset of patients with intermediate uveitis when a white opacity (commonly called "snowbank") occurs over the pars plana and the ora serrata. Although pars planitis probably does not represent a clinical entity distinct from intermediate uveitis, patients with pars planitis often have worse vitritis, more severe macular edema, and a worse prognosis compared with patients with intermediate uveitis who do not have a pars plana exudate.[6]

EPIDEMIOLOGY

Intermediate uveitis accounts for approximately 4% to 12% of cases of uveitis in a referral practice.[7-11] In approximately 15% of patients with uveitis referred to us at the National Institutes of Health (NIH), intermediate uveitis is diagnosed. In a retrospective, population-based cohort study, the incidence of pars planitis was 2.077 per 100,000 persons (95% confidence interval [CI]: 1.43–2.62).[12] Although the incidence of uveitis in children is low, intermediate uveitis may account for up to 25% of cases.[13] Intermediate uveitis has been reported in both young children and older adults, but it tends to mostly affect people from the teens to the 40s.[8] There appears to be no sex or race predilection.

There have been occasional reports of intermediate uveitis occurring in families, suggesting that either hereditary or environmental factors may predispose one to the disease. Human leukocyte antigen (HLA) associations have been identified in patients with multiple sclerosis and intermediate uveitis, but there is debate about the possibility of other HLA haplotypes being associated with intermediate uveitis.[14] In 1963, Kimura and Hogan[15] first reported multiple family members with intermediate uveitis. With a focus on the genetic associations of inflammatory diseases, a number of these families have been reported.[13,16-19] In one instance of familial pars planitis, the two affected brothers were not twins but had identical HLA haplotypes.[16] There have also been cases of intermediate uveitis of the pars planitis subtype in identical twins.[20] Some of the familial occurrences of intermediate uveitis are associated with demyelinating disease.[21,22] Studies have indicated a possible association of intermediate uveitis with HLA-A28, HLA-DR15, HLA-DR51, and HLA-DR17 haplotypes.[23-25] IL2RA gene variants were found to be associated with intermediate uveitis but not with HLA-B27 acute anterior uveitis.[26]

ETIOLOGY

The causes of intermediate uveitis and pars planitis have not been elucidated. Evidence suggests that all patients with intermediate uveitis probably do not have the same disease. Although intermediate uveitis

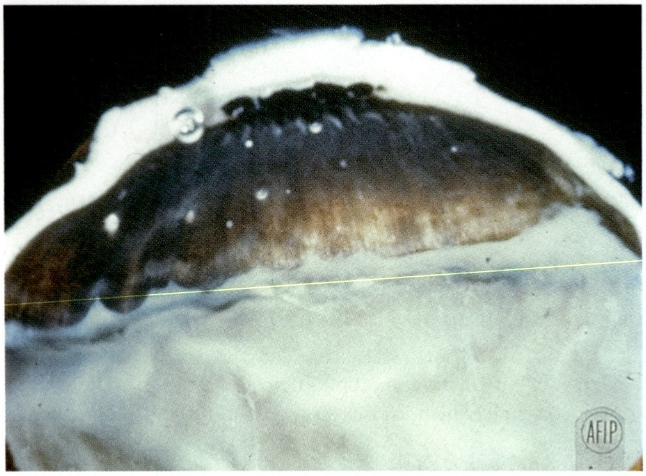

Fig. 22.1 Gross pathologic appearance of peripheral snowbank in patient with intermediate uveitis of pars planitis subtype. (Courtesy Lorenz Zimmerman, MD.)

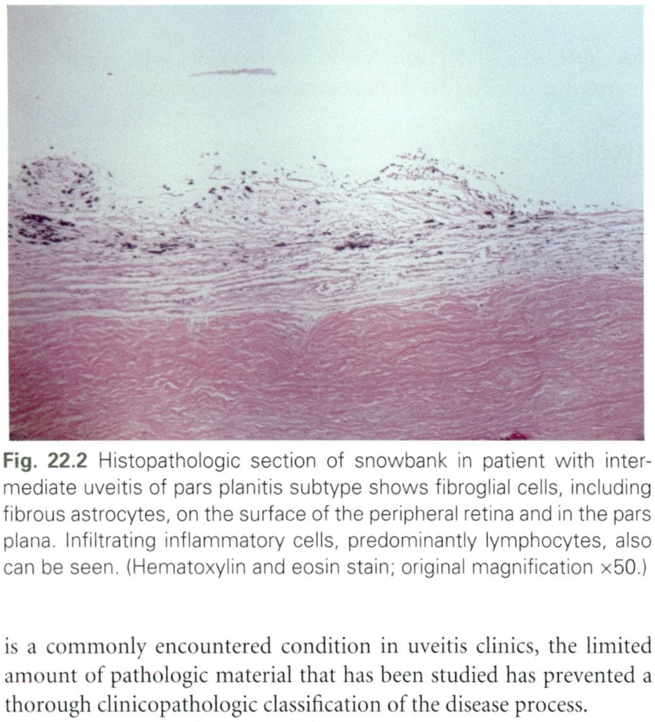

Fig. 22.2 Histopathologic section of snowbank in patient with intermediate uveitis of pars planitis subtype shows fibroglial cells, including fibrous astrocytes, on the surface of the peripheral retina and in the pars plana. Infiltrating inflammatory cells, predominantly lymphocytes, also can be seen. (Hematoxylin and eosin stain; original magnification ×50.)

is a commonly encountered condition in uveitis clinics, the limited amount of pathologic material that has been studied has prevented a thorough clinicopathologic classification of the disease process.

Exudate deposited in eyes with intermediate uveitis of the pars planitis subtype typically localizes to a broad area of the inferior pars plana (see Fig. 3.17). The inferior location of exudate is attributed to gravity. A diffuse phlebitis leads to breakdown of the blood–ocular barrier and release of inflammatory cells, cytokines, and other inflammatory mediators that settle inferiorly.[27] Gross pathologic examination of the peripheral snowbank in pars planitis shows exudate deposited on the peripheral retina and pars plana (Fig. 22.1). Histologic examination of this snowbank reveals collapsed vitreous; blood vessels; fibroglial cells, including fibrous astrocytes; and scattered inflammatory cells, predominantly lymphocytes (Fig. 22.2).[28] Peripheral veins show lymphocytic cuffing and infiltration. The vascular component of the snowbank is continuous with the retina in some cases; this suggests that the neovascularization associated with pars planitis may be the result of retinal vessels extending through breaks in the inner limiting membrane of the vitreous base.[28] Only mild inflammation is noted in the choroid and the ciliary body, suggesting that the inflammatory process in intermediate uveitis primarily involves the vitreous base and the peripheral retina, and not the uvea.

The vitreous snowballs in patients with intermediate uveitis are composed of epithelioid cells and multinucleated giant cells. Green et al.[29] noted that these cells are absent from the uvea, suggesting that the vitreous may be the primary site of inflammation. We had the opportunity to study an eye from a patient with familial pars planitis. Histologic examination revealed glial tissue in the snowbank and extensive peripheral vascular disease, with perivascular infiltration of lymphocytes and expression of major histocompatability complex (MHC) class II antigen on the vascular endothelium.[16] There was no substantial choroidal inflammation, again suggesting that pars planitis is a type of peripheral retinitis or vitritis, and not choroiditis. Studies of eyes with intermediate uveitis without pars plana exudate are sparse; this makes clinicopathologic correlation between the two disease types a difficult task.

The association between intermediate uveitis and autoimmune diseases, such as multiple sclerosis, suggests that at least some occurrences of the disorder are autoimmune in nature. Intermediate uveitis is thought to be a type of primary peripheral retinal perivasculitis. Once initiated, the process of vascular occlusion and inflammation may lead to vitritis and snowbank formation in some patients. Although others, such as Khodadoust et al.,[30] have hypothesized that intermediate uveitis is primarily vitreal inflammation, they have noted that the inflammation appears to start adjacent to the involved vascular tissue. Supporting the vascular etiology of the disease, Thorne et al.[31] demonstrated that current smoking was associated with a dose-dependent increase in cystoid macular edema complicating intermediate uveitis. Interestingly, in a study in monkeys, injection of hyaluronic acid into the vitreous induced a clinical picture similar to that of pars planitis.[32] Furthermore, Gartner[33] demonstrated that the vitreous contains cellular remnants that may be the antigenic stimulus in pars planitis. Bora et al.[34,35] noted a 36-kDa protein with sequence homology to a yeast nucleopore complex, which may be a marker for the disease, in the serum of patients with active intermediate uveitis.

However, none of these theories fully explains the familial association in intermediate uveitis; the association of this disorder with certain systemic diseases, such as sarcoidosis, inflammatory bowel disease, and multiple sclerosis; or the cause of cystoid macular edema. We think that the periphlebitis and breakdown of the blood–ocular barrier are the initiating events in many cases. Increased levels of immune markers, such as soluble interleukin (IL)-2 receptors and intercellular adhesion molecule-1 (ICAM-1), have been found in the serum of patients with intermediate uveitis.[36,37] Elevated levels of IL-6 in the vitreous humor of patients with pars planitis confirms the local immune activation in this disease.[38] However, the specific cause of this vascular disease is multifactorial and probably varies from patient to patient.

CLINICAL MANIFESTATIONS

Most patients present with blurred vision and/or floaters. Pain and photophobia are rare. Early in the course of the disease, visual acuity is often reduced to the 20/40 range as a result of moderate vitritis and cystoid macular edema. However, if inflammation is not well controlled, severe visual loss can ensue, associated with chronic cystoid macular edema, glaucoma, inflammatory changes in the retina, and retinal detachment. We have seen sudden loss of vision in several patients after vitreous hemorrhage. Bilateral involvement is seen in 70% to 80% of patients at the time of presentation, and bilateral involvement will occur in approximately one-third of patients who initially have unilateral disease experience.[6,8]

Most adults with intermediate uveitis have minimal anterior segment inflammation,[39] except those with intermediate uveitis associated with multiple sclerosis; these patients typically develop a granulomatous anterior uveitis with formation of mutton-fat keratic precipitates (KPs). Anterior segment inflammation is more common in pediatric uveitis, where there may be a moderate degree of anterior chamber cells with posterior synechiae. Brockhurst et al.[3] noted peripheral anterior synechiae in 24% of patients and posterior synechiae in 18%. Band keratopathy may be seen in children. Occasionally, patients may present with significant anterior segment inflammation with pain and photophobia and only later manifest signs typical of an intermediate uveitis.

Autoimmune endotheliopathy is a rare finding associated with pars planitis. Khodadoust et al.[30] reported four of 10 patients with pars planitis who demonstrated areas of peripheral corneal edema with KPs arranged linearly on the border between the edematous and normal areas of the cornea. This morphologic finding was reminiscent of a corneal graft endothelial rejection line. Although other investigators have not observed this finding as frequently as Khodadoust et al. did, the possible association of an autoimmune phenomenon is an intriguing notion.

Glaucoma has been described as a cause of severe visual loss in patients with intermediate uveitis. In a study of 182 eyes with intermediate uveitis, glaucoma was diagnosed in 15 (8%).[40] However, 11 of the 15 cases were thought to be related to corticosteroid use, and only 4 (2%) of the 182 eyes had disease-induced glaucoma. Cataract is a more common finding in these patients; it develops as a result of ocular inflammatory disease and corticosteroid therapy. Similar to other cataracts in patients with uveitis, posterior subcapsular cataract is the most common lenticular opacity found in patients with intermediate uveitis.

The most characteristic findings in this disease are in the vitreous and the peripheral retina. Cells are always present in the vitreous in active intermediate uveitis. Some patients may only have 1+ vitreous cells, but the absence of cellular activity in the vitreous precludes a diagnosis of active intermediate uveitis. White- and yellow-colored aggregates of inflammatory cells, called *vitreous snowballs,* tend to accumulate in the inferior vitreous. Occasionally, the vitritis is dense enough to obscure the retina entirely. This dense vitritis must be differentiated from vitreous hemorrhage that may also occur as a result of neovascularization, usually in the vitreous base or the peripheral retina.

Brockhurst et al.[3] described the early stages of peripheral uveitis as the accumulation of yellow-gray exudates at the ora serrata. Although this clinical finding is not required for a diagnosis of intermediate uveitis, it is the major clinical feature in the subset of intermediate uveitis that we call *pars planitis.* Not all patients with intermediate uveitis have a snowbank, and because some patients may have it in one eye only, the inferior white snowbank is an important finding but not an absolute requirement. Brockhurst et al. noted that as the disease progresses, these exudates coalesce to form the material commonly referred to as a "snowbank." This is usually located inferiorly only, but in rare patients, it can extend to 360 degrees. The snowbank may be discontinuous. It may form a fine band along the ora serrata or be broad and extend onto both the peripheral retina and the pars plana. It can be dense and extend several millimeters into the vitreous and is usually best seen with scleral depression (see Fig. 3.17). However, a high, dense snowbank on the pars plana can often be better seen with the indirect ophthalmoscope without using the 20-diopter lens while the patient looks down. Although this material has been termed *exudate,* it is probably a fibroglial mass and not true protein exudate, as will be discussed later. When a snowbank is observed, the area should be carefully examined for the presence of neovascularization because these areas are a source of potential vitreous hemorrhage.

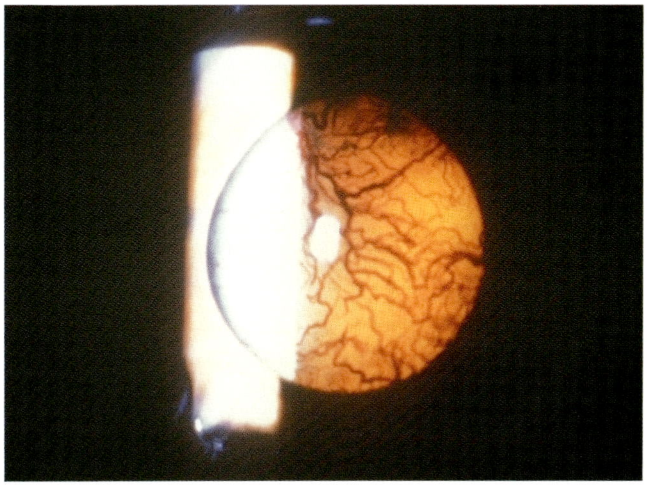

Fig. 22.3 Retroillumination photograph demonstrates a vascular cyclitic membrane in a patient with intermediate uveitis of the pars planitis subtype. (Courtesy Rubens Belfort, Jr., MD.)

The peripheral retinal vascular abnormalities may be obscured by the dense vitreal inflammation in some patients. When the vitreous is fairly clear, sheathing or obliteration of the small peripheral venules can be seen. Periarteritis of the small arteries is found less commonly. The perivasculitis is often associated with whitish infiltrates of the peripheral retina. In rare cases, the peripheral neovascularization can evolve into a vascular cyclitic membrane (Fig. 22.3).

Many patients have a mild course of intermediate uveitis or pars planitis and have no loss of visual acuity and may not require treatment. However, when visual acuity does decrease early in the disease process, cystoid macular edema is the most common cause; these patients usually require therapy. Fluorescein angiography or clinical examination frequently reveals cystoid macular edema. In addition, there is often diffuse retinal vascular leakage and optic disk edema when the disease is active. Interestingly, optic disk edema occurs in 50% of children with this entity.[41]

Vitreous hemorrhage resulting from peripheral neovascularization may occur in a small percentage of patients.[3] It occurs more frequently in intermediate uveitis of the pars planitis subtype and appears to be more common in children, occurring in 28% of children compared with 6% of adults, as found in one case series.[42] Vitreous hemorrhage has also been reported as a characteristic finding of intermediate uveitis associated with multiple sclerosis.[43] In many eyes, the hemorrhage will resolve, but some will require surgical intervention to remove persistent vitreous hemorrhage. In one patient, we observed the neovascularization extending well into the posterior pole, leading to recurrent vitreous hemorrhages (Fig. 22.4). Rhegmatogenous retinal detachment can occur as a result of vitreoretinal traction; it was reported in 3.7% to 22% of patients in different published series.[3,8] In our experience, rhegmatogenous retinal detachment is an uncommon complication of intermediate uveitis and occurs in less than 3% of patients. Retinal detachments, when they occur, tend to develop later in the disease process because persistent vitreal inflammation leads to vitreal contraction and retinal traction. In addition to rhegmatogenous retinal detachments, Brockhurst et al.[3] described nonrhegmatogenous retinal detachments associated with choroidal detachments.

Although macular edema is the most common cause of visual loss in patients with intermediate uveitis and is present in most of the patients who are referred to us, other series have reported an incidence of macular edema ranging from 28% to 50%.[6,8,44] Epiretinal membranes have been reported in 36% of eyes with intermediate

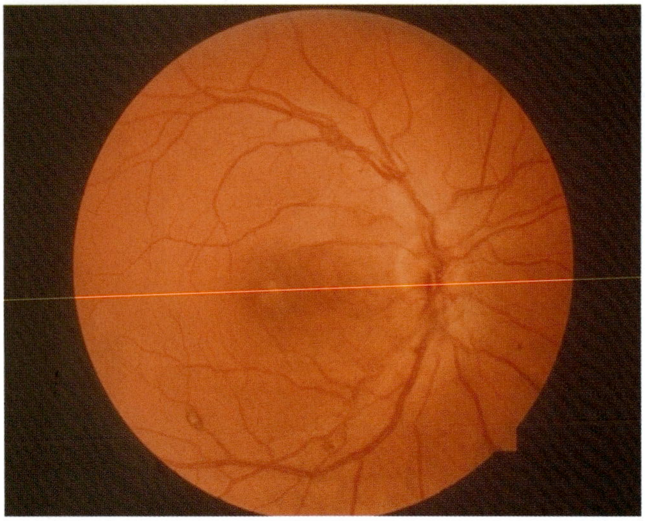

Fig. 22.4 Retinal photograph demonstrates small areas of neovascularization in the posterior pole in a patient with pars planitis and recurrent vitreous hemorrhages.

BOX 22.1 Differential Diagnosis of Intermediate Uveitis

Sarcoidosis
Multiple sclerosis
Inflammatory bowel disease
Lyme disease
Toxocariasis
Intraocular lymphoma
Retinoblastoma
Whipple disease
Iridocyclitis
Multifocal choroiditis
Irvine-Gass syndrome
Amyloidosis
Interstitial nephritis and uveitis syndrome
Human T-cell lymphoma virus type 1 (HTLV-1) infection
Cat scratch disease
Hepatitis C
Crohn disease

uveitis.[45] Long-standing macular edema can lead to stippling of the retinal pigment epithelium (RPE) in the macula and may be a subtle sign of previous edema in patients with chronic intermediate uveitis. Unfortunately, this postcystoid macular degeneration can cause severe visual loss in these patients.

Disk edema, optic atrophy, and optic disk neovascularization have been reported in patients with intermediate uveitis. Neovascularization of the disk is associated with severe retinal ischemia but responds to panretinal laser photocoagulation.[46] Phthisis bulbi may be the final outcome for an eye with chronic, poorly controlled intermediate uveitis. These eyes have often had total retinal detachments, proliferative vitreoretinopathy, or a cyclitic membrane leading to ciliary body traction and hypotony.[28]

DIAGNOSIS

Although intermediate uveitis may exist as an isolated idiopathic disorder, a number of underlying diseases are associated with this condition. Evidence of systemic disorders can be found in up to one-third of patients with intermediate uveitis, depending on the study.[47] In one study of 83 patients, 10 had presumed sarcoidosis, six had multiple sclerosis, two had optic neuritis, two had inflammatory bowel disease, four had thyroid abnormalities, and two had histories consistent with Epstein-Barr virus (EBV) infection.[47] In a study performed in the United Kingdom, a systemic diagnosis was associated with the disease in 36.1% of patients: 23% of patients had sarcoidosis, 4.6% had multiple sclerosis, 2.6% had HLA-B27–positive disease.[48] In a study performed in Saudi Arabia, 42% of patients with intermediate uveitis seen at a referral clinic had systemic disease: 22% had asthma, 8% had multiple sclerosis, 6% had presumed ocular tuberculosis, and 2% each had inflammatory bowel disease, non-Hodgkin lymphoma, and sarcoidosis.[49] Infectious diseases have also been associated with intermediate uveitis. It has been reported in patients with Lyme disease,[50,51] human T-cell lymphoma virus type 1 (HTLV-1) infection,[52] cat scratch disease,[53] and hepatitis C.[54] The diagnoses associated with intermediate uveitis are listed in Box 22.1. Many of these disorders are discussed in detail elsewhere in this text. Sarcoidosis is discussed in Chapter 23, Lyme disease in Chapter 11, toxocariasis in Chapter 17, intraocular lymphoma in Chapter 31, and iridocyclitis with Irvine-Gass syndrome in Chapter 19. Intermediate uveitis associated with multiple sclerosis is discussed later in this chapter. Other autoimmune disorders, including Crohn disease, can cause an intermediate uveitis.[55] Although specific diseases associated with intermediate uveitis can be identified in many patients, clinical investigation often fails to yield an exact diagnosis despite clinical findings that may suggest a unique condition. We reported 19 patients with phakia with vitritis, cystoid macular edema, and retinal periphlebitis, and in whom no specific disease could be discerned and there was good visual outcome.[56]

Our diagnostic evaluation of patients with intermediate uveitis includes a thorough evaluation for sarcoidosis, including chest x-ray, a serum angiotensin-converting enzyme (ACE) level, serum calcium level, pulmonary function testing, and gallium scanning. Patients with a history of chronic or bloody diarrhea are referred to a gastroenterologist for evaluation for inflammatory bowel disease. Neurologic history and examination are performed and magnetic resonance imaging (MRI) is performed in patients suspected of having multiple sclerosis. For patients with a history of a rash who live in an area endemic for Lyme disease, especially those with a history of chronic arthritis, a serologic test for Lyme disease is performed. If the inflammation is unilateral, a serologic test for *Toxocara* is performed, especially in younger patients. When intraocular lymphoma is suspected in older patients, they undergo MRI of the brain, a lumbar puncture for cytologic evaluation of cerebral spinal fluid, and diagnostic vitrectomy. Other tests are requested on the basis of a clinical suspicion of a specific disorder.

We usually request for fluorescein angiography or optical coherence tomography (OCT) angiography for these patients for two reasons: (1) to assess the presence and extent of cystoid macular edema, and (2) to examine the retinal vasculature for signs of perivasculitis, including staining of the vessel wall and vascular leakage of dye (Fig. 22.5). Ultrasonography can demonstrate cyclitic membranes or the extent of vitreous debris when the view of the posterior pole is obscured by cataract. Ultrasound biomicroscopy may reveal vitreoretinal adhesions that are not observed clinically.[57] OCT can be useful to assess macular edema and to monitor treatment effect. In addition, OCT angiography and swept-source wide-field OCT angiography have demonstrated reduced vascular density in the choroid and the choriocapillaris and may aid in diagnosis, prognosis, and monitoring of treatment effects.[58,59]

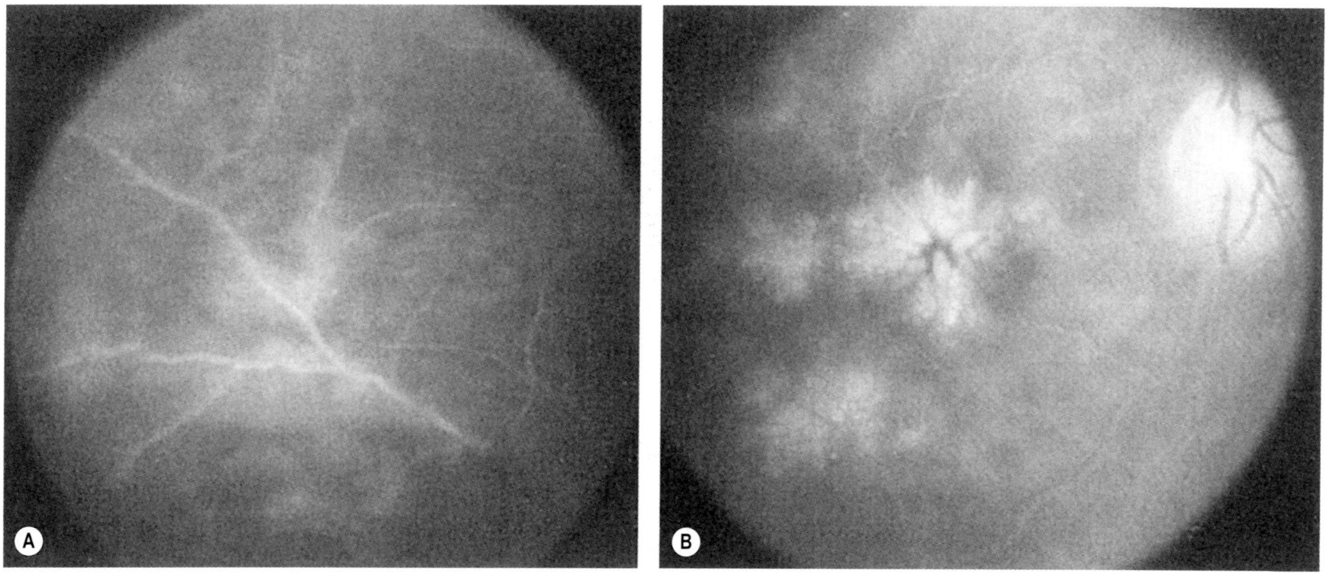

Fig. 22.5 (A) Late-phase fluorescein angiogram from a patient with intermediate uveitis shows substantial leakage of dye from peripheral retinal vessels. (B) Late-phase fluorescein angiogram from a patient with pars planitis shows vascular leakage and prominent cystoid macular edema.

MULTIPLE SCLEROSIS

Intermediate uveitis may occur in patients with multiple sclerosis. Although some authors initially classified multiple sclerosis as a masquerade syndrome, we prefer to consider it a cause of uveitis, like other uveitides with both central nervous system (CNS) and ocular manifestations, such as Vogt-Koyanagi-Harada (VKH) syndrome. Optic neuritis is a frequent finding in patients with multiple sclerosis, and Rizzo and Lessell[60] showed that within 15 years, multiple sclerosis develops in greater than 50% of patients with optic neuritis. Multiple sclerosis was first associated with inflammatory eye disease in the early 1900s, and Breger and Leopold[61] found uveitis in 14 of 52 patients with multiple sclerosis. In a meta-analysis of the literature, Marrie et al. suggested an increased risk of inflammatory bowel disease, a likely increased risk of uveitis, and a possible increased risk of pemphigoid in patients with multiple sclerosis.[62] In a review of large retrospective studies, the prevalence of uveitis among patients with multiple sclerosis was found to be about 1% and its prevalence among patients with uveitis also about 1%, which is higher than that in the general population.[63] The most common ocular findings in patients with multiple sclerosis include intermediate uveitis, anterior uveitis, and periphlebitis, and the uveitis may precede or follow the occurrence of multiple sclerosis. In one study, the diagnosis of multiple sclerosis preceded the onset of uveitis in 56% of patients, followed it in 25%, and was made concurrently in 19% of cases.[64] In a series of 113 patients (196 eyes) with uveitis, 73% were female, and the mean age at presentation was 40.6 years.[65] In this study, the majority (80%) presented with intermediate uveitis, and the clinical course of intermediate uveitis in these patients was similar to that in patients without multiple sclerosis. However, in a study of uveitis in patients with multiple sclerosis in clinical trials of fingolimod, patients with uveitis had a significantly shorter time to first relapse (mean 2.11 versus 8.12 years) and a significantly higher annualized relapse rate.[66]

Studying the pathogenesis of multiple sclerosis and associated uveitis can provide insight into the pathogenic causes of uveitis. Reich et al. reviewed the pathology and pathogenesis of multiple sclerosis and demonstrated that better understanding of the mechanisms of that disease could lead to new therapeutic approaches (Fig. 22.6).[67] From an ocular standpoint, Ohguro et al.[68] showed that eight of 14 patients with multiple sclerosis had serum antibodies to arrestin (retinal S-antigen [S-Ag]), although none of them had uveitis. In addition, antibody titers were higher during relapses than during remissions. These findings suggest that antibodies reactive with arrestin may be related to the clinical course of multiple sclerosis. Also, because arrestin is found in the eye, antiarrestin antibodies may explain the development of uveitis in some patients with multiple sclerosis.

The uveitis associated with multiple sclerosis has been treated with corticosteroids and immunosuppressive agents similar to other causes of intermediate uveitis. Interferon is used to treat multiple sclerosis and may have a beneficial effect on the uveitis associated with this disease.[69] A number of other biologic agents have been approved specifically for the treatment of multiple sclerosis. Fingolimod, an oral disease-modifying agent, has been approved for the treatment of relapsing–remitting multiple sclerosis but has been associated with the development of macular edema.[70]

TREATMENT

Because intermediate uveitis is a disorder associated with a number of underlying diseases, the first step in the treatment is to exclude the possibility of an underlying infectious disease or malignancy. A number of infectious diseases, such as Lyme disease, and malignancies, such as intraocular lymphoma, are included in the differential diagnosis of intermediate uveitis. It is critical to exclude infection or malignancy before immunosuppressive therapy is begun. The second step is to decide whether therapy is needed. There is ongoing debate regarding the usefulness of treating eyes with minimal inflammation and relatively good visual acuity.[71] Eyes with extensive neovascularization of the peripheral snowbank or with substantial vasculitis are often treated despite good vision. Nevertheless, we have seen a number of patients with intermediate uveitis with mild vitritis and periphlebitis, and in these patients, good vision has been maintained for years without therapy and the resultant side effects. Whether these patients are, in the long run, better served by more aggressive anti-inflammatory therapy early on is unknown; however, we treat patients who develop macular edema or other complications of inflammatory disease more aggressively. Other complications, including glaucoma, need to be recognized and treated promptly.

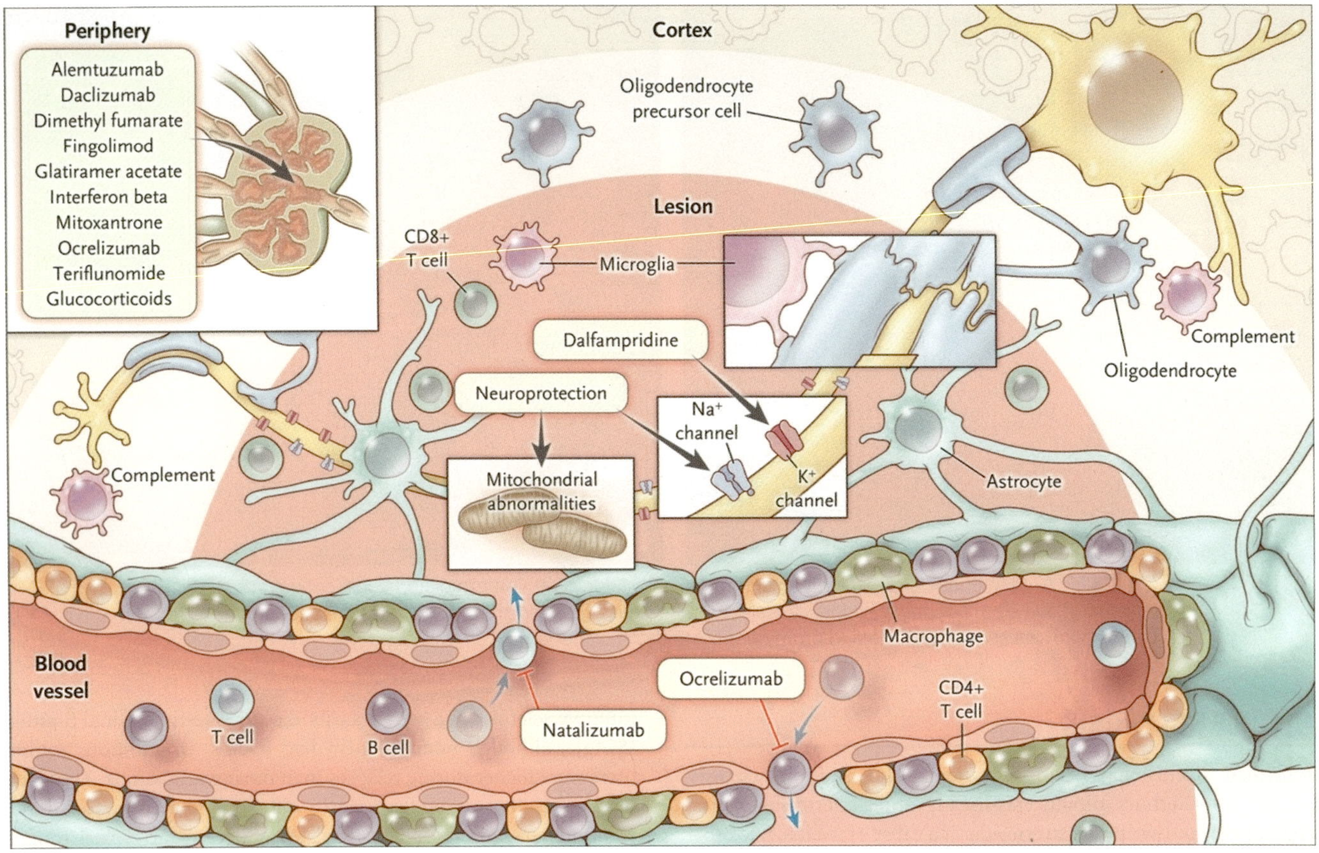

Fig. 22.6 Cells, molecules, and therapies for multiple sclerosis. (From Reich DS, Lucchinetti CF, Calabresi PA. Multiple sclerosis. *N Engl J Med.* 2018;378:169–180.)

Corticosteroids

Corticosteroids are the mainstay of therapy, as they are for most forms of uveitis. Although topical corticosteroids are effective in the treatment of anterior uveitis, we have found them to be ineffective in the treatment of intermediate uveitis in patients with phakia. In those without phakia, large doses of topical corticosteroids may yield a high enough concentration of the drug in the vitreous to treat mild disease. Most patients, however, will require either systemic therapy or local injections (Case 22.1). Periocular corticosteroids are effective in treating many patients with intermediate uveitis, especially those with uniocular disease. We prefer to use injections of 40 mg triamcinolone given retroseptally through the lower lid or into the sub-Tenon space supertemporally. We emphasize that two or three injections given over a 6- to 8-week period should be tried before the technique is deemed ineffective. We have also given bilateral periocular corticosteroid injections to children and some adults with intermediate uveitis under general anesthesia and have found this approach to be quite helpful. Intravitreal corticosteroids can be used to treat intermediate uveitis. Intravitreal triamcinolone has been found to be effective in reducing macular edema, even in patients resistant to previous therapy.[72] Sustained-release intravitreal corticosteroid implants are now approved by the U.S. Food and Drug Administration (FDA), the European Medicines Agency (EMA), and other regulatory agencies for the treatment of uveitis affecting the posterior segment of the eye. In a study of the dexamethasone intravitreal implant for noninfectious uveitis, greater than 80% of patients had a diagnosis of intermediate uveitis and the implant was effective in decreasing vitreous haze and improving visual acuity through week 26.[73] Cataract and elevated intraocular pressure (IOP) were noted as adverse effects of therapy. In a study of an injectable fluocinolone acetonide insert in patients with noninfectious uveitis affecting the posterior segment, uveitis recurrence rates were significantly lower in those receiving the fluocinolone insert compared with those receiving a sham at 6 months, with efficacy maintained through month 12 and prevention of vision loss.[74] Cataract and glaucoma were reported as the adverse effects of this therapy.

Systemic corticosteroid therapy is used in most patients with bilateral intermediate uveitis or uniocular disease resistant to periocular corticosteroid treatment. Initially we give patients 0.5 to 1 mg/kg/day of prednisone and taper it on the basis of the clinical response. Patients

CASE 22.1

An 8-year-old boy presented with a 1-year history of progressive unilateral visual loss. Examination revealed a visual acuity of 20/100, 2+ vitreous cells and haze, and pars plana exudate (snowbank); the diagnosis was intermediate uveitis of the pars planitis subtype. The patient received cryopexy to the snowbank and a periocular injection of 40 mg methylprednisolone acetate (Depo-Medrol). Over the next 2 weeks, his visual acuity improved from 20/100 to 20/30, with a concurrent reduction in inflammation. Visual acuity remained stable for the next 9 months, but intraocular inflammation began to recur. One year after the first cryopexy and periocular injection with corticosteroids, vision decreased to 20/80. The patient was treated with a second cryopexy procedure and periocular injection of corticosteroids. Vision again improved to 20/30, but 1 year later the vision again decreased to 20/80. A third cryopexy procedure and periocular corticosteroid injection had no effect. However, two additional periocular injections led to decreased ocular inflammation and improvement of vision to 20/30.

CASE 22.2

An 11-year-old girl presented with bilateral intermediate uveitis with pars plana exudates, resulting in reduced vision in both eyes. She was treated with systemic prednisone, and visual acuity improved. The patient, however, experienced intolerable weight gain, mood changes, and gastrointestinal distress, and the prednisone therapy was discontinued. She received three periocular injections of corticosteroids without improvement in vision. Cryotherapy to one eye similarly had no effect. Two years after the onset of the disease, the patient was left with bilateral cystoid macular edema, moderate vitritis, and visual acuity of 20/50 in the right eye and 20/80 in the left eye.

Therapy with cyclosporin at a dose of 4 mg/kg daily and bromocriptine at 10 mg/day was begun. Over the next 2 months, the vitreal inflammation and cystoid macular edema resolved, and visual acuity improved to 20/20 in the right eye and 20/32 in the left eye. The patient tolerated these medications without problems, and this therapeutic regimen was maintained thereafter.

should have a purified protein derivative (PPD) test before immunosuppressive therapy is started to determine whether antituberculosis medications are needed. In addition, patients should receive an antiulcer medication, such as a proton pump inhibitor.

Immunosuppressive Agents

For patients who have disease resistant to corticosteroid therapy or who require chronic corticosteroid treatment, we add an immunosuppressive agent. In the past, we used cyclosporin as our first-line steroid-sparing agent because it has been demonstrated to have good therapeutic efficacy in patients with intermediate uveitis (Case 22.2). The major side effects of cyclosporin include renal toxicity and hypertension (see Chapter 8); however, by carefully watching for signs of toxicity and adjusting the dose as needed, we have been able to maintain cyclosporin therapy in patients for up to 10 years. Other immunosuppressive agents that have been used for treating intermediate uveitis include azathioprine, methotrexate, cyclophosphamide, and mycophenolate mofetil. We prefer to avoid the use of cyclophosphamide for the treatment of this disorder because of the significant adverse effects associated with its use, such as bladder cancer. Biologics, including anti–tumor necrosis factor (TNF) monoclonal antibodies and daclizumab, a monoclonal antibody against IL-2 receptor, have been used to treat intermediate uveitis. Adalimumab, an antibody against TNF-α, has been approved by the FDA, the EMA, and other global regulatory authorities for the treatment of posterior segment uveitis, including intermediate uveitis. Adalimumab has been found to significantly decrease the median time to treatment failure compared with placebo, with greater improvements in vitreous haze and improvements in visual acuity.[75]

Surgery

Two surgical procedures have been used in the treatment of intermediate uveitis: cryotherapy and vitrectomy. Cryotherapy applied to the pars plana exudate is thought to be effective in the treatment of pars planitis. The rationale for cryotherapy is that it destroys the vascular component of peripheral retinitis or vitritis and eliminates the entrance site for inflammatory mediators into the eye.[41] Cryotherapy is often combined with periocular corticosteroid injections. The effect of cryotherapy is evident within several weeks and lasts for 3 to 6 months. A second treatment may be given if the first is effective.

Well-controlled, masked clinical trials of cryotherapy are lacking in the literature. Devenyi et al.[76] reported the use of cryotherapy in 27 eyes with steroid-resistant intermediate uveitis and neovascularization of the vitreous base. Patients were followed up for 2 to 12 years, and vitritis was eliminated in 78%. In addition, cryotherapy eliminated the need for corticosteroid therapy in 90% of eyes. Complications included transient increased vitreal inflammation, reduced accommodation, cataract, and hyphema. Others have reported that cryotherapy reduced vitritis, neovascularization of the vitreous base, and clinically apparent cystoid macular edema, but they also noted an increase in epiretinal membranes.[77] In a retrospective study of 186 eyes treated with peripheral cryoablation for active pars planitis, visual acuity improved over time in the cryotherapy group without significant complications, suggesting that the therapy is an effective treatment for active pars planitis and even suggested that it could be better than conventional corticosteroid therapy for induction of remission.[78] Some specialists, however, have stopped using cryotherapy for the treatment of intermediate uveitis because of a reported increase in the incidence of posttreatment retinal detachment. We now limit its use to patients with intermediate uveitis, neovascularization of the vitreous base, and a history of vitreous hemorrhage.

Reduced inflammatory disease has been reported after pars plana vitrectomy for chronic inflammation in patients with intermediate uveitis, possibly because the inflammatory mediators were removed from the eye.[79] Bacskulin and Eckardt[80] reported significant improvement in 12 of 19 eyes with chronic uveitis treated with vitrectomy. Cystoid macular edema was reduced in seven of eight eyes, and in two-thirds of eyes, the intensity of the inflammation decreased so much that the dose of corticosteroids could be reduced postoperatively. Miller et al.[81] reported significant visual improvement in patients undergoing vitrectomy for intermediate uveitis. However, six eyes (50%) required further surgery after the development of retinal detachment, recurrent vitreous hemorrhage, or cataract formation. Two case series also reported improvement in cystoid macular edema after vitrectomy.[82,83] However, there is potential for bias in all retrospective studies. First, additional anti-inflammatory therapy is usually given before, during, and after vitrectomy surgery. Second, patients tend to be much more compliant in taking medications after they have had surgery for their eye disease. In a small pilot study, patients with intermediate uveitis were randomly assigned to pars plana vitrectomy or immunomodulatory therapy.[84] Patients treated with vitrectomy had numeric improvement in uveitis compared with the immunomodulatory therapy group; however, larger randomized controlled trials (RCTs) are needed to discern the risks and benefits of vitrectomy for intermediate uveitis. We therefore tend to reserve vitrectomy for patients with persistent vitreous hemorrhage or dense vitreous debris that does not resolve with medical therapy or for those with disease that is clearly resistant to medical therapy.

Cataracts are a frequent complication of intermediate uveitis, resulting from both chronic inflammation and corticosteroid therapy. Extreme vigilance in controlling ocular inflammation preoperatively is a key to successful and safe cataract extraction in these patients.[85] The use of systemic corticosteroids is also required after surgery. Patients with intermediate uveitis often experience exacerbation of inflammatory activity starting about 3 days postoperatively. It is therefore necessary to see these patients almost daily in the early postoperative period so that increased inflammatory activity can be promptly recognized and appropriately treated.

Should patients with intermediate uveitis who are undergoing cataract surgery have intraocular lens placement? Michelson et al.[86] reported on 15 eyes in eight patients with intermediate uveitis who were undergoing cataract extraction with intraocular lens placement. Despite having quiescent disease for at least 6 months before surgery, 40% had a final visual acuity worse than 20/40. Complications included debris on the intraocular lens requiring multiple YAG (yttrium–aluminum–garnet) laser procedures to clear off the anterior surface. Although most patients with intermediate uveitis, without active inflammation at the time of surgery, and appropriate postoperative management of inflammation do well with intraocular lens implantation, it is our opinion that some patients with intermediate uveitis characterized by chronic relapsing inflammatory disease, cystoid macular edema, and substantial posterior synechiae are better served by correction of aphakia or by the use of contact lenses rather than intraocular lenses.

PROGNOSIS

Brockhurst et al.[3] originally described five groups with possible types of intermediate uveitis. The first group, which comprised 28% of their patients, had a benign course during which the inflammation subsided with good visual outcome. In fact, Schlaegel[7] stated that 80% of patients with intermediate uveitis of the pars planitis subtype need no therapy, and we have seen a number of patients with intermediate uveitis, with or without pars plana exudates, presenting with low-grade inflammation, but never macular edema or decreased visual acuity. However, in the second group of patients in the Brockhurst et al. study, choroidal and serous retinal detachments developed. In patients in the third group, vascularized high snowbanks developed and eventually formed cyclitic membranes that led to retinal detachments or glaucoma. Patients in the fourth group had significant vascular obliteration that led to visual field loss and optic atrophy. In the fifth group, which accounted for 46% of Brockhurst et al.'s patients, chronic smoldering inflammation developed.

In a later article, Brockhurst and Schepens[87] condensed the classification into four groups: benign (31%), mild chronic (49%), severe chronic (15%), and relentlessly progressive (10%). In an article published 5 years later, Smith et al.[8] found that 19% of patients with intermediate uveitis had mild disease, 42% had moderate inflammation, and 39% had severe inflammation. Clearly, the exact percentage of patients in any given category depends on the patient populations of the institutions in which the studies are performed. Tertiary referral centers will see more patients with severe disease compared with primary care institutions. For example, Brockhurst and Schepens[87] reported retinal detachments in 50% of their patients; however, patients with intermediate uveitis and retinal detachments were probably preferentially referred to their retina practice. We have found that retinal detachment occurs rarely in patients with intermediate uveitis, but this may reflect the positive effect of therapy with corticosteroids.

Long-term prognosis varies greatly, depending on treatment and development of complications, including epiretinal membrane and glaucoma. At the time of presentation, one-half of patients have a visual acuity of 20/30 or better.[6] Nevertheless, the disease can produce long-term visual disability in more than one-third of patients.[8] Schlaegel and Weber[88] found that two-thirds of eyes in patients treated with corticosteroids maintained visual acuity of 20/40 or better, and other studies have noted that the long-term prognosis for vision is often good with strict control of inflammation and proper management of complications.[89] In a 20-year cohort study, mean visual acuity after 10 years of follow-up was 20/30, with 75% of patients maintaining visual acuity of 20/40 or better.[90] One-third of patients in this study maintained normal visual acuity without treatment. In a cross-sectional study of 305 patients with intermediate uveitis, visual acuity at referral, RPE atrophy, and macular scarring were associated with increased risk of moderate visual loss; and visual acuity at referral, local therapy, macular scarring, retinal detachment, and hypotony and phthisis were associated with increased risk of severe visual loss.[48] The presence of pars plana exudation or snowbanks may be of some prognostic value. Henderly et al.[6] observed that eyes with pars plana exudates had more vitritis and macular edema, although the difference was not statistically significant. In addition, severity of disease appears to be related more to visual outcome than to the duration of disease.[8,91]

Although inflammatory disease does remit in some patients, Smith et al.[8] found only a 5% remission rate in patients followed up for 4 to 26 years. Similarly, Hogan et al.[1] reported only one remission in 56 patients followed up for 1 to 9 years. Patients with intermediate uveitis are often told that their disease will "burn out" after a number of years, and although many patients may maintain useful vision, the disease is usually characterized by either a chronically active course or a course of exacerbations interrupted by apparent remissions. In fact, Aaberg[41] stated that ophthalmologists rarely observe permanent spontaneous resolution of the disease. Subsequently, in a retrospective cohort study of 849 eyes with intermediate uveitis, the incidence of intermediate uveitis remission was 8.6 per 100 eye-years.[92] Factors that predicted disease remission included prior pars plana vitrectomy versus no vitrectomy, diagnosis within the last year versus greater than 5 years ago, age 45 years or greater, female sex, and Hispanic race/ethnicity versus white race. Presence of a systemic inflammatory disease was not associated with remission incidence.

REFERENCES

1. Hogan MJ, Kimura SJ, O'Connor GR, et al. Peripheral retinitis and chronic cyclitis in children. *Trans Ophthalmol Soc UK*. 1965;85:39–52.
2. Schepens CL. L'inflammation de la region de l'ora serrata et ses sequelles. *Bull Soc Ophthalmol Fr*. 1950;73:113–124.
3. Brockhurst RJ, Schepens CL, Okamura ID. Uveitis. II. Peripheral uveitis: clinical description, complications and differential diagnosis. *Am J Ophthalmol*. 1960;49:1257–1266.
4. Welch RB, Maumenee AE, Wahlen HE. Peripheral posterior segment inflammation, vitreous opacities, and edema of the posterior pole. *Arch Ophthalmol*. 1960;64:540–549.
5. Jabs DA, Nussenblatt RB, Rosenbaum JT. Standardization of Uveitis Nomenclature Working Group. Standardization of uveitis nomenclature for reporting clinical data. Results of the First International Workshop. *Am J Ophthalmol*. 2005;140:509–516.
6. Henderly DE, Haymond RS, Rao NS, et al. The significance of the pars plana exudate in pars planitis. *Am J Ophthalmol*. 1987;103:669–671.
7. Schlaegel TF Jr. Differential diagnosis of uveitis. *Ophthalmol Digest*. 1973;35:34.
8. Smith RE, Godfrey WA, Kimura SJ. Chronic cyclitis. I. Course and visual prognosis. *Trans Am Acad Ophthalmol Otolaryngol*. 1973;77:760–768.
9. Van Metre TE. Role of the allergist in diagnosis and management of patients with uveitis. *JAMA*. 1966;195:167–172.
10. McCannel CA, Holland GN, Helm CJ, et al. Causes of uveitis in the general practice of ophthalmology. UCLA Community-Based Uveitis Study Group. *Am J Ophthlamol*. 1996;121:35–46.
11. Engelhard SB, Patel V, Reddy AK. Intermediate uveitis, posterior uveitis, and panuveitis in the Mid-Atlantic USA. *Clin Ophthalmol*. 2015;9:1549–1555.
12. Donaldson MJ, Pulido JS, Herman DC, et al. Pars planitis: a 20-year study of incidence, clinical features, and outcomes. *Am J Ophthalmol*. 2007;144:812–817.
13. Giles CL. Uveitis in childhood. In: Tasman W, Jaeger EA, eds. *Duane's Clinical Ophthalmology*. Philadelphia: JB Lippincott; 1981:1–8.
14. Arocker-Mettinger E, Mayr WR, Huber SV, et al. Do HLA antigens play a role in intermediate uveitis? *Vox Sang*. 1992;63:282–284.
15. Kimura SJ, Hogan MJ. Chronic cyclitis. *Arch Ophthalmol*. 1964;71:193–201.
16. Wetzig RP, Chan CC, Nussenblatt RB, et al. Clinical and immunopathological studies of pars planitis in a family. *Br J Ophthalmol*. 1988;72:5–10.
17. Culbertson WW, Giles CL, West CW, et al. Familial pars planitis. *Retina*. 1983;3:179–181.
18. Augsburger JJ, Annesley WH, Sergott RC, et al. Familial pars planitis. *Ann Ophthalmol*. 1981;13:553–557.
19. Fitt A, Harrison RJ. Familial intermediate uveitis: a case report of two brothers. *Eye*. 1999;13:808–809.

20. Biswas J, Raghavendran SR, Vijaya R. Intermediate uveitis of pars planitis type in identical twins: report of a case. *Int Ophthalmol.* 1998;22:275–277.
21. Haimovici R, Lightman SL, Bird AC. Familial pars planitis and dominant optic atrophy. *Ophthalmic Genet.* 1997;18:43–45.
22. Lee AG. Familial pars planitis. *Ophthalmic Genet.* 1995;16:17–19.
23. Martin T, Weber M, Schmitt C, et al. Association of intermediate uveitis with HLA-A28: definition of a new systemic syndrome? *Graefes Arch Clin Exp Ophthalmol.* 1995;233:269–274.
24. Tang WM, Pulido JS, Eckels DD, et al. The association of HLA-DR15 and intermediate uveitis. *Am J Ophthalmol.* 1997;123:70–75.
25. Oruc S, Duffy BF, Mohanakumar T, et al. The association of HLA class II with pars planitis. *Am J Ophthalmol.* 2001;131:657–659.
26. Linder E, Weger M, Ardjomand N, et al. Associations of independent *IL-2RA* gene variants with intermediate uveitis. *PLoS One.* 2015;10:e0130737.
27. Deschenes J, Freeman W, Char DH, et al. Lymphocyte subpopulations in uveitis. *Arch Ophthalmol.* 1986;104:233–236.
28. Pederson JE, Kenyon KR, Green WR, et al. Pathology of pars planitis. *Am J Ophthalmol.* 1978;86:762–774.
29. Green WR, Kincaid MC, Michels GG, et al. Pars planitis. *Trans Ophthalmol Soc UK.* 1981;101:361–367.
30. Khodadoust AA, Karnama Y, Stoessel KM, et al. Pars planitis, an autoimmune endotheliopathy. *Am J Ophthalmol.* 1986;102:633–639.
31. Thorne JE, Daniel E, Jabs DA, et al. Smoking as a risk factor for cystoid macular edema complicating intermediate uveitis. *Am J Ophthalmol.* 2008;145:841–846.
32. Hultsch E. Peripheral uveitis in the owl monkey. *Mod Probl Ophthalmol.* 1977;18:247–251.
33. Gartner J. The vitreous base of the human eye and "pars planitis": electron microscopic observations. *Mod Probl Ophthalmol.* 1972;10:250–255.
34. Bora NS, Bora PS, Tandhasetti MT, et al. Molecular cloning, sequencing, and expression of the 36 kDa protein present in pars planitis: sequence homology with yeast nucleopore complex protein. *Invest Ophthalmol Vis Sci.* 1996;37:1877–1883.
35. Bora NS, Bora PS, Tandhasetti MT, et al. Molecular cloning, sequencing, and expression of the 36 kDa protein present in pars planitis. Sequence homology with yeast nucleopore complex protein. *Invest Ophthalmol Vis Sci.* 1996;37:2363–2364.
36. Murray PI, Young DW. Soluble interleukin-2 receptors in retinal vasculitis. *Curr Eye Res.* 1992;11(Suppl):193–195.
37. Arocker-Mettinger E, Steurer-Georgiew L, Steurer M, et al. Circulating ICAM-1 levels in serum of uveitis patients. *Curr Eye Res.* 1992;11(Suppl):161–166.
38. Perez VL, Papaliodis GN, Chu D, et al. Elevated levels of interleukin 6 in the vitreous of patients with pars planitis and posterior uveitis: the Massachusetts Eye & Ear experience and review of previous studies. *Ocul Immunol Inflamm.* 2004;12:193–201.
39. Capone A Jr, Aaberg TM. Intermediate uveitis. In: Albert DM, Jacobiec FA, eds. *Principles and Practice of Ophthalmology.* Philadelphia: WB Saunders; 1994:423–442.
40. Smith RE, Godfrey WA, Kimura SJ. Complications of chronic cyclitis. *Am J Ophthalmol.* 1976;82:277–282.
41. Aaberg TM. The enigma of pars planitis. *Am J Ophthalmol.* 1987;103:828–830.
42. Lauer AK, Smith JR, Robertson JE, et al. Vitreous hemorrhage is a common complication of pediatric pars planitis. *Ophthalmology.* 2002;109:95–98.
43. Valentincic NV, Kraut A, Rothova A. Vitreous hemorrhage in multiple sclerosis-associated uveitis. *Ocul Immunol Inflamm.* 2007;15:19–25.
44. Hogan MJ, Kimura SJ, O'Connor GR. Peripheral retinitis and chronic cyclitis in children. *Trans Ophthalmol Soc UK.* 1965;85:39–52.
45. Donaldson MJ, Pulido JS, Herman DC, et al. Pars planitis: a 20-year study of incidence, clinical features, and outcomes. *Am J Ophthalmol.* 2007;144:812–817.
46. Felder KS, Brockhurst RJ. Neovascular fundus abnormalities in peripheral uveitis. *Arch Ophthalmol.* 1982;100:750–754.
47. Boskovich SA, Lowder CY, Meisler DM, et al. Systemic diseases associated with intermediate uveitis. *Cleve Clin J Med.* 1993;60:460–465.
48. Niederer RL, Sharief L, Bar A, et al. Predictors of long-term visual outcome in intermediate uveitis. *Ophthalmology.* 2017;124:393–398.
49. Shoughy SS, Kozak I, Tabbara KF. Associations of systemic diseases with intermediate uveitis. *Ophthalmic Epidemiol.* 2016;23:27–31.
50. Breeveld J, Rothova A, Kuiper H. Intermediate uveitis and Lyme borreliosis. *Br J Ophthalmol.* 1992;76:181–182.
51. Guex CY, Herbort CP. Lyme disease in Switzerland: ocular involvement. *Klin Monatsbl Augenheilkd.* 1992;200:545–546.
52. Mochizuki M, Watanabe T, Yamaguchi K, et al. Uveitis associated with human T-cell lymphotropic virus type I. *Am J Ophthalmol.* 1992;114:123–129.
53. Soheilian M, Markomichelakis N, Foster CS. Intermediate uveitis and retinal vasculitis as manifestations of cat scratch disease. *Am J Ophthalmol.* 1996;122:582–584.
54. Perez-Alvarez AF, Jimenez-Alonso J, Reche-Molina I, et al. Retinal vasculitis and vitreitis in a patient with chronic hepatitis C virus. *Arch Intern Med.* 2001;161:2262.
55. Rosenbaum JT, Kurz D. An old crone finds a new home: Crohn's disease and pars planitis. *Ocul Immunol Inflamm.* 2002;10:157–160.
56. Park DW, Folk JC, Whitcup SM, et al. Phakic patients with cystoid macular edema, retinal periphlebitis, and vitreous inflammation. *Arch Ophthalmol.* 1998;116:1025–1029.
57. Haring G, Nolle B, Wiechens B. Ultrasound biomicroscopic imaging in intermediate uveitis. *Br J Ophthalmol.* 1998;82:625–629.
58. Wintergerst MWM, Pfau M, Muller PL, et al. Optical coherence tomography angiography in intermediate uveitis. *Am J Ophthalmol.* 2018;194:35–45.
59. Tian M, Tappeiner C, Zinkernagel MS, et al. Evaluation of vascular changes in intermediate uveitis and retinal vasculitis using swept-source wide-field optical coherence tomography angiography. *Br J Ophthalmol.* 2019;103(9):1289–1295.
60. Rizzo JF, Lessell S. Risk of developing multiple sclerosis after uncomplicated optic neuritis. *Neurology.* 1988;38:185–190.
61. Breger BC, Leopold IH. The incidence of uveitis in multiple sclerosis. *Am J Ophthalmol.* 1966;62:540–545.
62. Marrie RA, Reider N, Cohen J, et al. A systematic review of the incidence and prevalence of autoimmune disease in multiple sclerosis. *Mult Scler.* 2015;21:282–293.
63. Olsen TG, Frederiksen J. The association between multiple sclerosis and uveitis. *Surv Opththalmol.* 2017;62:89–95.
64. Zein G, Berta A, Foster CS. Multiple sclerosis-associated uveitis. *Ocul Immunol Inflamm.* 2004;12:137–142.
65. Messenger W, Hilderbrandt L, Mackensen F, et al. Characterisation of uveitis in association with multiple sclerosis. *Br J Ophthalmol.* 2015;99:205–209.
66. Lim LL, Silva DG, Lo TC, et al. Uveitis in patients with multiple sclerosis in clinical trials of fingolimod. *Ophthalmology.* 2018;126:438–444.
67. Reich DS, Lucchinetti CF, Calabresi PA. Multiple sclerosis. *N Engl J Med.* 2018;378:169–180.
68. Ohguro H, Chiba S, Igarashi Y, et al. β-Arrestin and arrestin are recognized by autoantibodies in sera from multiple sclerosis patients. *Proc Natl Acad Sci U S A.* 1993;90:3241–3245.
69. Becker MD, Heiligenjaus A, Hudde T, et al. Interferon as a treatment for uveitis associated with multiple sclerosis. *Br J Ophthalmol.* 2005;89:1254–1257.
70. Comi G, O'Connor P, Montaban X, et al. Phase II study of oral fingolimod (FTY720) in multiple sclerosis: 3-year results. *Mult Scler.* 2010;16:197–207.
71. Kaplan HJ. Intermediate uveitis (pars planitis, chronic cyclitis)—a four step approach to treatment. In: Saari KM, ed. *Uveitis Update.* Amsterdam: Excerpta Medica; 1984:169–172.
72. Young S, Larkin G, Branley M, et al. Safety and efficacy of intravitreal triamcinolone for cystoid macular oedema in uveitis. *Clin Exp Ophthalmol.* 2001;29:2–6.
73. Lowder C, Belfort R Jr, Lightman S, et al. Ozurdex HURON Study Group. Dexamethasone intravitreal implant for non-infectious intermediate or posterior uveitis. *Arch Ophthalmol.* 2011;129:545–553.

74. Jaffe GJ, Foster CS, Pavesio CE, et al. Effect of an injectable fluocinolone acetonide insert on recurrence rates in chronic non-infectious uveitis affecting the posterior segment: twelve-month results. *Ophthalmology*. 2019;126(4):601–610.
75. Jaffe GJ, Dick AD, Brezin AP, et al. Adalimumab in patients with active non-infectious uveitis. *N Engl J Med*. 2016;375:932–943.
76. Devenyi RG, Mieler WF, Lambrou FH, et al. Cryopexy of the vitreous base in the management of peripheral uveitis. *Am J Ophthalmol*. 1988;106:135–138.
77. Pulido JS, Mieler WF, Walton D, et al. Results of peripheral laser photocoagulation in pars planitis. *Trans Am Ophthalmol Soc*. 1998;96:127–137.
78. Sohn EH, Chaon BC, Jabs DA, et al. Peripheral cryoablation for treatment of active pars planitis: long-term outcomes of a retrospective study. *Am J Ophthalmol*. 2016;162:35–42.
79. Kaplan HJ. Surgical treatment of intermediate uveitis. *Dev Ophthalmol*. 1992;23:185–189.
80. Bacskulin A, Eckardt C. Results of pars plana vitrectomy in chronic uveitis in childhood. *Ophthalmologe*. 1993;90:434–439.
81. Miller WF, Will BR, Lewis H, et al. Vitrectomy in the management of peripheral uveitis. *Ophthalmology*. 1988;95:859–864.
82. Wiechens B, Nolle B, Reichelt JA. Pars-plana vitrectomy in cystoid macular edema associated with intermediate uveitis. *Graefes Arch Clin Exp Ophthalmol*. 2001;239:474–481.
83. Stavrou P, Baltatzis S, Letko E, et al. Pars plana vitrectomy in patients with intermediate uveitis. *Ocul Immunol Inflamm*. 2001;9:141–151.
84. Quinones K, Choi JY, Yilmaz T, et al. Pars plana vitrectomy versus immunomodulatory therapy for intermediate uveitis: a prospective, randomized pilot study. *Ocul Imunol Inflamm*. 2010;18:411–417.
85. Foster CS. Vitrectomy in the management of uveitis. *Ophthalmology*. 1988;95:1011–1012.
86. Michelson JB, Friedlander MH, Nozik RA. Lens implant surgery in pars planitis. *Ophthalmology*. 1990;97:1023–1026.
87. Brockhurst RJ, Schepens CL. Uveitis. IV. Peripheral uveitis: the complications of retinal detachment. *Arch Ophthalmol*. 1968;80:747–753.
88. Schlaegel TF, Weber JC. Corticosteroids for pars planitis. *Surv Ophthalmol*. 1977;22:120–130.
89. Bonfioli AA, Damico FM, Curi AL, Orefice F. Intermediate uveitis. *Semin Ophthalmol*. 2005;20:147–154.
90. Donaldson MJ, Pulido JS, Herman DC, et al. Pars planitis: a 20-year study of incidence, clinical features, and outcomes. *Am J Ophthalmol*. 2007;144:812–817.
91. Chester GH, Blach RK, Cleary PE. Inflammation in the region of the vitreous base: pars planitis. *Trans Ophthalmol Soc UK*. 1976;96:151–157.
92. Kempen JH, Gewaily DY, Newcomb CW, et al. Remission of intermediate uveitis: incidence and predictive factors. *Am J Ophthalmol*. 2016;164:110–117.

23

Sarcoidosis

Scott M. Whitcup

KEY CONCEPTS

- Sarcoidosis is a multisystem granulomatous disease that can affect almost every organ in the body in people of all racial and ethnic groups.
- The cause of sarcoidosis remains unknown, but a number of studies have elucidated the immunologic basis for the disease pathogenesis, with the macrophage playing a central role.
- Most patients with sarcoidosis present with respiratory symptoms, although some present with generalized symptoms, such as fever, fatigue, or weight loss.
- Many patients with sarcoidosis are asymptomatic at the time of diagnosis, and it is only recognized after an abnormal chest x-ray or laboratory test result. Uveitis may be the initial manifestation of the disease.
- Definitive diagnosis is made on the basis of biopsy in patients with radiographic evidence of disease and associated clinical findings.
- Ophthalmic findings, including anterior and posterior uveitis, dry eye, conjunctival nodules, retinal vasculitis, and optic nerve disease, are seen in one-third of patients.
- Systemic corticosteroids and immunosuppressive agents, including the biologics, are used to treat the disease, and with early diagnosis and appropriate treatment, sarcoid uveitis is associated with a favorable visual prognosis.
- Secondary glaucoma is a common cause of vision loss in eyes with sarcoidosis.

Sarcoidosis is a multisystem granulomatous disease that can affect almost every organ in the body in people of all racial and ethnic groups. The organs most commonly involved are the lungs, thoracic lymph nodes, and skin. The adrenal glands, which produce corticosteroids, are the only organs consistently spared by this disease. Sarcoidosis was initially described as a dermatologic disease by Hutchinson in 1869, and Boeck used the term *sarkoid* to describe skin biopsy specimens that had a histologic appearance similar to that of sarcomas.[1] Uveitis was described in patients with sarcoidosis in the early 1900s, and in 1936, sarcoid uveitis associated with a facial nerve palsy and uveoparotid fever was termed *Heerfordt syndrome*.[2] Although the cause of sarcoidosis remains unknown, progress has been made in understanding the immunologic features of the disease supporting the use of new immunotherapies for treatment. Despite advances in both diagnosis and therapy, sarcoidosis remains a diagnosis of exclusion and significant morbidity and mortality can occur when the disease is unrecognized, undiagnosed, and improperly treated. Therefore it is important to make the diagnosis of sarcoidosis in patients with uveitis not only to provide appropriate therapy for the eye disease but also to alert the patient's physician to the possible systemic manifestations that may also require treatment.

EPIDEMIOLOGY

Epidemiologic studies of sarcoidosis are prone to considerable error because of variability in the criteria for diagnosis. Nevertheless, there are substantial differences in the yearly incidence rate in different parts of the world, from 0.2 per 100,000 in Japan and Spain to 64 per 100,000 in Sweden.[3,4] In one study, the age-adjusted annual incidence in African Americans was 82 per 100,000 and in whites 8 per 100,000.[5] In another study, the adjusted annual incidence of sarcoidosis among African Americans was 35.5 per 100,000, compared with 10.9 per 100,000 in white Americans.[6] More recent epidemiologic studies report a low incidence of 0.73 per 100,000 in Japanese males[7] to a high of 71 per 100,000 in African American females.[8] African Americans with chronic sarcoidosis may be more likely to develop ocular manifestations compared with whites.[9] There are conflicting data in the literature regarding sarcoidosis being more common in females.[9,10] A study on the epidemiology of sarcoidosis from 1946 to 2013 showed that the incidence of the disease increased among females from 1950 to 1960 and that the peak age at incidence increased in males from 30 to 49 years to 40 to 59 years in 2010 and in females from 40 to 59 years to 50 to 69 years in 2010.[11] The overall annual incidence of sarcoidosis in this study was 10 per 100,000 population.

ETIOLOGY

Although the cause of sarcoidosis remains unknown, a number of studies have elucidated the immunologic basis for the pathogenesis of this disease (Fig. 23.1).[12] It is hypothesized that the macrophage, acting as an antigen-presenting cell, initiates the inflammatory response in sarcoidosis.[13-16] Possibly in response to presentation of an unknown antigen, macrophages are thought to release cytokines, such as tumor necrosis factor (TNF)-α and interleukin (IL)-12 that cause the infiltration of helper T (Th) lymphocytes. These lymphocytes will also release cytokines and recruit other inflammatory cells to the site of inflammation. In response to these events, granulomas are formed, and immunoglobulins are produced in large quantities by stimulated B lymphocytes and released into the circulation. The immunohistochemical staining of one eye with sarcoidosis showed granulomas in the choroid and the anterior uvea composed of macrophages and Th cells.[17]

The primary involvement of the lungs in sarcoidosis suggests sensitization and a resultant immune response to an endogenous lung antigen or an inhaled infectious agent or other antigen. Frequent involvement of the eye and the skin also supports this hypothesis. A number of epidemiologic studies have reported associations between environmental exposure and sarcoidosis. Early studies suggested an association between sarcoidosis and exposure to tree pollen and smoke from wood-burning stoves in rural areas.[18] Other environmental associations with sarcoidosis include mold and insecticides.[19] Microbial triggers have also been described in sarcoidosis.[20] The development of sarcoidosis has been associated with interferon (IFN)-α treatment for hepatitis, although the association may be related to the underlying hepatitis C infection.[21]

Additional data have suggested that sarcoidosis is an abnormal immune response directed against one of many different antigens in a patient with a hereditary or acquired abnormality of the immune system. Cytokine dysregulation may be involved in the development of inflammatory disease.[22] There does appear to be some genetic predilection for the disease. Sarcoidosis has been reported more commonly in monozygotic twins than in dizygotic twins.[23] Furthermore, there have been associations between both class I antigens (human leukocyte antigen [HLA]-B8)[24] and class II antigens (HLA-DRB1).[25] Paradoxically, patients with sarcoidosis have a number of immune defects. Despite the inflammatory response seen in multiple tissues, delayed-type hypersensitivity is depressed, causing anergy on skin testing, and a generally depressed cellular immunity can occur.

CLINICAL MANIFESTATIONS

Most patients with sarcoidosis present with respiratory symptoms, although some have generalized symptoms, such as fever, fatigue, or weight loss. However, many patients are asymptomatic at the time of diagnosis, and sarcoidosis is only recognized after an abnormal chest x-ray or laboratory test result. Ocular disease can be the initial manifestation of the disease. Sarcoid uveitis is diagnosed when ocular inflammation is found in a patient with extraocular findings diagnostic of sarcoidosis. The definitive diagnosis of sarcoidosis requires the demonstration of a noncaseating, granulomatous, noninfectious inflammatory process on biopsy; however, a number of laboratory and other diagnostic tests can strongly support the diagnosis. Two-thirds of patients with sarcoidosis experience remission within a decade after diagnosis with minimal health consequences; however, one-third of patients have recurrent, progressive disease leading to significant organ damage.[12]

One report described ophthalmic involvement in 50% of patients with sarcoidosis,[26] but most series report eye findings in about 25% of patients.[9,27,28] The common ocular findings in patients with sarcoidosis are listed in Table 23.1. Of patients with chronic systemic sarcoidosis, 26% have ophthalmic involvement at some point during the course of their disease.[9] Ocular disease is usually bilateral, but unilateral or markedly asymmetric involvement can occur. It is important to examine both the conjunctiva and the lacrimal gland in patients with possible sarcoidosis. The palpebral conjunctiva should be carefully scrutinized for sarcoid granulomas (Fig. 23.2), which are seen in 7% to 17% of patients with ophthalmic involvement.[9,27,28] The lacrimal gland, which is clinically involved in 7% to 26% of patients with ocular sarcoidosis,[9,27,28] should also be examined for possible enlargement as a result of the disease. Although a positive conjunctival biopsy for sarcoidosis does not correlate with the presence of anterior uveitis in sarcoidosis,[29] the demonstration of a noncaseating granuloma in the conjunctiva can be diagnostic.

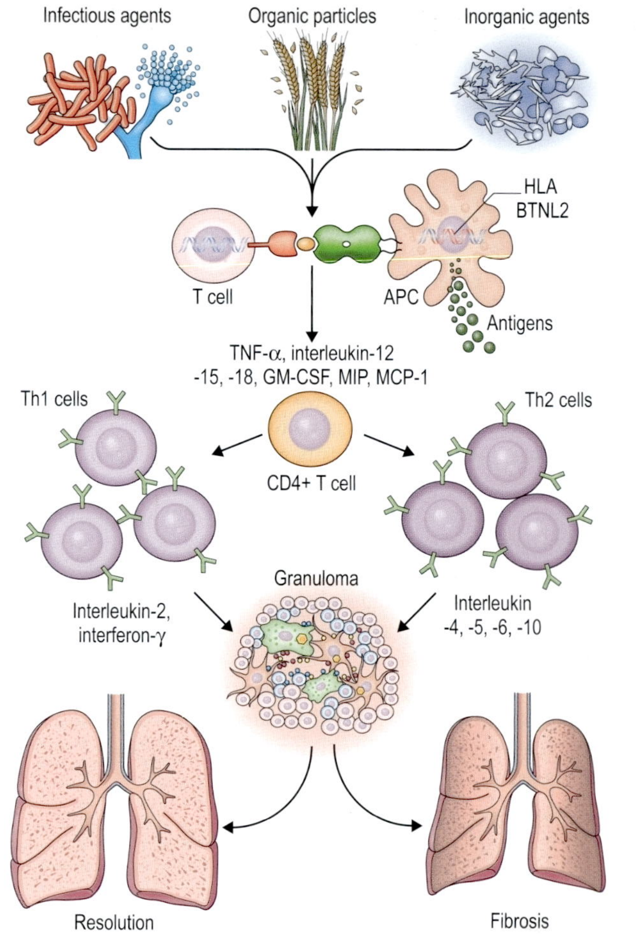

Fig. 23.1 Hypothesized immunopathogenesis of sarcoidosis. Infectious, organic, and inorganic agents are possible antigens in sarcoidosis. Any causative microbe, if present, is probably cleared, leaving behind an undegradable product or initiating a cross-reacting immune response to self-antigen. Antigen-presenting cells (APCs), in addition to producing high levels of tumor necrosis factor (TNF)-α, secrete interleukin (IL)-12, IL-15, and IL-18, macrophage inflammatory protein 1 (MIP-1), monocyte chemotactic protein 1 (MCP-1), and granulocyte–macrophage colony-stimulating factor (GM-CSF). A cardinal feature of sarcoidosis is the presence of CD4+ T cells that interact with APCs to initiate the formation and maintenance of granulomas. CD4+ T cells release IL-2 and interferon (IFN)-γ. Activated CD4+ cells differentiate into type 1 helper (Th1)-like cells and secrete predominantly IL-2 and IFN-γ. The efficiency of antigen processing, antigen presentation, and cytokine release is probably under genetic control; evidence strongly supports a role for macrophage human leukocyte antigen (HLA) and BTNL2 alleles in sarcoidosis susceptibility and phenotype.[86,87] However, T-cell genes that may confer a predisposition to sarcoidosis or affect the phenotype have not yet been identified. Sarcoidal granulomas are organized, structured masses composed of macrophages and their derivatives, epithelioid cells, giant cells, and T cells. Sarcoidal granulomas may persist, resolve, or lead to fibrosis. Alveolar macrophages activated in the context of a predominant type 2 helper (Th2) T-cell response appear to stimulate fibroblast proliferation and collagen production, leading to progressive fibrosis. (From Iannuzzi MC, Rybicki BA, Teirstein AS. Sarcoidosis. *N Engl J Med.* 2007;357:2153–2165. Copyright 2007 Massachusetts Medical Society. All rights reserved.)

TABLE 23.1 Uveitis Associated with Sarcoidosis

DIAGNOSTIC CRITERIA	
Suspected sarcoidosis	Hilar adenopathy, erythema nodosum, increased serum angiotensin-converting enzyme (ACE) level, positive lung or lacrimal or salivary gland gallium scan results, increased serum globulin level, increased serum or urinary calcium level, lymphadenopathy, decreased lung diffusing capacity
Definite sarcoidosis	Radiographic evidence, with characteristic clinical symptoms and histologic confirmation of noncaseating granulomas where other causes of granulomas have been ruled out
Associated findings	Uveitis, arthritis, neurologic signs and symptoms, anemia, decreased pulmonary function, lymphadenopathy
OCULAR FINDINGS	
Common	Acute nongranulomatous or chronic granulomatous iridocyclitis, cataract, vitritis, vitreal snowballs, macular edema, perivenous sheathing, small yellow choroidal, and patches of retinal pigment epithelium (RPE) inflammation, optic disk swelling, retinal neovascularization, elevated intraocular pressure and glaucoma
Rare	Large choroidal granulomas, subretinal neovascularization, optic neuropathy

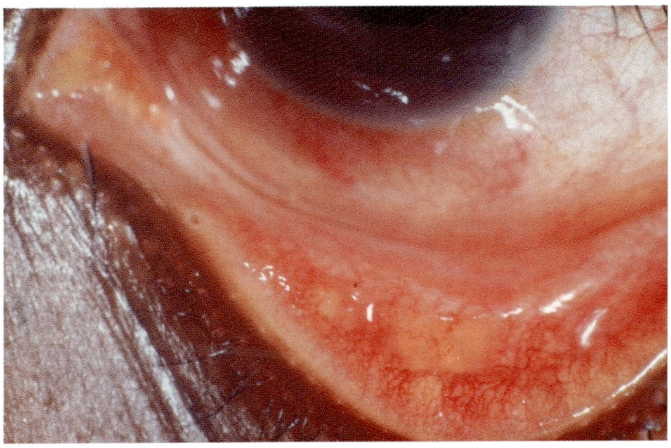

Fig. 23.2 Biopsy-proven conjunctival granulomas in a patient with sarcoidosis.

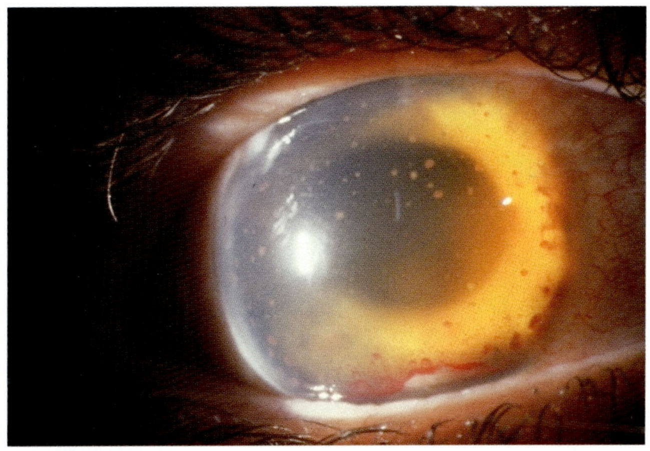

Fig. 23.3 Large granulomatous mutton-fat keratic precipitates in a patient with chronic uveitis and sarcoidosis.

Anterior Uveitis

Anterior uveitis is the most common ocular manifestation and occurs in almost two-thirds of patients with ocular sarcoidosis. Among patients with ocular sarcoidosis, 53% to 60% will have chronic granulomatous uveitis.[9,27,28] Most of these patients will have mutton-fat keratic precipitates (KPs) that may be extremely large and dense, as shown in Fig. 23.3. Patients with anterior uveitis may complain of redness, pain, photophobia, and blurred or diminished vision, but patients with more mild involvement can be asymptomatic. Iris nodules, albeit characteristic for granulomatous inflammation, occur in only 11% of all patients with ocular sarcoidosis (Fig. 23.4).[16] Occasionally, an iris nodule can enlarge to the point where it resembles a tumor. Although the presence of other signs of inflammation and the yellow color of the lesion may be reassuring, only a reduction in the size of the lesion after corticosteroid therapy can prove that the nodule is inflammatory and not malignant.

This chronic form of anterior inflammation generally occurs in patients with sarcoidosis in the fourth to sixth decades[28] and results in secondary damage to the eye, including cataract and glaucoma. The incidence of both of these complications is difficult to estimate on the basis of reports in the literature because there is an increasing incidence of both cataracts and glaucoma with increased duration of the chronic inflammation. The prevalence of cataracts in patients with chronic sarcoid uveitis is 8% to 17%, and the prevalence of glaucoma varies from 11% to 23%.[9,27,28] Both pupillary block and trabecular meshwork damage can cause glaucoma in these patients and may exist simultaneously. In contrast, chronic inflammation will occasionally lead to hypotony and phthisis.[17,30]

Acute iridocyclitis of limited duration associated with small, fine KPs occurs in 15% to 45% of patients with ocular sarcoidosis.[9,27,28] Even among patients with chronic systemic sarcoidosis, those with anterior iridocyclitis frequently have one attack early in the course of their disease and no further recurrences. Some will develop a pattern of acute recurrent uveitis without granulomatous signs. Therefore, although granulomatous uveitis is the more common presentation of ocular sarcoidosis, even a patient with recurrent anterior iritis may have sarcoidosis as an underlying cause. We have followed up several patients with recurrent anterior uveitis who developed mild vitritis years later, along with systemic manifestations of sarcoidosis. As will be discussed later, there is currently little proof that the lesions of acute iritis in patients with sarcoidosis are caused by the same pathologic process that is responsible for the noncaseating granulomas of the thorax.

Posterior Segment Findings

Inflammation of the vitreous, retina, and choroid is less common but more visually disabling than inflammation in the anterior segment, and occurs in 6% to 33% of patients with sarcoidosis.[9,27,28] Many of these patients also have anterior inflammation. The presence of

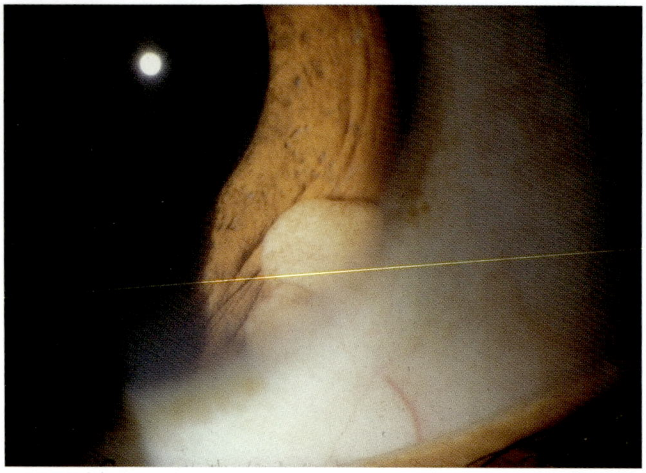

Fig. 23.4 Large iris granuloma in a patient with sarcoidosis associated with chronic anterior and posterior uveitis.

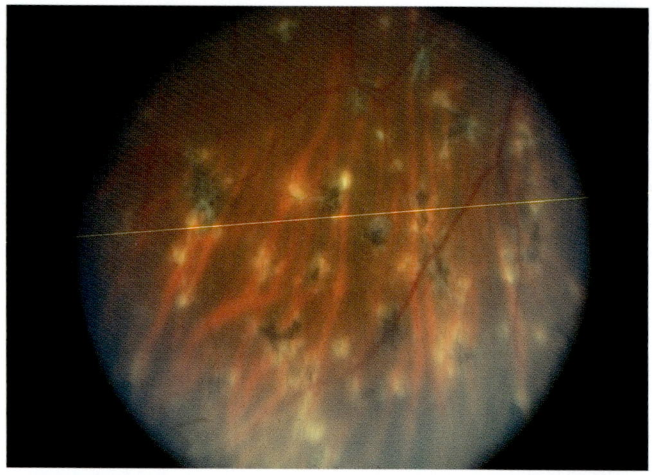

Fig. 23.6 Multiple Dalen-Fuchs nodules in patient with sarcoidosis.

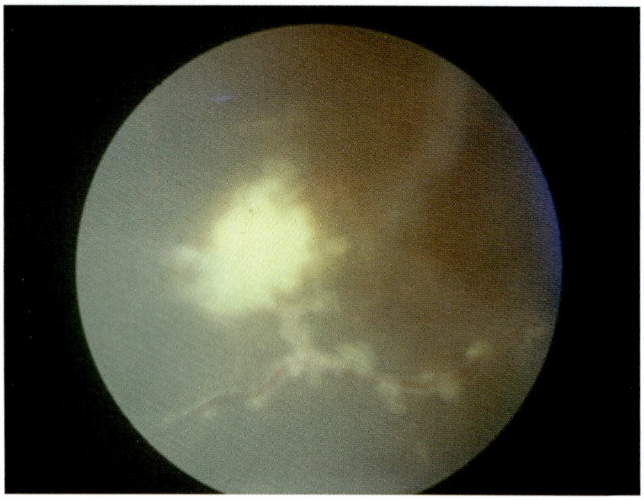

Fig. 23.5 Peripheral perivenous sheathing ("candle wax drippings") and peripheral retinal exudate in sarcoidosis.

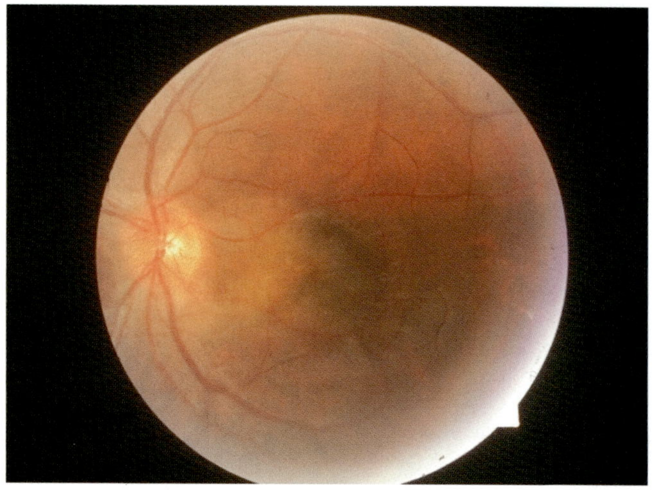

Fig. 23.7 Choroidal granuloma with associated serous retinal detachment in a patient with sarcoidosis.

clumps of cells and proteinaceous debris, called "snowballs," in the vitreous should suggest the diagnosis of sarcoidosis. These snowballs are often located inferiorly and lie on the retinal surface anterior to the equator. The classic "candle wax dripping" *(en taches de bougie)* along the retinal veins is not frequently seen (Fig. 23.5), but many patients with posterior inflammation will have perivenous sheathing.[27,31] In contrast, periarterial sheathing is rarely observed. Small areas of peripheral venous occlusion have been reported, but large vein occlusions are uncommon. Deep yellow choroidal lesions consistent with Dalen-Fuchs nodules and mottling of the retinal pigment epithelium (RPE) occur in 36% of these patients (Fig. 23.6) and are more common than true elevated choroidal granulomas.[31] These smaller lesions are probably small choroidal granulomas that evolve and lead to secondary RPE alterations. They are similar in appearance and histologic findings to the Dalen-Fuchs nodules of sympathetic ophthalmia, although the lesions may be somewhat larger in sarcoidosis than in sympathetic ophthalmia. Large granulomas of the choroid can also occur and may resemble choroidal tumors.[32,33] These appear as yellow-white or yellow-gray discrete elevated masses. Large granulomas can have overlying serous retinal detachments and will cause decreased acuity if they involve the fovea (Fig. 23.7). These lesions will block fluorescence in the early stages of fluorescein angiography and will stain in the late phase. If the lesions occur under the macula, one needs to be concerned about the development of a submacular neovascular net extending from the granuloma.

Chronic cystoid macular edema is usually the cause of decreased visual acuity in patients with posterior uveitis and sarcoidosis. However, opacities in the vitreous can occasionally be sufficiently dense in this disease to cause the decrease in visual acuity. Nevertheless, we have been surprised that visual acuity is only minimally affected in most patients with uveitis even in spite of dense opacity as long as the macula and the optic nerve are uninvolved. Neovascularization of the optic disk occurs in approximately 15% of patients with posterior uveitis related to sarcoidosis.[31] In our experience, prompt steroid therapy frequently leads to involution of these vessels, suggesting that the ischemic stimulus that promoted the neovascularization is reversible and related to the inflammation. If there is significant peripheral vascular ischemia or neovascularization, therapy with anti-inflammatory drugs may not be adequate, and photocoagulation may be indicated.

In contrast to retinal neovascularization, subretinal neovascularization in sarcoidosis is much less common and does not respond to anti-inflammatory therapy.[30,34,35] Case reports usually describe

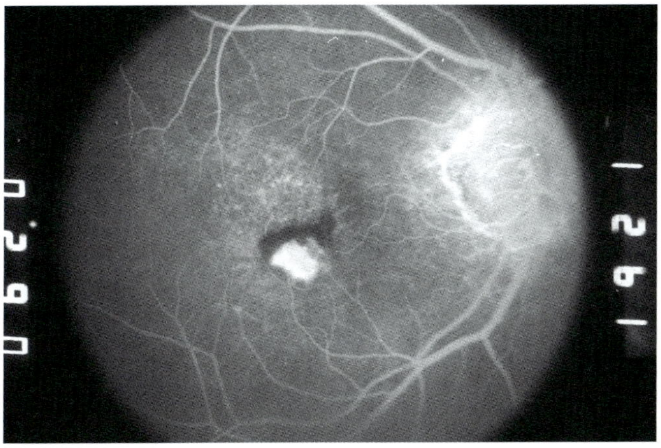

Fig. 23.8 Fluorescein angiogram of subretinal neovascular membrane in patient with sarcoidosis.

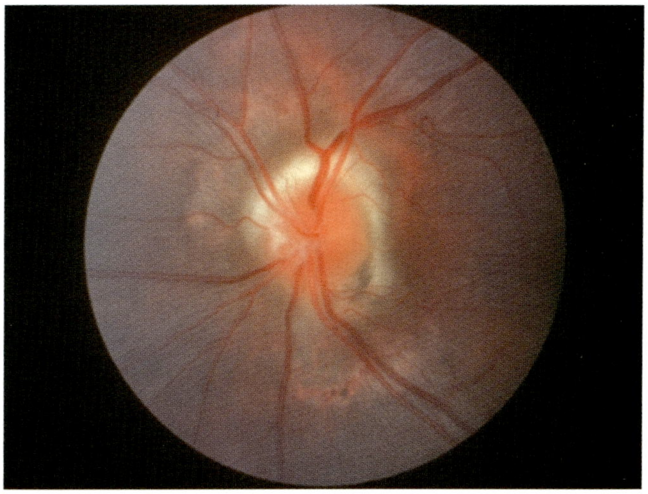

Fig. 23.9 Optic disk hyperemia and peripapillary fibrous ring in a patient with sarcoidosis and a history of optic disk swelling.

a peripapillary or macular subretinal neovascular membrane (Fig. 23.8). It is likely that choroidal inflammation with secondary RPE damage leads to breaks in the Bruch membrane, permitting the development of the neovascular net. The natural course of these vascular abnormalities is not well defined, but they probably have a prognosis similar to that for subretinal membranes because of other causes, such as age-related macular degeneration. Some reports have suggested that anti-vascular endothelial growth factor (VEGF) agents can be beneficial in the treatment of neovascularization,[36] but only limited data are available.

Optic disk swelling occurs in 39% of patients with posterior uveitis but is usually mild and not associated with visual dysfunction.[31] The optic disk may also be hyperemic. Papilledema can occur as a result of sarcoid granulomas that invade the optic nerve, but it is probably not the common cause of disk swelling because the swelling follows a course that parallels the severity of the posterior uveitis.[31] After the disk edema resolves, a peripapillary fibrous ring may remain (Fig. 23.9). Retrobulbar neuritis without intraocular signs of inflammation has also been reported and is presumably related to direct involvement of the optic nerve by granulomatous inflammation.[37]

Orbital involvement, including that of extraocular muscles, can occur.[38] Because skin lesions are common in sarcoidosis, it is not surprising that the eyelids can be involved. Dry eye disease, including Sjögren disease, occurs in patients with sarcoidosis. Scleritis has also been reported in patients with ocular sarcoidosis.[39]

Systemic Involvement

Sarcoidosis is a systemic disease, and the other organ systems involved in this disease are listed in Table 23.2. In a retrospective study of patients with uveitis and presumed or biopsy-proven sarcoidosis, uveitis was the initial presentation of sarcoidosis in 79% of patients, and 16% had concurrent undiagnosed systemic disease.[40] Lung involvement is common, and the disease is often recognized when pulmonary abnormalities are detected on a chest radiograph.[12] Although these pulmonary findings may be noted during routine physical examination, pulmonary symptoms, including cough and shortness of breath, can occur.

Skin lesions are common (Fig. 23.10), and biopsy of granulomatous lesions can be diagnostic. Both erythema nodosum and granulomatous sarcoid nodules of the skin have been described. Erythema nodosum is a nodular subcutaneous inflammation that presents on the lower extremities and occasionally on the upper extremities or face. The nodules are elevated, red, and tender. It is a hypersensitivity reaction and occurs in drug allergies and in some diseases, such as streptococcal infection, colitis, Behçet disease, and sarcoidosis. The lesions of erythema nodosum are not granulomatous, and the condition is generally self-limiting. It usually occurs in women with sarcoidosis in the second and third decades and is frequently associated with an acute presentation of sarcoidosis that also includes fever, arthralgia, hilar adenopathy, and iritis.[5] The granulomatous nodules of sarcoidosis in the skin appear as movable, nontender, subcutaneous nodules, usually on the lower extremities. Biopsy of these lesions often reveals noncaseating granulomas, which are diagnostic of sarcoidosis.

TABLE 23.2 Systemic Involvement of Sarcoidosis

Locus	Occurrence (%)
Hilar adenopathy	74
Lung parenchyma	46
Lymphadenopathy	28
Skin lesions (excluding erythema nodosum)	18
Erythema nodosum	15
Splenomegaly	10
Bone	4
Parotid	6
Central nervous system	5

Modified from Siltzbach LE, James DG, Neville E, et al. Course and prognosis of sarcoidosis around the world. *Am J Med*. 1974;57:847–852.

The arthritis of sarcoidosis can be either acute or chronic in nature. Of North American whites with sarcoidosis, 21% have joint symptoms,[41] and the rate in African Americans may be somewhat higher. Arthritis is most common during acute sarcoidosis but rarely becomes chronic in these patients. Although granulomas may be seen in the joint synovium, mild nongranulomatous synovitis is more common. Arthritis occurs less frequently in patients with chronic sarcoidosis, but these patients are more likely to have synovial granulomas.

A wide range of neurologic signs and symptoms, including cranial nerve palsies, neuropathy, myopathy, and aseptic meningitis, can result from the meningoencephalitis of sarcoidosis. Overall, the

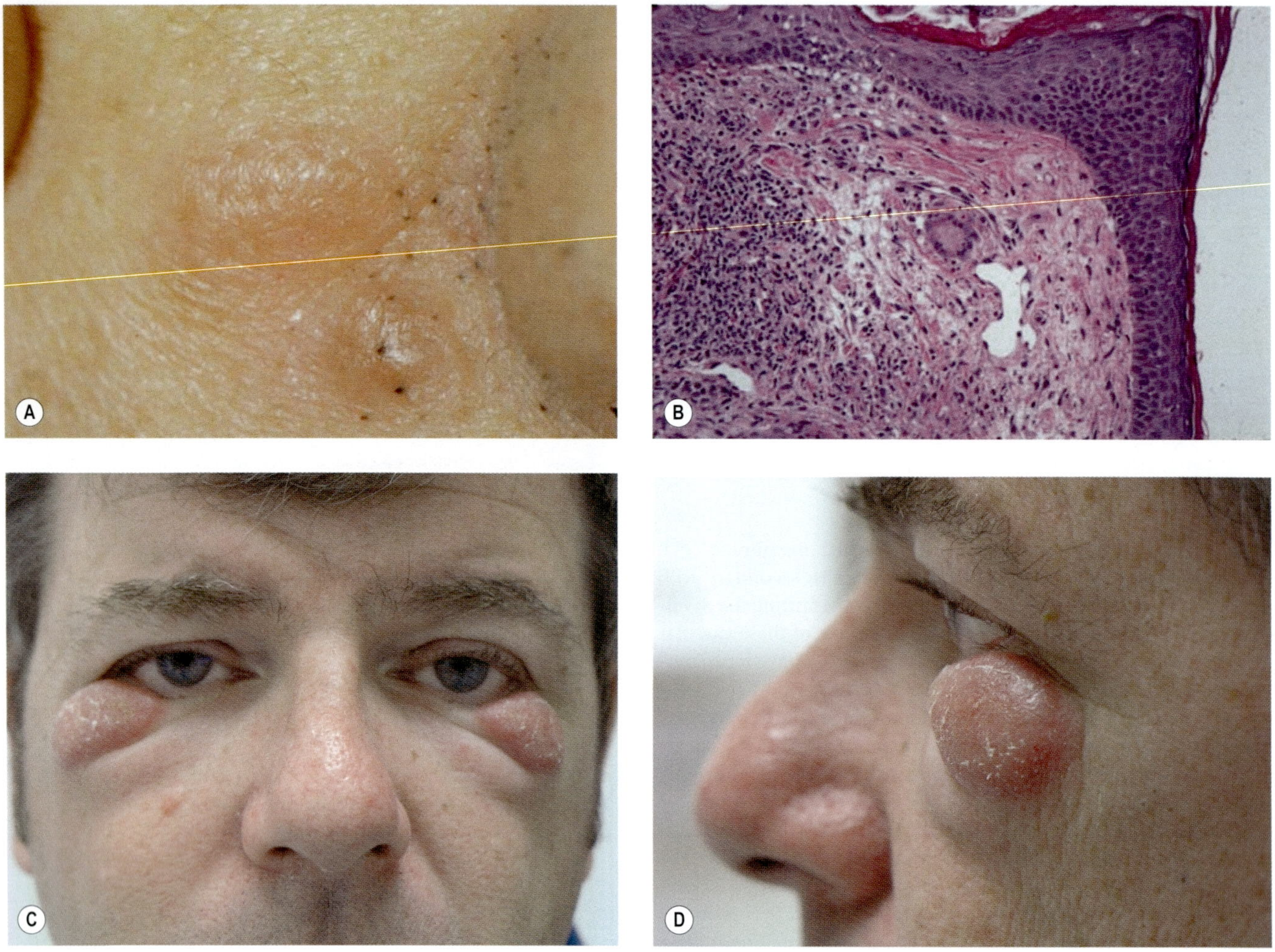

Fig. 23.10 (A) Two flesh-colored, slightly erythematous, minimally elevated plaques. (B) Biopsy of the lesion shown in (A) shows typical noncaseating granuloma consistent with the diagnosis of sarcoidosis. (C and D) Thick, erythematous, scaling plaques in the inferior periorbital area in a patient with sarcoidosis. (A and B, Courtesy Chi-Chao Chan, MD; C and D, Courtesy Teresa Soriano, MD.)

central nervous system (CNS) is involved in up to 25% of patients.[12] Lumbar puncture and CNS imaging studies are important to define the nature of the neurologic involvement that occurs in these patients.[5] Sarcoidosis that involves the base of the brain and the chiasm may be clinically difficult to prove without biopsy. The facial nerve is the cranial nerve most commonly involved in patients with sarcoidosis. Because Lyme disease is also a cause of facial nerve paresis, arthralgias, rash, and uveitis, it should be considered in the differential diagnosis of patients with these findings.

Other organs are frequently involved in sarcoidosis. Although hilar adenopathy is a more frequent finding in sarcoidosis, splenomegaly and lymphadenopathy, respectively, occur in 10% and 28% of patients with sarcoidosis.[5] These findings are detectable on physical examination and should be looked for in patients with possible sarcoidosis. Enlarged lymphoid organs are unusual in most types of endogenous uveitis and point to a clinical diagnosis of sarcoidosis. Liver involvement is also common. Approximately 10% of patients have elevated liver enzymes, and hepatic lesions can be detected on computed tomography (CT) scans in about 5% of patients.[42] Renal involvement can occur as a result of hypercalciuria. Importantly, cardiac granulomas are found at autopsy in about 25% of patients with sarcoidosis but are clinically apparent in only about 5% of all patients.[12] Furthermore, mortality from sarcoidosis frequently occurs as a result of end-stage pulmonary disease, neurologic disease, or cardiac complications, including arrhythmias or cardiomyopathy. The arrhythmias may present as sudden death. The diagnosis of sarcoidosis as a cause of uveitis is important, so the patient should be thoroughly evaluated and treated for these potentially life-threatening manifestations. Electrocardiography can help detect cardiac involvement in patients with presumed sarcoidosis during the evaluation for uveitis.[43]

Although less common in the pediatric population, sarcoidosis is a cause of uveitis in children younger than 5 years of age. In these cases, the disease is typically characterized by granulomatous anterior uveitis, polyarticular arthritis, rash, and lymphadenopathy.[44] Posterior uveitis and orbital disease also occur in children. Pulmonary disease occurs in only one-third of younger patients, but these children often have skin and joint diseases.[45] Finding anterior uveitis and arthritis in a young child with a normal chest x-ray result often leads to the misdiagnosis of juvenile rheumatoid arthritis. Intermittent fever and synovial swelling can delay the diagnosis of sarcoidosis in young children.[46] In infants, sarcoidosis may present more as a multisystem illness.[47] Nevertheless, as in the case of anterior uveitis seen in patients with juvenile rheumatoid arthritis, permanent loss of vision may occur, especially in young children susceptible to the development of amblyopia. In these

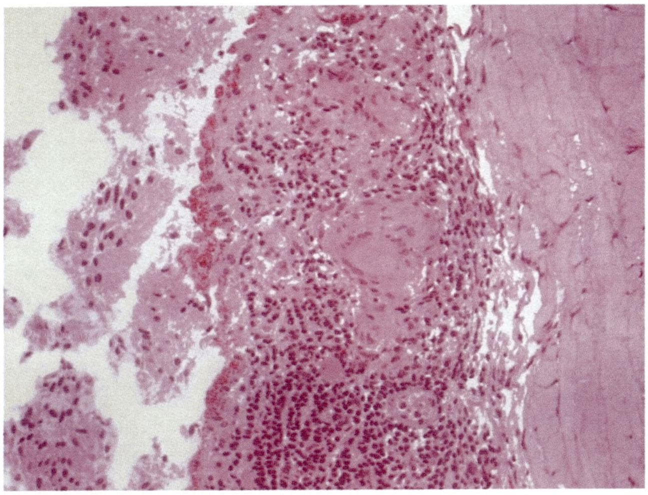

Fig. 23.11 Chorioretinal biopsy specimen from a patient with sarcoidosis shows inflammatory cell infiltration into retina with noncaseating granuloma. (Hematoxylin & eosin; original magnification ×400.) (Courtesy Chi-Chao Chan, MD.)

children especially, aggressive therapy is often warranted. In older children, the presentation and course of sarcoidosis more closely parallel those in adults.

One genetic disease that occurs in children that can mimic sarcoidosis is *Blau syndrome,* a disorder characterized by familial granulomatosis, arthritis, uveitis, and skin rash.[48] Although some of these patients may have elevated serum angiotensin-converting enzyme (ACE) levels, the disorder is otherwise clinically distinct. Patients with Blau syndrome may have camptodactyly and do not have pulmonary disease, hypercalcemia, or positive reactions to Kveim skin testing. The disease has been associated with *CARD15* gene mutations.[49] Blau syndrome may be misdiagnosed as early-infantile sarcoidosis.[50]

Although many patients with sarcoid uveitis maintain good visual acuity, permanent visual loss can occur despite appropriate therapy. In our patients with biopsy-proven ocular sarcoidosis, 14 of 21 (67%) had a visual acuity of 20/40 or worse in at least one eye. Visual acuity worse than 20/200 was most often found to be caused by secondary glaucoma, and aggressive treatment of this complication is therefore warranted.

PATHOLOGY

The definitive diagnosis of sarcoidosis requires the finding of noncaseating epithelioid cell granulomas on biopsy. The typical sarcoid granuloma consists of whorls of epithelioid cells surrounding multinucleated giant cells (Fig. 23.11). Mononuclear cells, fibroblasts, and lymphocytes may be found at the periphery of these nodules, and surrounding areas of fibrosis are common. True caseation, however, is absent. Although suggestive of sarcoidosis, these pathologic findings are nonspecific, and the presence of infectious agents or foreign bodies should be excluded. This may be accomplished with the use of cultures, special stains, and microscopic examination for foreign bodies under polarized light. Several types of inclusion bodies have been noted in biopsy specimens of sarcoid granulomas. Asteroid bodies composed of vimentin intermediate filaments, Schaumann bodies composed of aggregates of basophilic material, and crystalline inclusions containing calcium carbonate crystals have all been described.

Sarcoidosis is thought to be a Th1-driven inflammatory process. Activated Th1-type CD4+ T lymphocytes are fundamental to the development of the disease, including granuloma formation.[51] A number of Th1 cytokines have also been associated with disease activity. A reduced expression of regulatory T-cell–associated forkhead box P3 *(FoxP3)* genes in CD4+ T cells obtained from bronchoalveolar lavage fluid of patients with sarcoidosis suggests a possible defect in regulatory T cells with disease pathogenesis.[52]

Most histologic specimens from enucleated eyes have shown granulomas of the retina, the choroid, or the region of the RPE.[17,53] Histologic examination of the vitreous and perivascular and retinal infiltrates have revealed epithelioid cells.[53] The deeper lesions at the level of the RPE are granulomas, such as the Dalen-Fuchs nodules of sympathetic ophthalmia. Choroidal involvement is infrequent, and Gass and Olson[53] reported that many lesions that have been called "focal choroiditis" in sarcoidosis may be granulomas below the RPE and not discretely involving the choroid. However, large choroidal granulomas do occur (see Fig. 23.7).

The pathologic findings of the acute iritis of sarcoidosis can resemble erythema nodosum rather than the pulmonary granulomas that are prominent and diagnostic of sarcoidosis. Some suggest that iritis may be a hypersensitivity reaction of the eye that occurs in a number of diseases of diverse cause in a manner similar to the occurrence of erythema nodosum in association with a variety of unrelated diseases. It is clear that the granulomatous reaction that is characteristic of sarcoidosis is not necessarily the cause of some of the clinical pathologic conditions but, rather, a secondary response to underlying immune sensitization.

DIAGNOSIS

It is important to think of sarcoidosis as a specific cause of idiopathic uveitis, especially because sarcoidosis is associated with potentially life-threatening organ involvement. In a retrospective study of patients with active uveitis, chest radiography results were abnormal in 15% of patients, and a majority of these had findings consistent with sarcoidosis.[54]

Although the definitive diagnosis of sarcoidosis requires biopsy confirmation, a presumptive diagnosis of sarcoidosis can be made in patients with a characteristic clinical presentation. A diagnosis of sarcoidosis when chest radiographic evidence is accompanied by compatible clinical features and noncaseating granulomas on biopsy, when other causes of granulomas have been ruled out.[12] Typical findings on chest radiography in patients with pulmonary sarcoidosis include hilar adenopathy (Fig. 23.12A) and reticulonodular pulmonary infiltrate, often at the base of the lungs (see Fig. 23.12B). Biopsy should be performed in patients presumed to have sarcoidosis, with the exception of patients with Lofgren syndrome. Asymptomatic patients age 20 to 40 years with bilateral symmetric hilar and paratracheal lymphadenopathy are likely to have sarcoidosis. This likelihood is increased in patients who also have arthralgias, erythema nodosum, or associated uveitis. However, in most patients, biopsy is needed to make the diagnosis.

At the International Workshop on Ocular Sarcoidosis (IWOS), seven clinical signs consistent with the diagnosis were determined: (1) mutton-fat KPs, small granulomatous KPs, and/or iris nodules; (2) trabecular meshwork nodules and/or tent-shaped peripheral anterior synechiae; (3) vitreous opacities displaying "snowballs" or "strings of pearls"; (4) multiple active or atrophic chorioretinal peripheral lesions; (5) nodular and/or segmental periphlebitis; (6) optic disk nodules or a solitary choroidal nodule; and (7) bilateral disease.[55] The diagnostic criteria also included laboratory and biopsy criteria.

Our diagnostic approach is to closely examine the skin, conjunctiva, and lacrimal glands for nodular lesions and obtain biopsy specimens. Biopsy of nodular skin lesions can show granulomas diagnostic for sarcoidosis; however, biopsy of erythema nodosum lesions shows nonspecific vasculitis and is not useful. The incidence

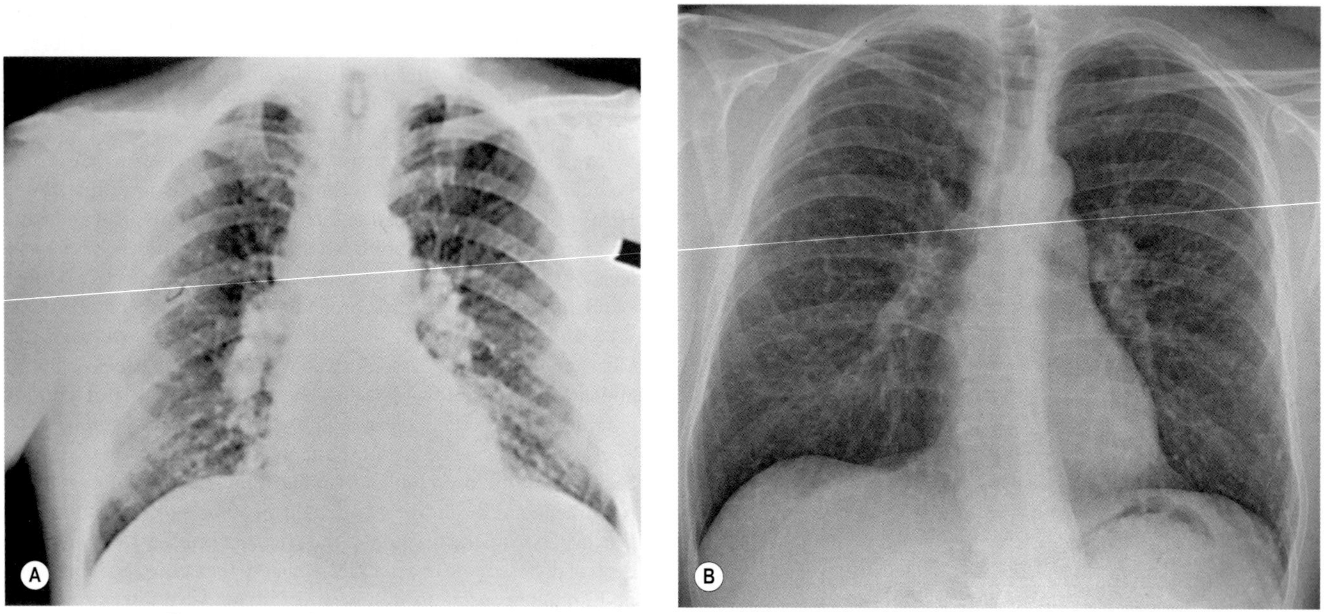

Fig. 23.12 (A) Chest radiograph showing the characteristic features of stage II sarcoidosis. Bilateral hilar adenopathy and diffuse interstitial lung disease are seen. (B) Chest radiograph from a patient with verified sarcoidosis showing hilar adenopathy and a nodular infiltrate, predominantly at the base of the lungs. (A, From Weinberger SE. *Principles of Pulmonary Medicine,* p 164. Copyright 2003 Elsevier. B, From Wikimedia Commons.)

of positive conjunctival biopsy results in patients with biopsy-proven sarcoidosis but no discrete conjunctival lesions is 27% to 55% but falls to 12% in patients with suspected sarcoidosis.[29] Granulomas have been found on biopsy of the lacrimal gland in 22% of patients with presumed ocular sarcoidosis.[56] The diagnostic yield of lacrimal gland biopsy is improved if there is increased uptake on a gallium scan or if the gland is clinically enlarged. The presence of specific inflammatory markers on biopsies of the conjunctiva and the lacrimal gland may also improve the sensitivity and the specificity of these biopsies. We studied lacrimal gland biopsy specimens from 14 patients with sarcoidosis.[57]Although few biopsies showed the classic histopathologic findings of noncaseating granuloma, immunohistochemical staining showed consistent preponderance of infiltrating activated CD4+ T cells and macrophages. In addition to the presence of TNF-α, we noted increased expression of the major histocompatibility complex (MHC) antigens HLA-DR and HLA-DQ and the cell adhesion molecules intercellular adhesion molecule-1 (ICAM-1) and lymphocyte function–associated antigen-1 (LFA-1).

Of patients with sarcoidosis, 90% have an abnormal chest x-ray result (see Fig. 23.12), and transbronchial biopsy is often a sensitive and specific diagnostic test. Approximately 60% of patients with sarcoidosis are found to have granulomas on transbronchial lung biopsy, even those with normal chest radiography results (stage 0 disease).[3] When a parenchymal abnormality is present on the chest film, almost 90% of patients will be found to have granulomas on transbronchial lung biopsy. However, some patients do require multiple biopsies for the correct diagnosis to be made. Some data suggest that CT of the chest may be useful in diagnosing sarcoidosis because it is more sensitive than conventional chest radiography. In a retrospective cohort study of 300 patients, chest CT was suggestive of sarcoidosis in 29%.[58] Kosmorsky et al.[59] reported that chest CT showed mediastinal lymphadenopathy in two older patients with uveitis. Subsequent lymph node biopsy with the use of mediastinoscopy demonstrated sterile noncaseating granulomas consistent with the diagnosis of sarcoidosis. Endoscopic ultrasound-guided fine-needle aspiration of intrathoracic lymph nodes was reported to have a diagnostic yield of 82% in one series.[60]

Laboratory testing may be useful in the diagnosis of sarcoidosis. Transbronchial lung biopsy cannot be performed on all patients with uveitis compatible with ocular sarcoidosis, and diagnostic tests can help determine which of these patients should undergo more invasive diagnostic procedures. ACE is predominantly produced in pulmonary macrophages and the vascular endothelium, and serum ACE levels are elevated in 60% to 90% of patients with sarcoidosis with active disease.[61] Unfortunately, serum ACE levels may be normal in patients with quiescent or isolated disease. In addition, ACE is produced by the epithelioid cells present in granulomas associated with a number of diseases, including tuberculosis, leprosy, silicosis, primary biliary cirrhosis, asbestosis, and histoplasmosis. ACE levels may be elevated in the aqueous humor of patients with ocular sarcoidosis[62] or in the cerebrospinal fluid (CSF) of patients with neurosarcoidosis. ACE levels may be high even in healthy children and are more difficult to interpret as a diagnostic indicator.

Serum lysozyme levels may also be elevated in patients with sarcoidosis but are less specific than ACE and hence rarely obtained. Hypercalcemia and hypercalciuria occur in some patients as a result of increased calcium absorption after increased production of 1,25-dihydroxycholecalciferol; they can be detected on routine laboratory tests. Lymphopenia and elevated liver enzymes, particularly alkaline phosphatase, may also occur. Serum-soluble IL-2 receptor levels are elevated in some patients with sarcoidosis and may have slightly better diagnostic value than ACE.[63]

In the past, the Kveim skin test was an accepted method to diagnose sarcoidosis. Kveim antigen is prepared from the spleens of patients with proven sarcoidosis and is then injected intradermally into a patient with suspected sarcoidosis.[41] The presence of granulomatous inflammation on skin biopsy performed 6 weeks after the injection was considered to be diagnostic for sarcoidosis. Although Kveim test results are positive in about 80% of patients with sarcoidosis, negative test results can occur in those with more limited disease.[64] In addition, the risk of transmission of infectious agents has led to the reduced use of the test, and there is still no commercial preparation of Kveim antigen for clinical use. Anergy on skin testing is also seen in about one-half of patients with sarcoidosis and may help support the diagnosis.

Gallium scanning, which detects concentrated radioactive gallium in areas of inflammation, can be useful for showing involvement of organs, such as the lungs, lacrimal glands, and parotid glands (Fig. 23.13).[30,65] Cardiac magnetic resonance imaging (MRI) and positron emission tomography (PET) can provide complementary value for estimating the likelihood of cardiac sarcoidosis and guiding therapy.[66] Bronchoalveolar lavage (BAL) may show lymphocytosis in patients with sarcoidosis. However, because BAL findings are not diagnostic of sarcoidosis, it is not commonly performed in the evaluation of patients with sarcoidosis. Pulmonary function tests can be useful in evaluating patients with suspected sarcoidosis. Limited diffusing capacity, noted as diminished carbon monoxide diffusion in the lungs, can occur before abnormalities are seen on chest x-ray. Diminished lung volumes are later seen with the development of restrictive lung disease and reduced forced expiratory volume in 1 second (FEV_1) are also noted. We retrospectively reviewed at the National Institutes of Health the records of 46 patients with biopsy-proven sarcoidosis. Of these patients, 21 had uveitis; 61% of the patients with sarcoid uveitis had an abnormal chest x-ray result, and only 36% had an elevated serum ACE level. The most sensitive diagnostic test in our patients was measurement of pulmonary diffusing capacity, which was diminished in 78% of the patients tested. Interestingly, there was no statistical difference in test results between patients with sarcoidosis with uveitis and those without. Our current diagnostic approach is to obtain pulmonary consultation for transbronchial biopsy in patients who have suspected ocular sarcoidosis and reduced diffusing capacity, especially if other diagnostic tests support the diagnosis.

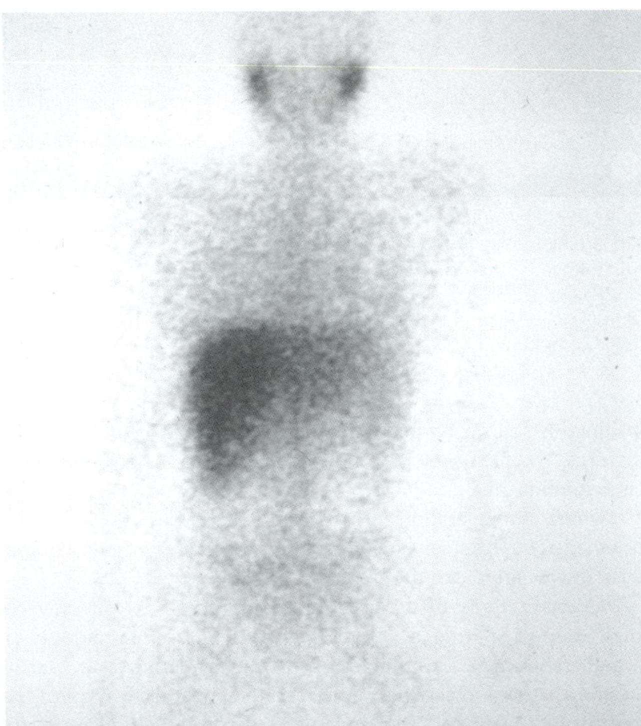

Fig. 23.13 Gallium scan of the upper torso and head of a patient with active systemic sarcoidosis demonstrates uptake in the parotid gland.

TREATMENT

Asymptomatic patients with hilar adenopathy do not require therapy and can be monitored. Treatment is usually reserved to prevent organ damage. Two main indications for therapy in patients with sarcoidosis are symptomatic pulmonary disease and uveitis. The mainstay of therapy for both systemic and ocular sarcoidosis is administration of corticosteroids.[5,30] Clinicians must rely on a number of indicators of disease activity to guide therapy. Doses of corticosteroids are adjusted, depending on clinical symptoms and signs and on the results of pulmonary function tests, chest x-ray, serum ACE measurement, and, occasionally, BAL. In a Cochrane Review of nine randomized controlled trials (RCTs) examining the use of corticosteroids for pulmonary sarcoidosis, the reviewers concluded that oral steroids improved the chest x-ray findings, symptoms, and spirometry results over 6 to 24 months.[67] However, they noted little evidence of an improving lung function.

The ophthalmologist is fortunate in being able to judge the severity of disease on the basis of clinical examination findings, and as described in Chapter 8, therapy must be tailored to the severity of the ocular disease. Acute anterior inflammation is best managed with topical corticosteroids, but frequently, periocular injections of corticosteroids are needed to control severe anterior uveitis complicated by iris nodules and glaucoma.

The treatment of chronic anterior or posterior uveitis is more difficult. Systemic therapy is often required for bilateral chronic uveitis, and patients with chronic ocular inflammatory disease frequently require higher daily doses of oral corticosteroid compared with those with chronic sarcoid pulmonary disease. However, sarcoidosis is often responsive to corticosteroids, and the use of high initial doses with slow tapering is effective in managing most cases (Case 23.1). Two or three high doses of intravenous pulse corticosteroids (1 g methylprednisolone) on consecutive days may induce more rapid remission.

CASE 23.1

A 78-year-old white woman presented with floaters and blurry vision in both eyes. On examination, the visual acuity was 20/80 in the right eye and 20/40 in the left eye, with vitreous cells and mild vitreous haze in both eyes. Fundus examination revealed yellow infiltrative retinal lesions in both eyes (Fig. 23.14A). Laboratory evaluation, including tests for syphilis and magnetic resonance imaging (MRI) of the brain, yielded normal results. The patient refused to undergo lumbar puncture. The patient had an unremarkable past medical history and no signs of pulmonary disease, and skin testing for tuberculosis was negative. Fluorescein angiography showed hyperfluorescent lesions in the areas of retinal infiltration with some late staining (see Fig. 23.14B). The patient underwent diagnostic vitrectomy to rule out primary intraocular lymphoma. Cytology (see Fig. 23.14C) demonstrated small, reactive lymphocytes with nests of macrophages and giant cells (see arrow in the figure) consistent with granulomatous inflammation. Cytokine analysis on the vitreous sample revealed an interleukin (IL)-10 level below 23.4 pg/mL (below detectable) and an IL-6 level of 226.8 pg/mL, suggestive of an inflammatory process rather than intraocular lymphoma. The patient was successfully treated with a short course of oral corticosteroids with reduction in the inflammation and improvement in visual acuity (see Fig.23.14D). On subsequent follow-up, the patient had hilar lymphadenopathy on chest x-ray and chest computed tomography (CT), and positron emission tomography (PET) showed increased uptake in the hilar lymph nodes, mediastinum, and thyroid gland, consistent with a diagnosis of sarcoidosis.

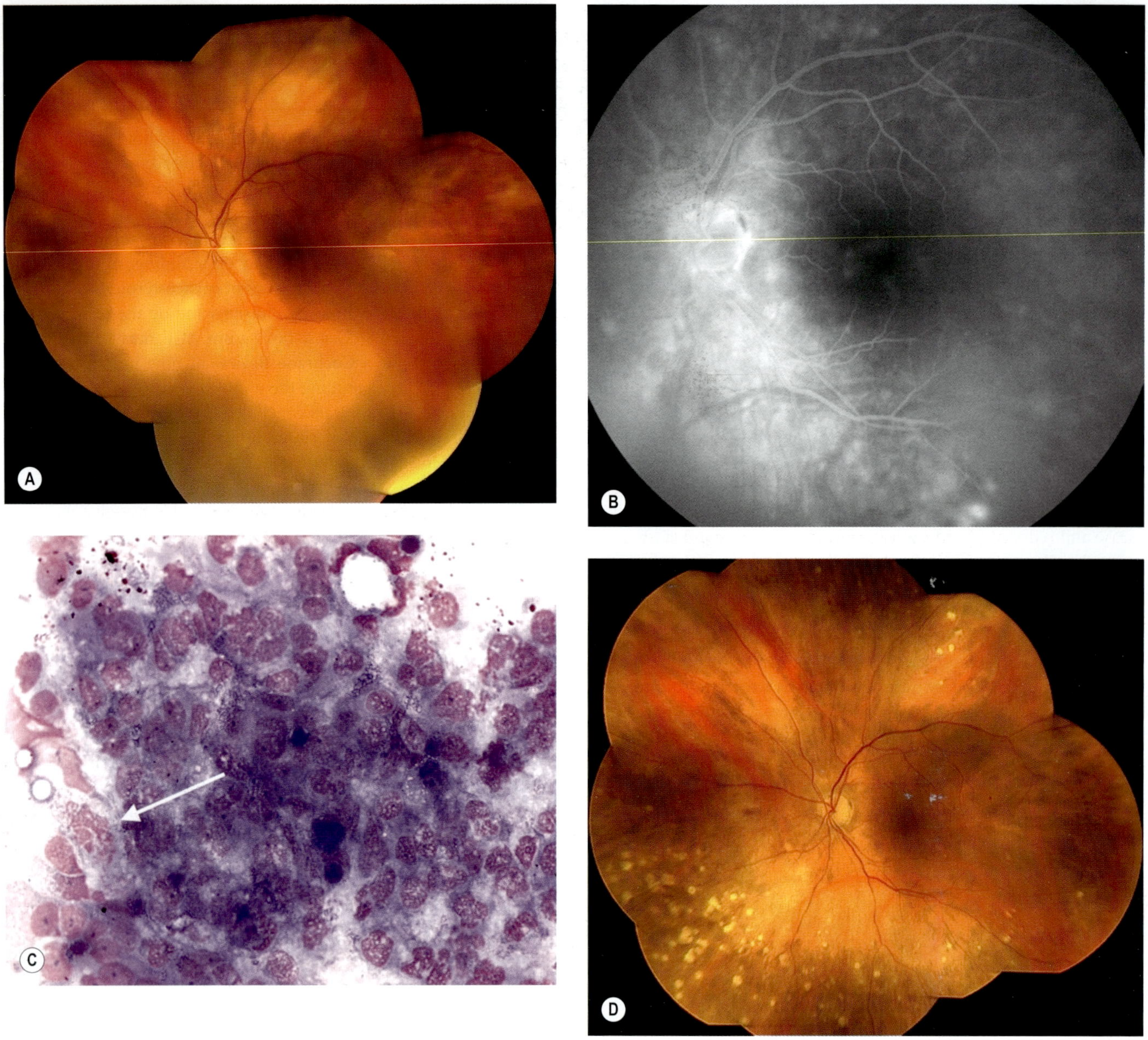

Fig. 23.14 (A) A retinal montage of the left eye showing yellow, exudative infiltrative lesions predominantly in the midperipheral and peripheral retina. Dalen-Fuchs nodules are also seen in the peripheral retina. (B) Fluorescein angiography showing hyperfluorescent lesions, some with late staining. (C) Cytology specimen from the vitreous showing multiple small, reactive lymphocytes and giant cells *(arrow)* consistent with a diagnosis of ocular sarcoidosis. (D) A retinal montage after therapy with oral corticosteroids showing resolution of the exudative lesions and revealing multiple Dalen-Fuchs nodules, predominantly in the inferior retina.

Sustained-release intravitreal corticosteroid implants containing dexamethasone or fluocinolone can be useful in the management of posterior segment inflammation.[68,69]

In patients with chronic sarcoidosis requiring prolonged systemic corticosteroid therapy, side effects often necessitate the addition of a steroid-sparing drug. Cyclosporin and other immunosuppressive agents have had therapeutic effects in patients with sarcoidosis, although most of the data are anecdotal, coming from case series. A Cochrane Review of immunosuppressive and cytotoxic therapy for pulmonary sarcoidosis concluded that evidence supporting the use of these therapies is limited and that side effects with some of the therapies were severe.[70] We have observed improvement in both the ocular and systemic manifestations of sarcoidosis after cyclosporin therapy,[30] but there is still no optimal safe long-term approach for the use of this drug. Supplementation with periocular steroids and pulse systemic steroids can assist in keeping the dose of cyclosporin low. Local intravitreal administration of corticosteroids as an injection or in a sustained-release implant may be useful, especially for patients with active disease limited to the eye.

Methotrexate is being used more frequently as an effective corticosteroid-sparing agent in the treatment of sarcoidosis. In a small randomized, double-masked trial of methotrexate versus placebo, patients receiving methotrexate appeared to require less prednisone to control their disease.[71] Low-dose methotrexate also appeared to be an effective and safe adjunctive therapy in patients with sarcoid-associated panuveitis.[72] In this retrospective case series, 100% of patients requiring oral corticosteroids were able to reduce their corticosteroid dosage from a mean initial dose of 26.6 mg/day to 1.5 mg/day, and 86% completely discontinued oral corticosteroids after receiving methotrexate. However, one must remember that up to 6 months may be required for methotrexate to take effect.

Treatments targeting TNF have been shown to be effective in treating some patients with chronic sarcoidosis. TNF-α appears to be important in the pathogenesis of the disease. The administration of infliximab, a chimeric monoclonal antibody that inhibits TNF-α, led to significant improvement in chronic pulmonary sarcoidosis in three patients.[73] However, an RCT in 138 patients reported only a small increase in forced vital capacity in patients treated with infliximab compared with placebo.[74] Biologic agents are being used more in the treatment of uveitis, including ocular inflammation associated with sarcoidosis. Most of the clinical trials of biologics for the treatment of sarcoid uveitis have focused on TNF inhibitors. Infliximab may help decrease ocular inflammation in patients with sarcoidosis.[75,76] Other TNF-α inhibitors, including adalimumab, etanercept, and golimumab, have also been used.[77,78] In a multicenter observational study of 160 patients with refractory uveitis (6% with sarcoidosis), anti-TNF treatment was effective in treating uveitis, and infliximab and adalimumab appeared to be equivalent in terms of efficacy.[79]

Paradoxical increases in inflammatory disease have been reported in some patients receiving anti-TNF therapy.[80] These cases are rare, and inflammation can decrease with continued use. Although the use of biologics for treating uveitis associated with sarcoidosis is increasing, they are not usually used as first-line therapy, especially in adults.

Other treatments are needed for some patients with resistant disease. Hydroxychloroquine can be an effective treatment for skin disease, CNS involvement, and some cases of pulmonary sarcoidosis. Sarcoidosis involving the CNS may be resistant to treatment, and radiotherapy has been tried for unresponsive disease. Gelwan et al.[81] have reported the use of radiotherapy for cases of sarcoidosis involving the anterior visual pathway. Lung, heart, and liver transplantations have been performed in patients with sarcoidosis, with results similar to those seen in other diseases.[12] Finally, there is some evidence that Janus kinase (JAK)–signal transducer and activator of transcription (STAT) signaling plays some role in the pathogenesis of sarcoidosis. A patient with cutaneous sarcoidosis was successfully treated with the oral JAK inhibitor tofacitinib[82]; however, additional research is needed to confirm the safety and efficacy of this class of drugs for treating the disease.

Sarcoidosis produces a high incidence of glaucoma and cataract, and surgical intervention is frequently required. Because of the changes in the anterior segment and the substantial opacities in the vitreous that often occur in sarcoidosis, some uveitis specialists prefer to use pars plana lensectomy to remove the cataract. However, there are no data on the relative benefits of this procedure compared with those of extracapsular cataract extraction in patients with sarcoidosis. Patients with sarcoidosis frequently have severe exacerbations of their ocular inflammation in the immediate postoperative period, and the optic disk may not be seen for the first few days. This occurs with both pars plana lensectomy and extracapsular cataract extraction. This inflammatory response peaks about 48 hours after surgery and lasts for 5 or 6 days, and patients with sarcoidosis should therefore be treated with high doses of systemic corticosteroids for the first week. The patient's immediate postoperative vision may be greatly reduced because of vitreous haze, but it will improve as vitritis resolves. The retinal and optic disk neovascularization that occurs in sarcoidosis frequently responds to oral corticosteroid therapy.[31] Laser photocoagulation has been used for subretinal neovascularization if it is in a treatable location.[30] Intravitreal injections of anti-VEGF therapy are now used in treating choroidal and subretinal neovascularization in patients with sarcoidosis.[83]

PROGNOSIS

Fortunately, many patients with sarcoidosis experience complete remission of their disease after several years. If sarcoidosis regresses spontaneously, it rarely recurs. In all patients with ocular manifestations of sarcoidosis, the goal is to control the inflammatory disease, thereby preventing permanent visually impairing changes, such as photoreceptor damage caused by chronic cystoid macular edema. With early diagnosis and prompt and appropriate therapy, visual outcomes can be good. Edelsten et al. noted that after 10 years, 54% of patients retained normal visual acuity and 4.6% had lost vision to less than 6/36 in both eyes.[84] However, vision loss can occur in chronic uveitis associated with sarcoidosis. In a study of 60 patients with sarcoid-associated uveitis, factors most significantly associated with a final visual acuity of worse than 20/40 included delay in presentation to a subspecialist, total duration of uveitis, development of cystoid macular edema or glaucoma, presence of intermediate or posterior uveitis, and systemic steroid use.[85]

The ideal therapy for all forms of sarcoidosis remains to be discovered; however, advances in the therapy of ocular sarcoidosis should follow improved understanding of the cause of systemic sarcoidosis and a clear insight into the relationship between ocular manifestations and the systemic inflammatory disease. As new biologic agents are being developed, their potential role in the treatment of uveitis associated with sarcoidosis should be tested in clinical trials so that improvements in visual outcomes can continue to be made.

REFERENCES

1. Hunter DG, Foster CS. Systemic manifestations of sarcoidosis. Albert DA, Jakobiec FA, eds. *Principles and Practice of Ophthalmology*. Philadelphia: WB Saunders; 1994:3132–3142.
2. Bruins Slot WJ. Ziekte van Besnier-Boeck en Febris uveoparotidea (Heerfordt). *Ned Tijdshr Geneeskd*. 1936;80:2859–2870.
3. Fanburg BL. Sarcoidosis. Wyngaarden JB, Smith LH Jr, Bennett JC, eds. *Cecil Textbook of Medicine*. 19th ed. Philadelphia: WB Saunders; 1992:430–435.
4. Bresnitz EA, Strom BL. Epidemiology of sarcoidosis. *Epidemiol Rev*. 1983;5:124–156.
5. Siltzbach LE, James DG, Neville E, et al. Course and prognosis of sarcoidosis around the world. *Am J Med*. 1974;57:847–852.
6. Rybicke BA, Major M, Popovich J Jr, et al. Racial differences in sarcoidosis incidence: a 5-year study in a health maintenance organization. *Am J Epidemiol*. 1997;145:234–241.
7. Morimoto T, Azuma A, Abe S, et al. Epidemiology of sarcoidosis. *Eur Resp J*. 2008;31. 372–329.
8. Cozier YC, Berman JS, Palmer JR, et al. Sarcoidosis in black women in the United States: data from the black women's health study. *Chest*. 2011;139:144–150.
9. Jabs DA, Johns CJ. Ocular involvement in chronic sarcoidosis. *Am J Ophthalmol*. 1986;102:297–301.
10. Ungprasert P, Carmona EM, Utz JP, et al. Epidemiology of sarcoidosis 1946–2013: a population based study. *Mayo Clin Proc*. 2016;2:183–188.
11. Milman N, Selroos O. Pulmonary sarcoidosis in the Nordic countries 1950–1982: epidemiology and clinical picture. *Sarcoidosis*. 1990;7:50–57.

12. Iannuzzi MC, Rybicki BA, Teirstein AS. Sarcoidosis. *N Engl J Med.* 2007;357:2153–2165.
13. Thomas PD, Hunninghake GW. Current concepts of the pathogenesis of sarcoidosis. *Am Rev Respir Dis.* 1987;135:747.
14. Crystal RG, Roberts WC, Hunninghake GW, et al. Pulmonary sarcoidosis: a disease characterized and perpetuated by activated lung T-lymphocytes. *Ann Intern Med.* 1981;94:73–94.
15. Hunninghake GW, Crystal RG. Pulmonary sarcoidosis: a disorder mediated by excess helper T-lymphocyte activity at sites of disease activity. *N Engl J Med.* 1981;305:429–434.
16. Sememzato G, Pezzutto A, Pizzolo G. Immunohistological study in sarcoidosis: evaluation at different sites of disease activity. *Clin Immunol Immunopathol.* 1984;30:29–40.
17. Chan CC, Wetzig RP, Palestine AG, et al. Immunohistopathology of ocular sarcoidosis: report of a case and discussion of immunopathogenesis. *Arch Ophthalmol.* 1987;105:1398–1402.
18. Bresnitz EA, Strom BL. Epidemiology of sarcoidosis. *Epidemiol Rev.* 1983;5:124–156.
19. Newman LS, Rose CS, Bresnitz EA, et al. A case control etiologic study of sarcoidosis: environmental and occupational risk factors. *Am J Respir Crit Care Med.* 2004;170:1324–1330.
20. Haijzadeh R, Sato H, Carlisle J, et al. *Mycobacterium tuberculosis* antigen 85A induces Th-1 immune responses in systemic sarcoidosis. *J Clin Immunol.* 2007;27:445–454.
21. Hwang CJ, Gausas RE. Sarcoid-like granulomatous orbital inflammation induced by interferon-alpha treatment. *Ophthalm Plast Reconstruct Surg.* 2008;24:311–313.
22. Ahmadzai H, Huang S, Steinfort C, et al. Sarcoidosis: a state of the art review from the Thoracic Society of Australia and New Zealand. *Med J Aust.* 2018;208(11):499–504.
23. Familial associations in sarcoidosis: a report to the Research Committee of the British Thoracic and Tuberculosis Association. *Tubercle.* 1973;54:87–98.
24. Brewerton DA, Cockburn C, James DC, et al. HLA antigens in sarcoidosis. *Clin Exp Immunol.* 1977;27:227–229.
25. Rossman MD, Thompson B, Frederick M, et al. HLA-DRB1*1101: a significant risk factor for sarcoidosis in blacks and whites. *Am J Hum Genet.* 2003;73:720–735.
26. Crick RP, Hoyle C, Smellie H. The eyes in sarcoidosis. *Br J Ophthalmol.* 1961;45:461–481.
27. Obenauf CD, Shaw HE, Sydnor CF, et al. Sarcoidosis and its ophthalmic manifestations. *Am J Ophthalmol.* 1978;86:648–655.
28. James DG, Neville E, Langley DA. Ocular sarcoidosis. *Trans Ophthalmol Soc UK.* 1976;96:133–139.
29. Nichols CW, Eagle RC, Yanoff M, et al. Conjunctival biopsy as an aid in the evaluation of the patient with suspected sarcoidosis. *Ophthalmology.* 1980;87:287–291.
30. Palestine AG, Nussenblatt RB, Chan CC. Treatment of intraocular complications of sarcoidosis. *Ann NY Acad Med.* 1986;465:564–573.
31. Spalton DJ, Sanders MD. Fundus changes in histologically confirmed sarcoidosis. *Br J Ophthalmol.* 1981;65:348–358.
32. Marcus DF, Bovino JA, Burton TC. Sarcoid granuloma of the choroid. *Ophthalmology.* 1982;89:1326–1330.
33. Campo RV, Aaberg TM. Choroidal granuloma in sarcoidosis. *Am J Ophthalmol.* 1984;97:419–427.
34. Frank KW, Weiss H. Unusual clinical and histopathologic findings in ocular sarcoidosis. *Br J Ophthalmol.* 1983;67:8–16.
35. Gragoudas ES, Regan CDJ. Peripapillary subretinal neovascularization in presumed sarcoidosis. *Arch Ophthalmol.* 1981;99:1194–1197.
36. Konidaris VE, Empeslidis T. Ranibizumab in choroidal neovascularisation associated with ocular sarcoidosis. *BMJ Case Rep.* 2013;2013. bcr2013010288.
37. Rush JA. Retrobulbar optic neuropathy in sarcoidosis. *Ann Ophthalmol.* 1980;12:390–394.
38. Mavrikakis I, Rootman J. Diverse clinical presentation of orbital sarcoid. *Am J Ophthalmol.* 2007;144:769–775.
39. Dursun D, Akova YA, Bilezikci B. Scleritis associated with sarcoidosis. *Ocul Immunol Inflamm.* 2004;12:143–148.
40. Ma SP, Rogers SL, Hall AJ, et al. Sarcoidosis-related uveitis: clinical presentation, disease course, and rates of systemic disease progression after uveitis diagnosis. *Am J Ophthalmol.* 2019;198:30–36.
41. Mitchell DN, Scadding JG, Heard BE, et al. Sarcoidosis: histopathological definition and clinical diagnosis. *J Clin Pathol.* 1977;30:395–408.
42. Scott GC, Berman JM, Higgins JL Jr. CT patterns of nodular hepatic and splenic sarcoidosis: a review of the literature. *J Comput Assist Tomogr.* 1997;21:369–372.
43. Han YS, Rivera-Grana E, Salek S, et al. Distinguishing uveitis secondary to sarcoidosis from idiopathic disease: cardiac implications. *JAMA Ophthlamol.* 2018;136(2):109–115.
44. Hoover DL, Khan JA, Giangiacomo J. Pediatric ocular sarcoidosis. *Surv Ophthalmol.* 1986;30:215.
45. Perruquet JL, Harrington TM, Davis DE, et al. Sarcoid arthritis in a North American Caucasian population. *J Rheumatol.* 1984;11:521–525.
46. Yotsumoto S, Takahashi Y, Takei S, et al. Early onset sarcoidosis masquerading as juvenile rheumatoid arthritis. *J Am Acad Dermatol.* 2000;43:969–971.
47. Roy M, Sharma OP, Chan K. Sarcoidosis presenting in infancy: a rare occurrence. *Sarcoidosis Vasc Diffuse Lung Dis.* 1999;16:224–227.
48. Raphael SA, Blau EB, Zhang WH, et al. Analysis of a large kindred with Blau syndrome for HLA, autoimmunity, and sarcoidosis. *Am J Dis Child.* 1993;147:842–848.
49. Schurmann M, Valentonyte R, Hampe J, et al. CARD15 gene mutations in sarcoidosis. *Eur Respir J.* 2003;22:748–754.
50. Manouvrier-Hanu S, Puech B, Piette F, et al. Blau syndrome of granulomatous arthritis, iritis, and skin rash: a new family and review of the literature. *Am J Med Genet.* 1998;76:217–221.
51. Grunewald J, Eklund A. Role of CD4+ T cells in sarcoidosis. *Proc Am Thorac Soc.* 2007;4:461–464.
52. Idali F, Wahlström J, Müller-Suur C, et al. Analysis of regulatory T cell associated forkhead box P3 expression in the lungs of patients with sarcoidosis. *Clin Exp Immunol.* 2008;152(1):127–137.
53. Gass JDM, Olson CL. Sarcoidosis with optic nerve and retinal involvement. *Arch Ophthalmol.* 1976;94:945–950.
54. Groen F, van Laar AJM, Rothova A. Chest radiographic screening for sarcoidosis in the diagnosis of patients with active uveitis. *Ann Am Thorac Soc.* 2017;14:912–918.
55. Herbort CP, Rao NA, Mochizuki M. Members of Scientific Committee of First International Workshop on Ocular Sarcoidosis. International criteria for the diagnosis of ocular sarcoidosis: results of the first International Workshop on Ocular Sarcoidosis (IWOS). *Ocul Immunol Inflamm.* 2009;17:180–189.
56. Cohen KL, Peiffer RL, Powell DA. Sarcoidosis and ocular disease in a young child. *Arch Ophthalmol.* 1981;99:422–424.
57. Smith JA, Chan CC, Egwuagu CE, et al. Immunohistochemical examination of lacrimal gland tissue from patients with ocular sarcoidosis. *Adv Exp Med Biol.* 1998;438:599–602.
58. Hadjadj J, Dechartes A, Chapron T, et al. Relevance of diagnostic investigations in patients with uveitis: retrospective cohort study on 300 patients. *Autoimmun Rev.* 2017;16:504–511.
59. Kosmorsky GS, Meisler DM, Rice TW, et al. Chest computed tomography and mediastinoscopy in the diagnosis of sarcoidosis-associated uveitis. *Am J Ophthalmol.* 1998;126:132–134.
60. Annema JT, Veselic M, Rabe KF. Endoscopic ultrasound-guided fine-needle aspiration for the diagnosis of sarcoidosis. *Eur Respir J.* 2005;25:405–409.
61. Lieberman J. Enzymes in sarcoidosis: angiotensin converting enzyme (ACE). *Clin Lab Med.* 1989;9:745.
62. Weinreb RN, Sandman R, Ryder MI, et al. Angiotensin converting enzyme activity in human aqueous humor. *Arch Ophthalmol.* 1985;34:103.
63. Groen-Hakan F, Eurelings L, ten Berge JC, et al. Diagnostic value of serum-soluble interleukin 2 receptor levels vs angiotensin-converting enzyme in patients with sarcoidosis-associated uveitis. *JAMA Ophthalmol.* 2017;135:1352–1358.
64. Munro CS, Mitchell DN. The Kveim response: still useful, still a puzzle. *Thorax.* 1987;42:321.
65. Weinreb RN. Diagnosing sarcoidosis by transconjunctival biopsy of the lacrimal gland. *Am J Ophthalmol.* 1984;97:573–576.

66. Vita T, Okada DR, Veillet-Chowdhury M, et al. Complementary value of cardiac magnetic resonance imaging and positron emission tomography/computed tomography in the assessment of cardiac sarcoidosis. *Circ Cardiovasc Imaging*. 2018;11:007030.
67. Paramothayan NS, Jones PW. Corticosteroids for pulmonary sarcoidosis. *Cochrane Database Syst Rev*. 2005;2:CD001114.
68. Myung JS, Aeker GD, Kiss S. Treatment of non-infectious posterior uveitis with dexamethasone intravitreal implant. *Clin Ophthalmol*. 2010;4:1423–1426.
69. Cunningham ET Jr, de Smet MD, Yeh S, et al. Sustained-release corticosteroids for uveitis. *Ocular Immunol Inflamm*. 2015;23:421–424.
70. Paramothayan S, Lasserson TJ, Walters EH. Immunosuppressive and cytotoxic therapy for pulmonary sarcoidosis. *Cochrane Database Syst Rev*. 2006;3:CD003536.
71. Baughman RP, Winget DB, Lower EE. Methotrexate is steroid sparing in acute sarcoidosis: results of a double blind, randomized trial. *Sarcoidosis Vasc Diffuse Lung Dis*. 2000;17:60–66.
72. Dev S, McCallum RM, Jaffe GJ. Methotrexate treatment for sarcoid-associated panuveitis. *Ophthalmology*. 1999;106:111–118.
73. Baughman RP, Lower EE. Infliximab for refractory sarcoidosis. *Sarcoidosis Vasc Diffuse Lung Dis*. 2001;18:70–74.
74. Baughman RP, Drent M, Kavuru M, et al. Infliximab therapy in patients with chronic sarcoidosis and pulmonary involvement. *Am J Respir Crit Care Med*. 2006;174:795–802.
75. Lindstedt EW, Baarsma GS, Kuijpers RW, et al. Anti-TNF-alpha therapy for sight threatening uveitis. *Br J Ophthalmol*. 2005;89:533–536.
76. Saurenmann RK, Levin AV, Rose JB. Tumour necrosis factor alpha inhibitors in the treatment of childhood uveitis. *Rheumatology*. 2006;45:982–989.
77. Riancho-Zarrabeitia L, Calvo-Rio V, Blanco R, et al. Anti-TNF-alpha therapy in refractor uveitis associated with sarcoidosis: multicenter study of 17 patients. *Semin Arthritis Rheum*. 2015;45:361–368.
78. Erckens RJ, Mostard RL, Wijnen PA, et al. Adalimumab successful in sarcoidosis patients with refractory chronic non-infectious uveitis. *Graefes Arch Clin Exp Ophthalmol*. 2012;250:713–720.
79. Vallet H, Seve P, Biard L, et al. Infliximab versus adalimumab in the treatment of refractory inflammatory uveitis: a multicenter study from the French Uveitis Network. *Arthritis Rheumatol*. 2016;68:1522–1530.
80. Ramos-Casals M, Roberto-Perez-Alvarez, Diaz-Lagares C, BIOGEAS Study Group, et al. Autoimmune diseases induced by biologic agents: a double-edged sword. *Autoimmun Rev*. 2010;9:188–193.
81. Gelwan MJ, Kellen RI, Burde RM, et al. Sarcoidosis of the anterior visual pathway: successes and failures. *J Neurol Neurosurg*. 1988;51:1473.
82. Damsky W, Thakral D, Phil M, et al. Tofacitinib treatment and molecular analysis of cutaneous sarcoidosis. *N Engl J Med*. 2018;379:2540–2546.
83. Konidaris VE, Empeslidis T. Ranibizumab in choroidal neovascularisation associated with ocular sarcoidosis. *BMJ Case Rep*. 2013;2013. bcr2013010288.
84. Edelsten C, Pearson A, Joynes E, et al. The ocular and systemic prognosis of patients presenting with sarcoid uveitis. *Eye (Lond)*. 1999;13:748–753.
85. Dana MR, Merayo-Lloves J, Schaumberg DA. Prognosticators for visual outcome in sarcoid uveitis. *Ophthalmology*. 1996;103:1846–1853.
86. Valentonyte R, Hampe J, Huse K, et al. Sarcoidosis is associated with a truncating splice site mutation in BTNL2. *Nat Genet*. 2005;37:357–364 (Erratum, Nat Genet 2005;37:652).
87. Rybicki BA, Walewski JL, Maliarik MJ, Kian H, Iannuzi MC. The BTNL2 gene and sarcoidosis susceptibility in African Americans and whites. *Am J Hum Genet*. 2005;77:491–499.

24

Sympathetic Ophthalmia

H. Nida Sen

KEY CONCEPTS

- Sympathetic ophthalmia (SO) is a bilateral condition.
- SO is now more commonly seen after vitrectomy than after accidental injury.
- Dalen-Fuchs nodules are commonly seen in the retinal periphery of eyes with SO, but they are not pathognomonic for the disease.

Sympathetic ophthalmia (SO) probably is the intraocular inflammatory condition best known to health care practitioners outside of ophthalmology. It has been suggested that although SO was not yet defined at that time, the famous composer J.S. Bach's poor vision after couching for cataracts may have resulted from this disorder.[1] It has also stimulated enormous interest within our field since its clinical description by MacKenzie[2] early in the nineteenth century. The annual incidence rate of SO is relatively small, but the dread of losing not only the involved eye but the contralateral, untouched eye as well in a potentially sight-threatening process is, indeed, great.

CLINICAL APPEARANCE AND PREVALENCE

SO is bilateral granulomatous uveitis that occurs after either intentional or unintentional penetrating trauma to one eye. Trauma to one eye (the exciting eye) will result in an inflammatory response not only in that eye but also in the contralateral eye (the sympathizing eye). SO is a disease that was known to the ancient Greeks and was referred to in the teachings of Hippocrates.[3] It was recognized also during the early and late Middle Ages and into the eighteenth and nineteenth centuries, as found in MacKenzie's full clinical description. Fuchs[4] published the classic description of the disease in 1905, establishing it as a separate entity. The disease can begin as early as several days after the penetrating insult or occur decades later, with the clinical diagnosis becoming apparent in 80% of patients some 3 months after injury to the exciting eye[5] and in 90% within 1 year of trauma.[6,7] SO occurs more often after nonsurgical trauma. Liddy and Stuart[8] found the disorder in 0.2% of eyes with nonsurgical wounds, and Holland[9] in 0.5% of eyes with nonsurgical trauma. Marak[5] estimated the incidence of this disease to be fewer than 10 cases in 100,000 surgical penetrating wounds. In a review by Gass,[10] in which 26 eye pathology laboratories were surveyed for a 5-year period from 1975 through 1980, sympathetic ophthalmia was diagnosed in 53 eyes (two of every 1000 eyes examined); 55% of these were posttraumatic occurrences. In the same survey, a survey of 34 retinal surgeons who had performed 14,915 vitrectomies reported SO in nine eyes (incidence rate of 0.06%), with vitrectomy performed as the only operative procedure in one eye (incidence rate of 0.01%). Since 2000 studies have suggested that ocular surgery, particularly vitreoretinal surgery, is the major initiating factor for this disorder.[11,12] This trend is being seen worldwide. In a review of 10 cases of SO in Singapore from 1993 to 2003,[13] the authors reported that the disease occurred in three patients after trauma, and in seven patients after surgery. Of those seven, four were seen after vitreoretinal surgery, two after diode laser cyclophotoablation, and one after neodymium:yttrium–aluminum–garnet (Nd:YAG) laser cyclotherapy. In their commentary, Kilmartin et al.[11] calculated the risk of sympathetic ophthalmia to be 1 per 1152 retinal surgical procedures, perhaps even as much as 1 per 800.[14] If this calculation reflects a true trend, the risk would be twice that reported previously for vitrectomy (0.06%).[10] The authors of this study raise the issue as to whether patients should be informed of this risk in the consent form because the calculated risk is more than twice the 0.05% risk of infectious endophthalmitis after vitrectomy (Table 24.1). It is interesting to note that no cases of SO were reported in the 467 perforated globes observed by the U.S. military during World War II, the Korean War, and the Vietnam War.[15] However, only one case of a soldier injured in the Iraq conflict has been reported.[16] These findings are in contrast to the earlier reports in the twentieth century, which suggested an incidence of about 2%,[7] and it was believed that 16% of ocular injuries during the American Civil War resulted in SO. In a prospective surveillance study in the United Kingdom and the Republic of Ireland,[12] which included 59 million citizens, 17 patients with newly diagnosed SO were reported in a 12-month period, and a minimum estimated incidence of 0.03 in 100,000 was calculated.

SO is thought to occur more commonly in males, children, and older adults—likely because of presumed higher incidence of ocular trauma in these groups—but this demographic is changing as the causes of SO are changing (see below), with no sex predilection and a lower incidence among children.

We reviewed 32 patients with SO seen at the National Eye Institute (NEI) during a 10-year period.[17] These patients represented 1.4% of the 2287 patients with uveitis seen by us during that period. There was no sex preponderance (16 males and 16 females), and in 23 of the 32 patients, the disease developed after accidental injury. Patient age ranged from 3 years to 80 years. In our group of patients, SO developed within 1 year of injury in 56%, with the disease developing in approximately 31% of them between 2 weeks and 3 months after an ocular insult; in one patient, the disease developed some 46 years later. Hakin et al.[18] reported their experience with 18 patients: 15 of their cases occurred after trauma, 11 of which after a known penetrating wound and the other four after a posterior scleral rupture. Three cases occurred after retinal detachment, with patients receiving, on average. three surgical interventions (Fig. 24.1). Castiblanco et al. performed a systematic review and identified 86 patients with SO. In 44%, ocular surgery was the inciting event, and 21% of the surgeries were vitrectomies.[19] However, according to a retrospective cohort study of 175 SO cases from India conducted by Tyagi et al., vitreoretinal surgery accounted for only 9.1% of all SO cases, and SO developed in only

TABLE 24.1 **Changes in Sympathetic Ophthalmia (SO) Trends Worth Taking Into Consideration**

Trend	Historical	Current
Cause	Post trauma	Post surgery (especially vitreoretinal)
Patients	Males and children (reflecting trauma peaks)	No gender predilection (reflects positive effect of injury prevention programs) and increasingly older patients (reflects effect of ocular surgery)
Incidence	Considered disappearing 30 years ago	Probably increasing (underdiagnosed in the past?)
Onset	For 65% within 2–8 weeks (for 90%, onset <1 year from trauma or most recent surgery)	Many delayed presentations (for significant percentage onset >1 year from trauma or most recent surgery)
Presentation	Granulomatous panuveitis	Any clinical uveitis
Outcome	Enucleation within 2 weeks for prevention of SO	Enucleation solely of SO prevention questionable
Visual prognosis	Poor	Reasonable because of modern immunosuppression

From Vote BJ, Hall A, Cairns J, et al. Changing trends in sympathetic ophthalmia. *Clin Exp Ophthalmol.* 2004;32:542–545.

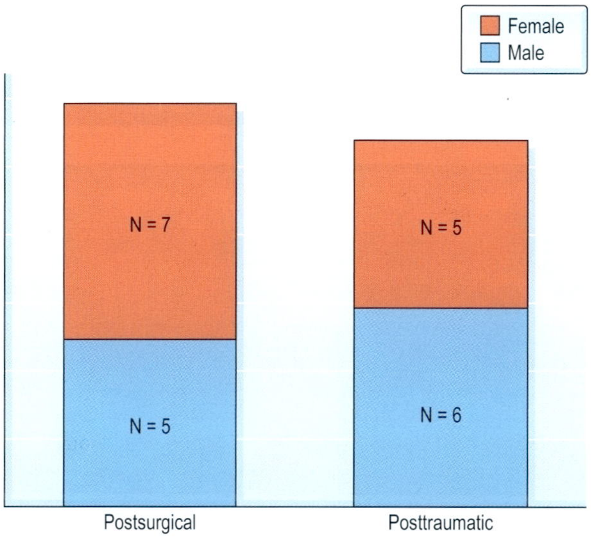

Fig. 24.1 Distribution of patients at the National Eye Institute in whom sympathetic ophthalmia developed after surgery and after trauma. Although these data were collected in the early 1990s, the number of postsurgical occurrences is interesting. (From Chan C, Roberge RG, Whitcup SM, et al. Thirty two cases of sympathetic ophthalmia examined at the National Eye Institute. A retrospective study at the National Eye Institute, Bethesda, MD, from 1982 to 1992. *Arch Ophthalmol.* 1995;113:597–600. Copyright © 1995, American Medical Association. All rights reserved.)

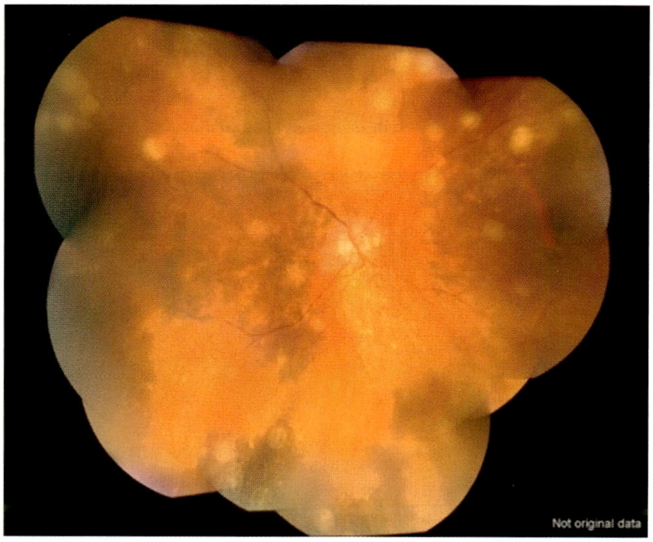

Fig. 24.2 Multiple cream-colored lesions that correspond to histologic diagnosis of Dalen-Fuchs nodules. Characteristically they tend to be strewn throughout the periphery and can extend to the disk and at times into the posterior pole. Initially, they appear to have "substance" to them, raising the overlying retina. With time they appear atrophic (Case 24.2).

0.038% of all pars plana vitrectomy cases.[20] Surgical trauma, particularly vitrectomy,[21] is well recognized as an antecedent event to SO, and, as mentioned earlier, it appears to be more common as the initiating event compared with accidental trauma, at least in some countries.[10,22-24]

Classic Presentation

In the classic presentation of SO, the inflammatory response seen in the anterior chamber is granulomatous, with mutton-fat keratic precipitates (KPs) on the corneal endothelium and findings of acute anterior uveitis. However, the anterior chamber inflammatory response can be relatively mild, with the inflammation taking on a nongranulomatous appearance as well. There is generally moderate to severe vitritis accompanied by multiple white-yellow lesions in the periphery, which sometimes become confluent (Fig. 24.2). These represent the clinical appearance of a Dalen-Fuchs nodule, a histologic finding. Swelling of the disk (papillitis) can be prominent, and circumpapillary choroidal lesions can also occur (Fig. 24.3). Retinal involvement is not an uncommon finding in SO and has been amply corroborated by histologic findings (see later discussion). Although rare, subretinal neovascularization has been reported to occur in SO,[25] as it has been in the Vogt-Koyanagi-Harada (VKH) syndrome (see Chapter 25). In a systematic review of 86 SO cases, the most common clinical features were intraocular inflammation in 83%—with anterior uveitis (55%) being slightly more common than vitritis (47.0%)—and Dalen-Fuchs nodules in 33.3%. Optic disk swelling (20%), serous retinal detachment (11.7%), and choroiditis (8.3%) were present less frequently.[19] Galor et al. evaluated 85 patients with SO from three academic centers and found that the majority of patients were males (60%) and white (57%); median age at presentation was 44 years; and median time to SO from trauma/surgery was 0.82 years. The etiology was trauma in 62% and surgery in 38%; in 52%, SO developed within the first year.[26] Active intraocular inflammation was present in 74% of sympathizing eyes (44% in inciting eyes), and exudative retinal detachment (RD) was present in 10% of sympathizing eyes (18% in inciting eyes). In a large multicenter retrospective study from the United Kingdom, Singapore, and India, the findings were similar in 130 patients with SO: the majority of patients were males (62%), and median patient age was 48 years.[27] In a series of 14 children with mostly traumatic SO (93%), 71% had

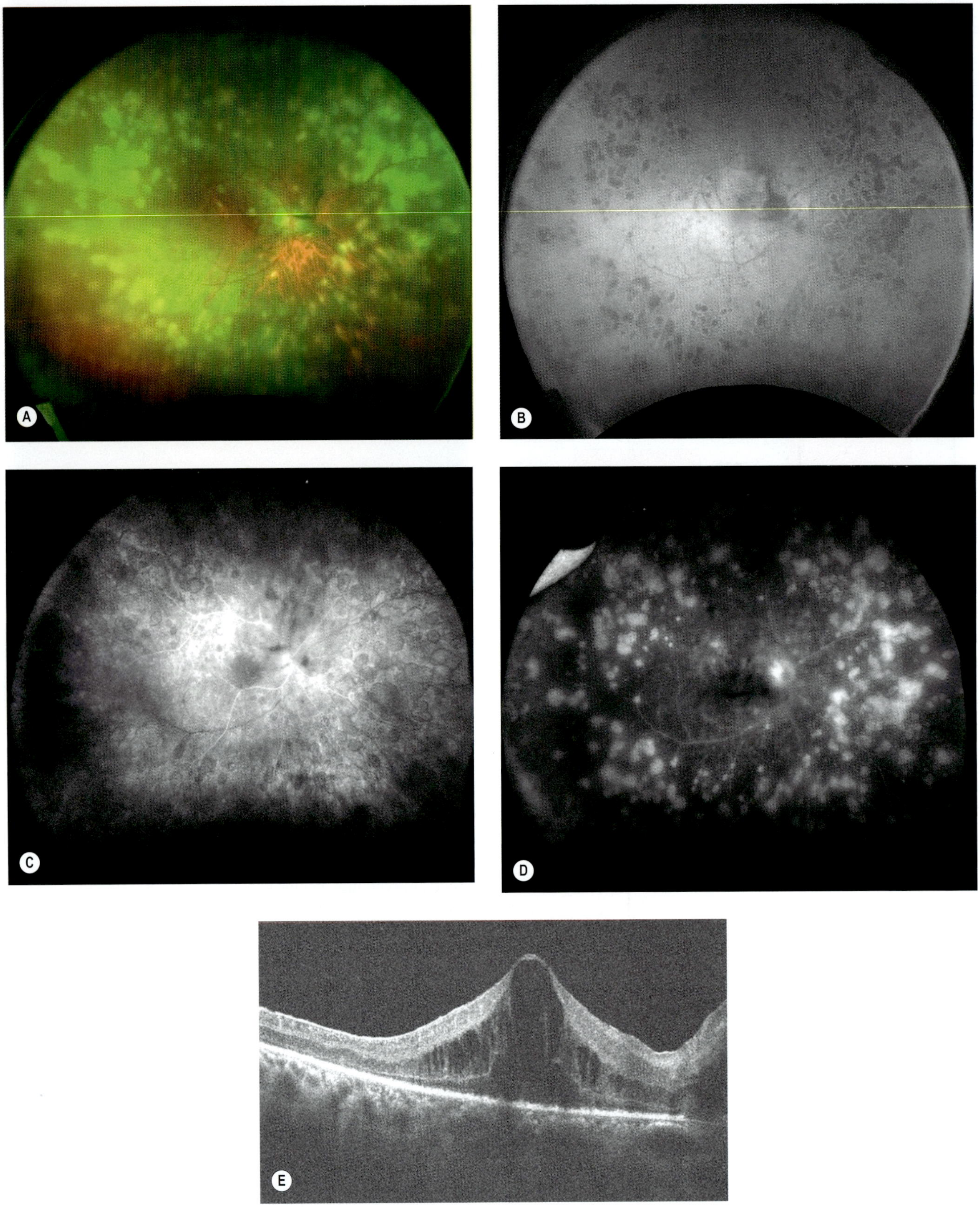

Fig. 24.3

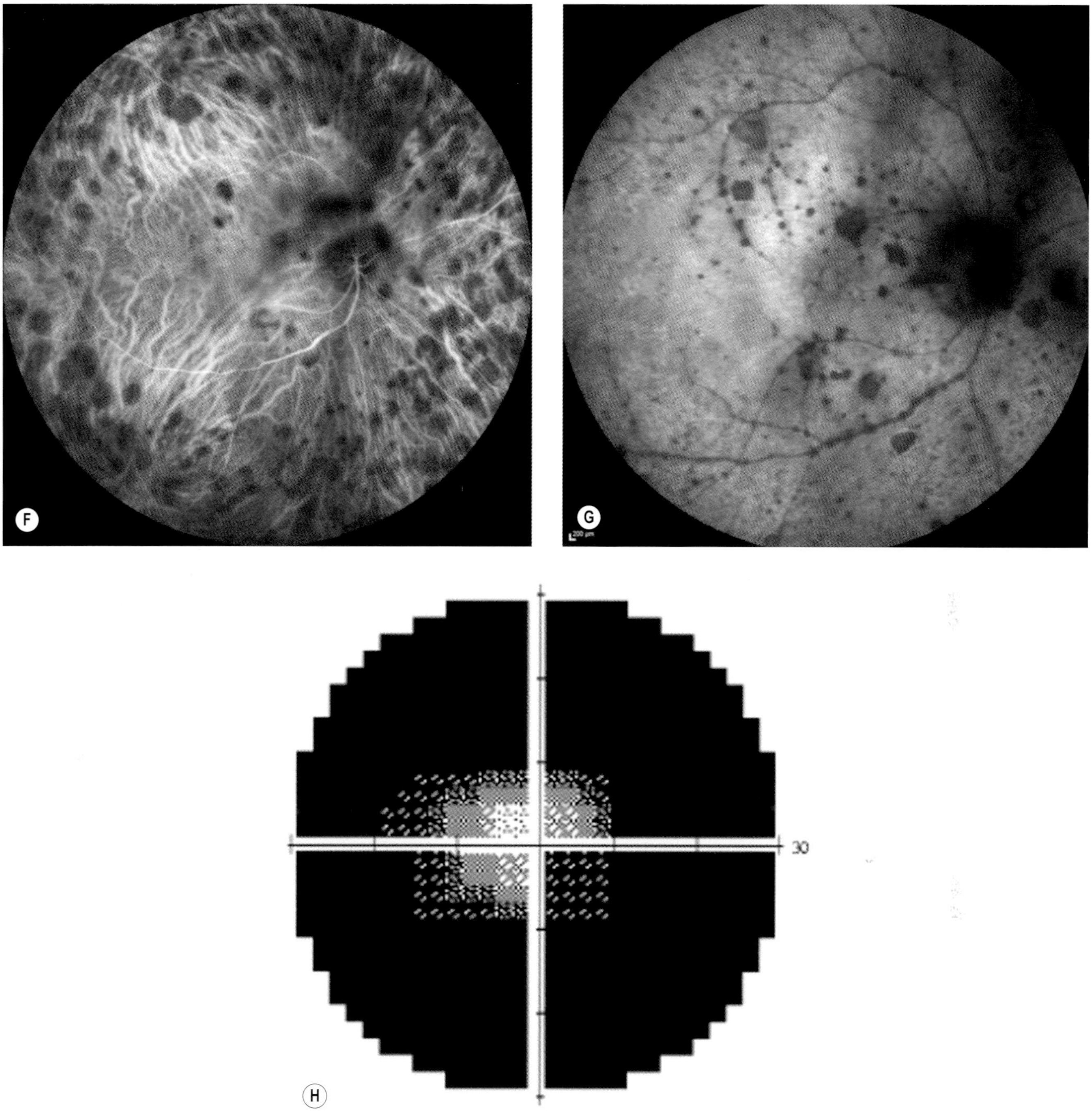

Fig. 24.3, cont'd Sympathetic ophthalmia developed in this eye after multiple retinal detachment surgeries and vitrectomy in the left eye. Multiple choroidal lesions at different stages throughout the posterior pole and periphery (A). Fundus autofluorescence shows mostly hypoautofluorescent lesions caused by atrophy or blockage, some surrounded by hyperautofluorescent margins (B). Fluorescein angiogram shows early blockage with late staining of choroidal lesions (C, D). Macular optical coherence tomography (OCT) reveals significant macular edema along with optic nerve edema (E). Indocyanine green (ICG) angiography shows hypocyanescent choroidal lesions more numerous than can be appreciated on clinical examination (F). Late ICG angiography shows lesions that are atrophic or are associated with retinal pigment epithelium (RPE)/ outer retinal damage (G). A Humphrey visual field testing using Stim III showed essentially extinguished visual fields with only less than 10 degrees of central field (H).

active anterior chamber inflammation, 50% had vitritis, 36% had disk edema, 71% had exudative retinal detachment, and 77% had thickened choroid on ultrasonography. Four had phthisis at presentation. Cataract was present in 21% at baseline, and 50% had 20/200 or worse vision in the sympathizing eye.[28] All patients were treated with systemic steroids, and 50% received immunosuppressives that included antimetabolites, cyclosporine, and alkylating agents, resulting in visual acuity gain.

A small number of patients with SO report or demonstrate extraocular findings not dissimilar from those seen in VKH syndrome (see Chapter 25), such as cells in cerebrospinal fluid (CSF pleocytosis);

hearing disturbances, such as high-frequency deafness[29]; and hair and skin changes (poliosis and vitiligo). These extraocular findings are rare in SO, unlike in VKH syndrome, in which they are fairly common and are important indicators in making the diagnosis. They are also important in the conceptualization of autoimmune diseases because SO is the only disease that is known to be associated with a specific event leading to autosensitization. The development of extraocular signs must be secondary to ocular immunization in the case of SO.

It should be noted that the clinical appearance of sympathetic ophthalmia comprises a spectrum of symptoms ranging from very mild to severe. Lewis et al.[30] reported a case of SO developing after trauma and vitrectomy confined to the posterior segment, with the SO resembling the focal lesions of acute posterior multifocal placoid pigment epitheliopathy (APMPPE) (see Chapter 30). Mild anterior uveitis has also been reported. Carrying the concept to the extreme, some have proposed the notion of unilateral SO. It is quite possible that the sympathizing response may be so mild as to disappear with minimal or no sequelae, and the spectrum of the histologic response seen would support this concept. However, if no inflammatory disease is noted, or if none is seen on a histologic specimen, it seems inappropriate to use the term *SO* to describe the disease under consideration. Marak[5] described a phenomenon he called *sympathetic irritation,* which occurs in the fellow eye after injury to or disease in one eye. About one-third of these patients may have cells and flare in the anterior chamber, with 67% of patients complaining of photophobia and a smaller number having perilimbal injection, conjunctival injection, or both. The distinction between this entity and "mild" SO seems unclear. There has been a suggested variant of SO with diffuse subretinal fibrotic changes. In one report, SO developed after multiple operations for the repair of retinal detachment, and there was fast deterioration of vision with the fibrotic changes becoming more extensive. This eye had many CD20+ cells (B cells) along with CD3+ (T cells) and CD68+ cells (macrophages).[31] In another report of multifocal granuloma and fibrosis, polymerase chain reaction (PCR) testing yielded negative results for herpes viruses, and types III, IV, V, and VI collagens were noted in the fibrosis; antibodies to photoreceptors were also seen.[32]

Several ocular entities have been associated with SO. Phacoanaphylaxis has been observed,[33] and Blodi[34] noted its occurrence in 23% of eyes with SO. He believed that the presence of the two entities in the same eye reflected the fact that these patients have a predisposition for autoimmune phenomena. In their excellent review of 105 cases, Lubin et al.[6] found an incidence of 46%. It should be noted that both entities can be found in the sympathizing (noninjured) eye as well,[35] and the phacoanaphylaxis can be a confounding element while attempting to diagnose SO (see later discussion).

Malignant melanoma or its treatment has also been associated with SO.[36-38] In 400 cases of SO evaluated by Easom and Zimmerman[39] at the Armed Forces Institute of Pathology, malignant melanoma was involved in seven. Fries et al.[40] reported SO after helium ion irradiation of a choroidal melanoma, whereas Margo and Pautler[41] reported the development of granulomatous bilateral uveitis after therapy with proton-beam irradiation. In the latter case, the authors stressed the fact that the sutures securing the four tantalum rings to the sclera did not penetrate the uvea.

SO has been reported to occur after cyclocryotherapy.[42] Harrison[43] discussed the development of SO in a patient who underwent cyclocryotherapy for neovascular glaucoma. No penetration of the sclera was noted in that patient. However, in one case of SO after cyclocryotherapy, it was felt that the procedure resulted in microperforations, with inflammatory cells and uveal pigment found in the subconjunctival space.[44] Edward et al.[45] reported a case after noncontact Nd:YAG laser cyclotherapy. Lam et al.[46] reported three others, and the problem was discussed by Tessler et al.[47] There may still be the rare case of no obvious clinical penetration into the globe, such as a case of penetrating trauma resulting in hyphema.[48] Of course, it is possible that a micropenetrating wound did occur.

Cataract surgery has been mentioned rarely as a cause of this entity.[49] In one report,[50] the disease occurred 3 months after intracapsular cataract extraction and anterior chamber lens placement; in this case, immediate postoperative problems, including flat chamber, pupillary block, and wound dehiscence, occurred, with one of the haptics protruding into the subconjunctival space. Vitrectomy and removal of the lens resulted in control of the disease and improvement of vision. A similar case was reported by Abu El-Asrar and Al-Obeidan.[51]

Sequelae

The sequelae of the inflammation noted in SO are quite variable, depending on the severity of the ocular inflammation and whether therapy has been instituted (see later discussion of therapy). Secondary glaucoma and cataract can result from the inflammatory process and from retinal and optic atrophy in association with retinal detachment and/or subretinal alterations, such as fibrosis and underlying choroidal atrophy. Disk neovascularization, which initially regressed with steroid therapy but was finally stabilized only with the addition of methotrexate, has been reported.[52] In their series of 85 patients with SO, Galor et al. noted that 47% of patients had ocular complications at presentation and that new complications occurred at a rate of 40% per person-year. The most common complications at presentation were hypotony, cataract, phthisis, and macular edema. Epiretinal membrane, choroidal neovascularization, and ocular hypertension were less common. Of the eyes with SO, 92% of inciting eyes and 26% of sympathizing eyes had 20/200 or worse vision at presentation; during follow-up, 59% maintained visual acuity of 20/50 or better. Traumatic etiology was more likely to be associated with vision loss. Active inflammation, cataract, and optic nerve abnormality were the most common factors associated with poor visual outcomes.[26] In a pediatric cohort of mostly trauma-associated SO, the common complications were phthisis (57%), cataract, and vitreous hemorrhage.

TESTS AND IMMUNOLOGIC CHARACTERISTICS

Clinical testing of patients will help put into perspective the severity of SO and identify subclinical choroidal lesions. Fluorescein angiography is useful in evaluating the degree of posterior segment disease. Spitznas[53] noted that fluorescein angiography performed during the acute stage of SO can demonstrate an exudative process, with multiple subretinal enlarging hyperfluorescent spots and pooling of dye (see Fig. 24.3). This observation is further validated with optical coherence tomography (OCT). Abu El-Asrar et al.[54] reported the presence of multiple exudative retinal detachments and areas of hyperreflectivity at the level of the retinal pigment epithelium (RPE). Early in the course of the disease, multiple progressive pinpoint leaks that evolve into pooling in areas of serous detachment are observed. Mild to moderate optic nerve leakage may be present. Patchy filling of choroid can also be seen.[55] Fluorescein angiographic findings in SO can be very similar to those in VKH syndrome. Although Spitznas thought that the retinal vasculature was not involved, retinal vasculitis (late staining or leakage) can rarely be seen in SO.[56,57] During the cicatricial phase, there is a coarsening of the pigment pattern in the fundus. The areas that are believed to correspond to Dalen-Fuchs nodules will, in the later stages of the disease, become atrophic and appear on the angiogram as window defects.

SO has been studied by using indocyanine green (ICG) angiography.[58] In the active stage, multiple hypocyanescent spots that

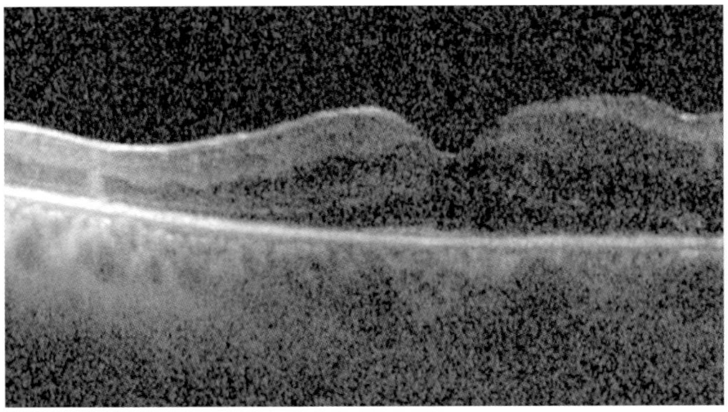

Fig. 24.4 Spectral domain optical coherence tomography (SD-OCT) shows significant disruption and loss of outer retinal structures and the presence of intraretinal fluid.

correspond to hyperfluorescent areas on fluorescein angiography are believed to represent focal choroidal inflammatory infiltrates (see Fig. 24.3).[55,59,60] Notably, these hypocyanescent spots diminish or resolve with successful corticosteroid therapy.[61] Two patterns of fluorescence have been observed. The first is a pattern of hypofluorescence in the intermediate phase of angiography, followed by a fading; and the second is a hypofluorescent pattern that persists throughout the course of the study. The first is interpreted as showing active lesions, whereas the persistent pattern is that of a cicatricial or atrophic lesion. Saatci et al.[62] used ICG angiography to monitor the therapeutic response of a patient with SO that developed after perforation of the anterior staphyloma. During active disease, there were multiple hyperfluorescent dots that coalesced; with adequate therapy, minimal residual dots were noted.[62]

Spectral domain (SD) and enhanced depth OCT can be helpful in identifying shallow serous detachments and choroidal thickening. Vascular lacunae normally present in the Sattler and Haller layers may not be visualized in SO. Dalen-Fuchs nodules may appear as small hyperreflective RPE detachments with disruption of the inner segment–outer segment junction on SD-OCT, which may resolve with treatment (Fig. 24.4).[55,63]

As might be expected, findings on both electroretinography and electrooculography can be affected by the disease. Dreyer et al.[64] observed changes in the photopic cone b-wave amplitudes and scotopic rod b-wave amplitudes during acute disease, with improvement in these functions after successful therapy. Visual fields can also be affected significantly (see Fig. 24.3H).

The immunogenetics of the disease has been studied and appears to be identical to those of VKH syndrome. In a small series of patients with SO, Davis et al.[65] reported human leukocyte antigen (HLA) typing results that appeared to be the same as those in the larger VKH syndrome group. The haplotypes HLA-DR4, DRw53, and DQw3 were found more often in both groups than in control subjects. Further work using high-resolution deoxyribonucleic acid (DNA)–based HLA typing has been done. In a study reported by Kilmartin et al.,[66] the highest relative risk was found for the haplotype HLA-DRB1*0404-DQA1*0301. Patients with that haplotype were more prone to SO developing earlier and needed more immunosuppressive therapy to control the disease. It is significant that this association appears to be the same in both Japanese patients[67] and those of European origin. Further research suggests that there was a significant association between the interleukin (IL)-10–1082 single-nucleotide polymorphism (SNP) and disease recurrence, whereas the GCC IL-10 promoter haplotype (IL-10–1082G, –819C, and –592C) was seen to be protective against disease recurrence.[68] Of interest, yet another SNP of IL-10 (–1082A) was found to be associated with unremitting SO.[69]

The histologic features of SO, which are rather distinctive, were first described by Fuchs in 1905.[4] In full-blown SO, the choroid is markedly thickened by a sea of lymphocytes, with a granulomatous nonnecrotizing reaction as the predominant feature (Fig. 24.5). In general, the choriocapillaris tends to be spared, although this is not always the case. The infiltrate in the choroid can also have large numbers of eosinophils. Although plasma cell infiltration into the choroid was not thought to be a part of the disease, these cells were noted in 85.7% of the cases reviewed by Lubin et al.[6] Marak et al.[70] reported the presence of more choroidal granulomas and eosinophils in African Americans than in whites, but no differences have been noted between patients in China and those in the United States.[71] As already noted, retinal changes are not rare. Croxato et al.[72] described retinal detachment and retinal perivasculitis in 50% of the 100 eyes with SO they examined, whereas 18% had mild inflammatory infiltrates into the retina.

Dalen-Fuchs Nodules

A typical, but by no means pathognomonic, finding in SO is Dalen-Fuchs nodules (see Fig. 24.5), which occur in about one-third of eyes with SO.[2,6] On fluorescein angiography, the lesion may block early (i.e., become hypofluorescent) and then stain late (i.e., hyperfluorescence).[73] As the lesions mature, with ultimate disruption of the RPE and probably a decrease in the inflammatory process, these lesions may simply appear as window defects. These lesions were thought by Fuchs[4] to represent RPE cells that had migrated and transformed. Although early Dalen-Fuchs nodules may represent such a phenomenon,[74] Jakobeic et al.[75] and Chan et al.[76,77] used monoclonal antibodies and structural analysis to demonstrate that Dalen-Fuchs nodules were made up of a mixture of Ia+, OKM1+ cells (presumably histiocytes), and depigmented RPE cells, which were Ia– and OKM1–. These authors' conclusions, which were similar for the epithelioid cells seen in the choroid itself, were corroborated by Rao et al.[78] The subsets of infiltrating lymphocytes into the choroid have been identified with the use of immunohistochemical techniques. Jakobeic et al.[75] noted that the predominant T cell was of the CD8+ subset (suppressor/cytotoxic cell) in the choroid of an eye removed 1.5 years after the initial surgical trauma. Chan et al.[79] evaluated an eye enucleated to treat SO only a few months after the initial nonsurgical trauma and found that the predominant T cell was the CD4 (Leu-3a) subset, the helper/inducer subset. The sympathizing eye of the same patient was eventually studied,[79] and in this eye, the predominant T-cell subset had changed to the suppressor/cytotoxic (CD8+) subset, as had been seen in the study by Jakobeic et al.[75] The interpretation of these observations is that the human eye's inflammatory response in this disease parallels that seen in the experimentally induced uveitis model in lower mammals (see Chapter 1)—that is, there is a dynamic, changing cellular immune response initiated by helper T cells. As the disease progresses, the body attempts to downregulate the immune response, and this is done by an influx of large numbers of the suppressor subset of T cells. Others have emphasized the presence of B cells in the infiltrate, found in more chronic conditions.

Chemokines that have been found in SO include matrix metalloproteinase-9, stromal cell–derived factor-1, and monocytic chemotactic protein-1.[80] This is not surprising because all these chemokines are found in the context of an inflammatory response.

Preservation of the Choriocapillaris

One of the classic findings in both SO and VKH syndrome is the preservation of the choriocapillaris. This is seen even when the choroid is filled with inflammatory cells. It has been suggested that the RPE can play both a proinflammatory role and an anti-inflammatory role in the eye.[81] Although RPE cells in culture may generate proinflammatory cytokines, such as IL-1 and IL-6, they may suppress the inflammatory response by releasing factors such as RPE-protective protein, which is believed to suppress neutrophil superoxide generation.[82,83]

The foregoing scenario, however, may not explain all cases. Several authors[72,77,84,85] have stressed the fact that the classic findings outlined represent one point in the spectrum in the disease recognized clinically as SO. An immunohistochemical study was completed in 29 patients with SO.[86] In 20 eyes, T cells predominated in the choroidal infiltration, whereas in four eyes, all from male patients, B cells were predominantly found. The presence of B cells correlated with long-term disease (> 9 months) and phthisical changes. It has classically been taught that the presence of B cells in the choroid of an eye with SO is extremely rare. The authors of this study suggested that these findings may reflect a secondary pathologic process. They further speculated on these findings from a therapeutic point of view. It could be argued that in light of these observations, cytotoxic agents, rather than the more T cell–specific drugs, such as cyclosporin, tacrolimus (FK506), or perhaps daclizumab, may be a more logical choice for patients whose disease does not respond to steroid therapy.

There is no established and accepted laboratory test for SO. Sen et al.[87] measured the level of serum β_2-microglobulin levels in the

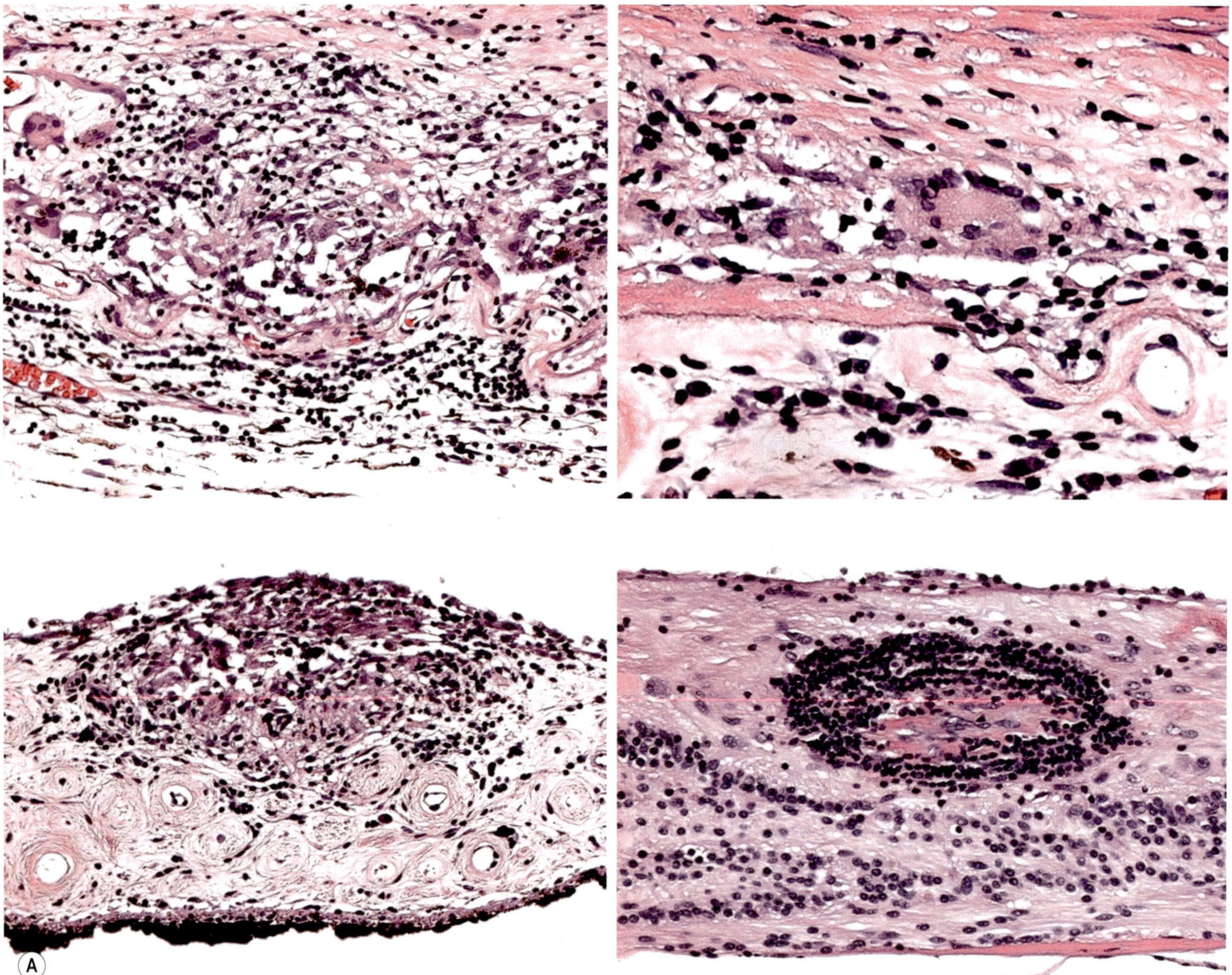

Fig. 24.5 Hematoxylin and eosin (H&E) staining of the iris, retina, and choroid of an enucleated inciting eye (A). The upper left shows granulomatous inflammation, with many giant cells in the choroid; the upper right shows a large giant cell in the retina, loss of RPE, Bruch membrane with remaining RPE pigments, and the choroid with mild chronic inflammation. The lower left taken from the iris shows a granuloma; the lower right taken from the retina shows vascular inflammation with mainly lymphocytes.

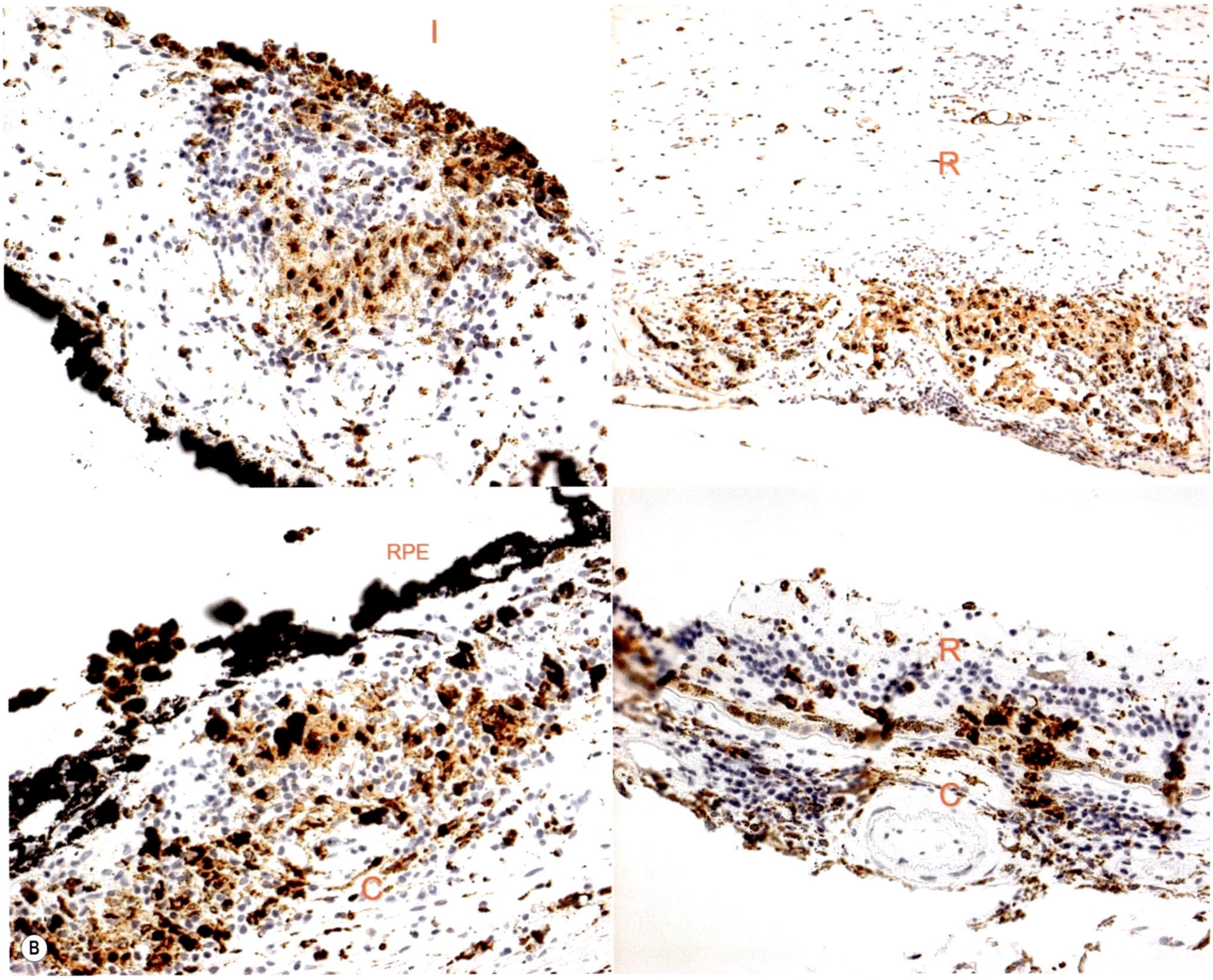

Fig. 24.5, cont'd CD68 staining (B) shows macrophage infiltration in the iris (I), retina (R), and choroid (C) showing both well-formed and ill-formed granulomas in the uvea. (Courtesy Chi Chao Chan, MD, National Eye Institute) (Case 24.2).

blood of patients with SO. They found the levels to be high in these patients compared with those with traumatic uveitis and control subjects. The levels appeared to be higher in the initial stages and reflected the severity of the disease. These results need to be corroborated. Immunohistochemistry performed on eight eyes with SO showed an increased expression of tumor necrosis factor (TNF)-α in the photoreceptor layer, whereas inducible nitric oxide synthase (iNOS) was found in the mitochondria, suggesting that photoreceptor oxidative stress occurs in the absence of leukocyte infiltrate and that this may lead to vison loss.[88] Chan et al. showed the presence of IL-17 in the macrophages and granuloma of eyes with SO. This is in agreement with the concept that IL-17 is a major player in propagating chronic inflammatory disease.[89]

Sympathetic Ophthalmia and Vogt-Koyanagi-Harada Syndrome

The question is whether SO can be distinguished histologically from VKH syndrome because they may be the same entity from an immunogenetic perspective. It would appear that both represent a spectrum of very similar inflammatory responses.[7] It is thought that "classic" SO neither involves the choriocapillaris nor has chorioretinal scarring, and both these are common in VKH syndrome. Although these changes can be seen in sympathetic ophthalmia,[5] they probably occur in fewer patients. In addition, the lack of chorioretinal scarring and obliteration of the choriocapillaris in eyes with SO (a phenomenon seen late) may reflect the fact that eyes with SO are usually removed early in the course of the inflammatory disease. In contrast, eyes with VKH syndrome that have been studied were removed late in the course of the disease. Is the inflammatory response seen in SO unique to this entity? Chan et al.[77] evaluated the cellular composition of the granulomas of SO and sarcoidosis. Most of the cells within the lesions were found to be identical and were mainly cells from bone-derived monocytes (Table 24.2). It has been suggested that in sarcoidosis, Dalen-Fuchs nodules are larger. A complicating factor is the presence of phacoanaphylaxis. Easom and Zimmerman[39] reported cases in which the clinical diagnosis in the exciting eye was thought to be SO, but histologic confirmation could not be obtained; the so-called sympathizing eye showed evidence only of phacoanaphylaxis, rather than the alterations typical of the suspected disorder. Although it is not always true, de

TABLE 24.2 Sympathetic Ophthalmia versus Sarcoidosis

Disease	Uveitis	Dalen-Fuchs Nodules	Other		
HISTOPATHOLOGY					
Sarcoidosis	Focal or diffuse granulomatous	Some larger	"Snowbanking" conjunctival and iris nodules		
Sympathetic ophthalmia	Diffuse granulomatous	Many	Sparing of choriocapillaris; retina may not be involved		
Disease	T cells	T helper cells	T suppressor cells	B cells	Macrophages
IMMUNOPATHOLOGY					
Sarcoidosis	Majority	Many	Some	A few	In granuloma and Dalen-Fuchs nodules
Sympathetic ophthalmia	Majority	Early—more; late—less	Early—less; late—more	Some	In granuloma and Dalen-Fuchs nodules

Veer[33] emphasized that in phacoanaphylaxis, disease in the first eye involved has already become quiescent by the time the second eye is involved. This is in contrast to SO, in which both eyes are inflamed at the same time. A history of penetrating trauma is imperative. If this is not available or if it is not clear whether ocular penetration occurred, then the diagnosis becomes even more difficult. VKH syndrome and sarcoidosis perhaps most resemble the disorder, but the diagnosis of localized posterior segment disorders, such as APMPPE (see Chapter 30), must also be considered.

The concept that an autoimmune inflammatory response is the basis of SO is not new, having been proposed by Elschnig in 1910.[90] For many years, the notion was that uveal pigment was the antigenic stimulus for this disease. A report by Woods[91] in 1921 outlined the interesting observation that patients who had sustained ocular trauma without resultant SO had circulating antibodies to uveal pigment, but that in all patients with SO, circulating antibodies were absent. Furthermore, in one of these latter type of patients, a cellular immune response to uveal pigment was seen, as measured with an intradermal skin test. These observations are striking, considering our knowledge of the predominant T-cell response in the eye. In vitro cell-culturing techniques have been used to evaluate cell-mediated anamnestic responses of lymphocytes from patients with SO, and in these patients, a positive response to uveal or uveoretinal preparations was seen.[92,93]

Of interest were the observations of Marak et al.[94] that blastogenic activity of lymphocytes from a small group of patients with SO could be elicited only with RPE and retinal antigens, but not with antigens from the choroid. De Smet et al.[95] tested two patient populations, one from the NEI's clinic and the other from a uveitis clinic in Japan. Patients with SO were tested for their cellular immune response to both S-antigen (S-Ag) and interphotoreceptor retinoid-binding protein (IRBP). These patients' lymphocytes were found to respond to several autoantigens and to several fragments. Chan et al.,[96] using enzyme-linked immunosorbent assay (ELISA), found no circulating antiretinal S-Ag antibodies. However, when serum from patients with SO was placed over normal human retinal tissue, a few showed antiretinal antibodies directed against the outer segments of the photoreceptors and against Müller cells. However, the titers of the antiretinal antibodies and the number of patients with these circulating antibodies were considerably higher in the VKH syndrome group than in the SO group. An association between HLA-A11 and SO has been suggested by Reynard et al.[97] However, this study reported the results in a multiethnic and multiracial population, making the validity of the results difficult to evaluate. As mentioned before, Davis et al.[65] found a strong association between the HLA-DR4, DRw53, and Bw54 haplotypes and both VKH syndrome and SO, but the small number of patients in the latter group precluded statistical analysis.

No exact experimental model for SO exists. The induction of uveitis with the ocular antigens IRBP and S-Ag will produce in monkeys and mice a disease with many of the characteristics of SO, including Dalen-Fuchs nodules (see Fig. 24.5). However, although there may some choroidal involvement, the disease induced in these animals is essentially retinal in nature. Another important factor in the development of the human disorder is the fact that penetrating trauma may lead to the development of intraocular lymphatics and the presentation of ocular antigens to the systemic immune system in an unusual manner.[85]

Is it then possible to develop a working hypothesis to explain the development of SO? The dominant T-cell response certainly seems clear. But what of the precipitating factors leading to the disease? The possibility of an autoimmune role still seems quite attractive, based on the type of disease that is induced with retinal antigens in the monkey model. It is possible to hypothesize that the perforating injury permits several events to take place. The first is that drainage of antigen from the eye can occur via the lymphatics, an event that does not occur under normal conditions. The second is that small amounts of adjuvant, such as bacterial cell wall or other immunostimulators, might now enter the eye. These products may come from already killed bacteria on the skin (e.g., *Propionibacterium acnes*), and therefore active proliferation of the organism is not significant to the hypothesis. Rather, these products may profoundly "upgrade" the local immune response, causing it to bypass certain inherent suppressor mechanisms in genetically prone persons. This then leads to the inflammatory kinetic process that we ultimately recognize as SO.

THERAPY

Enucleation of an injured eye before the sympathizing eye becomes involved is the only known way to prevent SO. Enucleation has traditionally been thought to have no effect on the course of the sympathizing eye once the disease has begun. However, on rare occasions, this may not be true. Bellan[98] reported the case of a patient who suffered penetrating trauma to one eye and underwent enucleation of the nonseeing eye 5 days after his injury. At the time of enucleation, his remaining eye was reported to be normal. Three months later, presumed SO developed in his remaining eye (although it was not histologically proven). Indeed, experience in the era before steroids suggested that enucleation did not help improve the patient's ultimate visual outcome.[99] However, a review by Lubin et al.[6] suggested that enucleation within 2 weeks of the initiation of the inflammatory response may beneficially affect the visual outcome of the remaining eye. Reynard et al.,[100] in their retrospective clinicopathologic study, also noted that enucleation within 2 weeks of the beginning of symptoms resulted in a fairly benign course. However, in a retrospective study by Chan et al.[17] and a prospective study reported by Kilmartin et al.,[12] enucleation was not seen to correlate with a better visual outcome. Indeed, in our experience, it appears that adequate and rapid immunosuppressive therapy was the most important factor in achieving good vision. Bellan[98] questioned the need for prophylactic enucleation, given the high treatment-to-benefit ratio in this disorder.[98] Therefore, we would hesitate to suggest early enucleation of an eye with any prognosis for useful vision. It is possible that the exciting eye's visual acuity could be superior to that obtained in the sympathizing eye. Brackup et al.[101] evaluated 50 eyes that had global rupture and were not removed within 2 weeks of injury and did not have visual acuity of no better than hand motion. Seventeen of the eyes were later removed, nine of them because of pain. The other 33 eyes were not removed and remained comfortable for a mean follow-up period of 66 months. Of interest was the fact that there were no cases of SO. An interesting point was raised by Hollander et al.[102]: In their discussion of penetrating injuries to an already blind eye, they suggested that enucleation, instead of a primary repair, could have a role. Determining when to treat a patient with SO with immunosuppressive therapy usually is not problematic. At initial presentation, the patient is seen to have marked, bilateral inflammation and a decrease in vision. On rare occasions, although an inflammatory response can be observed, the patient's vision remains good, and the practitioner may need to use other parameters, such as changing visual fields, to decide whether a therapeutic intervention is indicated.

There is an ongoing debate regarding the need to choose evisceration or enucleation. Many have claimed that evisceration carries a risk for the development of SO. Du Toit et al.[103] reviewed the cases of 1392 patients with penetrating eye trauma at the Groote Schuur Hospital in South Africa: 491 (35.5%) had primary evisceration, and no cases of SO were seen in this group. However, in rare cases, SO can occur after this procedure, as in the case of the patient from the Iraq conflict who underwent evisceration.[16]

Corticosteroids

If the decision has been made to intervene with anti-inflammatory therapy, the initial approach, in most cases, should be the use of systemic corticosteroids. They should be given at a dose of at least 1 to 1.5 mg/kg of prednisone or equivalent on a daily basis. Some practitioners recommend even higher doses, from 100 to 200 mg/day of prednisone.[5] To deal with a particularly severe inflammatory process, intravenous pulse steroid therapy can be employed,[104] but this needs to be invariably followed by daily administration of immunosuppressive agents. The practitioner must set both clinical guidelines and a time frame in which to see the patient. Usually, 3 months may be a reasonable time frame in which to evaluate whether a therapeutic approach has worked. More frequently, a second immunosuppressive agent is added at the time or soon after the oral prednisone is begun. At 3 months, a slow taper of the steroid should definitely be initiated. In the long-term follow-up (average 10.6 years) of patients with SO treated with steroids, Makley and Azar[105] noted that 65% of eyes had 20/60 or better visual acuity. Relapses were common, and secondary glaucoma, cataract, retinal detachment, and choroidal scarring were noted as sequelae. Reynard et al.[100] also found that corticosteroid therapy was associated with a good visual outcome. Jonas and Spandau[106] reported giving repeated intravitreal triamcinolone acetonide injections to a patient with SO. This approach is problematic because of complications secondary to steroid injection, lack of treatment of the other eye, and the fact that this cannot be a long-term strategy, which is what is needed for these patients. Mahajan et al. also reported eight cases of SO treated with fluocinolone acetonide intravitreal implant (Retisert). In all eight patients, concomitant systemic immunosuppressives could be reduced, with control of inflammation and maintenance or improvement of vision; two patients had recurrence and required the addition of a systemic immunosuppressive.[107]

Galor et al. found that 79% of their patients were treated with corticosteroids and 43% with immunomodulatory therapy, which included antimetabolites (methotrexate, azathioprine, mycophenolate mofetil), cyclosporine, alkylating agents, and infliximab. Time to disease inactivity was shorter, and the likelihood of inactive disease was significantly higher (11-fold) among those started on systemic prednisone.[26] In another large multicenter retrospective study (N = 130) by Tan et al. systemic steroids were used in almost all patients (97%), and 70.7% required additional immunosuppressive therapy.[27]

In some patients, however, the disease will not remain quiescent with prednisone dosage reduction. One should try to avoid higher doses of oral prednisone (>15 mg daily) beyond 3 months. If it is clear that a lower dose of steroid is not a reasonable goal and a second agent was not added at the start of therapy, another agent in addition to the steroid and even a third should be started. Spitznas[53] found that transitory hyperopia was an indicator of disease activity, and Schaelgel[108] suggested that the degree of papillitis is also an excellent indicator of activity. Imaging studies, such as SD-OCT (showing thickened choroid), fluorescein angiography (showing disk leakage), and ICG angiography (showing increasing choroidal lesions), can also help guide treatment.[109] OCT angiography can also be helpful in monitoring the response of choriocapillaris flow voids to treatment.[110] Hyperreflective changes at the level of the RPE, corresponding to Dalen-Fuchs nodules in the active stage, may or may not resolve with treatment.[63,111]

The International Uveitis Study Group suggested that cytotoxic agents may be appropriate for patients with steroid-resistant SO, but this was before the advent of many of the biologics, which have made this approach less popular. Tessler and Jennings[112] suggested a high-dose short-term approach with chlorambucil, an alkylating agent. All five patients with SO experienced sustained remission after an average therapy duration of 11 weeks and a total average dosage of 0.9 g. In the relatively short follow-up period (mean 4.5 years), no malignant processes occurred.

Immunosuppressive Agents

We have used cyclosporin as a second-line drug in the treatment of SO—that is, after corticosteroids but before cytotoxic agents. Typically, it would be used in patients whose disease responds to steroid therapy but in whom the maintenance dosage needed to maintain remission is quite high; those who need extended therapy (most do); or patients who cannot tolerate steroids (see Case 24.1). Generally, the inflammatory response appears to respond well to cyclosporin (see guidelines for therapy in Chapter 8). Kilmartin et al.[113] reported the case of a 3-year-old child with active refractory SO whose choroidal neovascular membrane resolved with cyclosporin therapy. On the basis of the immunohistochemical studies mentioned earlier[86] showing the presence of B cells in some patients with long-term disease, one could argue for the initial use of cytotoxic agents. However, cyclosporin is preferable because most of the specimens examined show predominance of T cells; patients have responded well to the steroid/cyclosporin regimen; and the potential for long-term side effects is arguably less with cyclosporin than with cytotoxic agents. An overall review of 32 patients at the NEI showed that 16 had a final visual acuity of 20/40 or better in at least one eye. A good visual outcome was associated with early aggressive immunotherapy. A poor visual outcome was associated with glaucoma, macular scarring, and persistent inflammation.[17]

In the series by Hakin et al.,[18] 18 patients with SO were treated with azathioprine or cyclosporin, or both were used in addition to steroids. Ten of the 18 patients had a visual acuity of 6/9 or better in their sympathizing eye. A poor visual outcome resulted from cystoid macular edema and lens opacities, and six patients needed antiglaucoma drugs during the course of their therapy.

In patients with difficult-to-control disease, triple immunosuppressive therapy can be considered, such as cyclosporin, an oral corticosteroid, and another nonbiologic immunosuppressive agent or a biologic. With the introduction of biologics, cytotoxic agents are rarely used or are used as a last resort; if they are used, it is imperative that they be used before irreversible changes in the eye occur.

Reports seem to indicate good results with the aggressive use of immunosuppressive agents. Gupta et al.[56] reviewed 40 cases between 1989 and 2000 and found that patients treated early tended to present early on with posterior segment findings and did better in the long term. A systematic review of the literature found that 95% of patients were treated with systemic corticosteroids and 75% received systemic immunomodulatory therapy; 70% of these patients experienced an improvement in their visual acuity.[19] Several cases of SO refractory to standard immunosuppressives were also successfully treated with the TNF inhibitors infliximab or adalimumab.[114-117] Payal and Foster reported drug-free remission for longer than 1 year in 5 of their 19 patients with SO after treatment with various biologic or nonbiologic immunosuppressives.[117] Tan et al.[27] reviewed 130 patients from three countries—the United Kingdom, Singapore, and India—and found that azathioprine and mycophenolate were the most commonly used first-line steroid-sparing agents; the biologics cyclophosphamide and tacrolimus were used infrequently. Only 14% required two or more immunosuppressives. Visual acuity improved in the majority of patients (80.8%). Younger age, Asian ethnicity, and lower visual acuity at presentation were associated with improvement in the visual acuity of the sympathizing eye. In this study, the authors also noted that patients from India were more likely to have used or needed steroid-sparing immunosuppressive therapy compared with those from the United Kingdom or Singapore.[27] Enucleation was done in 28% in this cohort, and no association between enucleation and visual outcomes were found.

Surgery will frequently be needed for eyes with SO. Probably most commonly performed surgery is for either glaucoma or cataract. Adequate immunosuppressive therapy is mandatory. It is important to ensure that the inflammatory process is controlled with medication and to wait as long as possible, ideally at least 3 months, before surgical intervention. DeAngelis et al.[118] reported performing cataract extraction by using phacoemulsification in a sympathizing eye and achieving a good result; and subsequently, a foldable lens was used. Ganesh et al.[119] reported the results of cataract extractions in 17 sympathizing eyes and one exciting eye. Three eyes had extracapsular cataract extractions followed by intraocular lens (IOL) placement; six eyes had the same procedure without IOL placement; and nine had phacoemulsification and IOL placement. The eyes endured the procedures reasonably well, and poor vision was often attributed to disruption of the posterior pole architecture. Photodynamic therapy has been used to treat choroidal neovascularization in a sympathizing eye with stabilization of the visual acuity.[120] Bom et al.[121-123] opted to remove a subfoveal choroidal neovascular membrane surgically, and this resulted in modest improvement in visual acuity and a diminution of visual distortions. Although successful in this case, this approach needs to be considered with great caution because it could cause adhesion of the membrane to the RPE or the retina, resulting in severe central vision impairment.

CASE 24.1

A 62-year-old man suffered a hunting injury that caused a bilateral inflammatory response several months after the trauma. Enucleation of the exciting eye demonstrated histologic alterations typical of SO. The patient's vision in the sympathizing eye was 20/200. His inflammatory disease responded to high-dose prednisone (80 mg/day), but he could not continue with this regimen because of side effects. At lower doses of prednisone, the disease recurred. A regimen of cyclosporin as the sole therapeutic agent was begun, and vision improved to 20/40. There was a slow reduction in the vision in the patient's eye because of a cataract. The patient underwent cataract extraction, and his vision stabilized at about 20/30. He had no major recurrence of his disease while receiving cyclosporin therapy. However, hypertension and renal toxicity developed as a result of the cyclosporin therapy.

CASE 24.2

A 70-year-old woman presented with panuveitis, which had developed in both eyes 4 months after retinal detachment surgery, vitrectomy, and scleral buckle in the left eye. The left eye, which had no light perception (NLP) vision, was eventually enucleated 1 month after the onset of panuveitis, before her visit to our center. At initial presentation, vision in the right eye was 20/40, and retinal examination showed multiple hypopigmented choroidal lesions and vitritis (see Fig. 24.2). The pathology slides were re-examined at the National Institutes of Health (NIH) for confirmation and showed ill-formed and well-formed granulomas in the iris and the choroid (see Fig. 24.5). The patient was successfully treated with prednisone taper and antimetabolites.

REFERENCES

1. Zegers RH. The eyes of Johann Sebastian Bach. *Arch Ophthalmol.* 2005;123(10):1427–1430.
2. MacKenzie W. *A Practical Treatise on Disease of the Eye*. London: Longmans; 1830.
3. Albert D, Diaz-Rohena R. A historical review of sympathetic ophthalmia and its epidemiology. *Surv Ophthalmol.* 1989;34:1–14.
4. Fuchs E. Über sympathislerende Entzündung zuerst Bemerkungeen über seröse traumatische Iritis. *Albrect Von Graefes Arch Ophthalmol.* 1905;61:365–456.
5. Marak GJ. Recent advances in sympathetic ophthalmia. *Surv Ophthalmol.* 1979;24:141–156.
6. Lubin J, Albert D, Weinstein M. Sixty-five years of sympathetic ophthalmia. A clinicopathologic review of 105 cases (1913–1978). *Ophthalmology.* 1980;87:109–121.
7. Goto H, Rao N. Sympathetic ophthalmia and Vogt-Koyanagi-Harada syndrome. *Int Ophthalmol Clin.* 1990;30:279–285.
8. Liddy N, Stuart J. Sympathetic ophthalmia in Canada. *Can J Ophthalmol.* 1972;7:157–159.
9. Holland G. About the indication and time for surgical removal of an injured eye. *Klin Monatsbl Augenheilkd.* 1964;145:732–740.
10. Gass J. Sympathetic ophthalmia following vitrectomy. *Am J Ophthalmol.* 1982;93:552–558.
11. Kilmartin D, Dick A, Forrester J. Commentary. Sympathetic ophthalmia risk following vitrectomy: should we counsel patients? *Br J Ophthalmol.* 2000;84:448–449.
12. Kilmartin D, Dick A, Forrester J. Prospective surveillance of sympathetic ophthalmia in the UK and Republic of Ireland. *Br J Ophthalmol.* 2000;84:259–263.
13. Su DH, Chee SP. Sympathetic ophthalmia in Singapore: new trends in an old disease. *Graefes Arch Clin Exp Ophthalmol.* 2006;244(2):243–247.
14. Vote BJ, Hall A, Cairns J, et al. Changing trends in sympathetic ophthalmia. *Clin Exp Ophthalmol.* 2004;32(5):542–545.
15. Hoefle F. Initial treatment of eye injuries. *Arch Ophthalmol.* 1968;79: 33–35.

16. Freidlin J, Pak J, Tessler HH, et al. Sympathetic ophthalmia after injury in the Iraq war. *Ophthalm Plast Reconstruct Surg*. 2006;22(2):133–134.
17. Chan C, Roberge RG, Whitcup SM, et al. Thirty two cases of sympathetic ophthalmia examined at the National Eye Institute. A retrospective study at the National Eye Institute, Bethesda, MD, from 1982 to 1992. *Arch Ophthalmol*. 1995;113:597–600.
18. Hakin K, Pearson R, Lightman S. Sympathetic ophthalmia: visual results with modern immunosuppressive therapy. *Eye*. 1992;6:453–455.
19. Castiblanco CP, Adelman RA. Sympathetic ophthalmia. *Graefes Arch Clin Exp Ophthalmol*. 2009;247(3):289–302.
20. Tyagi M, Agarwal K, Reddy Pappuru RR, et al. Sympathetic ophthalmia after vitreoretinal surgeries: incidence, clinical presentations and outcomes of a rare disease. *Semin Ophthalmol*. 2019;34(3):157–162.
21. Pollack A, McDonald HR, Ai E, et al. Sympathetic ophthalmia associated with pars plana vitrectomy without antecedent penetrating trauma. *Retina*. 2001;21:146–154.
22. Smith R, Webb R, van Heusen W. Sympathetic ophthalmia as a complication of pars plana vitrectomy. *Perspect Ophthalmol*. 1978;2:117–120.
23. Green W, Maumenee A, Sanders T. Sympathetic uveitis following evisceration. *Trans Am Acad Ophthalmol Otolaryngol*. 1972;76:625–644.
24. Awan K. Sympathetic uveitis in intraocular implant surgery. *J Ocul Ther Surg*. 1984;3:134–135.
25. Carney M, Tessler HH, Peyman GA, et al. Sympathetic ophthalmia and subretinal neovascularization. *Ann Ophthalmol*. 1990;22:184–186.
26. Galor A, Davis JL, Flynn HW Jr, et al. Sympathetic ophthalmia: incidence of ocular complications and vision loss in the sympathizing eye. *Am J Ophthalmol*. 2009;148(5):704–710.e2.
27. Tan XL, Seen S, Dutta Majumder P, et al. Analysis of 130 cases of sympathetic ophthalmia—a retrospective multicenter case series. *Ocul Immunol Inflamm*. 2019;27(8):1259–1266.
28. Kumar K, Mathai A, Murthy SI, et al. Sympathetic ophthalmia in pediatric age group: clinical features and challenges in management in a tertiary center in southern India. *Ocul Immunol Inflamm*. 2014;22(5):367–372.
29. Comer M, Taylor C, Chen S, et al. Sympathetic ophthalmia associated with high frequency deafness. *Br J Ophthalmol*. 2001;85:496–503.
30. Lewis M, Gass J, Spencer W. Sympathetic uveitis after trauma and vitrectomy. *Arch Ophthalmol*. 1978;96:263–267.
31. Lim WK, Chee SP, Sng I, et al. Immunopathology of progressive subretinal fibrosis: a variant of sympathetic ophthalmia. *Am J Ophthalmol*. 2004;138(3):475–477.
32. Wang RC, Zamir E, Dugel PU, et al. Progressive subretinal fibrosis and blindness associated with multifocal granulomatous chorioretinitis: a variant of sympathetic ophthalmia. *Ophthalmology*. 2002;109(8):1527–1531.
33. de Veer J. Bilateral endophthalmitis phacoanaphylactica. *Arch Ophthalmol*. 1953;49:607–632.
34. Blodi F. Sympathetic uveitis as an allergic phenomenon. *Trans Am Acad Ophthalmol Otolaryngol*. 1959;63:642–649.
35. Allen J. Sympathetic uveitis and phacoanaphylaxis. *Am J Ophthalmol*. 1967;63:280–283.
36. Romaine H. Malignant melanoma of the choroid with sympathetic ophthalmia. *Arch Ophthalmol*. 1949;42:102–103.
37. Melanowski W. Contribution to the pathogenesis of sympathetic ophthalmia: a case of sympathetic ophthalmia due to intraocular melanosarcoma. *Klin Monatsbl Augenheilkd*. 1936;97:52–59.
38. Garcia-Arumi J, Gil MM, Palau MM, et al. Sympathetic ophthalmia after surgical resection of iridociliary melanoma. A case report. *Graefes Arch Clin Exp Ophthalmol*. 2006;244:1353–1356.
39. Easom H, Zimmerman L. Sympathetic ophthalmia and bilateral phacoanaphylaxis. A clinicopathologic correlation of the sympathogenic and sympathizing eyes. *Arch Ophthalmol*. 1964;72:9–15.
40. Fries P, Char DH, Crawford JB, et al. Sympathetic ophthalmia complicating helium ion irradiation of a choroidal melanoma. *Arch Ophthalmol*. 1987;105:1561–1564.
41. Margo C, Pautler S. Granulomatous uveitis after treatment of a choroidal melanoma with proton-beam irradiation. *Retina*. 1990;10:140–143.
42. Sabates R. Choroiditis compatible with the histopathological diagnosis of sympathetic ophthalmia following cyclocryotherapy of neovascular glaucoma. *Ophthalmic Surg*. 1988;19:176–182.
43. Harrison T. Sympathetic ophthalmia after cyclocryotherapy of neovascular glaucoma without ocular penetration. *Ophthalmic Surg*. 1993;24:44–46.
44. Biswas J, Fogla R. Sympathetic ophthalmia following cyclocryotherapy with histopathologic correlation. *Ophthalmic Surg Lasers*. 1996;27:1035–1038.
45. Edward D, Brown SV, Higginbotham E, et al. Sympathetic ophthalmia following neodymium:YAG cyclotherapy. *Ophthalmic Surg*. 1989;20:544–546.
46. Lam S, Tessler HH, Lam BL, et al. High incidence of sympathetic ophthalmia after contact and non-contact neodymium:YAG cyclotherapy. *Ophthalmology*. 1992;99:1818–1822.
47. Tessler H, Lam S, Wilensky J, et al. Sympathetic ophthalmia after non-contact neodymium:YAG cyclotherapy. In: Dernouchamps J, et al., ed. *Recent Advances in Uveitis: Proceeding of the Third International Symposium on Uveitis*. Amsterdam: Kugler Publications; 1993:201–202.
48. Bakri SJ, Peters GB 3rd. Sympathetic ophthalmia after a hyphema due to nonpenetrating trauma. *Ocul Immunol Inflamm*. 2005;13(1):85–86.
49. Glavici M. Sympathetic ophthalmia after a cataract operation. *Oftalmologia*. 1992;36:397–401.
50. Lakhanpal V, Dogra M, Jacobson M. Sympathetic ophthalmia associated with anterior chamber intraocular lens implantation. *Ann Ophthalmol*. 1991;23:139–143.
51. Abu El-Asrar A, Al-Obeidan S. Sympathetic ophthalmia after complicated cataract surgery and intraocular lens implantation. *Eur J Ophthalmol*. 2001;11:193–196.
52. Sampangi R, Venkatesh P, Mandal S, et al. Recurrent neovascularization of the disc in sympathetic ophthalmia. *Indian J Ophthalmol*. 2008;56(3):237–239.
53. Spitznas M. Fluorescein angiography of sympathetic ophthalmia. *Klin Monatsbl Augenheilkd*. 1976;169:195–200.
54. Abu El-Asrar AM, Al Kuraya H, Al-Ghamdi A. Sympathetic ophthalmia after successful retinal reattachment surgery with vitrectomy. *Eur J Ophthalmol*. 2006;16(6):891–894.
55. Mahajan S, Invernizzi A, Agrawal R, et al. Multimodal imaging in sympathetic ophthalmia. *Ocul Immunol Inflamm*. 2017;25(2):152–159.
56. Gupta V, Gupta A, Dogra MR. Posterior sympathetic ophthalmia: a single centre long-term study of 40 patients from North India. *Eye (Lond)*. 2008;22(12):1459–1464.
57. Kadayifçilar S, Irkeç M, Eldem B. Sympathetic ophthalmia associated with ocular and cerebral vasculitis: an angiographic and radiologic study. *Eur J Ophthalmol*. 2003;13(6):584–587.
58. Bernasconi O, Auer C, Zografos L, et al. Indocyanine green angiographic findings in sympathetic ophthalmia. *Graefes Arch Clin Exp Ophthalmol*. 1998;236:635–638.
59. Kodati S, Burke S, Albini T. Indocyanine green angiography in uveitis. In: Sen HN, Read RW, eds. *Multimodal Imaging in Uveitis*. New York: Springer; 2018:25–36.
60. Casella AM, Farah ME, Martins MC, et al. Sympathetic ophthalmia—histopathological correlation with fluorescein and indocyanine green angiography: case report. *Arq Bras Oftalmol*. 2008;71:886–889.
61. Rua D, Pohlmann D, Pleyer U. Sympathetic Ophthalmia - a Contribution to Immunology, Clinic and Current Imaging. *Klin Monbl Augenheilkd*. 2020 Sep;237(9):1060–1069. English, German. https://doi.org/10.1055/a-1245-4373.
62. Saatci AO, Paşa E, Söylev MF, et al. Sympathetic ophthalmia and indocyanine green angiography. *Arch Ophthalmol*. 2004;122(10):1568–1569.
63. Muakkassa NW, Witkin AJ. Spectral-domain optical coherence tomography of sympathetic ophthalmia with Dalen-Fuchs nodules. *Ophthalmic Surg Lasers Imaging Retina*. 2014;45(6):610–612.
64. Dreyer WJ, Zegarra H, Zakov ZN, et al. Sympathetic ophthalmia. *Am J Ophthalmol*. 1981;92:816–823.
65. Davis J, Mittal KK, Freidlin V, et al. HLA associations and ancestry in Vogt–Koyanagi–Harada disease and sympathetic ophthalmia. *Ophthalmology*. 1990;97:1137–1142.
66. Kilmartin D, Wilson D, Liversidge J, et al. Immunogenetics and clinical phenotype of sympathetic ophthalmia in British and Irish patients. *Br J Ophthalmol*. 2001;85:281–286.
67. Shindo Y, Ohno S, Usui M, et al. Immunogenetic study of sympathetic ophthalmia. *Tissue Antigens*. 1997;49(2):111–115.

68. Atan D, Turner SJ, Kilmartin DJ, et al. Cytokine gene polymorphism in sympathetic ophthalmia. *Invest Ophthalmol Vis Sci.* 2005;46(11):4245–4250.
69. Glover N, Ah-Chan JJ, Frith P, et al. Unremitting sympathetic ophthalmia associated with homozygous interleukin-10–1082A single nucleotide polymorphism. *Br J Ophthalmol.* 2008;92(1):155–156.
70. Marak G, Font R, Zimmerman L. Histologic variations related to race in sympathetic ophthalmia. *Am J Ophthalmol.* 1974;78:935–938.
71. Kuo P, Lubin JR, Ni C, et al. Sympathetic ophthalmia: a comparison of the histopathological features from a Chinese and American series. *Int Ophthalmol Clin.* 1982;22:125–139.
72. Croxato J, Rao NA, McLean IW, et al. Atypical histopathologic features in sympathetic ophthalmia. A study of a hundred cases. *Int Ophthalmol.* 1981;3:129–135.
73. Allinson R, Le TD, Kramer TR, et al. Fluorescein angiographic appearance of Dalen-Fuchs nodules in sympathetic ophthalmia. *Ann Ophthalmol.* 1993;25:152–156.
74. Font R, Fine BS, Messmer E, et al. Light and electron microscopic study of Dalen-Fuchs nodules in sympathetic ophthalmia. *Ophthalmology.* 1983;90:66–75.
75. Jakobeic F, Marboe CC, Knowles DM, et al. Human sympathetic ophthalmia. An analysis of the inflammatory infiltrate by hybridoma-monoclonal antibodies, immunochemistry, and correlative electron microscopy. *Ophthalmology.* 1983;90:76–95.
76. Chan C, BenEzra D, Hsu SM, et al. Granulomas in sympathetic ophthalmia and sarcoidosis. Immunohistochemical study. *Arch Ophthalmol.* 1985;103:198–202.
77. Chan C, Nussenblatt RB, Fujikawa LS, et al. Sympathetic ophthalmia. Immunohistochemical study of epithelioid and giant cells. *Ophthalmology.* 1986;93:690–695.
78. Rao N, Xu S, Font R. Sympathetic ophthalmia. An immunohistochemical study of epithelioid and giant cells. *Ophthalmology.* 1985;92:1660–1662.
79. Chan C, Benezra D, Rodrigues MM, et al. Immunohistochemistry and electron microscopy of choroidal infiltrates and Dalen-Fuchs nodules in sympathetic ophthalmia. *Ophthalmology.* 1985;92:580–590.
80. Abu El-Asrar AM, Struyf S, Van den Broeck C, et al. Expression of chemokines and gelatinase B in sympathetic ophthalmia. *Eye.* 2007;21(5):649–657.
81. Rao N. Mechanisms of inflammatory response in sympathetic ophthalmia and VKH syndrome. *Eye.* 1997;11:213–216.
82. Wu G, Rao N. A novel retinal pigment epithelial protein suppresses neutrophil superoxide generation. I. Characterization of the suppressive factor. *Exp Eye Res.* 1996;63:713–725.
83. Wu G, Swiderek K, Rao N. A novel retinal pigment epithelial protein suppresses neutrophil superoxide generation. II. Purification and microsequencing analysis. *Exp Eye Res.* 1996;63:727–737.
84. Kaplan H, Waldrep JC, Chan WC, et al. Human sympathetic ophthalmia. Immunologic analysis of the vitreous and uvea. *Arch Ophthalmol.* 1986;104:240–244.
85. Rao N, Robin J, Hartmann D, et al. The role of the penetrating wound in the development of sympathetic ophthalmia. Experimental observations. *Arch Ophthalmol.* 1983;101:102–104.
86. Shah D, Piacentini MA, Burnier MN Jr, et al. Inflammatory cellular kinetics in sympathetic ophthalmia. A study of 29 traumatized (exciting) eyes. *Ocul Immunol Inflamm.* 1993;1:255–262.
87. Sen D, Sarin G, Mathur M. Serum beta-2 microglobulin level in sympathetic ophthalmitis. *Acta Ophthalmol (Copenh).* 1990;68:200–204.
88. Parikh JG, Saraswathy S, Rao NA. Photoreceptor oxidative damage in sympathetic ophthalmia. *Am J Ophthalmol.* 2008;146:866–875.
89. Furusato E, Shen D, Cao X, Furusato B, Nussenblatt RB, Rushing EJ, Chan CC. Inflammatory cytokine and chemokine expression in sympathetic ophthalmia: a pilot study. *Histol Histopathol.* 2011 Sep; 26(9):1145–51.
90. Elschnig A. Studies in sympathetic ophthalmia. II. The antigenic effect of eye pigments. *Albrecht von Graefes Arch Ophthalmol.* 1910;76:509–546.
91. Woods A. Immune reactions following injuries to the uveal tract. *JAMA.* 1921;77:1317–1322.
92. Wong V, Anderson R, O'Brien P. Sympathetic ophthalmia and lymphocyte transformation. *Am J Ophthalmol.* 1971;72:960–965.
93. Hammer H. Cellular hypersensitivity to uveal pigment confirmed by leucocyte migration tests in sympathetic ophthalmitis and the Vogt-Koyanagi-Harada syndrome. *Br J Ophthalmol.* 1974;58:773–776.
94. Marak GJ, Font RL, Johnson MC, et al. Lymphocyte-stimulating activity of ocular tissues in sympathetic ophthalmia. *Invest Ophthalmol Vis Sci.* 1971;10:770–774.
95. de Smet M, Yamamoto JH, Mochizuki M, et al. Cellular immune responses of patients with uveitis to retinal antigens and their fragments. *Am J Ophthalmol.* 1990;110:135–142.
96. Chan C, Palestine AG, Nussenblatt RB, et al. Anti-retinal auto-antibodies in Vogt-Koyanagi-Harada syndrome, Behçet's disease, and sympathetic ophthalmia. *Ophthalmology.* 1985;92:1025–1028.
97. Reynard M, Shulman IA, Azen SP, et al. Histocompatibility antigens in sympathetic ophthalmia. *Am J Ophthalmol.* 1983;95:216–221.
98. Bellan L. Sympathetic ophthalmia: a case report and review of the need for prophylactic enucleation. *Can J Ophthalmol.* 1999;34:95–98.
99. Winter F. Sympathetic uveitis. A clinical and pathologic study of the visual result. *Am J Ophthalmol.* 1955;101:102–104.
100. Reynard M, Riffenburgh R, Maes E. Effect of corticosteroid treatment and enucleation on the visual prognosis of sympathetic ophthalmia. *Am J Ophthalmol.* 1983;96:290–294.
101. Brackup A, Carter KD, Nerad JA, et al. Long-term follow-up of severely injured eyes following globe rupture. *Ophthalmol Plast Reconstruct Surg.* 1991;7:194–197.
102. Hollander DA, Jeng BH, Stewart JM. Penetrating ocular injuries in previously injured blind eyes: should we consider primary enucleation? *Br J Ophthalmol.* 2004;88(3):438.
103. du Toit N, Motala MI, Richards J, et al. The risk of sympathetic ophthalmia following evisceration for penetrating eye injuries at Groote Schuur Hospital. *Br J Ophthalmol.* 2008;92(1):61–63.
104. Hebestreit H, Huppertz HI, Sold JE, et al. Steroid-pulse therapy may suppress inflammation in severe sympathetic ophthalmia. *J Pediatr Ophthalmol Strabismus.* 1997;34:124–126.
105. Makley T, Azar A. Sympathetic ophthalmia. A long term follow up. *Arch Ophthalmol.* 1978;96:257–262.
106. Jonas JB, Spandau UH. Repeated intravitreal triamcinolone acetonide for chronic sympathetic ophthalmia. *Acta Ophthalmol Scand.* 2006;84(3):436.
107. Mahajan VB, Gehrs KM, Goldstein DA, Fischer DH, Lopez JS, Folk JC. Management of sympathetic ophthalmia with the fluocinolone acetonide implant. *Ophthalmology.* 2009;116(3):552–557.e1.
108. Schaelgel T, Azar A. Uveitis of suspected viral origin. In: Duane T, ed. *Clinical Ophthalmology.* Hagerstown, MD: Harper and Row; 1978.
109. Raven ML, Ringeisen AL, Yonekawa Y, Stem MS, Faia LJ, Gottlieb JL. Multi-modal imaging and anatomic classification of the white dot syndromes. *Int J Retina Vitreous.* 2017;3:12.
110. Brar M, Sharma M, Grewal SPS, Grewal DS. Treatment response in sympathetic ophthalmia as assessed by widefield OCT angiography. *Ophthalmic Surg Lasers Imaging Retina.* 2018;49(9):726–730.
111. Agrawal R, Jain M, Khan R, Jaisankar D, Xin W, Ding J, Testi I, Raman R, Biswas J. Choroidal Structural Changes in Sympathetic Ophthalmia on Swept-Source Optical Coherence Tomography. *Ocul Immunol Inflamm.* 2019 Nov;19:1–6.
112. Tessler H, Jennings T. High-dose short-term chlorambucil for intractable sympathetic ophthalmia and Behçet's disease. *Br J Ophthalmol.* 1990;74:353–357.
113. Kilmartin D, Forrester J, Dick A. Cyclosporine-induced resolution of choroidal neovascularization associated with sympathetic ophthalmia. *Arch Ophthalmol.* 1998;116:249–250.
114. Menghini M, Frimmel SA, Windisch R, Meier FM. Efficacy of infliximab therapy in two patients with sympathetic ophthalmia. *Klin Monbl Augenheilkd.* 2011;228(4):362–363.
115. Gupta SR, Phan IT, Suhler EB. Successful treatment of refractory sympathetic ophthalmia in a child with infliximab. *Arch Ophthalmol.* 2011;129(2):250–252.

116. Kim JB, Jeroudi A, Angeles-Han ST, Grossniklaus HE, Yeh S. Adalimumab for pediatric sympathetic ophthalmia. *JAMA Ophthalmol.* 2014;132(8):1022–1024.
117. Payal AR, Foster CS. Long-term drug-free remission and visual outcomes in sympathetic ophthalmia. *Ocul Immunol Inflamm.* 2017;25(2):190–195.
118. DeAngelis D, Gupta N, Howcroft M, et al. Cataract extraction by phacoemulsification in a sympathizing eye. *Can J Ophthalmol.* 2000;35:26–28.
119. Ganesh SK, Sundaram PM, Biswas J, et al. Cataract surgery in sympathetic ophthalmia. *J Cataract Refract Surg.* 2004;30(11):2371–2376.
120. Kinge B, Syrdalen P, Bjornsson OM. Photodynamic therapy for choroidal neovascularization secondary to sympathetic ophthalmia. *Retina.* 2005;25(3):375–377.
121. Bom S, Young S, Gregor Z, et al. Surgery for choroidal neovascularization in sympathetic ophthalmia. *Retina.* 2002;22(1):109–111.
122. Buller AJ, Doris JP, Bonshek R, et al. Sympathetic ophthalmia following severe fungal keratitis. *Eye.* 2006;20(11):1306–1307.
123. Jonas JB, Rensch F. Intravitreal steroid slow-release device replacing repeated intravitreal triamcinolone injections for sympathetic ophthalmia. *Eur J Ophthalmol.* 2008;18(5):834–836.

25

Vogt-Koyanagi-Harada Syndrome

H. Nida Sen

KEY CONCEPTS

- Vogt-Koyanagi-Harada (VKH) syndrome is a systemic autoimmune disease, which targets melanin containing cells.
- Typical manifestations include uveitis with exudative retinal detachments, headache, tinnitus, poliosis, and vitiligo.
- Posterior pole disease should be treated very aggressively.

Vogt-Koyanagi-Harada (VKH) syndrome is a systemic disorder involving many organ systems with melanin containing cells, including the eyes, ears, skin, and meninges. It includes a constellation of clinical signs and symptoms, and no definitive confirmatory diagnostic tests are available. In the twelfth century, a physician from the Arab world, Mohammad-al-Ghafiqi, described a disease with poliosis, neuralgias, and hearing changes.[1] In more modern times, in 1906, Vogt[2] presented one case in Basel, Switzerland, and in 1929, Koyanagi[3] described in detail six patients with bilateral nontraumatic chronic iridocyclitis associated with poliosis, vitiligo, and dysacousia. In 1926, Harada[4] described essentially posterior uveitis with an exudative retinal detachment associated with a pleocytosis in cerebrospinal fluid (CSF). As more of these cases were recognized, it became clear that many of the features seen in each of these entities overlapped. Babel[5] suggested that these symptoms were manifestations of the same underlying disorder and that only intensity and distribution varied from one patient to the next; it therefore seemed appropriate to call the entity the Vogt-Koyanagi-Harada syndrome, although it sometimes appears in the literature under other names, for example, *uveomeningitis.*

CLINICAL ASPECTS

Although VKH syndrome has been reported throughout the world, its appearance seems to be concentrated in certain racial and ethnic groups. The diagnostic criteria for VKH syndrome have been revised (Box 25.1). It is a common type of endogenous uveitis in Japan, constituting at least 8% of these cases.[6] The same holds true for certain parts of Latin America, particularly Brazil. It is, however, relatively uncommon in the United States and seems to be an exceedingly unusual diagnosis in persons of northern European extraction. Patients diagnosed with VKH syndrome in France have all been of Mediterranean origin.[7] At the National Eye Institute (NEI), examinations of 75 patients with VKH syndrome revealed that most patients (79%) were females.[8] However, Ohno et al.,[9] in their series of 186 patients, reported that the disease occurred in more males than females. In the NEI cohort, 44% of the patients were African American, 37% were white, 11% were Hispanic, and 6% were Asian. Interestingly, a high percentage of the patients with VKH syndrome seen at the NEI reported having Native American heritage, albeit a sometimes distant one. This observation is very significant because this certainly may be the unifying genetic bond between patients in the United States and those in Asia. VKH syndrome is commonly seen in the Hispanic population of Southern California, an ethnic group often with Native American ancestry, as well.[10] VKH is generally a disease of persons in the second to fourth decades of life, although the disease has been reported in children.[11-16] The proportion of pediatric cases among cohorts with VKH syndrome ranges from 3% to 15%. The visual prognosis is generally favorable.[16]

Systemic Findings

VKH syndrome is a systemic disorder, and the extraocular findings are most important in confirming the diagnosis. Perry and Font[17] stressed that in patients with the Harada form of the disease, some extraocular findings, such as hair and skin alterations, are uncommon.

VKH syndrome is nontraumatic bilateral panuveitis associated with integumentary, neurologic, or auditory signs, according to the revised diagnostic criteria proposed by the American Uveitis Society.[18] On the basis of the revised criteria, typical ocular involvement with only integumentary features or neurologic or auditory manifestations is considered *incomplete* VKH syndrome, and ocular involvement without extraocular manifestations is categorized as *probable* VKH syndrome. The incomplete or probable forms of the disease can account for up to 45% to 58% of patients.[19]

VKH syndrome is a multistage disease with prodromal, acute, chronic convalescent, and chronic recurrent stages. Ocular disease can be preceded by the *prodromal stage,* in which the patient may complain of headache, photophobia, orbital pain, stiff neck, scalp or skin sensitivity, vertigo, and rarely focal neurologic deficits (e.g., cranial nerve palsies). Fever may also be present. In the study by Beniz et al.,[20] in a group of mostly Hispanic patients, headache was, by far, the most common neurologic complaint. Others[21,22] have reported presentation with mild facial weakness, migraine-like headaches with a sensorimotor hemisyndrome, and cognitive dysfunction.

The patient complaining of central nervous system (CNS) symptoms needs to be evaluated immediately. Lumbar puncture will reveal pleocytosis in 84%,[9] with mostly lymphocytes and monocytes present. The CSF glucose level should show a normal relationship to the serum glucose level. The lumbar puncture result will be abnormal early in the course of the disease because pleocytosis will ultimately disappear, even though the inflammatory disease in the eye may continue. These CSF findings were central to the diagnosis criteria proposed by Sugiura[23] but not to the revised criteria. The CSF pleocytosis and the number of cells noted are significantly higher in those patients who develop a "sunset glow" fundus (see later discussion). Furthermore, this finding is occasionally very helpful in terms of determining the severity of the disease and the aggressiveness of the therapeutic approach.

BOX 25.1 Revised Criteria for Diagnosis of Vogt-Koyanagi-Harada Syndrome*

Complete VKH: Criteria 1–5 must be present
Incomplete VKH: Criteria 1–3 and either 4 or 5 must be present
Probable VKH (isolated ocular disease): Criteria 1–3 must be present

1. No history of penetrating ocular trauma or surgery preceding the initial onset of uveitis
2. No clinical or laboratory evidence suggestive of other ocular disease entities
3. Bilateral ocular involvement (a or b must be met, depending on the stage of disease when the patient is examined)
   a) Early manifestations of disease
      (1) Evidence of diffuse choroiditis (with or without anterior uveitis, vitreous inflammatory reaction or optic disc hypermia) which may manifest as (a) focal areas of subretinal fluid or (b) bullous serous retinal detachments
   b) Late manifestations of disease
      (1) History suggestive of prior presence of early findings noted in 3a and one or more of the late chronic signs below.
      (2) Ocular depigmentation (Sunset glow fundus or Sugiura sign), nummular chorioretinal depigmented scars or (b) retinal pigment epithelium clumping and/or migration or recurrent or chronic anterior uveitis
4. Neurological/auditory findings (may resolve by time of evaluation)
   (a) Meningismus (malaise, fever, headache, nausea, abdominal pains, stiffness of the neck and back or a combination of these factors); Note that headache alone is not sufficient to meet the definition of meningismus
   (b) Tinnitus
   (c) Cerebrospinal fluid pleocytosis
5. Integumentary finding (not preceding onset of central nervous system or ocular disease)
   (a) Alopecia, or
   (b) Poliosis, or
   (c) Vitiligo

* Modified from Read et al. Revised diagnostic criteria for Vogt-Koyanagi-Harada disease: report of an international committee on nomenclature. Am J Ophthalmol. 2001 May;131(5):647-52.

On occasion, it can aid in diagnosis; for example, melanin-laden macrophages in the CSF specimen helped make the diagnosis in a patient with titers positive for syphilis.[24]

The auditory difficulties associated with this disorder are central and will often occur concurrently with the ocular disease. The auditory disorder may, however, be the presenting problem. The hearing loss usually involves the higher frequencies and may affect more than three-quarters of patients with the disorder. Dysacousia, which was observed in 74% of patients in one study,[9] may resolve after several months; however, we and others have noted that it persists for years in some cases. Some patients will have tinnitus without an objective decrease in hearing. When we reviewed 24 patients, we noted that some may, indeed, present with tinnitus and even sudden hearing loss. However, audiologic examinations have revealed many more with hearing alterations.[25] Detailed auditory testing, carried out by competent professionals, is important to rule out a noncentral reason for the reduction in hearing.

Skin lesions may also be a prominent part of the disease complex. Approximately 72% of patients[9] report sensitivity to touch of both hair and skin during the active phase of their disease. Vitiligo and poliosis occur in a large number of patients (63% and 90%, respectively) during the convalescent stage, whereas alopecia was reported in 70% to 73% of one group with VKH syndrome[26,27] (Fig. 25.1). It should be noted that different ethnic groups may manifest different systemic symptoms, as suggested by the findings of Beniz et al.[20] These authors found dermatologic involvement only rarely in the group of mostly Hispanic patients with VKH syndrome who were followed up. One area frequently overlooked during an examination for such changes is the axilla.

Ocular Findings

VKH syndrome is a bilateral ocular condition. Although only one eye may be inflamed initially, in 94% of patients, the disease involves the second eye within 2 weeks. Optic disk hyperemia is a frequent presentation in acute VKH syndrome. In the acute stage, 94% of patients have disk leakage ("hot disk") on fluorescein angiography.[28] There is a tendency for the ocular disease to occur in the spring and autumn seasons.[9] The acute stage is characterized by panuveitis with exudative retinal detachments. The inflammatory disease is granulomatous in nature, with mutton-fat keratic precipitates (KPs) on the corneal endothelium. Perilimbal vitiligo (Sugiura sign) may be a striking feature, occurring in 85% of Asian patients.[9] The inflammatory activity can be quite severe and involves both the anterior chamber and the anterior vitreous in about 56% of patients. Nodules may be noted on the pupillary margin and in the iris stroma (Fig. 25.2). An early finding in the disease is the shallowing of the anterior chamber and a moderate increase in intraocular pressure (IOP).[29] This appears to be related to swelling of the ciliary processes, which has been noted to occur early in this disease.[30] This finding is apparent only with careful gonioscopic evaluation. Other patients, however, may have hypotony, probably as a result of edema of the ciliary body. A high incidence of neovascularization of the angle in the acute stage has been reported by one group of Japanese investigators.[31] The glaucoma associated with VKH syndrome can be difficult to control. In a series reported by Forster et al.,[32] 16 of 42 patients with VKH syndrome required either surgical or medical therapy for their glaucoma, with nine having open-angle glaucoma and seven having angle closure caused by pupillary block. A thickened iris is commonly noted in this disease. This is important for at least two reasons. The first is that laser iridotomy is very difficult to perform and the hole created by the laser often closes quickly. The second is that the patient may experience angle closure with a plateau iris, which often adheres completely to the lens, making it impossible to bow forward as one would expect in a more typical case of iris bombé. A rare presentation in dark-skinned persons is scleral perforation, presumably at the site of emergence of the scleral nerves, which are involved as innocent bystanders in the immune response directed against the melanocytes surrounding them[33] (Fig. 25.3).

Severe and rather characteristic changes are noted to occur in the posterior portion of the eye as this disorder evolves. A swelling of the optic nerve head is seen early in 87% of patients[9]; this usually occurs concurrently with a severe vitreous inflammatory response. In addition, retinal edema may be one of the first signs of the disease and may be seen in the posterior pole. As the disease process continues, exudative retinal detachment, an important diagnostic finding, may occur. The inferior portion of the retina is most frequently involved. In the periphery of the retina, yellow-white, well-circumscribed lesions may appear, similar to those seen in sympathetic ophthalmia (SO) (see Chapter 24). In the past, it was thought that these lesions were the clinical equivalent of Dalen-Fuchs nodules. The diffuse choroidal thickening that can be seen on ultrasonography or enhanced depth imaging optical coherence tomography (OCT) occurs during the acute phase of VKH syndrome and may correlate with diffuse granulomatous choroiditis and Dalen-Fuchs nodules.[34]

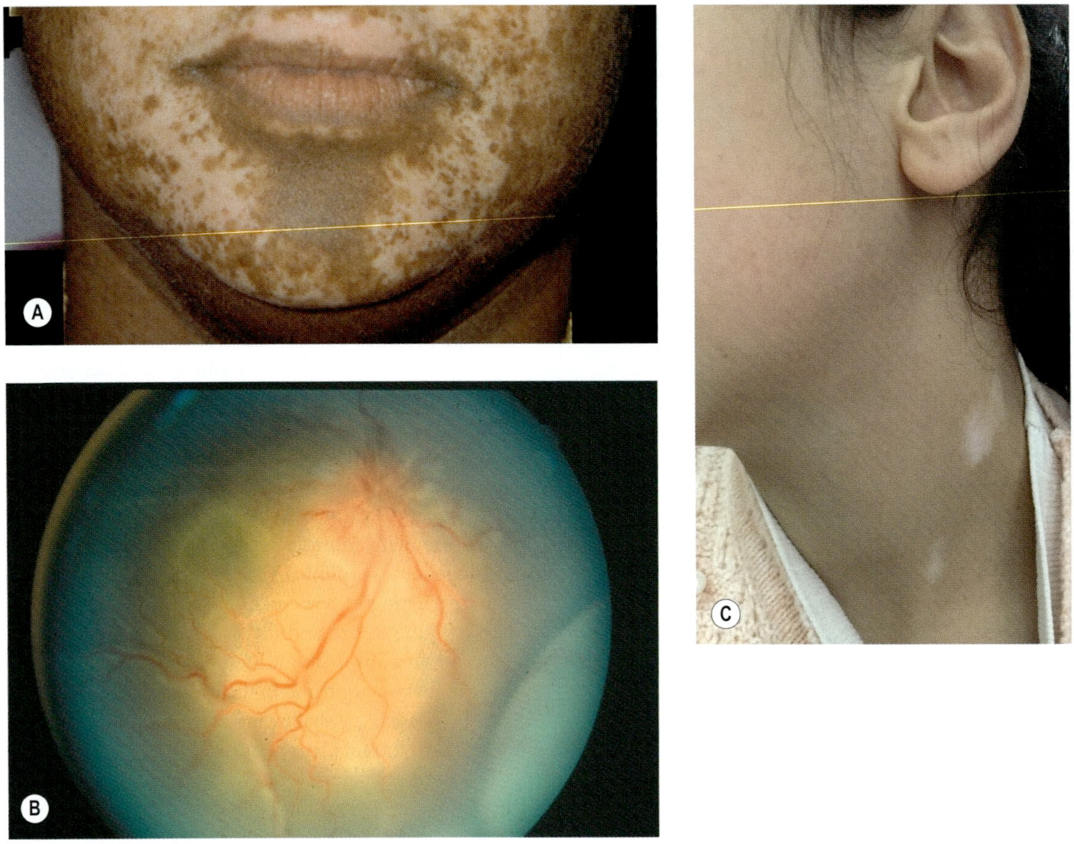

Fig. 25.1 (A) Widespread areas of vitiligo on the face of an African American patient with Native American heritage who has Vogt-Koyanagi-Harada (VKH) syndrome. (B) Fundus photo of the same patient shows extensive exudative retinal detachment and optic nerve edema. (C) Vitiligo on the neck of a Turkish patient. (Courtesy Didar Ucar, MD.)

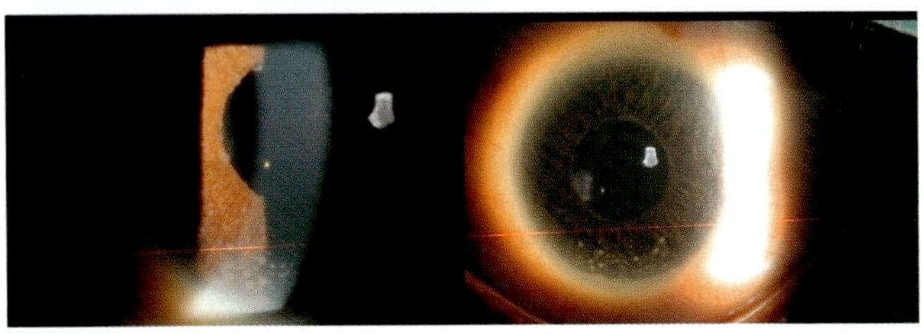

Fig. 25.2 Iris nodules at the pupillary border and mutton-fat keratic precipitates in a patient with Vogt-Koyanagi-Harada (VKH) syndrome.

Several structural complications occur as the disease process continues. Macular edema, although relatively rare (5%), is seen in eyes with more protracted inflammation in the chronic stage, in those with recurrent disease, or in those that have epiretinal membranes.[35,36] Neovascularization of the retina and the optic nerve can be seen, with subsequent recurrent and clinically significant vitreous hemorrhages. Subretinal neovascularization of the macula can also occur. In a large retrospective cohort of 2364 eyes (1357 patients) with posterior uveitis or panuveitis, but free of choroidal neovascularization (CNV) at the time of cohort entry, VKH syndrome was associated with a higher risk of incident CNV (hazard ratio [HR] 3.37; 95% confidence interval [CI] 1.52–7.46) only second to punctate inner choroidopathy (PIC).[37] Similarly, a higher incidence of retinal neovascularization with VKH syndrome (1% per eye-year) was reported in the same cohort.[38] Also, extramacular disciform lesions have been reported,[39] presumably in

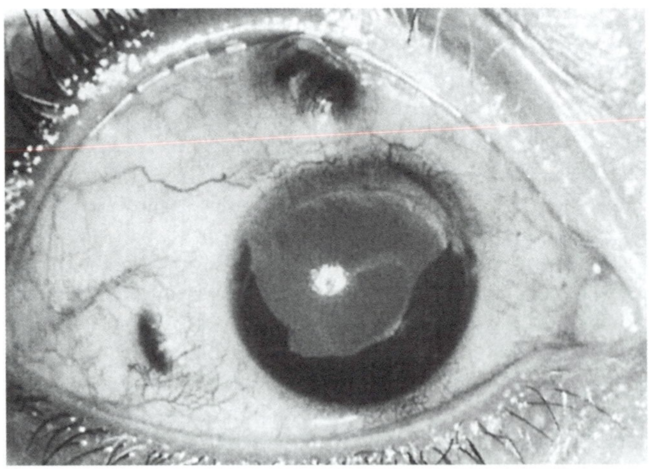

Fig. 25.3 Vogt-Koyanagi-Harada (VKH) syndrome with areas of focal scleritis and thinning of sclera anterior to insertion of rectus muscles. There is a large sector iridectomy superiorly. (Reproduced with permission from Tabbara KF. Scleromalacia associated with Vogt-Koyanagi-Harada syndrome. *Am J Ophthalmol.* 1988;105:694–695.)

areas of reactive proliferation of the retinal pigment epithelium (RPE) and perturbation of the Bruch membrane. Moorthy et al.[40] reported that subretinal neovascular membranes developed in seven of 58 patients with VKH syndrome who were followed up. These authors found that the seven affected patients showed more anterior and vitreous inflammation and more pigmentary disturbances in the fundus. As expected, the visual outcomes for these patients were also significantly poorer than those for patients with less severe alterations.

The exudative detachments frequently do not persist after the initial presentation, although other signs of inflammation continue to be present, for example, "demarcation lines" representing the extent of previous detachments. Rhegmatogenous detachments may also occur in these eyes, and constant surveillance for such changes therefore is vital.

Diagnostic criteria for both the complete and incomplete forms of the disease have been published (see Box 25.1). The study by Gaspar et al.[41] in Brazil reported 100% concordance in a retrospective review of 67 patients, 46 of whom were in the early phase of the disease. Rao et al.[19] reported a very good concordance rate as well when the criteria were applied retrospectively. However, Yamaki et al.[42] found that the criteria were effective for the final diagnosis but not for diagnosis in the early stage of the disease. These authors felt that it would be better to apply the criteria suggested by Sugiura, namely, pleocytosis in CSF and human leukocyte antigen (HLA) typing. Retrospective studies are helpful as starting points, but prospective studies are very much needed to effectively evaluate the usefulness of any criteria.

The chronic convalescent stage occurs 3 to 4 months after disease onset. This stage is characterized by nongranulomatous panuveitis, poliosis of the eyebrows and eyelashes, vitiligo, and alopecia. As the disease process begins to wane, a characteristic depigmentation of the posterior portion of the globe occurs. This "sunset glow" appearance to the fundus (Fig. 25.4), which reflects loss of pigment at the level of the RPE or choroid, is seen commonly in Asian patients. Keino et al.[43] found that the "sunset glow" fundus was more commonly seen in eyes with chronic inflammation persisting for months. At times, profound changes, such as subretinal fibrosis, disciform scars, RPE migration, and neovascularization, can be quite striking (Figs. 25.5 and 25.6).

Mondkar et al.[44] reported their experience with VKH syndrome in India, which represented only 2.2% of referrals. Extraocular manifestations were seen in 64% of patients at the time of presentation. Greater than 95% of these patients had meningismus. In the 78 patients with VKH syndrome seen at the NEI, the disease manifested predominantly as posterior pole changes. There were no patients with only anterior segment disorders.

Chronic recurrent stage starts 6 to 9 months after the onset of disease and can occur in 17% to 79% of patients.[43,45,46] This stage is characterized by recurrent granulomatous anterior uveitis and choroidal thickening.[47] Subretinal fibrosis can also occur in the chronic recurrent stage and may be a result of long uncontrolled inflammation and exudative detachment. Subretinal fibrosis appears to occur more frequently (13%) and earlier in patients of Hispanic ethnicity compared with Chinese patients, with less than 2% of the latter having subretinal fibrosis.[10,48-50]

Course of Disease

The clinical course of VKH syndrome is quite varied. In the typical patient, severe acute findings are present. The acute phase is followed by a period of quiescence, during which there is depigmentation of tissue, and a later stage with recurrent anterior segment inflammation. In some patients, there may be a limited period of severe ocular inflammatory activity, followed by rapid depigmentation and no further episodes. Other patients, however, continue to have ongoing, chronic disease. It is this group that requires constant monitoring. Anterior segment alterations, such as cataract and secondary glaucoma, occur in about one-third of patients. Peripapillary atrophy greater than 2 disk diopters was associated with greater visual dysfunction, and interestingly, in a multivariate analysis steroid treatment was the main determinant for peripapillary atrophy.[51,52] With aggressive therapy, exudative detachment will resolve. Depending on the time elapsed, reattachment usually results in reasonably good vision. However, close evaluation of the retina will demonstrate changes, such as preretinal membranes, RPE stippling, extensive posterior pole atrophy,[53] and subtle folds in the retina precluding return to previous levels of vision and subretinal fibrosis.[48] In a report of 75 patients seen at the NEI,[54] 30 (40%) had subretinal fibrosis, and 14.7% of eyes had CNV. The subretinal fibrosis was associated with longer duration of disease and worse visual acuity. The disease in children appears to be aggressive. Tabbara et al.[13] reported that 61% of children with VKH syndrome versus 17% of adults needed cataract surgery and that the final visual acuity in those children needing surgery was worse than that seen in

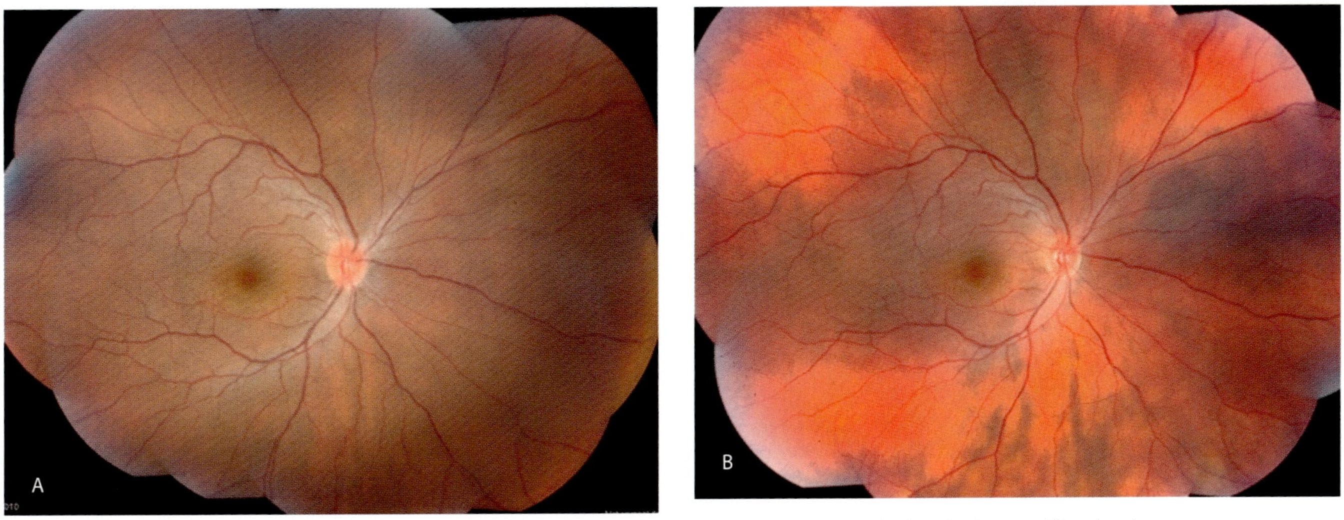

Fig. 25.4 A 24-year-old Hispanic man with sudden-onset blurred vision, headache, tinnitus, and hearing loss was diagnosed with Vogt-Koyanagi-Harada (VKH) syndrome and referred to the National Eye Institute (NEI). Fundus photos taken 1 month after the onset of symptoms (A) highlight the "sunset glow" fundus (B), which developed more than 6 months later.

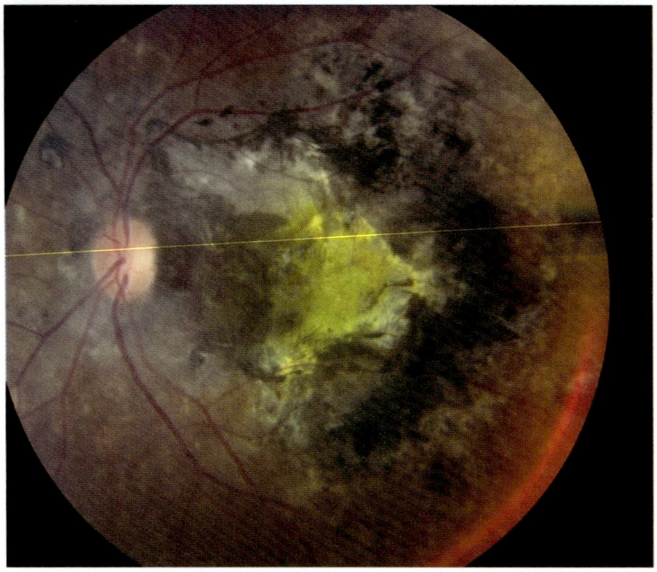

Fig. 25.5 Dramatic retinal pigment epithelium (RPE) changes and subretinal alterations with subretinal fibrosis can occur in severe and uncontrolled cases.

adults. Rathinam et al.[15] found that all of their small number of pediatric patients with VKH syndrome had cataracts. Clinical findings at presentation, the duration of the disease, and the development of extraocular manifestations are all prognostic factors relating to final visual acuity and recurrent inflammation.[55]

When the classic manifestations of acute VKH syndrome are present, there is little difficulty in making the diagnosis. However, when the patient is examined at a later stage of the disease, the sequelae of the inflammatory disease cannot reliably aid in determining what the original problem had been, particularly if nonocular findings are absent. The problems in diagnosing this condition were described by Kayazawa and Takahashi,[56] in their report on two patients with multiple yellow-white placoid lesions and a decrease in vision. On the basis of fluorescein angiography findings, one patient was believed to have acute posterior multifocal placoid pigment epitheliopathy. However, the fluorescein angiography findings in the other patient showed multiple pinpoint leaks, and later the fundus developed a "sunset glow" appearance. Rao and Marak[57] reported on four patients with SO, all of whom had penetrating wounds, and two or more extraocular manifestations usually associated with VKH syndrome, that is, vitiligo, poliosis, dysacousia, and meningitis (see Chapter 24). Other disorders that can mimic VKH syndrome include sarcoidosis (see Chapter 23)

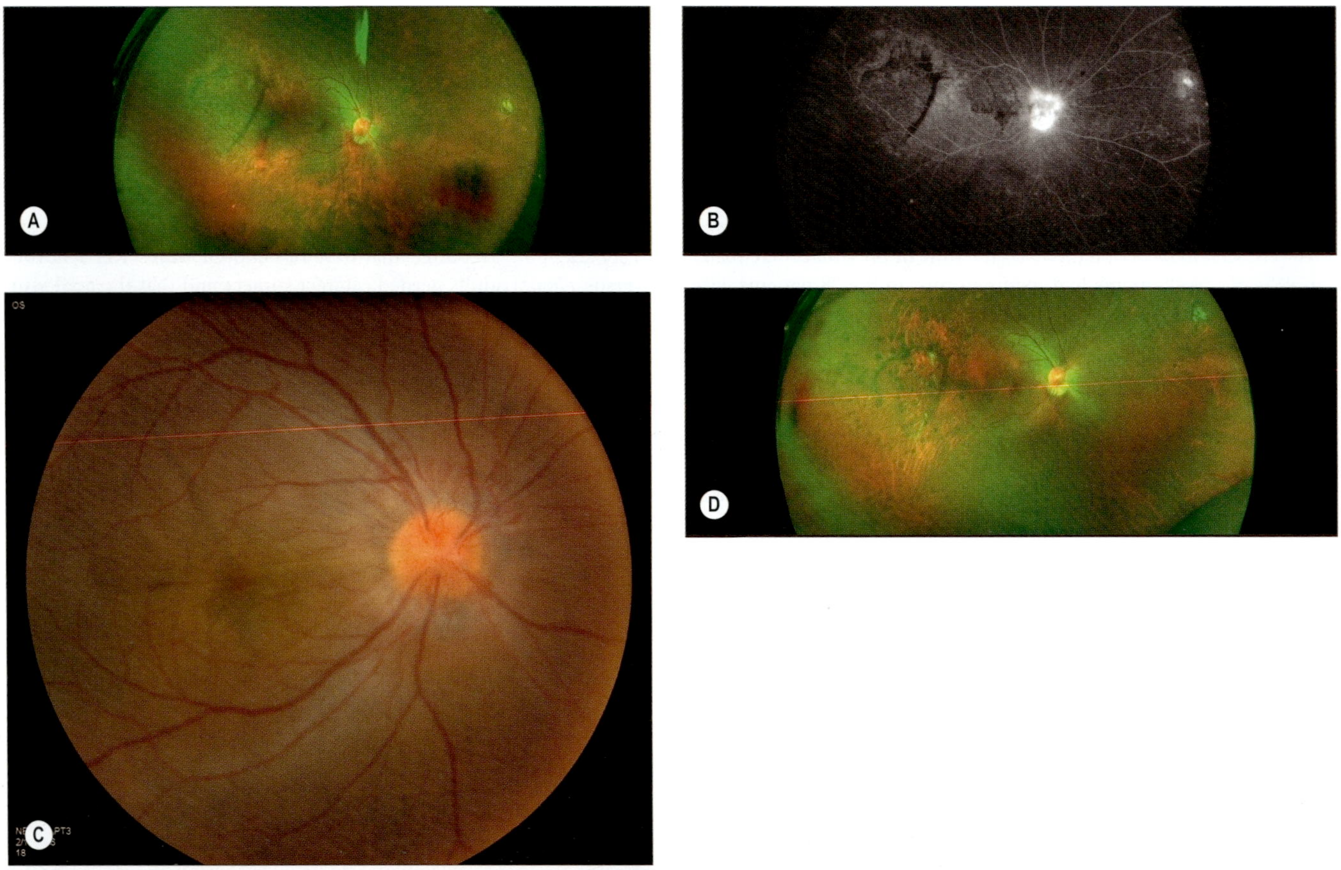

Fig. 25.6 (A–D) In a Hispanic man with chronic Vogt-Koyanagi-Harada (VKH) syndrome, neovascularization of the disk (NVD) and retina developed, with resultant vitreous hemorrhage (inferonasally) in the right eye (A). Wide-angle fluorescein angiography (B) shows late leakage from the NVD. Topcon color fundus photograph illustrates choroidal folds and the extent of NVD (C) in the same patient. After treatment with systemic corticosteroids, antimetabolites, tumor necrosis factor (TNF) inhibitors, intraocular anti–vascular endothelial growth factor (VEGF), and peripheral laser photocoagulation, the NVD in the right eye regressed (D).

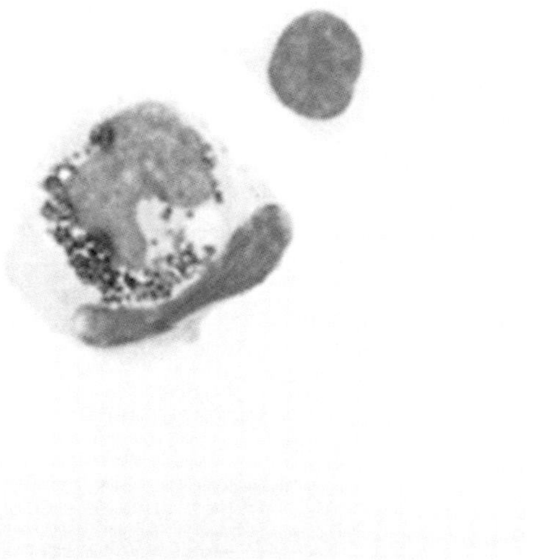

Fig. 25.7 Basophilic granules in a melanin-laden macrophage taken from the cerebrospinal fluid of a patient with VKH. (Reproduced with permission from Kamondi A, Szegedi A, Papp A, et al. Vogt-Koyanagi-Harada disease presenting initially as aseptic meningoencephalitis. *Eur J Neurol.* 2000;7:719–722.)

(particularly if there is choroidal involvement and subretinal changes) and some of the white-dot syndromes (see Chapter 30). One patient was reported as presenting with aseptic meningitis (Fig. 25.7), with the ocular findings typical of VKH only manifesting many months later.[58] Kouda et al.[59] reported on a patient with VKH syndrome who first presented with unilateral posterior scleritis and was found to have bilateral, severe granulomatous uveitis 12 months later. Other diseases may rarely mimic the fundus picture seen in VKH syndrome. *Bartonella* infection has been reported to present as unilateral VKH syndrome.[60] In addition, another patient, who had an indocyanine green (ICG) angiography and intravenous fluorescein angiography results compatible with VKH syndrome, ultimately was diagnosed with intravascular lymphoma.[61] Admittedly, these are rare occurrences. A short note to alert the treating physician: Interferon (IFN) therapy given for other indications (e.g., hepatitis) can induce serous detachment simulating VKH IVFA.[62] Although this possible complication has been recognized, some have argued that the positive therapeutic value of IFN outweighs any possible negative adverse effects.[63]

The observer should set minimal ocular criteria for the diagnosis of VKH syndrome because diagnosis is mainly a clinical decision. The revised diagnostic criteria are helpful in making the clinical diagnosis in most cases. Diffuse bilateral choroiditis with or without inflammation of the anterior chamber, vitreous, or optic nerve and the presence of acute exudative retinal detachment and typical pinpoint leakage at the level of the RPE early on, as noted on fluorescein angiography, are highly suggestive of the diagnosis, especially in the absence of a history of ocular trauma or surgery and laboratory or clinical evidence suggestive of other clinical entities. The presence of neurologic or auditory findings and integumentary changes would confirm the diagnosis of complete VKH syndrome (see Box 25.1). The presence of disk edema (and leakage seen on fluorescein angiography) is an important confirmatory sign, and many patients will have CNS pleocytosis early in the disease. The presence of other extraocular findings discussed earlier is helpful, but these may be missed late in the disease. Patient history of Native American heritage is helpful information. The Sugiura sign does not seem to occur in white patients with this disease.

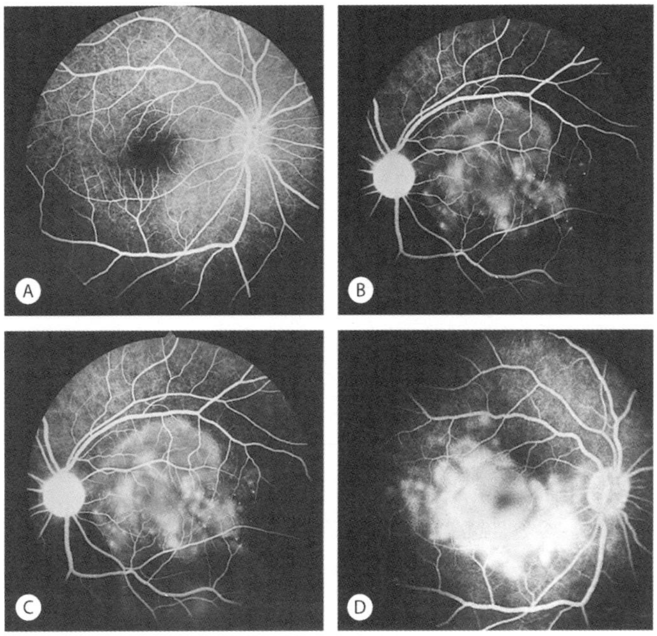

Fig. 25.8 Fluorescein angiograms of the right eye (A and D) and the left eye (B and C) of a patient with Vogt-Koyanagi-Harada (VKH) syndrome, demonstrating pinpoint subretinal leakage, which later coalesced into a large area of leakage.

LABORATORY TESTS, ETIOLOGY, AND HISTOPATHOLOGY

Several tests can be performed to evaluate the alterations occurring in the eye as a result of the inflammatory disease. The use of fluorescein angiography is helpful in evaluating the extent of the disease in the posterior segment of the globe. In the venous phase of fluorescein angiography, delayed filling of the choroid can be observed in the acute stage. Early in the disease, multiple pinpoint areas of leakage are noted at the level of the RPE. These can appear as a "starry sky," which is highly suggestive of VKH syndrome. The later frames from angiography may show large confluent areas of leakage (Figs. 25.8 and 25.9), and late leakage of the disk usually occurs. Disk leakage occurs in 94% in the acute stage and in 6% in the chronic stage of the disease. In the chronic stage, spotty areas of hyperfluorescence, caused by RPE window defect, and hypofluorescence, caused by blockage by RPE migration, can be observed.[28] Subretinal neovascularization can be evaluated best with fluorescein angiography. Manger and Ober[64] reported the presence of retinal arteriovenous anastomoses in a young woman with VKH syndrome. By using fluorescein angiography, these authors noted that these vessels were collaterals that had developed in areas of damaged RPE. Changes on both fluorescein angiography and ICG angiography findings have been well described. Herbort et al.[65] describe four general findings in VKH syndrome: (1) early large choroidal stromal vessel hyperfluorescence; (2) patchy hypofluorescence in the early phase of ICG angiography in the posterior pole and periphery presumed to be caused by delayed choroidal perfusion; (3) a diffuse fuzzy vascular pattern to the presumed large stromal vessel leakage; and (4) hypofluorescent dark dots in the intermediate phase of ICG angiography. Unlike the normally hypofluorescent appearance of the disk, in patients with VKH syndrome, disk hyperfluorescence can be observed on ICG angiography. With adequate immunosuppressive therapy, the dark dots will resolve. Others have used ICG angiography to examine the peripheral lesions usually identified as Dalen-Fuchs nodules.[66] These authors found one group of patients with nodules—which were

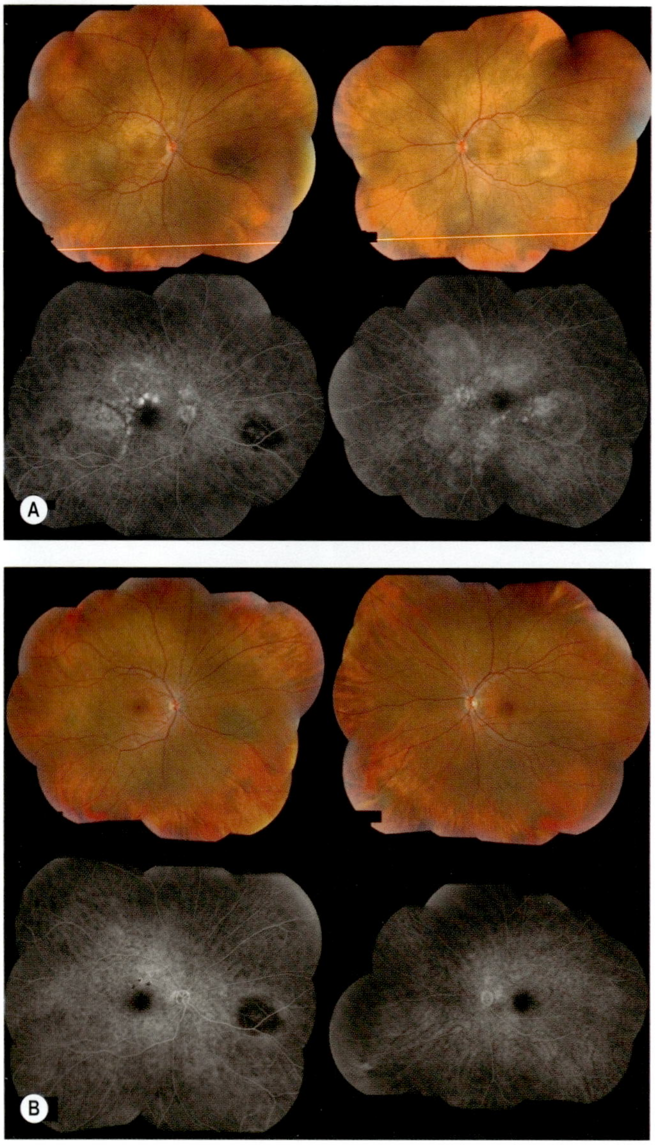

Fig. 25.9 (A) Fundus of a female patient from Nepal with VKH presenting with acute disease and visual acuity of 20/125 in the right eye and 20/40 in the left eye (top frames). Fluorescein angiogram shows typical pinpoint leakage with pooling in both eyes (bottom frames) in the acute phase. (B) Appearance of fundus approximately 6 weeks after high dose oral prednisone shows resolution of subretinal fluid and leakage and pooling on FA but with resultant RPE changes. Vision improved to 20/20 in both eyes.

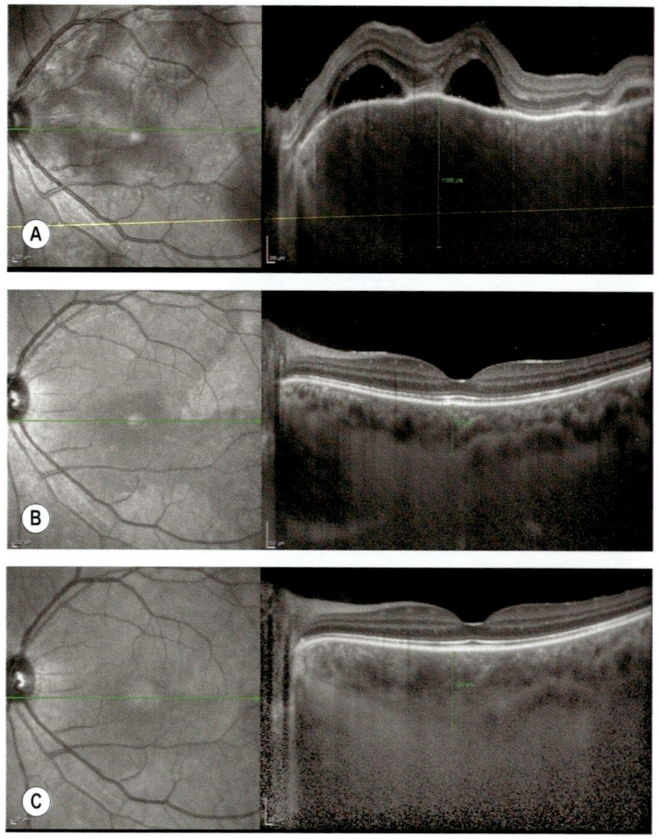

Fig. 25.10 (A–C) Enhanced depth imaging optical coherence tomography (EDI-OCT) of the left eye in acute stage of the same patient in Fig. 25.9 shows significantly thickened choroid along with large subretinal fluid pockets. After oral prednisone treatment and resolution of inflammation and of subretinal fluid, choroidal thickness normalized (B); however, reactivation with anterior and vitreous cells occurred in the absence of any subretinal fluid (C), which was accompanied by thickening of the choroid. Note the reconstitution of ellipsoid zone with time and treatment (A through C).

more common inferiorly and temporally—to be hyperfluorescent in the early phase and then becoming hypofluorescent in the later frames, and the authors felt that these patients had a shorter disease course. Those with nodules that showed small, round, hypofluorescent lesions early had a longer disease course. However, ICG angiography findings have not been particularly useful for prognostication, and it can be difficult to distinguish acute choroiditis from stromal scarring.[67]

Fundus autofluorescence (FAF) can show different patterns at different stages of VKH syndrome, ranging from hypoautofluorescent areas corresponding the subretinal fluid in the early stages to evolving placoid hyperautofluorescence in the convalescent stage and stippled areas of hyper- and hypoautofluorescent spots in the chronic phase with scarring and changes in the RPE. A peripheral lattice-like pattern has been reported. Early treatment may result in complete resolution of abnormal FAF patterns. Some of these changes may be more apparent on infrared FAF.[68,69] Patients with granular hyperautofluorescence on near-infrared were more likely to have "sunset glow" fundus.[70] In 2019, Nakamura et al. noted hyperreflective lesions on adaptive optics imaging corresponding to areas of near-infrared hyperautofluorescence and elevated RPE lesions on spectral domain OCT (SD-OCT).[71]

OCT has permitted the clinician to observe changes in this disorder more precisely.[72] It has been used to document anterior segment changes in the acute glaucoma that can be seen in VKH syndrome.[73] SD-OCT allows for visualization of exudative detachments, intraretinal edema, RPE undulations, and choroidal folds. Subretinal fibrinous septae can also be seen on OCT.[74] Enhanced depth imaging OCT (EDI-OCT) can show hyperreflective choroidal spots, which often resolve with treatment[75,76] (Fig. 25.10). Choroidal folds are not unusual in the eyes of patients with VKH syndrome, with one study reporting the finding in 12% of patients, often with hypofluorescent bands radiating from the optic disk.[77] Miura et al. found melanin accumulation at the RPE–Bruch membrane band by using multichannel OCT (MC-OCT), which corresponded to the areas of granular hyperautofluorescent lesions on near-infrared FAF.[70] These authors also showed that melanin loss was associated with "sunset glow" fundus by using polarization sensitive OCT.[70]

Electroretinography and electrooculography findings show varying degrees of abnormality, depending on the ocular disease. Studies have shown that multifocal electroretinography responses in patients can be severely altered, and that with therapy, there is a delayed but limited recovery of macular function over several months.[78] It is important to note that improvement in the results of both tests may occur during certain time points of the clinical course, with worsening associated with recurrence.[79] During the convalescent stage, foveal cone photoreceptor regeneration and recovery are delayed in VKH syndrome.[80] An image analyzer, measuring the ratio of red pixels to the total number of pixels, has been used to determine "sunset glow" changes early in the disease.[81]

Antigen-Specific and Immune Responses

Much attention has been focused on defining the immunoregulatory alteration that leads to VKH syndrome. Monoclonal antibodies directed to cell surface markers of various components of the immune system and to markers of cellular activation that appear at times have been used to study this disorder. In early studies, Okubo et al.[82] evaluated the various cellular immune components of seven patients with VKH syndrome who had active uveitis compared with those of 98 control subjects. They noted that the numbers of total T cells (OKT3+), helper T (Th) cells (OKT4+), and putative suppressor cells (OKT11+) were lower in patients than in control subjects. Liu and Sun[83] reported that the CD4/CD8 ratio was increased in patients whose disease recurred, as observed previously by us when patients with uveitis were evaluated in the United States. However, in the study by Okubo et al.[82] the number of cells bearing the antigen defined by the OK1a antibody was elevated. Ia or DR expression can be taken as a sign of immune system activation. DR expression can be enhanced by T-cell products released during the lymphokine cascade. In particular, IFN-γ is a powerful stimulus for DR activation on cell-surface membranes and does not have antiviral activity. The presence of circulating IFN-γ was evaluated in patients with VKH syndrome. Significantly increased IFN levels were detected in the blood of patients with VKH types 1 and 2 months after the initiation of ocular symptoms; further evaluation of the IFN present revealed it to be IFN-γ. IFN-γ could not be detected in CSF in those patients whose blood samples showed positivity.[84] Similar observations have been made in diseases of putative autoimmune origin, such as systemic lupus erythematosus, rheumatoid arthritis, and Sjögren syndrome.[85] Sakaguchi et al.[86] established nine T-cell clones from patients with VKH syndrome and found that all of them spontaneously produced greater amounts of IFN-γ, interleukin (IL)-6, and IL-8 than were produced by cells from control subjects. Imai et al.[87] repeatedly saw high IFN-γ levels produced by T-cell clones obtained from patients with VKH syndrome. The evaluation of cell-surface markers on lymphocytes in VKH syndrome has shown that CD3+ T cells are more commonly seen in the aqueous and CSF than in peripheral blood.[88] CD45+Ro+ cells (i.e., memory cells) were seen in a higher percentage in the aqueous and CSF than in peripheral blood, with Fas+ cells seen more in the aqueous than in CSF. In patients with VKH syndrome, CSF has been reported to have high amounts of the chemokine CXCL10 and lower amounts of CXCL17 than in serum, whereas CCL2/MCP-1 is lower in the CSF of patients with VKH syndrome than in controls.[89] These findings are similar to those seen in the CSF of patients with multiple sclerosis. Several studies have attempted to evaluate the presence of other markers of immune activation or immunoregulation. Li et al.[90] reported the upregulation of t-bet ribonucleic acid (RNA) expression in the peripheral blood of patients with VKH syndrome. T-bet is involved in the differentiation of T cells into Th1 cells. They also found that these cells, when stimulated, produced large amounts of IFN-γ, which is not surprising if they are Th1 cells. It has been suggested at least one source of immunoregulatory cells (i.e., those that can suppress or "modulate" the immune response) is found in a subgroup of CD4+ cells that bear large numbers of receptors for IL-2 (the receptor is called *CD25*), and therefore they are labeled as CD4+CD25high cells. Chen et al.[91] reported that the frequency of these cells was reduced in the peripheral blood of patients with VKH syndrome and that another marker for immunoregulatory cells, FoxP3, was also low. Chi et al.[92] reported that higher levels of IL-23, a lymphokine associated with IL-17, were seen in patients with VKH syndrome and that there was increased production of IL-17 in the peripheral blood cells, when stimulated polyclonally. This finding is not surprising. Along those lines, leptin, which is structurally similar to IL-6, IL-12, and IL-15, was seen to be elevated in the serum of these patients.[93] Furthermore, when peripheral blood mononuclear cells were cultured in the presence of leptin, there was proliferation of the cells and an increase in the secretion of IL-17 and IFN. In 2019, Urzua et al. suggested that glucocorticoid receptor isoforms (α and β) and mitogen-activated protein kinase phosphatase-1 (MKP-1) could be potential biomarkers for steroid resistance and disease activity.[94]

The notion that a specific antigen-driven immune response is occurring in this disorder remains an intriguing possibility. Initial hypotheses centered on the role of pigment as the antigen driving the immune response. Several reports observed positive in vitro immune phenomena when patients' lymphocytes were placed in an environment containing uveal extracts or pigment.[95] Most of these reports used a nonhuman, usually bovine, source for antigen, thereby raising the possibility that the positive test results were caused by sensitization against bovine antigens in meat-eating humans. Yuasa et al.,[96] however, used human uveal preparations. They observed that 13 of 30 patients tested had positive macrophage migration inhibition test results, evidence that the immune system is capable of a memory response to the antigen(s). Maezawa et al.[97] evaluated the role of cytotoxic T cells in this disorder and how they may react against melanocyte-associated antigens. They noted that in the six patients with VKH they studied, the cytotoxic T-cell component of the immune repertoire appeared to demonstrate specific killing against a P-36 melanoma cell line, which bears cross-reactive antigens with normal melanocytes. Furthermore, they demonstrated that the monoclonal antibody Leu-2a, specifically directed against the cytotoxic T-cell subset, blocked this reaction. They observed that the cytotoxic activity depended on the presence of DR+-adherent cells and that the activity could be augmented by the addition of interleukins into the in vitro system.[98] Tyrosinase family proteins have also been implicated. Yamaki et al.[99] demonstrated that a 30-mer sequence from the tyrosinase family induced a proliferative response in lymphocytes taken from patients with VKH syndrome. Sugita et al.[100] reported that that CD4+ cells infiltrating the eyes responded to tyrosinase and gp100 peptide, producing RANTES and IFN-γ. Additionally, when injected into Lewis rats, these antigens induced both ocular and extraocular disease (skin and meninges) approximately 12 days after immunization.[101] Gocho et al.[102] were able to establish 28 T-cell clones directed against tyrosinase and another 34 directed against tyrosinase-related protein 1. Yamada et al.[103] reported a higher prevalence of immunoglobulin G (IgG) antilens epithelium-derived growth factor in patients with VKH syndrome. A rather interesting example of the power of these autoaggressive immune cells was demonstrated in the study by Yeh et al.,[104] in which a patient with systemic melanoma received tumor infiltrating cells (TILs) with IL-2 therapy, resulting in the development of VKH syndrome. This suggests the fine balance between autoaggressive cells being therapeutically positive in preventing tumor spread and inducing an autoimmune response.

Immune responses directed against the retina can also be seen. Patients with VKH syndrome have circulating lymphocytes that have been noted to have in vitro proliferative responses to the retinal S-antigen (S-Ag),[105] although this finding is, by no means, unique to this disorder. Chan et al.,[106] however, noted that sera from these patients had particularly unique properties. Using the avidin–biotin–peroxidase technique for the detection of retinal antibodies, they found particularly large titers of antiretinal antibodies in these patients' sera directed against the outer segments of photoreceptors and Müller cells. Considerably lower titers were found in some patients with Behçet disease and in a few with SO. Whether this finding is reflective of a primary immune process or a result of the severe posterior pole disease seen in these patients still remains to be evaluated. It is also of interest that nonspecific triggering mechanisms can lead to the full disease. Several years ago, we followed up a patient in whom typical VKH syndrome developed after the purified protein derivative (PPD) skin test (see Case 25.2). Rathinam et al.[107] reported three patients who developed VKH syndrome after cutaneous injury, with the skin initially becoming vitiliginous. It is interesting to speculate on the role of other exogenous triggering factors. Tattoo-associated choroiditis and VKH syndrome–like findings have also been reported.[108]

Because of the increased prevalence of this disorder in certain ethnic groups, it is logical to hypothesize an immunogenetic basis for this disease. Cases of this disorder in siblings and monozygotic twins have been reported.[109,110] Ohno[84] evaluated the frequency of HLA antigens in Japanese patients with this disease compared with that in control subjects. HLA-DR4 was present in 88% of patients but in only 32% of controls, with a calculated relative risk of 15.2. All the patients had the supertypical DR antigen MT3 (HLA-B53), compared with 53% of the control subjects, with a resultant relative risk of 74.5. Kunikane[111] reported an association between HLA-DQWa and Harada disease in Japanese patients (relative risk 5.17), confirming the findings in Ohno's previous work with the same antigen. However, using two-dimensional electrophoresis and restriction fragment length polymorphism analysis, Kunikane noted that these antigen molecules differed in Japanese and white subjects tested. In typing 25 Han Chinese with VKH syndrome, Zhao et al.[112] found an association between HLA-DR4 (relative risk 16.0) and HLA-Dw53 (relative risk 34.2), similar to that seen in Japan. Zhang et al.[113] reported a strong association between VKH syndrome and HLA-DR4, with a calculated relative risk of 10.0, whereas a reduced frequency of HLA-DQw1 was seen in fewer patients. Numaga et al.,[114] using a polymerase chain reaction (PCR) technique, demonstrated that the HLA-DR β1 in 19 of 20 patients had a specific amino acid sequence in positions 70 and 71. However, Yu et al.[115] found an association with HLA-B22, with a relative risk calculated at 8.69. Kim et al.[116] reported an association between VKH syndrome and HLA-DRB1*0405 or the HLA-DRB1*0405-DQA1*0302-DQB1*0401 haplotype in Korean patients.

Davis et al.[117] evaluated the HLA associations with VKH syndrome in 23 American patients. A strong association was found with HLA-DR4 and HLA-DRw53. HLA-DQw3 was strongly associated with this disease because this antigen was in linkage disequilibrium with DR4. An interesting report by Rutzen et al.[118] described the development of VKH syndrome in monozygotic twins of Vietnamese ancestry. HLA typing disclosed HLA-DR4 positivity. In addition, the anecdotal association between VKH syndrome and Native American ancestry was confirmed. In the report by Martinez et al.[119] on North American patients of Cherokee Indian ancestry with VKH syndrome, assay results in seven patients showed the HLA-DRw52 haplotype. Five of these patients were homozygous for this allele, whereas patients in Mexico of Mestizo background had DRB1*04 on their cells.[120] Levinson et al. reported an increase in combined DR4 alleles in Mestizo patients with VKH syndrome in Southern California,[121] and these authors also reported a trend toward B KIR haplotypes, a finding similar to those in other autoimmune disorders.[122]

Others have examined whether other specific gene alleles or single nucleotide polymorphisms (SNPs) might be associated with VKH syndrome. Horie et al.[123] investigated possible relationships between the tyrosinase gene family TYR and dopachrome tautomerase. Although a very strong association was noted between VKH syndrome and HLA-DRB1*0405, no risk was identified with the tyrosinase gene family; nor did the group identify a genetic susceptibility with VKH syndrome and the *IFN-γ* gene.[124] Du et al.[125] reported an association between the cytotoxic lymphocyte-associated antigen-4 (CTLA-4), a negative regulator of T-cell responses, and VKH syndrome; however, the odds ratio was not very impressive.

The concept that this disorder is of viral origin has been an attractive one for many, and numerous attempts have been made to substantiate this theory. However, studies aimed at isolating virus from either the eye[126] or CSF[127] have not been successful. Sunakawa and Okinami[128] determined anti–Epstein-Barr virus antibody levels in control subjects and in patients with panuveitis, including patients with VHK syndrome, and found that the frequency of elevated titers was lower in the patients than in the controls. In the work by Sugita et al.,[100] mentioned earlier, CD+ ocular infiltrating cells recognizing tyrosinase were found, and these authors also recognized the cytomegalovirus envelope glycoprotein H, which has a high amino acid homology to tyrosinase. However, Ye et al. showed a distinct gut microbial signature in patients with VKH syndrome compared with healthy controls.[129] They were also able to show distinct microbial groups to be associated with treatment response.

Moreover, transfer of gut microbiota from patients with VKH syndrome exacerbated disease activity clinically and histopathologically in experimental autoimmune uveitis models.

Vogt-Koyanagi-Harada Syndrome versus Sympathetic Ophthalmia

Histologic evaluations of VKH syndrome in several patients have been reported in the literature.[6] A major discussion point has been how this disorder differs from SO (see Chapter 24). As in SO, in VKH syndrome, there is marked thickening of the choroid with macrophages, lymphocytes, and epithelioid cells that contain melanin. Unlike in SO, in VKH syndrome, plasma cells are readily observed. Dalen-Fuchs nodules are present, and involvement of the choriocapillaris is more common, unlike the classic "sparing" of this portion of the choroid in SO. Although much has been said about the histologic differences between SO and VKH syndrome, it is clear that both are entities on a spectrum of the same disease and that standard histologic evaluation of the posterior globe often cannot definitively differentiate one from the other. An interesting note about sparing of the choriocapillaris is that, as suggested by Rao,[130] this sparing results from the production of anti-inflammatory molecules by the RPE, which produces both transforming growth factor (TGF)-β and RPE-protective protein, which would suppress the generation of superoxides by phagocytes. A report by Rao[131] challenged another notion about VKH syndrome. In chronic VKH syndrome, the peripheral fundus scars are not Dalen-Fuchs nodules but areas of focal chorioretinal atrophy with loss of the RPE (Fig. 25.11). In the chronic stage of the disease, the histology takes on a nongranulomatous appearance, and there is involvement of the choriocapillaris; finally, in the chronic recurrent stage, the disease appears to become granulomatous again. This may indicate different mechanisms of immune response during different stages of the disease course.

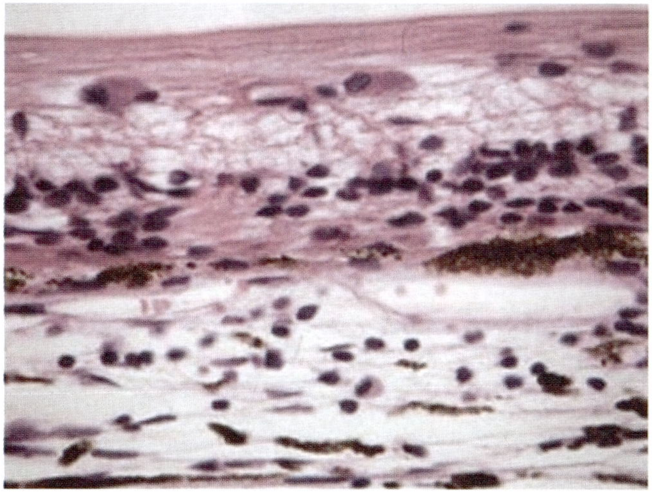

Fig. 25.11 Chronic stage of Vogt-Koyanagi-Harada (VKH) syndrome with atrophic lesion that was thought in the past to have been a Dalen-Fuchs nodule. (With kind permission of Springer Science & Business Media. Rao NA. Pathology of Vogt-Koyanagi-Harada's disease. *Int Ophthalmol.* 2007;27:81.)

THERAPY

Medical management is the main therapeutic approach to VKH syndrome. The initial drug of choice remains a corticosteroid. Usually given systemically (sometimes given intraocularly) for this bilateral condition, the dosage needed to achieve a positive therapeutic result may be high. Oral steroid administration (especially doses ≥40 mg/day) has been associated with reducing the loss of vision associated with this disorder.[132] The disease is particularly responsive to corticosteroids (Figs 25.9 and 25.10). In patients with severe disease, with bilateral retinal detachments and a dramatic drop in visual acuity, intravenous steroids or a higher starting dose of prednisone can be used. Hayasaka et al.[133] reported using drip infusions of 200 mg of prednisolone per day. They reported resolution of both intraocular and extraocular symptoms in most patients treated in this fashion. Their suggestion is that less steroid may be needed for the Harada type of the disease than for the Vogt-Koyanagi component. In patients with particularly severe ocular disease, some practitioners use intravenous high-dose pulse steroid therapy (up to 1 g/day of methylprednisolone given for 3 days), followed by oral prednisone at levels of about 1 mg/kg/day. Nakayama et al. reported successful control of inflammation in 111 patients treated with intravenous pulse steroids. Recurrence (22.5%), complication (21%), and immunosuppressive (cyclosporine) use (15%) were low. However, early recurrences were treated with a second course of intravenous pulse steroids (44%).[134] Pregnancy, which is a state of immunotolerance, should theoretically make the inflammatory disease less severe, as usually seen by us. However, Doi et al.[135] reported the need for high-dose steroid treatment in a 26-year-old Japanese woman with VKH syndrome just after the 18th week of pregnancy, whereas others have reported both mild and severe disease states.[136] Periocular or intravitreal corticosteroid injections have also been used to treat particularly severe acute retinal disease or frequently as an adjunct to systemic therapy.[137,138] Although in some instances, such local therapy may be useful, repeated injections are problematic. Aggressive therapy does seem to make a difference in the long-term outcome in these cases.[139] Miyanaga et al.[140] examined the visual outcomes in patients who were referred to them long after the onset of disease and were treated with low-dose steroid or only topical agents, and compared

CASE 25.1

A 39-year-old white woman of Native American ancestry developed bilateral posterior uveitis with serous retinal detachments. Her vision declined to 20/400 in both eyes (OU). She began to have severe headaches. Lumbar puncture was performed, and 25/mm^3 mononuclear cells were noted. Soon after, profound hearing loss developed in both ears, as documented on audiography. The patient was given high-dose oral prednisone for 1 month, and cyclosporin was added. The response in both eyes was slow, but a constant reduction in inflammatory disease was followed by a gradual improvement in visual acuity OU. Her vision eventually reached 20/40 OU. Several months after her vision was stabilized, an attempt was made to reduce and then stop cyclosporin. Recurrent intraocular inflammatory disease was observed. The patient's condition was stabilized with a dose of 10 mg of prednisone coupled with 2 to 3 mg/kg/day of cyclosporin.

these outcomes to those in patients who had undergone CSF examination and early pulse steroid therapy. They found that those with early and aggressive therapy had less integumentary involvement and less recurrent uveitis. All patients in that group had a vision of 0.8 or better, whereas 55% of those in the delayed treatment group did not. Read et al.[141] collected data from nine clinics and compared the results of patients with VKH syndrome who received oral steroid alone with those of patients receiving oral steroids plus intravenous pulse steroid therapy. No differences were seen in changes in visual acuity or in fundus changes.

The duration of treatment and the rate of therapy taper must be individualized for each patient. Rubsamen and Gass[142] treated patients with steroid therapy for 6 months, on average, and longer if the disease became chronic. In the past, steroids were given as the sole agent for extended periods (1 year), but adding a second or even a third immunosuppressive agent to reduce or eliminate the steroid dose sooner has now become the standard. Paredes et al.[143] reported that those patients with VKH syndrome receiving early immunosuppressive therapy did better in the long term with regard to their vision compared with those receiving steroid alone. Bykhovskaya et al. also found immunosuppressive use to be associated with decreased risk of vision loss.[132] This may reflect the fact that steroids cannot be maintained at an adequate dose to treat the inflammation effectively.[144]

Recurrences are possible, and patients need to be monitored. The presence of new inflammatory cells in the vitreous or extraocular complaints, such as headache, should arouse the physician's suspicion that the disorder may be recurring. However, continued RPE perturbation or increased prominence of peripheral white spots may or may not represent true disease activity. Visual field testing can be helpful in such cases. Cytotoxic agents have not been used widely in the treatment of this disorder, but a positive therapeutic response to their administration has been reported.[145] We have noted that cyclosporin has been effective in the treatment of patients with VKH syndrome who had posterior pole involvement and were not able to continue systemic corticosteroid therapy because of side effects or the extremely high doses needed to maintain good vision (see Case 25.1).[146] Wakatsuki et al.[147] reported that the combination of cyclosporin and prednisone was effective in a patient who required 200 mg or more of prednisone to control the disease, paralleling our experience. Others used prednisone and cyclosporin combined with azathioprine,[148] and Kim et al.[149] suggested the use of low-dose azathioprine. Others have also reported its therapeutic efficacy but stressed the secondary effects and the possibility of disease relapse with drug withdrawal.[150] Abu El-Asrar et al. reported a reduced rate of complications and improved visual outcomes with the use of cyclosporin and mycophenolate mofetil as first-line therapy.[151] Yang et al. reported successful inflammation control in greater than 97% of their 998 patients with VKH

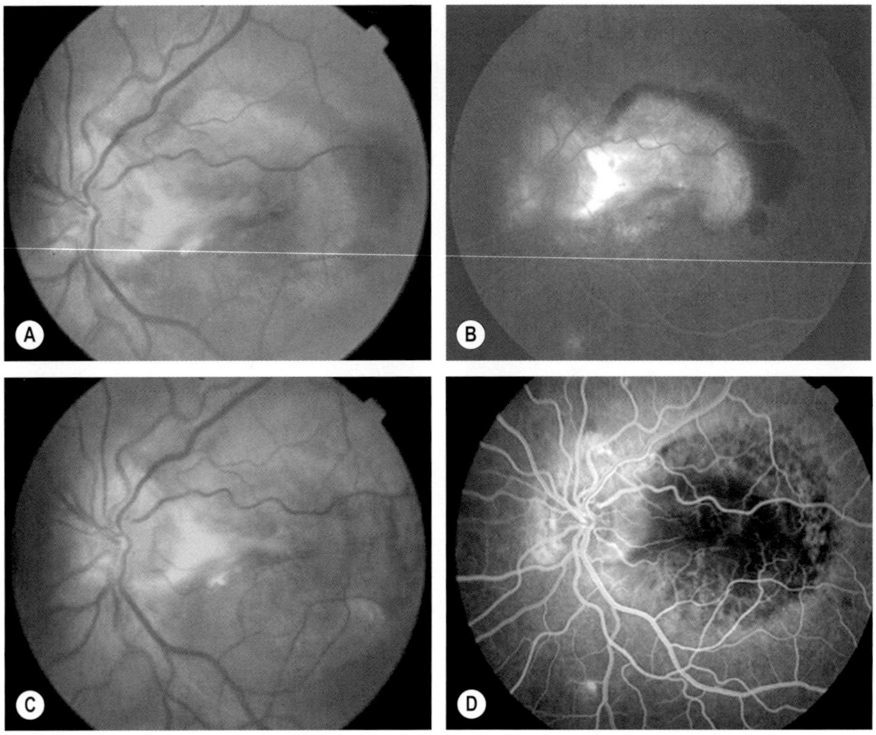

Fig. 25.12 A and B, A 10-year-old girl with VKH and a large subretinal neovascular membrane involving her whole posterior pole. Vision was 20/800. C and D, Photodynamic therapy was given, and vision stabilized at 20/320. (Courtesy of Rubens Belfort Jr, MD, and Cristina Muccioli, MD, São Paulo, Brazil.)

syndrome with the use of low-dose systemic corticosteroids combined with immunosuppressives, including cyclosporin, cyclophosphamide, methotrexate, and azathioprine. This regimen resulted in visual stability or improvement in greater than 88% of their cohort.[152] The combination of cyclosporine and azathioprine was suggested to induce remission faster compared with the combination of cyclosporine and mycophenolate in a small cohort.[153] Arevalo et al. noted that all of their 154 patients with VKH syndrome were treated with oral prednisone, with 31% also having received intravenous pulse steroids at disease onset. In this cohort, the authors reported a higher proportion of patients requiring immunosuppressive medications (76.6%), and the most commonly used immunosuppressives were cyclosporin in almost half (48.8%), followed by azathioprine, mycophenolate mofetil, and methotrexate.[154] Tacrolimus (FK506)[155] has been used in a small number of patients with VKH syndrome, resulting in a positive therapeutic response but with numerous adverse effects. TNF inhibitors, such as infliximab (Remicade) and adalimumab (Humira), have also been successfully used for the treatment of VKH syndrome in both adults and children.[156-158]

Subretinal neovascular membranes can occur in VKH syndrome and need to be treated (Fig. 25.12). Photodynamic therapy (PDT) was used in six eyes, with five demonstrating recent classic lesions and five having active inflammation.[159] The results appeared to be mixed. Although PDT appeared to control the membrane, subretinal fibrosis developed. Anti–vascular endothelial growth factor (VEGF) therapies are preferred today, and have been reported to be effective in the treatment of neovascular membranes complicating VKH syndrome.[160]

REFERENCES

1. Herbort CP, Mochizuki M. Vogt-Koyanagi-Harada disease. Inquiry into the genesis of a disease name in the historical context of Switzerland and Japan. *Int Ophthalmol.* 2007;27(2–3):67–79.
2. Vogt A. Frühzeitiges Ergrauen der Zilien und Bemerkungen üben den sogannten plözlichen Eintritt dieser Veränderung. *Klin Monatsbl Augenheilkd.* 1906;44:228–242.
3. Koyanagi Y. Dysakusis, Alopecia un Poliosis bei schwerer Uveitis nicht traumatischen Ursprungs. *Klin Monatsbl Augenheilkd.* 1929;82:194–211.
4. Harada E. Clinical observations of nonsuppurative choroiditis. *Acta Soc Ophthalmol Jpn.* 1926;30:356.
5. Babel J. Syndrome de Vogt-Koyanagi. *Schweiz Med Wochenschr.* 1932;44:1136–1140.
6. Sugiura S. Vogt-Koyanagi-Harada disease. *Jpn J Ophthalmol.* 1978;22:9–35.
7. Abad S, Monnet D, Caillat-Zucman S, et al. Characteristics of Vogt-Koyanagi-Harada disease in a French cohort: ethnicity, systemic manifestations, and HLA genotype data. *Ocul Immunol Inflamm.* 2008;16(1):3–8.
8. Belfort Jr Rubens. *Personal communication*; 1995.
9. Ohno S, Minakawa R, Matsuda H. Clinical studies on Vogt-Koyanagi-Harada's disease. *Jpn J Ophthalmol.* 1988;32:334–343.
10. Sukavatcharin S, Tsai JH, Rao NA. Vogt-Koyanagi-Harada disease in Hispanic patients. *Int Ophthalmol.* 2007;27(2–3):143–148.
11. Garcia LA, Carroll MO, Garza Leon MA. Vogt-Koyanagi-Harada syndrome in childhood. *Int Ophthalmol Clin.* 2008;48(3):107–117.
12. Lacerda R. Sindrome de Vogt-Koyanagi-Harada: descrição de um caso especial em criança de sete anos de idade. *Arq Bras Oftal.* 1994;57:46–48.
13. Tabbara KF, Chavis PS, Freeman WR. Vogt-Koyanagi-Harada syndrome in children compared to adults. *Acta Ophthalmol Scand.* 1998;76:723–726.
14. Berker N, Ozdamar Y, Soykan E, et al. Vogt-Koyanagi-Harada syndrome in children: report of a case and review of the literature. *Ocul Immunol Inflamm.* 2007;15(4):351–357.
15. Rathinam SR, Vijayalakshmi P, Namperumalsamy P, et al. Vogt-Koyanagi-Harada syndrome in children. *Ocul Immunol Inflamm.* 1998;6:155–161.
16. Abu El-Asrar AM, Al-Kharashi AS, Aldibhi H, Al-Fraykh H, Kangave D. Vogt-Koyanagi-Harada disease in children. *Eye.* 2008;22(9):1124–1131. 31.
17. Perry H, Font R. Clinical and histopathologic observations in severe Vogt-Koyanagi-Harada syndrome. *Am J Ophthalmol.* 1977;83:242–254.

18. Read RW, Holland GN, Rao NA, et al. Revised diagnostic criteria for Vogt-Koyanagi-Harada disease: report of an international committee on nomenclature. *Am J Ophthalmol.* 2001;131(5):647–652.
19. Rao NA, Sukavatcharin S, Tsai JH. Vogt-Koyanagi-Harada disease diagnostic criteria. *Int Ophthalmol.* 2007;27(2–3):195–199.
20. Beniz J, Forster DJ, Lean JS, et al. Variations in clinical features of the Vogt-Koyanagi-Harada syndrome. *Retina.* 1991;11:275–280.
21. Ikeda M, Tsukagoshi H. Vogt-Koyanagi-Harada disease presenting meningoencephalitis. Report of a case with magnetic resonance imaging. *Eur Neurol.* 1992;32:83–85.
22. Katterer C, Kaeser H, Steiger U. Rare form of uveitis with neurological symptoms: the Vogt-Koyanagi-Harada uveomeningoencephalitic syndrome. *Schweiz Med Wochenschr.* 1992;33:281–292.
23. Sugiura S. Some observations on uveitis in Japan, with special reference to Vogt-Koyanagi-Harada and Behçet diseases (author's transl). *Nippon Ganka Gakkai Zasshi.* 1976;80(11):1285–1326.
24. Kim LA, Khurana RN, Parikh JG, et al. Melanin-laden macrophages in the CSF to diagnose Vogt-Koyanagi-Harada simulating ocular syphilis. *Ocul Immunol Inflamm.* 2008;16(1):59–61.
25. Ondrey FG, Moldestad E, Mastroianni MA, et al. Sensorineural hearing loss in Vogt-Koyanagi-Harada syndrome. *Laryngoscope.* 2006;116(10):1873–1876.
26. Rosen E. Uveitis, with poliosis, vitiligo, alopecia and dysacousia (Vogt-Koyanagi syndrome). *Arch Ophthalmol.* 1945;33:281–292.
27. Igawa K, Endo H, Yokozeki H, et al. Alopecia in Vogt-Koyanagi-Harada syndrome. *J Eur Acad Dermatol Venereol.* 2006;20(2):236–238.
28. Arellanes-Garcia L, Hernandez-Barrios M, Fromow-Guerra J, Cervantes-Fanning P. Fluorescein fundus angiographic findings in Vogt-Koyanagi-Harada syndrome. *Int Ophthalmol.* 2007;27(2–3):155–161.
29. Kimura R, Sakai M, Okabe H. Transient shallow anterior chamber as initial symptom in Harada's syndrome. *Arch Ophthalmol.* 1981;99:1604–1606.
30. Kimura R, Kasai M, Shoji K, et al. Swollen ciliary processes as an initial symptom in Vogt-Koyanagi-Harada syndrome. *Am J Ophthalmol.* 1983;95:402–403.
31. Okinami S, Ogino N, Matsumura M, et al. Neovascularization at the angle of anterior chamber in cases of uveitis—high incidence in Vogt-Koyanagi-Harada disease. *Nippon Ganka Gakkai Zasshi.* 1982;86:2186–2189.
32. Forster DJ, Rao NA, Hill RA, et al. Incidence and management of glaucoma in Vogt-Koyanagi-Harada syndrome. *Am J Ophthalmol.* 1993;100:613–618.
33. Tabbara KF. Scleromalacia associated with Vogt-Koyanagi-Harada syndrome. *Am J Ophthalmol.* 1988;105:694–695.
34. Oellers P, Jaffe GJ, Proia AD. Clinical-pathological correlation of Vogt-Koyanagi-Harada disease. *JAMA Ophthalmol.* 2016;134(3):343–345.
35. Rutzen AR, Ortega-Larrocea G, Frambach DA, et al. Macular edema in chronic Vogt-Koyanagi-Harada syndrome. *Retina.* 1995;15:475–479.
36. Yang P, Ye Z, Xu J, et al. Macular abnormalities in Vogt-Koyanagi-Harada disease. *Ocul Immunol Inflamm.* 2019;27(8):1195–1202.
37. Baxter SL, Pistilli M, Pujari SS, et al. Risk of choroidal neovascularization among the uveitides. *Am J Ophthalmol.* 2013;156(3):468–477. e2.
38. Patel AK, Newcomb CW, Liesegang TL, et al. Systemic Immunosuppressive Therapy for Eye Diseases Research Group. Risk of retinal neovascularization in cases of uveitis. *Ophthalmology.* 2016;123(3):646–654.
39. Ober R, Smith R, Ryan S. Subretinal neovascularization in the Vogt-Koyanagi-Harada syndrome. *Int Ophthalmol.* 1983;6:225–234.
40. Moorthy R, Chong LP, Smith RE, et al. Subretinal neovascular membranes in Vogt-Koyanagi-Harada syndrome. *Am J Ophthalmol.* 1993;116:164–170.
41. Gaspar FT, Da Silva C, Damico FM, et al. Revised diagnostic criteria for Vogt-Koyanagi-Harada disease: considerations on the different disease categories. *Am J Ophthalmol.* 2009;147(2):339–345.
42. Yamaki K, Hara K, Sakuragi S. Application of revised diagnostic criteria for Vogt-Koyanagi-Harada disease in Japanese patients. *Jpn J Ophthalmol.* 2005;49(2):143–148.
43. Keino H, Goto H, Usui M. Sunset glow fundus in Vogt-Koyanagi-Harada disease with or without chronic ocular inflammation. *Graefes Arch Clin Exp Ophthalmol.* 2002;240:878–882.
44. Mondkar SV, Biswas J, Ganesh SK. Analysis of 87 cases with Vogt-Koyanagi-Harada Disease. *Jpn J Ophthalmol.* 2000;44:296–301.
45. Sakata VM, da Silva FT, Hirata CE, et al. High-rate of clinical recurrence in patients with Vogt-Koyanagi-Harada disease treated with early high-dose corticosteroids. *Graefes Arch Clin Exp Ophthalmol.* 2015;253:785–790.
46. Chee SP, Jap A, Bascal K. Spectrum of Vogt-Koyanagi-Harada disease in Singapore. *Int Ophthalmol.* 2007;27:137–142.
47. Tanigawa M, Ochiai H, Tsukahara Y, Ochiai Y, Yamanaka H. Choroidal folds in acute-stage Vogt-Koyanagi-Harada disease patients with relatively short axial length. *Case Rep Ophthalmol.* 2012;3(1):38–45.
48. Kuo IC, Rechdouni A, Rao NA, Johnston RH, Margolis TP, Cunningham ET Jr. Subretinal fibrosis in patients with Vogt-Koyanagi-Harada disease. *Ophthalmology.* 2000;107(9):1721–1728.
49. Zhao C, Dong F, Gao F, et al. Longitudinal observation of subretinal fibrosis in Vogt-Koyanagi-Harada disease. *BMC Ophthalmol.* 2018;18(1):6.
50. Yang P, Ren Y, Li B, Fang W, Meng Q, Kijlstra A. Clinical characteristics of Vogt-Koyanagi-Harada syndrome in Chinese patients. *Ophthalmology.* 2007;114(3):606–614.
51. Chee SP, Luu CD, Cheng CL, et al. Visual function in Vogt-Koyanagi-Harada patients. *Graefes Arch Clin Exp Ophthalmol.* 2005;243(8):785–790.
52. Jap A, Luu CD, Yeo I, et al. Correlation between peripapillary atrophy and corticosteroid therapy in patients with Vogt-Koyanagi-Harada disease. *Eye.* 2008;22(2):240–245.
53. Sonoda S, Nakao K, Ohbo N. Extensive chorioretinal atrophy in Vogt-Koyanagi-Harada disease. *Jpn J Ophthalmol.* 1999;43:113–119.
54. Lertsumitkul S, Whitcup SM, Nussenblatt RB, et al. Subretinal fibrosis and choroidal neovascularization in Vogt-Koyanagi-Harada syndrome. *Graefes Arch Clin Exp Ophthalmol.* 1999;237:1039–1045.
55. Al-Kharashi AS, Aldibhi H, Al-Fraykh H, et al. Prognostic factors in Vogt-Koyanagi–Harada disease. *Int Ophthalmol.* 2007;27(2–3):201–210.
56. Kayazawa F, Takahashi H. Acute posterior multifocal placoid pigment epitheliopathy and Harada's disease. *Ann Opthalmol.* 1983;15:58–62.
57. Rao N, Marak G. Sympathetic ophthalmia simulating Vogt-Koyanagi-Harada's disease: a clinico-pathologic study of four cases. *Jpn J Ophthalmol.* 1983;27:506–511.
58. Kamondi A, Szegedi A, Papp A, et al. Vogt-Koyanagi-Harada disease presenting initially as aseptic meningoencephalitis. *Eur J Neurol.* 2000;7:719–722.
59. Kouda N, Sasaki H, Harada S, et al. Early Manifestation of Vogt-Koyanagi-Harada disease as unilateral posterior scleritis. *Jpn J Ophthalmol.* 2002;46:590–593.
60. Khurana RN, Albini T, Green RL, et al. *Bartonella henselae* infection presenting as a unilateral panuveitis simulating Vogt-Koyanagi-Harada syndrome. *Am J Ophthalmol.* 2004;138(6):1063–1065.
61. Pahk PJ, Todd DJ, Blaha GR, et al. Intravascular lymphoma masquerading as Vogt-Koyanagi-Harada syndrome. *Ocul Immunol Inflamm.* 2008;16(3):123–126.
62. Papastathopoulos K, Bouzas E, Naoum G, et al. Vogt-Koyanagi-Harada disease associated with interferon-A and ribavirin therapy for chronic hepatitis C infection. *J Infect.* 2006;52(2):e59–e61.
63. Touitou V, Sene D, Fardeau C, et al. Interferon-α2a and Vogt-Koyanagi-Harada disease: a double-edged sword? *Int Ophthalmol.* 2007;27(2–3):211–215.
64. Manger CI, Ober R. Retinal arteriovenous anastomoses in the Vogt-Koyanagi-Harada syndrome. *Am J Ophthalmol.* 1980;89:186–191.
65. Herbort CP, Mantovani A, Bouchenaki N. Indocyanine green angiography in Vogt-Koyanagi-Harada disease: angiographic signs and utility in patient follow-up. *Int Ophthalmol.* 2007;27(2–3):173–182.
66. Wu W, Wen F, Huang S, et al. Indocyanine green angiographic findings of Dalen-Fuchs nodules in Vogt-Koyanagi-Harada disease. *Graefes Arch Clin Exp Ophthalmol.* 2007;245(7):937–940.
67. Chee SP, Jap A, Cheung CM. The prognostic value of angiography in Vogt-Koyanagi-Harada disease. *Am J Ophthalmol.* 2010;150(6):888–893.
68. Heussen FM, Vasconcelos-Santos DV, Pappuru RR, Walsh AC, Rao NA, Sadda SR. Ultra-wide-field green-light (532-nm) autofluorescence imaging in chronic Vogt-Koyanagi-Harada disease. *Ophthalmic Surg Lasers Imaging.* 2011;42(4):272–277.

69. Koizumi H, Maruyama K, Kinoshita S. Blue light and near-infrared fundus autofluorescence in acute Vogt-Koyanagi-Harada disease. *Br J Ophthalmol.* 2010;94(11):1499–1505.
70. Miura M, Makita S, Azuma S, et al. Evaluation of retinal pigment epithelium layer change in Vogt-Koyanagi-Harada disease with multicontrast optical coherence tomography. *Invest Ophthalmol Vis Sci.* 2019;60(10):3352–3362.
71. Nakamura T, Hayashi A, Oiwake T. Long-term changes of retinal pigment epithelium in the eyes with Vogt-Koyanagi-Harada disease observed by adaptive optics imaging. *Clin Ophthalmol.* 2019;13:927–933.
72. Gallagher MJ, Yilmaz T, Cervantes-Castañeda RA, et al. The characteristic features of optical coherence tomography in posterior uveitis. *Br J Ophthalmol.* 2007;91(12):1680–1685.
73. Yamamura K, Mori K, Hieda O, et al. Anterior segment optical coherence tomography findings of acute angle-closure glaucoma in Vogt-Koyanagi-Harada disease. *Jpn J Ophthalmol.* 2008;52(3):231–232.
74. Yamaguchi Y, Otani T, Kishi S. Tomographic features of serous retinal detachment with multilobular dye pooling in acute Vogt-Koyanagi- Harada disease. *Am J Ophthalmol.* 2007;144(2):260–265.
75. Fong AH, Li KK, Wong D. Choroidal evaluation using enhanced depth imaging spectral-domain optical coherence tomography in Vogt-Koyanagi-Harada disease. *Retina.* 2011;31(3):502–509.
76. Zhao C, Zhang MF, Dong FT, et al. Spectral domain optical coherence tomography of Vogt-Koyanagi-Harada disease: novel findings and new insights into the pathogenesis. *Chin Med Sci J.* 2012;27(1):29–34.
77. Wu W, Wen F, Huang S, et al. Choroidal folds in Vogt-Koyanagi-Harada disease. *Am J Ophthalmol.* 2007;143(5):900–901.
78. Yang P, Fang W, Wang L, et al. Study of macular function by multifocal electroretinography in patients with Vogt-Koyanagi-Harada syndrome. *Am J Ophthalmol.* 2008;146(5):767–771.
79. Nagaya T. Use of the electro-oculogram for diagnosing and following the development of Harada's disease. *Am J Ophthalmol.* 1972;74:99–109.
80. Okamoto Y, Miyake Y, Horio N, et al. Delayed regeneration of foveal cone photopigments in Vogt-Koyanagi-Harada disease at the convalescent stage. *Invest Ophthalmol Vis Sci.* 2004;45(1):318–322.
81. Suzuki S. Quantitative evaluation of 'sunset glow' fundus in Vogt-Koyanagi–Harada disease. *Jpn J Ophthalmol.* 1999;43:327–333.
82. Okubo K, Kurimoto S, Okubo K, et al. Surface markers of peripheral blood lymphocytes in Vogt-Koyanagi-Harada disease. *J Clin Lab Immunol.* 1985;17:49–52.
83. Liu T, Sun S. Peripheral lymphocyte subsets in patients with Vogt-Koyanagi-Harada syndrome (VKH). *Chung Hua Yen Ko Tsa Chih.* 1993;29:138–140.
84. Ohno S. Immunological aspects of Behçet's and Vogt-Koyanagi-Harada's diseases. *Trans Ophthalmol Soc UK.* 1981;101:335–341.
85. Hooks J, Moutsopoulos HM, Geis SA, et al. Immune interferon in the circulation of patients with autoimmune disease. *N Engl J Med.* 1979;301:5–8.
86. Sakaguchi M, Sugita S, Sagawa K, et al. Cytokine production by T cells infiltrating in the eye of uveitis patients. *Jpn J Ophthalmol.* 1998;42:262–268.
87. Imai Y, Sugita M, Nakamura S, et al. Cytokine production and helper T cell subsets in Vogt-Koyanagi-Harada's disease. *Curr Eye Res.* 2001;22:312–318.
88. Ohta K, Yoshimura N. Expression of Fas antigen on helper T lymphocytes in Vogt-Koyanagi-Harada disease. *Graefes Arch Clin Exp Ophthalmol.* 1998;236:434–439.
89. Miyazawa I, Abe T, Narikawa K, et al. Chemokine profile in the cerebrospinal fluid and serum of Vogt-Koyanagi-Harada disease. *J Neuroimmunol.* 2005;158(1–2):240–244.
90. Li B, Yang P, Zhou H, et al. Upregulation of T-bet expression in peripheral blood mononuclear cells during Vogt-Koyanagi-Harada disease. *Br J Ophthalmol.* 2005;89(11):1410–1412.
91. Chen L, Yang P, Zhou H, et al. Diminished frequency and function of CD4+CD25high regulatory T cells associated with active uveitis in Vogt-Koyanagi-Harada syndrome. *Invest Ophthalmol Vis Sci.* 2008;49(8):3475–3482.
92. Chi W, Yang P, Li B, et al. IL-23 promotes CD4+ T cells to produce IL-17 in Vogt-Koyanagi-Harada disease. *J Allergy Clin Immunol.* 2007;119(5):1218–1224.
93. Liu L, Yang P, He H, et al. Leptin increases in Vogt-Koyanagi-Harada (VKH) disease and promotes cell proliferation and inflammatory cytokine secretion. *Br J Ophthalmol.* 2008;92(4):557–561.
94. Urzua CA, Chen P, Chaigne-Delalande B, et al. Glucocorticoid receptor-α and MKP-1 as candidate biomarkers for treatment response and disease activity in Vogt-Koyanagi-Harada disease. *Am J Ophthalmol.* 2019;207:319–325.
95. Momoeda S. Lymphocyte transformation test in Vogt-Koyanagi-Harada syndrome. *Acta Soc Ophthalmol Jpn.* 1976;80:491–495.
96. Yuasa T, Murai Y, Hoki T, et al. Lymphocyte transformation test and migration inhibition test of macrophages in Vogt-Koyanagi-Harada's syndrome. *Acta Soc Ophthalmol Jpn.* 1973;77:1652–1657.
97. Maezawa N, Yano A, Taniguchi M, et al. The role of cytotoxic T lymphocytes in the pathogenesis of Vogt-Koyanagi-Harada disease. *Ophthalmologica.* 1982;185:179–186.
98. Maezawa N, Yano A. Requirement of Ia-positive nylon wool adherent cells for the activation of cytotoxic T lymphocytes specific for melanocyte-associated antigens in patients with Vogt-Koyanagi-Harada's disease. *Jpn J Opthalmol.* 1988;32:348–357.
99. Yamaki K, Gocho K, Hayakawa K, et al. Tyrosinase family proteins are antigens specific to Vogt-Koyanagi-Harada disease. *J Immunol.* 2000;165:7323–7329.
100. Sugita S, Takase H, Taguchi C, et al. Ocular infiltrating CD4+ T cells from patients with Vogt-Koyanagi-Harada disease recognize human melanocyte antigens. *Invest Ophthalmol Vis Sci.* 2006;47(6):2547–2554.
101. Yamaki K, Kondo I, Nakamura H, et al. Ocular and extraocular inflammation induced by immunization of tyrosinase related protein 1 and 2 in Lewis rats. *Exp Eye Res.* 2000;71:361–369.
102. Gocho K, Kondo I, Yamaki K. Identification of autoreactive T cells in Vogt-Koyanagi-Harada disease. *Invest Ophthalmol Vis Sci.* 2001;42:2004–2009.
103. Yamada K, Senju S, Shinohara T, et al. Humoral immune response directed against LEDGF in patients with VKH. *Immunol Lett.* 2001;78:161–168.
104. Yeh S, Karne NK, Kerkar SP, et al. Ocular and systemic autoimmunity after successful tumor-infiltrating lymphocyte immunotherapy for recurrent, metastatic melanoma. *Ophthalmology.* 2009;116(5):981–989.
105. Nussenblatt R, Gery I, Ballintine EJ, et al. Cellular immune responsiveness of uveitis patients to retinal S-antigen. *Am J Ophthalmol.* 1980;89(2):173–179.
106. Chan C, Palestine AG, Nussenblatt RB, et al. Anti-retinal auto-antibodies in Vogt-Koyanagi-Harada syndrome, Behçet's disease, and sympathetic ophthalmia. *Ophthalmology.* 1985;92:1025–1028.
107. Rathinam SR, Namperumalsamy P, Nozik RA, et al. Vogt-Koyanagi-Harada syndrome after cutaneous injury. *Ophthalmology.* 1999;106:635–638.
108. Kesav NP, Kaplan AJ, Hwang CK, et al. Tattoo-associated cases of posterior segment uveitis with Vogt-Koyanagi-Harada disease-like features. Retin Cases Brief Rep. 2020 Jun 3. doi: 10.1097/ICB.0000000000001007. Epub ahead of print. PMID: 32502130.
109. Ashkenazi I, Gutman I, Melamed S, et al. Vogt-Koyanagi-Harada syndrome in two siblings. *Metab Pediatr Syst Ophthalmol.* 1991;14:64–67.
110. Itho S, Kurimoto S, Kouno T. Vogt-Koyanagi-Harada disease in monozygotic twins. *Int Ophthalmol.* 1992;16:49–54.
111. Kunikane H. Analysis of HLA-DQWa antigen ethnic polymorphism among a Japanese and Caucasian population and an association with Harada's disease. *Hokkaido Igaku Zasshi.* 1986;61:672–681.
112. Zhao M, Yougin J, Abrahams I. Association of HLA antigens with Vogt-Koyanagi–Harada syndrome in a Han Chinese population. *Arch Ophthalmol.* 1991;109:368–370.
113. Zhang X, Wang X, Hu T. Profiling human leukocyte antigens in Vogt-Koyanagi-Harada syndrome. *Am J Ophthalmol.* 1992;113:567–572.
114. Numaga J, Matsuki K, Tokunaga K, et al. Analysis of human leukocyte antigen HLA-DR beta amino acid sequence in Vogt-Koyanagi-Harada syndrome. *Invest Ophthalmol Vis Sci.* 1991;32:1958–1961.
115. Yu Q, Mao W, Xie C, et al. HLA antigens and Vogt-Koyanagi-Harada's disease. *Yen Ko Hsueh Pao.* 1991;7:3–5.

116. Kim MH, Seong MC, Kwak NH, et al. Association of HLA with Vogt-Koyanagi-Harada syndrome in Koreans. *Am J Ophthalmol.* 2000;129:173–177.
117. Davis J, Mittal KK, Freidlin V, et al. HLA associations and ancestry in Vogt-Koyanagi-Harada disease and sympathetic ophthalmia. *Ophthalmology.* 1990;97:1137–1142.
118. Rutzen A, Ortega-Larrocea G, Schwab IR, et al. Simultaneous onset of Vogt-Koyanagi-Harada syndrome in monozygotic twins. *Am J Opthalmol.* 1995;119:239–240.
119. Martinez J, Lopez PF, Sternberg P Jr, et al. Vogt-Koyanagi-Harada syndrome in patients with Cherokee Indian ancestry. *Am J Opthalmol.* 1992;144:615–620.
120. Alaez C, del Pilar Mora M, Arellanes L, et al. Strong association of HLA class II sequences in Mexicans with Vogt-Koyanagi-Harada's disease. *Hum Immunol.* 1999;60:875–882.
121. Levinson RD, See RF, Rajalingam R, et al. HLA-DRB1 and -DQB1 alleles in Mestizo patients with Vogt-Koyanagi-Harada's disease in Southern California. *Hum Immunol.* 2004;65(12):1477–1482.
122. Levinson RD, Du Z, Luo L, et al. KIR and HLA gene combinations in Vogt-Koyanagi-Harada disease. *Hum Immunol.* 2008;69(6):349–353.
123. Horie Y, Takemoto Y, Miyazaki A, et al. Tyrosinase gene family and Vogt-Koyanagi-Harada disease in Japanese patients. *Mol Vis.* 2006;12:1601–1605.
124. Horie Y, Kitaichi N, Takemoto Y, et al. Polymorphism of IFN-gamma gene and Vogt-Koyanagi-Harada disease. *Mol Vis.* 2007;13:2334–2338.
125. Du L, Yang P, Hou S, et al. Association of the CTLA-4 gene with Vogt-Koyanagi-Harada syndrome. *Clin Immunol.* 2008;127(1):43–48.
126. Morris W, Schlaegel TJ. Virus-like inclusion bodies in subretinal fluid in uveo-encephalitis. *Am J Opthalmol.* 1964;58:940–945.
127. Moreira M, Moreira C. Virus search in cerebrospinal fluid in Vogt-Koyanagi syndrome: report of a case. *Arq Neuropsiquiatr.* 1984;42:408–410.
128. Sunakawa M, Okinami S. Epstein-Barr virus-related antibody pattern in uveitis. *Jpn J Opthalmol.* 1985;29:423–428.
129. Ye Z, Wu C, Zhang N, et al. Altered gut microbiome composition in patients with Vogt-Koyanagi-Harada disease. *Gut Microbes.* 2020;11(3):539–555. 1-17.
130. Rao NA. Mechanisms of inflammatory response in sympathetic ophthalmia and VKH syndrome. *Eye.* 1997;11:213–216.
131. Rao NA. Pathology of Vogt-Koyanagi-Harada disease. *Int Ophthalmol.* 2007;27(2–3):81–85.
132. Bykhovskaya I, Thorne JE, Kempen JH, et al. Vogt-Koyanagi-Harada disease: clinical outcomes. *Am J Ophthalmol.* 2005;140(4):674–678.
133. Hayasaka S, Okabe H, Takahashi J. Systemic corticosteroid treatment in Vogt-Koyanagi-Harada disease. *Graefes Arch Clin Exp Ophthalmol.* 1982;218:9–13.
134. Nakayama M, Keino H, Watanabe T, Okada AA. Clinical features and visual outcomes of 111 patients with new-onset acute Vogt-Koyanagi-Harada disease treated with pulse intravenous corticosteroids. *Br J Ophthalmol.* 2019;103(2):274–278.
135. Doi M, Matsubara H, Uji Y. Vogt-Koyanagi-Harada syndrome in a pregnant patient treated with high-dose systemic corticosteroids. *Acta Ophthalmol Scand.* 2000;78:93–96.
136. Miyata N, Sugita M, Nakamura S, et al. Treatment of Vogt-Koyanagi-Harada's disease during pregnancy. *Jpn J Ophthalmol.* 2001;45:177–180.
137. Andrade RE, Muccioli C, Farah ME, et al. Intravitreal triamcinolone in the treatment of serous retinal detachment in Vogt-Koyanagi-Harada syndrome. *Am J Ophthalmol.* 2004;137(3):572–574.
138. Moreker MR, Lodhi SA, Pathengay A. Role of intravitreal triamcinolone as an adjuvant in the management of Vogt-Koyanagi-Harada disease. *Indian J Ophthalmol.* 2007;55(6):479–480.
139. Yang P, Ren Y, Li B, et al. Clinical characteristics of Vogt-Koyanagi-Harada syndrome in Chinese patients. *Ophthalmology.* 2007;114(3):606–614.
140. Miyanaga M, Kawaguchi T, Shimizu K, et al. Influence of early cerebrospinal fluid-guided diagnosis and early high-dose corticosteroid therapy on ocular outcomes of Vogt-Koyanagi-Harada disease. *Int Ophthalmol.* 2007;27(2–3):183–188.
141. Read RW, Yu F, Accorinti M, et al. Evaluation of the effect on outcomes of the route of administration of corticosteroids in acute Vogt-Koyanagi-Harada disease. *Am J Ophthalmol.* 2006;142(1):119–124.
142. Rubsamen P, Gass D, Vogt-Koyanagi-Harada syndrome. Clinical course, therapy, and long-term visual outcome. *Arch Ophthalmol.* 1991;109:682–687.
143. Paredes I, Ahmed M, Foster CS. Immunomodulatory therapy for Vogt-Koyanagi-Harada patients as first-line therapy. *Ocul Immunol Inflamm.* 2006;14(2):87–90.
144. Andreoli CM, Foster CS. Vogt-Koyanagi-Harada disease. *Int Ophthalmol Clin.* 2006;46(2):111–122.
145. Limon S, Girard R, Bloch-Michel E, et al. Les aspects actuels du syndrome du Vogt-Koyanagi-Harada. Apropos de 9 cas. *J Fr Opthalmol.* 1985;8:29–35.
146. Nussenblatt R, Palestine A, Chan C. Cyclosporin A therapy in the treatment of intraocular inflammatory disease resistant to systemic corticosteroids and cytotoxic agents. *Am J Ophthalmol.* 1983;96:275–282.
147. Wakatsuki Y, Kogure M, Takahashi Y, et al. Combination therapy of cyclosporin A and steroid in the severe case of Vogt-Koyanagi-Harada's disease. *Jpn J Ophthalmol.* 1988;32:358–360.
148. Agarwal M, Ganesh SK, Biswas J. Triple agent immunosuppressive therapy in Vogt-Koyanagi-Harada syndrome. *Ocul Immunol Inflamm.* 2006;14(6):333–339.
149. Kim SJ, Yu HG. The use of low-dose azathioprine in patients with Vogt-Koyanagi-Harada disease. *Ocul Immunol Inflamm.* 2007;15(5):381–387.
150. Wakefield D, McCluckey P. Cyclosporine: a therapy in inflammatory eye disease. *J Ocul Pharmacol.* 1991;7:221–226.
151. Abu El-Asrar AM, Al Tamimi M, Hemachandran S, Al-Mezaine HS, Al-Muammar A, Kangave D. Prognostic factors for clinical outcomes in patients with Vogt-Koyanagi-Harada disease treated with high-dose corticosteroids. *Acta Ophthalmol.* 2013;91(6):e486–e493.
152. Yang P, Ye Z, Du L, et al. Novel treatment regimen of Vogt-Koyanagi-Harada disease with a reduced dose of corticosteroids combined with immunosuppressive agents. *Curr Eye Res.* 2018;43(2):254–261.
153. Arcinue CA, Radwan A, Lebanan MO, Foster CS. Comparison of two different combination immunosuppressive therapies in the treatment of Vogt-Koyanagi-Harada syndrome. *Ocul Immunol Inflamm.* 2013;21(1):47–52.
154. Arevalo JF, Lasave AF, Gupta V, et al. Clinical outcomes of patients with Vogt-Koyanagi-Harada disease over 12 years at a tertiary center. *Ocul Immunol Inflamm.* 2016;24(5):521–529.
155. Mochizuki M, Masuda K, Sakane T, et al. A clinical trial of FK506 in refractory uveitis. *Am J Ophthalmol.* 1993;115:763–769.
156. Diaz Llopis M, Amselem L, Romero FJ, et al. Adalimumab therapy for Vogt–Koyanagi–Harada syndrome. *Arch Soc Esp Oftalmol.* 2007;82(3):131–132 [in German].
157. Khalifa YM, Bailony MR, Acharya NR. Treatment of pediatric Vogt-Koyanagi-Harada syndrome with infliximab. *Ocul Immunol Inflamm.* 2010;18(3):218–222.
158. Couto C, Schlaen A, Frick M, Khoury M, Lopez M, Hurtado E, Goldstein D. Adalimumab treatment in patients with Vogt-Koyanagi-Harada disease. *Ocul Immunol Inflamm.* 2018;26(3):485–489.
159. Nowilaty SR, Bouhaimed M. Photodynamic therapy for subfoveal choroidal neovascularisation in Vogt-Koyanagi-Harada disease. *Br J Ophthalmol.* 2006;90(8):982–986.
160. Wu L, Evans T, Saravia M, Schlaen A, Couto C. Intravitreal bevacizumab for choroidal neovascularization secondary to Vogt-Koyanagi-Harada syndrome. *Jpn J Ophthalmol.* 2009;53(1):57–60.

26

Birdshot Chorioretinopathy

H. Nida Sen

KEY CONCEPTS

- Human leukocyte antigen (HLA)-A29 is very strongly associated with birdshot chorioretinopathy.
- Birdshot chorioretinopathy can lead to severe visual handicap.
- Long-term therapy is often needed to control the disease.

The spectrum of posterior uveitic entities is quite broad, with similar or identical entities referred to by various names in the literature. Better definition of these entities is a constant goal. Birdshot chorioretinopathy (BCR) fits the aforementioned spectrum and fits into the broad scheme of "white-dot syndromes." However, this disorder seems to have better-defined boundaries compared with some of the others in the white-dot group. Laboratory tests, albeit not definitive, appear to help the clinician in making this diagnosis. The entity appears to have distinct clinical characteristics; it occurs more frequently in whites of northern European extraction and has a strong genetic association. Several reviews have described it.[1-4] Because this is a chronic, ongoing disease, we need to be cognizant of the fact that it has a significant effect on the patients' quality of life.[5]

CLINICAL MANIFESTATIONS

Birdshot chorioretinopathy was first described by Ryan and Maumenee[6] in 1980 and soon after by Gass in 1981,[7] who called it *vitiliginous chorioretinitis.* According to Gass, it is seen in healthy persons, more commonly women (54%–62%),[7] with an onset somewhat later than that of other uveitic entities—in the third to the sixth decades, with average age at onset being 48 to 53 years—although younger age at onset, as young as 15 years, has also been reported.[8,9] One report described a case of birdshot chorioretinopathy with coexisting psoriasis[10]; another reported a case of BCR with coexisting autoimmune sensorineural hearing loss.[11] However, these cases may be chance occurrences. This disorder affects a small percentage of patients with uveitis seen at most uveitis centers. The proportion of patients with birdshot chorioretinopathy among all uveitis cases ranges from 4.3% in European cohorts (7.2% of posterior and panuveitis) to 0.1% in other parts of the world.[12-15] In a cohort at the National Eye Institute (NEI), 58% of these patients were women, with average age being 48 years.[16] Patients report an increased number of floaters and often have difficulty with night vision or color distinctions. The key elements of the clinical presentation, as given in the original description by Ryan and Maumenee,[6] are outlined in Box 26.1. Fig. 26.1 shows the distribution of lesions over the fundus. The criteria that have been assembled for research purposes are not really different in any major way from the clinical presentation outlined (Box 26.2).

Fuerst et al.[17] believed that they could distinguish four patterns of birdshot-spot distribution in the nine patients they evaluated: (1) macular sparing; (2) macular predominance; (3) asymmetric, with a concentration of spots, particularly inferiorly; and (4) diffuse. In our experience, the lesions tend to be present in the posterior pole and extend to the equator, but not generally beyond that. The lesions themselves appear deep in the fundus, are circular or oval in shape, and are fairly large (at times 0.75 disk diameter in area). The edges of the lesions are usually not sharply defined and frequently do not stand out, particularly in a "blond" fundus. They are best observed with the indirect ophthalmoscope. The lesions themselves may have "substance" to them; we have interpreted this appearance as evidence of an active lesion, whereas with time, they may flatten out, giving a more atrophic appearance (Fig. 26.2). The lesions can eventually disappear. Usually, the lesions in the posterior pole do not have a significant amount of pigment surrounding them and those in the periphery perhaps have even less. The overlying retina may be quite normal, although an edematous or thinned retina can be perceived in more advanced disease. In the late stages, examination of the posterior segment reveals a strikingly blond fundus, suggestive of involvement of the outer retina and the retinal pigment epithelium (RPE). Rothova and von Schooneveld[18] reported end-stage findings in a patient who did not receive immunosuppressive therapy. Electroretinography (ERG) ultimately showed a flat pattern, and the retina resembled tapetoretinal dystrophy. On fundus autofluorescence (FAF), the hypopigmented lesions did not correspond to the white-cream-colored lesions.[19] Such lesions are, however, reflective of RPE damage or death and could explain the poor vision in some patients (Fig. 26.3).

Ocular Examination and Ancillary Clinical Tests

Ocular examination shows typical ovoid lesions, vitreous inflammation, and sometimes low-grade anterior chamber inflammation. A study from France with a cohort of 58 patients with birdshot chorioretinopathy showed that 72% of patients had typical fundus lesions, 58% had optic nerve swelling, and 81% had vasculitis on examination (86% had it on fluorescein angiography); the majority had some level of vitritis.[8] Patients with more overt signs of posterior segment inflammation (e.g., vitritis and vasculitis) are more likely to have received treatment earlier and do better. Examination of the macula is imperative because cystoid macular edema (CME) is a significant sequela of this disease. At the NEI, 41% of the eyes with BCR had CME.[16] Its presence is important in establishing the diagnosis and in deciding on a correct therapeutic approach. Monnet et al.[20] reported that CME was the most common cause of a drop in visual acuity in the 80 patients they studied. Thorne et al.[21] reported CME in 20% of their patient group, noting that the longer the patient had had the disease, the greater were the chances of CME and of a decrease in vision. Similarly, Touhami et al. reported that 25% of their patients had CME at presentation and that it was associated with a poorer visual prognosis.[8]

BOX 26.1 Findings Supporting Diagnosis of Birdshot Chorioretinopathy

Patient

White

Female

Late 40s to 50s

Ocular Examination Findings

Quiet anterior chamber

Vitreal inflammation, but no snowbanking

Retinal vascular leakage and cystoid macular edema

Deep, circular, cream-colored lesions, mostly in the posterior pole and surrounding areas

Bilateral

Low to moderate risk of subretinal neovascularization

Additional Tests

Abnormal electroretinography and electrooculography findings

Evidence of retinal autoimmunity

Human leukocyte antigen (HLA)-A29+

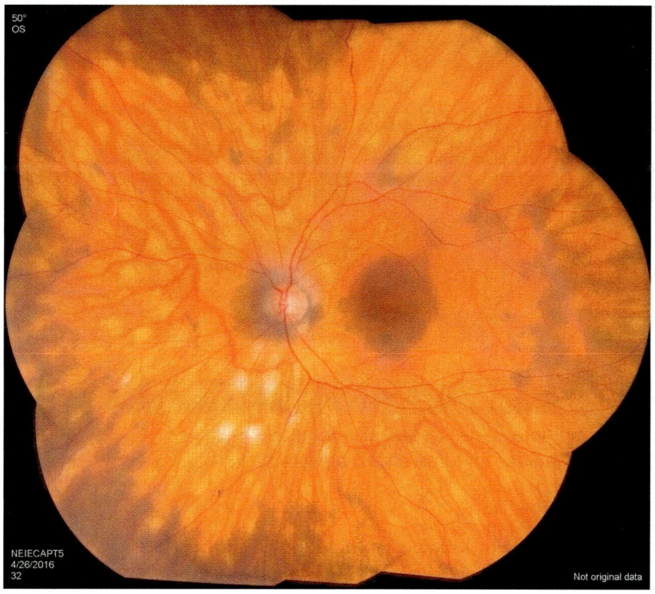

Fig. 26.1 Multiple cream-colored lesions, circular or oval, deep to the retina, are seen in birdshot chorioretinopathy. They tend to be clustered in the posterior pole but can extend out to the midperiphery.

Patients with BCR often have a vitreal reaction, although if CME is not present, visual acuity often is quite good despite the opacities present. The disease may initially be of a low grade, and patients may not be aware of visual alterations, with lesions being first noted on routine examination or after cataract surgery.[22,23]

The use of fluorescein angiography is helpful in delineating the degree of retinal vascular leakage and the severity of CME. This technique very dramatically underscores the rather marked retinal vascular component of this disease and the inflammatory disease affecting the optic nerve head (Fig. 26.4). However, as Gass first noted, as have all the investigators reporting their findings concerning this disease, the cream-colored lesions appear far more prominent when viewed through the ophthalmoscope than with fluorescein angiography. On fluorescein angiography, the characteristics of the lesion can vary

BOX 26.2 Birdshot Chorioretinopathy: Diagnostic Criteria for Research Purposes

Required Characteristics

1 Bilateral disease
2 Presence of at least three peripapillary "birdshot lesions"[a] inferior or nasal to the optic disk in one eye
3 Low-grade anterior segment intraocular inflammation (defined as ≤1 + cells in the anterior chamber)
4 Low-grade vitreous inflammatory reaction (defined as ≤2 + vitreous haze)

Supportive Findings

1 Human leukocyte antigen (HLA)-A29 positivity
2 Retinal vasculitis
3 Cystoid macular edema

Exclusion Criteria

1 Keratic precipitates
2 Posterior synechiae
3 Presence of infectious, neoplastic, or other inflammatory diseases that can cause multifocal choroidal lesions[b]

Adapted from Levinson RD, Brezin A, Rothova A, Accorinti M, Holland GN. Research criteria for the diagnosis of birdshot chorioretinopathy: results of an international consensus conference. Am J Ophthalmol. 2006 Jan;141(1):185-7.

[a] Cream-colored, irregular or elongated, choroidal lesions with indistinct borders, the long axis of which is radial to the optic disk. Typical lesions are illustrated in Fig. 26.1.

[b] Patient should be evaluated for the following disorders by appropriate history taking, physical examination, or laboratory tests: sarcoidosis with panuveitis or posterior uveitis; intraocular lymphoma; acute posterior multifocal placoid pigment epitheliopathy (APMPPE); multifocal choroiditis and panuveitis; punctate inner choroidopathy (PIC); multifocal evanescent white dot syndrome (MEWDS); pars planitis syndrome; posterior scleritis; sympathetic ophthalmia; Vogt-Koyanagi-Harada disease (chronic stage); syphilis; tuberculosis.

and depend on the age of the lesion or the phase of the procedure. Although mild hyperfluorescence may be noted in the later stage of fluorescein angiography, early angiograms may not demonstrate hypofluorescence or hyperfluorescence. Prolonged arteriovenous transit time has been reported and is believed to be caused by extreme leakage of fluorescein dye from the retinal arterioles into the surrounding tissue before entering the venous circulation[24] (Fig. 26.5).

Optical coherence tomography (OCT) is the best modality to determine the presence of CME and also to monitor for its disappearance (Fig. 26.6). Ultra-high-resolution OCT has provided a new and important view of the damage that can occur with the inflammatory disease of birdshot chorioretinopathy.[25] Monnet et al.[26] have corroborated what was described years ago—that a drop in visual acuity is associated with macular thickness rather than the area of fluorescein leakage. They reported that loss of the third highly reflective band (HRB) seen on OCT is associated with poorer visual acuity.[26] Forooghian et al.,[27] using high-definition OCT, showed that foveal atrophy was a complication of many uveitic syndromes, including BCR. Enhanced depth imaging OCT (EDI-OCT) can be helpful in assessing choroidal thickness in the active phase of the disease. Bousquet et al. showed in 80 patients with BCR that foveal choroidal thickness was lower in the patients with BCR compared with healthy controls. However, in patients with active BCR, the choroidal vascularity index was higher.[28] In a multicenter, cross-sectional study of 172 eyes of 86 individuals, Böni et al. showed that 63% of eyes showed one or more choroidal lesions defined as hyporeflective zones on EDI-OCT. These authors also noted that choroidal lesions on EDI-OCT did not always correspond to a clinically visible lesion. Use of

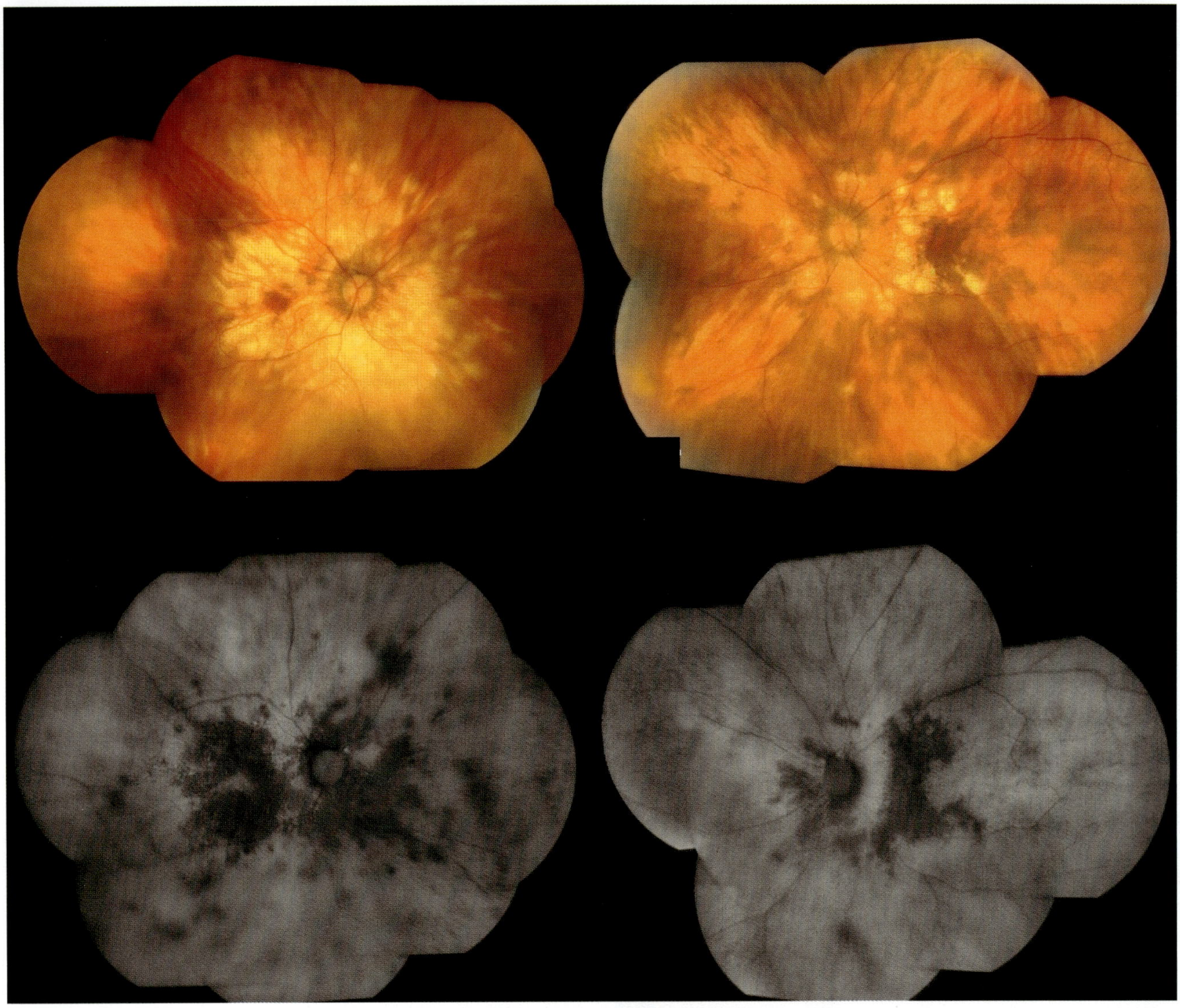

Fig. 26.2 Fundus photographs of lesions in long-standing disease. There is loss of retinal pigment epithelium and atrophic lesions *(top panel)* with corresponding hypoautofluorescence in some areas *(bottom panel)* and choroidal vessels are apparent.

immunomodulatory therapy was associated with a lower risk of abnormal choroidal thickness.[29] Birnbaum et al. also found that the presence of suprachoroidal fluid on EDI-OCT correlated with disease activity and photopsias.[30] OCT angiography (OCTA) is a newer approach to identifying vascular abnormalities in BCR. Pepple et al. was able to show choroidal flow voids in patients with active BCR near the large vessels in the Haller layer,[31] and Oberts et al. showed that retinal capillary density on OCTA was decreased in 21 patients with BCR compared with healthy controls and correlated with visual function.[32] Our group investigated the usefulness of OCT in assessing retinal vasculitis and retinal edema in patients with BCR by using montaged multifield OCT images. Perivascular thickening correlates with findings on fluorescein angiography and offers a noninvasive means of monitoring the posterior pole vessels.[33] We have also shown that choroidal lesions in patients with BCR can be differentially visualized by using multispectral widefield scanning laser ophthalmoscopy (Optos 532 nm and 635 nm lasers).[34]

Pohlmann et al. investigated multimodal imaging in patients with BCR and found capillary loops (58%) and telangiectatic vessels (44%) on OCTA. Altered superficial and deep capillary architecture significantly correlated with disease activity. In 72% of these patients, there was no fluorescein leakage on the peripheral or posterior pole retinal vessels, and macular leakage was present only in approximately 17%. FAF showed hypofluorescent dots in 67%, likely representing old, atrophic lesions, and indocyanine green (ICG) angiography showed hypocyanescent spots in 22%.[35]

Although ICG angiography (Fig. 26.7) has been used to elucidate more lesions than are seen clinically, early on in its use, it was suggested that it was not particularly useful in monitoring the disease course.[36] Herbort et al.[37] have shown that choroidal lesions evolve differently from retinal lesions, with the former seeming more responsive to immunosuppressive therapy. Lommatzsch et al.[38] studied choroidal blood flow by using perfusion-pressure videoangiography in a patient with BCR. They found that in this patient, fluorescein dye penetrated through the vessel walls of the large choroidal arterioles close to the short posterior ciliary arteries. ICG angiography can be sensitive for the diagnosis or management of patients with BCR. In patients with retinal vasculitis and low-grade inflammation and no apparent choroidal lesions on clinical examination, ICG angiography can help identify lesions.[39] ICG angiography has been suggested to be more sensitive than other modalities in detecting subclinical recurrences after a change in therapy.[40] In fact, as reported by

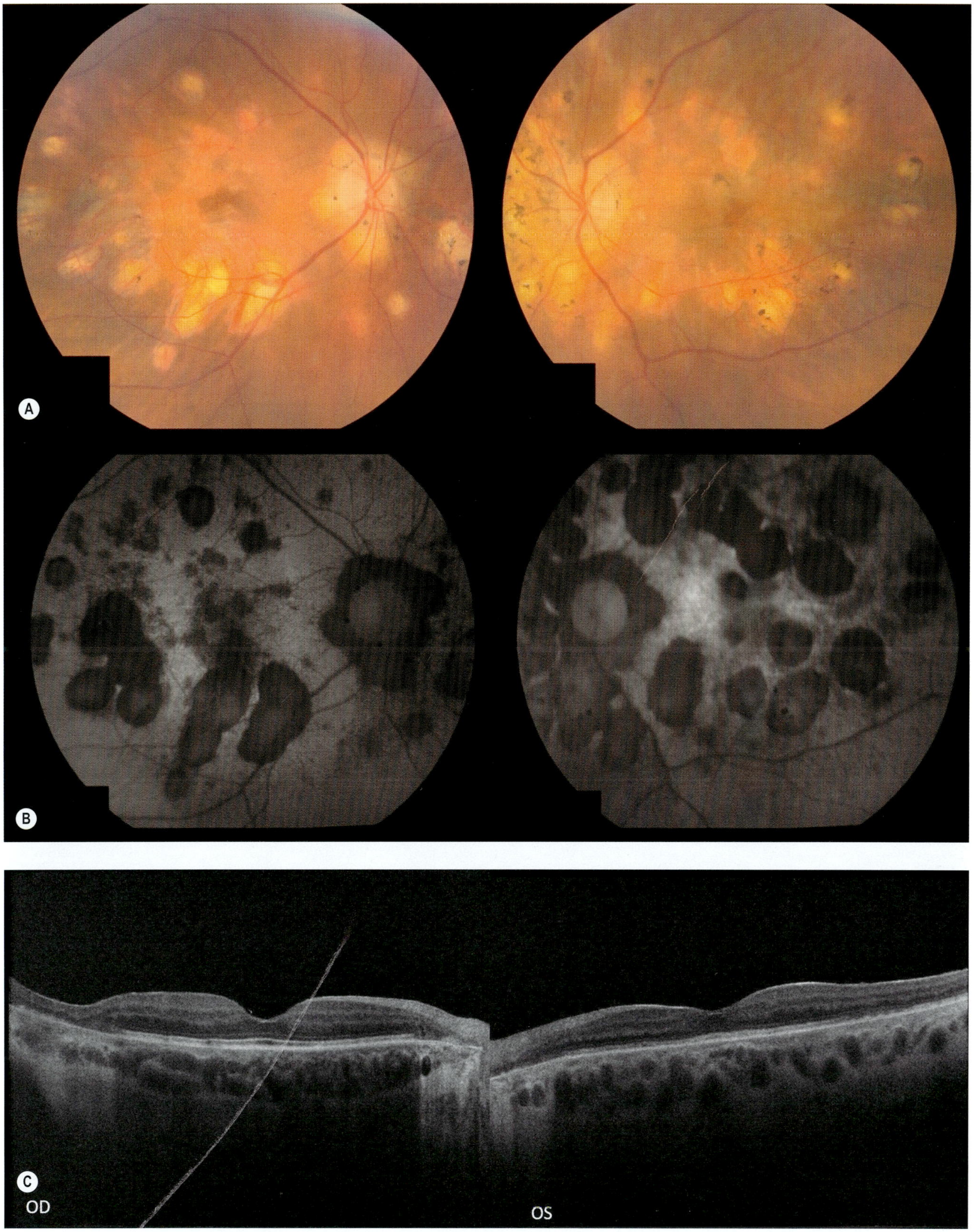

Fig. 26.3 Fundus autofluorescence in a patient with advanced birdshot chorioretinopathy. Note that the areas of fundus hypofluorescence indicating retinal pigment epithelium (RPE) atrophy (B) are larger and more numerous than visible lesions on color photography (A) and correspond to areas of outer retinal atrophy and retinal thinning on OCT (C).

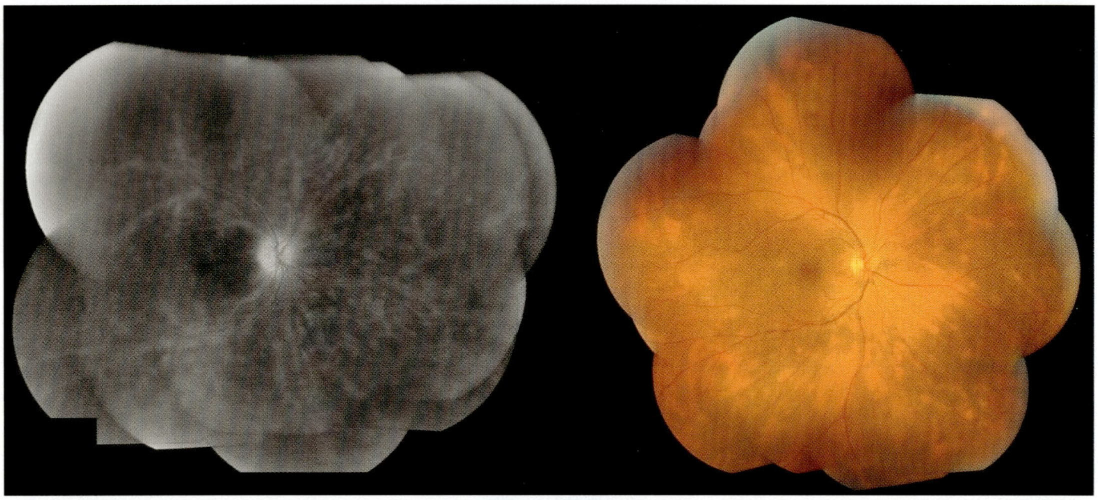

Fig. 26.4 Fluorescein angiogram from a patient with low lesion burden on examination, and the color fundus photo *(right)* shows extensive vascular leakage, emphasizing the vascular component of this disease.

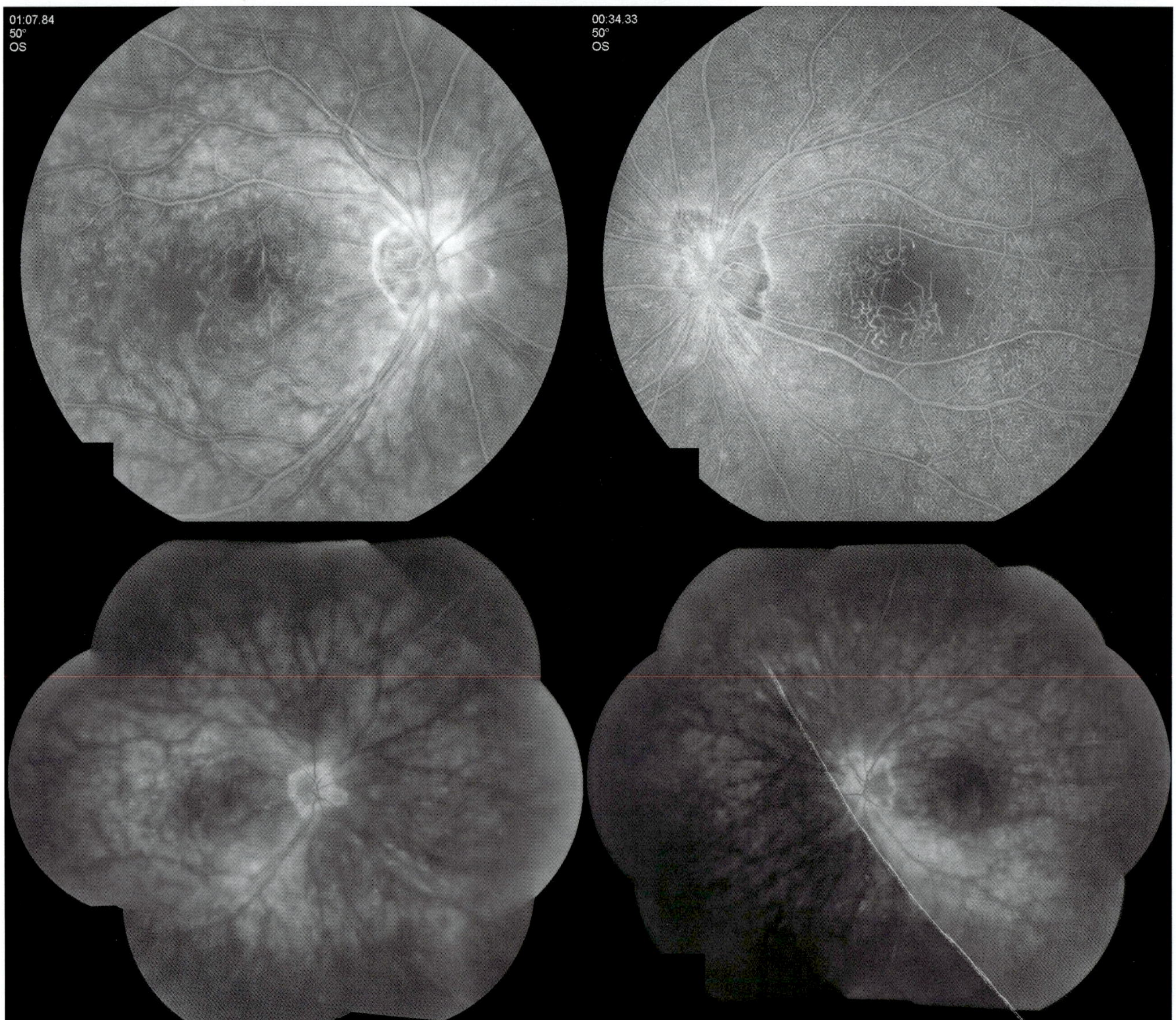

Fig. 26.5 Fluorescein angiogram changes in birdshot chorioretinopathy (BCR). Top panel shows pruning and telangiectatic vessels in the posterior pole during the early phase of angiography. Bottom panel is a montage from mid- to late phases showing "quenching" of the dye.

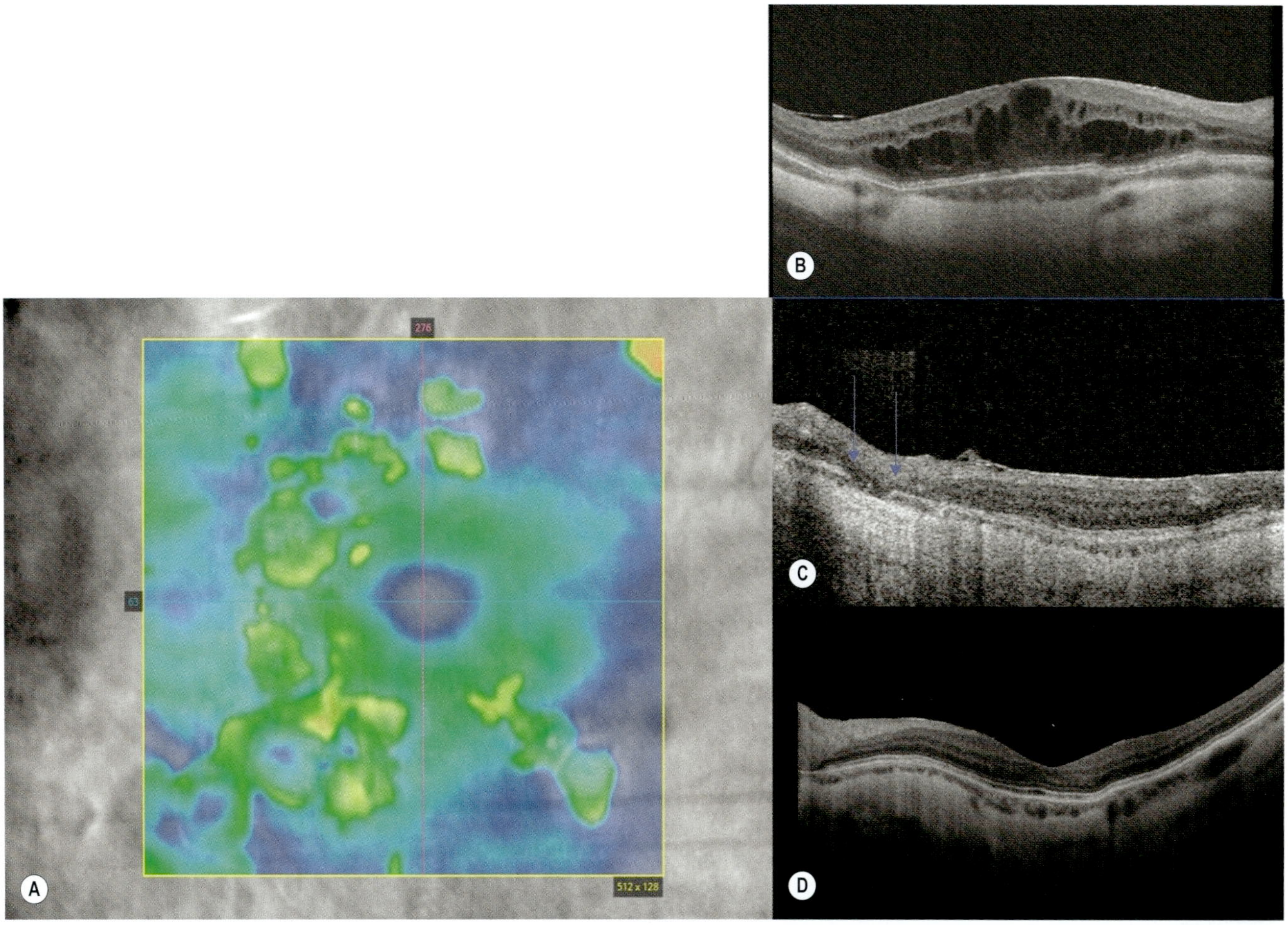

Fig. 26.6 Optical coherence tomography (OCT) from a patient with birdshot chorioretinopathy (BCR). The left eye shows atrophic lesions on en face images (A) that correspond to atrophy of the outer retina and retinal pigment epithelium (RPE) thinning on B-scans *(arrow)* (C). At presentation, the patient had significant cystoid macular edema (B), which resolved after treatment, but with residual ellipsoid zone atrophy (D). Note that the choroid is very thin throughout.

our group, in a BCR case treated with fluocinolone acetonide implants in both eyes, ICG angiography was the only modality that was able to detect the choroidal lesion burden after a change in therapy with systemic corticosteroids.[41] (Fig. 26.8). Importantly, many of the modalities are more useful in conjunction with another modality rather than as standalone testing. Multimodal imaging can help determine disease severity and titrate treatment because some of the changes can be reversible.[42]

Many of the patients with BCR show altered retinal function despite good visual acuity. The visual field and ERG results are two good ways to follow the course of disease in these patients. Visual field testing often reveals scotomata, even in patients with good vision and minimal ocular complaints.[43,44] In a report by Thorne et al.,[45] 75% of 48 eyes had abnormal I-4 changes on the visual field. Of the 28 eyes from patients receiving immunosuppression, the rate of visual field loss before therapy was 107 degrees per year for the I-4 isopter. After therapy was initiated, there was a rate of gain of 53 degrees per year for the isopter. Thus therapy may reverse the visual field loss. Problems with night vision and color discrimination are not uncommon in patients with BCR, sometimes despite excellent central visual acuity. These problems should not be taken lightly because alterations in retinal functions other than visual acuity can precede vision loss.

In reports investigating psychophysical and electrophysiologic testing of patients with this entity, disturbances in both the ERG and the electrooculography (EOG) have been noted. Fuerst et al.[17] reported reduction in b-wave amplitude and implicit time prolongation. We have seen abnormal ERG results in the majority of patients we have tested, similar to those reported by others[16] (Fig. 26.9). Several electrophysiologic changes have been reported. Holder et al.[46] reported that the cone-mediated flicker ERG responses are delayed before therapy initiation. Sobrin et al.[47] also saw cone b-wave flicker implicit time alterations as the most consistently affected parameter and that these alterations seemed to improve with therapy. Zacks et al.[48] suggested that the bright scotopic response amplitudes and the 30-Hz flicker implicit times were associated with recurrence of disease with tapering of immunosuppressive therapy. Regardless, in evaluating the significance of any change on ERG, one has to keep in mind that the intertest variability of ERG results among patients with BCR can be as high as 40%. Our group has shown that even in same-day testing on the same patient, the average variability was approximately 25%.[49] Robson et al.[50] suggested that postphototransduction involvement of the optic nerve pathway may be seen as well. Color-vision alterations can be found in patients with BCR, and some complain of colors being "washed out" or faded. Others may note a difference between the two eyes with regard to color discrimination. Holland et al,[51] by using the desaturated Lanthony 15-Hue test, showed that 49 of the 80 patients tested (61.3%) had abnormal color confusion scores, and this included patients with normal vision. Dark adaptation thresholds are invariably abnormal. Indeed, Kappel et al.[52] evaluated patients with BCR by using

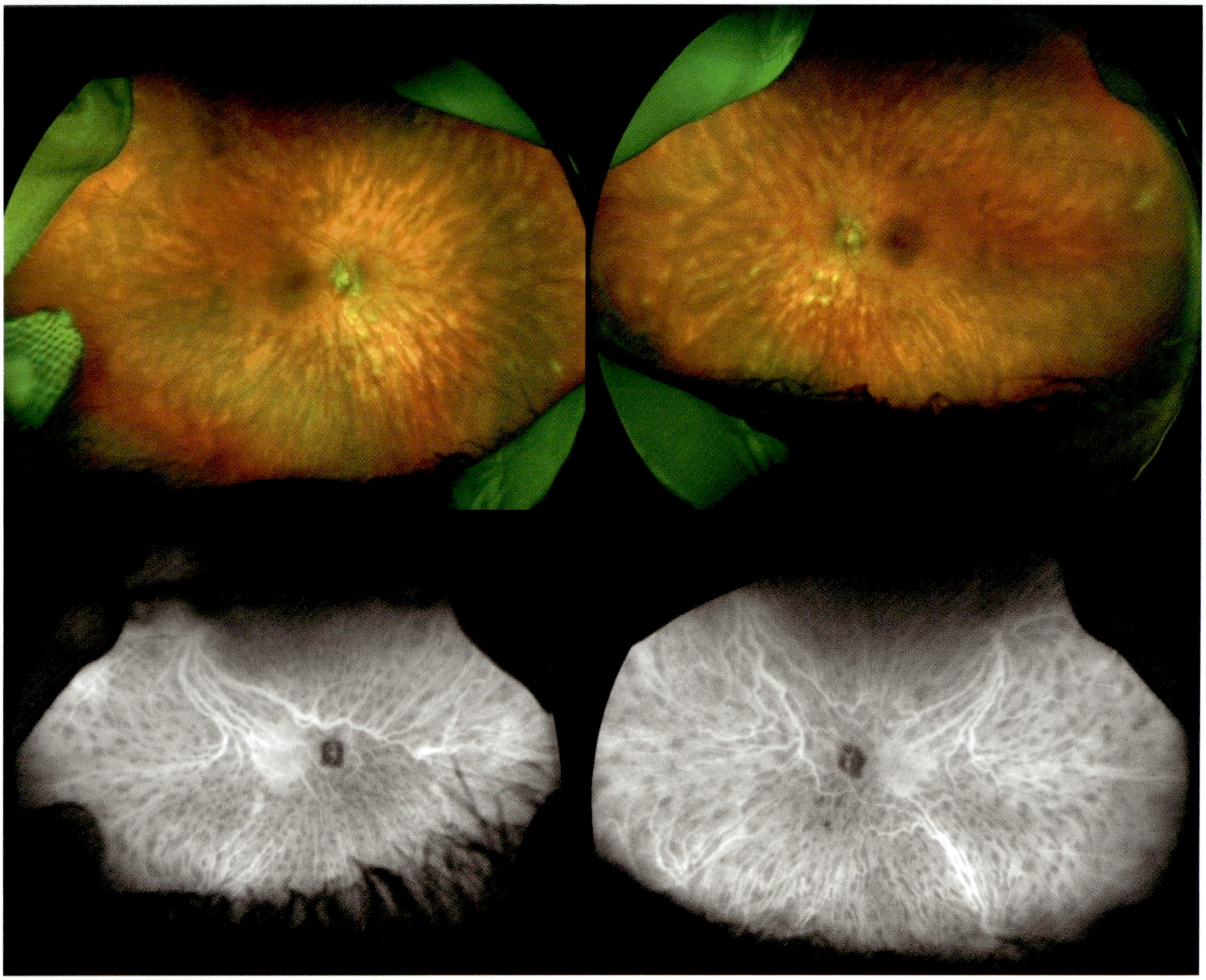

Fig. 26.7 Ultra-wide-field indocyanine green (ICG) angiography study of patient with birdshot chorioretinopathy (BCR). Top panel shows extensive burden of typical birdshot lesions distributed throughout the fundus on wide-field color fundus photography. Bottom panel shows spotty hypocyanescent areas corresponding to these lesions.

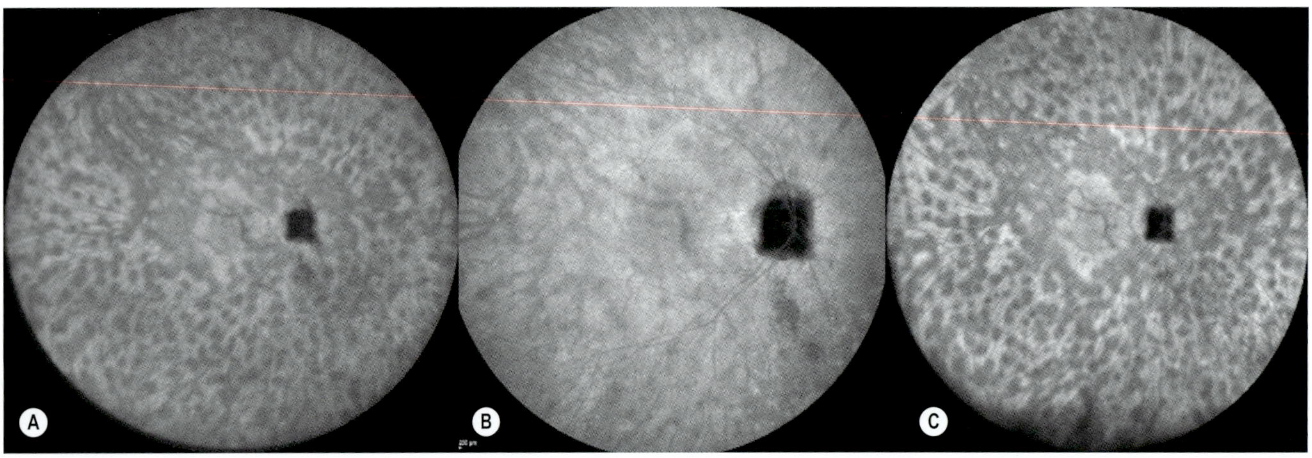

Fig. 26.8 Indocyanine green angiography of the same patient in Fig. 26.7, on the Heidelberg Spectralis, showing before (A), during (B), and after (C) systemic steroid use. Choroidal lesions disappear while the patient is on systemic steroids but reappear soon after it is tapered off.

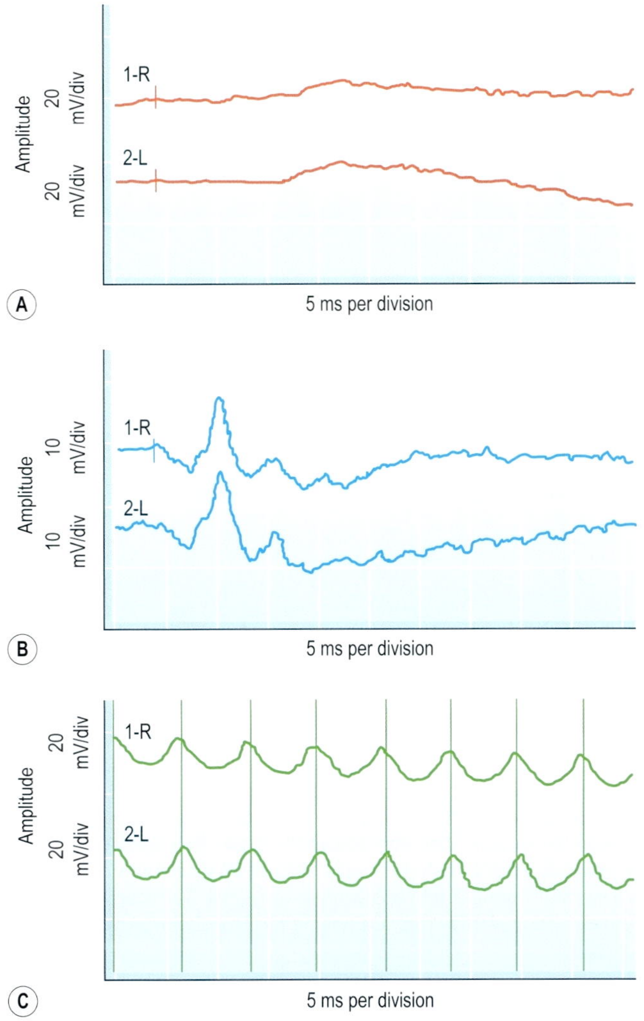

Fig. 26.9 Examples of rod- and cone-mediated electroretinograms, and flicker responses from the eye of a patient with birdshot chorioretinopathy (BCR). Rod responses (A) demonstrate markedly reduced amplitude, but cone responses (B) less so. Flicker responses (C), produced by cones, also have reduction of amplitude.(From Smith JA, Whitcup SM. Birdshot chorioretinopathy. *Br J Ophthalmol.* 1999;83:241–249, with permission from the BMJ Publishing Group.)

contrast sensitivity testing. Reduced contrast sensitivity is a common finding in these eyes, with 92% of 126 eyes tested showing abnormal results. Although these abnormal thresholds are often related to poor vision, Kappel et al. also found that of the 38 eyes with normal vision, 31 (82%) had abnormal contrast sensitivity.

Because the retinal lesions can be very striking, the diagnosis would appear to be relatively easy to make. However, as with all diseases, some occurrences fall within the "gray" zone. One should consider other diagnoses, such as multifocal choroiditis and panuveitis, described by Nozik and Dorsch[53] and also discussed by Dreyer and Gass.[54] The patients with the condition described by Nozik and Dorsch tend to be younger, have unilateral disease more often, have a greater degree of vitreous inflammation, and be less likely to have night blindness or abnormal ERG findings.[53] Furthermore, the lesions in this entity tend to become pigmented, smaller, and better defined than those seen in BCR. Sarcoidosis has been often considered as an alternative diagnosis in the patients we have seen and evaluated.[55] Brinkman and Rothova[56] reported on six patients with neurosarcoidosis and demonstrated multifocal chorioretinal lesions, optic nerve disease, and periphlebitis. In addition, multiple evanescent white-dot syndrome, described by Jampol et al.[57]; Waldenstrom macroglobulinemia[58]; and choroidal and vitreoretinal lymphoma should all be considered in the differential diagnosis. Noble and Greenberg[59] reported on a patient with myelodysplasia syndrome and fundus lesions resembling those of BCR. Cases of posterior scleritis with fundus lesions resembling BCR have been reported.[60] Lesions similar to those seen in BCR have also been seen in common variable immunodeficiency (CVID), sarcoidosis, and pembrolizumab use.[61-63] In the degenerative stage, BCR can look like inherited retinal dystrophies.[64] Sommer et al.[65] reported that the fundus appeared similar to that in BCR and that it was associated with tamoxifen toxicity.

The physician should consider an alternative diagnosis to BCR in nonwhite patients because this condition appears rarely, if at all, in nonwhites.[66] It was not reported in a survey of uveitis cases from a center in China, and, in Japan, it is very rare (see later discussion).[67] A Caucasian patient who was initially diagnosed with HLA-A29 negative BCR at the NEI was found to have Waldenstrom's Macroglobulinemia after an extensive evaluation. Therefore in atypical cases, particularly in HLA-A29 negative cases, it is critical to re-evaluate and rethink the diagnosis.

TESTS, HISTOLOGY, AND ETIOLOGY

The exact cause of BCR is unknown. However, observations have provided provocative hypotheses. We have found a strong correlation between BCR and HLA-A29 in white patients.[68] Of the patients tested, 80% showed HLA-A29 within their genetic makeup, whereas only 7% of control subjects had this antigen. This unusually high correlation yielded a relative risk of almost 50 (see discussion on HLA in Chapter 1). This finding suggests a strong genetic predisposition for this disease. Several other studies have demonstrated the same strong association with HLA-A29.[69-71] Le Hoang et al.[72] reported that 54 of 58 French patients with BCR showed HLA-A29 positivity (93.1%; relative risk 157.3) and that subtyping results for 33 of these patients showed the HLA-A29.2 subtype in all. HLA-A29.2 is considerably more common than HLA-A29.1. In the initial patient evaluation, the absence of the HLA-A29.1 subtype raised questions about a possible "resistance motif" in the HLA-A29.1 molecule. A single difference was found in the extracellular domain between the two HLA-A29 subtypes (i.e., A29.1 and A29.2). Because the HLA-A29.1 subtype contains a unique mutation, these authors hypothesized that the ancestral type was HLA-A29.2 and that the HLA-A29.1 mutation came later and conferred resistance to BCR. Work by Tabary et al.[73] showed that the sequence of HLA-A29.2 was identical in patients with BCR and in healthy controls. The position of the HLA-A29.1 mutation would not permit it to interact with the T-cell receptor; rather, it interacted with an accessory molecule, such as CD8.

De Waal et al.[74] examined the matter of HLA-A29 subtypes and found that in a white population from The Netherlands and Belgium, HLA-A29.2 was the more common subtype, being found in 90% of control subjects with HLA-A29. They found that the distribution of HLA-A29.2 versus that of HLA-A29.1 did not differ among the patients with BCR whom they had examined. Both subtypes were found, but HLA-A29.2 predominated, simply because it is almost 10 times more commonly seen, at least in this population. Others have reported the same findings.[75,76] In contrast to the northern European and American experiences, some Japanese and Brazilian observers are not sure that they have seen a classic case (Mochizuki and Belfort, personal communication, 1990). Saito et al.[77] reported a case in Japan, but neither the patient nor 10 other Japanese patients examined were HLA-A29 negative. All of our patients have been of European ancestry, except one with Hispanic ancestry. HLA-B12 has been found in 68%

of patients with BCR and has a relative risk of 6.15 (which is small compared with the calculated A29 relative risk).[78] This antigen is in linkage disequilibrium with HLA-A29. Levinson et al.[79] have evaluated the association between this entity and HLA class I specific killer cell immunoglobulin-like receptors (KIRs). KIRs are important receptors of human natural killer (NK) cells and CD8+ and CD4+ CD28 null cells. An association was noted between BCR and the *KIR2DS2/-S3/-S4* genes, which are associated with autoimmunity. It may be that these genes activate NK cells and T cells, perhaps to respond to intraocular self-antigens.

Additional information to support the notion that endogenous immune mechanisms play a role is the finding that patients' lymphocytes demonstrate an in vitro cell-mediated response to retinal antigens, most notably the retinal S-antigen (S-Ag)[68] (Fig. 26.10; Case 26.1). Nussenblatt et al.[68] and Le Hoang et al.[72] showed that lymphocytes from patients with BCR were reactive to S-Ag in 60% to 92%. Jobin et al.,[80] by using either lymphocyte proliferation assay or basophil degranulation, found that in vitro positivity to S-Ag appeared more frequently in the period preceding relapse of ocular inflammation. Furthermore, we have reported that the inflammatory response seen in one eye with BCR seemed directed to the photoreceptor region, the area from which the retinal S-Ag is isolated.[34] One report suggested that the major focus of the inflammatory response is situated in the choroid, with also a lymphocytic infiltrate around the retinal vasculature.[81] The collection of lymphocytes in the choroid could explain the white-cream-colored lesions. The striking number of patients with BCR who demonstrate evidence of retinal autoimmunity suggests that this mechanism is important in this disease. Furthermore, the disease elicited in monkeys immunized with the retinal S-Ag can take on certain characteristics not dissimilar to those seen in the human condition. The strong HLA association would add further support to the notion of an inbred error of immune regulation. In this disease, HLA-A29 positivity can be used as strong corroborative evidence to support the clinical diagnosis. One might expect a strong familial association with this disorder, but this has been rare, although familial cases have been reported.[82,83] However, Fich and Rosenberg[84] did report BCR in monozygotic twins. In this case, in one of the twins, the initial diagnosis was chorioretinal dystrophy.

To date, the exact pathogenic mechanism linking HLA-A29 to BCR is not known. It has been suggested that the disorder may be initiated by exogenous factors, such as a virus. One could conjecture that a viral antigen may bear sequences similar to an HLA sequence or that a new epitope consisting of a viral particle and the HLA motif becomes the target of the immune response. However, this does not completely explain the cell-mediated responsiveness against retinal antigens that has been noted in these patients. The report by Boisgérault et al.[85] offers another interesting explanation. These authors reported that two peptides from the carboxyl terminal sequence of the human retinal antigen bound efficiently to HLA-A29, suggesting a direct role for this HLA phenotype in the autoimmune response. Szpak et al.[86] created transgenic mice that expressed HLA-A29. Uveitis develops spontaneously in these animals, and the disease is similar to that seen in experimentally induced chorioretinitis (Fig. 26.11). However, it was not seen in all of them. The spontaneous disease was noted in 12 (80%) of 15 animals older than 12 months (aged mice).[87] The mechanisms leading to uveitis still need to be defined. In 2015, Kuiper et al. suggested that HLA-A29.02 may be functioning as a canonical antigen-presenting molecule for uveitogenic peptides.[88] They suggested that its role in viral-specific CD8+ T-cell activation may be related to disease pathogenesis. Kuiper et al. also identified ERAP2 as a susceptibility locus in a large genomewide association study across Europe.[89] ERAP2 plays a role in peptide trimming for antigen presentation; thus the authors suggested ERAP2 as a viable therapeutic target, particularly on the basis of the fact that 25% of whites lack ERAP2 without any functional impairment.

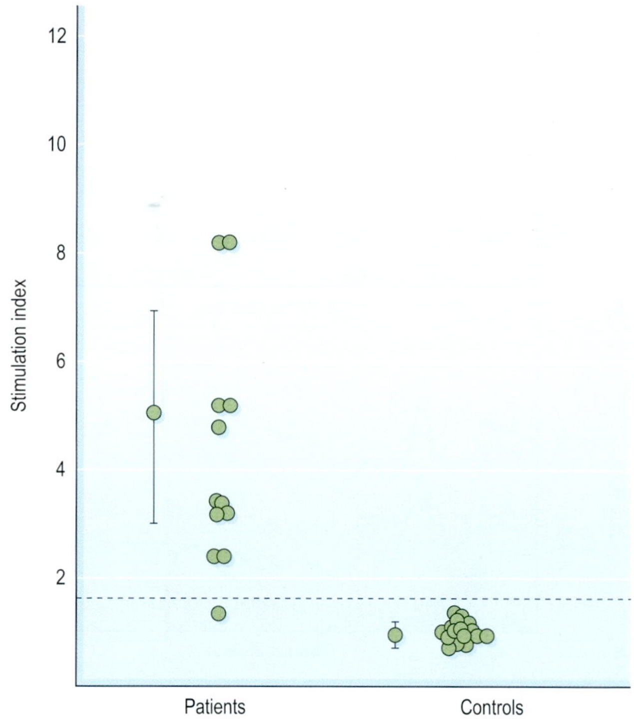

Fig. 26.10 Lymphocytes of patient with birdshot chorioretinopathy (BCR) demonstrate in vitro proliferative response to retinal S-antigen, whereas those of control subjects do not. This in vitro anamnestic response is thought to parallel what occurs in vitro when T cells (and other immune cells) become activated. (From Nussenblatt RB, Mittal KK, Ryan S, et al. Birdshot chorioretinopathy associated with HLA-A29 antigen and immune responsiveness to retinal S-antigen. *Am J Ophthalmol.* 1982;94:147–158. Copyright by The Ophthalmic Publishing Company.)

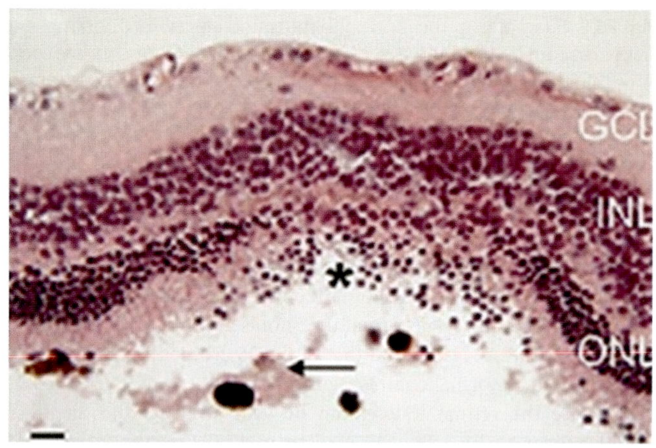

Fig. 26.11 Spontaneous uveitis in A29 transgenic mouse with destruction of the photoreceptor region noted. A serous detachment was also noted by the authors. (From de Kozak Y. Pathologic aspects of spontaneous uveitis and retinopathy in HLA-A29 transgenic mice and in animal models of retinal autoimmunity: relevance to human pathologies. *Ophthalmic Res.* 2008;40:175–180.)

Long-term studies of patients with retinal vasculitis have yielded interesting observations. In two patients with retinal vasculitis, Soubrane et al.[90] reported the appearance of typical lesions of BCR 7 and 8 years after the first symptoms. They suggested evaluating patients

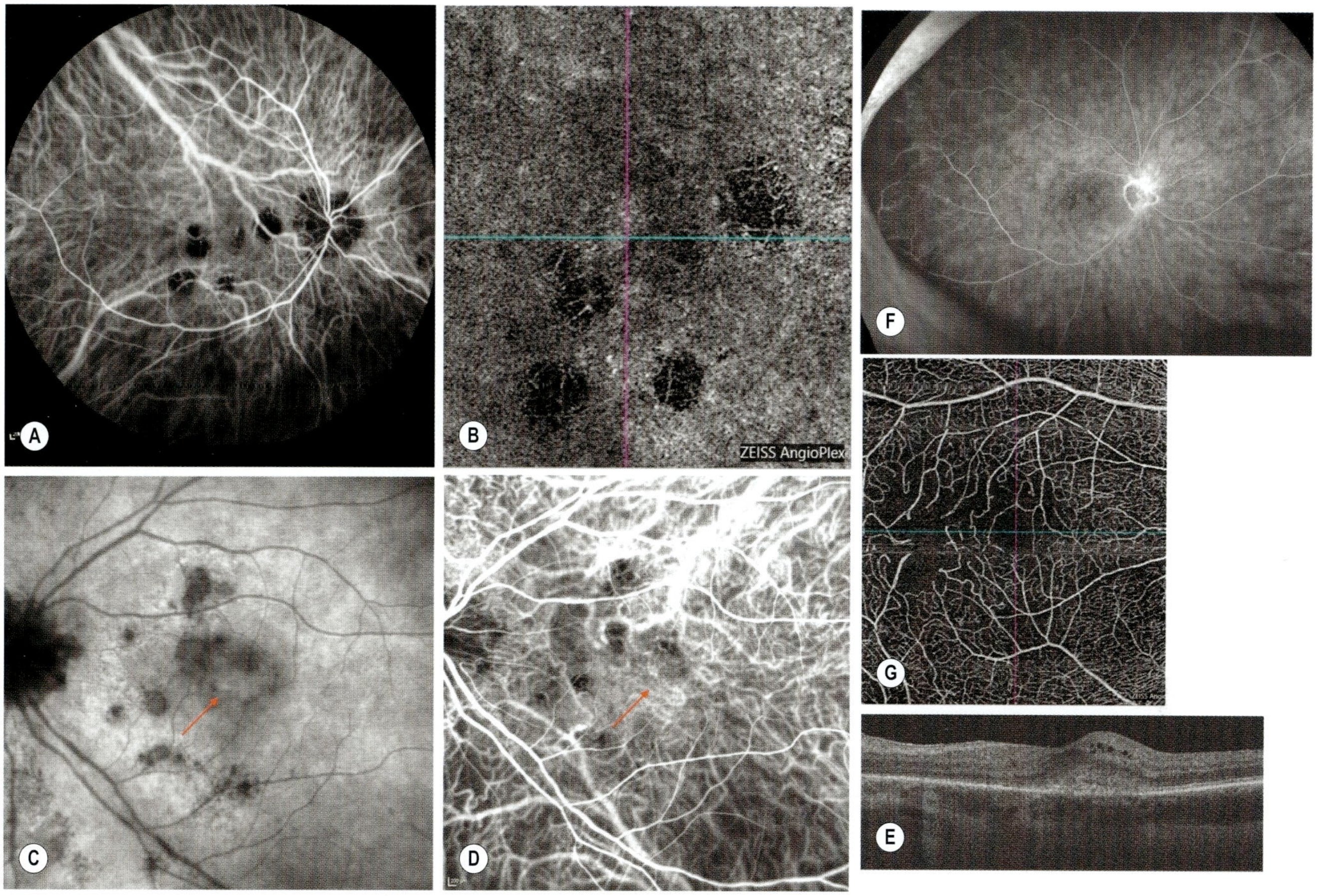

Fig. 26.12 Right eye of patient with birdshot chorioretinopathy (BCR) shows hypocyanescent spots in the posterior pole on indocyanine green (ICG) angiography (A), with corresponding flow deficits at the choriocapillaris level on optical coherence tomography angiography (OCTA) (B). The left eye of the same patient shows choroidal neovascularization at the border of one of the BCR lesions (C) with hypercyanescent spot in midphase *(arrow)* and a corresponding hypercyanescence on late ICG angiography (D; *arrow*). OCT of the left eye shows the area of central choroidal neovascularization (CNV) visualized as a hyperreflective area over the retinal pigment epithelium (RPE) with overlying intraretinal fluid (E). The fluorescein angiography (F) of another patient with BCR shows posterior pole and peripheral capillary dropout corroborated by areas of flow voids on superficial capillary plexus on OCTA (G).

for the presence of HLA-A29 even late in the course of retinal vasculitis. A similar evolution of clinical findings was reported by Godel et al.[91] An additional interesting observation was that by Bloch-Michel and Frau,[92] who reviewed the records of 20 patients with BCR and 36 with idiopathic retinal vasculitis. The HLA-A29 phenotype was seen in 95% of patients in the BCR group, as opposed to 61% in the other group. Long-term follow-up of patients with vasculitis showed that lesions compatible with BCR developed in only one patient. However, the HLA-A29 phenotype in the idiopathic vasculitis group was associated with more posterior pole involvement, a more severe disease course, and a poorer visual prognosis than in those without this phenotype. The authors suggested that the presence of this gene portends ill for its bearer, with or without lesions typical of BCR.

The role of T cells in BCR is implicated by their association with HLA and by the fact that choroidal lesions are predominantly infiltrated by T cells.[93] Additionally, vitreous samples obtained from patients with BCR were shown to contain almost exclusively CD4+ and CD8+ cells,[94] even though some of these T cells show reactivity to retinal/choroidal lysates; the exact antigen and the role of T cells in the pathogenesis of BCR are still unclear.

Humoral studies have not been particularly useful in further defining any underlying immunologic abnormality. This includes the absence of circulating anticardiolipin antibodies associated with thrombosis and diseases with a significant vascular component.[95] Kuhne et al.[96] reported two cases of retinal vasculitis associated with Q fever caused by *Coxiella burnetii*. One patient showed HLA-A29 positivity; although the authors speculated on the role of this agent in BCR, they were unable to show a definitive role for this organism.

THERAPY

A well-planned therapeutic regimen is required for the treatment of patients with BCR. Use of steroids still is the mainstay of therapy. The most common reason for decreased visual acuity is CME. CME is a harbinger of a long-term drop in visual acuity and therefore needs to be treated. Furthermore, ancillary testing mentioned earlier, such as ICG angiography, ERG, and visual field testing, supports the notion that there are physiologic changes even if visual acuity seems normal (see Case 26.3). The patient with good vision requires a full understanding of why treatment is being given. Rarely, one will see subretinal neovascular nets that need prompt attention (Fig. 26.12), with consideration of the use of anti–vascular endothelial growth factor (VEGF) injections along with appropriate anti-inflammatory therapy. A second agent needs to be added if it is clear that steroid therapy is needed for longer than 3 to 4 months. Others[97] have suggested using nonsteroidal anti-inflammatory agents, but we have not found them helpful, and they are not usually within our armamentarium for the treatment of this entity. Ladas et al.[98] reported that they were able to treat patients adequately after an initial prednisone dose of 1 mg/kg/day and then long-term (54–81 months) treatment with 5 mg or less. Zacks et al.[47] reported that abnormalities on ERG can be associated with recurrence of disease. Changes in the bright scotopic response amplitudes, particularly b-waves, and flicker implicit times were associated with recurrence. Thorne et al. showed that treatment with steroids and various immunosuppressives (cyclosporine, mycophenolate mofetil, methotrexate) were associated with improvements in visual fields[45] and that classic BCR spots can disappear with treatment.[41,99] Periocular or intraocular steroids can be used in patients with asymmetric disease severity or as adjunct treatment to systemic therapy. Martidis et al.[100] reported the use of intraocular triamcinolone acetonide for the treatment of cystoid edema. Bajwa et al. reported that in 11 patients with BCR disease was controlled by using the fluocinolone acetonide implant (Retisert), which also allowed for tapering of systemic immunosuppressives and resulted in improvement in CME.[101] Rush et al. similarly followed up 22 patients with BCR who received a fluocinolone acetonide implant and reported 100% resolution of vitreous haze by 1 year, along with significant improvement in visual acuity and reduction of CME. They also noted that systemic immunosuppressive use decreased from 82% to 5%.[102] In patients who have relatively good visual acuity and need occasional therapy, we really do not know whether these therapeutic approaches have a significant effect on the final visual outcome. It has been suggested that in approximately 15% of patients, BCR may be mild and may not need aggressive systemic therapy.[103] However, it is important to monitor these patients over the long term because the disease course may change, and silent loss of function can occur (see Case 26.2).

As with many uveitic entities, we do not know the natural history of this one. It has been the belief of some that the long-term visual prognosis for these patients is guarded, but others have thought that the disease has a tendency to stabilize. Our experience[16] has suggested that approximately 20% of patients appear to have self-limiting disease, maintaining good vision despite the fundus lesions. Some authors maintain that few eyes will maintain good vision, if left untreated.[104] In our published series,[16] 27 patients were followed up for 5 to 13 years: 52% had worsening of visual acuity, 30% had stable vision, and 18% had improved vision. A visual acuity of 20/40 or better was noted in at least one eye in two-thirds of these patients, whereas 22% had a visual acuity of <20/200 in the better eye.

Any patient requiring extended (>3 months) steroid therapy should also receive a steroid-sparing agent. Cyclosporine has been used in some patients, and we have seen good responses.[96] This finding has been corroborated by Le Hoang et al.[105] Vitale et al.[106] corroborated these earlier observations by using lower doses of the drug (2.5–5 mg/kg/day) as had been recommended because of concerns regarding renal toxicity. Some patients needed the addition of azathioprine (1.5–2 mg/kg/day). The investigators found that vitreous inflammation was controlled in 23 treated eyes (88.5%) and that stabilization or improvement in visual acuity occurred in 20 (83.3%).[106] These results are to be expected because this disorder appears to be mediated by T cells, and therefore an anti–T-cell agent should have a significant effect on the disease course. In the study by Kiss et al.,[107] the vast majority (93%) of patients receiving cyclosporine showed improvement or stabilization of visual acuity of over a median follow-up period of 81 months. A regression model has shown that patients treated with cyclosporin have better visual acuity compared with those treated with steroids.[2]

A disconcerting continued decrease in retinal function and retinal thinning and attenuation of the retinal vasculature may be seen even if the ocular inflammatory activity stabilizes. Rasquin and Pereleux[108] reported that a patient's fundus that began with BCR lesions looked, after 20 years, like tapetoretinal degeneration. This may have been caused by the triggering of apoptosis (programmed cell death) of the cells that constitute the retina. Because of these observations, the notion that cytotoxic agents should be given early in the disease has been entertained.

Other medications have been used in the treatment of BCR. Becker et al.[109] used a combination of immunosuppressive approaches and achieved control of the inflammatory response. Le Hoang et al.[110] conducted an interventional nonrandomized study involving 18 patients with BCR who received intravenous immunoglobulin (IVIg). Patients were given 1.6 g/kg of IVIg every 4 weeks for 6 months as sole treatment. Subsequently, they received injections of 1.2 to 1.6 g/kg at 6- to 8-week intervals. Mean period of follow-up was 39 months. Of the 26 eyes with vision less than 20/30, 14 improved by two lines or more, and vision decreased in two. Transient systemic hypertension, headache, eczematous lesions, and hyperthermia were reported to have occurred during the treatment period. Hesse et al.[10] described a patient with BCR and psoriasis in whom treatment with aromatic retinoids led to resolution of both the ocular and the dermatologic problems.

The use of biologics has entered into the therapeutic armamentarium for BCR as well, including anti–tumor necrosis factor (TNF)-α daclizumab, the anti–interleukin (IL)-2 receptor-blocking agent, and IL-6 inhibitors. In eight patients treated with daclizumab by Sobrin et al.,[111] resolution of vasculitis was noted in six, and there was stabilization of or improvement of vision and control of inflammation in seven. There was, however, a decline in ERG parameters in some despite control of the inflammation. This further supports the concept of an early therapeutic intervention for this disorder, as do the retinal physiologic observations in eyes that see well. In a large retrospective cohort of 132 patients with BCR, You et al. showed that long-term immunosuppressive use was associated with a low rate of disease exacerbation.[112] At 1 year, 40% of the eyes were quiet, whereas at 3, 5, and 8 years, greater than 70% were quiet. As expected, those that achieved quiescence had better visual field outcomes. Immunosuppressives used varied but included methotrexate, mycophenolate mofetil, cyclosporine, TNF inhibitors, and others; the cyclosporine and mycophenolate mofetil combination was the most commonly used. IL-6 inhibitors have also been used in smaller cohorts for the treatment of BCR and associated CME with good results, even in cases recalcitrant to TNF-inhibitors or interferon therapy.[113,114]

CASE 26.1

A 54-year-old white man was referred to the National Eye Institute with a complaint of increased floaters and shimmering. He was in good general health. His visual acuity was 20/32 in the right eye and 20/32-1 in the left eye. Both anterior chambers had an occasional cell, and the tensions were normal. The media had 1+ cells and 1+ haze in both eyes. Scattered yellow-white lesions were seen throughout the fundus, with more concentration in the posterior pole. The lesions appeared deep, probably at the level of the retinal pigment epithelium or photoreceptor region. There were occasional superficial retinal hemorrhages and faint, but not definitive, cystoid macular edema (CME) in the left eye. There was no snowbanking.

Fluorescein angiography demonstrated rather diffuse retinal vascular leakage, with staining of the disk in both eyes as well, and evidence of mild CME in the left eye. Goldmann fields were full, but there were patches of nonabsolute scotomas. Human leukocyte antigen (HLA) typing demonstrated the presence of HLA-A29. In vitro cell culturing showed an anamnestic response to the retinal S-antigen.

CASE 26.2

A 40-year-old white woman was diagnosed with human leukocyte antigen (HLA)-A29+ birdshot chorioretinopathy (BCR). She had been symptomatic with floaters only for approximately 2 years and subjective decrease in vision for 6 months. She had a relatively mild disease with modest lesion burden (Fig. 26.13A), minimal leakage on fluorescein angiography, and no cystoid macular edema on optical coherence tomography (OCT) but mild ellipsoid zone changes (see Fig. 26.13C). The patient had good visual acuity at 20/20 in the right eye and 20/25 in the left eye. Her visual fields and full-field electroretinography values were within the normal range. Given her symptoms, the mild changes on OCT, and her desire to be treated, she was started on azathioprine. Azathioprine was chosen as the immunomodulatory agent for family planning reasons. OCT showed some degree of reconstitution of the ellipsoid zone, and resolution of choroidal lesions was seen on examination (see Figs. 26.13B, D).

CASE 26.3

A 51-year-old white man had been experiencing floaters for 2.5 years before coming to the National Eye Institute. His vision was 20/20 in both eyes with normal intraocular pressure (IOP). Although the patient had no anterior segment inflammatory disease or vitritis, fundus examination showed cream-colored lesions typical of birdshot chorioretinopathy (BCR) and posterior vitreous detachment (Fig. 26.14, *top panel*). Fluorescein angiography showed no retinal vascular leakage but showed mild staining of the few BCR lesions. The patient had no macular edema, and testing revealed human leukocyte antigen (HLA)-A29 positivity. Visual fields and full-field electroretinography (ffERG) results were completely normal and stayed normal for a year (Fig. 26.15A, B). Close monitoring was recommended. The patient decided to continue treatment elsewhere and returned 10 years later with a history of a recent flare-up in the left eye that had been treated with periocular steroid injections. He complained of blurry vision and mild nyctalopia. His vision was 20/20 in the right eye (OD) and 20/32 in the left eye (OS), with normal IOP in both eyes (OU). Clinical examination showed atrophic BCR lesions, loss of retinal pigment epithelium (RPE) (see Fig. 26.14, *bottom panel*), and significant thinning and loss of the EZ zone on optical coherence tomography (OCT), OD > OS. His Goldmann visual fields (GVFs) revealed constricted I2e and I1e in both eyes, with multiple deep paracentral scotomas OS > OD, and Humphrey visual fields showed an enlarged blind spot OD, arcuate-like defects OS (see Fig. 26.15C and D). Full-field ERG showed a significant decline compared with the one performed 10 years prior (30%–50% loss on most amplitudes) with decreased dark adapted and light adapted responses, almost flat b-wave (OS >> OD), attenuated flicker responses, and prolonged implicit times, OS > OD. The patient was started on high-dose corticosteroids and mycophenolate mofetil, followed by addition of tumor necrosis factor (TNF) inhibitors. Despite seemingly good central visual acuity, there were extensive retinal structural and functional changes. Even though ERG and the visual field values eventually stabilized, it took time to control the loss of function despite aggressive therapy.

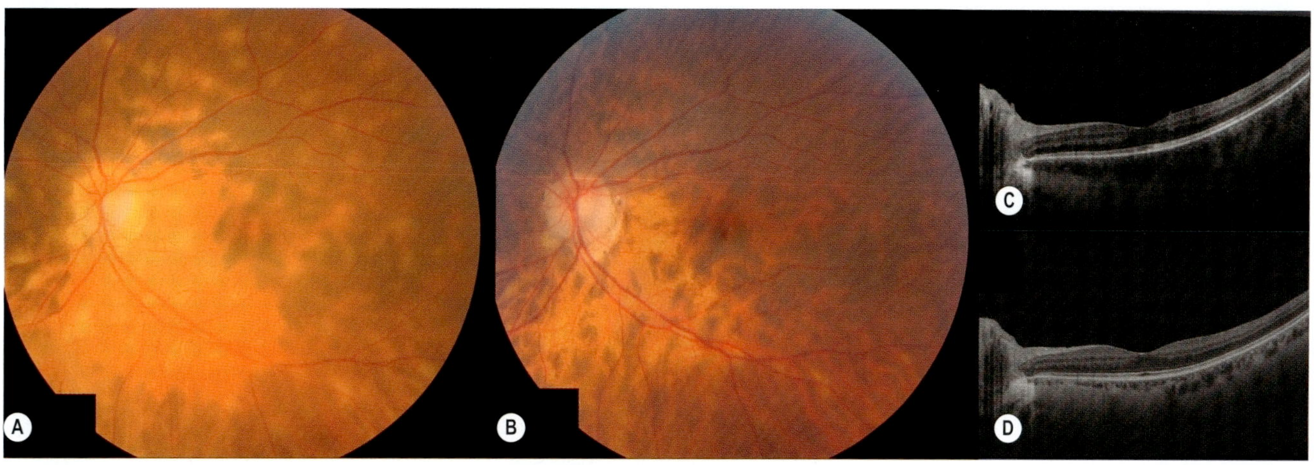

Fig. 26.13 A patient with birdshot chorioretinopathy with relatively modest lesion burden (A), minimal leakage on fluorescein angiography, and mild ellipsoid zone changes on optical coherence tomography (OCT) (C). Resolution of lesions on fundus photography (B) and some degree of reconstitution of the ellipsoid zone on OCT (D) can be seen after treatment (see Case 26.2).

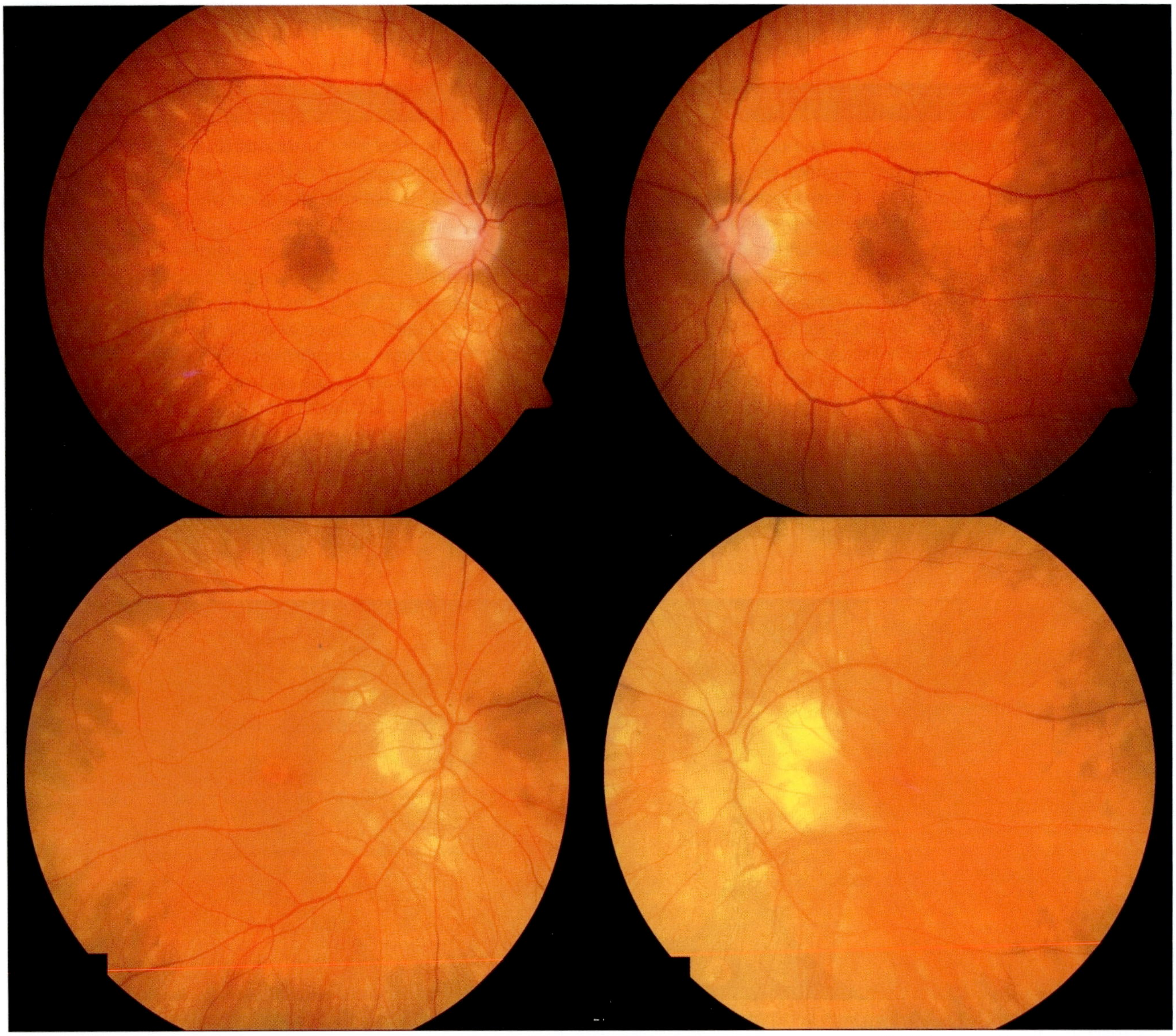

Fig. 26.14 Mild disease with low choroidal lesion burden in a human leukocyte antigen (HLA)-A29–positive patient with birdshot chorioretinopathy *(top panel)* at first visit; the patient returned 10 years later with advanced disease, atrophic lesions, and loss of retinal pigment epithelium (RPE) *(bottom panel)* (see Case 26.3).

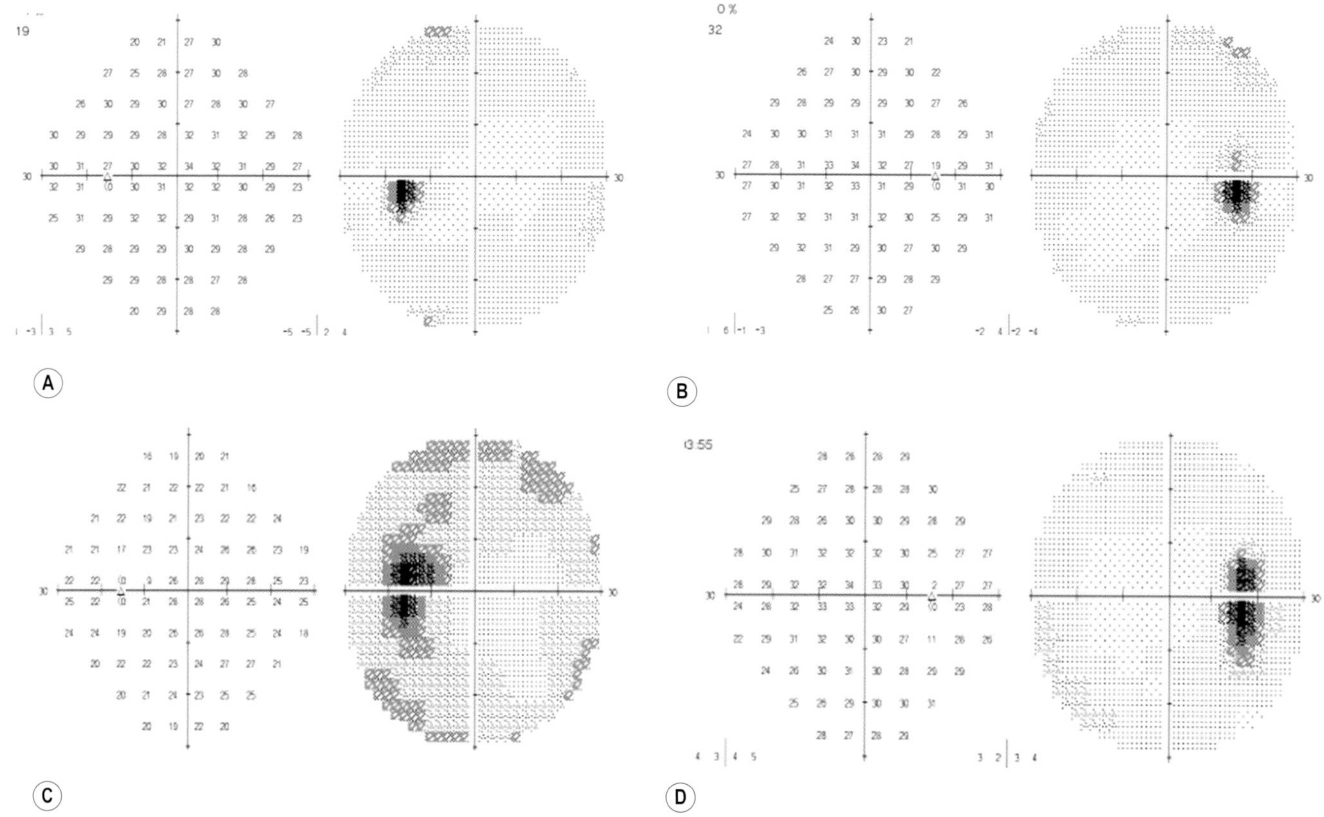

Fig. 26.15 Same patient as in Fig. 26.14 whose Humphrey visual fields were normal at first visit (A, B) but showed progression over 10 years with enlarged blind spot in the right eye, and arcuate-like defects in the left eye (C, D). Full-field electroretinography (ERG) also showed a significant decline compared with the one performed 10 years earlier.

REFERENCES

1. Cassoux N, Le Hoang P. Birdshot chorioretinopathy. *Ann Med Interne (Paris)*. 2000;151(Suppl 1):1S45–1S47.
2. Shah KH, Levinson RD, Yu F, et al. Birdshot chorioretinopathy. *Surv Ophthalmol*. 2005;50(6):519–541.
3. Kiss S, Anzaar F, Foster CS. Birdshot chorioretinopathy. *Int Ophthalmol Clin*. 2006;46(2):39–55.
4. Monnet D, Brezin AP. Birdshot chorioretinopathy. *Curr Opin Ophthalmol*. 2006;17(6):545–550.
5. Levinson RD, Monnet D, Yu F, et al. Longitudinal cohort study of patients with birdshot chorioretinopathy v. quality of life at baseline. *Am J Ophthalmol*. 2009;147(2):346–350.e2.
6. Ryan SJ, Maumenee AE. Birdshot chorioretinopathy. *Am J Ophthalmol*. 1980;89:31–45.
7. Gass J. Vitiliginous chorioretinitis. *Arch Ophthalmol*. 1981;99:1778–1787.
8. Touhami S, Fardeau C, Vanier A, et al. Birdshot retinochoroidopathy: prognostic factors of long-term visual outcome. *Am J Ophthalmol*. 2016;170:190–196.
9. Shah KH, Levinson RD, Yu F, et al. Birdshot chorioretinopathy. *Surv Ophthalmol*. 2005;50(6):519–541.
10. Hesse S, Berbis P, Chemila JF, et al. Psoriasis and birdshot chorioretinopathy: response to aromatic retinoids. *Dermatology*. 1993;187:137–139.
11. Heaton J, Mills R. Sensineural hearing loss associated with birdshot chorioretinopathy. *Arch Otolaryngol Head Neck Surg*. 1993;119:680–681.
12. Cimino L, Aldigeri R, Marchi S, et al. Changes in patterns of uveitis at a tertiary referral center in Northern Italy: analysis of 990 consecutive cases. *Int Ophthalmol*. 2018;38(1):133–142.
13. Mesquida VM, Sainz de la Maza M, Keller J, et al. Epidemiology of uveitis in a Western urban multiethnic population. The challenge of globalization. *Acta Ophthalmol*. 2015;93(6):561–567.
14. Gray CF, Quill S, Compton M, McAvoy CE, Williams MA. Epidemiology of adult uveitis in a Northern Ireland tertiary referral centre. *Ulster Med J*. 2019;88(3):170–173.
15. Kazokoglu H, Onal S, Tugal-Tutkun I, Batioglu F, Apaydin C. Demographic and clinical features of uveitis in tertiary centers in Turkey. *Ophthalmic Epidemiol*. 2008;15(5):285–293.
16. Gasch AT, Smith JA, Whitcup SM. Birdshot chorioretinopathy. *Br J Ophthalmol*. 1999;83:241–249.
17. Fuerst D, Tessler HH, Fishman GA, et al. Birdshot retinochoroidopathy. *Arch Ophthalmol*. 1984;102:214–219.
18. Rothova A, van Schooneveld MJ. The end stage of birdshot chorioretinopathy. *Br J Ophthalmol*. 1995;79(11):1058–1059.
19. Koizumi H, Pozzoni MC, Spaide RF. Fundus autofluorescence in birdshot chorioretinopathy. *Ophthalmology*. 2008;115(5):e15–e20.
20. Monnet D, Brézin AP, Holland GN, et al. Longitudinal cohort study of patients with birdshot chorioretinopathy. I. Baseline clinical characteristics. *Am J Ophthalmol*. 2006;141(1):135–142.
21. Thorne JE, Jabs DA, Peters GB, et al. Birdshot chorioretinopathy: ocular complications and visual impairment. *Am J Ophthalmol*. 2005;140(1):45–51.
22. Lim L, Harper A, Guymer R. Choroidal lesions preceding symptom onset in birdshot chorioretinopathy. *Arch Ophthalmol*. 2006;124(7):1057–1058.
23. Duprat F, Leveque Q, Le Hoang P. Birdshot chorioretinopathy: a case with delayed detection. *J Fr Ophtalmol*. 1998;21(7):525–528.
24. Guex-Crosier Y, Herbort CP. Prolonged retinal arteriovenous circulation time by fluorescein but not by indocyanine green angiography in birdshot chorioretinopathy. *Ocul Immunol Inflamm*. 1997;5:203–206.
25. Witkin AJ, Duker JS, Ko TH, et al. Ultrahigh resolution optical coherence tomography of birdshot chorioretinopathy. *Br J Ophthalmol*. 2005;89(12):1660–1661.

26. Monnet D, Levinson RD, Holland GN, et al. Longitudinal cohort study of patients with birdshot chorioretinopathy. III. Macular imaging at baseline. *Am J Ophthalmol*. 2007;144(6):818–828.
27. Forooghian F, Yeh S, Faia LJ, et al. Uveitic foveal atrophy: clinical features and associations. *Arch Ophthalmol*. 2009;127(2):179–186.
28. Bousquet E, Khandelwal N, Séminel M, et al. Choroidal structural changes in patients with birdshot chorioretinopathy. *Ocul Immunol Inflamm*. 2019:1–6. https://doi.org/10.1080/09273948.2019.1681472. Epub ahead of print.
29. Böni C, Thorne JE, Spaide RF, et al. Choroidal findings in eyes with birdshot chorioretinitis using enhanced-depth optical coherence tomography. *Invest Ophthalmol Vis Sci*. 2016;57(9):591–599.
30. Birnbaum AD, Fawzi AA, Rademaker A, Goldstein DA. Correlation between clinical signs and optical coherence tomography with enhanced depth imaging findings in patients with birdshot chorioretinopathy. *JAMA Ophthalmol*. 2014;132(8):929–935.
31. Pepple KL, Chu Z, Weinstein J, Munk MR, Van Gelder RN, Wang RK. Use of En Face Swept-Source Optical Coherence Tomography Angiography in Identifying Choroidal Flow Voids in 3 Patients With Birdshot Chorioretinopathy. *JAMA Ophthalmol*. 2018;136(11):1288–1292.
32. Oberts PK, Nesper PL, Goldstein DA, Fawzi AA. Retinal capillary density in patients wth birdshot chorioretinopathy. *Retina*. 2018;38(2):387–394.
33. Knickelbein JE, Tucker W, Kodati S, Akanda M, Sen HN. Non-invasive method of monitoring retinal vasculitis in patients with birdshot chorioretinopathy using optical coherence tomography. *Br J Ophthalmol*. 2018;102(6):815–820.
34. Knickelbein JE, Hasan J, Nussenblatt RB, Sen HN. Delineation of choroidal and retinal lesions in posterior uveitis by multispectral wide-field scanning laser ophthalmoscopy. *Retina*. 2016;36(11):2213–2219.
35. Pohlmann D, Macedo S, Stübiger N, Pleyer U, Joussen AM, Winterhalter S. Multimodal imaging in birdshot retinochoroiditis. *Ocul Immunol Inflamm*. 2017;25(5):621–632.
36. De Geronimo F, Glacet-Bernard A, Coscas G, et al. Birdshot chorioretinopathy: measurement of the posterior fundus spots and macular edema using a retinal thickness analyzer, before and after treatment. *Eur J Ophthalmol*. 2000;10(4):338–340.
37. Herbort CP, Probst K, Cimino L, et al. Differential inflammatory involvement in retina and choroid in birdshot chorioretinopathy. *Klin Monatsbl Augenheilkd*. 2004;221(5):351–356.
38. Lommatzsch P, Ulrich WD, Ulrich C, et al. Birdshot chorioretinopathy. Case report. *Fortschr Ophthalmol*. 1990;87:562–566.
39. Reddy AK, Gonzalez MA, Henry CR, Yeh S, Sobrin L, Albini TA. Diagnostic sensitivity of indocyanine green angiography for birdshot chorioretinopathy. *JAMA Ophthalmol*. 2015;133(7):840–843.
40. Elahi S, Gillmann K, Gasc A, Jeannin B, Herbort CP Jr. Sensitivity of indocyanine green angiography compared to fluorescein angiography and enhanced depth imaging optical coherence tomography during tapering and fine-tuning of therapy in primary stromal choroiditis: a case series. *J Curr Ophthalmol*. 2019;31(2):180–187.
41. Cheng SK, Thompson I, Okeagu C, Nida H. Choroidal lesions unresponsive to fluocinolone acetonide intravitreal implant in birdshot chorioretinopathy. *Retin Cases Brief Rep*. 2019 Oct 31. https://doi.org/10.1097/ICB.0000000000000909. Online ahead of print.
42. Teussink MM, Huis In Het Veld PI, de Vries LA, Hoyng CB, Klevering BJ, Theelen T. Multimodal imaging of the disease progression of birdshot chorioretinopathy. *Acta Ophthalmol*. 2016;94(8):815–823.
43. Gordon LK, Goldhardt R, Holland GN, et al. Standardized visual field assessment for patients with birdshot chorioretinopathy. *Ocul Immunol Inflamm*. 2006;14(6):325–332.
44. Gordon LK, Monnet D, Holland GN, et al. Longitudinal cohort study of patients with birdshot chorioretinopathy. IV. Visual field results at baseline. *Am J Ophthalmol*. 2007;144(6):829–837.
45. Thorne JE, Jabs DA, Kedhar SR, et al. Loss of visual field among patients with birdshot chorioretinopathy. *Am J Ophthalmol*. 2008;145(1):23–28.
46. Holder GE, Robson AG, Pavesio C, et al. Electrophysiological characterisation and monitoring in the management of birdshot chorioretinopathy. *Br J Ophthalmol*. 2005;89(6):709–718.
47. Sobrin L, Lam BL, Liu M, et al. Electroretinographic monitoring in birdshot chorioretinopathy. *Am J Ophthalmol*. 2005;140(1):52–64.
48. Zacks DN, Samson CM, Loewenstein J, et al. Electroretinograms as an indicator of disease activity in birdshot chorioretinopathy. *Graefes Arch Clin Exp Ophthalmol*. 2002;24:601–607.
49. Robson AG, Richardson EC, Koh AH, et al. Unilateral electronegative ERG of non-vascular aetiology. *Br J Ophthalmol*. 2005;89(12):1620–1626.
50. Knickelbein JE, Jeffrey BG, Wei MM, et al. Reproducibility of full-field electroretinogram measurements in birdshot chorioretinopathy patients: an intra- and inter-visit analysis. *Ocul Immunol Inflamm*. 2020 Jan 4:1–6. https://doi.org/10.1080/09273948.2019.1697824. Online ahead of print.
51. Holland GN, Shah KH, Monnet D, et al. Longitudinal cohort study of patients with birdshot chorioretinopathy II: color vision at baseline. *Am J Ophthalmol*. 2006;142(6):1013–1018.
52. Kappel PJ, Monnet D, Yu F, et al. Contrast sensitivity among patients with birdshot chorioretinopathy. *Am J Ophthalmol*. 2009;147(2):351–356.
53. Nozik R, Dorsch W. A new chorioretinopathy associated with anterior uveitis. *Am J Ophthalmol*. 1973;76:758–762.
54. Dreyer R, Gass J. Multifocal choroiditis and panuveitis. *Arch Ophthalmol*. 1984;102:1776–1784.
55. Brod R. Presumed sarcoid choroidopathy mimicking birdshot retinochoroidopathy. *Am J Ophthalmol*. 1990;109:357–358.
56. Brinkman C, Rothova A. Fundus pathology in neurosarcoidosis. *Int Ophthalmol*. 1993;17:23–26.
57. Jampol L, Sieving PA, Pugh D, et al. Multiple evanescent white dot syndrome. *Arch Ophthalmol*. 1984;102:671–679.
58. Kim JS, Jaworski L, Patel-Donnelly D, Nussenblatt RB, Sen HN. Waldenström's macroglobulinemia masquerading as birdshot chorioretinopathy. *Retin Cases Brief Rep*. 2017;11(2):152–155.
59. Noble KG, Greenberg J. Appearance of birdshot chorioretinopathy in a patient with myelodysplasia syndrome. *Am J Ophthalmol*. 1998;125:108–109.
60. Cunningham ET Jr, Sabrosa NA, Pavesio CE. Posterior scleritis mimicking birdshot chorioretinopathy. *Eye*. 2001;15(Pt 2):231–233.
61. Sullu Y, Yildiran A, Sullu Y, Helek D, Ozkaya O. Sarcoid uveitis simulating birdshot chorioretinopathy in a child. *Retin Cases Brief Rep*. 2012;6(1):7–10.
62. de Maeyer V, Leroy BP, Kerre T, et al. Birdshot-like chorioretinopathy in common variable immunodeficiency. *Retin Cases Brief Rep*. 2012;6(4):358–364.
63. Acaba-Berrocal LA, Lucio-Alvarez JA, Mashayekhi A, Ho AC, Dunn JP, Shields CL. Birdshot-like chorioretinopathy associated with pembrolizumab treatment. *JAMA Ophthalmol*. 2018;136(10):1205–1207.
64. Kellner U, Helbig H, Foerster MH. Phänokopien hereditärer Netzhautdegenerationen [Phenocopies of hereditary retinal degenerations]. *Ophthalmologe*. 1996;93(6):680–687.
65. Sommer S, Badet JC, Zaoui M, et al. Birdshot chorioretinopathy associated with tamoxifen retinal toxicity. *J Fr Ophtalmol*. 2000;23(5):494–497.
66. Knezevic A, Munk MR, Pappas F, Merrill PT, Goldstein DA. HLA-A29-positive birdshot chorioretinopathy in an African American patient. *Retin Cases Brief Rep*. 2016;10(3):201–204.
67. Yang P, Zhang Z, Zhou H, et al. Clinical patterns and characteristics of uveitis in a tertiary center for uveitis in China. *Curr Eye Res*. 2005;30(11):943–948.
68. Nussenblatt R, Mittal KK, Ryan S, et al. Birdshot chorioretinopathy associated with HLA-A29 antigen and immune responsiveness to retinal S-antigen. *Am J Ophthalmol*. 1982;94:147–158.
69. Le Hoang P, Donnefort N, Foucoult C, et al. Association between HLA-A29 antigen and birdshot chorioretinopathy. *Proceedings for the XXVth International Congress of Ophthalmology*. Rome: Kugler and Ghedini; 1986.
70. Baarmsa G, Kijlstra A, Oosterhuis JA, et al. Association of birdshot chorioretinopathy and HLA-A29 antigen. *Doc Ophthalmol*. 1986;61:267–269.
71. Baarsma G, Priem H, Kijlstra A. Association of birdshot chorioretinopathy and HLA-A29 antigen. *Curr Eye Res*. 1990;9(Suppl):63–68.
72. Le Hoang P, Mittal KK, Ryan S, et al. HLA-A29.2 subtype associated with birdshot chorioretinopathy. *Am J Ophthalmol*. 1992;113:33–35.
73. Tabary T, Prochnicka-Chalufour A, Cornillet P, et al. HLA-A29 subtypes and "birdshot" choroido-retinopathy susceptibility: a possible "resistance motif" in the HLA-As29.1 molecule. *C R Acad Sci III*. 1991;313:599–605.

74. de Waal L, Lardy NM, van der Horst AR, et al. HLA-A29 subtypes and birdshot chorioretinopathy. *Immunogenetics*. 1992;35:51–53.
75. Levinson RD, Rajalingam R, Park MS, et al. Human leukocyte antigen A29 subtypes associated with birdshot chorioretinopathy. *Am J Ophthalmol*. 2004;138(4):631–634.
76. Donvito B, Monnet D, Tabary T, et al. Different HLA class IA region complotypes for HLA-A29.2 and -A29.1 antigens, identical in birdshot chorioretinopathy patients or healthy individuals. *Invest Ophthalmol Vis Sci*. 2005;46(9):3227–3232.
77. Saito W, Yamamoto S, Mitamura Y, et al. Birdshot chorioretinopathy—a case report and a case study in Japanese patients. *J Jpn Ophthalmol Soc*. 2002;106:229–235.
78. Wee R, Papaliodis G. Genetics of birdshot chorioretinopathy. *Semin Ophthalmol*. 2008;23(1):53–57.
79. Levinson RD, Du Z, Luo L, et al. Combination of KIR and HLA gene variants augments the risk of developing birdshot chorioretinopathy in HLA-A*29-positive individuals. *Genes Immun*. 2008;9(3):249–258.
80. Jobin D, Thillaye B, de Kozak Y, et al. Severe chorioretinopathy: variations of humoral and cellular immunity to S-antigen in a longitudinal study. *Curr Eye Res*. 1990;9(Suppl):91–96.
81. Gaudio PA, Kaye DB, Crawford JB. Histopathology of birdshot chorioretinopathy. *Br J Ophthalmol*. 2002;86:1439–1463.
82. Tsui E, Takhar JS, Joye A, Ahmad TR, Acharya NR, Gonzales JA. High resolution DNA typing of human leukocyte antigen A29 in familial birdshot chorioretinopathy. 2019 Nov 13. *Ocul Immunol Inflamm*. 2019:1–4. https://doi.org/10.1080/09273948.2019.1682173. Online ahead of print.
83. Trinh L, Bodaghi B, Fardeau C, et al. Clinical features, treatment methods, and evolution of birdshot chorioretinopathy in 5 different families. *Am J Ophthalmol*. 2009;147(6):1042–1047. e1.
84. Fich M, Rosenberg T. Birdshot chorioretinopathy in monozygotic twins. *Acta Ophthalmol (Copenh)*. 1992;70(5):693–697.
85. Boisgérault F, Khalil I, Tieng V, et al. Definition of the HLA-A29 peptide ligand motif allows prediction of potential T-cell epitopes from the retinal soluble antigen, a candidate autoantigen in birdshot retinopathy. *Proc Natl Acad Sci USA*. 1996;93:3466–3470.
86. Szpak Y, Vieville JC, Tabary T, et al. Spontaneous retinopathy in HLA-A29 transgenic mice. *Proc Natl Acad Sci U S A*. 2001;98(5):2572–2576.
87. de Kozak Y, Camelo S, Pla M. Pathological aspects of spontaneous uveitis and retinopathy in HLA-A29 transgenic mice and in animal models of retinal autoimmunity: relevance to human pathologies. *Ophthalmic Res*. 2008;40(3–4):175–180.
88. Kuiper J, Rothova A, de Boer J, Radstake T. The immunopathogenesis of birdshot chorioretinopathy; a bird of many feathers. *Prog Retin Eye Res*. 2015;44:99–110.
89. Kuiper JJW, et al. A genome-wide association study identifies a functional ERAP2 haplotype associated with birdshot chorioretinopathy. *Hum Mol Genet*. 2014;23(22):6081–6087.
90. Soubrane G, Bokobza R, Coscas G. Late developing lesions in birdshot chorioretinopathy. *Am J Ophthalmol*. 1990;109:204–210.
91. Godel V, Baruch E, Lazar M. Late development of chorioretinal lesions in birdshot chorioretinopathy. *Ann Ophthalmol*. 1989;21:49–52.
92. Bloch-Michel E, Frau E. Birdshot chorioretinopathy and HLA-A29+ and HLA-A29- idiopathic retinal vasculitis: comparative study of 56 cases. *Can J Ophthalmol*. 1991;26:361–366.
93. Gaudio PA, et al. Histopathology of birdshot retinochoroidopathy. *Br J Ophthalmol*. 2002;86:1439–1441.
94. Kuiper JJW, Rothova A, Schellenkens PAW, Norel AO, Bloem AC, Mutis T. Detection of choroid- and retina-antigen reactive CD8(+) and CD4(+) T lymphocytes in the vitreous fluid of patients with birdshot chorioretinopathy. *Hum Immunol*. 2014;75:570–577.
95. Klok A, Geertzen R, Rothova A, et al. Anticardiolipin antibodies in uveitis. *Curr Eye Res*. 1992;11(Suppl):209–213.
96. Kuhne F, Morlat P, Riss I, et al. Is A29, B12 vasculitis caused by the Q fever agent *Coxiella burnetii? J Fr Ophthalmol*. 1992;15:315–321.
97. Hofmann H, Feicht B. Birdshot chorioretinopathy: systemic therapy with corticosteroids and nonsteroidal anti-inflammatory drugs. *Klin Monatsbl Augenheilkd*. 1990;197:159–161.
98. Ladas JG, Arnold AC, Holland GN. Control of visual symptoms in two men with birdshot chorioretinopathy using low-dose oral corticosteroid therapy. *Am J Ophthalmol*. 1999;128:116–118.
99. Leder HA, Galor A, Thorne JE, Jabs D. Disappearance of classic birdshot spots after immunosuppression with tacrolimus and mycophenolate mofetil. *Br J Ophthalmol*. 2008;92(2):291.
100. Martidis A, Duker JS, Puliafito CA. Intravitreal triamcinolone for refractory cystoid macular edema secondary to birdshot chorioretinopathy. *Arch Ophthalmol*. 2001;119:1380–1383.
101. Bajwa A, Aziz K, Foster CS. Safety and efficacy of fluocinolone acetonide intravitreal implant (0.59 mg) in birdshot retinochoroidopathy. *Retina*. 2014;34(11):2259–2268.
102. Rush RB, Goldstein DA, Callanan DG, Meghpara B, Feuer WJ, Davis JL. Outcomes of birdshot chorioretinopathy treated with an intravitreal sustained-release fluocinolone acetonide-containing device. *Am J Ophthalmol*. 2011;151(4):630–636.
103. Lages V, Skvortsova N, Jeannin B, Gasc A, Herbort CP. Low-grade "benign" birdshot retinochoroiditis: prevalence and characteristics. *Int Ophthalmol*. 2019;39(9):2111–2120.
104. Le Hoang P, Ryan SJ. Birdshot chorioretinopathy. In: Pepose JS, Holland GN, Wilhelmus KR, eds. *Ocular Infection and Immunity*. St. Louis: Mosby; 1995:570–578.
105. Le Hoang P, Girard B, Deray G, et al. Cyclosporine in the treatment of birdshot chorioretinopathy. *Transplant Proc*. 1988;20(3 Suppl 4):128–130.
106. Vitale A, Rodriguez A, Foster C. Low-dose cyclosporine therapy in the treatment of birdshot chorioretinopathy. *Ophthalmology*. 1994;101:822–831.
107. Kiss S, Ahmed M, Letko E, et al. Long-term follow-up of patients with birdshot chorioretinopathy treated with corticosteroid-sparing systemic immunomodulatory therapy. *Ophthalmology*. 2005;112(6):1066–1071.
108. Rasquin FA, Pereleux AA. Long term follow-up of birdshot chorioretinopathy. *Bull Soc Belge Ophtalmol*. 2004;293:25–33.
109. Becker MD, Wertheim MS, Smith JR, et al. Long-term follow-up of patients with birdshot chorioretinopathy treated with systemic immunosuppression. *Ocul Immunol Inflamm*. 2005;13(4):289–293.
110. Le Hoang P, Cassoux N, George F, et al. Intravenous immunoglobulin (IVIg) for the treatment of birdshot chorioretinopathy. *Ocul Immunol Inflamm*. 2000;8(1):49–57.
111. Sobrin L, Huang JJ, Christen W, et al. Daclizumab for treatment of birdshot chorioretinopathy. *Arch Ophthalmol*. 2008;126(2):186–191.
112. You C, Lasave AF, Kubaisi B, et al. Long-term outcomes of systemic corticosteroid-sparing immunomodulatory therapy for birdshot retinochoroidopathy. *Ocul Immunol Inflamm*. 2020;28(6):966-974.
113. Vegas-Revenga N, Calvo-Río V, Mesquida M, et al. Anti-IL6-receptor tocilizumab in refractory and noninfectious uveitic cystoid macular edema: multicenter study of 25 patients. *Am J Ophthalmol*. 2019;200:85–94.
114. Leclercq M, Le Besnerais M, Langlois V, et al. Tocilizumab for the treatment of birdshot uveitis that failed interferon alpha and anti-tumor necrosis factor-alpha therapy: two cases report and literature review. *Clin Rheumatol*. 2018;37(3):849–853.

27

Behçet Disease

H. Nida Sen

KEY CONCEPTS

- Behçet disease is a multisystem disease, with imminently vision-threatening posterior ocular complications.
- The posterior pole disease should not be treated with corticosteroids alone.
- Tumor necrosis factor (TNF) inhibitors have been suggested as first-line immunosuppressives for ocular Behçet disease.

Retinal vascular involvement is a common finding in many patients with posterior and intermediate uveitis. Behçet disease may be the best example of a disorder characterized mainly by its retinal vascular involvement, often with devastating effects on the patient's eyesight.

Behçet disease is a multisystem disorder named after the Turkish dermatologist, Hulusi Behçet (1889–1948),[1] who, in 1937, recognized and reported a triad of symptoms: recurrent intraocular inflammatory episodes with oral and mucosal ulcerations. These observations were based on three patients, two of whom had ocular symptoms. It should be noted that in the twentieth century, at least two other clinicians reported cases with similar findings earlier than Behçet did: Adamantiades in 1931 (publishing in the French literature)[2] and Shigeta from Japan in 1924.[3] However, their reports did not stimulate the universal interest that Behçet did, hence the commonly used term for the disease *Behçet disease.* The disease is believed to be known in ancient times, with Hippocrates probably being the first to describe an association between ocular inflammation and oral and genital lesions.[4] Familial occurrence is seen in 8% to 18% of Turkish patients with the disease, 15% of Koreans, and 13% of Jews, but much less in a Chinese population (2.6%).[5,6] In a study reviewing 761 patients in Turkey, almost 57% of patients with an identifiable diagnosis had Behçet disease, with 10.4% being of juvenile onset.[7] The prevalence has been calculated to be 80 to 370 per 100,000.[6] It is interesting to note that the frequency of the disease is 18-fold less in Turks living in Germany than in those in Turkey. In one center in the United States, Behçet disease constituted 2.5% of uveitis referrals.[8] One report from Iran[9] put the number of patients with Behçet disease seen at a uveitis clinic in Tehran at 8.6%, with more cases of ocular toxoplasmosis being seen. The complete form of Behçet disease is rare in Northern Italy, with a prevalence calculated at 3.8 per 100,000 (incidence of 0.24/100,000).[10] The disease has been noted to be especially common in the Far East and in the Mediterranean basin and is very frequently noted between 30° and 45° north latitude in Asian and European populations.[11] This corresponds to the old Silk Route used for centuries by traders making the dangerous passage from the East to the West (Fig. 27.1). The prevalence rate of Behçet disease ranges from 20 to 420 in 100,000 persons in Turkey to 0.63 in 100,000 in the United Kingdom.[12-14] It appears that the disease is changing in character, severity, and prevalence. About 40 years ago, Japan appeared to have the highest incidence of this disorder,[15] with an overall prevalence of 70 to 85 cases/1 million population, as calculated in the late 1970s.[16] In the early 1990s, it was estimated that the total number of patients with this disease in Japan was 16,570, with a prevalence of 135 cases/1 million population.[17] However, the northern portions of Japan have a higher incidence compared with the southern areas. Of the estimated 15,000 patients in Japan with Behçet disease in 1986, 11,000 were receiving treatment.[18] This diagnosis was applied to greater than 20% of the patients with uveitis seen in the uveitis clinic of the University of Tokyo's Department of Ophthalmology from 1965 through 1977.[16] Other studies have suggested a lower prevalence of 13.5 to 20/100,000 in Japan and Korea.[6]

This disorder may have devastating consequences for the eyes and has therefore attracted a great deal of attention. Insight into its mechanisms has led to improvement in the treatment of this disorder.

CLINICAL MANIFESTATIONS

The diagnosis of Behçet disease is based firmly on the presence of a constellation of clinical findings. Numerous sets of clinical criteria have been proposed for the diagnosis of Behçet disease.[19,20] For our service, we have adapted the criteria established by the Behçet Disease Research Committee of Japan (Box 27.1). As can be seen, these criteria include an additional major finding to the original three—that is, skin lesions. Furthermore, the presence of ocular inflammatory disease is given greater weight in the diagnosis. It should also be noted that the minor criteria are not considered in this grading system. The Behçet Disease Research Committee of Japan recognizes three special forms of the disease: intestinal Behçet disease, vasculo-Behçet disease, and neuro-Behçet disease (essentially the minor criteria). It has also specifically included three laboratory tests: a pathergy test (a skin-prick test), human leukocyte antigen (HLA) testing for HLA-B51, and screening for nonspecific factors indicative of immune system activation, such as an elevated erythrocyte sedimentation rate (ESR), positive results for cross-reactive protein (CRP), and an increase in the number of peripheral blood leukocytes.

Another system that the reader should be familiar with is the one suggested by the International Study Group for Behçet Disease,[21,22] which requires the presence of oral aphthous ulcers for the diagnosis in all patients (Box 27.2). These investigators emphasized the importance of oral aphthous ulcers as a sign of this disease on the basis of data collected from a large number of patients and control subjects; they found that 97% of patients with Behçet disease had oral aphthae.[22]

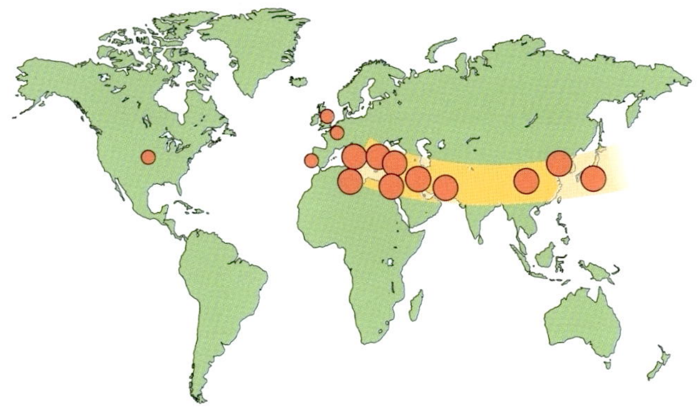

Fig. 27.1 Map of a broad band through Asia and Europe where Behçet disease is common. This coincides with the old Silk Route. (Courtesy S. Ohno, MD.)

BOX 27.1 Criteria for Diagnosis of Behçet Disease

Major Criteria

Recurrent aphthous ulcers of oral mucosa
Skin lesions
Erythema nodosum, acne, cutaneous hypersensitivity thrombophlebitis
Genital ulcers
Ocular inflammatory disease
Recurrent anterior and posterior

Minor Criteria

Arthritis
Intestinal ulcers
Epididymitis
Vascular disease
Obliteration, occlusion, aneurysm
Neuropsychiatric symptoms
Complete type
Four major symptoms simultaneously or at different times
Incomplete type
Three major symptoms simultaneously or at different times
or
Typical recurrent ocular disease with one other major criterion
Suspect type
Two major symptoms, excluding ocular
Possible type
One main symptom

Modified from Behçet's Disease Research Committee. Clinical research section recommendations. *Jpn J Ophthalmol.* 1974;18:291–294.

Many classification and diagnostic criteria have been established for Behçet disease since the 1940s. The most commonly used ones are the criteria developed by International Study Group (ISG) in 1990 and the Japanese Behçet Disease Research Committee in 1977 (see Boxes 27.1 and 27.2). Some systems have equated two of the minor criteria to one major criterion. Others have tried to introduce a standardized scoring system for all parts of the disease.[23] There is no question that some degree of uncertainty is inherent in any system because various symptoms may manifest at different times during the clinical course of the disease. The International Criteria for Behçet Disease (ICBD) was revised in 2014.[24]

BOX 27.2 Diagnostic Criteria of International Study Group for Behçet Disease

Recurrent Oral Ulceration

Minor or major aphthous lesions or herpetiform-like lesions should have been observed by the physician or patient at least three times within a 12-month period.

Presence of Two Other Criteria

Recurrent genital ulceration
Observation by the physician or the patient of aphthous ulceration or scar
Eye lesions
The ocular disease, including anterior and/or posterior uveitis, cells in the vitreous, or the presence of a retinal vasculitis
Skin lesions noted by the physician or the patient, including erythema nodosum, pseudofolliculitis, and papulopustular lesions; in addition, other lesions, including an acneiform nodule in postadolescent patients not receiving corticosteroid therapy
Positive pathergy test result read by physician at 24 to 48 hours

Modified from International Study Group for Behçet's Disease. Criteria for diagnosis of Behçet's disease. *Lancet.* 1990;335:1078–1080.

TABLE 27.1 Percentage of Patients Manifesting Criteria for Behçet Disease[a]

Criteria	Men	Women	Total
Major			
Ocular	86.2	67.8	78.6
Aphthae	97.9	98.8	98.3
Skin	89.8	91.3	90.4
Genital	76.8	83.8	79.8
Minor			
Arthritis	56.1	62.6	58.9
Intestinal	27.7	25.9	26.9
Vascular	8.7	6.3	7.7
Psychiatric	10.3	6.4	8.6

[a]At least 1700 patients were analyzed for each criterion.
Data from Mishima S, Masuda K, Izawa Y, et al. Behçet disease in Japan: ophthalmologic aspects. *Trans Am Ophthalmol Soc.* 1979;76:225–229.

In a 1991 survey of 3316 patients with Behçet disease in Japan, oral aphthae are the most frequently seen major symptom, occurring in 97.7%.[25] Other commonly seen problems were skin lesions (90.4%), with genital ulcers, and ocular attacks having a similar incidence (79.8% and 78.6%, respectively)[16] (Table 27.1). Oral aphthae are, by far, the most common symptom at presentation.[16] After oral aphthae, the order of appearance of the major symptoms is as follows: skin lesions; ocular symptoms (25.4% in males); genital ulceration in males; and ocular lesions in females (8.6%). With regard to the minor criteria, in Japan, the most frequently seen symptom is arthritis (see Table 27.1). The ratio of males to females with this disease in Japan has been reported as 1.2:1 in 1972 and 0.77:1 in 1981.[18] A study involving 25 eye centers and 14 countries identified 1465 patients with ocular lesions. Of those patients, 94.5% had oral ulcers, with skin lesions and genital ulcers found in greater than 60%. Behçet disease onset typically occurs in the third decade of life. The most common initial symptom is the presence of oral aphthae (82.1%), followed by genital ulcers (10%) and ocular lesions (uveitis and retinal vasculitis; 8.9%).[26] There are also

TABLE 27.2 Epidemiologic Changes in Behçet Disease in Japan from 1972 to 1991

	NO. MALES/ FEMALES		SEX RATIO	
Disease Type	**1972**	**1991**	**1972**	**1991**
Complete type	594/334	588/551	1.78	1.07
Incomplete type				
- With ocular disease	403/230	750/402	1.75	1.87
- Without ocular disease	172/298	300/725	0.58	0.41
Incomplete type				
- With genital ulcers	260/352	338/806	0.74	0.42
- Without genital ulcers	315/176	712/321	1.79	2.22
Incomplete type				
- With both ocular and genital	88/54	73/104	1.63	0.7
- Ocular without genital	315/176	674/298	1.79	2.26
- Genital without ocular	172/298	300/725	0.58	0.41

Reproduced with permission from Nakae K, Masaki F, Hashimoto T, et al. Recent epidemiologic features of Behçet's disease in Japan. In: Godeau P, Wechster B. *Behçet's Disease*. St. Louis: Elsevier; 1993. Copyright 1993 Elsevier.

TABLE 27.3 Comparison of Demographic Characteristics and Follow-Up Duration of Patients with Ocular Behçet Disease

Characteristic	**1960s**	**1980s**	**1990s**	**Total**
Total, n (%)	45 (38)	26 (21)	49 (41)	120 (100)
Sex, n (%)				
- Female	19 (42)	10 (38)	24 (49)	53 (44)
- Male	26 (58)	16 (62)	25 (51)	67 (56)
Race, n (%)				
- Caucasian	35 (78)	19 (73)	28 (57)	82 (68)
- African American	4 (9)	1 (4)	6 (12)	11 (9)
- Hispanic	2 (4)	2 (8)	2 (4)	6 (5)
- Asian	2 (4)	1 (8)	4 (8)	8 (7)
- American Indian	1 (2)	1 (4)	3 (6)	5 (4)
- Other/unknown	1 (2)	1 (4)	6 (12)	8 (7)
Age at diagnosis, median (years) (range)	28 (13–50)	28 (15–46)	30.5 (6–59)	28 (6–59)
Missing age at diagnosis, n	4	3	3	10
Follow-up, median (years) (range)	0.5 (0–9.3)	2.9 (0–16.8)	1.8 (0–13.1)	1.7 (0–16.8)
Period between ocular onset and first visit (years)	3.8	3.4	4.0	3.8

Reproduced with permission from Kump LI, Moeller KL, Reed GF, et al. Behçet's disease: Comparing 3 decades of treatment response at the National Eye Institute. *Can J Opthalmol.* 2008;43:468.

variable reports on male-to-female preponderance, with the majority of studies reporting a male preponderance.[26] In Turkey, the male-to-female ratio has been reported as 3.3:1.[18] More males have the complete form of the disease compared with females. Over a period of 20 years, differences have been noted in the various aspects of the disease and their presence in men and women (Table 27.2). In Israel, Krause et al.[27] evaluated 100 patients with Behçet disease, 66 of whom were of Jewish ethnicity (with origins from Iran, Turkey, and North Africa) and 34 of whom were of Arab ethnicity. The manifestation of the disease seemed to be the same, but the patients of Arab ethnicity appeared to have more serious eye disease. Muhaya et al.[28] compared 19 patients with the disease seen at Moorfields Hospital in London with 35 patients seen at the Kurume University Eye Clinic in southern Japan over the same period. The Japanese patients were older (average age 43 years) compared with those seen in London in the United Kingdom (average age 35 years). No significant differences were noted in the extraocular findings. More of the Japanese patients had acute uveitis and posterior pole disease and received treatment with topical steroids. The U.K. patients were more often treated with systemic steroids.

Although the onset of Behçet disease occurs in early adulthood, childhood onset has been reported in rare cases.[29,30] Laghmari et al.[31] studied 13 patients with childhood Behçet disease and found that familial Behçet disease and articular and digestive manifestations were more commonly seen in younger children, whereas neurologic and vascular involvement, including panuveitis, seemed to occur more frequently in older children. Ando et al.[32] compared patients seen in a Tokyo eye clinic from 1974 to 1983 with those seen from 1984 to 1993. The number of women presenting with the disease increased to about one-quarter of the patients. Initially, ocular symptoms manifested in 70% of patients (in their third and fourth decades), and by 1993, almost two-thirds of the patients seen at the clinic had the incomplete form of the disease. What was striking was the observation that the patients seen between 1984 and 1993 had a much better visual course, ascribed by the authors to better therapy (see later discussion). In one study of 520 patients with Behçet disease in North Africa,[33] 83% were males, and the mean age of patients was 20 years, which is a very young age, according to our experience. Eighty percent of the patients had ophthalmic involvement, with one-quarter losing sight because of their disease. Being male, initial presentation with poor visual acuity, and posterior or panuveitis were all associated with a poor visual outcome.[34,35] Being female and having the disease at a young age were associated with nonrecurrence of ocular involvement.[36]

The majority of 120 patients with Behçet disease seen at the National Eye Institute (NEI) over three decades were males.[37] During the same period, the majority (68%) of these patients were Caucasian, and the median age at diagnosis was remarkably similar over the three decades (Table 27.3); and 95% of the patients had bilateral disease. All the patients presented with oral ulcers, and genital and skin lesions were the next most common symptoms. Over the three decades, 8% to 22% of patients had central nervous system (CNS) disease (Table 27.4). The reader can find a comparison of the extraocular findings with the frequency of clinical findings and onset of manifestations reported in 661 Turkish patients in Table 27.5.[38] Table 27.6 provides a comparison of the therapies used over the three decades. We have seen a marked improvement in initial visual acuity in those patients treated in the 1990s and 2000s compared with the earlier groups. The mean inflammation score decreased as well.

Barra et al.,[39] in Brazil, reviewed 49 patients with Behçet disease, representing 2% of the total number of patients with uveitis they saw over a 16-year period. Of their patients, 71% were males, and more than three-quarters of all patients were white; in 34.5%, the ocular attack was the first symptom of the disease; overall, it took a little

TABLE 27.4 Comparison of Extraocular Manifestations of Behçet Disease over Three Decades[a]

Manifestation	1960s, n (%)	1980s, n (%)	1990s, n (%)	Total, n (%)
Total patients	45 (38)	26 (21)	49 (41)	120 (100)
Oral ulcers	45 (100)	26 (100)	49 (100)	120 (100)
Genital ulcers	32 (71)	16 (62)	35 (71)	83 (69)
Skin lesions	26 (58)	17 (65)	27 (55)	70 (58)
Arthritis	13 (29)	12 (46)	20 (41)	45 (38)
Central nervous system	10 (22)	5 (19)	4 (8)	19 (16)
Vascular lesions	3 (7)	–	3 (6)	6 (5)
Epididymitis	2 (4)	1 (4)	2 (4)	5 (4)

[a]No significant difference among decades (Fisher's exact test).
Reproduced with permission from Kump LI, Moeller KL, Reed GF, et al. Behçet's disease: comparing 3 decades of treatment response at the National Eye Institute. *Can J Opthalmol.* 2008;43:468.

TABLE 27.5 The Frequency of Clinical Findings and Onset Manifestations

Clinical Features	Patients (n = 661)	%
Oral ulcer	661	100
Genital ulcer	564	85.3
Papulopustular lesions	366	55.4
Erythema nodosum	292	44.2
Articular involvement	221	33.4
Ocular involvement	193	29.2
Thrombophlebitis	71	10.7
Vascular involvement	29	4.4
Neurologic involvement	20	3.0
Gastrointestinal involvement	11	1.6
Skin pathergy reaction	250	37.8
Onset lesions		
Oral ulcer	586	88.7
Genital ulcer	94	14.2
Erythema nodosum	38	5.7
Ocular involvement	28	4.2
Simultaneous occurrence of the symptoms (n = 79)		
Oral ulcer and genital ulcer	65	9.8
Oral ulcer and erythema nodosum	21	3.1
Oral ulcer and ocular involvement	15	2.2
Oral ulcer, genital ulcer, and erythema nodosum	16	2.4
Oral ulcer, genital ulcer, and ocular involvement	11	1.6

Reproduced with permission from Alpsoy E, Donmez L, Onder M, et al. Clinical features and natural course of Behçet's disease in 661 cases: a multicentre study. *Br J Dermatol.* 2007;157:901.

TABLE 27.6 Comparison of Systemic Treatment in Patients with Ocular Behçet Disease over Three Decades

Medication	1960s, n (%)	1980s, n (%)	1990s, n (%)	Total, n (%)
Total patients	45 (38)	26 (21)	49 (41)	120 (100)
Systemic corticosteroids	43 (96)	26 (100)	41 (84)	110 (92)
Systemic corticosteroids alone	31 (69)	2 (8)	8 (16)	41 (34)
Topical/periocular corticosteroids only	2 (4)	–	4 (8)	6 (5)
Cyclosporin	–	23 (89)	27 (55)	50 (42)
Daclizumab	–	–	15 (31)	15 (13)
Chlorambucil	6 (13)	4 (15)	4 (8)	14 (12)
Azathioprine	1 (2)	2 (8)	10 (20)	13 (11)
Methotrexate	2 (4)	–	8 (16)	10 (8)
Mycophenolate mofetil	–	–	8 (16)	8 (7)
Infliximab	–	–	7 (14)	7 (6)
Cyclophosphamide	2 (4)	3 (12)	2 (4)	7 (6)
Sirolimus	–	–	1 (2)	1 (1)
6-Mercaptopurine	1 (2)	–	–	1 (1)

Reproduced with permission from Kump LI, Moeller KL, Reed GF, et al. Behçet's disease: Comparing 3 decades of treatment response at the National Eye Institute. *Can J Opthalmol.* 2008;43:468.

longer than 3 years for the ocular symptoms to appear after the first manifestation of the disease. In a review of 31 French patients, an ocular manifestation was the first symptom in 29%.[40]

Oral Aphthous Ulcers

An almost universal finding in Behçet disease is the amount of discomfort the oral lesions can cause. The number of patients with oral aphthae in the general population is quite high. However, in our experience, the lesions in patients with Behçet disease can occur in clusters and may be found not only on the gums but also on the lips, posterior pharynx, uvula, palate, and tongue. They can be small but painful, and they recur (Fig. 27.2). They usually heal in 7 to 10 days without scarring, but scarring occurs in the case of a particularly large ulcer. It has been suggested that in contrast to the regular flat borders of the aphthae seen in this disorder, the lesions in Stevens-Johnson syndrome tend to be irregular, and in Reiter syndrome, they can have heaped-up edges.[41] In some patients, these lesions can be induced as a result of eating certain foods; however, Wray et al.[42] have shown that trauma to the oral mucosa can cause them, in a manner strikingly reminiscent of the prick test.

Skin Lesions

Erythema nodosum–like lesions are frequently noted on the anterior surface of the legs (Fig. 27.3) but can also be seen on the face, neck, buttocks, and elsewhere. These lesions involute without ulceration after several weeks.

Acne-like lesions and folliculitis are also common dermatologic lesions. They can appear on the back and the face and are histologically identical to those of the "typical" disorder. Thrombophlebitis is found usually in the extremities. This finding clearly denotes a more general vascular disease that can be life threatening (discussed later). The thrombophlebitis in the extremities can be migratory and can also occur after an injection or the taking of a blood sample.

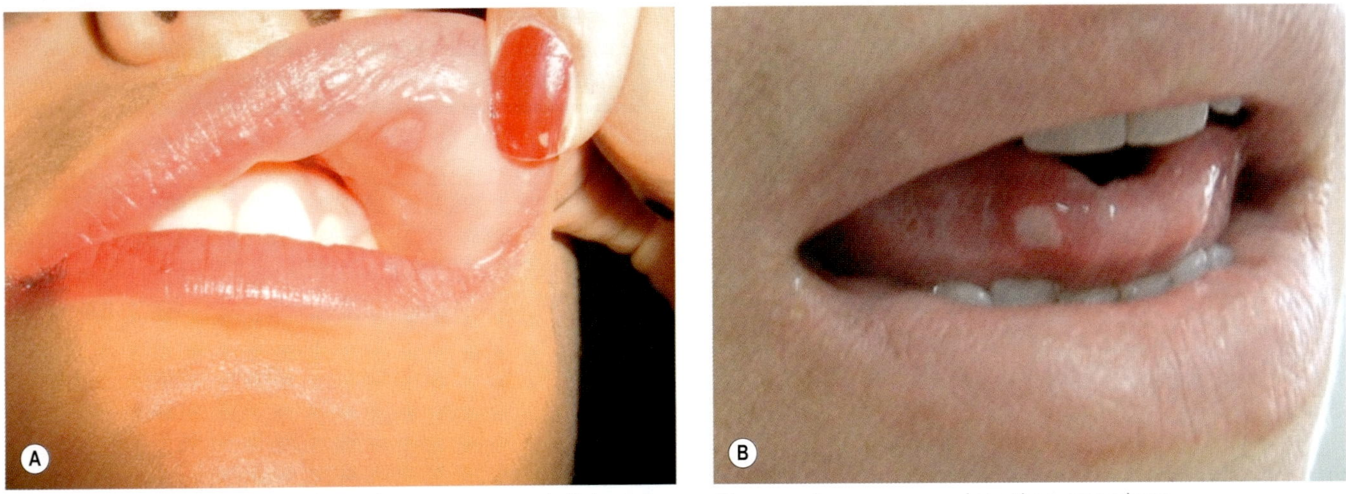

Fig. 27.2 Aphthous ulcers are common in Behçet disease. They usually appear several at a time, sometimes on common surfaces such as the mucosa of the lip (A), or on less common regions, such as the tongue (B). (Courtesy Dr. Murat Borlu, Turkey.)

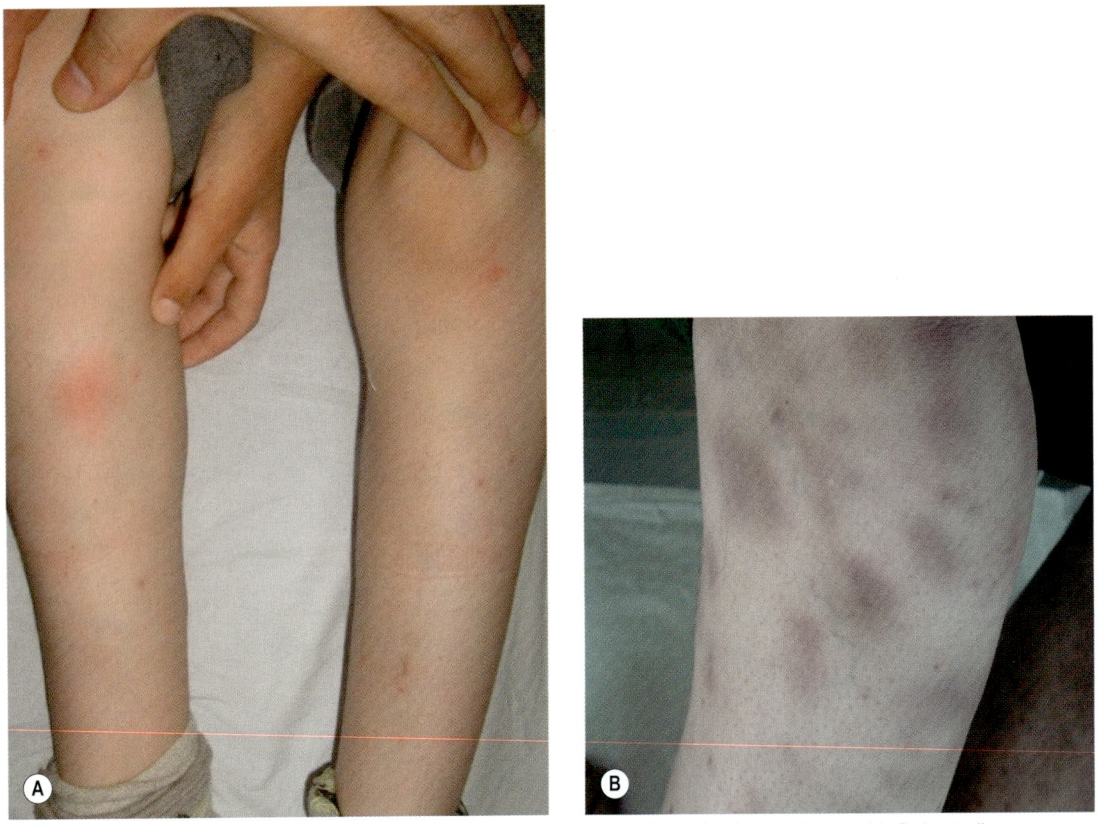

Fig. 27.3 Examination of the peripheral extremities is important in evaluating patients with Behçet disease. An area of erythema nodosum on the legs of a pediatric patient with Behçet disease (A) and an adult patient with Behçet disease (B). (Courtesy Dr. Murat Borlu, Turkey.)

Cutaneous hypersensitivity is a characteristic feature of Behçet disease. Dermatographism, a localized hive-like reaction occurring after a scratch on skin, can be observed in one-third to one-half of patients. Scratching the skin with a needle or taking a blood sample often causes a pustule at that site, called *pathergy*. This phenomenon has become the basis for the "prick" test, with some researchers believing that this is an important criterion that can be used in diagnosing the disease (discussed later), as first suggested by Curth.[43] Use of the pathergy test varies in different countries, and the rates of positivity can range from 8% to 65% in reports from different countries.[44] In our experience, this phenomenon seems to be less common in patients with Behçet disease.

Genital Ulcers

In males, the lesions may appear on the scrotum and the penis and therefore are quite evident, resulting in the patient seeking professional help early in the disease. Females usually have the lesions on the vulva or on the vaginal mucosae. Other lesions may be perianal.

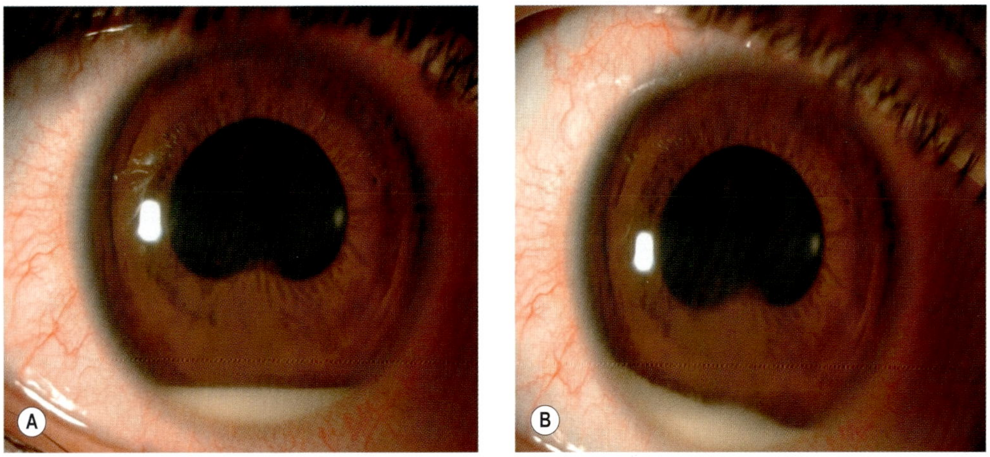

Fig. 27.4 Hypopyon is considered a classic symptom in Behçet disease (A). A shifting hypopyon is typical in Behçet disease and can shift freely with the head movement (B). However, it is not always present during anterior segment inflammation and sometimes can be seen only on gonioscopic examination. (Courtesy Dr. Didar Ucar, Turkey.)

Kobayashi et al.[45] reported that lesions on the vulva occur in the premenstrual part of the month. Genital lesions can be particularly painful and distressing and, initially, it is frequently misdiagnosed as being herpetic in origin.

The genital lesions can be deep and therefore leave scars. Thus an examination of the genital region in a patient with suspected Behçet disease can be useful because signs of earlier disease may be present.

Ocular Disease

The ocular manifestations in Behçet disease have serious implications for the patient. Mamo[46] estimated that vision would be lost 3.36 years after the onset of ocular symptoms. The ominous clinical course should make the clinician especially careful in evaluating these patients.

The disease can affect both the anterior and posterior segments, but certain characteristic signs can and should be looked for. Ocular involvement occurs in approximately 40% to 55.6% of patients.[44] Statistically, ocular disease manifests some 2 to 3 years after the initial symptoms are noted.[47] The disease is bilateral, with unilateral cases occurring rarely. One important aspect is the recurrent, explosive nature of the ocular disease. Patients do not have "chronic" ocular inflammatory disease, that is, a lingering inflammatory episode that can be noted over a long period. Rather, the disease appears, is floridly active for a set period (2–4 weeks), and then disappears, albeit after causing damage; the patient's ocular disease is quiescent for some time, whether one treats or not. Therefore therapeutic strategies and their evaluation must be undertaken with this in mind.

Anterior uveitis or iridocyclitis is seen frequently, with an associated hypopyon in about one-third of patients[11] (Fig. 27.4). Although a typical occurrence, it is not pathognomonic for the disease.[48] The hypopyon may not be visible to the naked eye but seen only with the slit lamp. On occasion, a small hypopyon can be seen cradled in the angle on gonioscopic examination. The inflammatory disease has a nongranulomatous appearance. The cells will move easily and slide over the corneal endothelium if the patient's head is tilted in the right direction. Using confocal microscopy, Mocan et al.[49] identified that the keratic precipitates (KPs) in Behçet disease are made up of small round cells, one of five types identified in ocular inflammatory disease. When the disease is particularly severe and long-standing, cyclitic membranes can form, putting these eyes at risk for phacoanaphylaxis.[50] Posterior synechiae can obscure the view of the posterior pole. In our experience, an isolated vitreous reaction is not characteristic of this disorder. We have observed this when a patient is receiving therapy that is insufficient to completely prevent ocular inflammation, and then a smoldering response ensues. Smoldering disease and impending reactivation remain significant problems. Although one does not measure acute activity by the flare in the anterior segment in patients who have had chronic or repeated attacks, Tugal-Tutkun et al.,[51] using the laser cell flare meter and examining a large number of patients with Behçet disease, felt that the eyes with flare measured at less than 6 photons/second had a higher risk of recurrence.

Retinal Disease

Retinal disease is the most disquieting aspect of Behçet disease and can ultimately lead to blindness. These recurrent retinal vaso-occlusive episodes ultimately cause irreversible alterations and vision loss. Macular ischemia, even bilateral, has been reported[52,53]; this leads to a severe decline in visual acuity, with a guarded prognosis for return of vision. Bilateral central retinal vein thrombosis has been described.[54] Funduscopic examination during the acute attack will, in addition, reveal areas of retinal hemorrhage and edema, accompanied by an inflammatory response in the vitreous humor. The retinitis can have the appearance of viral retinitis with surrounding hemorrhage, and the cause of the lesion usually is determined on the basis of the overall context in which it is being observed (Fig. 27.5). Indeed, the disease can readily mimic acute retinal necrosis.[55] The sequelae of the retinal vaso-occlusive episodes can be best seen with fluorescein angiography, which is a good modality to monitor disease activity (Fig. 27.6). Some of the changes can be extensive, far more so than estimated on clinical examination alone. Areas of capillary dropout and vascular-tree rearrangement are not uncommon. The loss of a clearly defined capillary-free zone is commonly seen but is not unique to this type of intraocular inflammation. In addition, fluorescein angiography may show diffuse retinal vascular leakage, late staining of the vasculature, leakage from the disk, and neovascularization. In the evaluation of a patient with Behçet disease, it is most important to consider performing fluorescein angiography because although the clinical examination may not demonstrate dramatic changes, angiography may show extensive changes (Fig. 27.7). It has been thought that the posterior pole disease is essentially a retinal disease. However, one can see evidence of choroidal, outer retinal, or retinal pigment epithelium (RPE) involvement, raising the notion that in some patients, choroidal involvement is probably of some importance. There are reports

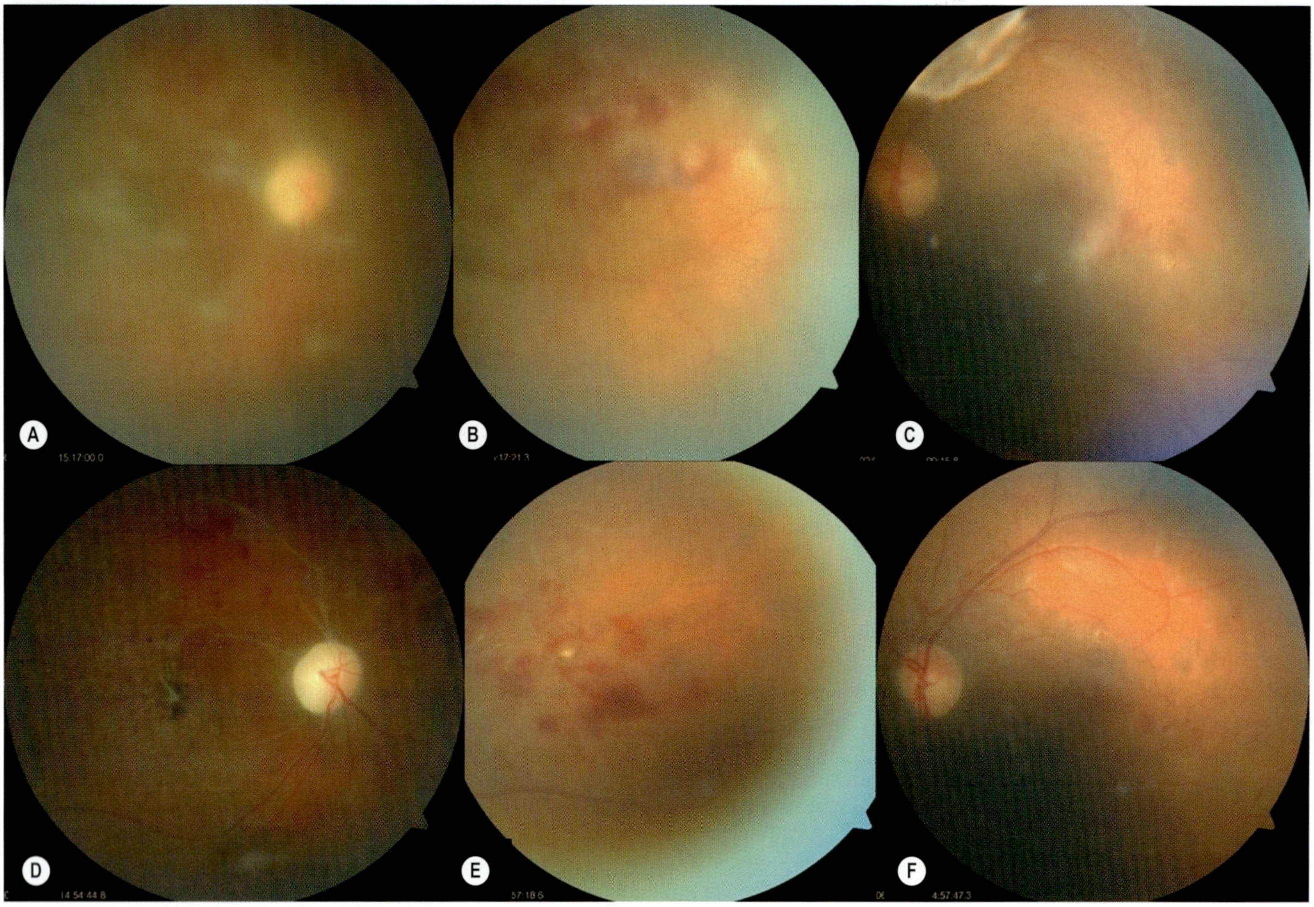

Fig. 27.5 Patient with Behçet disease with significant vitritis, retinitis, and retinal hemorrhages in the right eye posterior pole (A) and the nasal quadrant (B) than in the left eye (C). After systemic steroids and infliximab treatment, resolution of vitritis and improvement of hemorrhages in both eyes are seen (C, D, E). Note the resultant pale optic nerve, macular scar, and sclerotic vessels (C). (Courtesy Dr. Didar Ucar, Turkey.)

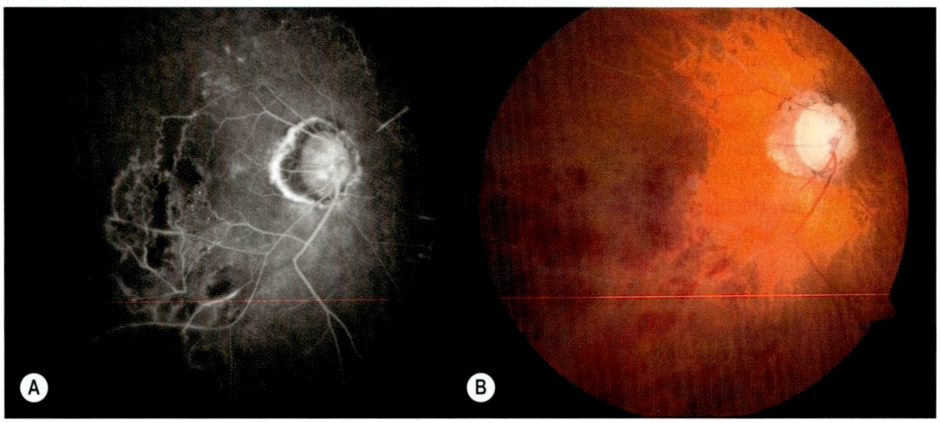

Fig. 27.6 Repeated vaso-occlusive episodes of the posterior pole resulting from Behçet disease can cause retinal hemorrhages (A), severe vascular dropout with large areas of nonperfusion on fluorescein angiography (B), and visual impairment (20/800 in this case).

of indocyanine green (ICG) angiography used in the evaluation of Behçet disease. In one study, Bozzoni-Pantaleoni et al.[56] noted several patterns of dye accumulation. In 50% of eyes, poorly defined areas of intermediate and late hyperfluorescence were seen. Atmaca et al.[57] reported choroidal areas of hyper- and hypofluorescence in 53 (76.8%) of the 69 eyes they studied. Therefore subretinal alterations are not a rare event. However, it still appears that the retinal alterations are the most damaging. In most studies, on ICG angiography, the presence of hyperfluorescent areas up to the late phase was related to disease duration. However, it is important to note that diagnostic criteria developed by Tugal-Tutkun et al. indicated that choroiditis and granulomatous anterior uveitis were highly unlikely to be associated with Behçet disease.[58]

Other ocular manifestations include episcleritis, filamentary keratitis, conjunctivitis, and subconjunctival hemorrhages.[59] Extraocular muscle paralysis may be a result of neuro-Behçet disease.[15]

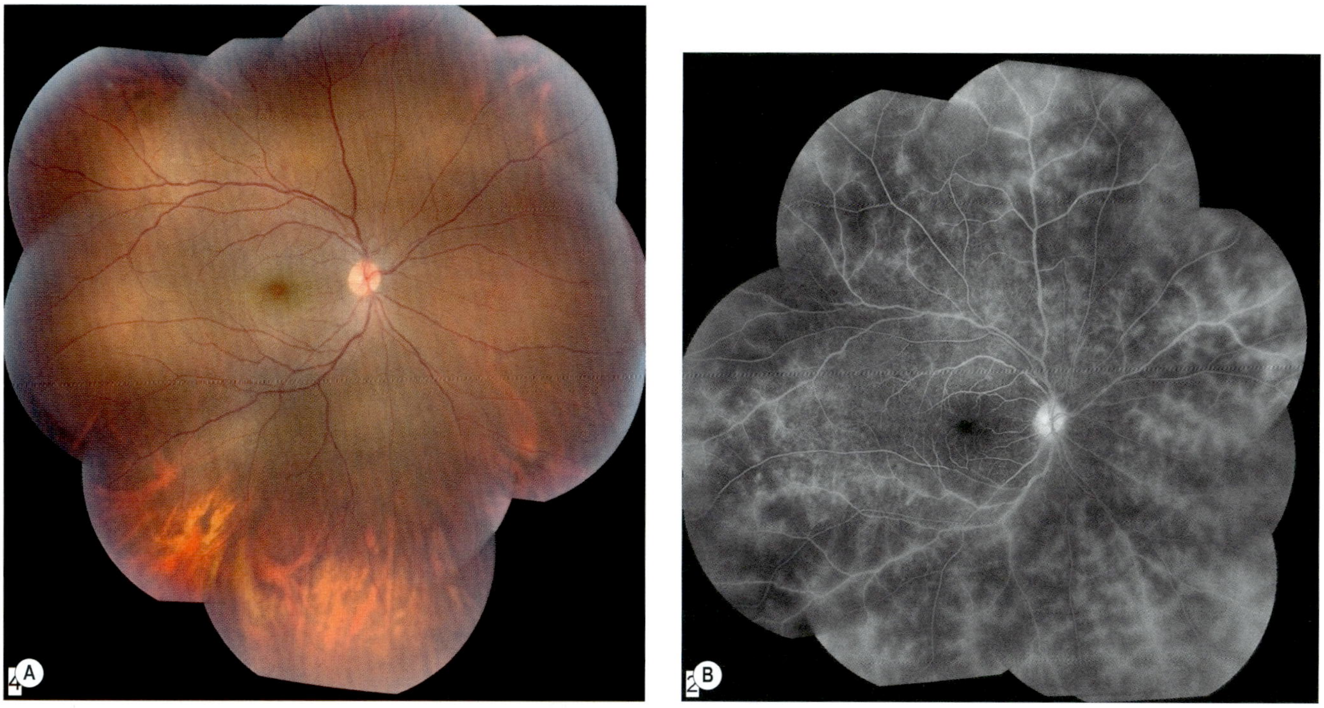

Fig. 27.7 This 23-year-old woman with Behçet disease had bouts of anterior uveitis, but at presentation, she was complaining of minor visual alterations. (A) The fundus examination result was not particularly alarming. (B) Fluorescein angiography demonstrated diffuse retinal vascular leakage.

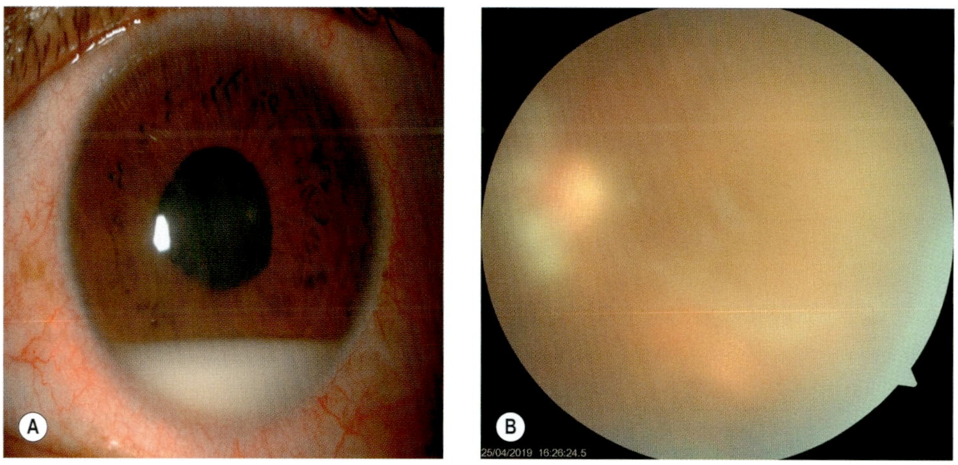

Fig. 27.8 New-onset Behçet disease presenting with severe hypopyon, with retinitis and severe vitritis at the same time. (Courtesy Dr. Didar Ucar, Turkey.)

Complications

The complications of repeated inflammatory bouts are of major concern and depend somewhat on where the inflammation is located. Anterior segment inflammation can lead to glaucoma, particularly angle-closure glaucoma. Iris atrophy may be seen as well. Cataract formation is not unusual, because of the inflammation or the medications used to treat the condition. Iris neovascularization and secondary glaucoma are ominous findings and can accompany recurrent posterior globe inflammatory episodes. The visual prognosis for a patient with anterior segment uveitis is thought to be good only in Behçet disease. More women than men in the Japanese experience have been found to have this type of disease, and therefore their visual prognosis is less guarded than that for men. In our experience, the disease most frequently involves both segments of the eye (Fig. 27.8). The reader can see that the ocular complications, as seen over three decades, have been relatively similar in percentage distribution (Table 27.7).

The posterior segment sequelae of Behçet disease can lead to serious visual handicap (Fig. 27.9). Sakamoto et al.[60] studied 51 patients with Behçet disease and found that in addition to posterior pole attacks, skin lesions and arthritis were associated with loss of vision. In women with the disease, anterior segment attacks and increased intervals between attacks were related to retention of vision. Retinal atrophy is the end result of multiple ocular inflammatory episodes. With this, there will be associated optic atrophy and often markedly attenuated retinal vessels. In a percentage of patients, an associated neovascular component will be seen, leading to recurrent vitreous hemorrhages, subsequent vitreal contraction, and retinal detachment.

In patients with typical Behçet disease, there is little problem in establishing this clinical diagnosis. However, as with all entities, there is overlap in clinical presentations. Furthermore, because parts of the disease spectrum may have occurred sometime before presentation and cannot be verified, some uncertainty may exist. The anterior uveitis can mimic almost any severe recurrent process, and particularly the HLA-B27–associated entities, because hypopyon uveitis is seen with these disorders as well. However, these diseases are unilateral in their presentation, whereas in Behçet disease, unilateral presentation occurs only in a small number of patients. Sarcoidosis can mimic some of the posterior pole lesions. However, the clinical course of sarcoidosis is generally more indolent than the explosive episodes seen in Behçet disease. The retinitis of Behçet disease in its most florid form is highly suggestive of viral retinitis, which should certainly be included in the differential diagnosis.

TABLE 27.7 Comparison of Ocular Complications in Patients with Ocular Behçet Disease over Three Decades

Complication	1960s, n (%)	1980s, n (%)	1990s, n (%)	Total, n (%)
Total patients	45 (38)	26 (21)	49 (41)	120 (100)
Cataract	19 (42)	11 (42)	15 (31)	45 (38)
Macular edema	13 (29)	9 (35)	16 (32)	38 (32)
Optic atrophy	13 (29)	8 (31)	9 (18)	30 (25)
Epiretinal membrane	8 (18)	5 (19)	8 (16)	21 (18)
Glaucoma	7 (16)	5 (19)	6 (12)	18 (15)
Papillitis	13 (29)	8 (31)	2 (4)	23 (19)
Intra-/subretinal hemorrhage	10 (22)	5 (19)	3 (6)	18 (15)
Intravitreal hemorrhage	5 (11)	6 (23)	3 (6)	14 (12)
Branch retinal vein occlusion	9 (20)	3 (12)	3 (6)	15 (13)
Maculopathy	5 (11)	2 (8)	3 (6)	10 (8)
Retinal detachment	2 (4)	2 (8)	3 (6)	7 (6)
Disk/retinal neovascularization	1 (2)	3 (12)	1 (2)	5 (4)
Phthisis bulbi	2 (4)	1 (4)	–	3 (2.5)
Corneal ulcer	2 (4)	–	–	2 (2)
Macular hole	–	1 (4)	1 (2)	2 (2)

Reproduced with permission from Kump LI, Moeller KL, Reed GF, et al. Behçet's disease: Comparing 3 decades of treatment response at the National Eye Institute. *Can J Opthalmol.* 2008;43:468.

Minor Criteria

As previously mentioned, the symptoms associated with Behçet disease are legion. As was so aptly emphasized by Geraint James and Spiteri,[61] patients with Behçet disease may first be seen by practitioners in many different medical disciplines. Although these symptoms are called "minor," it should be stressed that the descriptive term refers only to their importance in the determination of the diagnosis. Three of these minor criteria deserve comment.

Arthritis

At least in half the patients with Behçet disease, a nonmigrating, nondestructive arthritis manifests, with the knee being the most common joint affected. The arthritis is often linked to a general systemically active state of the disease, accompanied, at times, by other symptoms, such as fever, skin lesions, acute-phase reactants, and, on occasion, ocular lesions. One of our patients could predict an ocular attack whenever his joints became involved, signaling to him general activation of his disease. Firestein et al.[62] reported the coexistence of relapsing polychondritis and Behçet disease, in which inflamed cartilage was noted.

Vascular Alterations

Vessels of all sizes can be involved in this disorder, and angiographic Behçet and cardio-Behçet disease (aortitis) are associated with a poor prognosis.[63,64] Müftüoglu et al.[65] observed vascular involvement, mostly deep and superficial thrombophlebitis of the legs, in 24% of the 531 patients they reviewed. These thrombo-occlusive episodes can cause elevation of the ESR. Aneurysms are not uncommon, and their rupture can be the cause of death. Furthermore, deep vessel thrombosis may occur, often involving the large vessels of the body, such as the vena cava.[66] Vasculitis of the small veins may also occur, as in the case of gastrointestinal involvement. The ileocecal region is most commonly involved and can become perforated, with rare esophageal and gastric ulcerations. Computed tomography (CT) will demonstrate bowel wall thickening initially.[67]

Neurologic Involvement (Neuro-Behçet Disease)

This grave complication may affect about 8% of Japanese patients with Behçet disease.[16] Of interest, Inaba[68] reported that most patients who had neuro-Behçet disease did not have ocular disease, with 83.9% of them having the incomplete form of the disease and 90.4% having no ocular disease during the clinical course of their disease. In 68 autopsies, Inaba found that the thalamus, the basal ganglia, and the brainstem were involved in 85% to 95%. In addition to the neurologic ones, Behçet disease can also induce frank psychiatric symptoms.

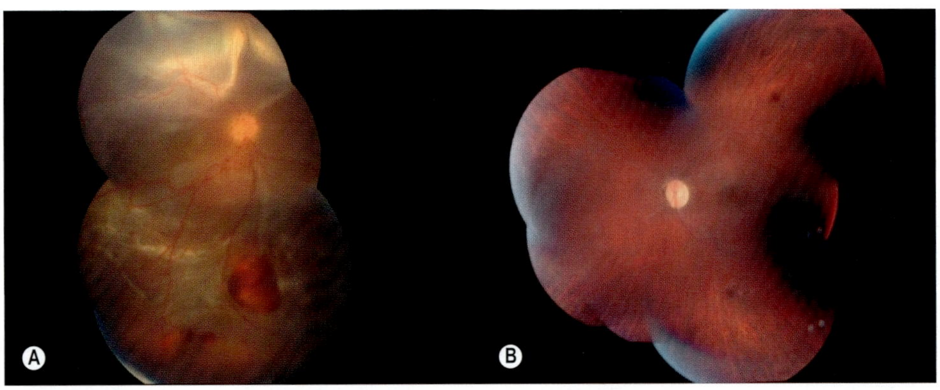

Fig. 27.9 End stage of repeated Behçet disease attacks of the posterior pole with multiple retinal detachment surgeries after an initial diagnostic vitrectomy in the right eye (A). The left eye (B) shows attenuated and sclerotic vessels and optic nerve pallor despite good central visual acuity (see Case 27.2).

In patients with neuro-Behçet disease, cerebrospinal fluid (CSF) shows evidence of pleocytosis. During the acute stage, neutrophils may predominate, leading to a possible diagnosis of aseptic meningitis, whereas in other patients, mononuclear cells may predominate. Inaba[68] reported predominance of OKT4+ T cells in CSF, and the α_2-macroglobulin levels were markedly increased. Of interest, the β_{1A} fraction of C3 was found to be greatly increased during the active stage, suggesting that the alternative pathway of the complement system may be involved. Oligoclonal banding is usually not seen, but Sharief et al.[69] have reported the presence of immunoglobulin A (IgA) and immunoglobulin M (IgM) oligoclonal bands in the CSF of patients with active neuro-Behçet disease and documented the disappearance of the bands with remission of neurologic disease. Wang et al.[70] found that levels of anticardiolipin antibodies (particularly the IgM isotype) and interleukin (IL)-6 were elevated in the CSF of patients with neuro-Behçet disease and the levels fell as disease activity abated.

CT of the brain shows defects in a large number of patients, as does electroencephalography (EEG), but some lesions may not be seen well with these types of studies. The use of gadolinium–diethylenetriamine pentaacetic acid–enhanced magnetic resonance imaging (MRI) is another modality that appears to provide good definition of CNS lesions. Of interest, the studies by Ogawa and Sawada[71] and Edem et al.[72] found that the unenhanced MRI images continued to show lesions even after therapy initiation and resolution of clinical disease, whereas the enhanced images showed resolution (Fig. 27.10). Alkan et al.,[73] showed reduced perfusion in the brains of neuro-Behçet patients and suggested that brain perfusion MRI can be helpful in the diagnosis of MRI negative neuro-behcet cases.

IMMUNOLOGIC AND HISTOLOGIC CONSIDERATIONS

The histopathologic appearance of the lesions seen in Behçet disease is that of perivasculitis associated with tissue destruction (Fig. 27.11).

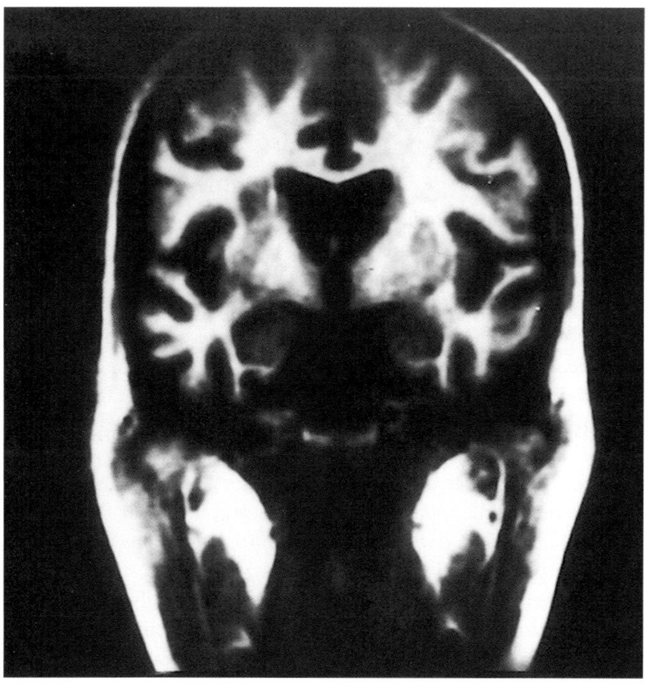

Fig. 27.10 Magnetic resonance imaging (MRI) brain scan of a patient with neuro-Behçet disease. Gray-matter lesions are interpreted to be evidence of central nervous system (CNS) activity of disease. This patient also had retinal vasculitis.

In a case from the NEI, nongranulomatous uveitis with CD4+ T lymphocytes and some B cells and plasma cells infiltrated the eye. There was extensive expression of adhesion molecules on the vascular endothelium.[74] Winter and Yukins[75] believed that the underlying lesion was obliterative vasculitis. Mullaney and Collum[76] noted necrotizing arteriolitis and phlebitis with thromboses in an eye they examined. Mural IgG, immunoglobulin A (IgA), and C3 deposits were noted in the episclera and some choroidal veins, but not in the retina. The notion has been that the underlying mechanism leading to this histologic alteration was immune complex deposition.[41] Indeed, the deposition of complement components has been reported in some lesions.[77] This notion has been supported by the presence of circulating immune complexes (CICs) in patients with Behçet disease[78] and neutrophils in the aqueous of eyes with hypopyon uveitis. Increased chemotactic activity of neutrophils has been observed in Behçet disease.[79,80] Some reports describing histologic findings in Behçet eyes are listed in Table 27.8. Neurologic lesions include perivascular cuffing with mononuclear cells, focal necrosis, demyelinization, and gliosis.[80]

Some observers have suggested that other mechanisms may be at play in this disorder. Kasp et al.[81] noted that of 32 patients with Behçet disease, only one-third had elevated CIC levels. Furthermore, the presence of CICs was associated with quiescent periods, suggesting that CICs may play a beneficial role in the course of the disease (see Chapter 1).

Role of T Cells

The role of T cells in the underlying mechanism of Behçet disease is stressed by many. Recent immunohistologic studies of recurrent mouth ulcers seen in Behçet disease have demonstrated that most of the lymphocytes infiltrating the lesion were DR-negative T cells, whereas the macrophages were DR positive.[82] We have seen predominance of T cells, rather than neutrophils, in the recurrent hypopyon uveitis of a patient with Behçet disease. In 1982, Cogan reviewed 18 eyes for a joint Japanese–American workshop on Behçet disease. Although perivasculitis was noted, evidence of typical fibrinoid changes associated with immune complex–mediated disease was not present (personal communication, 1984). Charteris et al.[83] carried out a postmortem examination of the eyes of a patient with Behçet disease who had suffered from severe recurrent retinal vasculitis. These authors found hyaline thickening of the retinal vessels, with perivascular infiltrate made up of mostly CD4+ T cells bearing large numbers of IL-2 receptors. In another study of five enucleated eyes from patients with Behçet disease, Charteris et al.[84] again found predominance of CD4+ T cells, with no complement or immunoglobulin deposits. The notion that T cells in the eyes of patients with Behçet disease are expanded by specific antigen-driven stimulation is supported by the findings of Keino et al.,[85] who showed a restricted number of T-cell receptors (BV3, BV5, and BV7) in a patient's eye.

Indeed, perturbations of the systemic T-cell circuitry can be found in patients with Behçet disease. Valesini et al.[86] noted in the blood of patients with Behçet disease with ocular involvement an increase in the number of T4 (CD4) cells and an elevated CD8 fraction, thereby lowering the CD4:CD8 ratio, a finding also noted in other ocular inflammatory conditions. Essentially the same observations have been noted in Japan by Kikkawa and Shirotsuki,[87] who studied 11 patients with Behçet disease and uveitis. Other evidence for an intrinsic T-cell problem comes from the work of Sakane et al.,[88] in which they noted a defect in a T-cell-mediated suppressor system. Furthermore, interferon (IFN)-γ, a T-cell product, was detected at a higher level in the sera of patients with Behçet disease than in sera of control subjects,[89] particularly during the convalescent stage of the disease. Serum IL-2 levels of patients with Behçet disease with ocular involvement were elevated compared with those of

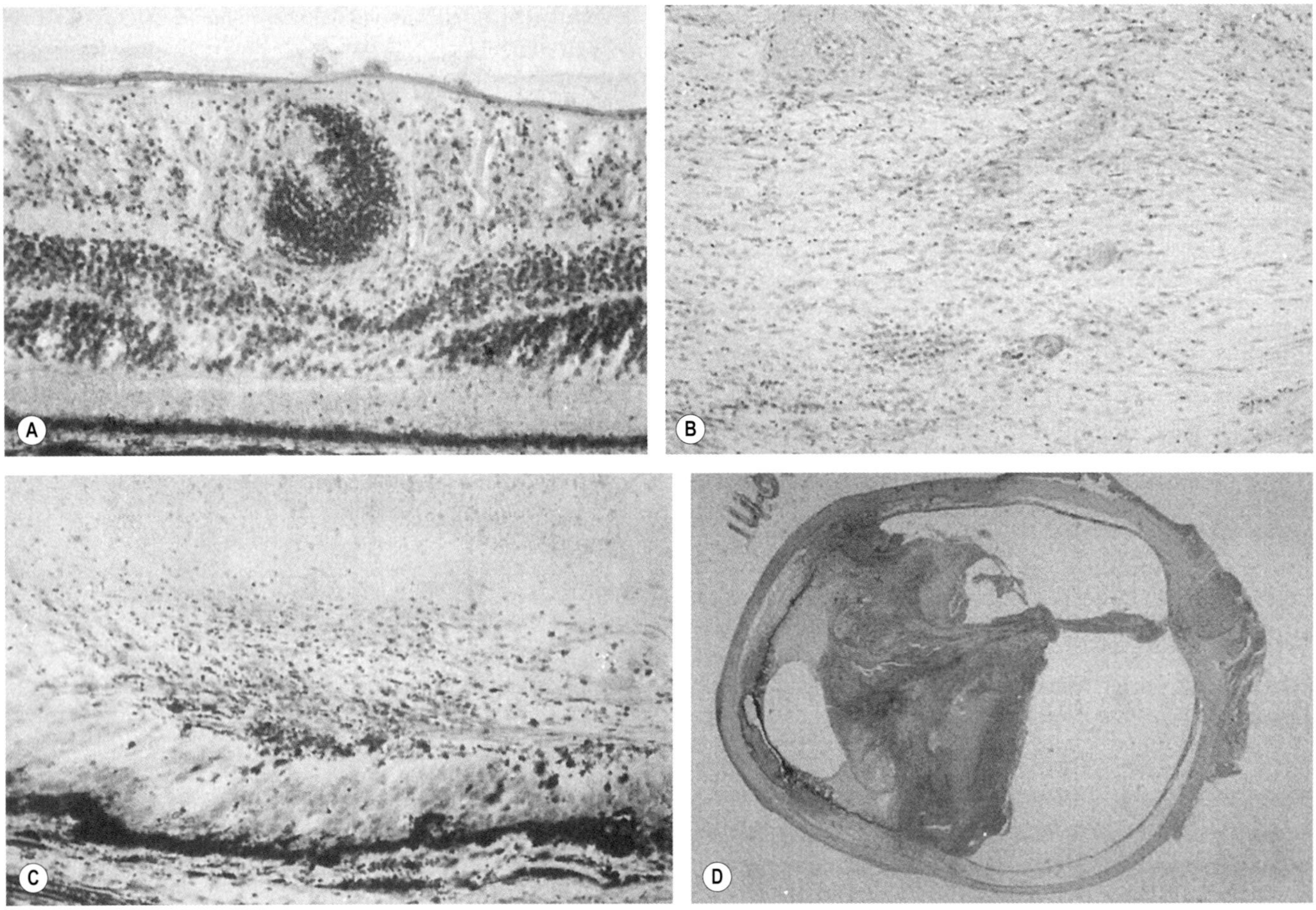

Fig. 27.11 (A) Retinal vasculitis in Behçet disease. Note periarteriolar infiltrate and other lymphocytes diffusely spread throughout the inner layer of the retina. (B) Occlusive retinitis in the retinal vessels of a 37-year-old with long-standing complete Behçet disease. (C) Early stage of ocular disease in a patient with neuro-Behçet disease, with severe pars plana inflammation, macrophages, and lymphocytes, and fibrous proliferation. (D) Enucleated eye of a 37-year-old patient with complete Behçet disease shows complete detachment of the sensory retina with preretinal and subretinal granulation tissue. (Courtesy Professor J. Inomata, Fukuoka, Japan. From Vasculitis and intraocular neovascularization in Behçet's disease: histopathology of the early and advanced late stages. In: Dernouchamps JP, Verougstraete C, Caspers-Velu L, et al., eds. *Recent Advances in Uveitis* [Proceedings of the Third International Symposium on Uveitis, Brussels, Belgium, May 24–27, 1992]. Amsterdam: Kugler; 1993.)

control subjects and patients with intermediate uveitis.[90] We also found elevated serum levels of IL-17 in patients with uveitis, including those with Behçet disease as well.[91] Others have reported an increase in TNF-α, soluble IL-1 receptor, IL-6, and IL-8 levels.[92] Bonacini et al. showed IL-2, IL-8, IL-13, TNF-α, eotaxin, and IL-1ra to be higher in aqueous samples of patients with Behçet disease.[93] As with other patients whose uveitis involves the posterior segment, patients with Behçet disease demonstrate evidence of cell-mediated responses to uveitogenic antigens and to their fragments.[94] Other antigens to which patients with Behçet disease have cell-mediated or humoral responses include resistin[95] (adipocyte hormones antagonize insulin action), selenium,[96] and α-tropomyosin.[97] These responses could be blocked by the addition of anti-CD4, anti-HLA, and anti-CD11a antibodies.[98] Yamamoto et al.[99] were able to establish S-antigen (S-Ag)–specific CD4+ and CD8+ clones from the blood of a patient with Behçet disease. Intraocularly, much evidence suggests a strong helper T cell type 1 (Th1) profile. Ahn et al.[100] found that TNF-α was higher in the aqueous of patients with Behçet disease than in the aqueous of other patients with uveitis, whereas IFN-α was high in the aqueous of patients with Behçet disease as well. No IL-10 was noted. Ahn et al.[101] also reported that $CD8^{bright}CD56+$ cytotoxic effector cells, producing IFN-α and high amounts of preformed perforin, were seen in the aqueous of these patients. Yu et al.[102] reported similar findings, with CD8+ cells predominating in patients with Behçet disease, whereas CD4+ cells predominated in the aqueous of other patients with uveitis; also, natural killer (NK) CD3+ CD56+ T cells were higher in the blood and aqueous of patients with Behçet disease.

Our experience and those of others with cyclosporin further support the role of T cells in this disease because the disease appears to be effectively controlled in many patients with this anti–T-cell medication (see later discussion). Although there is overwhelming evidence incriminating T cells in this disease, it is clear that there is a rather general and severe immune alteration. Perhaps under T-cell control in the beginning, the immune system's delicate checks and balances seem to have gone awry almost universally. Indeed, one finds alterations in many parts of the immune system, including the CICs. Neutrophils and neutrophil extracellular traps (NETs) have also been implicated.[103] Polymorphonuclear lymphocytes in the peripheral blood of patients with Behçet disease appear to undergo less spontaneous apoptosis in the remission phase of the disease[104]; however, the reason for this is unclear.

TABLE 27.8 Histologic Reports Describing the Ocular Complications of Behçet Disease

Authors	No. Reports	Findings
Fenton and Easom[a]	4	Lymphocytes, PMNs, macrophages
Winter and Yukins[75]	2	Lymphocytes, macrophages
Green and Koo[a]	1	PMNs, lymphocytes, macrophages
Kaneko et al.[a]	1	Round cells
Okabe and associates[210]	2	Macrophages, lymphocytes
Mullaney et al.[a]	1	Lymphocytes, plasma cells, PMNs, IgG, IgA, C3
Charteris et al.[83]	2	CD4 T cells, HLA-DR+ cells
Charteris et al.[84]	5	T cells, macrophages, PMNs, HLA-DR+ cells
Inomata et al.[a]	25	Lymphocytes, macrophages, PMNs
George et al.[74]	1	T and B cells, plasma cells, macrophages, PMNs, HLA-DR+ cells, HLA-DQ+ cells, ICAM-1, LFA-1, VCAM, E-selectin

ICAM-1, intercellular adhesion molecule-1; *LFA-1,* lymphocyte function antigen-1; PMN, polymorphonuclear leukocytes; *VCAM,* vascular cell adhesion molecule.

[a]Fenton R, Easom H. Behçet's syndrome. *Arch Ophthalmol.* 1964;72:71–81; Green WR, Koo BS. Behçet's disease: a report of ocular histopathology of one case. *Surv Ophthalmol.* 1967;12:324–332; Kaneko H, Nakajima H, Okamura A, et al. Histopathology of Behçet's disease. Review of literature with a case report. *Acta Pathol Jpn.* 1976;26:765–779; Mullaney J, Collum LM. Ocular vasculitis in Behçet's disease. A pathologic and immunohistochemical study. *Int Ophthalmol.* 1985;7:183–191; Inomata H, Kohno T, Rao NA, et al. Vasculitis and intraocular neovascularization in Behçet's disease. Histopathology of the early and advanced late stages. In: Dernouchamps JP, Verougstraete C, Caspers-Verlu L et al., eds. *Recent Advances in Uveitis.* Amsterdam: Kugler; 1992.

Complete elaboration of all the immune system alterations that have been reported in Behçet disease is beyond the scope of this chapter.

Genetics

HLA typing has proven helpful in the diagnosis of Behçet disease. HLA-B51, a split product of HLA-B5, has been found to be associated with the disease in Japanese patients,[11] with a calculated relative risk of 9.4. The frequency of this antigen in control subjects was 12%, whereas in patients, it was 57% (58% in patients with the complete form of the disease versus 54% in those with the incomplete form). A study using polymerase chain reaction (PCR)–restriction fragment length polymorphism methodology to evaluate 90 Japanese patients yielded a relative risk for HLA-B51 of 7.9.[105] Some disagreement has arisen as to the strength of these observations when applied to non-Japanese patients. Most of these studies were performed before the "B5" antigen was split. Godeau et al.[106] found an incidence of 54% of HLA-B5 in patients with Behçet disease (most of Mediterranean origin) versus 13% in the control population. Several other studies, from Israel,[66] Turkey,[107] and Greece,[108] have supported the HLA-B5 association. Further support for the association of HLA-B51 and this disorder came with a publication by Villanueva et al.[109] These investigators reported on three siblings, all females, with Behçet disease, including the ocular manifestations. They all had the same HLA phenotype, which included HLA-B51. Gül et al.[110] found no association between HLA-B51 positivity and severity of disease. However, in a German study, those with HLA-B51 were more likely to have ocular involvement (63% versus 43%), and in addition those of German descent (as opposed to Turkish) with the disease were less likely to bear B51 on their cells.[111] In familial Behçet disease[112] parent–child involvement was more common in patients without ocular lesions than in those with them.

However, O'Duffy et al.[113] found no such association in the 26 patients they typed in the United States, nor did Ohno et al.,[114] who typed six white patients. The reason for this may be lack of association; however, it may reflect the different criteria for diagnosis used in these American studies as opposed to the Japanese studies. In a study from the southwestern United States, of the 63 patients with Behçet disease, 49.2% were Hispanic, 31.7% were non-Hispanic European, 14.3% were Native Americans, and only 4.7% were ancestrally from the Middle East and the Silk Route through Asia, and HLA-B51 was positive in 74.2%, 42.1%, 89%, and 100%, respectively.[115] In an effort to explain this lack of association with B51 in some ethnic groups, it has been suggested that the HLA-B exon sequence that encodes B51 is the real pathogenic factor.[116] HLA-26 has also been proposed as a risk factor, especially for ocular involvement, both in Japanese and Greek cohorts, and perhaps a more severe course[117-119] (see Case 27-1).

In addition to HLA typing and polymorphisms, there has been much interest in evaluating single-nucleotide polymorphisms (SNPs) of various mediators of the immune response. One study evaluated 102 patients of Middle Eastern descent with Behçet disease for a possible link between a specific tumor necrosis factor SNP and the disease. Although HLA-B51 was again found to be strongly linked with the disease, no TNF gene polymorphisms were found to be associated.[120] TNF-α SNP–1031C was found to be associated with the disease in a study performed in the United Kingdom.[121] In Turks, an association with the disease has been reported with the IL-1A–889 allele and the IL-1B +5887 haplotype.[122] Another portion of the genome that has been investigated has been a novel family of the major histocompatibility complex (MHC) class I genes, located near the HLA-B gene and termed *MIC* (MHC class I chain-related genes). Yabuki et al.[123] reported an association between one MICA (one of the transmembrane regions) microsatellite polymorphism A6 in patients with Behçet disease compared with control subjects (86.8% versus 50%). However, Salvarani et al.[124] did not find such a linkage. No association was seen in cytotoxic T-lymphocyte associated antigen 4 (CTLA-4), an adhesion molecule important in cell trafficking SNPs distributions between controls and patients with Behçet disease.[125] In 2010, Remmers et al. studied 1215 patients with Behçet disease and 1278 healthy controls from Turkey. They confirmed disease association with HLA-B51 but also found an independent association within the MHC class I region, at IL-10. Furthermore, they combined five cohorts and confirmed associations with IL-10 (rs1518111), where the disease-associated variant was associated with decreased messenger ribonucleic acid (mRNA) expression and lower protein production, and the IL-23R–IL-12RB2 locus (rs924080).[126] In a large genomewide association study of 1209 Turkish patients with Behçet disease and 1278 controls, Kirino et al. found new associations at CCR1, STAT4, and KLRC4 in addition to two SNPs in ERAP1.[127] They also found epistasis between HLA-B51 and ERAP1.

Various investigators have attempted to identify an exogenous cause, particularly a viral one, for Behçet disease. The incidence of the disease is greater in the northern portions of Japan, although there is no known genetic difference, such as a higher incidence of HLA-B51, between the people in the north of Japan as opposed to those in the south. A somewhat dated report emphasized that there had been no documented cases of the disease in Nisei living in Hawaii,[128] suggesting that an exogenous source may, indeed, act at least as a triggering mechanism.

The search for the presence of live virus in the retina has not been successful, and therapeutic approaches with this concept as its underlying logic have not been rewarding (see later discussion). Denman et al.[129] offered a more interesting theory on the role of viruses in this disorder. They noted that mononuclear cells from patients with Behçet disease have a high concentration of the IFN-induced enzyme 2′,5′-oligoadenylate synthetase, which is suggestive, but not confirmatory, of a viral infection.[130] They speculated that the virus may act as a "promoter" by stimulating the expansion of clones of abnormal lymphocytes that will induce disease. Bonass et al.,[131] using DNA dot-blotting techniques, found evidence of the presence of herpes simplex virus type 1 DNA in a high percentage of patients with Behçet disease. Several studies have centered on the possible role of streptococcal-related antigens as an etiologic agent of this disease. Hirohata et al.[132] showed that when *Streptococcus sanguis*–related antigens (RRE KTH-1 antigens) were added to T cells of patients with Behçet disease in in vitro cultures, the amount of IL-6, an "inflammatory" cytokine, is higher than that produced by T cells from control subjects stimulated in a similar fashion. This suggests that a hypersensitivity response to these bacterial antigens could be a triggering mechanism for this disease. Tanaka et al.[133] reported finding titers of the 65-kDa heat shock protein of *Streptococcus* in patients with Behçet disease. Pervin et al.[134] demonstrated the responsiveness of T-cell clones from patients with Behçet disease to four peptide determinants within the 65-kDa heat shock proteins derived from *Mycobacterium tuberculosis.* The inflammatory response seen in these patients could, in part, be attributed to a heightened response to bacterial antigens.[135] The potential role of these findings still needs to be elucidated. Kurhan-Yavuz et al.[136] showed an association with an endogenous antigen, which is a common sequence found in various HLA-B molecules and is shared by HLA-B7 and HLA-B51 (B27PD). Increased amounts of IL-2 and TNF-2 were seen in the supernatants from lymphocytes of patients with Behçet disease after stimulation with this molecule.

No truly specific tests for the diagnosis of Behçet disease exist. The skin-prick test looking for evidence of pathergy has been suggested to be highly diagnostic for Behçet disease by some, particularly Turkish researchers. Skin hyperreactivity has not been a markedly striking feature in the patients we have seen in the United States. Wechsler et al.[137] have applied immunofluorescence techniques to skin biopsy specimens obtained after an intradermal injection of distilled water. About 60% of patients thought to have Behçet disease had complement and/or IgM deposition, compared with 14% of control subjects. There was no concordance with HLA-B5. Dogan et al.[138] found that total serum sialic acid levels and the proportion of total serum sialic acid to total protein levels can help distinguish Behçet disease from other uveitic entities. Michaelson et al.[139] investigated the presence of anticytoplasmic antibodies in this disease by means of an indirect immunofluorescence technique with the use of a guinea pig lip as the tissue substrate. Although all eight American patients with Behçet disease had positive test reactions, only 10 of 16 Turkish patients showed positivity. Anticardiolipin antibodies, which have been observed in several patients with systemic lupus erythematosus accompanied by retinal vascular disease, were reported to be present in high serum titers in one patient with neuro-Behçet disease.[140] These antibodies were looked for in patients with Behçet disease with uveitis, and no correlation could be made by Efthimiou et al.,[141] but Bergman et al.[142] claimed that IgM isotypes were increased in these patients. However, Aydintug et al.[143] found no evidence of anticardiolipin or antineutrophil cytoplasmic antibodies in 72 Turkish patients they screened. Rather, they found that 18% had evidence of antiendothelial cell antibodies (AECAs), which did not induce complement-mediated cytotoxicity; nor was the binding caused by the immune complexes. However, those authors did find that patients with evidence of AECAs were more apt to develop acute thrombotic events and retinal vasculitis.

THERAPY

Because of the difficulty in treating the posterior pole aspects of Behçet disease, numerous therapies have been proposed. Despite these sometimes intensive attempts, loss of useful visual acuity may occur in about three-quarters of the eyes 6 to 10 years after the initiation of ocular symptoms.[144] The visual course of the patient is often a major factor in evaluating whether therapy is successful or should be altered or stopped.

The most commonly used agents in the past have been systemic corticosteroids, cytotoxic agents (alkylating agents), colchicine, and cyclosporin and tacrolimus (FK506). Posterior segment involvement requires systemic immunosuppression. The advent of biologics has significantly improved the outcomes for patients with Behçet disease.[145] Since early 2000s, IFN-α and anti-TNF therapy have begun to be used more frequently. It is important to remember that few medications have been evaluated in randomized studies, and even fewer in the ocular realm. An evaluation of evidenced-based studies shows many randomized controlled trials (RCTs) (Table 27.9).

Systemic Corticosteroids

Although Behçet disease may initially respond to systemic corticosteroids, it will invariably become "resistant," with a further drop in vision and the need to use additional therapeutic modes.[144] Reed[146] reported the use of high-dose intravenous methylprednisolone, followed by oral immunosuppressive therapy, to rapidly reverse retinal disease. Mohammadi et al. randomized 34 patients with ocular Behçet disease to intravenous pulse methylprednisone versus placebo in addition to standard therapy with intravenous cyclophosphamide, azathioprine, and prednisolone for 6 months. These authors concluded that the group that received induction intravenous pulse steroids did better than the group that only received the standard combination therapy.[147]

Cytotoxic Agents and Antimetabolites

In several reports from countries in the Mediterranean basin, the efficacy of cytotoxic agents (particularly alkylating agents) in the treatment of the ocular component of Behçet disease has been demonstrated.[148-150] Mamo[148] noted no ocular recurrences in most patients treated. In a retrospective clinical study, Pivetti-Pezzi et al.[151] found that the visual prognosis for patients treated with chlorambucil early in their disease course was considerably better than that for those treated early with steroids. A reappraisal of the role of chlorambucil in the treatment of this disorder by Tabbara[152] found chlorambucil considerably less favorable. He underlined the significant side effects seen with the drug and noted that three-quarters of the eyes studied had a visual acuity of 20/200 or less when chlorambucil was used as the sole therapeutic agent. Kazokoglu et al.[153] evaluated the long-term effects of cyclophosphamide and colchicine and concluded that in their 64 patients, there was no statistically significant positive change in visual acuity or the attack rate compared with the posttreatment period. These observations essentially corroborated those of BenEzra and Cohen[144] and ours. A disturbing report by Takeuchi and Takeuchi[154] found an increased

TABLE 27.9 A Review of Several Randomized Controlled Studies in Behçet Disease

Trial	Agent	Duration	Patient Selection	Comments
Mohammadi M et al. (2017)	Intravenous (IV) pulse methylprednisone vs placebo for 3 days; both groups received combination therapy with IV cyclophosphamide, azathioprine, and prednisolone	6 months	17 (13 males [M], 4 females [F]) patients with new-onset or recurrent posterior uveitis and/or retinal vasculitis	Visual acuity improved significantly more in the IV pulse methylprednisone group. Other inflammatory outcome measures improved in both groups.
Davatchi F et al. (2010)	Rituximab and methotrexate and prednisolone versus placebo added to cyclophosphamide, azathioprine, and prednisolone	6 months	20 (13 M, 7 F) patients with long-standing ocular disease with retinal vasculitis	Total adjusted disease activity index (TADAI) improved more in the rituximab arm. Other inflammatory indices improved more in the rituximab group than in the cyclophosphamide group, but the difference was not significant.
Buggage RR et al.[199] (2007)	Daclizumab (1 mg/kg) infusions monthly vs. placebo added to immunosuppressive therapy	15 month median	17 (8 M, 9 F) patients with recurrent ocular attacks	No suggestion that daclizumab was beneficial. However, low attack rate for both arms limited the ability to make a definitive comparison.
Mat CM et al.[211] (2006)	Methylprednisolone acetate 40 mg intramuscular (IM) three times weekly versus placebo	27 weeks	86 (43 M, 43 F) patients with mainly genital ulcers	Effective for erythema nodosum in females but not in males. The drug is more effective in females, similar to the colchicine trial.
Melikoglu M et al.[212] (2005)	Etanercept 25 mg subcutaneous (SC) 2 times weekly versus placebo	4 weeks	40 males with positive pathergy, monosodium urate tests, and mucocutaneous lesions	No effect on pathergy and monosodium urate tests, but effective for oral ulcers, nodular lesions, and papulopustular lesions.
Alpsoy E et al.[213] (2002)	Interferon (IFN)-α2a 6 million units three times weekly versus placebo	3 months	50 (31 M, 19 F) with mucocutaneous lesions	Favorable effects on oral and genital ulcers and papulopustular lesions. Adverse effects and high cost limit its use.
Sharquie KE et al.[214] (2002)	Dapsone 100 mg daily versus placebo	3 months	20 patients with mucocutaneous lesions	Favorable effect on mucocutaneous lesions.
Yurdakul S et al.[164] (2001)	Colchicine 1–2 mg daily versus placebo	2 years	116 (60 M, 56 F) with active mucocutaneous lesions	Effective for genital ulcers, erythema nodosum, and arthritis in females, but only for arthritis in males.
Hamuryudan V et al.[215] (1998)	Thalidomide 100 mg or 300 mg daily versus placebo	24 weeks	96 male patients with active mucocutaneous lesions	Both dosages are effective for oral and genital ulcers and follicular lesions. Polyneuropathy and teratogenesis limit its use.
Moral F et al.[216] (1995)	Azapropazone 300 mg daily versus placebo	3 weeks	63 with acute arthritis	No difference from placebo on arthritis.
Yazici H et al.[156] (1990)	Azathioprine 2.5 mg/kg body weight daily versus placebo	2 years	73 males (48 with and 25 without eye disease)	Effective for the preservation of visual acuity and for the prevention of the emergence of new eye disease, mucocutaneous lesions, and arthritis.
Masuda K et al.[174] (1989)	Cyclosporin 10 mg/kg body weight daily versus colchicine 1 mg daily	16 weeks	96 patients with active eye disease	Cyclosporin is more effective for eye and mucocutaneous lesions compared with colchicine.
Davies UM et al.[193] (1988)	Acyclovir 4 g, then 800 mg daily versus placebo	12 weeks	22 (7 M, 15 F) patients with mainly mucocutaneous lesions	No difference in the frequency of orogenital lesions between groups.
Aktulga E et al.[163] (1980)	Colchicine 0.5 mg daily versus placebo	6 months	35 patients with mainly mucocutaneous lesions	Beneficial for erythema nodosum and arthralgia.
Denman AM et al.[217] (1979)	Transfer factor versus placebo	6 months	20 (11 M, 9 F) patients with mainly mucocutaneous lesions	No difference between the groups.

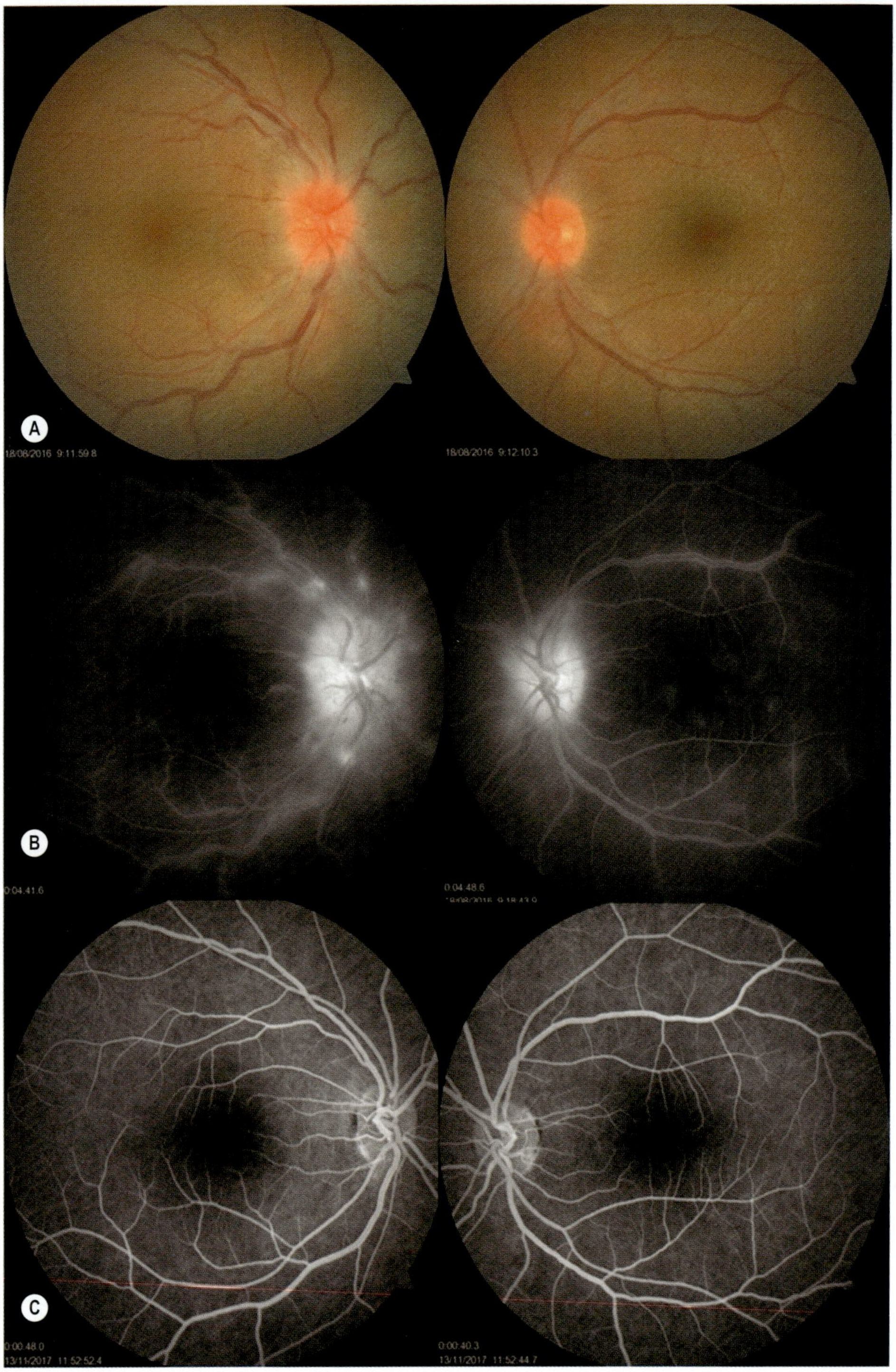

Fig. 27.12 A 23-year-old Turkish woman with new-onset Behçet disease presented with mild vitritis, significant optic nerve edema, and inflammation (A) and retinal vascular leakage, as seen on fluorescein angiography (B). The patient's vision was 20/63 and 20/50 in the right and left eye, respectively. After treatment with prednisone, azathioprine, and cyclosporine, the inflammation resolved completely (C), and vision improved to 20/20 in both eyes. (Courtesy Dr. Didar Ucar, Turkey.)

frequency of chromosomal aberrations (dicentrics) in patients with Behçet disease treated with cytotoxic agents in combination with colchicine. Another approach similar to that used for severe renal disease has been to use intravenous pulse cyclophosphamide therapy (which may have fewer side effects) to treat Behçet disease. Our experience with this method has not been especially promising, whereas Hamza et al.[155] reported some advantage with this method over pulse steroid therapy. Yazici et al.[156] reported that azathioprine was superior to placebo in the treatment of this disease. Although any RCT deserves attention, it has been noted that maintenance of visual acuity was a goal that was met with only modest success.[157,158] (Fig. 27.12). However, long-term results demonstrated that maintenance of visual acuity was better achieved in the azathioprine-treated group than in the control group.[159] Greenwood et al.[160] reported their experience with the use of azathioprine in treating the ocular manifestations of Behçet disease and found that it was only partially effective in reducing the steroid dosage and, overall, was not overwhelmingly effective. Davatchi et al. showed significant improvement in inflammatory activity and visual acuity in a longitudinal cohort by using combination azathioprine and intravenous cyclophosphamide.[161] They also found, in a separate study, that long-term methotrexate combined with prednisone was a successful regimen in patients with posterior uveitis but to a lesser extent in patients with retinal vasculitis.[161]

Colchicine

Because the results of leukocyte migration studies showed abnormalities, the use of colchicine was thought ideal because it would inhibit such migration.[162] Most practitioners use it to prevent recurrences, not to treat active disease. Hijikata et al.[150] found that the visual prognosis for patients receiving colchicine was better than that for those receiving steroids. A masked, randomized study in Turkey, in which patients received colchicine or placebo, demonstrated no differences between the groups.[163]

An RCT (colchicine versus placebo)[164] on the treatment of active mucocutaneous disease demonstrated that the colchicine-treated group had a reduced incidence of genital ulcers, erythema nodosum, and arthritis. This effect was seen particularly in women. This medication is being used less and less because other medications, at least for ocular disease, seem to give better control.

Interferon-α

IFN-α has been shown to be effective for mucocutaneous lesions in Behçet disease in an RCT.[165] The use of IFN-α in the treatment of the ocular complications of Behçet disease has been reported by many. Kotter et al.[166] used an initial dose of 6×10^6 units subcutaneously daily and then 3×10^6 units every day for 1 month, followed by 3×10^6 units subcutaneously every other day. This group saw an improvement in all seven patients treated. Pivetti-Pezzi et al.[167] and Wechsler et al.[168] used a dose of 3×10^6 units three times a week. Pivetti-Pezzi and associates saw a 50% reduction of ocular relapses.[167] In two patients, the medication was stopped, and there was a recurrence of disease. All patients had a flu-like illness during therapy. A review of literature by Kotter et al., in 2004, showed that the use of IFN-α resulted in partial or complete remission in 95% of patients, and drug-free long-term remission was achieved in 56%.[169] Sakane and Takeno[170,171] stressed the potential secondary effects of this therapy, such as immune reactivity, thyroiditis, and a Behçet disease–like retinopathy, all having been associated with IFN-α therapy. Other dose-limiting side effects include depression, neutropenia, alopecia, elevated liver enzymes, and the risk of suicide[172] (Fig. 27.13).

Cyclosporin and Tacrolimus (FK506)

Observations at the NEI early on in the use of cyclosporin suggested clearly that patients with Behçet disease appeared to have a particularly positive therapeutic response to this agent.[173] These observations were confirmed in a randomized, double-masked multicenter study in Japan, in which cyclosporin was found to be superior to the original standard therapy.[174] In their report, Ando et al.[32] noted: "The introduction of cyclosporin in 1985 is probably responsible for the improvement of the visual prognosis in Behçet disease patients." Observations have been made in Israel, where the drug was compared with cytotoxic agents in a masked study,[175] and in Turkey.[176] Ozyazgan et al.,[177] in a single masked study, compared 5 mg/kg/day of cyclosporin with intravenous administration of 1 g cyclophosphamide (Cytoxan) per month. In this small study of 23 patients, they found that the cyclosporin group had a significantly marked improvement of their vision compared with the other group, but at 24 months, it was not clear whether this improvement was sustained, leaving the observers with the call for further long-term studies. Kotake et al.[178] treated 20 Japanese patients with Behçet disease with low doses of cyclosporin (5 mg/kg/day), and found it to be effective in 70%. Chavis et al.[179] in Saudi Arabia reported a salutary effect of cyclosporin on loss of vision as a result of papillitis, optic neuritis, macular neuroretinitis, and retinal phlebitis, but not with retinal arteritis. Their different approach involves an intermittent low-dose therapy, as opposed to continuous low-dose cyclosporin therapy as described previously. Whitcup et al. reported their long-term results with cyclosporin in 19 patients with Behçet disease.[180] They found that combination therapy with cyclosporin and prednisone appeared to be effective in treating Behçet disease. The combination permits the use of lower doses of both medications, thereby helping reduce the possibility of untoward secondary effects. Also of interest was the positive therapeutic effect of cyclosporin therapy reported by Elidan et al.[181] on the hearing loss that occurred in their patients with Behçet disease.

Because of its mechanism that is essentially the same as that of cyclosporin, it is logical to assume that tacrolimus would be a useful therapy for Behçet disease. It has been used in the treatment of presumed pulmonary vasculitis caused by Behçet disease, with resolution of the pulmonary lesion and alleviation of uveitis.[182]

Anti–Tumor Necrosis Factor Therapy

Infliximab, a chimeric monoclonal antibody directed against TNF-α, was reported to be effective in treating five patients with Behçet disease. When one dose was given at the last relapse, remission was evident within 24 hours. Abu El-Asrar et al.[183] reported that the response persisted over a relatively long period (16–36 months). When given at 5 mg/kg at time 0, week 2, and then week 6, followed by every 8 weeks, they found that three of six patients were attack free but that positive antinuclear antibodies (ANAs) developed in two. Sfikakis et al. reported long-term outcomes after short-term infliximab use and suggested that infliximab may induce long-term remission in patients with ocular Behçet disease.[184] It is important to remember that infliximab is a chimeric antibody (see Chapter 8) and therefore more prone to the development of drug reactions and antidrug antibodies; it is often given in conjunction with methotrexate to minimize these responses. Furthermore, it is contraindicated in patients with suspected multiple sclerosis,[185] and there is an increased risk of systemic infection (tuberculosis and fungal disease). Like many of the biologics, infliximab is expensive, with the annual cost for rheumatoid arthritis treatment estimated at £11,000 sterling.[186] Adalimumab (Humira), however, is a fully human TNF inhibitor approved by the U.S. Food and Drug Administration (FDA) for the treatment of posterior segment uveitis. It has also been used to treat uveitis associated with Behçet disease.[187,188] Martín-Varillas reported 87% remission rate after 6 months of adalimumab therapy in an open label study.[187] In a large registry-based study of 177 patients with Behçet disease–related uveitis refractory to conventional nonbiologic treatment, Atienza-Mateo et al. compared 103 patients who received infliximab and 74 who received adalimumab for a year. Inflammation control was comparable between the two groups, whereas visual acuity improvement was better in those treated with adalimumab. The drug retention rate was also higher in the adalimumab group.[189] Yalçindag et al. compared 20 patients treated with infliximab and 33 patients treated with IFN and found 80% and 85% remission rates, respectively. Both treatment approaches resulted in comparable inflammation control and visual improvement.[190] In a systematic review that included 378 patients treated with biologic or nonbiologic immunosuppressives, Urruticoechea-Arana et al. found that infliximab was more effective than cyclosporin, and rituximab was similar to cytotoxic drugs. Adalimumab reduced the risk of flare-up and visual impairment[191] (Fig. 27.14).

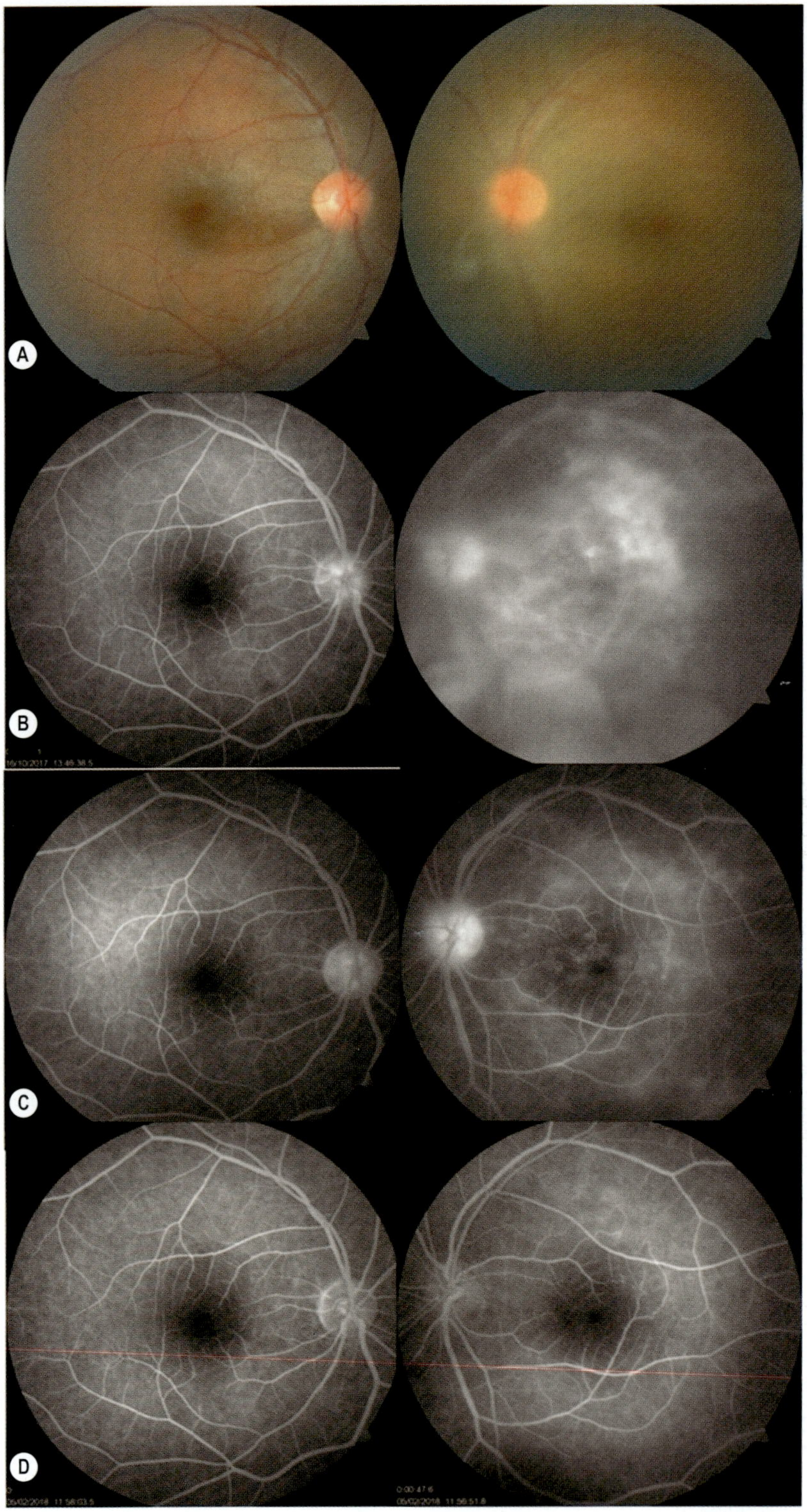

Fig. 27.13 A 33-year-old Turkish man who was in remission on cyclosporine and azathioprine presented with a flare-up in his left eye with vitritis on examination (A) and retinal vasculitis on fluorescein angiogram (B). His vision was 20/20 in the right eye and 20/63 in the left eye. Interferon (IFN)-α was added to his regimen, with modest improvement in retinal vascular leakage (C) and visual acuity (20/32). The patient was switched to the tumor necrosis factor (TNF) inhibitor infliximab for residual leakage and intolerance to IFN, with resultant resolution of retinal vascular leakage in the left eye (D) and improvement in visual acuity to 20/20. (Courtesy Dr. Didar Ucar, Turkey.)

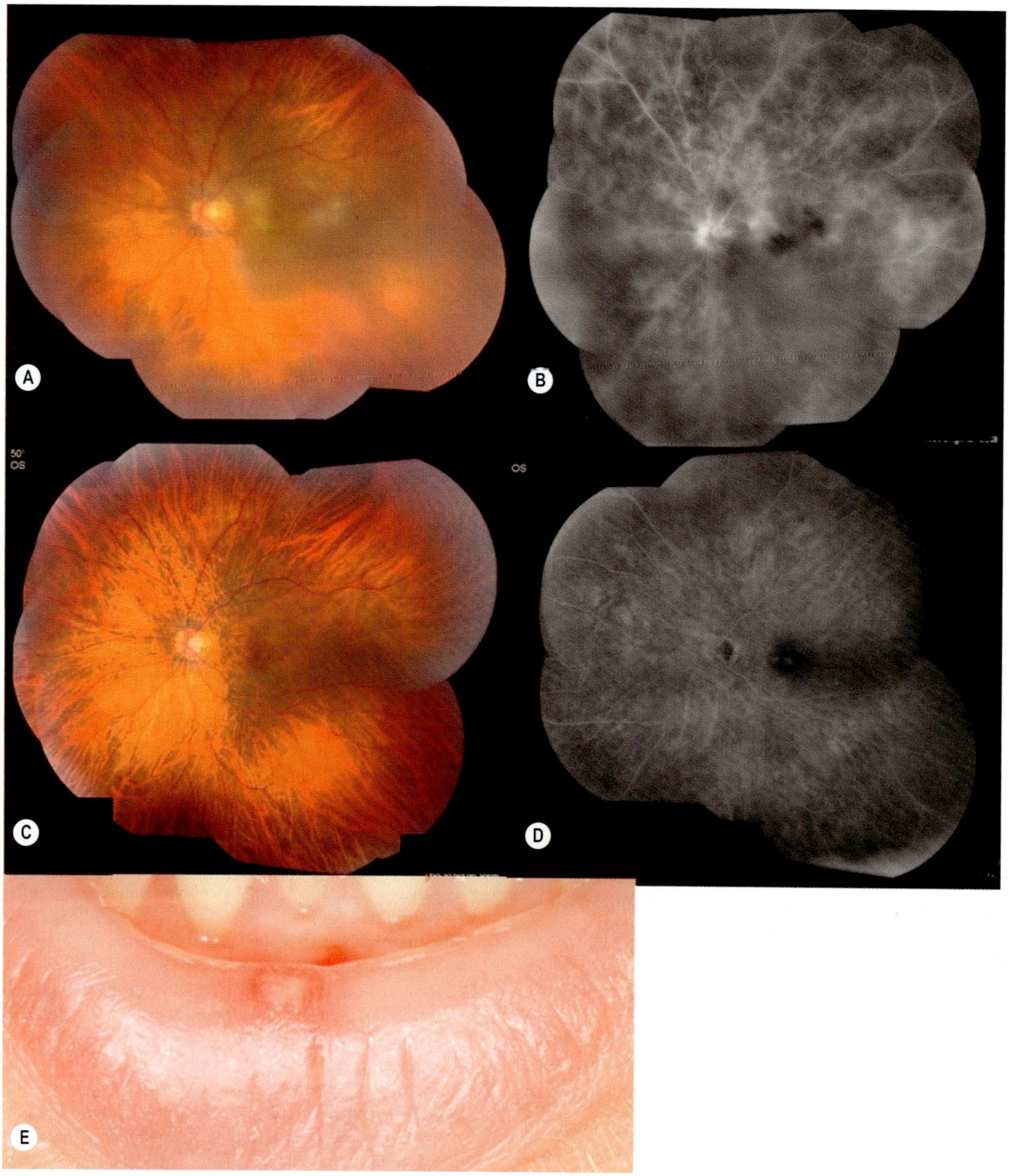

Fig. 27.14 Macular retinitis, vitritis (A), and vasculitis (B) in a patient with Behçet disease, which resolved after intravenous pulse steroids and infliximab infusions (C, D). Oral ulcers (lower lip, E) developed while the patient was on maintenance dose of infliximab and cyclosporine.

Other Approaches

Brief comments should be made about some of the other therapeutic approaches suggested for Behçet disease. Bonnet et al.[192] treated seven patients with plasma exchange to remove circulating immune complexes (CICs) and simultaneously gave high doses of acyclovir, with very discouraging results. The use of antiviral agents has not been useful. A randomized study using acyclovir for the treatment of Behçet disease showed no value in the treatment, at least with regard to the orogenital ulcers.[193] Some centers, both inside and outside the United States, have used thalidomide to treat various components of Behçet disease in the past. Although some aspects of the disease may respond positively to this approach,[194] the ocular lesions do not seem to be particularly amenable.[195] Rituximab, an antibody directed against CD20, a marker for B cells, induced a 24-month remission in one patient.[196] In a single-masked small RCT of 20 patients, Davatchi et al. found that 6-month treatment with rituximab was significantly better compared with cytotoxic combination therapy in terms of the total adjusted disease activity index (TADAI) and inflammatory markers of posterior uveitis.[197] Additionally, a clinical trial using Campath-1H directed at the CD52 marker, a marker for T cells, induced tolerance in the majority of 18 patients with Behçet disease.[198] A randomized study looking at the usefulness of daclizumab in treating the ocular manifestations of the disease did not show it to be effective when used as a sole agent.[199] Therapeutic agents targeting IL-1 have also been tried in Behçet disease.

Fabiani et al.[200] investigated 19 consecutive patients treated with anakinra, a recombinant human IL-1 receptor antagonist, or canakinumab, a long-acting human anti-IL-1β monoclonal antibody. They reported a significant decrease in ocular inflammatory episodes and the need for concomitant corticosteroid use after treatment.[200] The same group also found that the presence of uveitis and long-standing disease was particularly associated with a positive response.[201] Our group also investigated the effectiveness of anakinra and found it partially effective in the treatment of oral and genital ulcers in Behçet disease. Only three of the six patients had ocular disease, but it was not active or imminently vision threatening in any of them.[202]

A novel IL-1β inhibitor, gevokizumab, appeared promising in a small open-label pilot study in 2012 in patients with ocular Behçet disease.[203] However, this drug failed to reach its primary endpoint in a phase III RCT (EYEGUARD-B). Other TNF inhibitors (e.g., golimumab) and tocilizumab have also been used successfully in a small number of patients.[204] Eser Ozturk et al. found tocilizumab to be effective in controlling inflammation in five patients with Behçet disease–associated uveitis.[205] Tocilizumab was also found to be particularly useful in treating macular edema in a number of uveitic conditions, including Behçet disease.[206]

In patients with Behçet disease with severe ocular involvement, it is important to institute an aggressive long-term immunosuppressive therapy regimen that ideally includes TNF inhibitors. After all, an expert panel did recommend that TNF inhibitors, infliximab or adalimumab, be considered as first-line immunosuppressives in Behçet disease.[207]

It must be stressed that many agents that are used have not been approved by the FDA for the treatment of this disorder in the United States, but certainly some have become the standard of care. The patient must be made fully aware of the side effects of these drugs. Some practitioners have reported the use of intravitreal triamcinolone injections, which are often given repeatedly.[208,209] This approach should not be considered for long-term treatment but can be used to deal with acute problems needing immediate action.

CASE 27.1

A 26-year-old Jewish man had a history of idiopathic chronic panuveitis with macular edema for 2 years in both eyes. He had been treated with local corticosteroid injections in the right eye for active uveitis and macular edema in the past, with resultant poor vision, cataract, and macular atrophy. His visual acuity at presentation was 20/250 in the right eye and 20/20 in the left eye. He was placed on systemic prednisone and cyclosporine. Mycophenolate mofetil was added to the regimen to allow successful prednisone taper. His condition was stable on this regimen for several years, but a flare-up of macular retinitis in the left eye occurred, and his vision dropped to 20/640 (see Figs. 27.14A, B).

The patient initially denied any genital or oral ulcers. He was human leukocyte antigen (HLA)-B51 negative but HLA-A26 positive. Nevertheless, a diagnosis of Behçet disease–like retinitis was made on the basis of clinical appearance, and the patient was treated with intravenous pulse corticosteroids followed by oral prednisone taper and infliximab 5 mg/kg infusions in addition to mycophenolate and cyclosporine. His vision recovered to 20/50 within 2 months (see Figs. 27.14C,D), and he was continued on infliximab and cyclosporine; mycophenolate had to be stopped because of bone marrow suppression. Interestingly, 3 years into this regimen, the patient developed painful oral ulcers that lasted more than a week, although they were negative for herpes, as demonstrated by polymerase chain reaction testing (Fig. 27.14E), and his condition remained stable.

CASE 27.2

A 34-year-old Italian American man was diagnosed with Behçet disease at age 14 years with findings of severe bilateral panuveitis and oral ulcers. His history included diagnostic vitrectomy, which was followed by retinal detachment that led to treatment with pars plana vitrectomy, scleral buckle, and silicone oil. His vision was hand motion in the right eye and 20/63 in the left eye. Examination revealed vitritis, retinal vasculitis, and retinitis in the left eye. He was treated with oral prednisone, cyclosporine, mycophenolate mofetil, and chlorambucil, all of which either failed or he was intolerant to. At age 17 years, the patient was started on infliximab before infliximab became the standard of care for Behçet disease. Around the same time, the disease course was complicated by tractional retinal detachment, which led to more surgeries in the right eye (see Fig. 27.9A). The patient's vision was hand motion in the right eye and 20/25 in the left eye. He was continued on infliximab for approximately 6 years and was switched to mycophenolate mofetil. Eventually, phthisis developed in the right eye. However, the patient's condition has remained stable, with quiet uveitis and retinal vasculitis with residual sclerotic and attenuated retinal vessels and modest cataract in the left eye (see Fig. 27.9B). Despite his very severe disease and its complicated course, the patient continues to maintain 20/25 vision in the left eye.

REFERENCES

1. Behçet H. Ueber rezideivierende, aphthöse, durch ein Virus verursachte Geschwüre am Mund, am Auge und an den Genitalien. *Dermatol Wochenschr.* 1937;46:414–419.
2. Adamantiadis B. Sur un cas d'iritis a hypopyon recidevante. *Ann Ocul.* 1931;168:271–274.
3. Shigeta T. Recurrent iritis with hypopyon and its pathological findings. *Acta Soc Ophthalmol Jpn.* 1924;28:516–521.
4. Feigenbaum A. Description of Behçet's syndrome in the Hippocratic third book of endemic diseases. *Br J Ophthalmol.* 1956;40:355–357.
5. Onal S, Tugal-Tutkun I, Urgancioglu M, et al. Clinical course of ocular Behçet's disease in siblings. *Ocular Immunology and Inflammation.* 2001;9:111–124.
6. Fietta P. Behçet's disease: familial clustering and immunogenetics. *Clin Exp Rheumatol.* 2005;23(4 Suppl 38):S96–105.
7. Kazokoglu H, Onal S, Tugal-Tutkun I, et al. Demographic and clinical features of uveitis in tertiary centers in Turkey. *Ophthalmic Epidemiol.* 2008;15(5):285–293.
8. Rodriguez A, Calonge M, Pedroza-Seres M, et al. Referral patterns of uveitis in a tertiary eye care center. *Arch Ophthalmol.* 1996;114:593–599.
9. Soheilian M, Heidari K, Yazdani S, et al. Patterns of uveitis in a tertiary eye care center in Iran. *Ocul Immunol Inflamm.* 2004;12(4):297–310.
10. Salvarani C, Pipitone N, Catanoso MG, et al. Epidemiology and clinical course of Behçet's disease in the Reggio Emilia area of Northern Italy: a seventeen-year population-based study. *Arthritis Rheum.* 2007;57(1):171–178.
11. Ohno S, Matsuda H. Studies of HLA antigens in Behçet's disease in Japan. In: Lehner T, Barnes C, eds. *Recent Advances in Behçet's Disease.* London, UK: Royal Society of Medicine Services; 1986:11–16.
12. Cakir N, Dervis E, Benian O, et al. Prevalence of Behçet's disease in rural western Turkey: a preliminary report. *Clin Exp Rheumatol.* 2004;22:S53–S55.
13. Azizlerli G, Kose AA, Sarica R, et al. Prevalence of Behçet's disease in Istanbul, Turkey. *Int J Dermatol.* 2003;42:803–806.
14. Seaman G, Pearce RA. Behçet's disease manifestation in a population drawn from the UK Behçet's syndrome society. In: Hamza M, ed. *Behçet's Disease.* Tunisia: Pub Adhoua; 1997:196–199.
15. Bietti G, Bruna F. An ophthalmic report on Behçet's disease. In: Monacelli M, Nazzaro P, eds. *Behçet's Disease.* Basel: Karger; 1966:79.
16. Mishima S, Masuda K, Izawa Y, et al. Behçet's disease in Japan: ophthalmologic aspects. *Trans Am Ophthalmol Soc.* 1979;76:225–279.
17. Nakae K, Masaki F, Hashimoto T, et al. Recent epidemiological features of Behçet's disease in Japan. In: Godeau P, Wechsler B, eds. *Behçet's Disease.* St. Louis: Elsevier Science Publishers; 1993:145–151.

18. Ohno S. Behçet's disease in the world. In: Lehner T, Barnes C, eds. *Recent Advances in Behçet's*. London, UK: Royal Society of Medicine Services; 1986:181–186.
19. Dilsen N, Konice M, Aral O. Our diagnostic criteria of Behçet's disease – an overview. In: Lehner T, Barnes C, eds. *Recent Advances in Behçet's Disease*. London, UK: Royal Society of Medicine Services; 1986:177–180.
20. Barnes CG. Behçet's syndrome—classification criteria. *Ann Med Interne*. 1999;150(6):477–482.
21. ISGBD, International Study Group for Behçet's Disease. Criteria for diagnosis of Behçet's Disease. *Lancet*. 1990;335:1078–1080.
22. ISGBD, The International Study Group for Behçet's Disease. Evaluation of diagnostic ("classification") criteria in Behçet's disease—towards internationally agreed criteria. *Br J Rheumatol*. 1992;31:299–308.
23. Bhakta BB, Brennan P, James TE, et al. Behçet's disease: evaluation of a new instrument to measure clinical activity. *Rheumatology*. 1999;38: 728–733.
24. International Team for the Revision of the International Criteria for Behcet's Disease (ITR-ICBD), Davatchi F, Assaad-Khalil S, Calamia KT, et al. The International Criteria for Behcet's Disease (ICBD): a collaborative study of 27 countries on the sensitivity and specificity of the new criteria. *J Eur Acad Dermatol Venereol*. 2014;28:338–347.
25. Nakae K, Masaki F, Inaba G, et al. *A nation-wide epidemiological survey on Behçet's disease, report 2: association of HLA-B51 with clinico-epidemiological features. Report of Behçet's Disease Research Committee*. Japan: Ministry of Health and Welfare; 1993.
26. Davatchi F, Chams-Davatchi C, Shams H, et al. Behcet's disease: epidemiology, clinical manifestations, and diagnosis. *Expert Rev Clin Immunol*. 2017;13(1):57–65.
27. Krause I, Mader R, Sulkes J, et al. Behçet's disease in Israel: the influence of ethnic origin on disease expression and severity. *J Rheumatol*. 2001;28:1033–1036.
28. Muhaya M, Lightman S, Ikeda E, et al. Behçet's disease in Japan and in Great Britain: a comparative study. *Ocul Immunol Inflamm*. 2000;8: 141–148.
29. Hafner R, Truckenbrodt H. Behçet's syndrome with childhood onset. *Acta Univ Carol [Med] (Praha)*. 1991;37:25–30.
30. Losieau-Corvez M, de Kerdanet MM, Chevrant-Breton J, et al. Phlebothrombosis revealing Behçet's disease in a 13-year-old adolescent. *Arch Fr Pediatr*. 1992;49:815–817.
31. Laghmari M, Karim A, Allali F, et al. La maladie de Behçet chez l'enfant, aspects cliniques et evolutifs. A propos de 13 cas. *J Fr Ophthalmol*. 2002;25:904–908.
32. Ando K, Fujino Y, Hijikata K, et al. Epidemiological features and visual prognosis of Behçet's disease. *Jpn J Ophthalmol*. 1999;43:312–317.
33. El Belhadji M, Hamdani M. L'attente ophtalmologique dans la maladie de Behçet. A propos de 520 cas. *J Francais D'ophtalmologie*. 1997;20:592–598.
34. Cho YJ, Kim WK, Lee JH, et al. Visual prognosis and risk factors for Korean patients with Behçet uveitis. *Ophthalmologica*. 2008;222(5):344–350.
35. Kitaichi N, Miyazaki A, Iwata D, et al. Ocular features of Behçet's disease: an international collaborative study. *Br J Ophthalmol*. 2007;91(12):1579–1582.
36. Matsuo T, Itami M. Recurrent versus non-recurrent or no eye involvement in Behçet's disease. *Ocul Immunol Inflamm*. 2005;13(1):73–77.
37. Kump LI, Moeller KL, Reed GF, et al. Behçet's disease: comparing 3 decades of treatment response at the National Eye Institute. *Can J Ophthalmol*. 2008;43(4):468–472.
38. Alpsoy E, Donmez L, Onder M, et al. Clinical features and natural course of Behçet's disease in 661 cases: a multicentre study. *Br J Dermatol*. 2007;157(5):901–906.
39. Barra C, Belfort R Jr, Abreu MT, et al. Behçet's disease in Brazil – a review of 49 cases with emphasis on ophthalmic manifestations. *Jpn J Ophthalmol*. 1991;35:339–346.
40. Cochereau-Massin I, Wechsler B, Le Hoang P, et al. Ocular prognosis in Behçet's disease. *J Fr Ophthalmol*. 1992;15:343–347.
41. Michaelson J, Chisari F. Behçet's disease. *Surv Ophthalmol*. 1982;26: 190–203.
42. Wray D, Graykowski E, Notkins A. Role of mucosal injury in initiating recurrent aphthous stomatitis. *Br Med J [Clin Res]*. 1981;283:1569–1570.
43. Curth H. Behçet's syndrome, abortive form (?): recurrent aphthous oral lesions and recurrent genital ulcerations. *Arch Dermatol Syphilol*. 1946;54:179–196.
44. Hatemi G, Seyahi E, Fresko I, Talarico R, Hamuryudan V. One year in review 2019: Behçet's syndrome. *Clin Exp Rheumatol*. 2019;37(Suppl 121[6]):3–17.
45. Kobayashi T, Matsumaya E, Sugimoto T. Gynecological aspect of mucocutaneous–ocular syndromes. *World Obstet Gynecol*. 1959;11:995–999.
46. Mamo J. The rate of visual loss in Behçet's disease. *Arch Ophthalmol*. 1970;84:451–452.
47. Imai Y. Studies on prognosis and symptoms of Behçet's disease in long-term observation. *Jpn J Clin Ophthalmol*. 1971;25:665–694.
48. Ramsay A, Lightman S. Hypopyon uveitis. *Surv Ophthalmol*. 2001;46: 1–18.
49. Mocan MC, Kadayifcilar S, Irkec M. Keratic precipitate morphology in uveitic syndromes including Behçet's disease as evaluated with in vivo confocal microscopy. *Eye*. 2008;23:1221–1227.
50. Inomata H, Yoshikawa H, Rao NA. Phacoanaphylaxis in Behçet's disease: a clinicopathologic and immunohistochemical study. *Ophthalmology*. 2003;110(10):1942–1945.
51. Tugal-Tutkun I, Cingü K, Kir N, et al. Use of laser flare-cell photometry to quantify intraocular inflammation in patients with Behçet uveitis. *Graefes Arch Clin Exp Ophthalmol*. 2008;246(8):1169–1177.
52. Yilmaz G, Akova Y, Aydin P. Macular ischaemia in Behçet's disease. *Eye*. 2000;14(Pt 5):717–720.
53. Garcher C, Bielefeld P, Desvaux C, et al. Bilateral loss of vision and macular ischemia related to Behçet's disease. *Am J Ophthalmol*. 1997;124:115–117.
54. Abu El-Asrar AM, al-Momen AK, Alamro SA, et al. Bilateral central retinal vein thrombosis in Behçet's disease. *Clin Rheumatol*. 1996;15: 511–513.
55. Balansard B, Bodaghi B, Cassoux N, et al. Necrotising retinopathies simulating acute retinal necrosis syndrome. *Br J Ophthalmol*. 2005;89(1): 96–101.
56. Bozzoni-Pantaleoni F, Gharbiya M, Pirraglia MP, et al. Indocyanine green angiographic findings in Behçet's disease. *Retina*. 2001;21:230–236.
57. Atmaca LS, Sonmez PA. Fluorescein and indocyanine green angiography findings in Behçet's disease. *Br J Ophthalmol*. 2003;87(12):1466–1468.
58. Tugal-Tutkun I, Onal S, Stanford M, et al. An Algorithm for the diagnosis of Behçet disease uveitis in adults. *Ocul Immunol Inflamm*. 2020 Apr 14:1–10. https://doi.org/10.1080/09273948.2020.1736310. Online ahead of print.
59. Furusawa T. A clinical study on mucocutaneous ocular syndrome. *Gank Rinsho Iho*. 1958;52:1143–1146.
60. Sakamoto M, Akazawa K, Nishioka Y, et al. Prognostic factors of vision in patients with Behçet's disease. *Ophthalmology*. 1995;102:317–321.
61. Geraint James D, Spiteri M. Behçet's disease. *Ophthalmology*. 1982;89:1279–1284.
62. Firestein G, Gruber H, Weisman MH, et al. MAGIC syndrome: mouth and genital ulcers with inflamed cartilage. In: Lehner T, Barnes C, eds. *Recent Advances in Behçet's Disease*. London, UK: Royal Society of Medicine Services; 1986:275–280.
63. Shimizu T, Ehrlich GE, Inaba G, et al. Behçet's disease (Behçet's syndrome). *Semin Arthritis Rheum*. 1979;8:223–260.
64. Tai Y, Fong PC, Ng WF, et al. Diffuse aortitis complicating Behçet's disease leading to severe aortic regurgitation. *Cardiology*. 1991;79:156–160.
65. Müftüoglu U, Yurdakul S, Yurdakul S, et al. Vascular involvement in Behçet's disease—a review of 129 cases. In: Lehner T, Barnes C, eds. *Recent Advances in Behçet's Disease*. London, UK: Royal Society of Medicine Services; 1986:255–260.
66. Chajek T, Fairnau M. Behçet's disease. Report of 41 cases and a review of the literature. *Medicine*. 1975;54:179–196.
67. Ebert EC. Gastrointestinal manifestations of Behçet's disease. *Dig Dis Sci*. 2008;103(3):776–787.
68. Inaba G. Clinical features of neuro-Behçet's syndrome. In: Lehner T, Barnes C, eds. *Recent Advances in Behçet's Disease*. London, UK: Royal Society of Medicine Services; 1986:235–246.

69. Sharief M, Hentges R, Thomas E. Significance of CSF immunoglobulins in monitoring neurologic disease activity in Behçet's disease. *Neurology.* 1991;41:1398–1401.
70. Wang C, Chuang C, Chen C. Anticardiolipin antibodies and interleukin-6 in cerebrospinal fluid and blood of Chinese patients with neuro-Behçet's syndrome. *Clin Exp Rheumatol.* 1992;10:599–602.
71. Ogawa M, Sawada T. Sequential gadolinium-DTPA enhanced MRI studies in neuro-Behçet's disease. *Neuroradiology.* 1991;33:136–139.
72. Edem E, Carlier R, Idir AB, et al. Gadolinium-enhanced MRI in central nervous system Behçet's disease. *Neuroradiology.* 1993;35:142–144.
73. Alkan A, Goktan A, Karincaoglu Y, Kamisli S, Dogan M, Oztanir N, Turan N, Kocakoc E. Brain perfusion MRI findings in patients with Behcet's disease. ScientificWorldJournal. 2012;2012:261502. doi: 10.1100/2012/261502. Epub 2012 Apr 30. PMID: 22654579; PMCID: PMC3361152.
74. George RK, Chan CC, Whitcup SM, et al. Ocular immunopathology of Behçet's disease. *Surv Ophthalomol.* 1997;42:157–162.
75. Winter F, Yukins R. The ocular pathology of Behçet's disease. *Am J Ophthalmol.* 1966;62:257–262.
76. Mullaney J, Collum L. Ocular vasculitis in Behçet's disease. A pathological and immunohistochemical study. *Int Ophthalmol.* 1985;7:183–191.
77. Gamble C, Wiesner KB, Shapiro RF, et al. The immune complex pathogenesis of glomerulonephritis and pulmonary vasculitis in Behçet's disease. *Am J Med.* 1979;66:1031–1039.
78. Levinsky R, Lehner T. Circulating soluble immune complexes in recurrent oral ulceration and Behçet's syndrome. *Clin Exp Immunol.* 1978;32:193–198.
79. Matsumura N, Mizushima Y. Leucocyte movement and colchicine treatment in Behçet's disease. *Lancet.* 1975;2:813.
80. Fukuda Y, Hayashi H. *Pathologic Studies on Neuro-Behçet's Disease.* Japan: Annual Report of Behçet's Disease Research Committee; 1980.
81. Kasp E, Graham EM, Stanford MR, et al. Retinal autoimmunity and circulating immune complexes in ocular Behçet's disease. In: Lehner T, Barnes C, eds. *Recent Advances in Behçet's Disease.* London, UK: Royal Society of Medicine Services; 1986:67–72.
82. Poulter L, Lehner T, Duke O. Immunohistological investigation of recurrent oral ulcers and Behçet's disease. In: Lehner T, Barnes C, eds. *Recent Advances in Behçet's Disease.* London, UK: Royal Society of Medicine Services; 1986:123–128.
83. Charteris D, Barton K, McCartney AC, et al. CD4+ lymphocyte involvement in ocular Behçet's disease. *Autoimmunity.* 1992;12:201–206.
84. Charteris D, Champ C, Rosenthal AR, et al. Behçet's disease: activated T lymphocytes in retinal perivasculitis. *Br J Ophthalmol.* 1992;76:499–501.
85. Keino H, Sakai J, Nishioka K, et al. Clonally accumulating T cells in the anterior chamber of Behçet's disease. *Am J Ophthalmol.* 2000;130:243–245.
86. Valesini G, Pivetti-Pezzi P, Mastrandrea F, et al. Evaluation of T cell subsets in Behçet's syndrome using anti-T cell monoclonal antibodies. *Clin Exp Immunol.* 1985;60:55–60.
87. Kikkawa T, Shirotsuki H. Imbalance in T lymphocyte subsets in panuveitis type of Behçet's disease. *J Eye.* 1984;1:1007–1010.
88. Sakane T, Kotani H, Takada S, et al. Functional aberration of T cell subsets in patients with Behçet's disease. *Arthritis Rheum.* 1982;25:1343–1351.
89. Ohno S, Kato F, Matsuda H, et al. Studies on spontaneous production of gamma-interferon in Behçet's disease. *Ophthalmologica.* 1982;185:187–192.
90. BenEzra D, Maftzir G, Kalichman I, et al. Serum levels of interleukin-2 receptor in ocular Behçet's disease. *Am J Opthalmol.* 1993;115:26–30.
91. Jawad S, Liu B, Agron E, Nussenblatt RB, Sen HN. Elevated serum levels of interleukin-17A in uveitis patients. *Ocul Immunol Inflamm.* 2013;21(6):434–439.
92. Evereklioglu C, Er H, Türköz Y, et al. Serum levels of TNF-alpha, sIL-2R, IL-6, and IL-8 are increased and associated with elevated lipid peroxidation in patients with Behçet's disease. *Mediators Inflamm.* 2002;11(2):87–93.
93. Bonacini M, Soriano A, Cimino L, et al. Cytokine profiling in aqueous humor samples from patients with non-infectious uveitis associated with systemic inflammatory diseases. *Front Immunol.* 2020;11:358.
94. Yamamoto J, Minami M, Inaba G, et al. Cellular autoimmunity to retinal specific antigens in patients with Behçet's disease. *Br J Ophthalmol.* 1993;77:584–589.
95. Yalçindag FN, Yalçindag A, Batioglu F, et al. Evaluation of serum resistin levels in patients with ocular and non-ocular Behçet's disease. *Can J Ophthalmol.* 2008;43(4):473–475.
96. Okunuki Y, Usui Y, Takeuchi M, et al. Proteomic surveillance of autoimmunity in Behçet's disease with uveitis: selenium binding protein is a novel autoantigen in Behçet's disease. *Exp Eye Res.* 2007;84(5): 823–831.
97. Mahesh SP, Li Z, Buggage R, et al. Alpha tropomyosin as a self-antigen in patients with Behçet's disease. *Clin Exp Immunol.* 2005;140(2):368–375.
98. Hamzaoui K, Mili Boussen E, Hamzaoui A, et al. Cellular autoimmunity to retinal specific antigens in Behçet's disease. *Soc Tunisienne Sci Med Tunis.* 1998;76:66–70.
99. Yamamoto JH, Fujino Y, Lin C, et al. S-antigen specific T cell clones from a patient with Behçet's disease. *Br J Ophthalmol.* 1994;78:927–932.
100. Ahn JK, Yu HG, Chung H, et al. Intraocular cytokine environment in active Behçet's uveitis. *Am J Ophthalmol.* 2006;142(3):429–434.
101. Ahn JK, Chung H, Lee DS, et al. $CD8^{bright}CD56+$ T cells are cytotoxic effectors in patients with active Behçet's uveitis. *J Immunol.* 2005;175(9):6133–6142.
102. Yu HG, Lee DS, Seo JM, et al. The number of CD8+ T cells and NKT cells increases in the aqueous humor of patients with Behçet's uveitis. *Clin Exp Immunol.* 2004;137(2):437–443.
103. Le Joncour A, Martos R, Loyau S, et al. Critical role of neutrophil extracellular traps (NETs) in patients with Behçet's disease. *Ann Rheum Dis.* 2019;78:1274–1282.
104. Fujimori K, Oh-i K, Takeuchi M, et al. Circulating neutrophils in Behçet's disease is resistant for apoptotic cell death in the remission phase of uveitis. *Graefes Arch Clin Exp Ophthalmol.* 2008;246(2):285–290.
105. Mizuki N, Inoko H, Mizuki N, et al. Human leukocyte antigen serologic and DNA typing of Behçet's disease and its primary association with B51. *Invest Ophthalmol Vis Sci.* 1992;33:3332–3340.
106. Godeau P, Torre D, Campanchi R, et al. HLA-B5 and Behçet's disease. In: Dausset J, Svejgaard A, eds. *HLA and Disease.* Paris: PUB; 1976:101.
107. Ersoy F, Berkel I, Firat T, et al. HLA antigens associated with Behçet's disease. In: Dausset J, Svejgaard A, eds. *HLA and Disease.* Paris: PUB; 1976:100.
108. Palimeris G, Papakonstantinov P, Mantas M. The Adamantiadis–Behçet syndrome in Greece. In: Saari K, ed. *Uveitis Update*Amsterdam: Excerpta Medica; 1984:321.
109. VIllaneuva J, Gonzalez-Dominguez J, Gonzalez-Fernandez R, et al. HLA antigen familial study in complete Behçet's syndrome affecting three sisters. *Ann Rheum Dis.* 1993;52:155–157.
110. Gül A, Uyar FA, Inanc M, et al. Lack of association of HLA-B*51 with a severe disease course in Behçet's disease. *Rheumatology.* 2001;40:668–672.
111. Krause L, Köhler AK, Altenburg A, et al. Ocular involvement is associated with HLA-B51 in Adamantiades–Behçet's disease. *Eye.* 2009;23(5):1182–1186.
112. Nishiyama M, Nakae K, Umehara T. A study of familial occurrence of Behçet's disease with and without ocular lesions. *Jpn J Ophthalmol.* 2001;45:313–316.
113. O'Duffy J, Taswell H, Elveback L. HL-A antigens in Behçet's disease. *J Rheumatol.* 1976;3:1–3.
114. Ohno S, Char DH, Kimura SJ, et al. Studies on HLA antigens in American patients with Behçet's disease. *Jpn J Ophthalmol.* 1978;22:58–61.
115. Muruganandam M, Rolle NA, Sibbitt WL Jr, et al. Characteristics of Behçet's disease in the American Southwest. *Semin Arthritis Rheum.* 2019;49:296–302.
116. Sano K, Yabuki K, Imagawa Y, et al. The absence of disease-specific polymorphisms within the HLA-B51 gene that is the susceptible locus for Behçet's disease. *Tissue Antigens.* 2001;58(2):77–82.
117. Kato H, Takeuchi M, Horita N, et al. HLA-A26 is a risk factor for Behçet's disease ocular lesions. *Mod Rheumatol.* 2020 Jan 4:1–5. https://doi.org/10.1080/14397595.2019.1705538. Online ahead of print.

118. Kuroyanagi K, Sakai T, Kohno H, et al. Association between the major histocompatibility complex and clinical response to infliximab therapy in patients with Behçet uveitis. *Jpn J Ophthalmol.* 2015;59(6):401–408.
119. Mizuki N, Ohno S, Ando H, et al. A strong association between HLA-B*5101 and Behçet's disease in Greek patients. *Tissue Antigens.* 1997;50(1):57–60.
120. Verity DH, Wallace GR, Vaughan RW, et al. HLA and tumour necrosis factor (TNF) polymorphisms in ocular Behçet's disease. *Tissue Antigens.* 1999;54:264–272.
121. Ahmad T, Wallace GR, James T, et al. Mapping the HLA association in Behçet's disease: a role for tumor necrosis factor polymorphisms? *Arthritis Rheum.* 2003;48(3):807–813.
122. Karasneh J, Hajeer AH, Barrett J, et al. Association of specific interleukin 1 gene cluster polymorphisms with increased susceptibility for Behçet's disease. *Rheumatology (Oxford).* 2003;42(7):860–864.
123. Yabuki K, Mizuki N, Ota M, et al. Association of MICA gene and HLA-B*5101 with Behçet's disease in Greece. *Invest Ophthalmol Vis Sci.* 1999;40:1921–1926.
124. Salvarani C, Boiardi L, Mantovani V, et al. Association of MICA alleles and HLA-B51 in Italian patients with Behçet's disease. *J Rheumatol.* 2001;28:1867–1870.
125. Bye L, Modi N, Stanford MR, et al. CTLA-4 polymorphisms are not associated with ocular inflammatory disease. *Tissue Antigens.* 2008;72(1):49–53.
126. Remmers EF, Cosan F, Kirino Y, et al. Genome-wide association study identifies variants in the MHC class I, IL10, and IL23R-IL12RB2 regions associated with Behçet's disease. *Nat Genet.* 2010;42(8):698–702.
127. Kirino Y, Bertsias G, Ishigatsubo Y, et al. Genome-wide association analysis identifies new susceptibility loci for Behçet's disease and epistasis between HLA-B*51 and ERAP1. *Nat Genet.* 2013;45(2):202–207.
128. Hirohata T, Kuratsume M, Nomura A. Prevalence of Behçet's syndrome in Hawaii. *Hawaii Med J.* 1975;34:244–246.
129. Denman A, Hylton W, Pelton BK, et al. The viral aetiology of Behçet's disease. In: Lehner T, Barnes C, eds. *Recent Advances in Behçet's Disease.* London, UK: Royal Society of Medicine Services; 1986:23–30.
130. Hylton W, Cayley J, Dore C, et al. 2′5′-oligoadenylate synthetase induction in lymphocytes of patients with connective tissue diseases. *Ann Rheum Dis.* 1986;45:220–224.
131. Bonass W, Bird-Stewart JA, Chamberlain MA, et al. Molecular studies in Behçet's syndrome. In: Lehner T, Barnes C, eds. *Recent Advances in Behçet's Disease.* London, UK: Royal Society of Medicine Services; 1986:37–42.
132. Hirohata S, Oka H, Mizushima Y. Streptococcal-related antigens stimulate production of IL6 and interferon gamma by T cells from patients with Behçet's disease. *Cell Immunol.* 1992;140:410–419.
133. Tanaka T, Yamakawa N, Koike N, et al. Behçet's disease and antibody titers to various heat-shock protein 60s. *Ocul Immunol Inflamm.* 1999;7:69–74.
134. Pervin K, Childerstone A, Shinnick T, et al. T cell epitope expression of mycobacterial and homologous human 65-kilodalton heat shock protein peptides in short term cell lines from patients with Behçet's disease. *J Immunol.* 1993;151:2273–2282.
135. Evereklioglu C. Current concepts in the etiology and treatment of Behçet's disease. *Surv Ophthalmol.* 2005;50(4):297–350.
136. Kurhan-Yavuz S, Direskeneli H, Bozkurt N, et al. Anti-MHC autoimmunity in Behçet's disease: T cell responses to an HLA-B-derived cross-reactive with retinal-S antigen in patients with uveitis. *Clin Exp Immunol.* 2000;120:162–166.
137. Saadoun D, Wechsler B. Behçet's disease. Orphanet J Rare Dis. 2012 Apr 12;7:20. doi: 10.1186/1750-1172-7-20. PMID: 22497990; PMCID: PMC3472229.
138. Dogan H, Pasaoglu H, Ekinciler OF, et al. A comparative study of total protein, total and lipid associated serum sialic acid levels in patients with Behçet's disease and control groups. *Acta Ophthalmol (Copenh).* 1992;70:790–794.
139. Michaelson J, Chisari F, Kansu T. Antibodies to oral mucosa in patients with ocular Behçet's disease. *Ophthalmology.* 1985;92:1277–1281.
140. Salvarani C, Massai G, Macchioni P, et al. Anticardiolipin antibodies in a case of neuro-Behçet's with superior vena caval obstruction. *Clin Rheumatol.* 1987;6:88–91.
141. Efthimiou J, Cambridge G, Harris EN, et al. Anticardiolipin antibodies and vascular complications in Behçet's syndrome. In: Lehner T, Barnes C, eds. *Recent Advances in Behçet's Disease.* London, UK: Royal Society of Medicine Services; 1986:151–154.
142. Bergman R, Lorber M, Lerner M, et al. Anticardiolipin antibodies in Behçet's disease. *J Dermatol.* 1990;17:164–167.
143. Aydintug A, Tokgöz G, D'Cruz DP, et al. Antibodies to endothelial cells in patients with Behçet's disease. *Clin Immunol Immunopathol.* 1993;67:157–162.
144. BenEzra D, Cohen E. Treatment and visual prognosis in Behçet's disease. *Br J Ophthalmol.* 1986;70:589–592.
145. Benitah NR, Sobrin L, Papaliodis GN. The use of biologic agents in the treatment of ocular manifestations of Behcet's disease. *Semin Ophthalmol.* 2011;26:295–303.
146. Reed JB, Morse LS, Schwab IR. High-dose intravenous pulse methylprednisolone hemisuccinate in acute Behçet's retinitis. *Am J Ophthalmology.* 1998;125:410–411.
147. Mohammadi M, Shahram F, Shams H, Akhlaghi M, Ashofteh F, Davatchi F. High-dose intravenous steroid pulse therapy in ocular involvement of Behcet's disease: a pilot double-blind controlled study. *Int J Rheum Dis.* 2017;20(9):1269–1276.
148. Mamo J. Treatment of Behçet's disease with chlorambucil. *Arch Ophthalmol.* 1976;94:580–583.
149. Tricoulis D. Treatment of Behçet's disease with chlorambucil. *Br J Ophthalmol.* 1976;60:55–57.
150. Hijikata K, Masuda K. Visual prognosis in Behçet's disease: effects of cyclophosphamide and colchicine. *Jpn J Ophthalmol.* 1978;22:506–519.
151. Pivetti-Pezzi P, Gasparri V, De Liso P, et al. Prognosis in Behçet's disease. *Ann Ophthalmol.* 1985;17:20–25.
152. Tabbara K. Chlorambucil in Behçet's disease. A reappraisal. *Ophthalmology.* 1983;90:906–908.
153. Kazokoglu H, Saatçi O, Cuhadaroglu H, et al. Long-term effects of cyclophosphamide and colchicine treatment in Behçet's disease. *Ann Ophthalmol.* 1991;23:148–151.
154. Takeuchi F, Takeuci A. Chromosome aberration in lymphocytes from Behçet's disease. *J Rheumatol.* 1991;18:1207–1210.
155. Hamza M, Meddeb S, Mili I, et al. Bolus of cyclophosphamide and methylprednisolone in uveitis in Behçet's disease. Preliminary results with the use of new criteria of evaluation. *Ann Med Interne (Paris).* 1992;143:438–441.
156. Yazici H, Pazarli H, Barnes CG, et al. A controlled trial of azathioprine in Behçet's syndrome. *N Engl J Med.* 1990;322:281–285.
157. O'Duffy JD. Behçet's syndrome. *N Engl J Med.* 1990;322(5):326–328.
158. Tabbara K. Azathioprine in Behçet's syndrome. *N Engl J Med.* 1990;322:326–328.
159. Hamuryudan V, Ozyazgan Y, Hizli N, et al. Azathioprine in Behçet's syndrome. Effects on long-term prognosis. *Arthritis Rheum.* 1997;40:769–774.
160. Greenwood AJ, Stanford MR, Graham EM. The role of azathioprine in the management of retinal vasculitis. *Eye.* 1998;12(Pt 5):783–788.
161. Davatchi F, Sadeghi Abdollahi B, Shams H, et al. Combination of pulse cyclophosphamide and azathioprine in ocular manifestations of Behçet's disease: longitudinal study of up to 10 years. *Int J Rheum Dis.* 2014;17(4):444–452.
162. Lange U, Schumann C, Schmidt KL. Current aspects of colchicine therapy classical indications and new therapeutic uses. *Eur J Med Res.* 2001;6:150–160.
163. Aktulga E, Altaç M, Müftüoglu A, et al. A double blind study of colchicine in Behçet's disease. *Haematologica.* 1980;65:399–402.
164. Yurdakul S, Mat C, Tüzün Y, et al. A double-blind trial of colchicine in Behçet's syndrome. *Arthritis Rheum.* 2001;44:2686–2692.
165. Warde N. Therapy: Behçet uveitis: good results for IFN-alpha-2a. *Nat Rev Rheumatol.* 2010;6:437.
166. Kotter I, Eckstein AK, Stübiger N, et al. Treatment of ocular symptoms of Behçet's disease with interferon alfa 2a: a pilot study. *Br J Ophthalmol.* 1998;82:488–494.
167. Pivetti-Pezzi P, Accorinti M, Pirraglia MP, et al. Interferon alpha for ocular Behçet's disease. *Acta Ophthalmol Scand.* 1997;75:720–722.
168. Wechsler B, Bodaghi B, Huong DL, et al. Efficacy of interferon alfa-2a in severe and refractory uveitis associated with Behçet's disease. *Ocul Immunol Inflamm.* 2000;4:293–301.

169. Kotter I, Gunaydin I, Zierhut M, Stubiger N. The use of interferon α in Behçet disease: review of the literature. *Semin Arthritis Rheum.* 2004;33:320–335.
170. Sakane T, Takeno M. Interferon therapy in Behçet's disease. *Intern Med (Tokyo).* 2000;39:604–605.
171. Sakane T, Takeno M. Novel approaches to Behçet's disease. *Exp Opin Invest Drugs.* 2000;9:1993–2005.
172. Mesquida M, Molins B, Llorenç V, et al. Current and future treatments for Behçet's uveitis: road to remission. *Int Ophthalmol.* 2014;34(2):365–381.
173. Nussenblatt R, Palestine AG, Chan CC, et al. Effectiveness of cyclosporin therapy for Behçet's disease. *Arthritis Rheum.* 1985;28:671–679.
174. Masuda K, Nakajima A, Urayama A, et al. Double-masked trial of cyclosporin versus colchicine and long-term open study of cyclosporin in Behçet's disease. *Lancet.* 1989;1(8647):1093–1096.
175. BenEzra D, Brodsky M, Pe'er J, et al. Ciclosporin (CyA) versus conventional therapy in Behçet's disease. Preliminary observations of a masked study. In: Schindler R, ed. *Ciclosporin in Autoimmune Diseases.* Berlin: Springer-Verlag; 1985:158–161.
176. Assuman U, Müftüoglu H. Treatment of ocular involvement in Behçet's disease with ciclosporin A (preliminary report). In: Schindler R, ed. *Ciclosporin in Autoimmune Diseases.* Berlin: Springer-Verlag; 1985:147–151.
177. Ozyazgan Y, Yurdakul S, Yazici H, et al. Low dose cyclosporin A versus pulsed cyclophosphamide in Behçet's syndrome: a single masked trial. *Br J Ophthalmol.* 1992;76:241–243.
178. Kotake S, Ichiishi A, Kosaka S, et al. Low dose cyclosporin treatment for ocular lesions of Behçet's disease. *Nippon Ganka Gakkai Zasshi.* 1992;96:1290–1294.
179. Chavis P, Antonio S, Tabbara K. Cyclosporine effects on optic nerve and retinal vasculitis in Behçet's disease. *Doc Ophthalmol.* 1992;80:133–142.
180. Whitcup S, Salvo EJ, Nussenblatt R. Combined cyclosporine and corticosteroid therapy for sight threatening uveitis in Behçet's disease. *Am J Ophthalmol.* 1994;118:39–45.
181. Elidan J, Levi H, Cohen E, et al. Effect of cyclosporine A on the hearing loss in Behçet's disease. *Ann Otol Rhinol Laryngol.* 1991;100:464–468.
182. Koga T, Yano T, Ichikawa Y, et al. Pulmonary infiltrates recovered by FK506 in a patient with Behçet's disease. *Chest.* 1993;104:309–311.
183. Abu El-Asrar AM, Abboud EB, Aldibhi H, et al. Long-term safety and efficacy of infliximab therapy in refractory uveitis due to Behçet's disease. *Int Ophthalmol.* 2005;26(3):83–92.
184. Sfikakis PP, Arida A, Ladas DS, Markomichelakis N. Induction of ocular Behçet's disease remission after short-term treatment with infliximab: a case series of 11 patients with a follow-up from 4 to 16 years. *Clin Exp Rheumatol.* 2019;37(Suppl 121[6]):137–141.
185. van Oosten BW, Barkhof F, Truyen L, et al. Increased MRI activity and immune activation in two multiple sclerosis patients treated with the monoclonal anti-tumor necrosis factor antibody cA2. *Neurology.* 1996;47:1531–1534.
186. Murray PI, Sivaraj RR. Anti-TNF-alpha therapy for uveitis: Behçet and beyond. *Eye.* 2005;19(8):831–833.
187. Martín-Varillas JL, Calvo-Río V, Beltrán E, et al. Successful optimization of adalimumab therapy in refractory uveitis due to Behçet's disease [published correction appears in *Ophthalmology.* 2019;126(1):177]. *Ophthalmology.* 2018;125(9):1444–1451.
188. Fabiani C, Vitale A, Emmi G, et al. Efficacy and safety of adalimumab in Behçet's disease-related uveitis: a multicenter retrospective observational study. *Clin Rheumatol.* 2017;36(1):183–189.
189. Atienza-Mateo B, Martín-Varillas JL, Calvo-Río V, et al. Comparative study of infliximab versus adalimumab in refractory uveitis due to Behçet's disease: national multicenter study of 177 cases. *Arthritis Rheumatol.* 2019;71(12):2081–2089.
190. Yalçindag N, Köse HC. Comparison of the treatment results for Behçet uveitis in patients treated with infliximab and interferon. *Ocul Immunol Inflamm.* 2020;28(2):305–314.
191. Urruticoechea-Arana A, Cobo-Ibáñez T, Villaverde-García V, et al. Efficacy and safety of biological therapy compared to synthetic immunomodulatory drugs or placebo in the treatment of Behçet's disease associated uveitis: a systematic review. *Rheumatol Int.* 2019;39(1):47–58.
192. Bonnet M, Ouzan D, Trepo C. Plasma exchange and acyclovir in Behçet's disease. *J Fr Ophthalmol.* 1986;9:15–22.
193. Davies UM, Palmer RG, Denman AM. Treatment with acyclovir does not affect orogenital ulcers in Behçet's syndrome: a randomized double-blind trial. *Br J Rheumatol.* 1988;27(4):300–302.
194. Allen B. The use of thalidomide in orogenital ulceration: an overview. In: Lehner T, Barnes C, eds. *Recent Advances in Behçet's Disease.* London, UK: Royal Society of Medicine Services; 1986:355–358.
195. Hamza M. Treatment of Behçet's disease with thalidomide. *Clin Rheumatol.* 1986;5:365–371.
196. Sadreddini S, Noshad H, Molaeefard M, et al. Treatment of retinal vasculitis in Behçet's disease with rituximab. *Mod Rheumatol.* 2008;18(3):306–308.
197. Davatchi F, Shams H, Rezaipoor M, et al. Rituximab in intractable ocular lesions of Behçet's disease; randomized single-blind control study (pilot study). *Int J Rheum Dis.* 2010;13(3):246–252.
198. Lockwood CM, Hale G, Waldman H, et al. Remission induction in Behçet's disease following lymphocyte depletion by the anti-CD52 antibody CAMPATH 1-H. *Rheumatology (Oxford).* 2003;42(12):1539–1544.
199. Buggage RR, Levy-Clarke G, Sen HN, et al. A double-masked, randomized study to investigate the safety and efficacy of daclizumab to treat the ocular complications related to Behçet's disease. *Ocul Immunol Inflamm.* 2007;15(2):63–70.
200. Fabiani C, Vitale A, Emmi G, et al. Interleukin (IL)-1 inhibition with anakinra and canakinumab in Behçet's disease-related uveitis: a multicenter retrospective observational study. *Clin Rheumatol.* 2017;36(1):191–197.
201. Fabiani C, Vitale A, Rigante D, et al. The presence of uveitis is associated with a sustained response to the interleukin (IL)-1 inhibitors anakinra and canakinumab in Behçet's disease. *Ocul Immunol Inflamm.* 2020;28(2):298–304.
202. Grayson PC, Yazici Y, Merideth M, et al. Treatment of mucocutaneous manifestations in Behçet's disease with anakinra: a pilot open-label study. *Arthritis Res Ther.* 2017;19(1):69.
203. Gül A, Tugal-Tutkun I, Dinarello CA, Reznikov L, Esen BA, Mirza A, et al. Interleukin-1beta-regulating antibody XOMA 052 (gevokizumab) in the treatment of acute exacerbations of resistant uveitis of Behçet's disease: an open-label pilot study. *Ann Rheum Dis.* 2012;71(4):563–566.
204. Santos-Gómez M, Calvo-Río V, Blanco R, et al. The effect of biologic therapy different from infliximab or adalimumab in patients with refractory uveitis due to Behçet's disease: results of a multicentre open-label study. *Clin Exp Rheumatol.* 2016;34(6 Suppl 102):S34–S40.
205. Eser Ozturk H, Oray M, Tugal-Tutkun I. Tocilizumab for the treatment of Behçet uveitis that failed interferon alpha and anti-tumor necrosis factor-alpha therapy. *Ocul Immunol Inflamm.* 2018;26(7):1005–1014.
206. Vegas-Revenga N, Calvo-Río V, Mesquida M, et al. Anti-IL6-receptor tocilizumab in refractory and noninfectious uveitic cystoid macular edema: multicenter study of 25 patients. *Am J Ophthalmol.* 2019;200:85–94.
207. Levy-Clarke G, Jabs DA, Read RW, Rosenbaum JT, Vitale A, Van Gelder RN. Expert panel recommendations for the use of anti-tumor necrosis factor biologic agents in patients with ocular inflammatory disorders. *Ophthalmology.* 2014;121(3):785-96.e3. doi:10.1016/j.ophtha.2013.09.048.
208. Ohguro N, Yamanaka E, Otori Y, et al. Repeated intravitreal triamcinolone injections in Behçet disease that is resistant to conventional therapy: one-year results. *Am J Ophthalmol.* 2006;141(1):218–220.
209. Atmaca LS, Yalçindag FN, Ozdemir O. Intravitreal triamcinolone acetonide in the management of cystoid macular edema in Behçet's disease. *Graefes Arch Clin Exp Ophthalmol.* 2007;245(3):451–456.
210. Okabe S, Matsuo N, Okamoto S, et al. Electron microscopic studies on retinochoroidal atrophy in the human eye. *Acta Med Okayama.* 1982;36:11–21.
211. Mat C, Yurdakul S, Uysal S, et al. A double-blind trial of depot corticosteroids in Behçet's syndrome. *Rheumatology (Oxford).* 2006;45(3):348–352.
212. Melikoglu M, Fresko I, Mat C, et al. Short-term trial of etanercept in Behçet's disease: a double blind, placebo controlled study. *J Rheumatol.* 2005;32(1):98–105.

213. Alpsoy E, Durusoy C, Yilmaz E, et al. Interferon alfa-2a in the treatment of Behçet's disease: a randomized placebo-controlled and double-blind study. *Arch Dermatol.* 2002;138(4):467–471.
214. Sharquie KE, Najim RA, Abu-Raghif AR. Dapsone in Behçet's disease: a double-blind, placebo-controlled, cross-over study. *J Dermatol.* 2002;29(5):267–279.
215. Hamuryudan V, Mat C, Saip S, et al. Thalidomide in the treatment of the mucocutaneous lesions of the Behçet syndrome. A randomized, double-blind, placebo-controlled trial. *Ann Intern Med.* 1998;128(6):443–450.
216. Moral F, Hamuryudan V, Yurdakul S, et al. Inefficacy of azapropazone in the acute arthritis of Behçet's syndrome: a randomized, double blind, placebo controlled study. *Clin Exp Rheumatol.* 1995;13(4):493–495.
217. Denman AM, Hollingworth P, Webster ADB, et al. Failure of transfer factor in the treatment of Behçet's syndrome: a double-blind trial. In: Lehner T, Barnes CG, eds. *Behçet's Syndrome.* London, UK: Academic Press; 1979.

28

Retinal Vasculitis

Alan G. Palestine

KEY CONCEPTS

- Retinal vascular changes can be seen in many ocular inflammatory entities; some are associated with systemic diseases.
- Fluorescein angiography is very important to evaluate the full extent of the vascular disease.
- Therapy for the ocular disease needs to be coordinated with the clinicians treating an associated systemic illness.

Retinal vascular inflammatory involvement is a common occurrence in many cases of posterior and intermediate uveitis. Retinal vasculitis has been poorly defined in the ophthalmic literature. In the past, the term *vasculitis* suggested that the underlying mechanism leading to these alterations is a type III hypersensitivity reaction, that is, one of immune complexes. However, evidence from experimental models and from eyes evaluated through histologic examinations suggests that this is not the case. In one sense, anytime a retinal vessel is leaking, it is appropriate to consider it inflamed and thus use the term *vasculitis.* Alternatively, this vascular leakage only could be considered a sign of vascular permeability alterations and not true inflammation of the vessel, and we could restrict the term *vasculitis* to actual inflammation of the retinal vessel itself. In a similar manner, we would not consider cystoid macular edema to be retinal vasculitis, although the retinal vessels show leakage, but if the inflammation caused retinal vascular occlusion, we would be more certain that the retinal vessel was inflamed in a manner that caused pathologic alterations in the retina. In the case of macular edema, we consider this to be a secondary effect of inflammation within the eye and not the primary site of the inflammation. However, even when the vessel wall appears to be clinically inflamed, as shown by staining on fluorescein angiography, and there is vascular sheathing, the available pathologic data indicate that the most accurate term for these entities perhaps is *perivasculitis* or, in most cases, *phlebitis.* Although there are conditions in which the retinal vascular component is the predominant feature of the ocular disease, the ubiquitous nature of these retinal vascular alterations indicates that "retinal vasculitis" can also be a clinical sign. Behçet disease is perhaps the sine qua non of retinal vasculitis (see Chapter 27); however, numerous disorders can have a similar presentation. It has been suggested that the retinal veins are involved in Behçet disease, tuberculosis, sarcoidosis, multiple sclerosis, pars planitis, Eales disease, and the ocular manifestations of human immunodeficiency virus (HIV). Arteriolar involvement is more common in systemic disorders with predominantly arterial involvement, such as polyarteritis nodosa and systemic lupus erythematosus (SLE).[1] Lymphoma, albeit rare, should always be considered as a possible underlying cause of retinal vasculitis.[2]

Because of lack of clear understanding of the process of retinal vascular inflammation, we should therefore divide clinical retinal vascular inflammation into three groups: (1) those cases where there is occlusive retinal vasculitis and loss of retinal perfusion, (2) those cases where there is retinal vascular staining and leakage on fluorescein angiography of vessels other than retinal capillaries, and (3) those cases where the leakage is primarily confined to the retinal capillaries. This last form of leakage has been termed ferning when observed on widefield angiography and is most commonly seen in pars planitis and non-pars planitis intermediate uveitis.

Retinal vasculitis needs to be monitored because it is an excellent indicator of inflammatory activity and can be objectively assessed by using fluorescein angiography. Furthermore, vasculitis can lead to occlusive vasculitis, which can then cause sudden vision loss, including macular infarcts, optic nerve infarction, and retinal ischemia. Because these sequelae can predispose the patient to neovascularization of the retina and the iris, awareness of retinal vascular inflammation is important in the management of many types of ocular inflammation.

CLINICAL CHARACTERISTICS

Although this chapter deals with multiple mechanisms, patients with retinal vasculitis most often report a painless decrease in vision or a marked loss of vision; this may, at times, be accompanied by floaters. There can also be large areas of scotomata relating to the areas of ischemia. If the retinal vascular changes occur in the periphery of the fundus, then patients may report minimal symptoms or none at all in spite of marked changes noted on ocular examination.

Examination of the retina shows striking vascular alterations, sometimes best seen with fluorescein angiography. Active vascular disease is characterized by sheathing of the vessels or, in some conditions, such as sarcoidosis, an immense inflammatory response, described as "candle wax drippings," around the vessels. Sheathing can skip along the length of a vessel. Although histologically, we can only presume what is occurring, it is thought that perivasculitis underlies what we describe clinically as "sheathing": large numbers of cells either leaving or entering the vessels. What is drawing the cells there? We do not know, and speculation abounds. It could be caused by expression of vascular endothelial antigens, the presence of adhesion molecules, simple passage of immune cells through the vessel wall to reach the retina and its immunogenic antigens, or a combination of all of these.

Another characteristic of retinal vasculitis is occlusive retinopathy, which can be prominent in some patients. Large areas of capillary

BOX 28.1 Disorders with Retinal Vasculitis as a Common Finding

Systemic Disorders
Behçet disease
Sarcoidosis
Systemic lupus erythematosus
Postvaccination inflammation
Multiple sclerosis
Wegener granulomatosis
Takayasu disease
Buerger disease
Polyarteritis nodosa
Polymyositis
Dermatomyositis
Whipple disease
Crohn disease
Sjögren A antigen
Kikuchi-Fujimoto disease
Susac syndrome

Infectious Disorders
Syphilis
Cat scratch fever
Hepatitis C
Chickenpox
Toxoplasmosis
Toxocariasis
Coccidioidomycosis
Tuberculosis
Cytomegalovirus infection
Herpes simplex
Herpes zoster
Rift Valley fever
West Nile virus infection
Acute retinal necrosis
Candidiasis
Leptospirosis
Rickettsia
Mediterranean spotted fever
Drucellosis
Amebiasis
Mononucleosis
Lyme disease
Hepatitis B

Ocular Disorders
Birdshot retinochoroidopathy
Pars planitis
Eales disease
Choroiditis
Retinal arteritis and aneurysms
Behçet retina without systemic disease
Vein occlusion

Neoplasms
Paraneoplastic syndromes
Ocular and systemic lymphoma
Acute leukemia

Reproduced with permission from Samuel MA, Equi RA, Chang TS, et al. Idiopathic retinitis, vasculitis, aneurysms, and neuroretinitis (IRVAN): new observations and a proposed staging system. *Ophthalmology.* 2007;114(8):1526–1529.

dropout are commonly seen. In many inflammatory conditions of the retina, the capillary-free zone takes on a markedly jagged and enlarged appearance. Often, in addition to capillary dropout, one sees vascular architectural alterations just temporal to the macula, sometimes manifesting as arteriolar/venular anastomoses and crossing of vessels over the horizontal raphe.

The involvement of primarily the retinal vasculature in an inflammatory disorder is seen rather commonly, the best example being Behçet disease (see Chapter 27). However, other well-recognized entities, such as birdshot retinochoroidopathy (see Chapter 26) and sarcoidosis (see Chapter 23), and infectious processes, have or can have marked involvement of the retinal vasculature, although we frequently do not think of these diseases in that sense. Indeed, the entities with a significant retinal vasculature component are listed in Box 28.1. It is important to note that noninflammatory conditions can also lead to what appears to be a retinal vasculitis. Venous obstruction, Coats disease, and diabetes mellitus can mimic the changes seen in an inflammation-driven process.

Although a systemic evaluation for the patient with ocular vasculitis being seen for the first time makes sense, we would like to present our experience to the reader. Rosenbaum reviewed 1390 patients with uveitis and found only 11 with systemic vasculitis.[3] In the National Eye Institute (NEI) report on 25 patients with "primary" ocular vasculitis, only one had a history suggestive of systemic disease (systemic lupus erythematosus [SLE]). False-positive diagnostic test results were obtained in five (20.8%) of 24 of these patients. No underlying disease was found in any of these patients at review some 4 years later.[4] Hence, although one should always look for systemic vasculitis that could be potentially life threatening, the results of this search are likely to be negative.

OCULAR VASCULITIS WITHOUT SYSTEMIC DISEASE

We have seen patients with ocular findings that are indistinguishable from those in patients with Behçet disease. These patients have none of the typical systemic findings and yet have recurrent episodes of retinal vasculitis. In addition, some of these persons show human leukocyte antigen (HLA)-B51 positivity. There is a strong possibility that Behçet disease may develop. However, on a statistical basis, one would expect other features of the disorder to develop within 3 years of the appearance of the first one, and this has not been the case. The recurrent episodes of retinal vasculitis (and retinitis) are frequently difficult to control and often require the use of other immunosuppressive agents in addition to prednisone. Lueck et al.[5] reported the case of a patient with recurrent steroid-sensitive uveitis and central nervous system (CNS) disease thought to be caused by sarcoidosis. Postmortem examination revealed a histologic picture compatible with that of Behçet disease despite the absence of any of the systemic stigmata associated with this diagnosis. The authors have called this entity Behçet MINUS (multifocal intermittent neurologic and uveitic syndrome).

We have seen other patients with severe retinal vasculitis that appears to be unassociated with systemic disease; attempts to identify an underlying abnormality (e.g., immune complexes or sedimentation rate) often prove fruitless. The disorder frequently may persist despite aggressive immunotherapy (Fig. 28.1).

Eales Disease

Although Eales disease had been discussed by others, the disorder is named after Henry Eales, who, in 1880,[6] described five young men with recurring vitreal and retinal hemorrhages associated with constipation and epistaxis. The definition of the condition has changed considerably over the years. The problem with this is that it is difficult to read the published reports and be sure that one report of a group of patients is really discussing the same disease as is another report. As Franceschetti wrote in 1962:

> The question naturally arises as to the necessity for naming a new retinal affliction when, since Leber (1916), everything seems to have been described and classified. It would seem to be reasonable that a nameless retinal affliction must be either a variant of a known one or an extremely rare entity. However, a rare affliction often becomes less rare when given an appropriate name.[7]

Eales disease can be defined as an idiopathic condition that manifests as obliterative perivasculitis (particularly involving the venule side) affecting the retina in multiple quadrants, starting at, or anterior to, the equator and progressing posteriorly. The disease sometimes is accompanied by neovascularization, without vitritis, obvious uveal inflammation, or obvious systemic disease. It is, in essence, a diagnosis of exclusion, and the patient population is probably heterogeneous, but it remains unclear whether all occlusive vasculitis without a systemic association should be called *Eales disease.* There is a strong association with purified protein derivative (PPD) skin test positivity,[8] and Moura et al.[9] reported that strongly positive Mantoux test results were found in 87% of 141 patients. Biswas et al.[10] published two reports of studies in India further evaluating the relationship between tuberculosis and Eales disease. In one study, polymerase

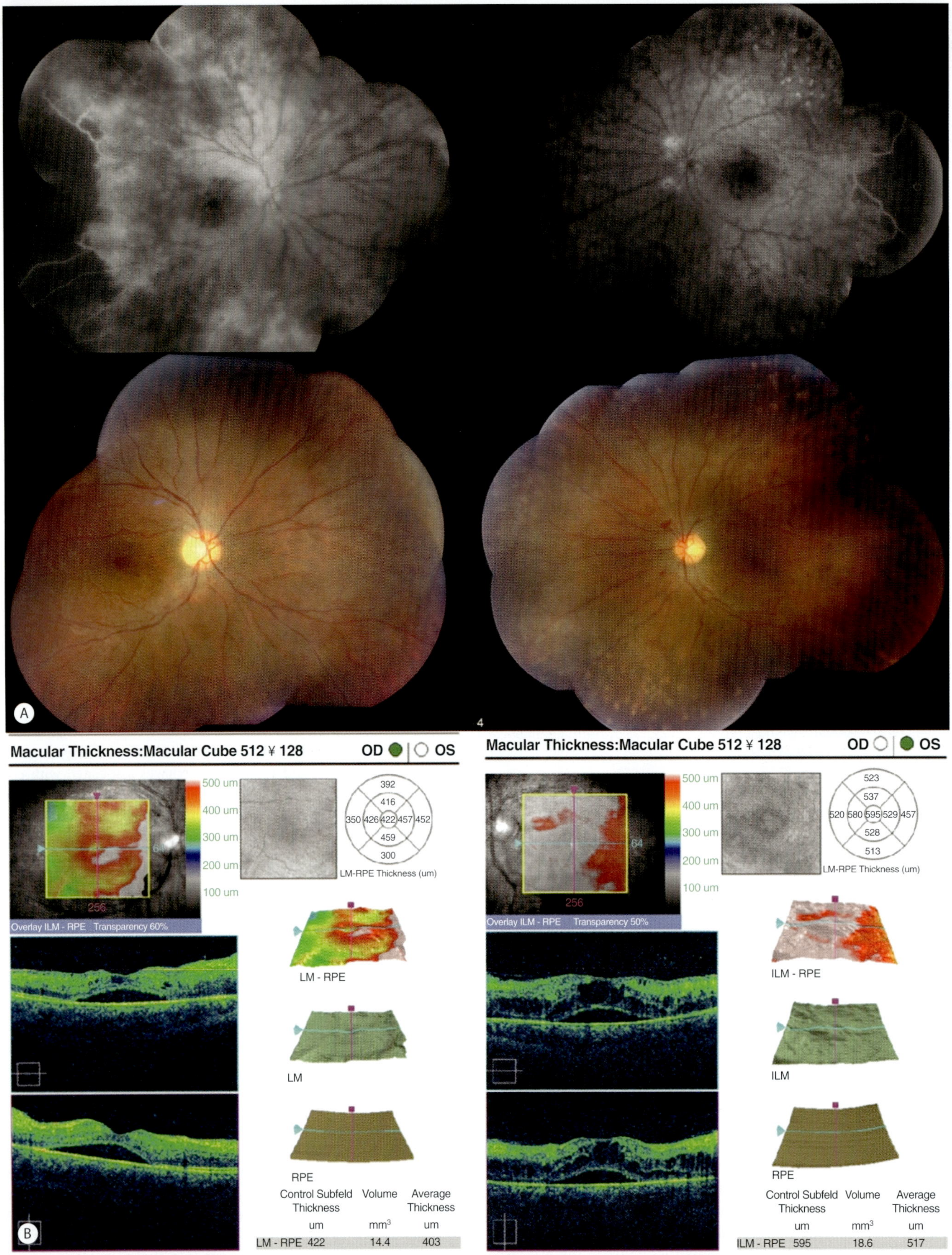

Fig. 28.1 This 17-year-old Hispanic woman complained of decreased vision. She was found to have a retinal vasculitis in both eyes. (A) Montage and fundus findings. Note the peripheral retinal capillary loss. Laser photocoagulation had been started in the periphery of the left eye (OS) before referral to the National Eye Institute (NEI). (B) Optical coherence tomography (OCT) of both eyes showing macular edema and subretinal fluid. An extensive evaluation revealed no systemic abnormality. She was stabilized on prednisone and cyclosporin in the short term.

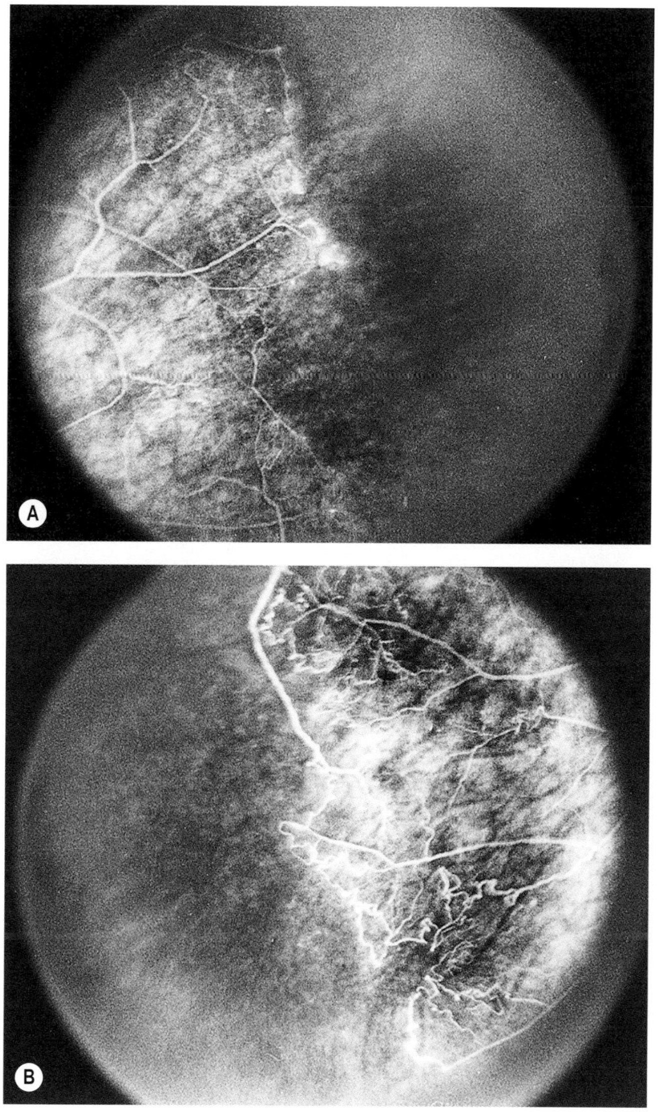

Fig. 28.2 (A and B) Peripheral retinal vaso-occlusive disease with neovascularization caused by Eales disease. (Courtesy R. Murphy, MD.)

chain reaction (PCR) was performed on 12 vitrectomy specimens from patients with Eales disease and on 45 specimens from patients without Eales disease. This methodology had the sensitivity to detect 2.5 pg of *Mycobacterium tuberculosis.* Five of the 12 specimens (41.6%) from the patients with Eales disease versus one of 45 specimens (2.2%) from the patients without Eales disease were positive for *M. tuberculosis.* In their second study,[11] 11 of 23 epiretinal membranes (47.8%) versus three of 27 control epiretinal membranes (11.1%) ($p = 0.001$) were positive for the *M. tuberculosis* genome. In another study from India, Therese et al.,[12] using PCR, reported finding *Mycobacterium fortuitum* and *Mycobacterium chelonae* in vitrectomy specimens, suggesting that other mycobacteria could initiate similar immune responses. The disease has been estimated to affect 1% of adult men in India and usually occurs in patients younger than 40 years of age. The disease process has minimal inflammation associated with it.

The disorder may start with retinal edema, followed by a progressive cuffing of the venules (periphlebitis) and then by peripheral retinal vascular nonperfusion and retinal neovascularization.[13] The condition affects the retinal periphery, but on occasion, it can begin at the optic nerve head, mimicking a venous occlusion. Only with the more characteristic peripheral retinal signs will the diagnosis become clear. The arteries are not involved. Unlike occlusions that result from arteriosclerotic plaques, this occlusion does not usually occur at an arteriovenous crossing. Periphlebitis may occlude substantial portions of a vein, but in an irregular fashion. Unlike venous occlusions in the posterior pole, those in the periphery will not cause cotton-wool spots.[14] The development of neovascularization may be rapid. Fluorescein angiography of the retinal vasculature may show nonperfusion, arteriovenous shunting, and neovascularization (Fig. 28.2). Recurrent vitreous hemorrhage, with ensuing vitreous contraction and retinal detachment, is a serious risk in this disorder. Although the disease is thought to be an ocular disorder, Biswas et al.[15] reported three patients with seizures and/or migraine. Magnetic resonance imaging (MRI) showed a putaminal infarct with white matter edema in two patients.

Although the disease may proceed to its full-blown clinical state, as described, in some patients, the process may spontaneously reverse itself. The visual prognosis in these patients is not totally hopeless. Elliot[16] reported that 25 of 46 eyes he monitored for, on average, 6 years had visual acuity of 20/50 or better, whereas 26% had visual acuity of 20/200 or worse. The exact role of the immune system remains unclear. However, Murugeswari et al.[17] have shown a correlation between vascular endothelial growth factor (VEGF) and interleukin-6 (IL-6) levels in the vitreous specimens of patients with Eales disease, with IL-8 and monocyte chemoattractant protein-1 (MCP-1) also being elevated compared with the levels in controls. This would suggest that at least locally active inflammatory factors are being produced. Part of the definition calls for minimal or no evidence of inflammatory disease. Muthukkaruppan et al.[18] found circulating immune complexes in these patients. Rennie et al.[19] have also noted vestibuloauditory problems associated with the ocular condition, suggesting that this is, indeed, a systemic disease. The notion that the disease is caused by tuberculosis hypersensitivity is difficult to support because it does not seem to be found in greater numbers of patients in countries where the population is actively immunized with Bacille Calmette-Guérin (BCG) vaccination. It may be that mycobacterial antigens are particularly good initiators of a still-undefined disease mechanism, but other antigens are probably capable of producing the same effect. Alternatively, a specific genetically determined immune background may put some patients at higher risk for this disease.

For patients with capillary dropout and neovascularization, laser ablation could be contemplated. Vitrectomy certainly plays a role in the management of patients who have recurrent vitreous hemorrhages. Dehghan et al.[20] observed that in their study of 67 eyes, vitrectomy and laser photocoagulation resulted in improved visual acuity and regression of neovascularization. Most other observers will consider other therapies. Some have resorted to systemic immunosuppression, including methotrexate,[21] and have reported an improvement in visual acuity. Others have used intravitreal injections of steroid. Ishaq et al.[22] observed reduction of leakage, but their follow-up period was short, whereas Agrawal et al.[23] reported a reduction in inflammatory activity in the eyes in two cases, in one of which there was recurrence of disease (Fig. 28.3). Others have reported the use of anti-VEGF therapies. Akova et al.[24] reported regression and no recurrence of disease after 12 months in a patient whose disorder was not responsive to panretinal photocoagulation and who received 1.25 mg of bevacizumab intravitreally. Kumar and Sinha[25] reported a similar positive result in a patient they had treated. Evaluation of these therapies is made very difficult by the natural history of the disease, which may regress by itself. Moreover, it appears that although many approaches may be valuable, the difficulty lies in choosing the best one for a specific patient.

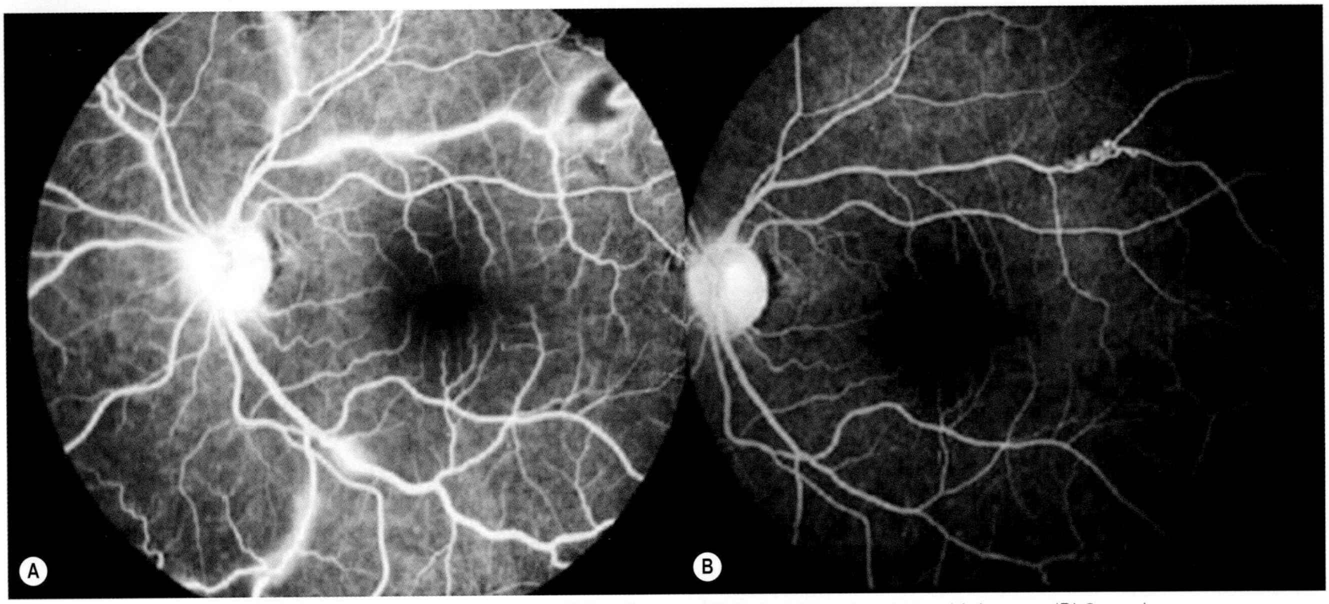

Fig. 28.3 Fundus photographs of eye with Eales disease. (A) Before intravitreal steroid therapy. (B) 8 weeks after the injection. (Reproduced with permission from Ishaq M, Feroze AH, Shahid M, et al. Intravitreal steroids may facilitate treatment of Eales' disease (idiopathic retinal vasculitis): an interventional case series. *Eye*. 2007;21(11):1403–1405.)

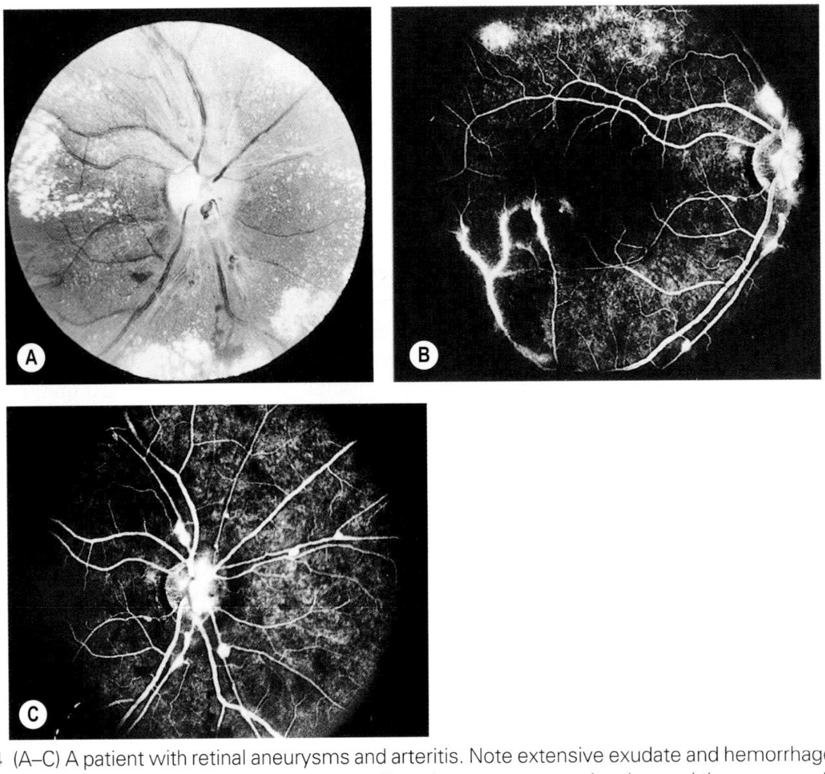

Fig. 28.4 (A–C) A patient with retinal aneurysms and arteritis. Note extensive exudate and hemorrhage, sheathing of vessels, and macroaneurysms. Extensive capillary dropout was seen just beyond these areas of exudate.

Idiopathic Retinal Vasculitis, Aneurysms, and Neuroretinitis (IRVAN Syndrome)

A rare condition with multiple saccular and fusiform aneurysms involving the larger arterioles, combined with peripheral vascular nonperfusion and uveitis, has been reported.[26,27] The degree of nonperfusion can be quite profound (Fig. 28.4). Neuroretinitis, retinal neovascularization, optic nerve head swelling, and anterior uveitis can all be associated with this disorder, which occurs in younger persons. The underlying nature of the disorder remains uncertain. It is interesting that the disease appears quite dynamic, with the aneurysms reported to regress and appear elsewhere sometimes quite rapidly.[28,29] It is not clear whether immunosuppressive agents are beneficial in treating this condition. Some suggest that it may be a matter of dosage. Ishikawa et al.[30] reported the case of a 15-year-old whose ocular disease did not respond to oral steroid, but did respond with 500

BOX 28.2 Ocular Findings in IRVAN

Stage	Findings
1	Macroaneurysms, exudation, neuroretinitis, retinal vasculitis
2	Capillary nonperfusion (angiographic evidence)
3	Posterior segment neovascularization of disc or elsewhere and/or vitreous hemorrhage
4	Anterior segment neovascularization (rubeosis iridis)
5	Neovascular glaucoma

From Samuel MA, Equi RA, Chang TS, et al. Idiopathic retinitis, vasculitis, aneurysms, and neuroretinitis (IRVAN): new observations and a proposed staging system. *Ophthalmology.* 2007;114(8):1526–1529.

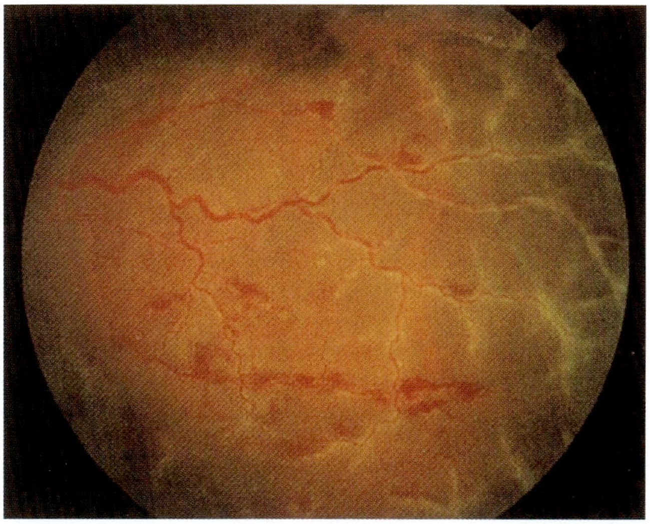

Fig. 28.5 Fundus of a young boy with idiopathic frosted branch angiitis. Yannuzzi has suggested that angiitis is seen in children, whereas periphlebitis generally is noted in young adults. (Courtesy L. A. Yannuzzi, MD.)

mg of intravenously administered prednisolone. This may indicate that the disease occurs at the level of the retinal vasculature rather than that of the immune system. In our experience, systemic immunosuppression with multiple agents can be useful in disease control, with mycophenolate and tumor necrosis factor (TNF) inhibitors being the most useful. Jampol et al.[31] reported a case of occlusive retinal arteriolitis with neovascularization. Although the disease course in the patient, who was a 34-year-old white woman, had some similarities to the entity just described, no aneurysms were noted. The disease has been seen in a pregnant woman in a hypercoagulable state,[32] and peripheral venule and arteriolar occlusions have been noted,[33] again suggesting the local, vascular element in the disorder. Laser photocoagulation has been shown to be beneficial in only a relatively small number of patients. Abu El-Asrar et al.[34] reported regression of IRVAN aneurysms in a patient with allergic fundal sinusitis, and Tomita et al.[35] reported that the regression remained long after photocoagulation of the nonperfused areas of the retina. Samuel et al.[36] reviewed 44 eyes with this condition and came up with a scoring system for the disease (Box 28.2). They conclude that retinal laser photocoagulation should be performed as early as possible if there are areas of widespread retinal nonperfusion.

Frosted Branch Angiitis

Frosted branch angiitis has been described by Walker et al.[37] as "florid translucent retinal perivascular sheathing." First reported in a 6-year-old boy, who had vessels resembling frosted branches,[38] this disease generally occurs in younger individuals. The disorder usually results in a severe drop in visual acuity, at least during the acute period. Although both

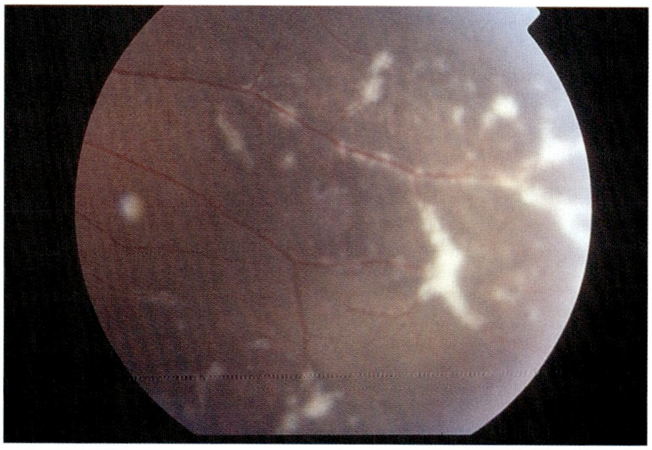

Fig. 28.6 Frosted branch angiitis in a pediatric human immunodeficiency virus (HIV)–positive patient.

arteries and veins may be involved, the venules tend to be more commonly affected (Fig. 28.5). About three-quarters of reported cases have been bilateral; the disease has no sex preference, and greater than 65% to 70% of patients have been reported to have retinal edema and intermediate uveitis. One case of macular choroidal neovascularization associated with the disorder has been reported.[39] Frosted branch angiitis is an ocular phenotype and not a specific disease entity and can have many causes, some of which are infectious. It has been reported to occur before and after the appearance of ocular toxoplasmosis[40,41] and after influenza A exposure,[42] but it can be idiopathic, with no obvious systemic cause.[43] One can speculate that it is an extreme example of diffuse perivasculitis. The "frosting" around the vessels could, in fact, be large numbers of inflammatory cells moving through the vascular wall into the retina. However, the appearance is distinctly different in that the vascular sheathing seen in sarcoidosis or the intermediate uveitis associated with multiple sclerosis seen in frosted branch angiitis is largely restricted to the posterior pole and the whitening extends far beyond the vessel walls.

The condition will disappear with proper and aggressive therapy, depending on the underlying disease pathology. Frosted branch angiitis has been associated with ocular cytomegalovirus (CMV) infection in patients with acquired immunodeficiency syndrome (AIDS). Resolution of symptoms in adults is seen with aggressive anti-CMV therapy. In one of our patients, an HIV-positive child, the angiitis persisted even after therapy with intravenous ganciclovir and foscarnet and resolution of antigenemia (Fig. 28.6).[44] This suggested that even in the context of HIV infection, CMV is not the sole cause of this ocular finding. Other infectious conditions in which this disease has developed include tuberculosis, syphilis, and herpes simplex virus type 2 (HSV-2) infection.[45] Others have found it to be associated with aseptic meningitis,[46] lymphoma, leukemia, sarcoidosis, multiple sclerosis, pars planitis, and SLE. Masuda et al.[47] reported a patient with frosted branch angiitis with yellow-white placoid lesions, and evaluation suggested occlusion of the choriocapillaris. Borkowski and Jampol[48] reported retinal and disk neovascularization in a patient with bilateral frosted branch angiitis who also had peripheral retinal ischemia. Retinal neovascularization was noted by Kleiner et al.[49] after multiple branch vein occlusions. Borkowski and Jampol's patient was treated with steroids and photocoagulation, with a good outcome. Responsiveness of this disorder to steroid therapy was also reported by Sykes and Horton[50] in a patient who also had Crohn disease.

Scleritis

Although scleritis certainly is not a disease of the retinal vasculature, it seems important to discuss it and how it may relate to intraocular inflammatory disease. Scleritis is more broadly discussed in Chapter 21. The vasculature near the scleritis appears to be integrally involved in the inflammatory/pathologic process, with medial necrosis, perivasculitis, or thrombosis often seen.[51,52] The inflammatory reaction associated with anterior scleritis can spill over into the eye, leading to anterior or even intermediate uveitis. Posterior scleritis is an entity that is frequently not included in the differential diagnosis of posterior pole lesions[53] (Fig. 28.7). This disorder may not be associated with anterior segment changes. Patients frequently report ocular pain, although the eye does not appear inflamed. At times, the conjunctiva may appear slightly boggy. There may be a mild vitreous inflammatory response associated with a decrease in visual acuity. Careful examination of the posterior segment may reveal choroidal folds or even thickening of the retina, although these processes are often subtle and difficult to determine. Ultrasound examination of the globe is very useful for diagnosis. In many patients, the disease responds to corticosteroid therapy, although relapse may occur once the dosage is reduced.

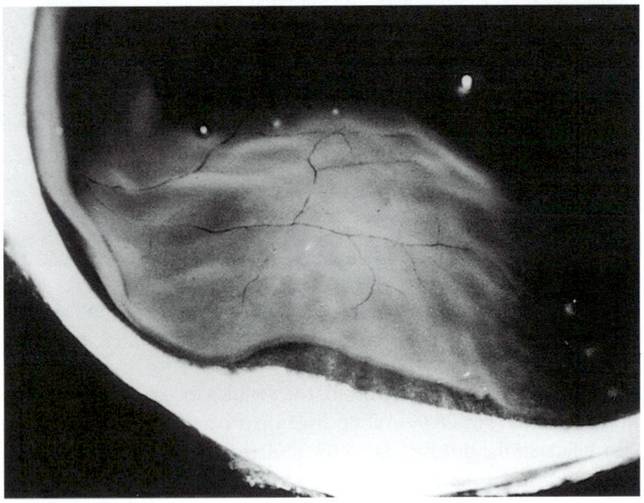

Fig. 28.7 Although not retinal vasculitis, posterior scleritis should be considered in patients with poor vision, pain, uveitis, and striae of choroid. (Courtesy David Cogan, MD.)

A note of caution is warranted. Although most cases of posterior scleritis are not associated with a systemic disorder, it is important to consider this possibility. The ophthalmologist always needs to be aware of the fact that this entity can manifest as a systemic disorder, and a careful rheumatologic evaluation seems warranted for most patients (see Chapter 21).

OCULAR VASCULITIS WITH SYSTEMIC DISEASE

Perhaps the most common systemic entities that we see with a marked vascular component are sarcoidosis (Fig. 28.8), Behçet disease, and multiple sclerosis. Although sarcoidosis is usually not thought of as the basis for retinal vasculitis, it can cause numerous ocular manifestations,

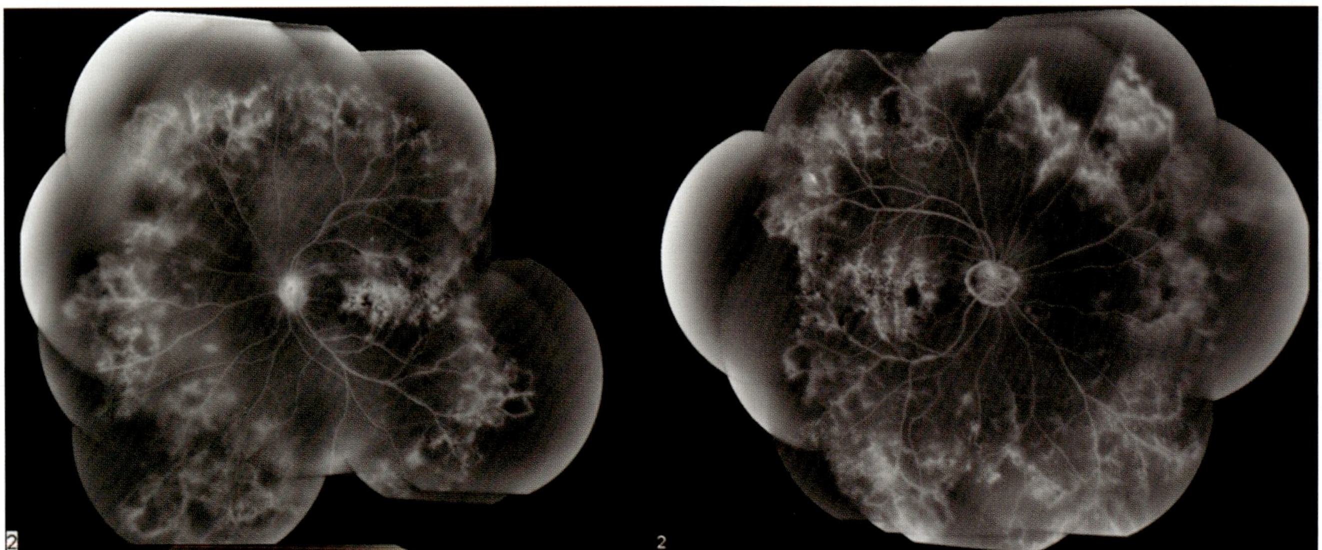

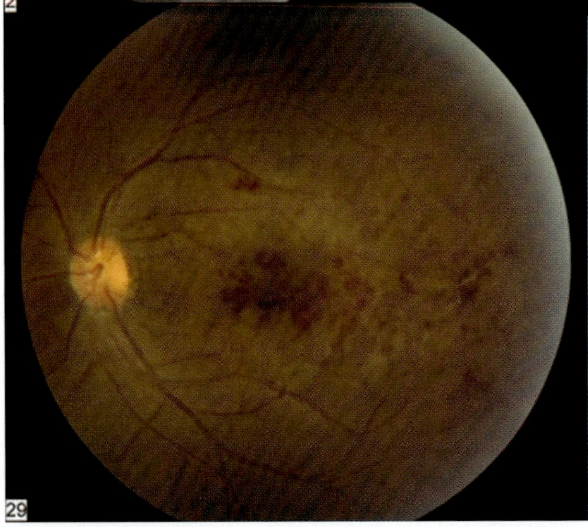

Fig. 28.8 A 50-year-old African American woman with sarcoidosis and marked pulmonary involvement presenting with a bilateral retinal vasculitis. The fundus picture of the left eye shows multiple retinal hemorrhages.

including severe involvement of the retinal vasculature (see Chapter 23). Multiple sclerosis was first associated with ocular inflammatory disease at the turn of the twentieth century. In an early article, Rucker[54] suggested that perhaps 20% of patients with multiple sclerosis may have retinal sheathing (i.e., vasculitis); others, such as Breger and Leopold,[55] reported this finding in an even higher percentage of patients (14 of 52 [27%]). In our experience, generally less than 5% to 8% of these patients seemed to have this complication.

Apart from the more common ocular entities, retinal vasculitis can be associated with several systemic entities, many of which are among the collagen-vascular group of disorders. A key point to consider in making these diagnoses is that usually the patient's complaints are associated with a subacute chronic disorder. The findings include malaise, weight loss, arthritis, fever, and rash. An important finding is mononeuritis multiplex. This is an acute neuropathy that begins at one named nerve root and then progresses to one or more other nerve roots, one at a time. It more commonly affects the nerve roots of the lower extremities and can have an abrupt, painful onset, with the patient reporting deep muscle pain. It is a common presenting sign in polyarteritis nodosa and occurs in a significant number of patients with SLE or rheumatoid arthritis later in the disease course. The ophthalmologist should be aware that other disorders, including diabetes, paraneoplastic syndromes, and even jellyfish stings, can cause mononeuritis multiplex.[56,57]

Some of the diseases that need to be considered in the search for a systemic cause for retinal vasculitis include those discussed in the sections below.

Systemic Lupus Erythematosus

SLE is a common systemic disorder that is diagnosed by use of a combination of clinical and laboratory criteria. A milder form of the ocular disease may have microangiopathy in which vaso-occlusion and vasculitis are less common. Retinal vasculitis can rarely be the presenting finding.[58] Histology has shown capillary lumen obliteration and deposition of immunoglobulin G (IgG) in these eyes.[59] Thought to be the classic immune complex disorder,[60] it affects the eye with severe intraocular complications in a relatively small number of patients. However, when it does, it can be extremely problematic because it is sometimes difficult to provide adequate therapy. Jabs et al.[61] reported on 11 patients with severe retinal vaso-occlusive disease and poor visual outcome often associated with CNS involvement in SLE (Figs. 28.9–28.11). Antiphospholipid antibodies are associated with vaso-occlusive ocular disease, leading, it is thought, to microthrombi.[62] Therefore anticoagulation must be considered in preventing further thrombosis. Proliferative retinopathy can be a serious problem as well.[63] It should be mentioned that antiphospholipid antibodies may cross-react with cardiolipin, which is used in some syphilis tests.[64] This condition raises an intellectually interesting, but also practically important, question: Should therapy consist of laser photocoagulation or systemic immunotherapy to stop the underlying inflammatory process that presumably induces the retinal vascular alterations? Although aggressive systemic immunosuppressive therapy is often needed, plasmapharesis[65] has been used acutely in conjunction with immunosuppression to reverse the ocular pathology.

Polyarteritis Nodosa

Polyarteritis nodosa was first described by Kussmaul and Maier in 1866. This necrotizing vasculitis involves the medium-sized muscular arteries and smaller arterioles. It can present as a bilateral iritis, vitritis, and retinal vasculitis involving both veins and arteries and can be very aggressive in nature,[66,67] with one reported case manifesting central retinal artery occlusion as well.[68] It has been estimated that up to 20% of these patients may have ocular involvement.[69] Mononeuritis multiplex, an acute neuropathy described earlier, has been estimated to develop in two-thirds of patients with polyarteritis nodosa. The most common sites are in the lower extremities. This is a potentially fatal disorder: 5-year survival is 13% with treatment versus 80% without treatment.[70] Current therapy usually consists of corticosteroids and cyclophosphamide.[24]

Wegener Granulomatosis

Wegener granulomatosis is characterized by necrotizing granulomatous vasculitis of the upper and lower respiratory tract, systemic small vessel vasculitis that can involve multiple organs, and focal necrotizing glomerulonephritis. Ocular complications, including uveitis, scleritis, and retinal vasculitis, can occur in 16% of patients.[71,72] One must remember that with the exception of mild anterior segment disease, eye diseases do not respond to topical medications and that systemic therapy usually indicated for the disease needs to be employed.[73] It is also important to remember that the antineutrophil cytoplasmic antibody (ANCA) test is highly specific for this disease. Soukasian et al.[74] reported that the ANCA test result was positive in seven patients with scleritis caused by Wegener granulomatosis but negative in 54 patients with ocular inflammatory disease caused by other conditions. Others have reported the usefulness of this test, not only for diagnosis but also for monitoring the course of the disease.[75,76] ANCAs are markers not only for Wegener granulomatosis but also for necrotizing vasculitis, Churg-Strauss syndrome, microscopic polyangiitis, and idiopathic crescentic glomerulonephritis. Indeed, Gallagher[77] reported observing microscopic polyangiitis in ANCA-positive patients with retinal vasculitis.

Two caveats should be kept in mind by the ophthalmologist. Two patterns of ANCA are reported: a cytoplasmic pattern (cANCA), which is believed to be more specific for Wegener granulomatosis, and a peripheral pattern (pANCA), which is less useful in making the diagnosis. Young,[78] in testing patients with uveitis, used the ANCA test and found positive results in those with chronic uveitis of various underlying causes. Because this test is interpreted manually and thus there can be great variation in the results, enzyme-linked immunosorbent assay (ELISA) directed toward proteinase 3 is now being used. The second caveat is that if a high suspicion remains in the physician's mind, it is useful to repeat the cANCA test because results may initially be negative in patients with Wegener granulomatosis localized to the orbit or the eye but will become positive with time.

Whipple Disease

Whipple disease, described by George Hoyt Whipple at the beginning of the twentieth century, is a multisystem disorder, usually manifesting as malabsorption, diarrhea, and polyarthritis.[79] The first report of a case with eye findings was ascribed to Jones and Paulley in 1949[80]; it has been estimated that less than 5% of patients will have uveitis. The disease is caused by the bacillus *Tropheryma whipplei,* which can be found in vitreous specimens by using electron microscopy and PCR, along with foamy macrophages.[81] In some patients, fluorescein angiography results show diffuse vasculitis with hemorrhages, exudates, retinal capillary occlusion, and choroidal folds.[82] Although gastrointestinal complaints are typically present, some authors have reported patients with minimal symptoms related to that organ system.[83] Bodaghi et al.[84] reported a similar constellation of problems caused by *Arthrobacter* infection. Lo Monaco et al.[85] highlighted neurologic signs found in one patient who had retinal vasculitis and was treated with high-dose steroid and cyclophosphamide. Chan et al.[86] emphasized the need for early diagnosis because early antibiotic therapy leads to a greater chance of resolution.

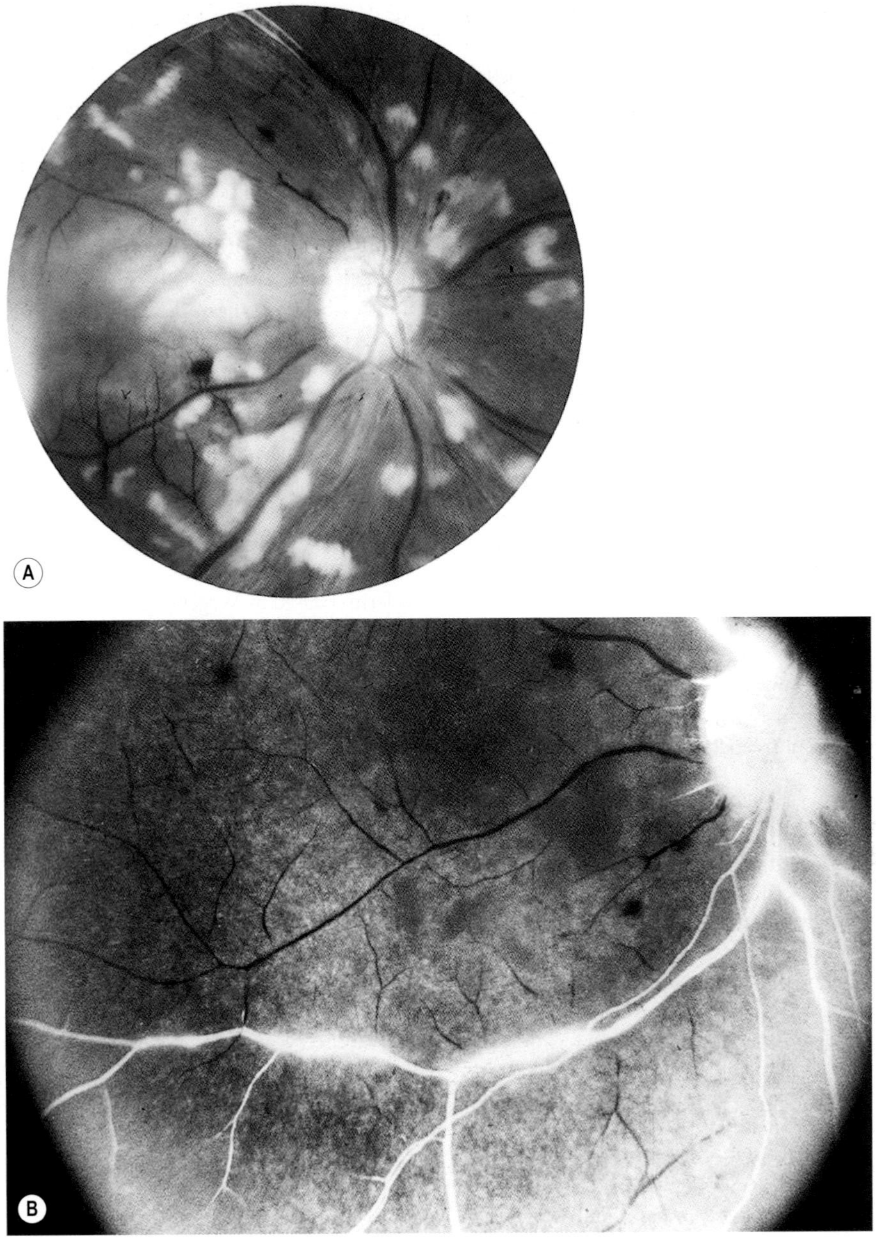

Fig. 28.9 Systemic lupus erythematosus. (A) Fundus shows multiple cotton-wool spots, arterial occlusion, vascular sheathing, and intraretinal hemorrhage. (B) Extensive nonperfusion, with staining of retinal vessels walls. (Courtesy D.A. Jabs, MD; from Jabs DA, Fine SL, Hochberg MC, et al. Severe retinal vaso-occlusive disease in systemic lupus erythematosus. *Arch Ophthalmol.* 1986;104:558–563. Copyright © 1986, American Medical Association. All rights reserved.)

Inflammatory Bowel Disease

Crohn disease commonly affects the eye in several ways, including uveitis (pars planitis), retinitis, scleritis, and keratitis. However, Duker et al.[87] reported the case of a patient with severe bilateral, obliterative retinal arteritis and phlebitis. There are case reports of both bilateral and unilateral retinal vasculitis occurring with Crohn disease.[88,89] The disorder appeared to respond to systemic corticosteroid and cyclophosphamide therapy. Ruby and Jampol[90] reported two cases of retinal vascular disease, with one patient having disease involving both retinal arteries and retinal veins, with apparent branch retinal artery occlusion. In one report, Felekis et al.[91] evaluated 60 patients with inflammatory bowel disease, and of these, 23 had Crohn disease. Only one case of retinal vasculitis was noted, and this was in a patient with ulcerative colitis.[91]

Autoantibodies to Sjögren Syndrome A Antigen

This SLE-like illness may be systemically mild, but retinal arteriolitis that leads to retinal ischemia, optic disk neovascularization, and retinal neovascularization may occur.[92]

Retinal Vein Occlusion

It is important to note that putative nonimmune mechanisms may lead to ophthalmoscopic findings that mimic an immune-driven

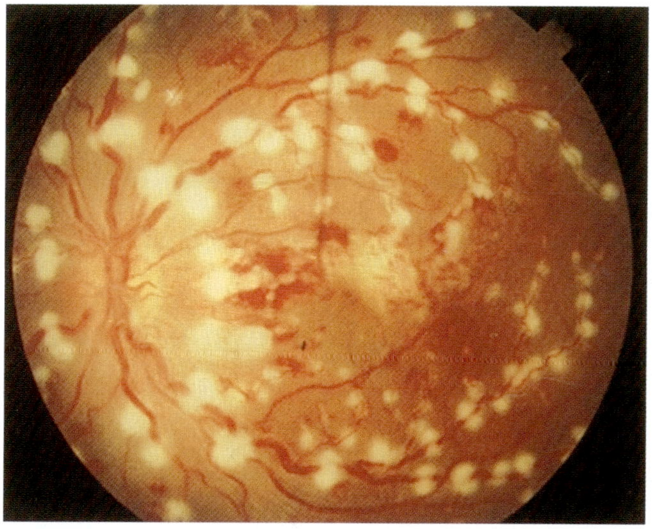

Fig. 28.10 Fundus of a young woman with difficult-to-control systemic lupus erythematosus. Extensive nerve fiber infarcts and hemorrhage create a dramatic picture, with maintenance of good visual acuity. Retinopathy resolved after disease was controlled.

pathologic condition,[93] such as retinal vein occlusion. After thrombosis, the vein occlusion can develop secondary perivasculitis.

Relapsing Polychondritis

Relapsing polychondritis is a systemic inflammatory disease of connective tissue that may have associated ocular manifestations. The diagnosis is characteristically made by observation of inflammation of the cartilage of the nose, earlobes, or trachea. Inflammation at two of these sites is sufficient for the diagnosis. Alternatively, inflammation of one such site combined with two of the associated signs is consistent with a diagnosis: hearing loss, vestibular imbalance, ocular inflammation, and rheumatoid factor–negative arthritis. In a review of 112 patients, Issak et al.[94] found ocular signs or symptoms in 21 of the patients at the time of diagnosis. Ocular involvement occurred in 57 of these patients at some time during the course of their disease. The most common ocular findings were episcleritis (39%) and scleritis (14%). Iridocyclitis has been observed in as many as 30% of patients with this disease[95] but was found in only 9% of patients in the series by Issak et al.[94] Retinopathy, primarily exudates, and hemorrhages were seen in 9% as well. Occasionally, retinal vascular occlusions, serous retinal detachments, and optic neuropathy develop. Systemic vasculitis was reported in 9% of patients,[94] demonstrating the systemic inflammatory nature

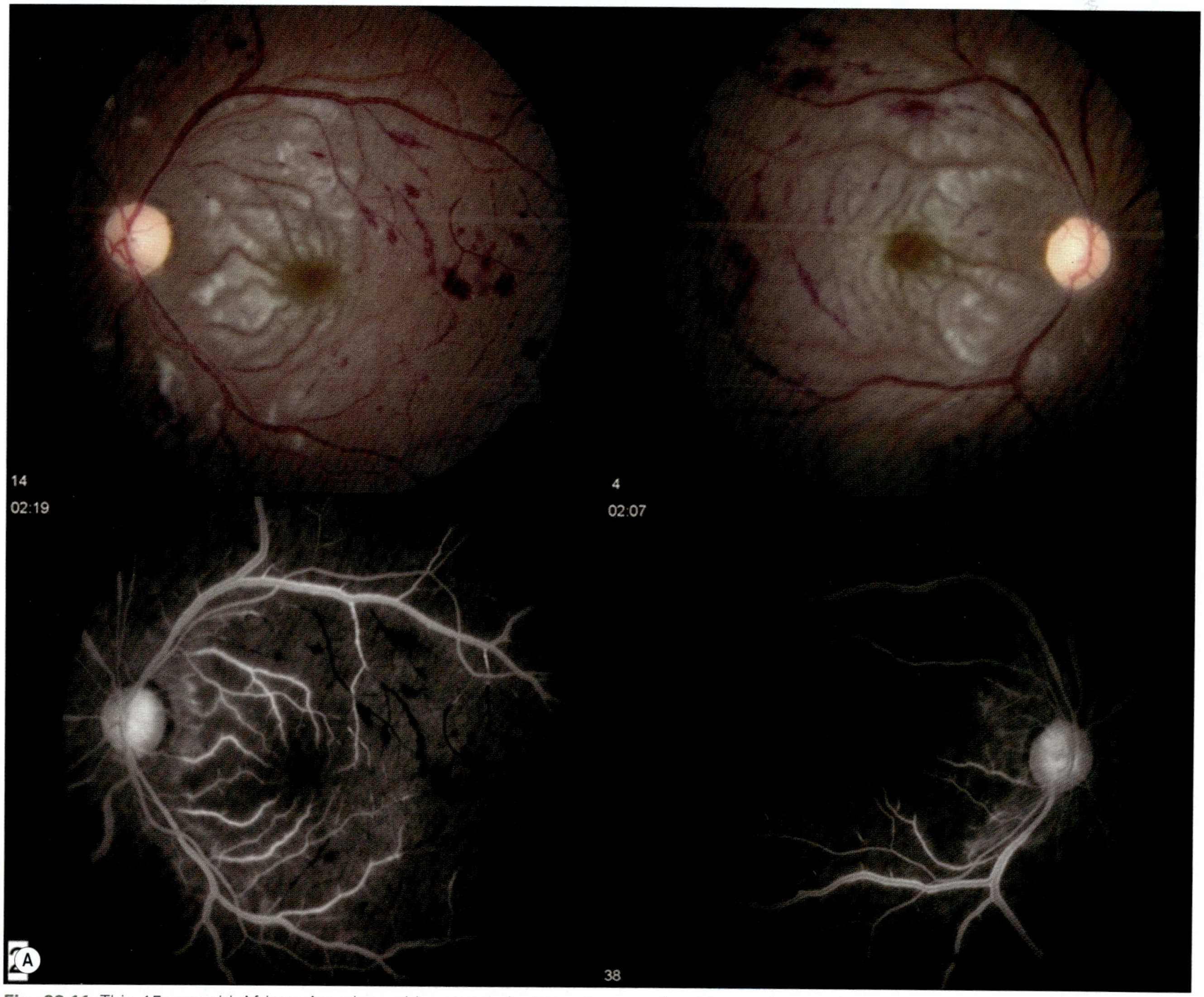

Fig. 28.11 This 15-year-old African American girl presented with a decrease in vision and systemic symptoms compatible with systemic lupus erythematosus (SLE). (A) The fundus as it appeared at the initial examination at the National Eye Institute (NEI). Note the retinal hemorrhages and remarkable degree of loss of vasculature seen on the angiogram.

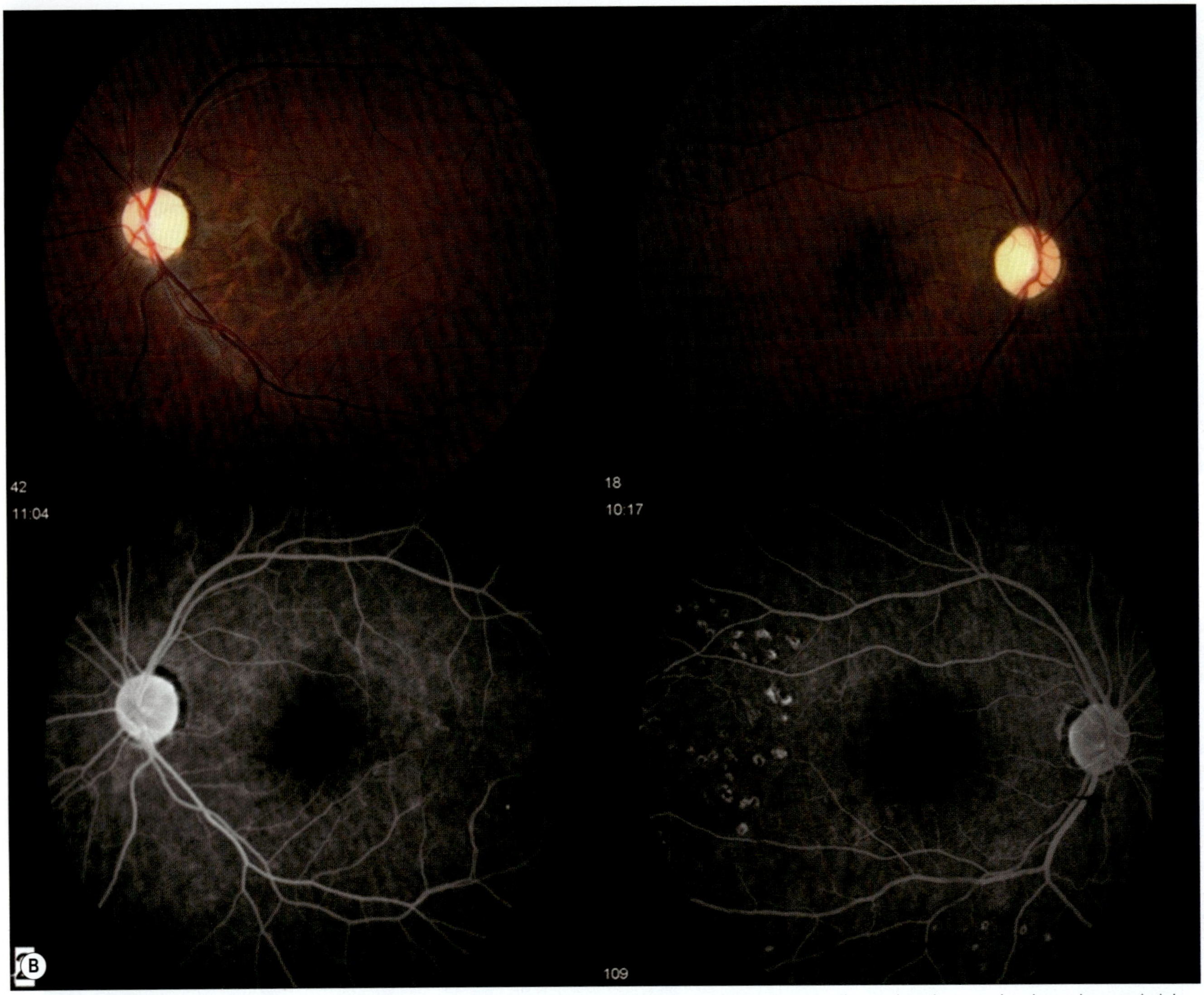

Fig. 28.11 cont'd (B) One year later, after systemic immunosuppressive therapy and laser therapy, the patient has retained good central vision, but the optic nerve changes continue to be disquieting.

of this syndrome. Vessels of any caliber may be involved. It is possible that although the episcleral/scleral involvement in this disease is immunologically similar to the mechanisms that lead to inflammation of the cartilage, other ocular manifestations are not tissue specific but are part of the varied accompanying systemic vascular involvement. For example, we reported a patient with polychondritis, with posterior scleritis being the important presenting sign.[96]

Viral Diseases

The exact role of viruses in the development of vasculitis of the retinal vasculature with no overt destruction of the retina itself remains to be defined. Some specific viral diseases that cause uveitis and vasculitis are discussed more extensively in other chapters. HIV/AIDS is discussed in Chapter 12, acute retinal necrosis (ARN) and progressive outer retinal necrosis (PORN) in Chapter 13, and other viral diseases in Chapter 14. It is clear that viruses can cause vascular endothelial cells to express receptors that might make them more susceptible to involvement in an immune event. Iwase et al.[97] reported on a 6-year-old child who first developed a dendritic corneal ulcer and iritis as a result of HSV-1 infection, followed by a drop in vision caused by retinal periphlebitis and a vitreal inflammatory reaction that responded to acyclovir therapy. Herpes zoster has been implicated in several cases. Retinal vasculitis has been reported in association with chickenpox.[98,99] Yet another patient had a unilateral retinal varicella zoster retinitis with no systemic symptomology, proven by PCR performed on the aqueous. The patient was treated with antiviral therapy.[100] Retinal vasculitis has been noted in a patient with chronic hepatitis C infection.[101]

Other viral entities that can present with a retinal vasculitis include Rift Valley fever, dengue, West Nile disease, and human T-cell lymphoma virus type 1 (HTLV-1) (Fig. 28.12). Dengue has been reported by observers in Southeast Asia. In a report from Singapore by Chan et al.,[102] 12 of 13 patients with dengue had central visual impairment, which seemed to coincide with the nadir of the patients' thrombocytopenia. All recovered vision to 20/30 or better. In a case report, a patient who suffered from a C4 deficiency that predisposes to autoimmune disorders presented with retinal vasculitis and macular detachment.[103] In addition, West Nile virus (WNV) infection can present with ischemic and hemorrhagic retinal vasculitis.[104,105] In a review of WNV cases in North America, Chan[106] described that of 14 eyes, 86% had multifocal chorioretinal changes, 43% had vitritis, and 29% had sheathing and vasculitis.

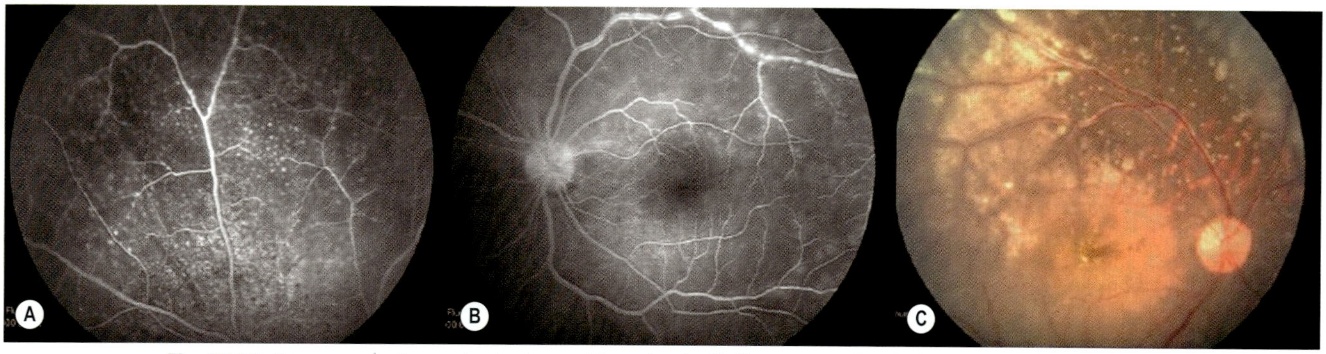

Fig. 28.12 A very rare instance of retinal vasculitis and retinal infiltrates associated with human T-cell lymphoma virus type 1 (HTLV-1) systemic disease. (A) Punctate hyperfluorescent subretinal infiltrates along with a retinal periphlebitis. (B) Subretinal infiltrates and superior temporal periphlebitis. (C) Fundus photograph showing subretinal infiltrates with periphlebitis and macular edema. (Reproduced with permission from Merle H, Donnio A, Gonin C, et al. Retinal vasculitis caused by adult T-cell leukemia/lymphoma. *Jpn J Ophthalmol*. 2005;49(1):41–45.)

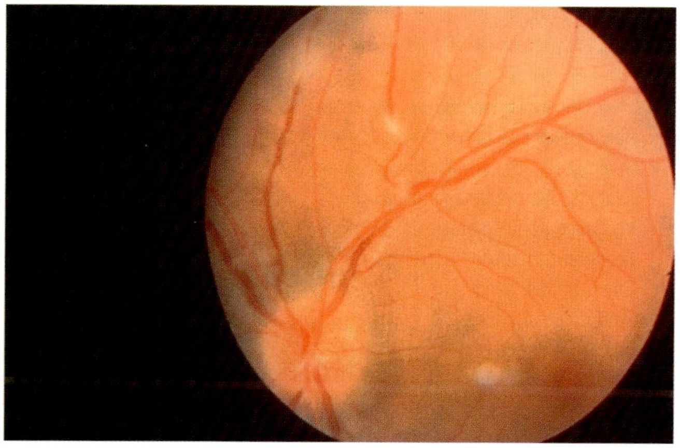

Fig. 28.13 Retinal vasculitis in a patient with tattoo-associated uveitis and sarcoidosis.

Multiple Sclerosis

It has been suggested that 9% to 23% of patients with multiple sclerosis will have peripheral uveitis and retinitis.[107] Although these numbers seem high, it is clear that it does happen. Friedman[108] reported a case of multiple scleritis in which retinal vasculitis was the initial finding.

Tuberculosis

Central retinal artery vasculitis leading to occlusion[109] (see Chapter 10) has been noted. In a study from India, 360 patients with uveitis with positive PPD results were found to have fewer recurrences (16% versus 47%) when their steroid treatment was combined with four-drug antituberculosis therapy.[110]

Rheumatoid Arthritis

In a report by Giordano et al.,[111] 11 (18.3%) of 60 patients with rheumatoid arthritis had fluorescein angiography evidence of retinal vasculitis. Matsuo et al.[112] reported the case of a 37-year-old woman who developed choroiditis and retinal vasculitis while receiving low-dose steroid therapy for her rheumatoid arthritis.

Kikuchi-Fujimoto Disease

This necrotizing lymphadenitis is usually self-limiting. Zou et al.[113] reported a case with bilateral occlusive retinal vasculitis with subsequent development of neovascularization. The patient was treated with methotrexate and prednisone.

Susac Syndrome

This syndrome is characterized by microangiopathy of the brain, retina, and cochlea. It mostly affects young women. In one reported case,[114] there were focal nonperfused retinal arterioles with staining of the vessel walls, but no intraocular inflammation was reported. The patient was treated with cyclophosphamide, and improved retinal perfusion was seen. The recurrent arterial occlusive disease accompanied by retinal vascular staining on fluorescein angiography can be indicative of CNS vasculitis as well. In general, Susac syndrome is best managed by using a combination of rituximab, mycophenolate, and (if needed) intravenous gamma globulin to prevent recurrent vascular occlusive episodes that lead to permanent CNS and retinal functional loss.[115]

Sweet Syndrome

Acute febrile neutrophilic dermatosis, or Sweet syndrome, is a skin disorder characterized by reddish papules and nodules, along with fever, circulating neutrophilia, and neutrophils infiltrating into the dermis.[116] Systemic corticosteroids are used to treat the disorder. Anterior segment problems, such as scleritis, glaucoma, and keratitis, have been reported, as has been choroiditis. It has been associated with Crohn disease and malignancies. It has been estimated that about a quarter of these patients will have ocular complications.[117] In addition, a bilateral retinal vasculitis has been described with this syndrome, which was treated with prednisone, colchicine, and diaphenylsulfone.[118]

Tattoo- and Drug-Induced Vasculitis

Moschos et al.[119] reported the case of a 21-year-old man who experienced retinal vasculitis and macular edema after receiving multiple tattoos. He was aggressively treated with immunosuppressive therapy. Another patient was reported to develop retinal vasculitis after trimethoprim sulfamethoxazole–induced urticaria.[120] The disease, however, manifested 2 years after the cutaneous problem began. It is possible to theorize that both tattooing and a severe enough cutaneous inflammatory reaction released skin antigens (perhaps melanin-like ones) that are shared with the eye. Most patients with tattoo-associated uveitis will either have, or go on to develop, systemic sarcoidosis (Fig. 28.13), and tattoo-associated uveitis may be related to sarcoid-like granuloma in reaction to the tattoo ink in patients who have sarcoidosis.

In summary, this group of disorders primarily affecting the retinal vasculature frequently presents great challenges to treating physicians. It is remarkable how many disorders can manifest as retinal vasculitis.[121,122] We are learning more about the underlying immune mechanisms of this group of diseases. Immune complexes have

BOX 28.3 Laboratory Tests

- Complete blood count (CBC), with differential
- Erythrocyte sedimentation rate (ESR)
- Cross-reactive protein (CRP)
- Serum chemistry panel, with tests for renal and liver functions
- Blood sugar
- Urinalysis
- Venereal Disease Research Laboratory (VDRL) test, fluorescent treponemal antibody absorption (FTA-ABS) test
- Tuberculin skin testing
- Toxoplasmosis serology
- Lyme disease serology
- Cat-scratch disease serology
- Human immunodeficiency virus (HIV), human T-cell lymphoma virus type 1 (HTLV-1), cytomegalovirus (CMV), herpes simplex virus (HSV), varicella zoster virus (VZV), hepatitis virus, and West Nile virus (WNV) serology
- Polymerase chain reaction (PCR) to identify pathogens in ocular specimens
- Serum angiotensin-converting enzyme (ACE)
- Rheumatoid factor (RF)
- Antinuclear antibody (ANA)
- Anti–deoxyribonucleic acid (DNA)
- Antineutrophil cytoplasmic antibody (ANCA)
- Antiphospholipid antibodies (lupus anticoagulants and anticardiolipin antibodies)
- Serum complement, CH50, AH50
- Extractable nuclear antigen
- Serum protein electrophoresis
- Serum cryoglobulins
- Human leukocyte antigen (HLA) testing
- Vitreous biopsy
- Cerebrospinal fluid cytology and cell count
- Imaging:
  - Fluorescein angiography
  - Optical coherence tomography (OCT)
  - Ultrasonography
  - Chest radiography
  - Computed tomography (CT)
  - Magnetic resonance imaging (MRI)
  - Gallium scanning
  - Sacroiliac radiography

From Abu El-Asrar AM, Herbort CP, Tabbara KF. Retinal vasculitis. *Ocul Immunol Inflamm.* 2005;13(6):415–433.

traditionally been hailed as the underlying cause, but we are now seeing alternative hypotheses. One example is the possible role of effector T cells and their ability to activate endothelial cells, leading to effector cell homing, whereas Müller cells may be attempting to modulate this response.[123] Wallace et al.[124] have reported a CX3CR1 genotype association (particularly the I249/M280 haplotype) in British patients with retinal vasculitis. These variants may be implicated in leukocyte migration and neuronal protection. We are beginning to learn more of the kinds of inflammatory cell products that are elevated in retinal vasculitis. Wallace et al.[124] reported that macrophage inflammatory protein (MIP)-1α and 1β were elevated in the sera of retinal vasculitis patients. Lee et al.[125] reported that interferon (IFN)-β was elevated in the sera of 47% of patients with retinal vasculitis and stayed elevated for 6 to 12 months; the level of E-selectin (an adhesion molecule) was also elevated.

The potential workup for these patients can be very long[126,127] (Boxes 28.3–28.5). For well-defined disorders, such as Behçet disease,

BOX 28.4 Disorders Associated with Retinal Vasculitis

Infectious Disorders

- Bacterial disorders (tuberculosis, syphilis, Lyme disease, Whipple disease, brucellosis, cat-scratch disease, endophthalmitis)
- Viral disorders (human T-cell lymphoma virus type 1, cytomegalovirus, herpes simplex virus, varicella zoster virus, Rift Valley fever virus, hepatitis, acquired immunodeficiency syndrome, West Nile virus infection)

Parasitic Disorders (Toxoplasmosis)

- Rickettsial disorders (Mediterranean spotted fever)

Neurologic Disorders

- Multiple sclerosis
- Microangiopathy of the brain, retina, and cochlea (Susac syndrome)

Malignancy

- Paraneoplastic syndromes
- Ocular lymphoma
- Acute leukemia

Systemic Inflammatory Disease

- Behçet disease
- Sarcoidosis
- Systemic lupus erythematosus
- Wegener granulomatosis
- Polyarteritis nodosa
- Churg-Strauss syndrome
- Relapsing polychondritis
- Sjögren A antigen
- Rheumatoid arthritis
- Human leukocyte antigen (HLA)-B27–associated uveitis
- Crohn disease
- Postvaccination inflammation
- Dermatomyositis
- Takayasu disease
- Buerger disease
- Polymyositis

Ocular Disorders

- Frosted branch angiitis
- Idiopathic retinal vasculitis, aneurysms, and neuroretinitis
- Acute multifocal hemorrhagic retinal vasculitis
- Idiopathic recurrent branch retinal arterial occlusion
- Pars planitis
- Birdshot retinochoroidopathy

aggressive therapy is imperative, with various options for immunosuppression available. Howe et al.[128] reported on the effectiveness of steroid therapy for retinal vasculitis. Of their patients, 29 were given 1 mg/kg or greater of prednisolone, and therapy was maintained at a dose of 40 mg or greater for at least 5 weeks. Of these 29 patients, 60% had an increase in visual acuity with therapy, and this number increased to 77% when other agents were added to the regimen in eight additional patients. Stanford and Verity[129] also reported that some patients with ischemic retinal vasculitis did not do well with steroid therapy.

However, some cases of retinal vascular disease may be quite severe but are neither associated with a systemic disorder nor well-characterized in the literature. Such an example is seen in Fig. 28.14, a patient with intermediate uveitis and severe retinal vascular disease. Not

BOX 28.5 Diagnostic Studies Performed on Patients with Retinal Vasculitis

Laboratory Tests

- Complete blood count (CBC) with differential
- Erythrocyte sedimentation rate (ESR)
- Cross-reactive protein (CRP)
- Serum chemistry panel, with tests for renal and liver functions
- Blood sugar
- Urinalysis
- Syphilis immunoglobulin G (IgG) enzyme-linked immunosorbent assay (ELISA), Venereal Disease Research Laboratory (VDRL) test, fluorescent treponemal antibody absorption (FTA-ABS) test
- Tuberculin skin testing
- Toxoplasmosis serology
- Lyme disease serology
- Cat-scratch disease serology
- Human immunodeficiency virus (HIV), human T-cell lymphoma virus type 1 (HTLV-1), cytomegalovirus (CMV), herpes simplex virus (HSV), varicella zoster virus (VZV), hepatitis virus, and West Nile virus (WNV) serology
- Polymerase chain reaction (PCR) to identify pathogens in ocular specimens
- Serum angiotensin-converting enzyme (ACE)
- Rheumatoid factor (RF)
- Antinuclear antibody (ANA)
- Anti–deoxyribonucleic acid (DNA)
- Antineutrophil cytoplasmic antibody (ANCA)/PR3/MPO
- Antiphospholipid antibodies (lupus anticoagulants and anticardiolipin antibodies)
- Serum complement, CH50, AH50
- Extractable nuclear antigen
- Serum protein electrophoresis
- Serum cryoglobulins
- Human leukocyte antigen (HLA) testing
- Vitreous biopsy
- Cerebrospinal fluid cytology and cell count

Imaging

- Fluorescein angiography
- Optical coherence tomography (OCT)
- Optical coherence tomography angiography (OCTA)
- Ultrasonography
- Chest radiography
- Computed tomography (CT)
- Magnetic resonance imaging (MRI)
- Gallium scanning
- Sacroiliac radiography

The diagnostic workup should be tailored according to the patient's medical history, review of systems, and physical examination.

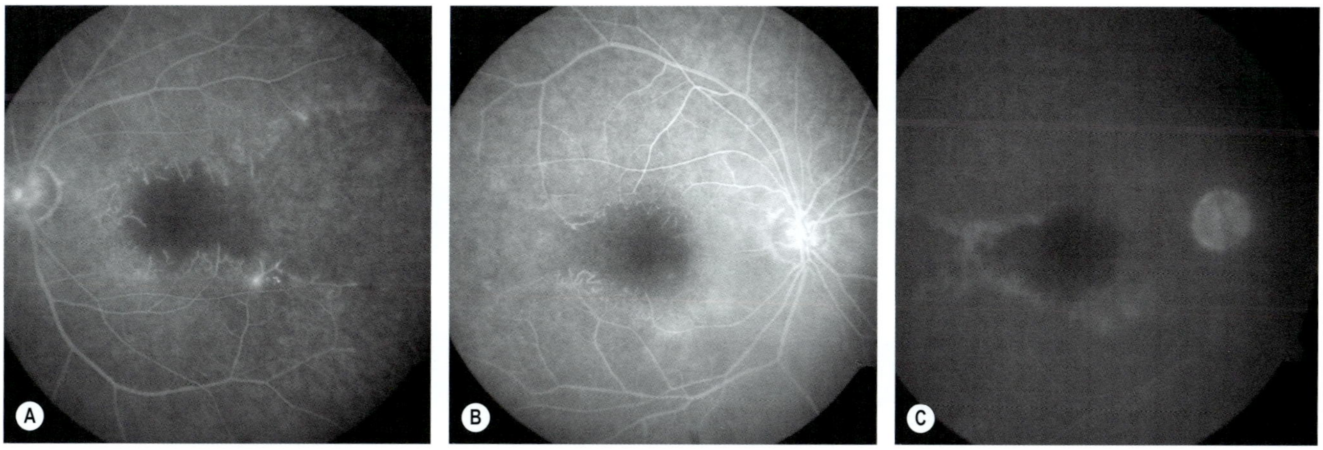

Fig. 28.14 (A and B) Fluorescein angiogram of the eyes of a middle-aged patient of Scandinavian background, who had moderate intermediate uveitis associated early on with macular edema. The fundus examination was not remarkable, and one needed to look carefully to perceive retinal vascular changes. However, the fluorescein angiogram shows striking symmetric loss of retinal vasculature, which extended into the periphery. (C) The edges of the areas of loss hyperfluoresced and then would appear to be pruned by the time the next angiography was performed. No systemic disease was ever found over the course of many years.

only is the natural history of severe retinal vascular disease unknown, but frequently, it is also not associated with impressive inflammatory disease (Figs. 28.15 and 28.16). The therapeutic approach in these cases is not dissimilar to that for other types of ocular inflammation, methotrexate or mycophenolate combined with anti-TNF therapy as the first choice, but is often compounded by the presence of neovascularization. Panretinal photocoagulation (PRP) may have a beneficial effect on the course of retinal vascular diseases, such as IRVAN syndrome or other diseases in which there is significant retinal nonperfusion. Indeed, this therapy seems to be the only modality that has been successful in some cases with severe occurrences of retinal vasculitis. The use of anti-VEGF therapies has opened up a new avenue for treatment of these patients. It should be added that we have seen severe inflammatory episodes apparently provoked by PRP. However, even with that risk, it may still be the indicated approach, if there is clear evidence of capillary dropout, as seen on angiography, but perhaps even if there is not.

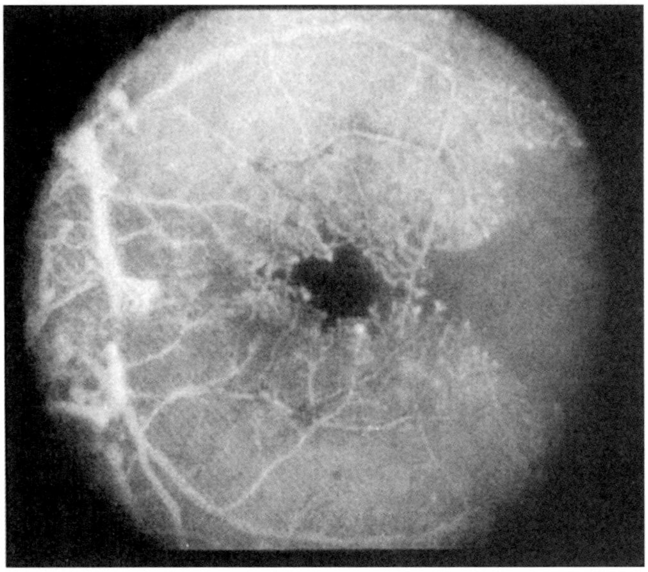

Fig. 28.15 Fluorescein angiogram of the left eye in a 16-year-old girl with decreased vision, who suffered from recurrent vitreous hemorrhages. Extensive workup failed to demonstrate any systemic disorder. High-dose oral prednisone was not successful in preventing progression of the disorder.

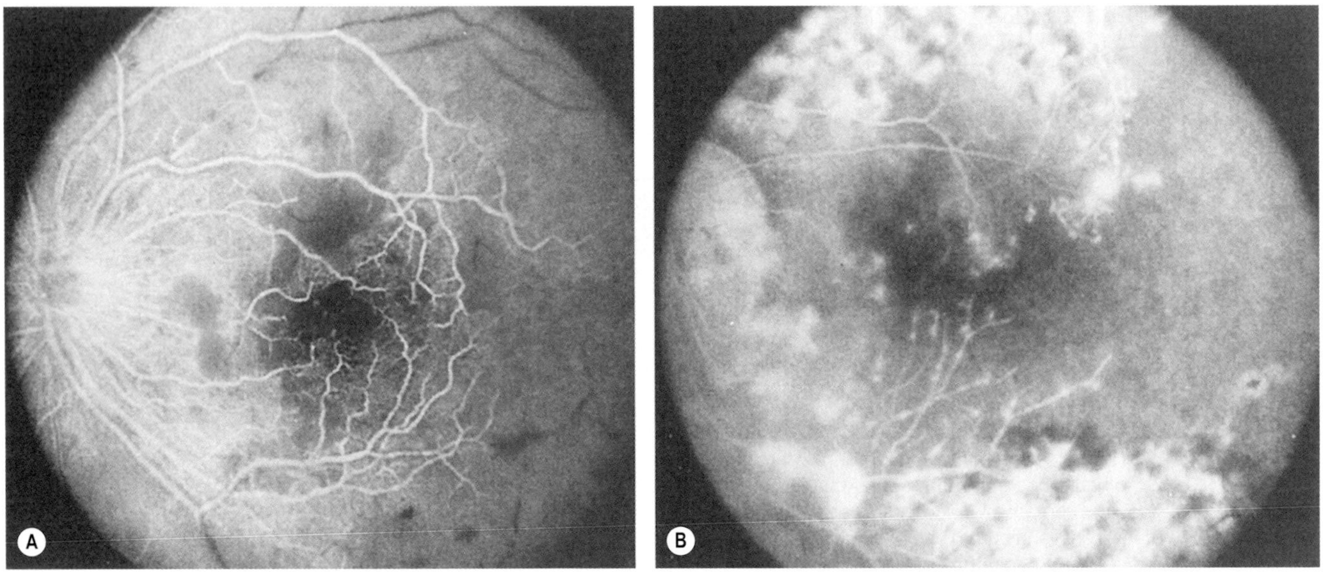

Fig. 28.16 (A) Fluorescein angiogram of a 46-year-old man who developed poor vision associated initially with a low-grade intraocular inflammatory response. Extensive systemic evaluation revealed no abnormalities. Note the extensive capillary loss involving a significant portion of the posterior pole and nonperfusion of larger vessels. Aggressive immunosuppression to the point of toxicity was initiated with no therapeutic effect. (B) Angiogram obtained 9 months later shows further loss of retinal vasculature. Areas of circular hyperfluorescence are from panretinal photocoagulation, which had been recently initiated, resulting in some stabilization of the disorder. However, with such extensive loss, long-term visual prospects are most guarded.

REFERENCES

1. Abu el-Asrar AM, Tabbara KF. Retinal vasculitis. *Curr Opin Ophthalmol.* 1997;8(3):68–79.
2. Merle H, Donnio A, Gonin C, et al. Retinal vasculitis caused by adult T-cell leukemia/lymphoma. *Jpn J Ophthalmol.* 2005;49(1):41–45.
3. Rosenbaum JT, Ku J, Ali A, Choi D, Suhler EB. Patients with retinal vasculitis rarely suffer from systemic vasculitis. *Semin Arthritis Rheum.* 2012;41(6):859–865.
4. George RK, Walton RC, Whitcup SM, et al. Primary retinal vasculitis. Systemic associations and diagnostic evaluation. *Ophthalmology.* 1996;103:384–389.
5. Lueck C, Pires M, McCartney AC, et al. Ocular and neurological Behçet's disease without orogenital ulceration? *J Neurol Neurosurg Psychiatry.* 1993;56:505–508.
6. Eales H. Cases of retinal hemorrhage associated with epistaxis and constipation. *Birmingham Med Rev.* 1880;9:262–273.
7. Franceschetti A. A curious affection of the fundus oculi: helicoid peripapillar chorioretinal degeneration. Its relation to pigmentary paravenous chorioretinal degeneration. *Doc Ophthalmol.* 1962;16:81–110.
8. Ashton N. Pathogenesis and aetiology of Eales's disease. In: *Proceedings of the 19th International Congress of Ophthalmology.* Bombay, India: Times of India Press; 1962.
9. Moura R, Orefice F. Retinal vasculitis. In: Orefice F, Belfort RJ, eds. *Uveitis.* São Paulo, Brazil: Roca; 1987:315–319.
10. Biswas J, Therese L, Madhavan HN. Use of polymerase chain reaction in detection of *Mycobacterium tuberculosis* complex DNA from vitreous sample of Eales' disease. *Br J Ophthalmol.* 1999;83:994–997.
11. Madhavan HN, Therese KL, Gunisha P, et al. Polymerase chain reaction for detection of *Mycobacterium tuberculosis* in epiretinal membrane in Eales' disease. *Invest Ophthalmol Vis Sci.* 2000;41:822–825.
12. Therese KL, Deepa P, Therese J, et al. Association of mycobacteria with Eales' disease. *Indian J Med Res.* 2007;126(1):56–62.
13. Das T, Biswas J, Kumar A, et al. Eales' disease. *Indian J Ophthalmol.* 1994;42:3–18.
14. Wise G, Dollery C, Henkind P. *The Retinal Circulation.* New York: Harper and Row; 1971.
15. Biswas J, Raghavendran R, Pinakin G, et al. Presumed Eales' disease with neurologic involvement. Report of three cases. *Retina.* 2001;21:141–145.
16. Elliot A. Recurrent intraocular hemorrhage in young adults (Eales' disease). *Trans Am Ophthalmol Soc.* 1954;52:811.
17. Murugeswari P, Shukla D, Rajendran A, et al. Proinflammatory cytokines and angiogenic and anti-angiogenic factors in vitreous of patients with proliferative diabetic retinopathy and Eales' disease. *Retina.* 2008;28(6):817–824.
18. Muthukkaruppan V, Rengarajan K, Chakkalath HR, et al. Immunological status of patients of Eales' disease. *Indian J Med Res.* 1989;90:351–359.
19. Rennie W, Murphy RP, Anderson KC, et al. The evaluation of patients with Eales' disease. *Retina.* 1983;3:243–247.
20. Dehghan MH, Ahmadieh H, Soheilian M, et al. Therapeutic effects of laser photocoagulation and/or vitrectomy in Eales' disease. *Eur J Ophthalmol.* 2005;15(3):379–383.
21. Bali T, Saxena S, Kumar D, et al. Response time and safety profile of pulsed oral methotrexate therapy in idiopathic retinal periphlebitis. *Eur J Ophthalmol.* 2005;15(3):374–378.
22. Ishaq M, Feroze AH, Shahid M, et al. Intravitreal steroids may facilitate treatment of Eales' disease (idiopathic retinal vasculitis): an interventional case series. *Eye.* 2007;21(11):1403–1405.
23. Agrawal S, Agrawal J, Agrawal TP. Intravitreal triamcinolone acetonide in Eales' disease. *Retina.* 2006;26(2):227–229.
24. Akova YA, Jabbur NS, Foster CS. Ocular presentation of polyarteritis nodosa. Clinical course and management with steroid and cytotoxic therapy. *Ophthalmology.* 1993;100(12):1775–1781.
25. Kumar A, Sinha S. Intravitreal bevacizumab (Avastin) treatment of diffuse diabetic macular edema in an Indian population. *Indian J Ophthalmol.* 2007;55(6):451–455.
26. Karel I, Peleska M, Divisova G. Fluorescence angiography in retinal vasculitis in children's uveitis. *Ophthalmologica.* 1973;166:251–264.
27. Kincaid J, Schatz H. Bilateral retinal arteritis with multiple aneurysmal dilations. *Retina.* 1983;3:171–178.
28. Yeshurun I, Recillas-Gispert C, Navarro-Lopez P, et al. Extensive dynamics in location, shape, and size of aneurysms in a patient with idiopathic retinal vasculitis, aneurysms, and neuroretinitis (IRVAN) syndrome. Idiopathic retinal vasculitis, aneurysms, and neuroretinitis. *Am J Ophthalmol.* 2003;135(1):118–120.
29. Sashihara H, Hayashi H, Oshima K. Regression of retinal arterial aneurysms in a case of idiopathic retinal vasculitis, aneurysms, and neuroretinitis (IRVAN). *Retina.* 1999;19(3):250–251.
30. Ishikawa F, Ohguro H, Sato S, et al. A case of idiopathic retinal vasculitis, aneurysm, and neuroretinitis effectively treated by steroid pulse therapy. *Jpn J Ophthalmol.* 2006;50(2):181–185.
31. Jampol L, Isenberg S, Goldberg M. Occlusive retinal arteriolitis with neovascularization. *Am J Ophthalmol.* 1978;81:583–589.
32. McDonald HR. Diagnostics and therapeutic challenges. IRVAN syndrome. *Retina.* 2003;23(3):392–399.
33. Venkatesh P, Verghese M, Davde M, et al. Primary vascular occlusion in IRVAN (idiopathic retinal vasculitis, aneurysms, neuroretinitis) syndrome. *Ocul Immunol Inflamm.* 2006;14(3):195–196.
34. Abu El-Asrar AM, Jestaneiah S, Al-Serhani AM. Regression of aneurysmal dilatations in a case of idiopathic retinal vasculitis, aneurysms and neuroretinitis (IRVAN) associated with allergic fungal sinusitis. *Eye.* 2004;18(2):197–199. Discussion 199–201.
35. Tomita M, Matsubara T, Yamada H, et al. Long term follow up in a case of successfully treated idiopathic retinal vasculitis, aneurysms, and neuroretinitis (IRVAN). *Br J Ophthalmol.* 2004;88(2):302–303.
36. Samuel MA, Equi RA, Chang TS, et al. Idiopathic retinitis, vasculitis, aneurysms, and neuroretinitis (IRVAN): new observations and a proposed staging system. *Ophthalmology.* 2007;114(8):1526–1529. e1.
37. Walker S, Iguchi A, Jones NP. Frosted branch angiitis: a review. *Eye.* 2004;18(5):527–533.
38. Ito Y, Nakano M, Kyu N, et al. Frosted branch angiitis in a child. *Jpn J Clin Ophthalmol.* 1976;30:797–803.
39. Liu Y, Ma Z, Tso MO, et al. Frosted branch angiitis secondary to macular choroidal neovascularization in a Chinese woman. *Jpn J Ophthalmol.* 2005;49(3):228–230.
40. Oh J, Huh K, Kim SW. Recurrent secondary frosted branch angiitis after toxoplasmosis vasculitis. *Acta Ophthalmol Scand.* 2005;83(1):115–117.
41. Díaz-Valle D, Díaz-Rodríguez E, Díaz-Valle T, et al. Frosted branch angiitis and late peripheral retinochoroidal scar in a patient with acquired toxoplasmosis. *Eur J Ophthalmol.* 2003;13(8):726–728.
42. Jo T, Mizota A, Hatano N, et al. Frosted branch angiitis-like fundus following presumed influenza virus type A infection. *Jpn J Ophthalmol.* 2006;50(6):563–564.
43. Taban M, Sears JE, Crouch E, et al. Acute idiopathic frosted branch angiitis. *J AAPOS.* 2007;11(3):286–287.
44. Fine HF, Smith JA, Murante BL, et al. Frosted branch angiitis in a child with HIV infection. *Am J Ophthalmol.* 2001;131:394–396.
45. Markomichelakis NN, Barampouti F, Zafirakis P, et al. Retinal vasculitis with a frosted branch angiitis-like response due to herpes simplex virus type 2. *Retina.* 1999;19(5):455–457.
46. Johkura K, Hara A, Hattori T, et al. Frosted branch angiitis associated with aseptic meningitis. *Eur J Neurol.* 2000;7:241.
47. Masuda K, Ueno M, Watanabe I. A case of frosted branch angiitis with yellowish-white placoid lesions: fluorescein and indocyanine green angiography findings. *Jpn J Ophthalmol.* 1998;42:484–489.
48. Borkowski LM, Jampol LM. Frosted branch angiitis complicated by retinal neovascularization. *Retina.* 1999;19(5):454–455.
49. Kleiner RC, Kaplan HJ, Shakin JL, et al. Acute frosted retinal periphlebitis. *Am J Ophthalmol.* 1988;106:27–33.
50. Sykes S, Horton JC. Steroid-responsive retinal vasculitis with a frosted branch appearance in Crohn's disease. *Retina.* 1997;17(5):451–454.
51. Watson P. The nature and treatment of scleral inflammation. *Trans Ophthalmol Soc UK.* 1982;102:257–281.
52. Watson P. Chapter 23: Diseases of the sclera and episclera. In: Duane T, Jaeger E, eds. *Clinical Ophthalmology.* Philadelphia: Harper and Row; 1987.

53. Benson W. Posterior scleritis. *Surv Ophthalmol.* 1988;32:297–316.
54. Rucker C. Sheathing of the retinal veins in multiple sclerosis. *JAMA.* 1945;127:970–973.
55. Breger B, Leopold I. The incidence of uveitis in multiple sclerosis. *Am J Ophthalmol.* 1966;62:540–545.
56. Hellman D, Laing TJ, Petri M, et al. Mononeuritis multiplex: the yield of evaluations for occult rheumatic diseases. *Medicine.* 1988;67:145–153.
57. Hellmann D. Mononeuritis multiplex. In: Klippel J, Dieppe P, eds. *Rheumatology.* London: Mosby-Yearbook-Europe Limited; 1991:6.26.2–6.26.5.
58. Bandyopadhyay SK, Moulick A, Dutta A. Retinal vasculitis – an initial presentation of systemic lupus erythematosus. *J Indian Med Assoc.* 2006;104(9):526–527.
59. Nag TC, Wadhwa S. Histopathological changes in the eyes in systemic lupus erythematosus: an electron microscope and immunohistochemical study. *Histol Histopathol.* 2005;20(2):373–382.
60. Nag TC, Wadhwa S. Vascular changes of the retina and choroid in systemic lupus erythematosus: pathology and pathogenesis. *Curr Neurovasc Res.* 2006;3(2):159–168.
61. Jabs D, Fine SL, Hochberg MC, et al. Severe retinal vaso-occlusive disease in systemic lupus erythematosus. *Arch Ophthalmol.* 1986;104:558–563.
62. Au A, O'Day J. Review of severe vaso-occlusive retinopathy in systemic lupus erythematosus and the antiphospholipid syndrome: associations, visual outcomes, complications and treatment. *Clin Exp Ophthalmol.* 2004;32(1):87–100.
63. Vine A, Barr C. Proliferative lupus retinopathy. *Arch Ophthalmol.* 1984;102:852–854.
64. Read RW. Clinical mini-review: systemic lupus erythematosus and the eye. *Ocul Immunol Inflamm.* 2004;12(2):87–99.
65. Papadaki TG, Zacharopoulos IP, Papaliodis G, et al. Plasmapheresis for lupus retinal vasculitis. *Arch Ophthalmol.* 2006;124(11):1654–1656.
66. Curi AL, Freeman G, Pavesio C. Aggressive retinal vasculitis in polyarteritis nodosa. *Eye.* 2001;15(Pt 2):229–231.
67. Morgan C, Foster C, Gragoudas E. Retinal vasculitis in polyarteritis nodosa. *Retina.* 1986;6:205–209.
68. Emad Y, Basaffar S, Ragab Y, et al. A case of polyarteritis nodosa complicated by left central retinal artery occlusion, ischemic optic neuropathy, and retinal vasculitis. *Clin Rheumatol.* 2007;2(5):814–816.
69. Stillermen M. Ocular manifestations of diffuse collagen disease. *Arch Ophthalmol.* 1951;45:239–250.
70. Leib ES, Restivo C, Paulus HE. Immunosuppressive and corticosteroid therapy of polyarteritis nodosa. *Am J Med.* 1979;67(6):941–947.
71. Fauci A, Haynes BF, Katz P, et al. Wegener's granulomatosis: Prospective clinical and therapeutic experience with 85 patients for 21 years. *Ann Intern Med.* 1983;98:76–85.
72. Mangouritsas G, Ulbig M. Cotton-wool spots as the initial ocular manifestation in Wegener's granulomatosis. *German J Ophthalmol.* 1994;3:68–70.
73. Pakrou N, Selva D, Leibovitch I. Wegener's granulomatosis: ophthalmic manifestations and management. *Semin Arthritis Rheum.* 2006;35(5):284–292.
74. Soukasian S, Foster CS, Niles JL, et al. Diagnostic value of anti-neutrophil cytoplasmic antibodies in scleritis associated with Wegener's granulomatosis. *Ophthalmology.* 1992;99:125–132.
75. Nolle B, Specks U, Ludemann J, et al. *Ann Intern Med.* 1989;111:28–40.
76. Cohen Tervaert J, van der Woude FJ, Fauci AS, et al. Association between active Wegener's granulomatosis and anticytoplasmic antibodies. *Arch Intern Med.* 1989;149:2461–2465.
77. Gallagher MJ, Ooi KG, Thomas M, et al. ANCA associated pauci-immune retinal vasculitis. *Br J Ophthalmol.* 2005;89(5):608–611.
78. Young D. The antineutrophil antibody in uveitis. *Br J Ophthalmol.* 1991;75:208–211.
79. Whipple GH. A hitherto undescribed disease characterized anatomically by deposits of fat and fatty acids in the intestinal and mesenteric lymphatic tissues. *Johns Hopkins Hosp Bull.* 1907;18:382–391.
80. Jones FA, Paulley JW. Intestinal lipodystrophy. *Lancet.* 1949;1:214–216.
81. Rickman LS, Freeman WR, Green WR, et al. Brief report: uveitis caused by *Tropheryma whipplei* (Whipple's bacillus). *N Engl J Med.* 1995;332:363–366.
82. Avila M, Jalkh AE, Feldman E, et al. Manifestations of Whipple's disease in the posterior segment of the eye. *Arch Ophthalmol.* 1984;102:384–390.
83. Nishimura JK, Cook BE, Pach JM. Whipple disease presenting as posterior uveitis without prominent gastrointestinal symptoms. *Am J Ophthalmol.* 1998;126:130–132.
84. Bodaghi B, Dauga C, Cassoux N, et al. Whipple's syndrome (uveitis, B27-negative spondyloarthropathy, meningitis, and lymphadenopathy) associated with *Arthrobacter* sp. infection. *Ophthalmology.* 1998;105:1891–1896.
85. Lo Monaco A, Govoni M, Zelante A, et al. Whipple disease: unusual presentation of a protean and sometimes confusing disease. *Semin Arthritis Rheum.* 2008;38:403–406.
86. Chan RY, Yannuzzi LA, Foster CS. Ocular Whipple's disease. *Ophthalmology.* 2001;108:2225–2231.
87. Duker J, Brown G, Brooks L. Retinal vasculitis in Crohn's disease. *Am J Ophthalmol.* 1987;103:664–668.
88. Garcia-Diaz M, Mira M, Nevado L, et al. Retinal vasculitis associated with Crohn's disease. *Postgrad Med J.* 1995;71(833):170–172.
89. Saatci OA, Koçak N, Durak I, et al. Unilateral retinal vasculitis, branch retinal artery occlusion and subsequent retinal neovascularization in Crohn's disease. *Int Ophthalmol.* 2001;24(2):89–92.
90. Ruby A, Jampol L. Crohn's disease and retinal vascular disease. *Am J Ophthalmol.* 1990;110:349–353.
91. Felekis T, Katsanos K, Kitsanou M, et al. Spectrum and frequency of ophthalmologic manifestations in patients with inflammatory bowel disease: a prospective single-center study. *Inflamm Bowel Dis.* 2009;15(1):29–34.
92. Farmer S, Kinyoun JL, Nelson JL, et al. Retinal vasculitis associated with autoantibodies to Sjögren's syndrome A antigen. *Am J Ophthalmol.* 1985;100:814–821.
93. Green W, Chan CC, Hutchins GM, et al. Central retinal vein occlusion: a prospective histopathologic study of 29 eyes in 28 cases. *Trans Am Soc Ophthalmol.* 1981;79:371–422.
94. Issak B, Liesegang T, Michet C. Ocular and systemic findings in relapsing polychondritis. *Ophthalmology.* 1986;93:681–689.
95. Matas B. Iridocyclitis associated with relapsing polychondritis. *Arch Ophthalmol.* 1970;84:474–476.
96. Rodríguez-Colón G, Palestine AG. Polychondritis with auricular and ocular involvement. *N Engl J Med.* 2015;373(26):2562.
97. Iwase K, Murao M, et al. A case of dendritic corneal ulcer associated with retinal periphlebitis and uveitis. A new diagnostic method and treatment. *Rinsho Ganka.* 1986;40:403–407.
98. Kuo Y-H, Yip Y, Chen S-N. Retinal vasculitis associated with chickenpox. *Am J Ophthalmol.* 2001;132:584–585.
99. Wolf AH, Thurau SR, Kook D, et al. Ocular manifestation of primary VZV infection in a splenectomized patient. *Ocul Immunol Inflamm.* 2008;16(4):199–201.
100. Wimmersberger Y, Gervaix A, Baglivo E. VZV retinal vasculitis without systemic infection: diagnosis and monitoring with quantitative polymerase chain reaction. *Int Ophthalmol.* 2010;30(1):73–75.
101. Perez-Alvarez AF, Jiménez-Alonso J, Reche-Molina I, et al. Retinal vasculitis and vitritis in a patient with chronic hepatitis C virus. *Arch Intern Med.* 2001;161(18):2262.
102. Chan DP, Teoh SC, Tan CS, et al. Ophthalmic complications of dengue. *Emerg Infect Dis.* 2006;12(2):285–289.
103. Chang PE, Cheng CL, Asok K, et al. Visual disturbances in dengue fever: an answer at last? *Singapore Med J.* 2007;48(3):e71–e73.
104. Garg S, Jampol LM, Wilson JF, et al. Ischemic and hemorrhagic retinal vasculitis associated with West Nile virus infection. *Retina.* 2006;26(3):365–367.
105. Garg S, Jampol LM. Systemic and intraocular manifestations of West Nile virus infection. *Surv Ophthalmol.* 2005;50(1):3–13.
106. Chan CK, Limstrom SA, Tarasewicz DG, et al. Ocular features of West Nile virus infection in North America: a study of 14 eyes. *Ophthalmology.* 2006;113(9):1539–1546.
107. Engell T, Anderson PK. The frequency of periphlebitis in multiple sclerosis. *Acta Neurol Scand.* 1982;65:601–608.

108. Friedman SM. Retinal vasculitis as the initial presentation of multiple sclerosis. *Retina*. 2005;25(2):218–219.
109. Fountain J, Werner R. Tuberculous retinal vasculitis. *Retina*. 1984;4:48–50.
110. Bansal R, Gupta A, Gupta V, et al. Role of anti-tubercular therapy in uveitis with latent/manifest tuberculosis. *Am J Ophthalmol*. 2008;146:772–792.
111. Giordano N, D'Ettorre M, Biasi G, et al. Retinal vasculitis in rheumatoid arthritis: an angiographic study. *Clin Exp Rheumatol*. 1990;8:121–125.
112. Matsuo T, Masuda I, Matsuo N. Geographic choroiditis and retinal vasculitis in rheumatoid arthritis. *Jpn J Ophthalmol*. 1998;42(1):51–55.
113. Zou W, Wen F. Bilateral occlusive retinal vasculitis in Kikuchi-Fujimoto disease. *Clin Exp Ophthalmol*. 2007;35(9):875–877.
114. Martinet N, Fardeau C, Adam R, et al. Fluorescein and indocyanine green angiographies in Susac syndrome. *Retina*. 2007;27(9):1238–1242.
115. Rennebohm RM, Asdaghi N, Srivastava S, Gertner E. Guidelines for treatment of Susac syndrome – an update. *Int J Stroke*. 2020;15(5):484–494.
116. Gottlieb CC, Mishra A, Belliveau D, et al. Ocular involvement in acute febrile neutrophilic dermatosis (Sweet syndrome): new cases and review of the literature. *Surv Ophthalmol*. 2008;53(3):219–226.
117. Fett DL, Gibson LE, Su WP. Sweet's syndrome: systemic signs and symptoms and associated disorders. *Mayo Clin Proc*. 1995;70(3):234–240.
118. Sato M, Kawamura T, Hase S, et al. A case of bilateral retinal vasculitis associated with Sweet syndrome. *Retina*. 2005;25(6):800–802.
119. Moschos MM, Guex-Crosier Y. Retinal vasculitis and cystoid macular edema after body tattooing: a case report. *Klin Monatsbl Augenheilkd*. 2004;221(5):424–426.
120. Batioglu F, Taner P, Aydintuğ OT, et al. Recurrent optic disc and retinal vasculitis in a patient with drug-induced urticarial vasculitis. *Cutan Ocul Toxicol*. 2006;25(4):281–285.
121. Abu El-Asrar AM, Herbort CP, Tabbara KF. Retinal vasculitis. *Ocul Immunol Inflamm*. 2005;13(6):415–433.
122. Herbort CP, Cimino L, Abu El Asrar AM. Ocular vasculitis: a multidisciplinary approach. *Curr Opin Rheumatol*. 2005;17(1):25–33.
123. Hughes EH, Dick AD. The pathology and pathogenesis of retinal vasculitis. *Neuropathol Appl Neurobiol*. 2003;29(4):325–340.
124. Wallace GR, Vaughan RW, Kondeatis E, et al. A CX3CR1 genotype associated with retinal vasculitis in patients in the United Kingdom. *Invest Ophthalmol Vis Sci*. 2006;47(7):2966–2970.
125. Lee MT, Hooper LC, Kump L, et al. Interferon-beta and adhesion molecules (E-selectin and s-intracellular adhesion molecule-1) are detected in sera from patients with retinal vasculitis and are induced in retinal vascular endothelial cells by Toll-like receptor 3 signalling. *Clin Exp Immunol*. 2007;147(1):71–80.
126. Levy-Clarke GA, Nussenblatt R. Retinal vasculitis. *Int Ophthalmol Clin*. 2005;45(2):99–113.
127. Walton RC, Ashmore ED. Retinal vasculitis. *Curr Opin Ophthalmol*. 2003;14(6):413–419.
128. Howe LJ, Stanford MR, Edelsten C, et al. The efficacy of systemic corticosteroids in sight-threatening retinal vasculitis. *Eye*. 1994;8(Pt 4):443–447.
129. Stanford MR, Verity DH. Diagnostic and therapeutic approach to patients with retinal vasculitis. *Int Ophthalmol Clin*. 2000;40(2):69–83.

29

Serpiginous Choroiditis

Scott M. Whitcup

KEY CONCEPTS

- Serpiginous choroiditis is a rare, clinically defined disorder characterized by a geographic pattern of choroiditis that typically extends from the juxtapapillary area and spreads centrifugally over time.
- The disease often involves both eyes and can cause irreversible retinal damage and permanent vision loss.
- No specific etiology can be identified in most cases, and the disease is thought to be autoimmune. As a result, the disorder often responds to treatment with immunosuppressive therapy.
- Infections, such as tuberculosis, herpes virus infection, and syphilis, should be ruled out because they can look like serpiginous choroiditis and require specific anti-infective therapy.

Serpiginous choroiditis (SC) is a clinically defined disorder characterized by destruction of the inner choroid and the retinal pigment epithelium (RPE) with secondary involvement of the overlying retina. The disease tends to involve the peripapillary choroid and then spreads centrifugally, with periods of disease quiescence and reactivation. In addition to being called *serpiginous choroiditis,* this disorder has been known by a multitude of other names, including *serpiginous choroidopathy, geographic choroiditis, geographic choroidopathy, geographic helicoid peripapillary choroidopathy, macular geographic helicoid choroidopathy,* and *multifocal serpiginoid choroiditis.*[1-6] Although it had been recognized as a distinct, but poorly defined, entity by the early part of the twentieth century,[7] our understanding of this disease remains limited. We cannot identify a specific cause in most patients with SC, although most cases are thought to be autoimmune in nature and respond to immunosuppressive therapy. Furthermore, SC overlaps with other forms of white-dot syndromes, including acute posterior multifocal placoid pigment epitheliopathy (APPMPE).

EPIDEMIOLOGY

As expected, the prevalence of SC in ophthalmology clinics varies, depending on the study. Because the disease can lead to severe and permanent vision loss, it is fortunate that the disorder is relatively rare. In a study of general ophthalmology practices in southern California, no cases of SC were reported out of 213 patients seen.[8] In an academic uveitis clinic, 14 cases of SC among 1417 cases of endogenous uveitis were reported.[9] In most case series, SC has accounted for well under 5% of cases of posterior uveitis.[10] Although the disease has been reported in patients of varying ethnic backgrounds, it may be seen more commonly in white persons. In some series, a slight male preponderance has been seen.[11]

CLINICAL FEATURES

SC was first described by Jonathan Hutchinson in 1900 as a distinctive pattern of choroidal inflammation with an intermittent progression and an appearance of the borders of a continent on a map.[12] The typical patient with serpiginous choroiditis is middle-aged and has no major underlying medical problems.

Patients usually report blurred vision or a central or pericentral scotoma in one eye, although examination usually reveals bilateral disease. SC primarily affects the choroid, choriocapillaris, and the RPE. The terms *serpiginous, helicoid,* and *geographic* describe the appearance of the chorioretinal disease, which progresses in a serpentine fashion, usually starting at the optic disk and winding through the posterior pole (Fig. 29.1). Acute lesions are gray-white or yellow in color and involve the choriocapillaris and the RPE. On careful examination, these new lesions appear to have "substance," and they subtly elevate the overlying retina. Acute lesions last up to several months, but over time, they become atrophic, with disappearance of the choriocapillaris and involvement of the larger underlying large choroidal vessels.[13] Thinning of the overlying neurosensory retina usually occurs after disease of the choroid and the RPE, and scarring with clumps of the RPE are common late in the course of the disease.

It is important to identify active lesions, especially if they threaten vision critical areas, such as the macula and the optic disk, because they warrant immediate and more aggressive therapy. Patients rarely have a solitary active lesion separate from other lesions. More typically, active lesions occur adjacent to an area of choroidal and RPE atrophy. An area of chorioretinal atrophy often can be found next to the optic disk in a symptom-free contralateral eye.

Prominent vitritis or anterior chamber inflammation are rare in SC. Hamilton and Bird[14] observed no inflammatory disease in the patients they studied. In our experience, however, a mild cellular reaction in the posterior vitreous can occur, especially in patients with acute lesions. In fact, mild vitritis has been reported in about one-third of patients.[15,16] Anterior uveitis has also been described in patients with SC but is rarer.[17]

Choroidal neovascularization (CNV) can also occur in SC. Gass[15] stated that CNV occurs in as many as 25% of patients, although we have observed it in fewer than 10% of our patients at the National Eye Institute (NEI). Blumenkranz et al.[11] reported active CNV in seven of 53 patients with the disease. CNV may be seen at the time the disease is diagnosed and, when located in the macula, may cause visual

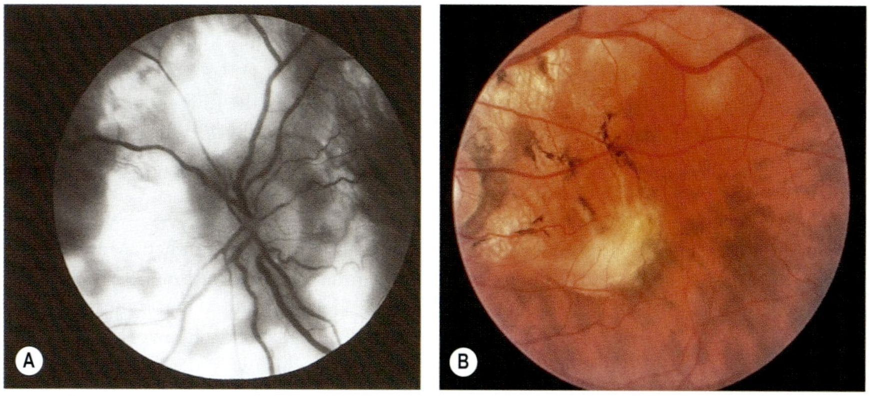

Fig. 29.1 (A) A large serpiginous lesion surrounding the optic disk. An active area is seen interior to the disk. Older atrophic regions can be seen both to right and left of the active lesion. Some choroidal vessels can be noted through the lesion. (B) A white active lesion is seen at the edge of an old atrophic area.

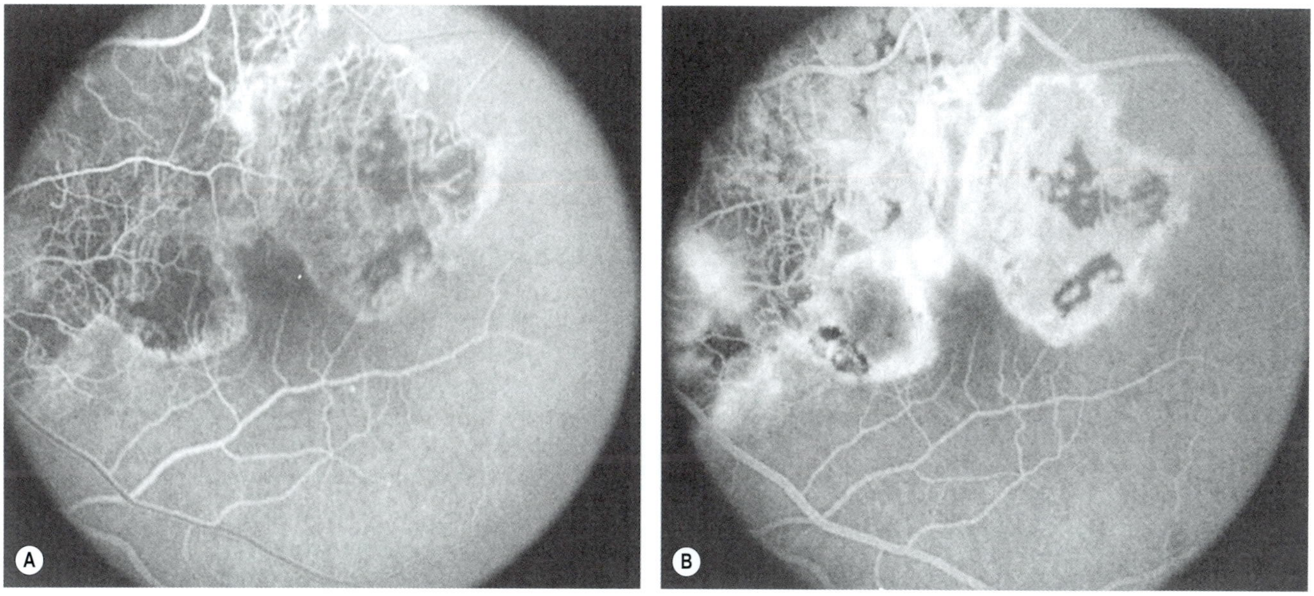

Fig. 29.2 Fluorescein angiograms showing a choroidal neovascular membrane in a patient with serpiginous choroiditis. (A) Early frame shows lacy hyperfluorescence. (B) Late frame shows late leakage in the area of the choroidal neovascular membrane.

disturbance (Fig. 29.2). Although the CNV may regress spontaneously in some patients,[18] neovascular membranes threatening the fovea probably warrant therapy. Serous detachments of the neurosensory retina and the RPE detachments have been reported in patients with SC.[17,19] Retinal vasculitis may also occur, and branch vein occlusions have been reported.[15,17]

As noted previously, SC usually begins near the disk, with new areas of activity occurring at the margin of older lesions. This centripetal or helicoid extension can continue for years. Laatikainen and Erkkilä[20] followed up 15 patients for a mean of 4.9 years and noted new lesions in eight. These acute lesions can cause a decrease in visual acuity that may return after a long recovery period. Weiss et al.[16] observed that visual acuity decreased in nine of 17 eyes after an acute inflammatory episode and that visual acuity returned to the preattack level once the inflammatory lesions resolved. They further noted that 15 of 17 eyes ultimately developed lesions involving the fovea, although this varies by report, and Laatikainen and Erkkilä[20] noted loss of central vision in only six of 28 eyes.

The diagnosis of SC is made primarily on the basis of clinical appearance; the common diagnostic features are listed in Box 29.1. Fluorescein angiography and serial fundus photography are also

BOX 29.1 Diagnostic Features of Serpiginous Choroiditis

Patient Demographics

White race

Both sexes, with slight male preponderance

Late teens to 60s

Ocular Findings

Mild anterior uveitis and vitritis

Gray-white geographic lesions that begin in the peripapillary region and progress in a centripetal or helicoid pattern

Active lesions

Bilateral asymmetric involvement

Diagnostic Tests

Early hypofluorescence of active lesions on fluorescein angiography, with hyperfluorescence in areas of chorioretinal atrophy

Absence of choriocapillaris on optical coherence tomography (OCT) angiography

OCT showing chorioretinal atrophy

helpful in monitoring the disease. Fluorescein angiography of an active lesion will show early blockage with late hyperfluorescent borders that spread toward the center of the lesion (Fig. 29.3). The early hypofluorescence of active lesions may be caused by blockage of the underlying choroidal fluorescence by swollen RPE cells but more likely represents the impaired choroidal vasculature. Old atrophic lesions demonstrate diffuse staining, and hyperfluorescence is noted in areas of RPE clumping. Late staining of the retinal vessels occurs in patients with vasculitis or perivasculitis. Indocyanine green (ICG) angiography may demonstrate additional lesions that are not seen on fluorescein angiography and may help better delineate the extent of the disease.[21-25] Fundus autofluorescence and optical coherence tomography (OCT)[26] can be useful in assessing SC. In one study reported by Cardillo-Piccolino et al.,[27] autofluorescence, OCT, and ICG angiography were used to monitor the disease course in two patients with SC. Interestingly, these authors found that fundus hyperautofluorescence was noted 2 to 5 days after the appearance of an active clinical lesion, defining an area of RPE damage. As the lesions became quiescent clinically, the previously hyperautofluorescent areas became hypoautofluorescence. OCT of active SC lesions can demonstrate photoreceptor layer disruption and hyperreflectivity of the choriocapillaris and outer retina.[28] Yeh et al. reported on 10 eyes of 5 patients with SC.[29] Hypoautofluorescence corresponded with areas of chorioretinal atrophy, and in three eyes, new areas of hyperautofluorescence appeared at the border of hypoautofluorescent areas and appeared to suggest areas of inflammatory activity.

PATHOLOGY

Unfortunately, few eyes with SC have been studied in the pathology laboratory. Histology reveals that the choriocapillaris and parts of the choroid are infiltrated by lymphocytes, supporting the inflammatory etiology of the disorder and the classification of this entity as choroiditis (Fig. 29.4).[15,30] Histologic examination of the retina shows an extensive loss of the RPE and destruction of the overlying retina. Areas of RPE hypertrophy and subretinal scarring have also been described.

ETIOLOGY

The cause of SC is unknown. Most data suggest that the disease is an inflammatory or autoimmune disorder in most patients. Laatikainen and Erkkilä[20] indicated that immune-mediated vasculitis might induce occlusion of the choroidal vessels. The finding of a lymphocytic infiltrate in the choroid and accompanying vitritis supports an inflammatory etiology. Some studies suggest a human leukocyte antigen (HLA) association with the disease. In one study, the incidence of HLA-B7 was higher in 15 Finnish patients with SC than in the control group (54.5% versus 24.3%, $P < 0.05$), but these results need to be confirmed in other independent trials.[31] It is important to recognize that a number of infectious diseases can lead to a clinical picture similar to that of SC. Data to support infectious etiologies are often circumstantial. These researchers further demonstrated that increased levels of antibacterial antibodies, such as antistreptolysin O, were found in eight of the patients with SC.[31] Other factors suggesting infection include the clinical course of the disease, with multiple recurrent inflammatory episodes, and compatibility with an infectious disease process, such as herpes virus infection. SC has been reported after viral meningitis, and some clinicians have given anecdotal reports of improvement after treatment with acyclovir. Nevertheless, firm evidence to suggest an infectious cause for most cases of SC is lacking. In a report by Akpek et al.,[30] no evidence of herpes simplex virus (HSV) P1/P2 (for HSV-1,

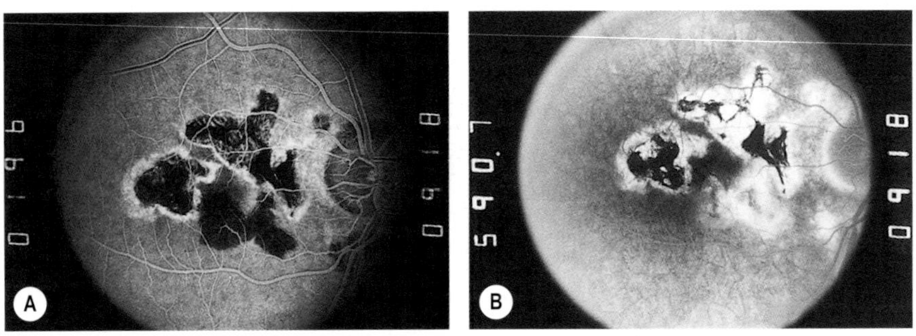

Fig. 29.3 Fluorescein angiogram of a serpiginous lesion. (A) Early frame showing central blockage of fluorescence. (B) Late frame demonstrating areas of diffuse hyperfluorescence with some areas of blocked fluorescence corresponding to clumping of the retinal pigment epithelium.

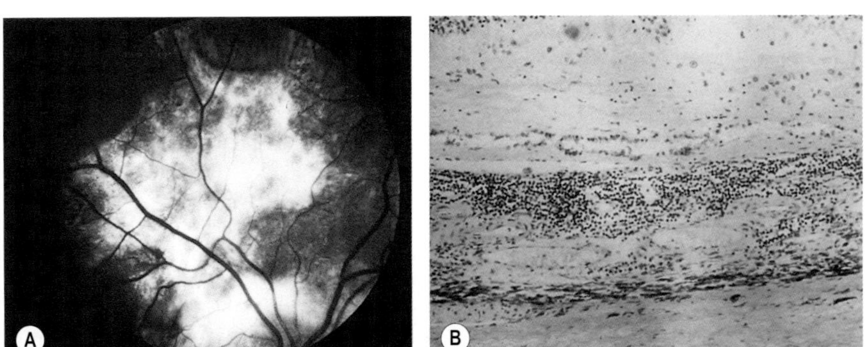

Fig. 29.4 (A) Clinical photograph of the eye of a young man with serpiginous choroiditis showing a typical choroidal lesion. (B) Photomicrograph of the eye showing marked lymphocytic infiltrate of the choroid. (Courtesy J.D.M. Gass, MD.)

HSV-2, Epstein-Barr virus [EBV], cytomegalovirus [CMV], human herpes virus [HHV]-8) and varicella-zoster virus (VZV) P1/P2 (for VZV, HHV-6, HHV-7) was demonstrated in the infiltrating lymphocytes or the choroidal tissue on polymerase chain reaction (PCR) analysis. Theoretically, it is possible that the inflammatory disease may be a secondary phenomenon unrelated to previous infection that may have originally been directed against a viral antigen. Retinal degeneration after the impairment of the choroidal vasculature could release potentially antigenic moieties, which, in genetically prone persons, leads to an inflammatory response.

Tuberculosis and syphilis have also been suggested as a cause of SC. However, as with the presumed viral etiologies of the disease, it may be better to consider these infectious conditions as disorders in the differential diagnosis of SC.

DIFFERENTIAL DIAGNOSIS

A number of disorders should be considered in the differential diagnosis of SC, and the major diseases are listed in Box 29.2. It is especially important to rule out the infectious causes of SC because these diseases are best treated with specific medications to treat the infection and because immunosuppressive therapy can exacerbate these conditions. Several authors have reported the association of SC-like lesions with tuberculosis. Gupta et al.[32] reported seven patients in India with choroidal tuberculosis that presented with a disorder that looked like SC. The clinical presentation included multifocal lesions that progressed to a wave-like confluence. Other lesions were described as plaque-like with an ameboid presentation. Teyssot et al.[33] reported on 14 patients with diseases involving the choroid, choriocapillaris, and the RPE and showed that they had a family history of tuberculosis or active infection. Mackensen et al.[34] performed a retrospective evaluation of German patients with an SC-like condition. Eleven of the 21 patients tested positive for tuberculosis on the QuantiFERON assay. Tuberculosis may also explain the relatively high percentage (19%) of patients with SC seen in a large uveitis center in India.[35]

Other infectious processes have been reported to present with SC-like lesions. Herpes virus infections have been associated with SC.[36] Syphilis, which can causes chorioretinitis, should always be ruled out in cases of SC. Finally, there are scattered reports of a plethora of other ocular infections with a clinical appearance similar to that of SC. Rarely, some diseases, such as ocular histoplasmosis and toxoplasmosis, can look like SC. As an example, there was a case of a 32-year-old woman presenting with blurred vision in her left eye. Fundus examination revealed extensive SC-like lesions (Fig. 29.5), and blood serology and PCR performed on the aqueous from her eye were positive for toxoplasmosis.[37]

APMPPE is one of the white-dot syndromes that can frequently appear similar to SC. Acute lesions in both diseases may have a yellow color and involve the choroid, choriocapillaris, and RPE. RPE clumping can be seen late in the course of both diseases. Furthermore, the acute lesions of both APMPPE and SC show early blockage of fluorescence and late hyperfluorescence on fluorescein angiography. However, unlike in SC, the acute lesions of APMPPE resolve within 2 weeks, and recurrence is uncommon. In addition, choroidal atrophy and CNV are atypical in APMPPE but common in SC, and the visual prognosis is far better for patients with APMPPE than for those with SC.

We have, however, seen a number of patients with a disease that falls between the classic findings of SC and APMPPE. We would frequently debate over our lunchtime case presentations whether these patients had SC or APMPPE. At one meeting where we could not decide, I said this patient has "APMPPiginous choroiditis" (Fig. 29.6). Since that time, Bob Nussenblatt and I informally called this condition "ampiginous choroiditis" and somehow the term has remained in the literature.[38] How does ampiginous choroiditis differ from SC? Patients with ampiginous choroiditis do not have the relentless, helical progression that is characteristic of SC and usually maintain good vision. However, in some patients, large portions of the retina may become involved.

Jones et al.[39] described a condition they called "relentless placoid chorioretinitis," similar to ampiginous choroiditis, but with a more prolonged and progressive clinical course with widespread lesions (Fig. 29.7). In their initial description of six patients, the authors noted retinal lesions similar to those of APMPPE or SC, but unlike the typical course of these two disorders, patients with relentless placoid chorioretinitis had evidence of numerous posterior and peripheral retinal lesions that predated or occurred simultaneously with macular involvement. In addition, the cases all demonstrated prolonged periods of activity resulting in the appearance of more than 50 and sometimes hundreds of lesions. Perhaps another variant of SC and ampiginous choroiditis is a condition termed *persistent placoid maculopathy*,[40] which presents as macular choroiditis, often with CNV (see Chapter 30 on white-dot syndromes). Whether these conditions are all varying presentations of the same underlying condition or separate diseases is unknown and will

BOX 29.2 Differential Diagnosis of Serpiginous Choroiditis

Infectious Diseases

- Syphilitic choroiditis
- Tuberculous choroiditis
- Herpes virus choroiditis
- Ocular histoplasmosis
- Ocular toxoplasmosis

Noninfectious Diseases

- Acute posterior multifocal placoid pigment epitheliopathy
- Ampiginous choroiditis
- Relentless placoid chorioretinitis
- Multifocal choroiditis
- Tumors (benign and malignant, ocular and metastatic)
- Posterior scleritis

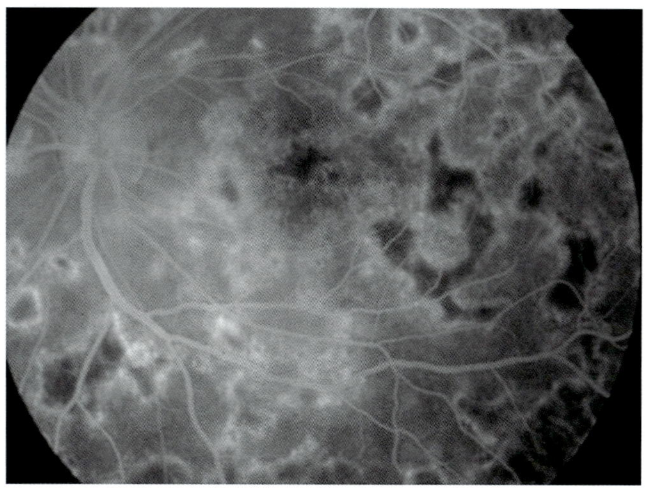

Fig. 29.5 A case of toxoplasmosis that resembles serpiginous choroiditis. (Reproduced with permission from Mahendradas P, Kamath G, Mahalakshmi B, et al. Serpiginous choroiditis-like picture due to ocular toxoplasmosis. *Ocul Immunol Inflamm.* 2007;15(2):127–130.)

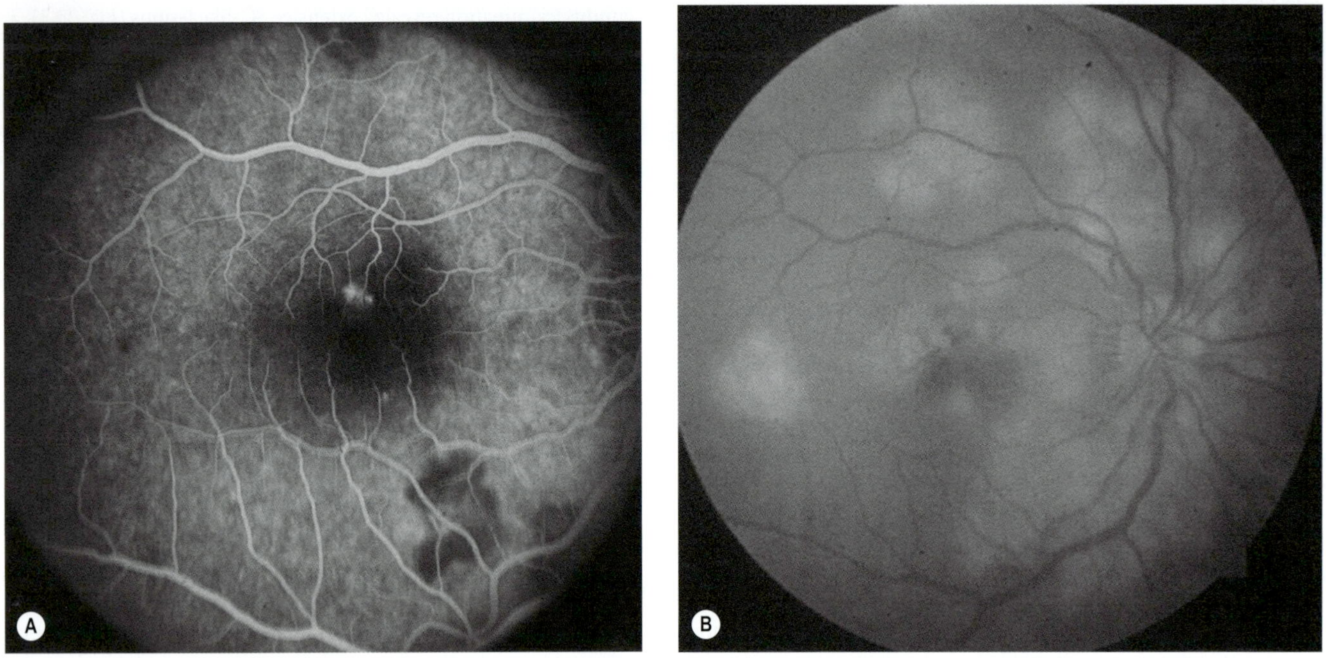

Fig. 29.6 Case of ampiginous choroiditis. This 32-year-old man presented with vague visual complaints. (A) At presentation, angiography showed areas of blockage of choroidal fluorescence in the macula with one small area of hyperfluorescence in the posterior pole. The patient was thought to have APMPPE. About 2 weeks later, he presented with new lesions and a drop in visual acuity (B). Multiple new choroidal lesions were noted and immunosuppressive therapy was started. Therapy was discontinued, and the disease recurred in the contralateral eye. Angiography demonstrated very extensive changes in the choroid. The clinical course and appearance of the disease were now more consistent with a diagnosis of serpiginous choroiditis, and a diagnosis of APPMPiginous (ampiginous choroiditis) was made. Seven years later, his vision was 20/40 + 2 in this eye.

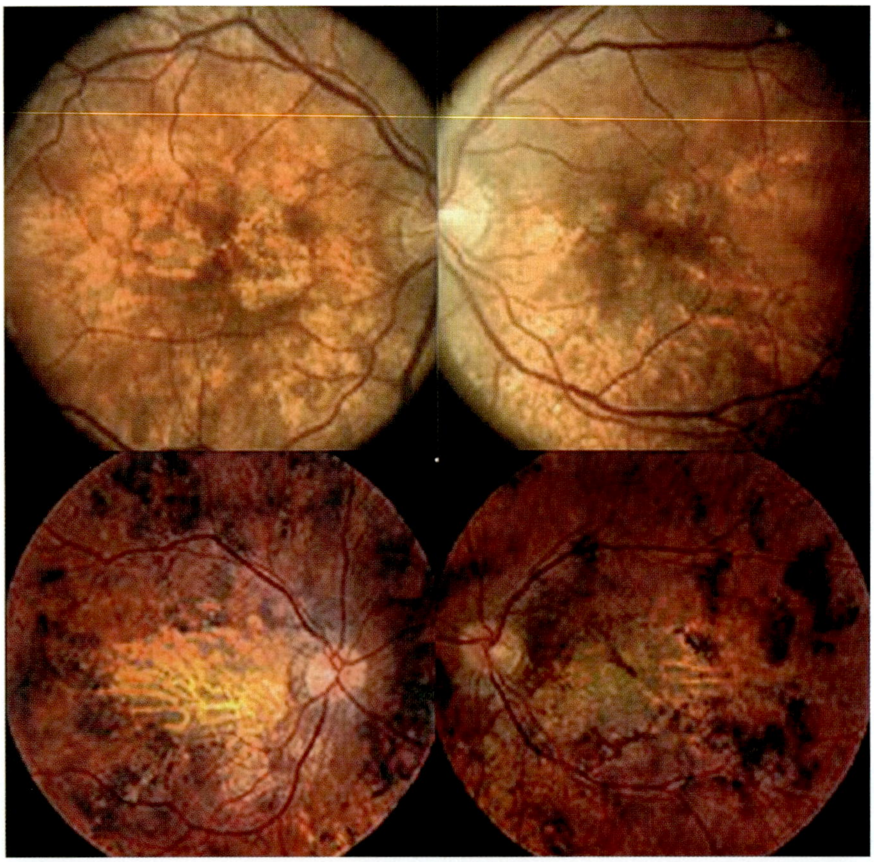

Fig. 29.7 A case of posterior placoid chorioretinitis. The top photos were taken as the new lesions developed. The bottom photos show the lesions after therapy and stabilization. Compare with the photo showing ampiginous choroiditis fundus (see Fig. 29.7). (Reproduced with permission from Yeh S, Lew JC, Wong WT, Nussenblatt RB. Relentless placoid chorioretinitis associated with central nervous system lesions treated with mycophenolate mofetil. *Arch Ophthalmol.* 2009;127(3):341–343.)

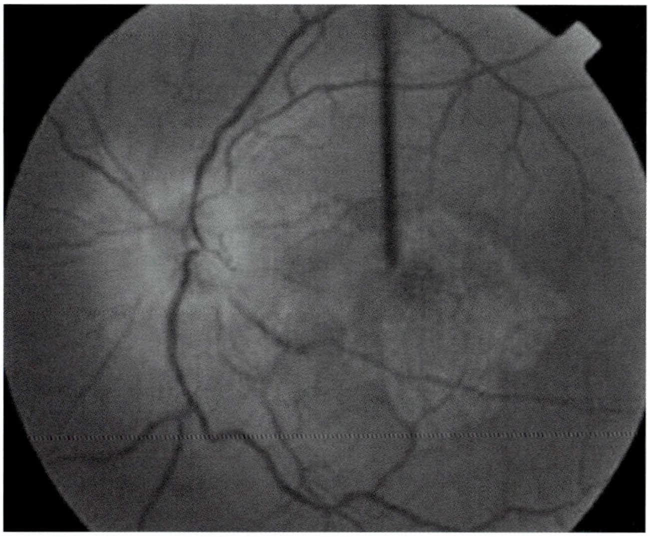

Fig. 29.8 Posterior scleritis resembling macular serpiginous choroiditis. (Reproduced with permission from Sonika, Narang S, Kochhar S, et al. Posterior scleritis mimicking macular serpiginous choroiditis. *Indian J Ophthalmol.* 2003;51(4):351–353.)

probably only be determined when the specific etiologies of these diseases are discovered.

Many other noninfectious conditions can look like SC. Posterior scleritis may mimic a macular serpiginous lesion (Fig. 29.8), although scleritis is often associated with pain.[41] Diseases that cause peripapillary chorioretinal scarring can be confused with SC. Age-related macular degeneration, angioid streaks, idiopathic CNV, and previous retinal laser photocoagulation are other entities to be considered in the evaluation of patients suspected of having SC. Edelstein et al.[42] described an unusual case of ocular sarcoidosis with manifestations similar to those of SC. Ocular malignancies and metastatic lesions to the choroid and retina may appear like SC. A patient with systemic non-Hodgkin lymphoma was reported to present with fundus lesions suggestive of SC.[43]

THERAPY

As with all patients with uveitis, infection should be considered and ruled out because specific anti-infective drugs are warranted for infectious causes of ocular inflammatory disease. In patients with a clinical appearance of SC, the two infections to most strongly consider are syphilis and tuberculosis. If diagnostic tests for syphilis are positive, antibiotic therapy is clearly beneficial (see Chapter 11). Although antituberculosis medications are not beneficial for most patients with SC,[13] these agents may be considered in patients with a history and clinical examination suggestive of possible underlying tuberculosis. Patients who present with more multifocal SC, especially in countries endemic for tuberculosis or where diagnostic testing supports the diagnosis of the disease, antituberculosis therapy should be considered.[44] Antiviral therapy has been used in patients suspected of having herpetic chorioretinitis.

If infection is unlikely, anti-inflammatory therapy is given to treat the associated vitritis and anterior uveitis and, more importantly, active lesions threatening the fovea. In our experience, patients with a significant inflammatory disease, including acute yellowish lesions and overlying vitritis, respond to corticosteroid therapy (Case 29.1). We have observed improvement in visual acuity in patients treated with oral prednisone, but there are no large randomized controlled trials (RCTs) investigating treatments for SC. In addition, we have treated one patient in whom an active lesion was threatening the fovea with pulse intravenous methylprednisolone at a dose of 1 g/day for 3 days. Markomichelakis et al.[45] also described their experience in the use of pulse methylprednisolone, reporting a positive therapeutic response within 10 days.

Because SC is usually bilateral with frequent disease reactivation, most uveitis specialists use immunosuppressive agents in the management of the disease (Cases 29.2 and 29.3). We have used cyclosporin in combination with corticosteroids to treat some patients with SC.[46]

CASE 29.1

A 64-year-old white man was referred to the National Eye Institute (NEI) because of gradual loss of vision in the right eye over the previous 6 months. The left eye was amblyopic. Visual acuity was 20/100 in the right eye and 20/200 in the left eye. There were 1+ cells and flare in both anterior chambers and 1+ vitreous cells in both eyes, with some strands. Choroidal, perifoveal lesions in both eyes were compatible with the diagnosis of serpiginous choroiditis (SC). The patient was treated with 50 mg prednisone/day for 1 week, with a slow taper to 20 mg/day over several months. His vision improved to 20/25 in the right eye after 3 weeks. We elected to keep treating the patient with low-dose prednisone (10–15 mg/day) for 1 year. Repeat fluorescein angiography showed no further progression of the lesion in that eye. Good vision in that eye has been maintained for 3 years after prednisone was discontinued.

CASE 29.2

A patient with serpiginous choroiditis (SC) was treated with a combination of oral prednisone and two immunosuppressive agents, with successful control of active posterior pole lesions (see Fig 29.9A). Despite aggressive therapy and an initial therapeutic response, the patient returned 1 month later with active disease involving a large part of the superior posterior pole (see Figs. 29.9B and C).

CASE 29.3

A 43-year-old man with an 11-year diagnosis of serpiginous choroiditis (SC) was referred to the National Eye Institute (NEI) with decreased vision that was worse in the right eye. He lost good central vision in the right eye despite previous medical and laser therapies. He had exacerbations of inflammatory disease in his left eye 8 and 10 years after the initial flare-up, each episode resolving after periocular injections of betamethasone. One year after the last flare-up, the patient was first seen at the NEI with no active disease. He returned with a flare-up of his disease about 5 months later, with complaints of metamorphopsia and changes on Amsler grid testing. Although his visual acuity remained 20/20, he was treated with periocular and systemic corticosteroids, and his vision returned to baseline. Ten months later, the patient returned with similar complaints of metamorphopsia. An active lesion with a cream-colored and slightly elevated border was noted on fundus examination. Fluorescein angiography showed blocked fluorescence in the early frames with late hyperfluorescence. Hyperfluorescence suggestive of a serious detachment of the retina adjacent to the lesion was also noted in the late frames (Figs. 29.10A and B).

The patient was treated with pulse intravenous methylprednisolone at a dose of 1 g/day for 3 days. He was then given a regimen of oral prednisone (20 mg/day) and cyclosporin (7 mg/kg body weight/day). Within the first 3 to 4 days, the patient noted diminished metamorphopsia, and angiography showed resolution of the area of blocked fluorescence (see Fig. 29.10B). The subsequent disease course has been characterized by development of a choroidal neovascular membrane (see Fig. 29.2), which was treated with laser photocoagulation. Subsequently the patient has developed inflammatory activity despite therapy with oral prednisone (60 mg/day) and cyclosporin (6 mg/kg of body weight/day). We have therefore added azathioprine to his therapeutic regimen.

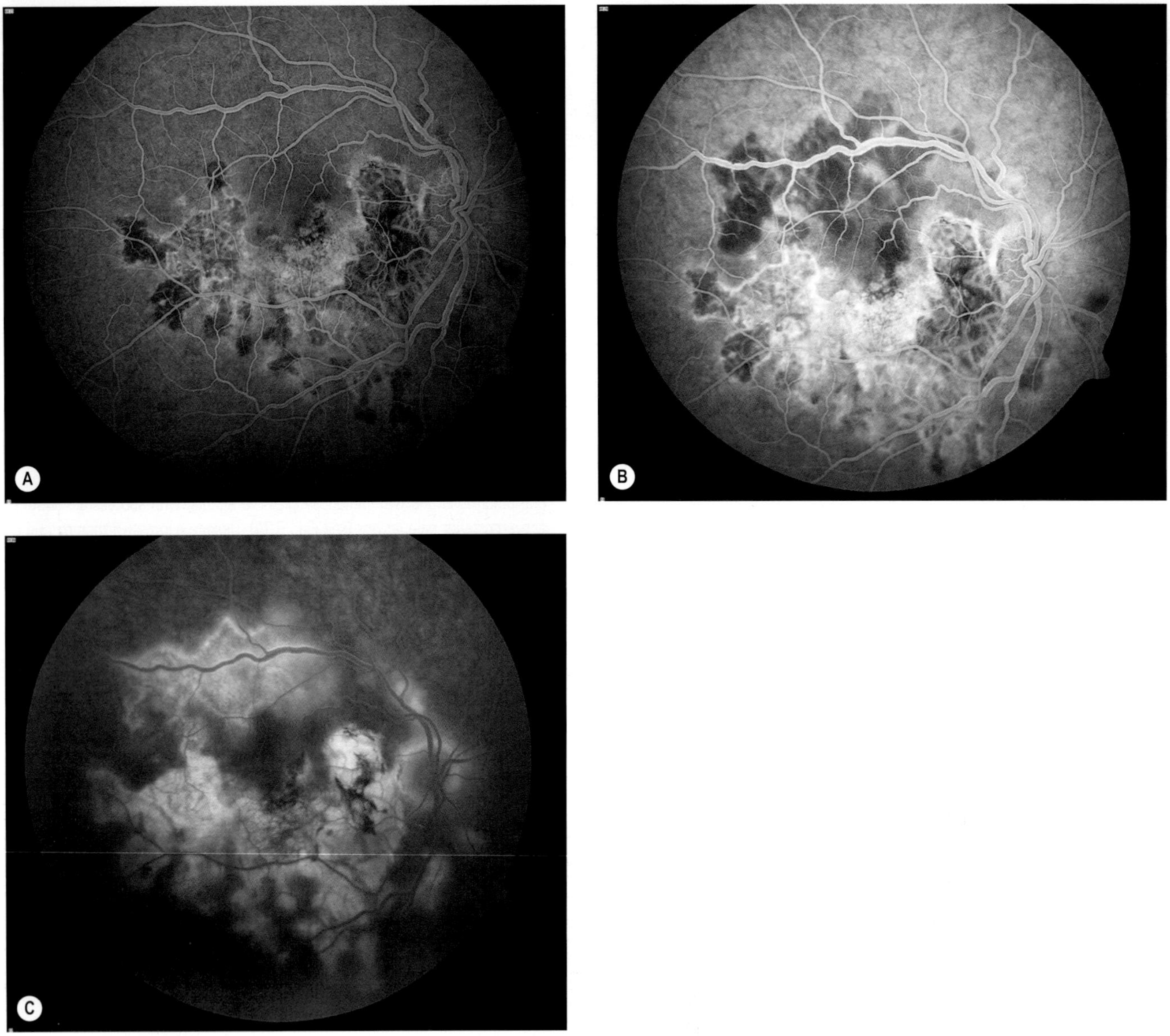

Fig. 29.9 Fluorescein angiograms from a patient with serpiginous choroiditis. The patient was treated with corticosteroids and immunosuppressive therapy, and the lesions were thought to be quiescent (A). The patient returned 1 month after therapy was started with a large recurrence involving the superior part of the posterior pole (B and C).

Araujo et al.[47] found that cyclosporin, given at 3 to 5 mg/kg/day, seemed to be safe and effective for SC, with remissions in six of seven patients in their series. However, there is variability in treatment response, and cyclosporin was not found to be successful in treating SC in other studies.[48] Multiple other immunosuppressive regimens, including corticosteroids and cytotoxic agents, have been used in treating SC.[49] Hooper and Kaplan[50] used the combination of azathioprine (1.5 mg/kg of body weight/day), cyclosporin (5 mg/kg/day), and prednisone (1 mg/kg/day) to treat patients with SC and observed rapid remission of active disease. However, they noted that the disease often recurred immediately after discontinuation of low-dose therapy but was then arrested when therapy was resumed. Vianna et al. reported that azathioprine (1.5–2.0 mg/kg/day) and prednisone (1 mg/kg) effectively controlled the disease.[51] Akpek et al.[52] reported the use of an alkylating agent (either chlorambucil or cyclophosphamide) to treat SC: seven of nine patients experienced long-term drug-free remissions. Side effects included bone marrow suppression (transient), nausea, and fatigue; carcinoma of the bladder occurred in one patient.

More recently, biologic agents have been used to treat SC. Sobaci et al.[53] reported on the beneficial effects of interferon (IFN)-α_{2a}, 4,500,000 units, three times a week for the first 3 months, followed by once a week for the next 3 months, in combination with corticosteroids as a treatment for SC. Anti–tumor necrosis factor-alpha (TNF-α) agents have also been tried in the treatment of this disease.[54] However, infection should be considered in these patient before immunosuppressive therapy is started. Cordero-Coma et al. reported disseminated tuberculosis after the use of anti-TNF therapy in a patient with SC-like fundus lesions, although initial findings on laboratory workup for tuberculosis had been negative.[55]

It is also difficult to decide how long to treat a patient with SC. As with other chronic forms of uveitis, therapy should always be based on the risk/benefit of treatment and patient desire and ability to comply with therapy and follow-up. Imaging technology, such as fundus autofluorescence, fluorescein angiography, and OCT, can help identify active lesions and response to therapy. Again, active inflammation and lesions threatening vision are key indications for more aggressive therapy.

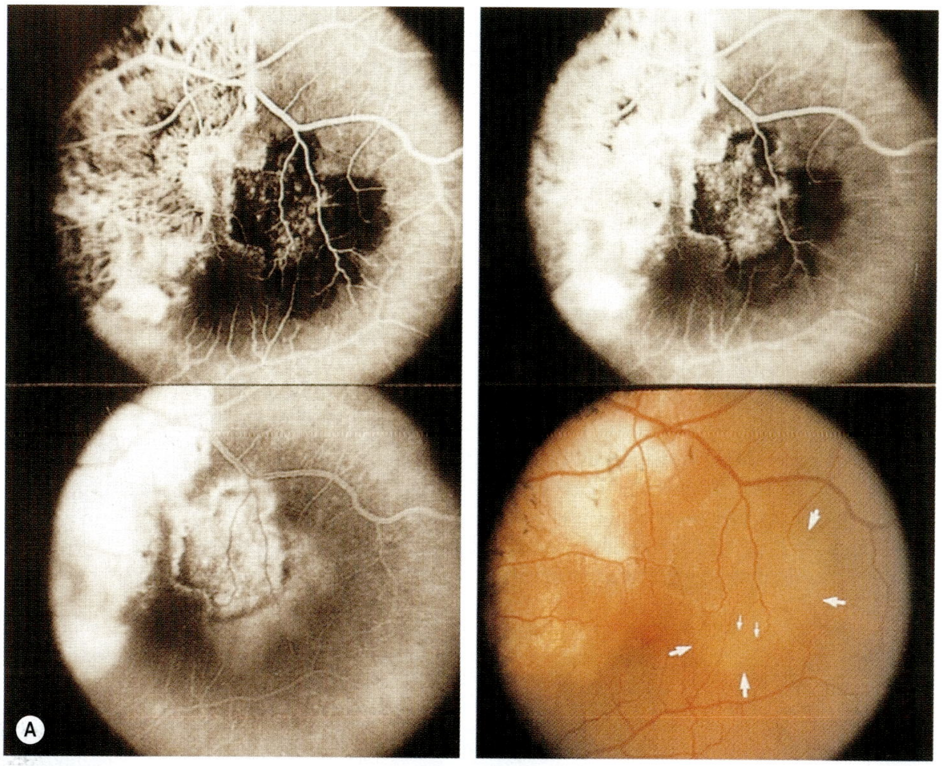

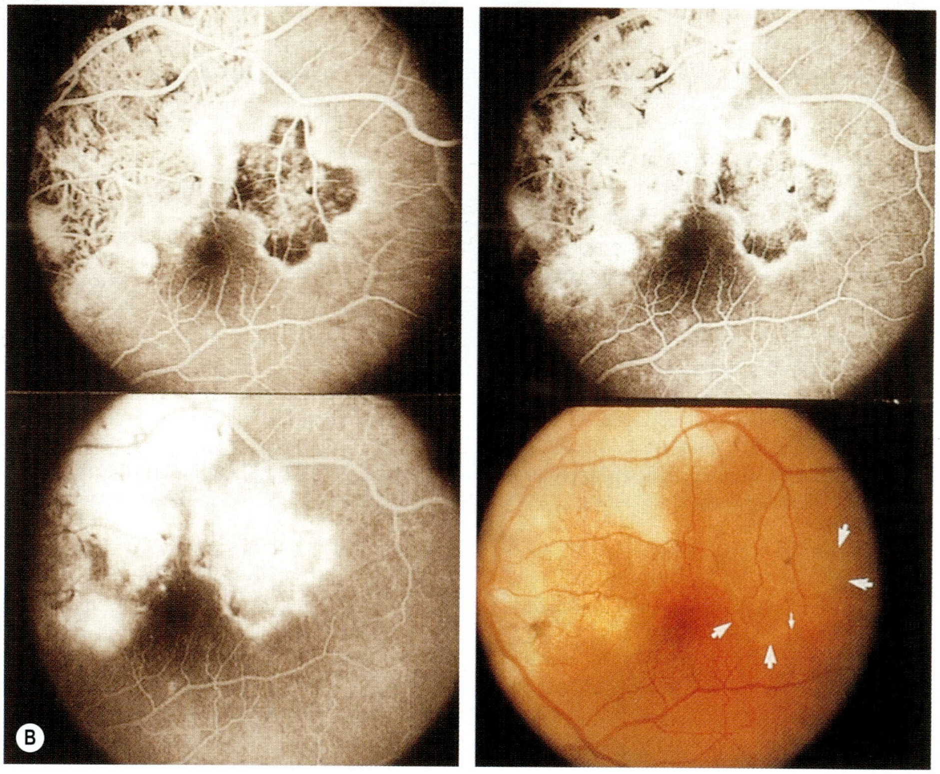

Fig. 29.10 (A) Fluorescein angiogram and fundus photograph from a patient with serpiginous choroiditis and complaints of slightly decreased visual acuity and metamorphopsia in the left eye. Early blocked fluorescence and late leakage are seen at the borders of active lesions. The late frame also shows late leakage compatible with serous detachment of adjacent retina *(arrows)*. (B) Fluorescein angiogram and fundus photograph of same patient 9 days after pulse intravenous methylprednisolone therapy. The patient had noted decreased metamorphopsia. Early blocked fluorescence is no longer seen at the border of the lesion, and the serous retinal detachment has resolved *(arrows)*. (Reproduced with permission from Hooper PL, Kaplan HJ. Triple agent immunosuppression in serpiginous choroiditis. *Ophthalmology.* 1991;98:948–952. Copyright Elsevier 1991.)

On the basis of therapeutic response, treatment can then be tapered and patients should then be followed up closely for signs of disease activity. There are patients with SC who are reported to do well for decades with only intermittent corticosteroid therapy for disease activity.[56]

Local injections of corticosteroid therapy have been used to treat the disease. Intravitreal triamcinolone has been used to treat this condition,[57] with one report suggesting that a single injection effectively controlled the active lesion.[58] Seth and Gaudio[59] reported that the use of a fluocinolone acetonide intravitreal implant controlled SC for over 14 months. Miserocchi et al. reported that the dexamethasone intravitreal implant controlled SC activity in eight eyes of seven patients with SC.[60]

Other treatments have been used to treat the complications of SC. Choroidal neovascular membranes occur with SC and can cause severe vision loss. Initially, these were treated with photodynamic therapy,[61] but more recently, the anti–vascular endothelial growth factor (VEGF) agents have been used to treat choroidal neovascular membranes in patients with SC.[62,63] Corticosteroids can successfully treat RPE detachment and serous detachment in SC.[64] Steinmetz et al.[65] reported that acetazolamide was useful in treating cystoid macular edema in one patient with SC.

PROGNOSIS

Vision loss is common in patients with SC. Because of the chronic course of the disease, with periodic inflammatory recurrences that involve the fovea and peripapillary area, it is not surprising that severe and permanent vision loss can occur in the disease. Mean final visual acuity has been reported to be 20/125, with a wide range from 20/20 to no light perception (NLP).[56,66,67] Lesions threatening the fovea, including choroidal neovascular membranes, are associated with worse vision. The hope is that the use of newer immunosuppressive agents and employing imaging technologies to better identify active lesions and response to therapy can improve the prognosis. Better treatments for the complications of SC, such as choroidal neovascular membranes, may also improve the visual outcomes in this disorder.

REFERENCES

1. Schatz H, Maumenee AE, Patz A. Geographic helicoid peripapillary choroidopathy: clinical presentation and fluorescein angiographic findings. *Trans Am Acad Ophthalmol Otolaryngol*. 1974;78:747–761.
2. Orth D, Daily MJ, Babb MF. Subretinal neovascularization with geographic (serpiginous) choroiditis. *Am J Ophthalmol*. 1979;88:683–689.
3. Bock CJ, Jampol LM. Serpiginous choroiditis. In: Albert DM, Jacobiec FA, eds. *Principles and Practice of Ophthalmology*. Philadelphia: Mosby; 1974:517–523.
4. Schatz H, McDonald HR. Geographic helicoid peripapillary choroidopathy (serpiginous choroiditis). In: Ryan SJ, et al., ed. *Retina*. St. Louis: Mosby; 1989.
5. Hardy RA, Schatz H. Macular geographic helicoid choroidopathy. *Arch Ophthalmol*. 1987;105:1237–1242.
6. Nazari H, Rao NA. Serpiginous choroiditis and infectious multifocal serpiginoid choroiditis. *Surv Ophthalmol*. 2013;58:203–232.
7. Junius P. Seltene augenspielgelbilder zum klinischen phanomen des retinitis exsuditiva Coats und der retinochoroiditis 'parapapillaris'. *Arch Augenheilkd*. 1932;106:475.
8. McCannel CA, Holland GN, Helm CJ, et al. Causes of uveitis in the general practice of ophthalmology. UCLA Community-Based Uveitis Study Group. *Am J Ophthalmol*. 1996;121:35–41.
9. Pivetti-Pezzi P, Accoriniti M, La Cava M, et al. Endogenous uveitis: an analysis of 1,417 cases. *Ophthalmologica*. 1996;210:234–238.
10. Chang JH, Wakefield D. Uveitis: a global perspective. *Ocul Immunol Inflamm*. 2002;10(4):263–279.
11. Blumenkranz MS, Gass JDM, Clarkson JG. Atypical serpiginous choroiditis. *Arch Ophthalmol*. 1982;100:1773–1775.
12. Huthinson J. Serpiginous chroiditis in scrofulous subjects: choroidal lupus. *Arch Surg (Lond)*. 1900;11:126–135.
13. Laatikainen I, Erkkilö H. Serpiginous choroiditis. *Br J Ophthalmol*. 1974;58:777–783.
14. Hamilton AM, Bird AC. Geographical choroidopathy. *Br J Ophthalmol*. 1974;58:784–797.
15. Gass JDM. *Stereoscopic Atlas of Macular Diseases: Diagnosis and Treatment*. St. Louis: Mosby; 1987:136.
16. Weiss H, Annesley WH Jr, Shields JA, et al. The clinical course of serpiginous choroidopathy. *Am J Ophthalmol*. 1979;87:133–142.
17. Masi RJ, O'Connor R, Kimura SJ. Anterior uveitis in geographic or serpiginous choroiditis. *Am J Ophthalmol*. 1978;86:228–232.
18. Laatikainen I, Erkkilä H. Subretinal and disc neovascularization in serpiginous choroiditis. *Br J Ophthalmol*. 1982;66:326–331.
19. Wojno T, Meredith TA. Unusual findings in serpiginous choroiditis. *Am J Ophthalmol*. 1982;94:650–655.
20. Laatikainen I, Erkkilä H. A follow-up study on serpiginous choroiditis. *Acta Ophthalmol (Copenh)*. 1981;59:707–718.
21. Salati C, Pantelis V, Lafaut BA, et al. A 8 months indocyanine angiographic follow-up of a patient with serpiginous choroidopathy. *Bull Soc Belge Ophtalmol*. 1997;265:29–33.
22. Squirrell DM, Bhola RM, Talbot JF. Indocyanine green angiographic findings in serpiginous choroidopathy: evidence of a widespread choriocapillaris defect of the peripapillary area and posterior pole. *Eye*. 2001;15(Pt 3):336–338.
23. Giovannini A, Ripa E, Scassellati-Sforzolini B, et al. Indocyanine green angiography in serpiginous choroidopathy. *Eur J Ophthalmol*. 1996;6:299–306.
24. Giovannini A, Mariotti C, Ripa E, et al. Indocyanine green angiographic findings in serpiginous choroidopathy. *Br J Ophthalmol*. 1996;80:536–540.
25. van Liefferinge T, Sallet G, De Laey JJ. Indocyanine green angiography in cases of inflammatory chorioretinopathy. *Bull Soc Belge Ophtalmol*. 1995;257:73–81.
26. Punjabi OS, Rich R, Davis JL, et al. Imaging serpiginous choroidopathy with spectral domain optical coherence tomography. *Ophthalmic Surg Lasers Imaging*. 2008;39(4 Suppl):S95–S98.
27. Cardillo Piccolino F, Grosso A, Savini E. Fundus autofluorescence in serpiginous choroiditis. *Graefes Arch Clin Exp Ophthalmol*. 2009;247(2):179–185.
28. Gallagher MJ, Yilmaz T, Cervantes-Casaneda RA, et al. The characteristic features of optical coherence tomography in posterior uveitis. *Br J Ophthalmol*. 2007;91:1680–1685.
29. Yeh S, Forooghian F, Wong WT, et al. Fundus autofluorescence imaging of the white dot syndromes. *Arch Ophthalmol*. 2010;128:46–56.
30. Akpek EK, Chan CC, Shen D, et al. Lack of herpes virus DNA in choroidal tissues of a patient with serpiginous choroiditis. *Ophthalmology*. 2004;111(11):2071–2075.
31. Erkkilö H, Laatikainen I, Jokinen E. Immunological studies on serpiginous choroiditis. *Graefes Arch Clin Exp Ophthalmol*. 1982;219:131–134.
32. Gupta V, Gupta A, Arora S, et al. Presumed tubercular serpiginous-like choroiditis: clinical presentations and management. *Ophthalmology*. 2003;110(9):1744–1749.
33. Teyssot N, Bodaghi B, Cassoux N, et al. Acute posterior multifocal placoid pigment epitheliopathy, serpiginous and multifocal choroiditis: etiological and therapeutic management. *J Fr Ophtalmol*. 2006;29(5):510–518.
34. Mackensen F, Becker MD, Wiehler U, Max R, et al. QuantiFERON TB-Gold—a new test strengthening long-suspected tuberculous involvement in serpiginous-like choroiditis. *Am J Ophthalmol*. 2008;146:761–767.
35. Biswas J, Narain S, Das D, et al. Pattern of uveitis in a referral uveitis clinic in India. *Int Ophthalmol*. 1996;20(4):223–228.
36. Priya K, Madhavan HN, Reiser BJ, et al. Association of herpesviruses in the aqueous humor of patients with serpiginous choroiditis: a polymerase chain reaction-based study. *Ocul Immunol Inflamm*. 2002;10:247–261.
37. Mahendradas P, Kamath G, Mahalakshmi B, et al. Serpiginous choroiditis-like picture due to ocular toxoplasmosis. *Ocul Immunol Inflamm*. 2007;15(2):127–130.

38. Lim WK, Buggage RR, Nussenblatt RB. Serpiginous choroiditis. *Surv Ophthalmol.* 2005;50(3):231–244.
39. Jones BE, Jampol LM, Yannuzzi LA, et al. Relentless placoid chorioretinitis. A new entity or an unusual variant of serpiginous chorioretinitis. *Arch Ophthalmol.* 2000;118:931–938.
40. Golchet PR, Jampol LM, Wilson D, et al. Persistent placoid maculopathy: a new clinical entity. *Ophthalmology.* 2007;114(8):1530–1540.
41. Sonika, Narang S, Kochhar S, et al. Posterior scleritis mimicking macular serpiginous choroiditis. *Indian J Ophthalmol.* 2003;51(4):351–353.
42. Edelstein C, Stanford MR, Graham EM. Serpiginous choroiditis: an unusual presentation of ocular sarcoidosis. *Br J Ophthalmol.* 1994;78:70–71.
43. Rattray KM, Cole MD, Smith SR. Systemic non-Hodgkin's lymphoma presenting as a serpiginous choroidopathy: report of a case and review of the literature. *Eye.* 2000;14:706–710.
44. Majumder PD, Biswas J, Gupta A. Enigma of serpiginous choroiditis. *Indian J Ophthalmol.* 2019;67:325 333.
45. Markomichelakis NN, Halkiadakis I, Papaeythymiou-Orchan S, et al. Intravenous pulse methylprednisolone therapy for acute treatment of serpiginous choroiditis. *Ocul Immunol Inflamm.* 2006;14(1):29–33.
46. Nussenblatt RB, Palestine AG, Chan CC. Cyclosporine A therapy in the treatment of intraocular inflammatory disease resistant to systemic corticosteroids and cytotoxic agents. *Am J Ophthalmol.* 1983;96:275–282.
47. Araujo AAQ, Wells AP, Dick AD, et al. Early treatment with cyclosporin in serpiginous choroidopathy maintains remission and good visual outcome. *Br J Ophthalmol.* 2000;84:979–982.
48. Laatikainen I, Tarkkanen A. Failure of cyclosporin A in serpiginous choroiditis. *J Ocul Ther Surg.* 1984;3:280–283.
49. Vonmoos F, Messerli J, Moser HR, et al. Immunosuppressive therapy in serpiginous choroiditis—case report and brief review of literature. *Klin Monatsbl Augenheilkd.* 2001;218:394–397.
50. Hooper PL, Kaplan HJ. Triple agent immunosuppression in serpiginous choroiditis. *Ophthalmology.* 1991;98:948–952.
51. Vianna RN, Ozdal PC, Deschênes J, et al. Combination of azathioprine and corticosteroids in the treatment of serpiginous choroiditis. *Can J Ophthalmol.* 2006;41(2):183–189.
52. Akpek EK, Jabs DA, Tessler HH, et al. Successful treatment of serpiginous choroiditis with alkylating agents. *Ophthalmology.* 2002;109:1506–1513.
53. Sobaci G, Bayraktar Z, Bayer A. Interferon alpha-2a treatment for serpiginous choroiditis. *Ocul Immunol Inflamm.* 2005;13(1):59–66.
54. Seve P, Mennesson E, Grange JD, et al. Infliximab in serpiginous choroiditis. *Acta Ophthalmol.* 2010;88:e342–e343.
55. Cordero-Coma M, Benito MF, Hernández AM, et al. Serpiginous choroiditis. *Ophthalmology.* 2008;115(9):1633. e1–e2.
56. Karagiannis DA, Sampat V, Dowler J. Serpiginous choroidopathy with bilateral foveal sparing and good visual acuity after 18 years of disease. *Retina.* 2007;27(7):989–990.
57. Pathengay AO. Intravitreal triamcinolone acetonide in serpiginous choroidopathy. *Indian J Ophthalmol.* 2005;53(1):77–79.
58. Adiguzel U, Sari A, Ozmen C, et al. Intravitreal triamcinolone acetonide treatment for serpiginous choroiditis. *Ocul Immunol Inflamm.* 2006;14(6):375–378.
59. Seth RK, Gaudio PA. Treatment of serpiginous choroiditis with intravitreous fluocinolone acetonide implant. *Ocul Immunol Inflamm.* 2008;16(3):103–105.
60. Miserocchi E, Berchicci L, Iuliano L, et al. Dexamethasone intravitreal implant in serpiginous choroiditis. *Br J Ophthalmol.* 2017;101:327–332.
61. Lim JI, Flaxel CJ, LaBree L. Photodynamic therapy for choroidal neovascularisation secondary to inflammatory chorioretinal disease. *Ann Acad Med Singapore.* 2006;35(3):198–202.
62. Parodi MB, Iacono P, Verbraak FD, et al. Antivascular endothelial growth factors for inflammatory chorioretinal disorders. *Dev Ophthalmol.* 2010;46:84–95.
63. Parodi MB, Iacono P, La Spina C, et al. Intravitreal bevacizumab for choroidal neovascularisation in serpiginous choroiditis. *Br J Ophthalmol.* 2014;98:519–522.
64. Hoyng C, Tilanus M, Deutman A. Atypical central lesions in serpiginous choroiditis treated with oral prednisone. *Graefes Arch Clin Exp Ophthalmol.* 1998;236:154–156.
65. Steinmetz RL, Fitzke FW, Bird AC. Treatment of cystoid macular edema with acetazolamide in a patient with serpiginous choroidopathy. *Retina.* 1991;11:412–415.
66. Christmas NJ, Oh KT, Oh DM, et al. Long-term follow-up of patients with serpiginous choroiditis. *Retina.* 2002;22:550–556.
67. Lampariello DA. Geographic (serpiginous) choroiditis. *J Am Optom Assoc.* 1992;63:112–116.

30

White-Dot Syndromes

Alan G. Palestine

KEY CONCEPTS

- White-dot syndromes include a group of posterior uveitides characterized by discrete, well-circumscribed white or yellow-colored lesions at the level of the outer retina, retinal pigment epithelium, or choroid. These lesions may have some degree of atrophy as well.
- The white-dot syndromes are inflammatory in mechanism and predominantly noninfectious, although the possibility of an underlying infectious cause should always be considered because the exact cause of many of these disorders remains unknown. In addition, clinical phenotypic presentation may result from multiple etiologic processes, and hence the classification of these diseases by clinical and imaging criteria may not reflect a homogenous cause of disease.
- Localized, well-circumscribed areas of inflammatory disease in the fundus are a common manifestation of many intraocular inflammatory disorders and are also discussed in other chapters. In addition, several entities occur with multiple white dots in the fundus, usually in the deeper layers of the posterior segment. They are grouped here because of their sometimes overlapping features and the belief by some that these disorders may represent the broad spectrum of one underlying entity[1] and that the underlying histopathologic lesion is a microgranuloma.[2] The desire to categorize these posterior uveitides into discrete diseases is balanced by others who suggest that many of these phenotypes are really the expression of one disease, as suggested many years ago by Gass.[3] Most occur acutely, at times leaving minimal or no permanent long-term visual loss. An infectious cause has been suggested for some,[3] although evidence does not support this theory, and other disorders resulting from presumed infectious causes may not easily fit into the better-defined entities.[4]

MULTIPLE EVANESCENT WHITE-DOT SYNDROME

Clinical Findings

Jampol et al.[5] reported on 11 patients in whom similar funduscopic changes were noted. The alterations are unilateral and are predominantly seen in young women. Numerous small (100–200 μm), discrete white lesions are noted deep in the retina or at the level of the retinal pigment epithelium (RPE) (Fig. 30.1). The lesions appear in the posterior pole and extend to the midperiphery. They tend to be concentrated in the perifoveal region but seem usually to spare the fovea itself. In addition, often the macula has a granular appearance. The granularity may take the appearance of tiny white or orange specks, which do not approach the size of the deeper circular lesions, and the lesions are sometimes described as wreath-like. The macular changes cause irregularity of the internal limiting membrane reflex. Other ocular findings include mild vitreous cells and occasional sheathing of the retinal venules (Box 30.1). There is usually no significant anterior chamber reaction. Although the lesions appear to fade with time, hence the term *multiple evanescent white-dot syndrome* (MEWDS), they can evolve into pigmented RPE stippling and scars.[6]

Approximately 50% of patients with MEWDS report a preceding flu-like episode, but this historical information is not completely reliable. The mean age at onset of symptoms is about 28 years,[5,7] but Lim et al.[8] reported two patients in their seventh decade. The decrease in visual acuity is usually quite sudden. The disease may cause a marked drop in visual acuity even to the level of 20/200, and an afferent pupillary defect may be noted. The disease runs its course over an average of 7 weeks, and a return to a visual acuity of between 20/20 and 20/40 usually ensues. The white lesions and macular granularity will fade with time, but subtle RPE alterations can be noted. Recurrences of the disorder are seen rarely.[9,10] Aaberg et al.[9] reported recurrence in a previously affected eye 3 years after the initial visual loss and recurrences in the contralateral eye. Although most reports are from North America, this disorder has been seen in Europe.[11] Asano et al.[12] found that the degree of myopia was statistically higher in Japanese patients than that seen in controls. It is usually not associated with systemic disease. Lu et al.[13] reported fundus lesions as seen in MEWDS after murine typhus, and Stangos et al.[14] reported similar fundus changes in a 50-year-old individual after vaccination for hepatitis A and yellow fever. An interesting observation was made by Landolfi et al.[15] in reporting a case of sympathetic ophthalmia that appeared to mimic MEWDS. In a patient whose eye was promptly repaired after a ruptured globe, a decrease in vision and 100- to 500-mm gray-white lesions developed in the other eye. MEWDS-like lesions have been described in a cohort of patients with pseudoxanthoma elasticum, further raising the possibility that clinical appearance may not totally reflect pathogenesis.[16] There is overlap between MEWDS and acute idiopathic blind spot enlargement (AIBSE), and the patient with AIBSE may also have subretinal spots and foveal granularity, but the visual field defect in AIBSE may not improve.[17] However, others have reported blind spot improvement,[18] and these two syndromes may be variants of one disease process.

Laboratory Findings

There appear to be neither systemic manifestations of MEWDS nor characteristic blood test abnormalities. Jampol et al.[5] reported collecting acute and convalescent sera for viral titers from one patient, but no antibody to a specific virus was identified.

Findings on electroretinography (ERG), early receptor potential (ERP), and visual pigment regeneration tests have been noted to be abnormal in these patients during the acute phase of the disease, with a return to normal during the recovery phase.[19] Indeed, during the acute phase, a wave of ERG and ERP amplitudes were markedly affected.

Feigl et al.[20] performed multifocal ERG on four patients with MEWDS. Although the results were varied, first-order kernel amplitudes seemed to reflect early disturbances of the photoreceptors. Van Meel et al.[21] performed scanning laser densitometry on a patient with MEWDS and noted small areas of absent visual pigment that did not correspond to the white fundic spots. Even with recovery, these abnormal areas of pigment loss were still faintly seen. The authors believed that their study supported the notion that this disorder is the result of a metabolic disturbance at the level of the RPE. MP1 mapping areas of retinal sensitivity can show enlarged blind spots in these patients.[22] Fundus autofluorescence (FAF) shows areas of hyperfluorescence. Yenerel et al.[23] reported that in their study, FAF showed the lesions before the clinical examination became apparent.

Fluorescein angiography frequently shows early hyperfluorescence with late staining. This is unlike the angiographic findings associated with acute posterior multifocal placoid pigment epitheliopathy (APMPPE) (see later discussion). There is staining also of the macula and late staining of the disk. Gross et al.[24] reported recognizing new angiographic features, that is, dots and spots, in a subgroup of patients with MEWDS. Small dots noted on fluorescein angiography were interpreted to be at the level of the inner retina or the RPE, whereas larger spots were more external, in the sub-RPE level. These findings would suggest varying degrees of choroidal and retinal involvement in this disorder. Indocyanine green (ICG) angiography shows hypofluorescent lesions throughout the posterior pole, which are more visible on ICG angiography than is apparent on clinical examination[25] and appear to be seen longer on ICG angiography than on clinical examination.[26]

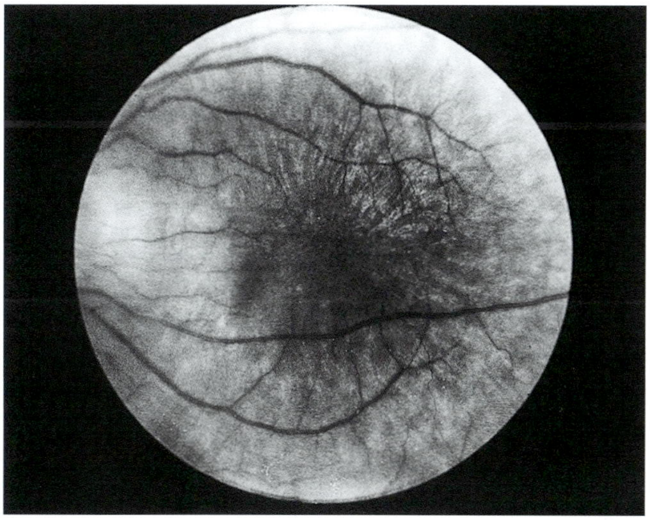

Fig. 30.1 Fundus photograph showing alterations noted in multiple evanescent white-dot syndrome (MEWDS).

BOX 30.1 Clinical Findings in Multiple Evanescent White-Dot Syndrome

- Sudden drop in visual acuity
- Patients are mostly young females
- Small discrete white dots at retinal pigment epithelium (RPE) level
- "Grainy" macula
- Electroretinography (ERG) changes that reverse after episode
- Minimal RPE perturbation after episode
- Condition rarely recurs
- Vision returns without medication

Optical coherence tomography (OCT) consistently shows changes in the outer retina.[27-29] What appears to be most often reported is loss of retinal photoreceptor inner and outer segments, which can return to a more normal appearance after the acute episode (Fig 30.2). There is disruption of the ellipsoid zone hyperreflective material in the RPE, ellipsoid zone, and outer nuclear layer in most cases.[30] It should be noted that Spaide et al.[29] found these changes in patients with various acute zonal occult outer retinopathy-complex diseases. Sikorski et al.[27] have suggested that spectral mapping indicates that the alterations noted are better explained by alterations in the RPE/photoreceptor juncture rather than sites of active inflammatory disease. These outer retinal abnormalities distinguish MEWDS from many of the other white-dot syndromes and suggest that the primary involved tissue is the outer retina.

Several entities have ocular manifestations similar to those seen in MEWDS. APMPPE is usually a bilateral disease with considerably larger lesions. With resolution, there is often considerable RPE perturbation in this disorder, whereas in MEWDS, the changes are more subtle. In APMPPE, the fluorescein angiography picture is one of initial blockage with late staining, unlike that seen in MEWDS. Multifocal

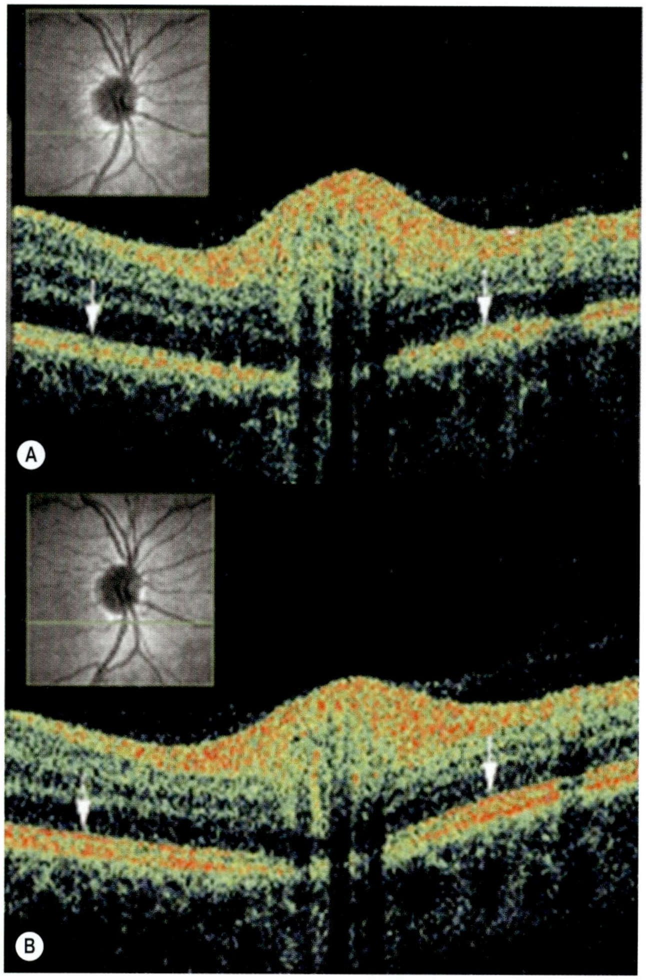

Fig. 30.2 (A) Case of multiple evanescent white-dot syndrome (MEWDS) with initial loss of inner segment/outer segment boundary (arrows). (B) Spontaneous resolution with segment boundary restored. (From Spaide RF, Koizumi H, Bailey Freund K. Photoreceptor outer segment abnormalities as a cause of blind spot enlargement in acute zonal occult outer retinopathy-complex diseases. *Am J Ophthalmol.* 2008;146:111–120. © 2008, Elsevier Inc.)

choroiditis, as first reported by Nozik and Dorsch,[31] can be distinguished from MEWDS on the basis of the more severe inflammatory response in the vitreous in some cases, cystoid macular edema (CME), and persistent lesions, which are often punched out and pigmented in appearance as they evolve. Birdshot retinochoroidopathy causes ERG and electrooculography (EOG) changes that do not improve with time, and the involvement of the retinal vasculature with CME is common (see Chapter 26). Sarcoidosis should be ruled out in all patients with posterior uveitis, including patients with MEWDS, because lesions that appear similar can be seen; however, sarcoid lesions tend to involve the choroid rather than the outer retina. Usually, the lesions of sarcoidosis are bilateral, have more associated vitritis, and cause more permanent RPE alterations compared with those seen in MEWDS. As mentioned earlier, some researchers, including Callanan and Gass,[1] have stressed the notion that there may be an overlap of symptoms in the white-dot syndromes. Furthermore, Bryan et al.[32] reported MEWDS occurring in the eyes of four patients with multifocal choroiditis. Gass and Hamed[33] reported MEWDS in an eye that had acute macular neuroretinopathy 5 years ago, with lesions in this entity being red-orange and some appearing in the central macula.

Therapy

To date, in cases of MEWDS, treatment has rarely been necessary. Sequelae to the acute episode seem to be minimal, with an expected return to near-preattack vision in about 7 weeks, on average.[5] However, some patients may experience recurrences. Figueroa et al.[34] used cyclosporin to treat one such patient who had multiple recurrences. The recurrences stopped while the patient was taking a therapeutic dose of the medication.

MULTIFOCAL CHOROIDITIS AND PANUVEITIS

Multifocal choroiditis with panuveitis (MFCPU) was the term initially used to differentiate this entity from presumed ocular histoplasmosis syndrome (POHS; see Chapter 16). This description was based on the report by Nozik and Dorsch[31] of two patients with bilateral uveitis associated with distinctive chorioretinopathy, but the disease was more completely defined by Dreyer and Gass.[35] The identification of patients with MFCPU is relevant because of the associated sequelae that may lead to irreversible visual impairment. It is still unclear whether all patients with this disease have true panuveitis, and it may be best to term the characteristic choroidal lesions as *multifocal choroiditis* and continue to use Dreyer and Gass's terminology (MFCPU) to refer to this disease entity. It is likely that all cases of MFCPU are not of uniform etiology, especially considering its varied clinical presentations and course. However, because no etiology has been defined, grouping patients with lesions in the 150- to 400-micron range is appropriate at this time. Features of MFCPU can overlap with those of punctate inner choroidopathy (PIC), and some patients may have findings of PIC in one eye and MFCPU in the other.

Clinical Findings

Patients have multifocal choroiditis that shares some clinical aspects of POHS (Fig. 30.3). However, they also can have significant vitritis and often anterior uveitis. Anterior and vitreous inflammation need not be present to make the diagnosis of MFCPU. The lesions, 150 to 400 micron in diameter, can be distributed throughout the fundus but, in our experience, are posterior to the equator. They often have a punched-out appearance with white centers and pigmented borders and appear to be at the level of the RPE or the inner choroid. At times, pigment is heaped around the edge of the lesion. The pigmentary changes around the disk that are associated with POHS can be seen here as well. The disorder is usually bilateral and occurs more frequently in women. In a review by Dreyer and Gass,[35] the median age at onset was 33 years, and in the group reported by Morgan and Schatz,[36] 28 years. Most of our group of 24 patients (19 females and five males; average age 52 years) were evaluated after they had had a long, chronic course of inflammation. Morgan and Schatz[36] found that all but one of the patients they examined had myopia. Patients with this disorder do not necessarily come from an area that is endemic for histoplasmosis, and a relatively low percentage show a response to the histoplasmin skin test or have calcific nodules on chest x-ray.[35] Notably, patients with POHS are usually diagnosed in regions that are endemic for histoplasmosis, whereas MFCPU is seen worldwide.

The inflammatory activity in the vitreous may be marked, and chorioretinal involvement can be noted on detailed examination. CME was found in 14% of the eyes studied by Dreyer and Gass,[35] whereas 41% of our patients had sequelae of this disorder. At least one-third of the eyes will ultimately have a subretinal neovascular membrane in the macula.[35] These choroidal neovascular membranes are similar to others removed from eyes with other entities and represent an end-stage response to inflammatory disruption of the choroid–RPE barrier; many have extra-domain B-containing fibronectin.[37] Mild disk edema can also be seen. However, acute and symptomatic blind-spot enlargements with no signs of optic nerve abnormalities have been reported by Khorran et al.,[38] who hypothesized that this could be a manifestation of peripapillary retinal

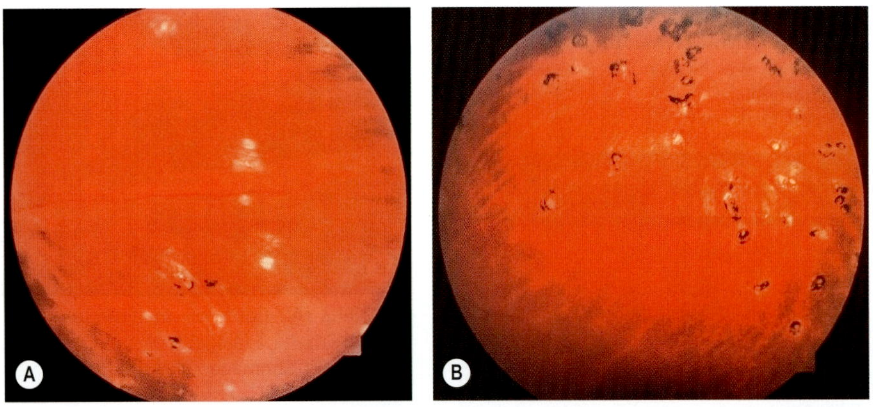

Fig. 30.3 (A and B) Multiple histoplasmosis-like lesions in periphery of patients with focal choroiditis and uveitis. These eyes, unlike those with ocular histoplasmosis syndrome, have a profound vitreous inflammatory response and cystoid macular edema. Both conditions carry the risk of subretinal neovascularization of the fovea.

dysfunction similar to the process in MEWDS and AIBSE. Callanan and Gass[1] also reported an acutely enlarged blind spot in seven of their patients. Also, in four of these, white dots similar to those in MEWDS were transiently noted, suggesting a similar cause for these two disorders. Peripheral chorioretinal streaks, once thought to be seen only in the POHS, were noted in three of 47 eyes with multifocal choroiditis.[39]

Laboratory Findings

Patients with multifocal choroiditis do not appear to originate from areas that are endemic for histoplasmosis. However, some provide a history of an antecedent febrile illness as is commonly reported in many cases of posterior uveitides.

Fluorescein angiography of the punched-out lesions shows early hyperfluorescence, typical of an RPE window defect. Morgan and Schatz[36] noted fuzzy hyperfluorescent leakage in the late phase of angiography in some lesions, and this may represent active choroidal lesions appearing to block fluorescence early and stain later. ICG angiography[40,41] tends to show more spots that appear as blockage of the fluorescence and are considered to be presumptive lesions that are not noted on a clinical examination or on fluorescein angiography. Electrophysiologic testing does not demonstrate typical findings in multifocal choroiditis. Indeed, the results of ERG will tend to be normal or borderline in most patients, suggesting that MFCPU does not diffusely involve the posterior segment.[13]

The disorders that need to be excluded when diagnosing MFCPU include many of those mentioned for MEWDS. One to note in particular is birdshot retinochoroidopathy (see Chapter 26). Human leukocyte antigen (HLA) typing has not been performed on many of these patients, and no information, to date, suggests any linkage, whereas HLA-A29 is strongly associated with birdshot retinochoroidopathy (see Chapter 26). In addition, the lesions in this entity tend to be smaller and more punched out or discrete in appearance than those in birdshot retinochoroidopathy. Birdshot retinochoroidopathy tends to occur in older persons who have less anterior segment inflammatory disease, more optic nerve involvement, and problems with night vision, photopsia, and color discrimination. The presence of CME appears to be as common in both entities in our experience, but the incidence of subretinal foveal neovascularization is higher in this condition. In presumed ocular histoplasmosis, vitreous cells should not be present, and the lesions may extend more peripherally. The incidence of subfoveal neovascular nets is higher in ocular histoplasmosis. Deutsch and Tessler[42] reported their observations in 28 patients with pseudohistoplasmosis syndrome; 43% of these patients were African Americans, and 32% had disciform scars. Furthermore, 32% of the patients were presumed to have sarcoidosis, 29% tuberculosis, and 11% syphilis. Multifocal, creamy choroidal infiltrates in older patients can be caused by masquerade syndromes including intraocular lymphoma (see Chapter 31).[43] Patients with familial juvenile systemic granulomatosis (Blau syndrome) have been shown to have multifocal choroiditis lesions[44] (Fig. 30.4). Patients with MEWDS will more often have unilateral disease, with yellow lesions at the level of the outer retina, and often experience spontaneous resolution.

Visual field changes need to be documented. Holz et al.,[45] in an early description of these patients, noted the presence of an enlarged blind spot and that the visual field alterations could not be explained on the basis of the fundus changes—that is, the field defects were larger than the spots. This could be used as evidence that both multifocal choroiditis and PIC are just one manifestation of acute zonal occult outer retinopathy (AZOOR), as has been suggested by some. However, one could argue that the spots are simply the tip of the iceberg, reflective of changes surrounding these funduscopically apparent lesions that disrupt the neighboring photoreceptors and the RPE.

A provocative hypothesis was that MFCPU is virally induced. Grutzmacher et al.[46] ascribed the RPE punched-out lesions to herpes retinitis in an otherwise healthy patient. Tiedeman[47] evaluated 10 patients with MFCPU for evidence of Epstein-Barr virus (EBV)–specific antibodies. These patients were noted to have antibodies directed against the viral capsid antigen (immunoglobulin [Ig] M) or the EBV early antigen. None of the control subjects tested was found to have these antibodies, but most did have viral capsid antigen IgG or EBV nuclear antigen antibodies, indicating previous exposure to this virus. Although none of the patients had overt systemic disease, it was hypothesized that these responses suggested an active or persistent state of viral infection and that the patients might be immunologically unable to clear the virus. Because we know that the ocular disease can continue for years, this hypothesis suggests that such persons would, in theory, have a higher risk for the systemic complications of EBV infection, an association that has not been made so far. Furthermore, chronic EBV infection has been reported by Wong et al.[48] to manifest as a different intraocular inflammatory disease that responds to treatment with acyclovir. However, acyclovir is not usually an active therapy for EBV infection. More studies have not borne out these observations. Spaide et al.[49] evaluated 11 patients with multifocal choroiditis and compared them with 11 sex- and age-matched control subjects for the presence of anti-EBV antibodies. They found no significant differences in the antiviral capsid antigen IgG and in the antinuclear antigen antibody titers between the two groups. None of the patients in either group had IgM antibodies to the antiviral capsid antigen. One patient with multifocal choroiditis and three control subjects had positive anti–early antigen antibody titers.

There is still debate as to whether PIC (discussed later) is a variant of MFCPU or a separate disease. This is, in part, an issue with defining disease by phenotypic clinical findings rather than etiologic mechanisms. For patients with the PIC subgroup of the disease, a novel, but unproven, mechanistic explanation was offered by Scheider.[50] He hypothesized that young women with myopia are more prone to this syndrome because of their tendency to have bacteremia, which, coupled with the attenuated choroidal vessels of myopia, would increase their risk of infectious thromboses.

Chorioretinal biopsies of the lesions in multifocal choroiditis have shown the presence not of a virus (see Case 30.2) but of a large number of B cells in the choroid.[51] Shimada et al.[52] reported the histopathology of choroidal neovascular lesions removed from 14 eyes with multifocal

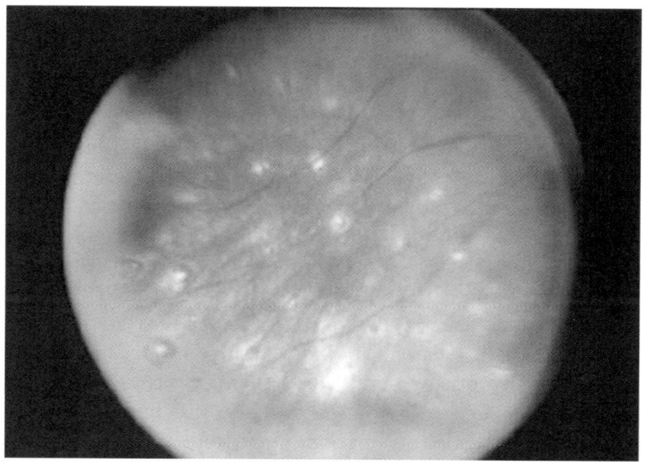

Fig. 30.4 Multifocal choroiditis in patient from family with familial juvenile systemic granulomatosis (Blau syndrome). (From Latkany PA, Jabs DA, Smith JR, et al. Multifocal choroiditis in patients with familial juvenile systemic granulomatosis. *Am J Ophthalmol.* 2002;134:897–904.)

choroiditis and PIC. Vascular endothelial growth factor (VEGF) was seen in all the specimens (no surprise), and in three of the eight multifocal choroiditis specimens, CD20+ B cells were noted. Overall, there appeared to be no real histopathologic differences between the specimens from the eyes with multifocal choroiditis and the eyes with PIC. These findings are in contrast to the report of Nölle and Eckardt[53] that in nine vitrectomy specimens from patients with multifocal choroiditis there were a large number of T cells—about one-third of the cell population being macrophages—and only rare B cells. Charteris and Lee[54] reported the necropsy results of eyes from a 59-year-old woman with this disorder. They noted that 70% to 80% of the lymphocytes were identified as T cells; less than 20% were B cells. In situ hybridization for identification of herpes simplex virus showed negative results. The finding of a large number of T cells, presumably in the choroid, in this study reflects the fact that different underlying mechanisms will result in similar clinical entities, which we had also seen with this entity[52] (see Case 30.2). An eye that was evaluated showed B cells and substantial numbers of CD3+ lymphocytes. No microgranulomas were noted.[55]

Therapy for multifocal choroiditis has centered on the use of immunosuppressive agents (see later discussion), with varying success. An interesting hypothesis is that an initial viral disorder may have triggered an immune response that no longer requires the presence of the virus but rather needs immunosuppressive therapy to be controlled.

Therapy

Periocular or systemic corticosteroids have been used to treat multifocal choroiditis during initial presentation. In the report by Dreyer and Gass,[35] six of 18 patients had improvement of vision with steroid therapy, whereas nine had no change, and in two, it was thought that this form of therapy halted a rapid decline in vision. Morgan and Schatz[36] reported that in their patients, the inflammatory disease responded very well to steroid therapy and that most patients were left with good vision, as reported by Levy et al. as well.[56] We studied 24 patients, and 10 of the 17 who needed steroid therapy had CME. We have seen a moderately good response to steroid therapy, but the disorder can become chronic, requiring consideration of the addition of other immunosuppressive agents. In our experience, the visual prognosis is guardedly optimistic. Of great interest was the report by Morgan and Schatz[36] that subretinal neovascular lesions regressed with steroid therapy. This was not seen by Dreyer and Gass[35] in one patient. We have not observed regression in our patients but have observed that the neovascular lesions remain quiet on immunosuppressive therapy once the patients have initially been treated with anti-VEGF injections. Michel et al.[57] reported their experience in treating 19 patients with multifocal choroiditis. In their series, no patient experienced visual loss after they were given immunosuppressive therapy. Laser ablation of the subretinal net may be indicated in extrafoveal lesions; however, several caveats apply. The first is that there is risk of an increase in the inflammatory response after such an intervention—something to avoid if we theorize that the inflammatory response is the underlying "initiator" of the neovascular net. Second, the experience of Dreyer and Gass suggests that laser ablation has not been particularly successful in preventing further deterioration of vision. The combination of photodynamic therapy (PDT) and intravitreal injection of triamcinolone has been reported to yield a positive therapeutic result.[58] Cirino et al.[59] reported resolution of a choroidal neovascularization (CNV) lesion secondary to PIC when a patient with multiple sclerosis began receiving regular therapy with interferon (IFN)-β_{1A}. It would seem reasonable to suppose that the CNV is driven by the inflammation in part, and therefore treating the inflammation and giving some agent directed against the neovascular component would be a good approach. Intravitreal anti-VEGF agents are also effective in treating subretinal neovascularization and are the preferred treatment in most cases. Unlike with age-related macular degeneration, these drugs can often be stopped once the inflammation is controlled.[60]

Nölle and Eckardt[53] saw no impressive therapeutic effect of vitrectomy in nine patients with multifocal choroiditis. We have limited experience with the removal of submacular neovascular nets in these patients, who often, unlike those with histoplasmosis syndrome, have a great deal of fibrosis associated with the net, making removal difficult, if at all possible. Spaide et al.[61] used PDT to treat seven patients with multifocal choroiditis with subretinal neovascular membranes. All had myopia, and in four of the seven, corticosteroid therapy was unsuccessful. The mean improvement in visual acuity was 0.86 line.

PUNCTATE INNER CHOROIDOPATHY

Watzke et al.[62] described a group of patients with a condition they termed *punctate inner choroidopathy* (PIC), which we consider to be a variant of multifocal choroiditis until proved otherwise. In their report of 10 women with moderate myopia, the ocular changes noted were essentially the same as those already described, except that there were no signs of ocular inflammation. The women had blurred vision associated with light flashes and paracentral scotomas. The lesions were 100 to 300 mm in diameter and initially appeared yellow. Reddy et al.[63] believed that PIC and multifocal choroiditis, although quite similar, can be differentiated. In multifocal choroiditis, there is vitreous inflammation, and the retinal lesions are less discrete and shallower, whereas PIC lesions are deep, punched out, and cylindrical. Also, new lesions can appear with multifocal choroiditis, which is unusual in PIC. In our mind, these distinctions are blurred, and thus we generally consider PIC as a subgroup of multifocal choroiditis. Although macular edema may be somewhat less common with PIC, both PIC and multifocal choroiditis are associated with the real risk of subretinal membranes. A comparison of 66 patients with multifocal choroiditis and 13 with PIC does suggest some differences clinically.[64] Those with PIC presented earlier with symptoms (29 years versus 45 years). At presentation, in the comparison reported, patients with PIC presented more frequently with CNV (76.9% versus 27.7%); however, they appeared to have fewer structural complications caused by intraocular inflammation, such as cataract, CME, and epiretinal membranes. Those with PIC also tended not to have as great a decrease in visual acuity. A questionnaire sent to members of the PIC Society essentially corroborated those clinical findings.[65] Those who responded confirmed the impression that the typical patient was a young, Caucasian woman with myopia. The self-reports of the members indicated that in most, CNV and subretinal fibrosis developed within the first year of diagnosis. Often observers are intoning a dual diagnosis; that is, an initial diagnosis of PIC is made, but with time and findings of unexplained visual field changes and sometimes electrophysiologic alterations, a diagnosis of AZOOR is then made.[66] This blurring of diagnoses can sometimes be a bit confusing unless one is convinced that these clinical disorders are really the same, a hypothesis that yet needs to be proved.

Laboratory Findings

There are no specific plasma tests that are useful in the diagnosis of PIC. Imaging is useful in diagnosis and in identification of new and progressive PIC lesions. FAF demonstrates hyperautofluorescence of active lesions and hypoautofluorescent/pigmented older lesions, and this is helpful in serially observing the patient for progression. Fluorescein angiography demonstrates early hyperfluorescence of active lesions with late staining. As expected, late-stage atrophic scars are seen as window defects on fluorescein angiography.[67] Similarly, ICG angiography demonstrates hypofluorescent lesions in the late stages of imaging, with more numerous lesions than can be seen on clinical examination. OCT demonstrates focal hyperreflective elevation of the RPE, with corresponding disruption of the interface of the inner and outer segment photoreceptors. RPE elevation on OCT may be a sign of an active PIC lesion.[68] Zhang et al. described the evolution of PIC lesions into five stages, beginning at the level of the RPE, breaking through into the outer retina, and then later regressing, leaving outer segment loss in the retina.[68] On OCT angiography, the CNV has been described as "having 'lacy wheel,' 'pruned large-trunk,' and 'dead tree aspect' vessel shapes with or without areas of nonperfusion" and flow voids can be seen in the inner choroid, corresponding to the spots seen on ICG angiography.[69,70]

Therapy

Patients with PIC are divided into three categories for possible therapy. The first group is of patients who have only a few PIC lesions with one or two episodes and may not require any treatment. The second group consists of patients who will continue to have recurrences that will cause progressive macular atrophy and should be treated with long-term immunosuppression. Most immunosuppressants have similar effectiveness, and an initial choice of methotrexate or mycophenolate is appropriate. A second agent, such as adalimumab or tacrolimus, can then be added if there is still evidence of progressive disease or recurrences. The third group of patients consists of those with development of CNV. Intravitreal anti-VEGF therapy is appropriate and usually effective. As with other inflammatory choroidal neovascular membranes, intravitreal injection can often be stopped if the patient's inflammation is controlled with systemic immunosuppression, thereby decreasing the inflammatory stimulus to the blood vessels and preventing new disruptions of the RPE.

ACUTE RETINAL PIGMENT EPITHELIITIS

Clinical Findings

Acute retinal pigment epitheliitis (ARPE) was first reported by Krill and Deutman,[71] who described a group of relatively young patients with fairly subtle alterations at the level of the RPE. The condition resulted in an acute drop in visual acuity or metamorphopsia. This appears to be an acute inflammation of the RPE, with a usually benign course. Some of the changes may be so mild that patients do not seek medical attention. Clusters of lesions, usually in the posterior pole, are noted. The lesions themselves are deep, fine, dark-gray or black spots, which, in their acute stage, are surrounded by a yellow halo. With resolution, the halo may disappear, and the lesions may appear darker in color. Fine subfoveal pigmentary clumping may be present and could be caused by inflammation of the neurosensory retina.[72,73]

Central serous retinopathy has been noted in this entity, presumably as a result of perturbation of the RPE. Retinopathy may be either bilateral or unilateral and can affect both sexes. A gradual resolution with complete or near-complete return to good vision occurs within 6 to 12 weeks.

As many disease processes can affect the RPE, it is difficult to know what appearance denotes a unique disease rather than a phenotypic variant. ARPE is much less common than the diseases discussed earlier but is likely a distinct entity, as indicated by the course of spontaneous remission. One example is the report by Hsu et al.[74] of their findings on OCT. They showed outer neurosensory retinal involvement rather than RPE changes (which is similar to MEWDS), suggesting that RPE alterations may be secondary. Advances in ophthalmic imaging will be helpful in understanding pathophysiology in white-dot syndromes.

Laboratory Findings

Fluorescein angiography will demonstrate an area of hypofluorescence surrounded by an area of hyperfluorescence. As ARPE progresses, it leaves a somewhat depigmented background, and a "lacy" hyperfluorescence may be noted. Central serous retinopathy may also be documented on angiographic examination.

Electrophysiologic testing may show abnormal EOG results during the acute phase of ARPE, with values returning to normal as the disorder wanes. The finding does, however, strongly suggest that the disorder affects the RPE in a far more widespread manner than is recognized on the basis of ophthalmoscopic observations. ERG results and visually evoked cortical responses have been reported as being normal.[75]

OCT has demonstrated abnormal reflectivity in the inner segment ellipsoid layer in most cases, with some patients showing disruption in the external limiting membrane and outer nuclear layer. Most of these imaging findings resolve over several months, but in those who do not recover vision fully, these changes remain.[76]

Because of the acute nature of the illness, it has been assumed that it is viral in origin. To date, however, no studies have corroborated this hypothesis. Zoledronate, a bisphosphonate used to treat tumor-induced hypercalcemia, was reported to induce acute retinal pigment epitheliitis in a patient (it has also been reported to induce uveitis).[77] Loh and Chee[78] reported ARPE-like changes in a patients with dengue fever.

Therapy

No therapy is generally called for because the disease should resolve spontaneously within 1 to 2 months. One patient was treated with nonsteroidal anti-inflammatory drugs, and vision returned to normal.[79]

ACUTE POSTERIOR MULTIFOCAL PLACOID PIGMENT EPITHELIOPATHY

The term *APMPPE* was first used by Gass in 1968[80] to describe a syndrome of multiple, large, plaque-like lesions at the level of the RPE associated with temporary visual loss. Although there is no histologic confirmation that this is an inflammatory disease, the transient nature of the lesions and a possible association with a viral prodrome have led most authors to consider APMPPE as a manifestation of inflammation or infection at the level of the RPE or the superficial choroid. It is probable that the clinical entity of benign diffuse external exudative retinitis first described by Scuderi et al.[81] in 1948 represents part of the clinical spectrum that we now include in the diagnosis of APMPPE.

Clinical Findings

The disease usually manifests with a sudden onset of visual blurring or flashing lights in a patient younger than 30 years of age.[82-84] There is no sex predilection. The disorder has been occasionally reported in older patients. In some patients, flashing lights precede visual loss by several weeks. Most cases are bilateral and appear simultaneously in both eyes. However, unilateral cases and a delay in the appearance of the disease in the second eye by several weeks have also been noted. The anterior segments may have no significant inflammation, or there may be a 1+ to 2+ nongranulomatous inflammation. The vitreous may also have a mild to moderate inflammatory response. The characteristic clinical finding is multiple flat, yellow-white (cream-colored) plaques at the level of the RPE (Fig. 30.5). These vary in size and are clearly defined. The placoid lesions typically begin in the macula or the posterior pole, with later-developing lesions noted more peripherally. The lesions do not extend beyond the equator. CME is not a prominent part of this syndrome and is rarely seen, if ever. In the acute phase, vision is often moderately decreased but rarely falls to less than 20/400. Some patients may have only a mild decrease, with vision in the 20/25 to 20/40 range. Visual field testing will demonstrate a central or pericentral scotoma.[85]

Papillitis is occasionally seen in association with this disease.[86,87] Characteristically, vision begins to improve spontaneously within a few weeks after onset of symptoms but may be somewhat slower in resolving.[82-85] Initial resolution of the cream-colored placoid lesions usually precedes the visual improvement by a few weeks. As the fundus lesions resolve, they lose their cream-colored appearance. Older lesions may resolve while new lesions are still appearing. There is often residual RPE stippling, mottling, and depigmentation (Fig. 30.6).

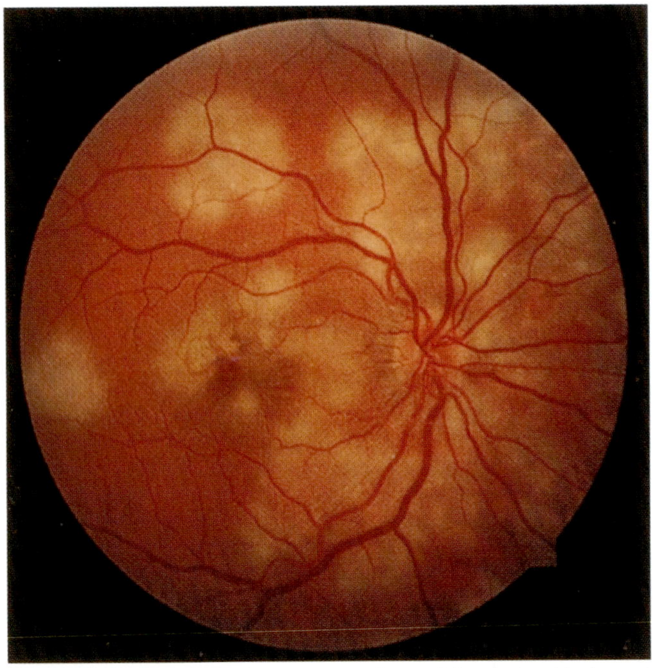

Fig. 30.5 Acute lesions of acute posterior multifocal placoid pigment epitheliopathy (APMPPE).

Vision usually returns to near-normal, but some patients may have mild residual visual deficits. Snellen acuity returns rapidly in most patients, but residual defects in visual fields, color vision, and the Stiles-Crawford effect may persist for up to a year. A few patients will have significant residual visual loss.[88]

Although APMPPE is thought to be a nonrecurrent disorder and the prognosis has been considered favorable, there are reports of recurrences. Of 13 patients in one study, five had late recurrences in previously unaffected eyes.[78] We observed one patient who had recurrent episodes of APMPPE leading to significant visual loss. We have seen disease beginning as what appears to be a severe form of APMPPE and take on characteristics similar to serpiginous choroidopathy and termed the condition *ampiginous choroiditis (AC)* (see Chapter 29). AC appears very similar to that described in the literature as *relentless placoid chorioretinitis (RPC)*.[89]

APMPPE typically occurs in otherwise healthy persons. There have been occasional reports associating it with systemic disorders, suggesting that as with many of these white-dot syndromes, they are not really one "disorder" but a sign of RPE/photoreceptor dysfunction induced by a number of factors. Fine et al.[90] reported APMPPE presenting after varicella vaccination. It has been reported to occur after swine flu, hepatitis B, and meningococcal C conjugate vaccination. Many authors have noted a viral prodrome in some patients,[82-84] and there is a report of APMPPE occurring after mumps.[91] Occasional reports of erythema nodosum,[66] episcleritis,[74] neurosensory hearing loss,[92] and cerebral vasculitis[93] associated with APMPPE have reinforced the concept that this is an immune-driven vascular alteration. Hsu et al.[74] reported APMPPE associated with systemic necrotizing vasculitis (there is another case associated with the more typical Wegener granulomatosis, mentioned later), and there is a report of fundus changes arising in a patient with clear cell renal cell carcinoma.[94] Bilateral central retinal vein occlusions have been associated with APMPPE as well, perhaps reflecting vasculitis of the ciliary vessels.[95] Others have reported neurosensory detachment, retinal vasculitis, and papillitis.[96] There is no coherent explanation for the development of this disease.

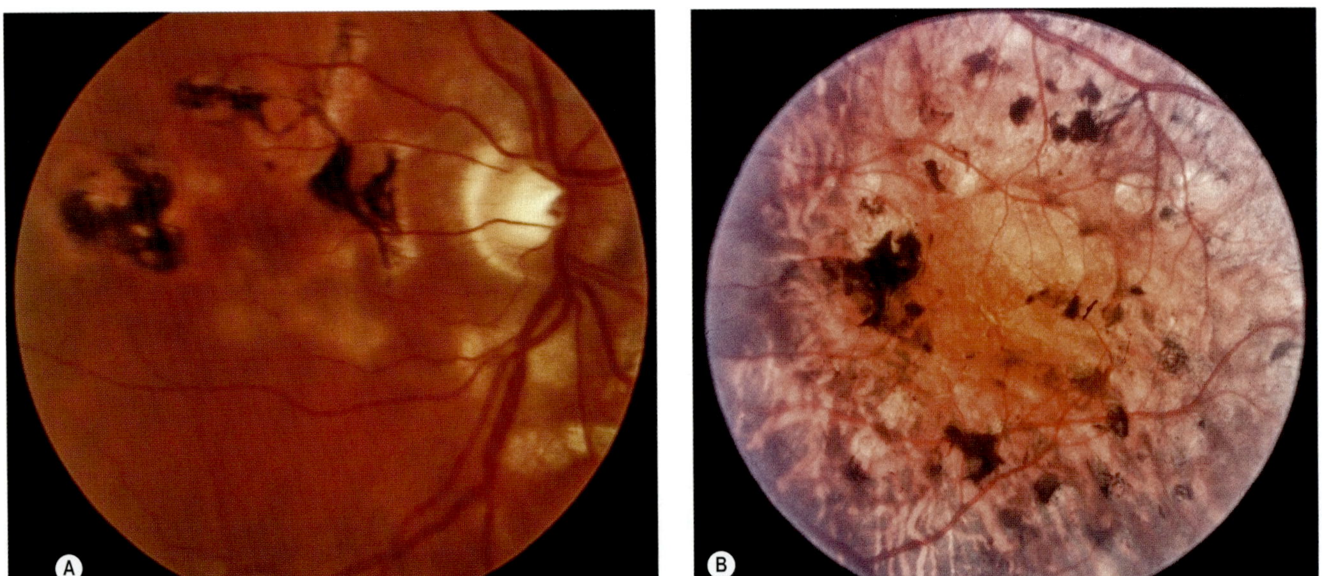

Fig. 30.6 (A) Reparative stage with retinal pigment epithelium (RPE) clumping. (B) Late stage of disease, showing a profound amount of RPE perturbation.

Laboratory Findings

In addition to the striking clinical appearance of the fundus, fluorescein angiography findings are characteristic in APMPPE[82-84,97] (Fig. 30.7). In the acute stage of the disease, during which there are active cream-colored lesions, the choroidal fluorescence is blocked in the early phases of angiography. In the late phases, there is staining of the lesions that had previously blocked fluorescence. Hypofluorescence followed by hyperfluorescence in combination with appropriately sized and colored fundic lesions is diagnostic of APMPPE. Fluorescein angiography findings in the late or resolved stage of the disease are less characteristic and demonstrate transmission defects in the RPE without leakage. There are hypofluorescent dots during the active stage, and these dots later become hyperfluorescent. Autofluorescence shows areas of hypofluorescence that do not always correlate with the fundus lesions that are visible (Fig. 30.8).

ICG angiography demonstrates hypocyanescent lesions, interpreted as choroidal hypoperfusion, corresponding to the lesions seen on fluorescein angiography.[98] However, ICG angiography shows lesions that may be more extensive than those seen on fluorescein angiography. OCT demonstrates disruption of photoreceptors acutely with outer retinal hyperreflectivity and sometimes subretinal fluid, but intraretinal edema is uncommon. On OCT angiography, there are flow voids at the level of the choriocapillaris, suggesting choroidal small vessel vasculitis or occlusion.[99]

Usually, APMPPE is limited to the eye. However, this disorder has been associated with cerebral vasculitis.[100] This can occur at the time of the ocular disease or months later. Pleocytosis may be seen in cerebrospinal fluid. In one report,[101] multifocal white-matter lesions were seen on magnetic resonance imaging (MRI), and the neurologic symptoms

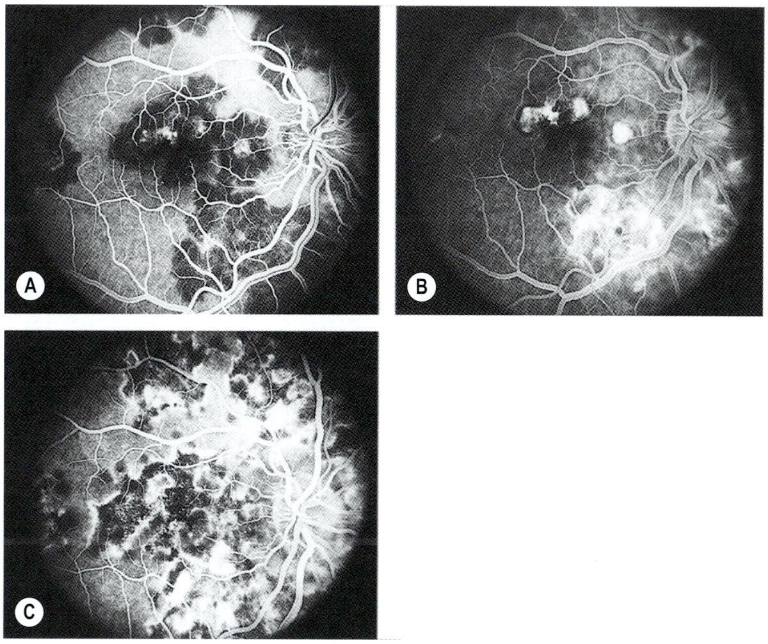

Fig. 30.7 (A) Early blockage of lesions seen on fluorescein angiography. (B) Late hyperfluorescence seen in the inferior portion of the same lesion. (C) Extensive hyperfluorescence seen in the angiogram of an eye with old acute posterior multifocal placoid pigment epitheliopathy (APMMPE).

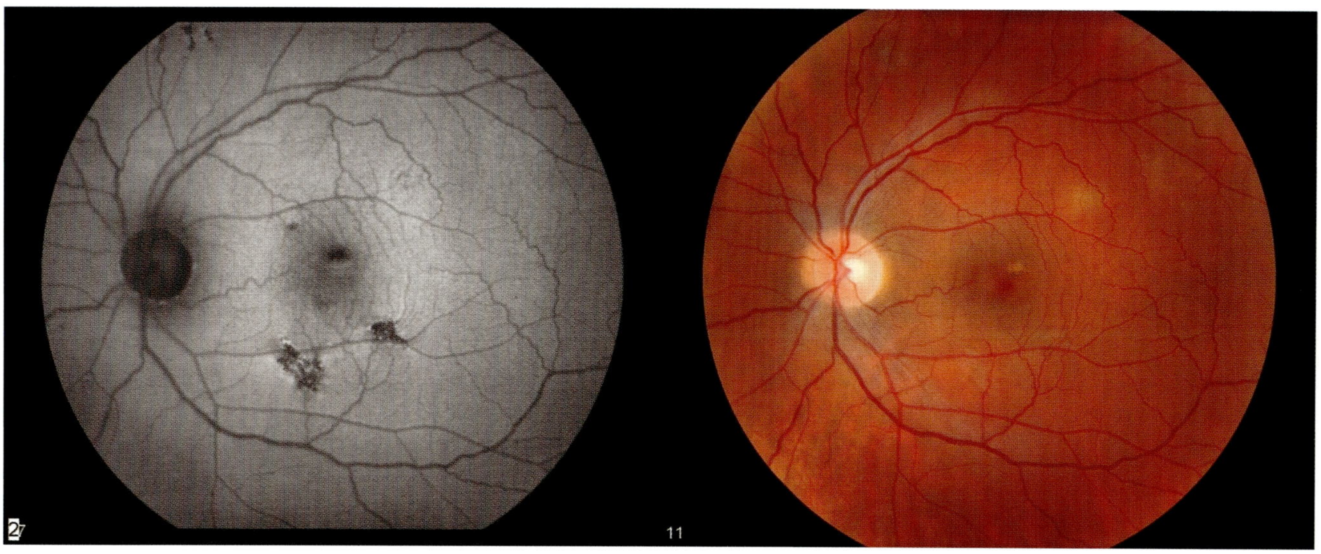

Fig. 30.8 An example of autofluorescence showing areas of hypofluorescence that do not correlate with the fundus lesions that are visible.

disappeared with steroid therapy. It has been associated with diseases that may have a significant vasculitis component, such as Wegener granulomatosis[102] and scleritis.[103] APMPPE has been diagnosed in a patient with juvenile rheumatoid arthritis and was treated with cyclosporin and prednisone.[104] APMPPE may not be a specific disease but rather a response of the RPE or the choroid to various disease processes (Fig. 30.9).

In his initial description, Gass[80] believed that the site of the lesion in APMPPE was at the level of the RPE or was caused by an abnormality in choroidal perfusion with secondary involvement of the RPE. EOG is markedly impaired during the acute phase of the disease, supporting the concept of RPE involvement.[85] Isolated areas of choroidal nonperfusion inside placoid lesions suggest that the primary lesion is impaired filling of the choroid,[97] perhaps as a result of choroidal vasculitis.[105] It is now thought that the choroidal vasculature is obstructed at the level of the precapillary arterioles. It is interesting to note that true vasculitis, such as Wegener granulomatosis, can produce ocular lesions that resemble those of APMPPE.[106] The varying sizes of the APMPPE lesions could support the hypothesis of choroidal hypoperfusion. It is possible that APMPPE is part of a spectrum of choroidal perfusion abnormalities, and, as Young et al.[97] suggested, patients with more confluent lesions may have a less favorable clinical course compared with those with APMPPE; yet the lesions appear to have the same root cause—choroidal ischemia with secondary involvement of the RPE. The photoreceptors are most likely involved in this ischemic process, accounting for the visual loss and the slow recovery of sensitive measures of photoreceptor function, such as the Stiles-Crawford effect.[85] Patients with unilateral lesions but bilateral perfusion abnormalities have been described, further supporting the choroidal location of the disease process. The variability in the degree of choroidal ischemia may explain some of the unusual sequelae of APMPPE, such as subretinal

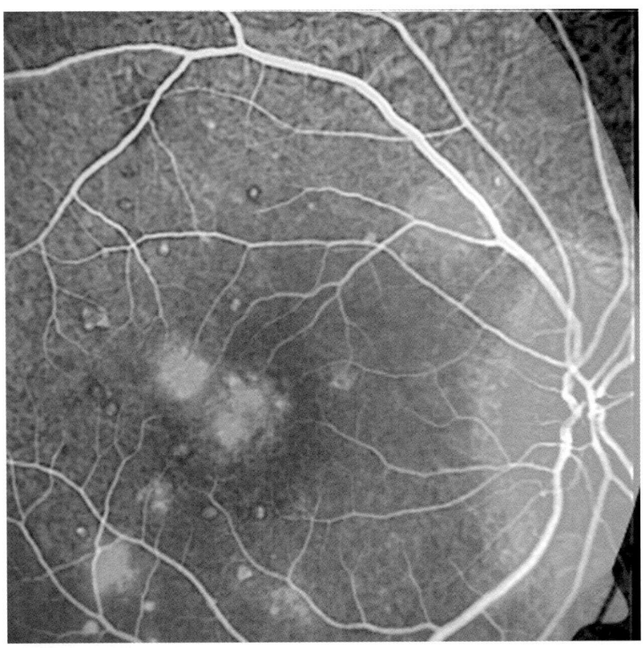

Fig. 30.9 Indocyanine green (ICG) angiogram superimposed on the fluorescein angiogram of a patient in the early stages of "ampiginous" choroiditis. "White" lesions are those seen on fluorescein angiography, and dark lesions are those seen on ICG angiography. Here, curiously, there is a good correlation between the two tests. This is unlike other observations, which found more lesions on ICG angiography than on fluorescein angiography. (Courtesy Ronald Buggage, MD, and Sunil Srivastava, MD.)

neovascular membranes. Preceding viral illnesses are certainly often reported and raise the possibility of a localized viral infection. Bodine et al.[107] reported one case they believed was associated with Lyme disease. A variant of APMPPE termed *panretinal APMPPE,* reported by Baxter and Opremcak in 2013, is linked to HLA-A3 and HLA-C7.[108] All patients had a viral prodrome and a characteristic 4- to 8-week course, as is common in APMPPE, but lesions that extended into the peripheral retina, as is seen in RPC and AC, as discussed later in the chapter.

Therapy

Most patients with APMPPE have a good visual prognosis and do not require therapy. Some authors have used systemic corticosteroid therapy, but it is difficult to assess its value in view of the overall favorable prognosis. In one study[109] in which patients with APMPPE were followed up for an extended period, lack of responsiveness to steroid therapy was corroborated, and more than one-quarter of the eyes had a vision of 6/24 or less. However, in one patient with CME secondary to APMPPE, intravitreal injection of steroid was reported to improve vision and cause regression of the CME.[110] In severe cases with papillitis and retinal vasculitis, we believe there is little harm in beginning a course of oral corticosteroid early in the course because it may lead to faster resolution of the lesions and hence less damage. The reported varying responses may reflect the fact that we are seeing a manifestation of many different inflammatory mechanisms, some that are short lived and clear without intervention and others that are chronic and need therapy.

SUBRETINAL FIBROSIS AND UVEITIS SYNDROME

Clinical Findings

Palestine et al. reported on the first three patients with subretinal fibrosis and uveitis syndrome.[111] This rare entity[112,113] is characterized by chronic inflammation in the vitreous, with whitish-yellow subretinal lesions that appear to be gliotic or fibrotic (Figs. 30.10A and B). These lesions can coalesce to form a large sheet of fibrotic-appearing material and progress to encompass the whole posterior pole, resulting in loss of vision. However, in some patients, the progression may not continue, and a steady state may be reached; or the lesion may encircle but not encroach on the macula (see Fig. 30.10C). Sometimes, although the macula is not directly involved, CME may result, with a subsequent drop in visual acuity. The vitreal inflammatory response may be quite marked, and there may be a low-to-moderate anterior chamber response. In our experience, patients with this syndrome mostly were young women, mostly African American; and in all but one, the disease was bilateral. The number of cases followed up is still too small to define the ultimate visual outcome in these patients. A similar clinical finding of progressive subretinal fibrosis has been seen after ocular surgery and has been hypothesized to be a variant of sympathetic ophthalmia.[114] Our patients had no such history. Subretinal fibrosis can be a sequela to almost any inflammatory condition stimulating the RPE region, particularly with retinal elevation. It has been noted in conjunction with multifocal choroiditis[115] and associated with longstanding ulcerative colitis.[116]

It is interesting to note that the entity may have been reported by Fuchs in his 1949 *Atlas of the Ocular Fundus.*[117] In it, Fuchs described an "extremely rare" bilateral condition in which there were large areas of connective tissue formation under the retina, leading to a severe drop in visual acuity.

Laboratory Findings

In patients with more advanced disease, ERG and EOG show markedly diminished values. ERG may show changes in both rod and cone functions. Fluorescein angiography shows predominantly subretinal alterations. In the early phase of angiography, one may see multiple areas of blockage of choroidal fluorescence and hyperfluorescence. In the later phase, staining of the lesions without leakage can be noted. In the acute phase of this disease, OCT shows subretinal fluid associated with the areas of fibrosis.

Laboratory testing does not appear to be contributory. Culturing of peripheral lymphocytes has not demonstrated an in vitro anamnestic response to retinal antigens, such as the S-antigen.

We performed immunohistochemical evaluation of two eyes with this entity[118,119] (Fig. 30.11) and observed a markedly inflamed choroid with a predominance of B cells and plasma cells. Complement and IgG were deposited above the Bruch membrane. In one eye, granulomatous lymphocytic infiltrate was present in the choroid. Of the T-cell subpopulations, there was a predominance of the helper/inducer subset. Müller cells expressed class II antigens. There were no circulating antiretinal antibodies, and virus could not be cultured from the specimen. The subretinal fibrosis contained islands of cells that were interpreted as originating from the RPE. The impression was that a dysregulation leading to a B-cell disorder with antibody and complement deposition occurs. This leads to retinal and RPE damage and to the development of fibrosis. Without any definitive data to date, one can only speculate as to what is at the basis of this B-cell dysregulation and whether the B cells are the cause of the fibrosis. One possible explanation is that the two are not related but rather cause a shift in T-cell subsets, from a helper T cell type 1 (Th1) response to a Th2 profile. Whereas Th1 cells would produce IFN and interleukin (IL)-2, Th2 inducer cells would produce a lymphokine cascade rich in IL-4, which could stimulate B cells, and transforming growth factor (TGF)-β, a lymphokine associated with scarring and fibrosis.

Although we believe that subretinal fibrosis and uveitis syndrome is a distinct condition, as do Cantrill and Folk,[120] several other conditions could mimic its clinical features. Long-standing retinal detachment can lead to subretinal fibrosis. Ocular inflammatory conditions to consider include sarcoidosis, ocular histoplasmosis syndrome, APMPPE, syphilis, tuberculosis, birdshot retinochoroidopathy, pathologic myopia, acute macular neuroretinopathy,[121] sympathetic ophthalmia, and toxoplasmosis.

Therapy

In the acute phase of subretinal fibrosis and uveitis syndrome, there is significant subretinal fluid and CME. The fluid seems to respond to corticosteroid therapy, resulting in an increase in visual

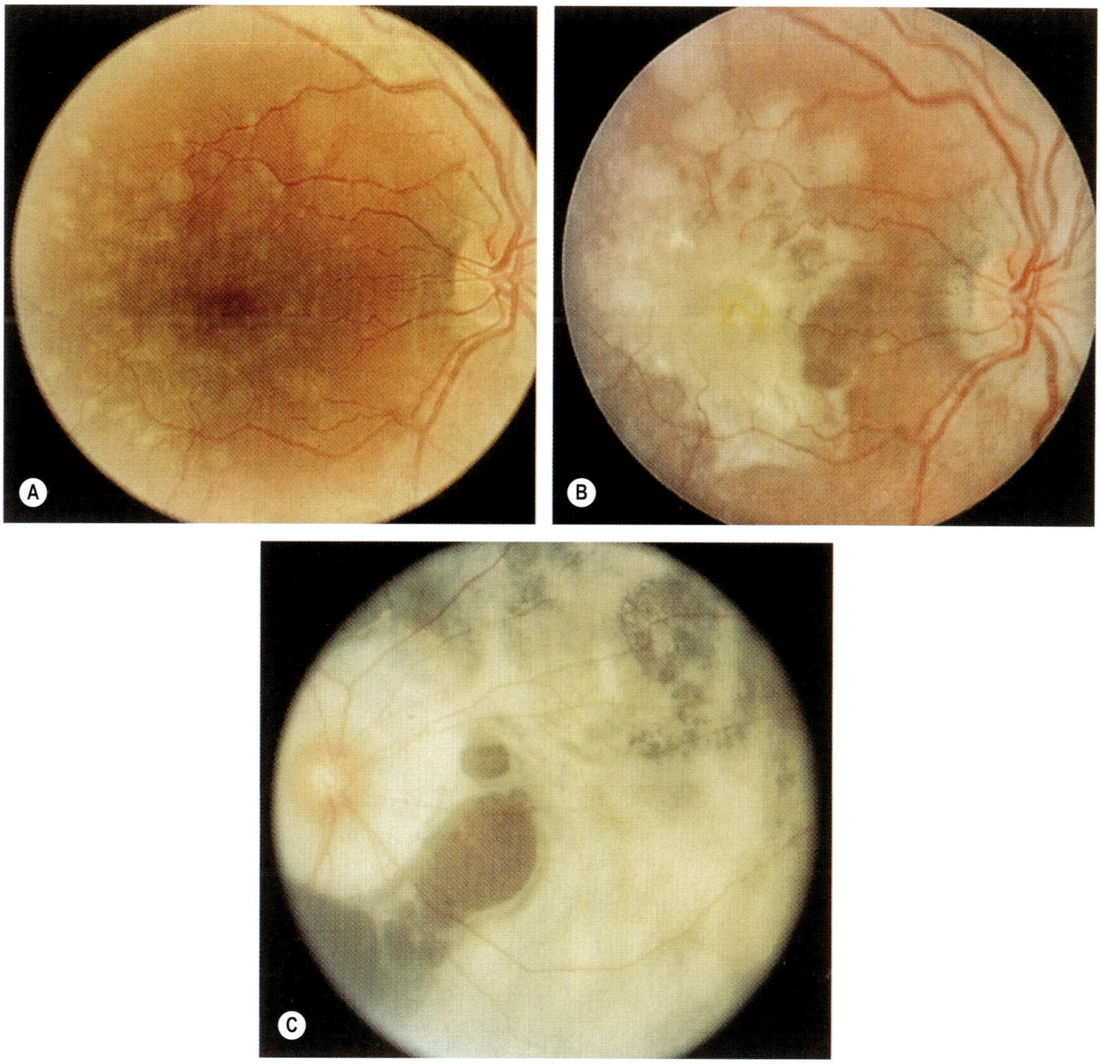

Fig. 30.10 (A) Early changes of subretinal fibrosis syndrome and uveitis. With time, these changes coalesced to form the picture seen in (B). (C) Extensive subretinal fibrosis involving the disk and then extending into the macular region.

acuity. However, we have not found that our therapeutic intervention has slowed or in any way altered the fibrotic changes, at least in the most advanced or fulminant cases. If diagnosed and treated early with systemic immunosuppression, disease progression can be halted. Fortunately, in some patients, the disease may progress very slowly or stop altogether. Initial corticosteroid therapy would seem appropriate in light of the B-cell nature of the disease. However, it is known that the factors stimulating fibroblast proliferation may not be affected by this kind of therapy. In one patient who was treated with aggressive cytotoxic therapy[107] (cyclophosphamide), the course of the disease was not altered. Cornish et al. reported success in two patients who, on the basis of predominance of B cells found on pathology, were treated with rituxan.[122] In one of our patients, the disease appeared to have been controlled with methotrexate.

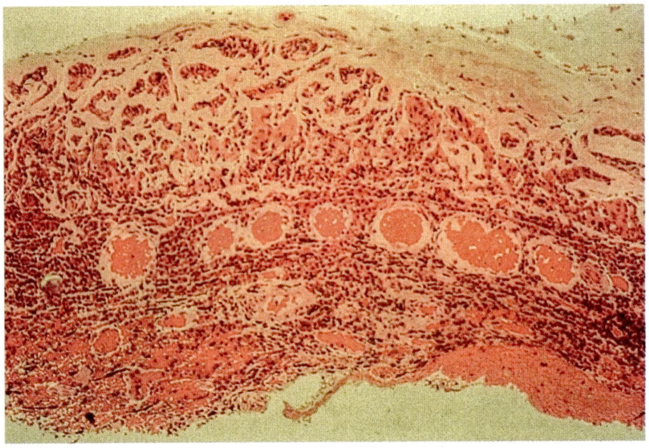

Fig. 30.11 Chorioretinal biopsy specimen from a patient with subretinal fibrosis and uveitis syndrome. There is marked choroidal infiltration by lymphocytes and replacement of normal retinal structures by islands of irregular cells and amorphous connective tissue. Electron microscopic examination revealed that the connective tissue consisted of collagen fibrils and these islands of cells had characteristics suggestive of retinal pigment epithelium (RPE). Both T and B lymphocytes were seen, but there was a differential increase in the number of B cells compared with that in peripheral blood. No virus or other organisms were found either on culture or electron microscopy. (From Palestine AG, Nussenblatt RB, Chan CC, et al. Histopathology of the subretinal fibrosis and uveitis syndrome. *Ophthalmology.* 1985;92:838–844.)

We have also used mycophenolate or methotrexate in combination with adalimumab with successful results in two patients. One report[123] suggested that infliximab was successful in treating one case. Although subretinal changes were seen in that case, it lacked the overwhelming fibrotic appearance that we have noted, but a spectrum of the disease exists.

ACUTE ZONAL OCCULT OUTER RETINOPATHY AND THE AZOOR COMPLEX DISEASES

Gass[124] reported on 13 patients, predominantly young women (77%), with a group of findings that he named *acute zonal occult outer retinopathy* (AZOOR). These changes include rapid loss of one or more large zones of outer retinal function, manifesting as progressive scotomata and photopsia (an important complaint), with minimal funduscopic changes, at least initially. There is little or no clinical evidence of inflammatory disease, but later there may be RPE atrophy. Thus the disorder is characterized by the development of one or more scotomas (readily documented with visual field testing), usually associated with photopsia, in one or both eyes. In spite of the initially minimal funduscopic changes, the ERG findings will be abnormal.[125] Francis et al.[126] suggested that in addition to the clinical findings, the diagnostic criteria should include electrophysiologic changes that show a consistent pattern of dysfunction both at the photoreceptor/RPE complex and at the inner retinal levels. In addition, they found a delayed 30 Hz flicker on ERG and a reduction in light rise on EOG. Full-field ERG performed by Zibrandtsen et al.[127] also revealed alterations in the 30 Hz flicker responses and subnormal photopic responses and a subnormal scotopic response in one case. These authors felt that the findings suggested photoreceptor atrophy. Multifocal electroretinography (mERG) revealed localized outer retinal dysfunction. Several groups have reported OCT abnormalities at the level of the inner and outer retinal segments, as seen in many of these white-dot syndromes.[29,128,129] With time, striking RPE changes occur (Fig. 30.12). Spaide[130] reported extensive autofluorescence and atrophy of the choriocapillaris seen on ICG angiography. During the early stage of the disease, a large number of disorders need to be excluded, including retrobulbar neuritis, a pituitary or an intracranial tumor, and cancer-associated retinopathy. Results of medical and neurologic investigations are usually unrewarding.[124] No autoantibodies to the photoreceptor region have been reported.[125] In the later disease stages, the differential diagnosis includes disorders that

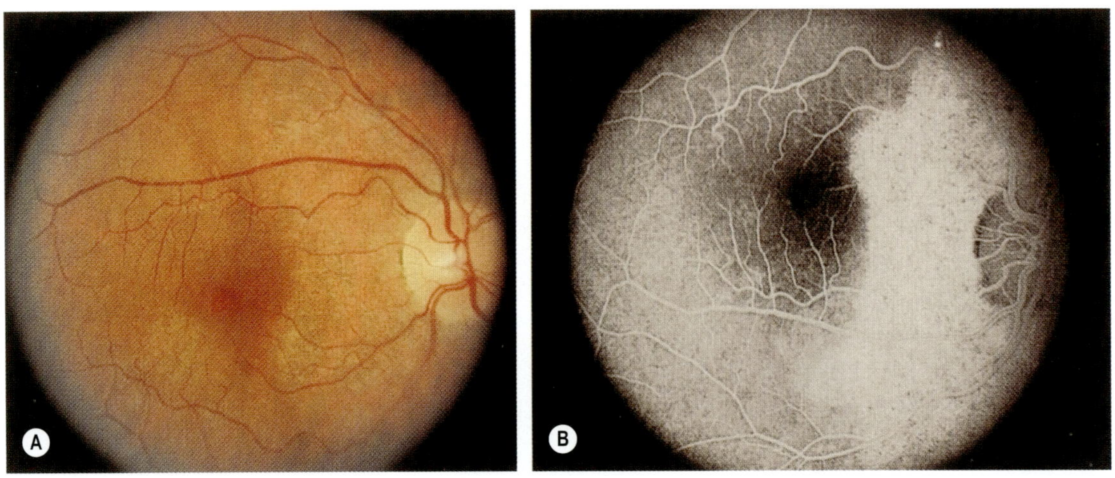

Fig. 30.12 (A) Fundus photograph. (B) Fluorescein angiogram from a patient with acute zonal occult outer retinopathy (AZOOR).

cause retinal vascular narrowing and RPE alterations, including syphilis, retinal vasculitis, and diffuse unilateral subacute neuroretinitis. In a long-term follow-up of 51 patients[131] (37 females and 14 males; average age 33 years), AZOOR was present in one eye in 31 patients (61%) and in both eyes in 20 patients (39%). Eighty-eight percent of patients presented with photopsias, and the fundus was deemed to be normal in 82 eyes. ERG showed depressed values in all eyes, and this finding has been seen by others as well.[132] In the long-term study by Gass (Table 30.1), visual field changes stabilized within 6 months in 37% of patients, progressed in 4%, and partially improved in 24%. A final visual acuity of 20/40 was seen in 68% of eyes, and 18% became legally blind. Changes at the level of the RPE were seen in 43 eyes (48%). Of the patients reviewed, 28% had an autoimmune disease. Immunosuppressive therapy and antiviral medication have been given. The results are difficult to assess, but it would appear that dramatic results have not been seen with these therapies (Table 30.2).

TABLE 30.1 Minimum 3-Year Follow-Up Study of 51 Patients with AZOOR (90 Eyes with 113 Eye Episodes of Visual Loss)

	Number of Patients	Number of Recurrences	Number of Eye Episodes
Duration of follow-up	51 (100)		
Median, 96 months			
Mean, 100 months			
Range, 36–420 months			
Sex			
Female	37 (73%)		
Male	14 (27%)		
Age at onset of AZOOR	51 (100%)		
Median, 33 years			
Mean, 36 years			
Range, 13–63 years			
Race (recorded in 43 patients)			
Caucasian	39 (91%)		
Hispanic	3 (7%)		
Asian	1 (2%)		
Unilateral involvement at onset[a]	31 (61%)		
Bilateral involvement at onset[b]	20 (39%)		
Unilateral at final examination	12 (24%)		
Bilateral at final examination	39 (76%)		
Delayed involvement in fellow eye			
Median, 31 months			
Mean, 50 months			
Range, 2–192 months			
Recurrence of AZOOR	16 (31%)	23	
Median time from onset of AZOOR			
39 months; mean 52 months			
Range, 12–156 months			
Course of visual field loss			
Improvement[c]	13 (20%)		21 (19%)
Stable within 6 months after onset	40 (78%)		87 (77%)
Stepwise progression of visual loss[d]	2 (4%)		4 (4%)
Follow-up <6 months	1 (2%)		1 (1%)
Totals	56[e]	23	113

[a]Monocular in one patient.
[b]Occult in one eye of five (25%) cases.
[c]One patient with improvement worsened after a recurrence and was stable thereafter. Improvement in the visual field in 12 patients persisted for duration of follow-up.
[d]Two patients with 3- and 10-year intervals between onset in the first and second eye had stepwise loss of vision in both eyes.
[e]Five patients had a different course in the two affected eyes.
AZOOR, acute zonal occult outer retinopathy.
Reproduced with permission from Golchet PR, Jampol LM, Wilson D, Yannuzzi LA, Ober M, Stroh E. Persistent placoid maculopathy: a new clinical entity. *Ophthalmology.* 2007;14(8):1530–1540.

A variant of AZOOR perhaps is acute idiopathic blind-spot enlargement syndrome.[17] Findings in this syndrome are similar to those in AZOOR, including photopsias, but the findings on ERG are usually normal and those on focal ERG are abnormal.

Gass described a group of entities identified as "AZOOR complex," which has been referred to as *AZOOR complex of diseases.* These include MEWDS, multifocal choroiditis and PIC, acute idiopathic blind spot enlargement, acute macular neuroretinopathy[124] (Fig. 30.13), acute annular outer retinopathy, and AZOOR. Gass believed that these diseases have an infectious cause.[3] There have been several reports describing patients with one of these entities, such as multifocal choroiditis, which then progresses to what the authors believed is AZOOR.[40,66] An interesting exchange between Gass on one side and Jampol and Becker on the other is found in the literature. Jampol and Becker[133] took the view that these entities are probably discrete but that patients with these diseases share

TABLE 30.2 Comparison of Three White-Dot Syndromes

	Persistent Placoid Maculopathy	Macular Serpiginous Choroiditis[4,6-9,11-13,23]	Acute Posterior Multifocal Placoid Pigment Epitheliopathy[8,18-21]
Lesion characteristics	Long-standing geographic central whitish plaques involving the fovea	Variable sizes and shapes; heal to scars and atrophy in weeks	Multiple postequatorial cream-colored placoid lesions of varying sizes; fade in 1–2 weeks
Visual acuity	Normal to mildly affected (20/20–20/60) with good prognosis for recovery unless complicated by CNV	Rapid decrease in central vision to counting fingers with poor prognosis for recovery	Sudden onset of moderate vision loss, photopsia, and scotomas with excellent prognosis for recovery
Sex	Only 6 patients	Male = female	Male = female
Laterality	Bilateral, symmetric (6/6 patients)	Eventually all bilateral, usually asymmetric	Usually bilateral and symmetric
FA characteristics	Early hypofluorescence, followed by partial filling-in in the late phase	Early hypofluorescence of the central portion of the lesion surrounded by progressive hyperfluorescence at the margins with eventual late staining	Early hypofluorescence, followed by late hyperfluorescence and staining; window defects appear in the quiescent stage
ICG angiography characteristics	Persistent hypofluorescence throughout angiography	Early hypofluorescence with some resolution in the late phase; no staining of lesion borders	Hypofluorescence of the active and healed lesions
Complications	CNV in 11 of 12 eyes, with 9 resulting in disciform macular scars so far; RPE mottling in 1 of 12 eyes	CNV and disciform macular scars in up to 35%; RPE mottling and subretinal scar formation common; RPE detachments and vein and artery occlusions described	Most patients spontaneously recover; rare cases of permanent loss of vision secondary to RPE alterations or CNV; also, reports of CME, papillitis, bilateral central vein occlusions, and associated CNS vasculitis
Clinical course	Persistent lesions with mild decrease in VA unless complicated by CNV or RPE damage	Multiple discrete recurrences usually adjacent to old lesions, variably spaced over many years	Acute transient decrease in VA associated with a viral prodrome and rare recurrences

CME, cystoid macular edema; *CNS,* central nervous system; *CNV,* choroidal neovascularization; *FA,* fluorescein angiography; *ICG,* indocyanine green; *RPE,* retinal pigment epithelium; *VA,* visual acuity.

From Golchet PR, Jampol LM, Wilson D, Yannuzzi LA, Ober M, Stroh E. Persistent placoid maculopathy: a new clinical entity. *Ophthalmology.* 2007;114(8):1530–1540.

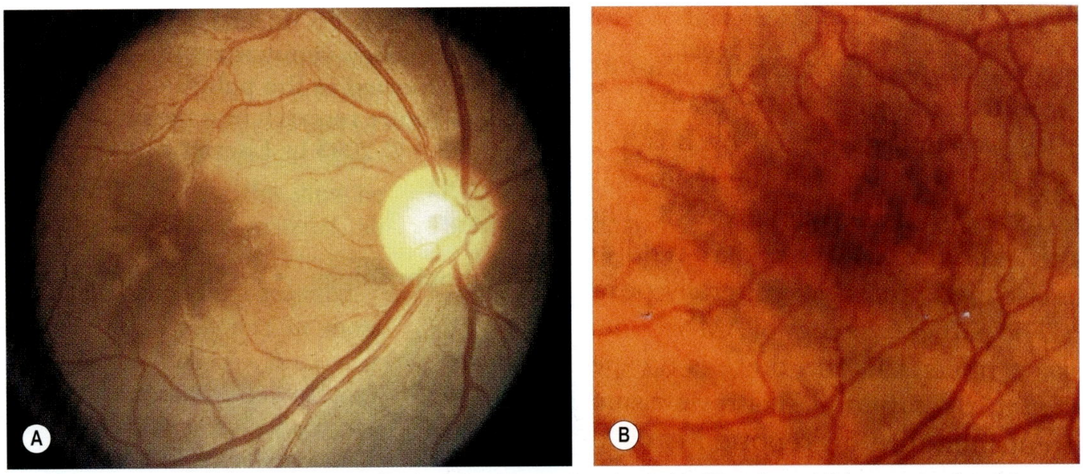

Fig. 30.13 (A and B) Two examples of acute macular neuroretinopathy. Note the reddish-orange color of the lesions. (Reproduced with permission from Turbeville SD, Cowan LD, Gass JD, et al. Acute macular neuroretinopathy, a review of the literature. *Surv Ophthamol.* 2003;48:1.)

common non–disease-specific genes and that environment and other factors trigger the manifestation of the disease seen clinically. We are beginning to see this appellation applied to many disorders in which the visual field alterations may not fit the clinical fundus appearance, moving away from Gass's original grouping of the disorders.[134] One example is AZOOR described as being associated with pars planitis.[135]

RELENTLESS PLACOID CHOROIDITIS, AMPIGINOUS CHOROIDITIS, AND PERSISTENT PLACOID MACULOPATHY

Clinical Findings

RPC, AC, and persistent placoid maculopathy (PPM) represent a spectrum of clinical appearances bridging the white-dot syndromes discussed in this chapter with serpiginous choroiditis (see Chapter 29). RPC was first described by Jones in 2000 as choroiditis with initial acute features similar to those of APMPPE but with lesions that continued to occur and progress and that also involved the more peripheral retina.[136] As noted earlier, AC is most likely the same clinical entity as RPC. PPM was first described in 2007 by Golchet as having some characteristic of serpiginous choroiditis, with a large posterior pole whitish plaque lesion and reasonably good vision in the early course until onset of CNV.[137] Imaging of and therapy for these entities are more completely discussed in Chapter 29, but the fact that there is an overlapping spectrum of clinical appearances among APMPPE, RPC, AC, PPM, and serpiginous choroiditis demonstrates that appearance alone, even when supplemented by current ophthalmic imaging, may not classify these diseases into categories that can be investigated for specific etiologies. These disease entities mentioned above may represent a pathologic response altered by other patient factors, such as genetics, and the appearance may not be specific to the etiology. Table 30.2 provides a comparison of three white-dot syndromes.

ONE DISEASE OR SEVERAL?

The entities discussed here have been discretely described in the past.[138-140] They are believed, by some, to be essentially one entity that expresses itself clinically in multiple ways, but it is our belief that they can be clinically differentiated. More importantly, some white-dot diseases, such as multifocal choroiditis, are much more likely to require long-term therapy compared with MEWDS or APMPPE. Furthermore, until we learn more about the underlying mechanisms, we cannot really speculate as to whether these are all separate entities or simply variations on a single theme. However, there are strong reasons to distinguish them on the basis of clinical findings because doing so is helpful in predicting the ultimate visual outcome in an individual patient. Because we are dealing with a range of disorders—from those that are not sight threatening and resolve without therapy to others for which we have no effective therapy and which have the potential to cause severe visual handicap—it would seem that their recognition on clinical grounds and their very different natural histories would justify our noting them as separate conditions. It is, however, important to remember that many believe that these disorders represent a spectrum of basically the same underlying disorder. Gass,[124] for instance, would place some disorders, such as MEWDS, multifocal choroiditis, and geographic atrophy of the RPE, under the rubric of AZOOR with focal fundus lesions. To date, no direct viral mechanism has been substantiated. It is also true that several reports seem to indicate various white-dot syndrome entities in the same eye at different points in time.[40,66] Even the presence of CNV may be the first manifestation of many of these white-dot syndromes, MEWDS, multifocal choroiditis, and PIC.[141] However, it may be that the eye can react at the level of the RPE in only a limited number of ways despite the fact that the initiating events may be quite different. AZOOR has been described to occur after a car accident.[142]

CASE 30.1

A 24-year-old Hispanic woman came to the eye clinic because of poor vision in her right eye for 3 months. Testing revealed hand motion vision in the right eye and 20/20 in the left eye.

Examination of the right eye showed extensive subretinal fibrosis, extending from around the disk and encompassing essentially all of the posterior pole. The left eye was normal. A workup was performed to rule out several disorders, including syphilis, tuberculosis, and sarcoid, and testing results supported none of these diagnoses. Results of the patient's toxoplasmosis titer were positive. She was thought to have subretinal fibrosis with uveitis syndrome. Because the right eye had such poor vision, it was decided not to treat her. She returned 3 months later with a complaint of decreased vision in the left eye. Visual acuity was hand motions in the right eye and 20/200 in the left eye. Patches of white subretinal fibrosis associated with a vitreal response were noted. The patient was prescribed a regimen of 80 mg prednisone daily, but her vision continued to diminish, and new lesions were noted. An alkylating agent was added to the prednisone. Despite this therapy, vision in the left eye continued to decrease until it reached that of the right eye.

Comment 30.1. Many cases of subretinal fibrosis will not proceed inexorably to poor vision. We have noted patients whose vision will stabilize, and a few of these had unilateral disease. However, the ideal therapy for this potentially sight-threatening, predominantly B-cell disease, is lacking.

CASE 30.2

A 53-year-old Japanese American woman with myopia had a small symptomatic retinal hole noted on a routine ocular examination. This was treated with laser therapy. Some months later, the patient noticed floaters and decreased visual acuity. She was found to have in the right eye 1+ vitreal cells and multiple creamy-white lesions strewn throughout the posterior pole and extending toward the equator. Despite prednisone therapy, her vision continued to decline in that eye. After a macular hemorrhage, her vision dropped to 20/400, and fibrosis ensued. Some months later, the same problem occurred in her left eye. The patient's vision decreased somewhat to 20/30, with multiple creamy-white lesions being seen in the fundus. She underwent an extensive evaluation to uncover the underlying reason for what was diagnosed as a multifocal choroiditis. Results of lumbar puncture were normal, as were those of gallium scanning and conjunctival biopsy. Of interest was the finding of elevated serum titers for herpes simplex 1 (1:2560), herpes simplex 2 (1:320), and herpes zoster (1:640). Because of this finding, the patient was given a short course of acyclovir, but the lesions continued to evolve, and new ones were seen. The progression in the left eye continued along the same course as that seen in the right, and neither antiviral nor immunosuppressive therapy was effective in altering the course of the disease.

Thus the ophthalmologist was presented with a diagnostic dilemma. Because the macula in the left eye was threatened, it was decided to perform chorioretinal biopsy. There was mild atrophy of the inner retinal layers. The choroid was filled with B cells and plasma cells. At the level of the retinal pigment epithelium (RPE), there were nodules resembling Dalen-Fuchs nodules but that were made up predominantly of B cells. Virus could not be detected by using immunofluorescence, electron microscopy, or culture. It was decided to treat the patient

Continued

CASE 30.2—cont'd

with cyclophosphamide. The reasons for this decision were that (1) there was no evidence of active infection and (2) with a predominantly B-cell infiltrate, cyclosporin—with its effect being essentially on the T-cell arm of the immune response—would not be indicated. The patient's ocular disease responded rapidly to cyclophosphamide (initial dose 2 mg/kg, then lowered) combined with 17.5 mg of prednisone. The lesions involuted, and cytotoxic medication was stopped after about 1 year. The patient's eyes have shown no inflammatory activity for more than 3 years after therapy was stopped. The patient required cataract extraction in the right eye, from which a biopsy specimen was obtained, but her visual acuity, 20/400 in the right eye and 20/30 in the left eye, has been maintained.

Comment 30.2. The white-dot syndromes still remain problematic. Chorioretinal biopsy helped enormously in determining a therapeutic approach. In addition, the finding of B cells in this disease was quite unexpected. We have seen a similar finding in a biopsy specimen of another patient with this disorder. It is interesting to note that T-cell infiltrates at this level of the eye can look clinically essentially the same.[31]

REFERENCES

1. Callanan D, Gass J. Multifocal choroiditis and choroidal neovascularization associated with the multiple evanescent white dot and acute idiopathic blind spot enlargement syndrome. *Ophthalmology*. 1992;99(11):1678–1685.
2. Ben Ezra D, Forrester JV. Fundal white dots: the spectrum of a similar pathological process. *Br J Ophthalmol*. 1995;79:856–860.
3. Gass JD. Editorial: Are acute zonal occult outer retinopathy and the white spot syndromes (AZOOR complex) specific autoimmune diseases? *Am J Ophthalmol*. 2003;135:380–381.
4. Grand MG, Storch GA. Presumed parvovirus B19-associated retinal pigment epitheliopathy. *Retina*. 2000;20:199–202.
5. Jampol L, Sieving PA, Pugh D, et al. Multiple evanescent white dot syndrome. I. Clinical findings. *Arch Ophthalmol*. 1984;102:671–674.
6. Kozielec GF, Wyhinny GJ, Jampol LM. Evolution of distinct chorioretinal scars in recurrent MEWDS. *Retina*. 2001;21:180–182.
7. Mamalis N, Daily M. Multiple evanescent white-dot syndrome. A report of eight cases. *Ophthalmology*. 1987;94:1209–1212.
8. Lim JI, Kokame GT, Douglas JP. Multiple evanescent white dot syndrome in older patients. *Am J Ophthalmol*. 1999;127:725–728.
9. Aaberg T, Campo R, Joffe L. Recurrences and bilaterality in the multiple evanescent white-dot syndrome. *Am J Ophthalmol*. 1985;100:29–37.
10. Meyer R, Jampol L. Recurrences and bilaterality in the multiple evanescent white-dot syndrome. *Am J Ophthalmol*. 1986;101:388–389.
11. Borruat F, Othenin-Girard P, Safran A. Multiple evanescent white dot syndrome. *Klin Monatsbl Augenheilkd*. 1991;198:453–456.
12. Asano T, Kondo M, Kondo N, et al. High prevalence of myopia in Japanese patients with multiple evanescent white dot syndrome. *Jpn J Ophthalmol*. 2004;48(5):486–489.
13. Lu TM, Kuo BI, Chung YM, et al. Murine typhus presenting with multiple white dots in the retina. *Scan J Infect Dis*. 1997;29:632–633.
14. Stangos A, Zaninetti M, Petropoulos I, et al. Multiple evanescent white dot syndrome following simultaneous hepatitis-A and yellow fever vaccination. *Ocul Immunol Inflamm*. 2006;14(5):301–304.
15. Landolfi M, Bhagat N, Langer P, et al. Penetrating trauma associated with findings of multiple evanescent white dot syndrome in the second eye: coincidence or an atypical case of sympathetic ophthalmia? *Retina*. 2004;24(4):637–645.
16. Gliem M, Birtel J, Müller PL, et al. Acute retinopathy in pseudoxanthoma elasticum. *JAMA Ophthalmol*. 2019 Aug 8. https://doi.org/10.1001/jamaophthalmol.2019.2910. Epub ahead of print.
17. Volpe NJ, Rizzo JF 3rd, Lessell S. Acute idiopathic blind spot enlargement syndrome: a review of 27 new cases. *Arch Ophthalmol*. 2001;119(1):59–63.
18. Trese MGJ, Cohen SR, Besirli CG. Recovery of outer retina in acute idiopathic blind spot enlargement (AIBSE). *Am J Ophthalmol Case Rep*. 2016;1:13–15.
19. Sieving P, Fishman GA, Jampol LM, et al. Multiple evanescent white dot syndrome. II. Electrophysiology of the photoreceptors during retinal pigment epithelial disease. *Arch Ophthalmol*. 1984;102:675–679.
20. Feigl B, Haas A, El-Shabrawi Y. Multifocal ERG in multiple evanescent white dot syndrome. *Graefes Arch Clin Exp Ophthalmol*. 2002;240:615–621.
21. van Meel G, Keunen JE, van Norren D, et al. Scanning laser densitometry in multiple evanescent white dot syndrome. *Retina*. 1993;(13):29–35.
22. Boscarino MA, Johnson TM. Microperimetry in multiple evanescent white dot syndrome. *Can J Ophthalmol*. 2007;42(5):743–745.
23. Yenerel NM, Kucumen B, Gorgun E, et al. Atypical presentation of multiple evanescent white dot syndrome (MEWDS). *Ocul Immunol Inflamm*. 2008;16(3):113–115.
24. Gross NE, Yannuzzi LA, Freund KB, et al. Multiple evanescent white dot syndrome. *Arch Ophthalmol*. 2006;124(4):493–500.
25. Ie D, Glaser BM, Murphy RP, et al. Indocyanine green angiography in multiple evanescent white-dot syndrome. *Am J Ophthalmol*. 1994;117:7–12.
26. Tsukamoto E, Yamada T, Kadoi C, et al. Hypofluorescent spots on indocyanine green angiography at the recovery stage in multiple evanescent white dot syndrome. *Ophthalmologica*. 1999;213:336–338.
27. Sikorski BL, Wojtkowski M, Kaluzny JJ, et al. Correlation of spectral optical coherence tomography with fluorescein and indocyanine green angiography in multiple evanescent white dot syndrome. *Br J Ophthalmol*. 2008;92(11):1552–1557.
28. Nguyen MH, Witkin AJ, Reichel E, et al. Microstructural abnormalities in MEWDS demonstrated by ultrahigh resolution optical coherence tomography. *Retina*. 2007;27(4):414–418.
29. Spaide RF, Koizumi H, Freund KB. Photoreceptor outer segment abnormalities as a cause of blind spot enlargement in acute zonal occult outer retinopathy-complex diseases. *Am J Ophthalmol*. 2008;146(1):111–120.
30. Marsiglia M, Gallego-Pinazo R, Cunha de Souza E, et al. Expanded clinical spectrum of multiple evanescent white dot syndrome with multimodal imaging. *Retina*. 2016;36:64–74.
31. Nozik R, Dorsch W. A new chorioretinopathy associated with anterior uveitis. *Am J Ophthalmol*. 1973;76:758–762.
32. Bryan RG, Freund KB, Yannuzzi LA, et al. Multiple evanescent white dot syndrome in patients with multifocal choroiditis. *Retina*. 2002;22:317–322.
33. Gass JD, Hamed LM. Acute macular neuroretinopathy and multiple evanescent white dot syndrome occurring in the same patients. *Arch Ophthalmol*. 1989;107:189–193.
34. Figueroa MS, Ciancas E, Mompean B, et al. Treatment of multiple evanescent white dot syndrome with cyclosporine. *Eur J Ophthalmol*. 2001;11:86–88.
35. Dreyer R, Gass J. Multifocal choroiditis and panuveitis. A syndrome that mimics ocular histoplasmosis. *Arch Ophthalmol*. 1984;102:1776–1784.
36. Morgan C, Schatz H. Recurrent multifocal choroiditis. *Ophthalmol*. 1986;93:1138–1147.
37. Nicolo M, Birò A, Cardillo-Piccolino F, et al. Expression of extradomain-B-containing fibronectin in subretinal choroidal neovascular membranes. *Am J Ophthalmol*. 2003;135:7–13.
38. Khorran K, Jampol L, Rosenberg M. Blind spot enlargement as a manifestation of multifocal choroiditis. *Arch Ophthalmol*. 1991;109:1403–1407.
39. Spaide R, Yannuzzi L, Freund K. Linear streaks in multifocal choroiditis and panuveitis. *Retina*. 1991;11:229–231.
40. Saito A, Saito W, Furudate N, et al. Indocyanine green angiography in a case of punctate inner choroidopathy associated with acute zonal occult outer retinopathy. *Jpn J Ophthalmol*. 2007;51(4):295–300.
41. Vadala M, Lodato G, Cillino S. Multifocal choroiditis: indocyanine green angiographic features. *Ophthalmologica*. 2001;215:16–21.
42. Deutsch T, Tessler H. Inflammatory pseudohistoplasmosis. *Ann Ophthalmol*. 1985;17:461–465.
43. Jakobiec F, Sacks E, Kronish JW, et al. Multifocal static creamy choroidal infiltrates. An early sign of lymphoid neoplasia. *Ophthalmology*. 1987;94(4):397–406.
44. Latkany PA, Jabs DA, Smith JR, et al. Multifocal choroiditis in patients with familial juvenile systemic granulomatosis. *Am J Ophthalmol*. 2002;134:897–904.

45. Holz FG, Kim RY, Schwartz SD, et al. Acute zonal occult outer retinopathy (AZOOR) associated with multifocal choroidopathy. *Eye*. 1994;8(Pt 1):77–83.
46. Grutzmacher R, Henderson D, McDonald PJ, et al. Herpes simplex chorioretinitis in a healthy adult. *Am J Ophthalmol*. 1983;(96):788–794.
47. Tiedeman J. Epstein–Barr viral antibodies in multifocal choroiditis and panuveitis. *Am J Ophthalmol*. 1987;103:659–663.
48. Wong K, D'Amico DJ, Hedges TR 3rd, et al. Ocular involvement associated with chronic Epstein-Barr virus disease. *Arch Ophthalmol*. 1987;105:788–792.
49. Spaide R, Sugin S, Yannuzzi LA, et al. Epstein-Barr virus antibodies in multifocal choroiditis and panuveitis. *Am J Ophthalmol*. 1991;112(4):410–413.
50. Scheider A. Multifocal inner choroiditis. *Ger J Ophthalmol*. 1993;2:1–9.
51. Martin D, Chan CC, de Smet MD, et al. The role of chorioretinal biopsy in the management of posterior uveitis. *Ophthalmology*. 1993;100:5.
52. Shimada H, Yuzawa M, Hirose T, et al. Pathological findings of multifocal choroiditis with panuveitis and punctate inner choroidopathy. *Jpn J Ophthalmol*. 2008;52(4):282–288.
53. Nölle B, Eckardt C. Vitrectomy in multifocal choroiditis. *Ger J Ophthalmol*. 1993;2:14–19.
54. Charteris D, Lee W. Multifocal posterior uveitis: clinical and pathological findings. *Br J Ophthalmol*. 1990;74:688–693.
55. Dunlop AAS, Cree IA, Hague S, et al. Multifocal choroiditis. clinicopathologic correlation. *Arch Ophthalmol*. 1998;116:801–803.
56. Levy J, Shneck M, Klemperer I, et al. Punctate inner choroidopathy: resolution after oral steroid treatment and review of the literature. *Can J Ophthalmol*. 2005;40(5):605–608.
57. Michel SS, Ekong A, Baltatzis S, et al. Multifocal choroiditis and panuveitis. *Ophthalmology*. 2002;109:378–383.
58. Chan WM, Shneck M, Klemperer I, et al. Combined photodynamic therapy and intravitreal triamcinolone for choroidal neovascularization secondary to punctate inner choroidopathy or of idiopathic origin: one-year results of a prospective series. *Retina*. 2008;28(1):71–80.
59. Cirino AC, Mathura JR Jr, Jampol LM. Resolution of activity (choroiditis and choroidal neovascularization) of chronic recurrent punctate inner choroidopathy after treatment with interferon B-1A. *Retina*. 2006;26(9):1091–1092.
60. D'Souza P, Ranjan R, Babu U, Kanakath AV, Saravanan VR. Inflammatory choroidal neovascular membrane: long-term visual and anatomical outcomes after intravitreal anti-vascular endothelial growth factor therapy. *Retina*. 2018;38(7):1307–1315.
61. Spaide RF, Freund KB, Slakter J, et al. Treatment of subfoveal choroidal neovascularization associated with multifocal choroiditis and panuveitis with photodynamic therapy. *Retina*. 2002;22:545–549.
62. Watzke R, Packer AJ, Folk JC, et al. Punctate inner choroidopathy. *Am J Ophthalmol*. 1984;98:572–584.
63. Reddy CV, Brown J Jr, Folk JC, et al. Enlarged blind spots in chorioretinal inflammatory disorders. *Ophthalmology*. 1996;103:606–617.
64. Kedhar SR, Thorne JE, Wittenberg S, et al. Multifocal choroiditis with panuveitis and punctate inner choroidopathy: comparison of clinical characteristics at presentation. *Retina*. 2007;27(9):1174–1179.
65. Gerstenblith AT, Thorne JE, Sobrin L, et al. Punctate inner choroidopathy: a survey analysis of 77 persons. *Ophthalmology*. 2007;114(6):1201–1204.
66. Taira K, Nakazawa M, Takano Y, et al. Acute zonal occult outer retinopathy in the fellow eye 5 years after presentation of punctate inner choroidopathy. *Graefes Arch Clin Exp Ophthalmol*. 2006;244(7):880–882.
67. Zarranz-Ventura J, Sim DA, Keane PA, et al. Characterization of punctate inner choroidopathy using enhanced depth imaging optical coherence tomography. *Ophthalmology*. 2014;121(9):1790–1797.
68. Zhang X, Zuo C, Li M, Chen H, Huang S, Wen F. Spectral-domain optical coherence tomographic findings at each stage of punctate inner choroidopathy. *Ophthalmology*. 2013;120(12):2678–2683.
69. Pohlmann D, Pleyer U, Joussen AM, Winterhalter S. Optical coherence tomography angiography in comparison with other multimodal imaging techniques in punctate inner choroidopathy. *Br J Ophthalmol*. 2019;103(1):60–66.
70. Kim EL, Thanos A, Yonekawa Y, Todorich B, Wolfe J, Randhawa S, Faia LJ. Optical coherence tomography angiography findings in punctate inner choroidopathy. *Ophthalmic Surg Lasers Imaging Retina*. 2017;48(10):786–792.
71. Krill A, Deutman A. Acute retinal pigment epitheliitis. *Am J Ophthalmol*. 1972;74:193–205.
72. Luttrull JK, Chittum ME. Acute retinal pigment epitheliitis. *Am J Ophthalmol*. 1995;120:389–391.
73. Lutrull JR, Chittum ME. Acute retinal pigment epitheliitis. *Am J Ophthalmol*. 1997;123:127–129.
74. Hsu CT, Harlan JB, Goldberg MF, et al. Acute posterior multifocal placoid pigment epitheliopathy associated with a systemic necrotizing vasculitis. *Retina*. 2003;23(1):64–68.
75. Deutman A, Oosterhuis JA, Boen-Tan TN, et al. Acute posterior multifocal placoid pigment epitheliopathy. *Br J Ophthalmol*. 1972;56:863–874.
76. Cho HJ, Han SY, Cho SW, Lee DW, Lee TG, Kim CG, Kim JW. Acute retinal pigment epitheliitis: spectral-domain optical coherence tomography findings in 18 cases. *Invest Ophthalmol Vis Sci*. 2014;55(5):3314–3319.
77. Gilhotra JS, Gilhotra AK, Holdaway IM, et al. Acute retinal pigment epitheliitis associated with intravenous bisphosphonate. *Br J Ophthalmol*. 2006;90(6):798–799.
78. Loh BK, Chee SP. Optical coherence tomography findings in acute retinal pigment epitheliitis. *Am J Ophthalmol*. 2007;143(6):1071. Author reply 1071.
79. Poyato P, et al. Acute retinal pigment epitheliitis: uncommon symptoms in a case report. *Arch Soc Esp Oftalmol*. 2000;1:51–54.
80. Gass J. Acute posterior multifocal placoid pigment epitheliopathy. *Arch Ophthalmol*. 1968;80:177–185.
81. Scuderi G, Recupero S, Valvo A. Acute posterior multifocal placoid pigment epitheliopathy. *Ann Ophthalmol*. 1977;9:189–194.
82. Ryan S, Maumenee A. Acute posterior multifocal placoid pigment epitheliopathy. *Am J Ophthalmol*. 1972;81:403–412.
83. Holt W, Regan A, Trempe C. Acute posterior multifocal placoid pigment epitheliopathy. *Am J Ophthalmol*. 1976;81:403–412.
84. Savino P, Weinberg RJ, Yassin JG, et al. Diverse manifestations of acute posterior multifocal placoid pigment epitheliopathy. *Am J Ophthalmol*. 1974;77:659–662.
85. Smith V, Pokorny J, Ernest JT, et al. Visual function in acute posterior multifocal placoid pigment epitheliopathy. *Am J Ophthalmol*. 1978;85:192–199.
86. Abu El-Asrar AM, Alijazairy AH. Acute posterior multifocal placoid pigment epitheliopathy with retinal vasculitis and papillitis. *Eye*. 2002;16:642–644.
87. Kirkham T, Ffytche T, Sanders M. Placoid pigment epitheliopathy with retinal vasculitis and papillitis. *Br J Ophthalmol*. 1972;56:875–880.
88. Damato B, Nanjiani M, Foulds W. Acute posterior multifocal placoid pigment epitheliopathy. A follow-up study. *Trans Ophthalmol Soc UK*. 1983;103:517–522.
89. Jones BE, Jampol LM, Yannuzzi LA, et al. Relentless placoid chorioretinitis. A new entity or an unusual variant of serpiginous chorioretinitis. *Arch Ophthalmol*. 2000;118:931–938.
90. Fine HF, Kim E, Flynn TE, et al. Acute posterior multifocal placoid pigment epitheliopathy following varicella vaccine. *Br J Ophthalmol*. 2010;94(3):282–283.
91. Borruat FX, Piguet B, Herbort CP. Acute posterior multifocal placoid pigment epitheliopathy following mumps. *Ocul Immunol Inflamm*. 1998;6:189–193.
92. Clearkin L, Hung S. Acute posterior multifocal placoid pigment epitheliopathy associated with transient hearing loss. *Trans Ophthalmol Soc UK*. 1983;103:562–564.
93. Kersten D, Lessell S, Carlow T. Acute posterior multifocal placoid pigment epitheliopathy and late-onset meningo-encephalitis. *Ophthalmology*. 1987;94:393–396.
94. Parmeggiani F, Costagliola C, D'Angelo S, et al. Clear cell renal cell carcinoma associated with bilateral atypical acute posterior multifocal placoid pigment epitheliopathy. *Oncology*. 2004;66(6):502–509.
95. Allee SD, Marks SJ. Acute posterior multifocal placoid pigment epitheliopathy with bilateral central retinal vein occlusion. *Am J Ophthalmol*. 1998;126:309–312.

96. Vedantham V, Ramasamy K. Atypical manifestations of acute posterior multifocal placoid pigment epitheliopathy. *Indian J Ophthalmol.* 2006;54(1):49–52.
97. Young N, Bird A, Sehmi K. Pigment epithelial diseases with abnormal choroidal perfusion. *Am J Ophthalmol.* 1980;90:607–618.
98. Mrejen S, Sarraf D, Chexal S, Wald K, Freund KB. Choroidal involvement in acute posterior multifocal placoid pigment epitheliopathy. *Ophthalmic Surg Lasers Imaging Retina.* 2016;47:20–26.
99. Furino C, Shalchi Z, Grassi MO, et al. OCT angiography in acute posterior multifocal placoid pigment epitheliopathy. *Ophthalmic Surg Lasers Imaging Retina.* 2018;50:428–436.
100. Althaus C, Unsöld R, Figge C, et al. Cerebral complications in acute posterior multifocal placoid pigment epitheliopathy. *Ger J Ophthalmol.* 1993;(2):150–154.
101. Stoll G, Reiners K, Schwartz A, et al. Acute posterior multifocal placoid pigment epitheliopathy with cerebral involvement. *J Neurol Neurosurg Psychiatry.* 1991;54(1):77–79.
102. Chiquet C, Lumbroso L, Denis P, et al. Acute posterior multifocal placoid pigment epitheliopathy associated with Wegener's granulomatosis. *Retina.* 1999;19:309–313.
103. Matsuo T, Horikoshi T, Nagai C. Acute posterior multifocal placoid pigment epitheliopathy and scleritis in a patient with pANCA-positive systemic vasculitis. *Am J Ophthalmol.* 2002;133:566–568.
104. Bridges WJ, Saadeh C, Gerald R. Acute posterior multifocal placoid pigment epitheliopathy in a patient with systemic-onset juvenile rheumatoid arthritis: treatment with cyclosporin A and prednisone. *Arthritis Rheum.* 1995;38:446–447.
105. Spaide R, Yannuzzi L, Slakter J. Choroidal vasculitis in acute posterior multifocal placoid epitheliopathy. *Br J Ophthalmol.* 1991;75:685–687.
106. Kinyoun J, Kalina R, Klein M. Choroidal involvement in systemic necrotizing vasculitis. *Arch Ophthalmol.* 1987;105:939–942.
107. Bodine S, Marino J, Camisa TJ, et al. Multifocal choroiditis with evidence of Lyme disease. *Am J Ophthalmol.* 1992;24:169–173.
108. Baxter KR, Opremcak EM. Panretinal acute multifocal placoid pigment epitheliopathy: a novel posterior uveitis syndrome with HLA-A3 and HLA-C7 association. *J Ophthalmic Inflamm Infect.* 2013;3(1):29.
109. Roberts TV. Acute posterior multifocal placoid pigment epitheliopathy: A long-term study. *Aust NZ J Ophthalmol.* 1997;25:277–281.
110. Yenerel NM, Gorgun E, Dinc UA, et al. Treatment of cystoid macular edema due to acute posterior multifocal placoid pigment epitheliopathy. *Ocul Immunol Inflamm.* 2008;16(1):67–71.
111. Palestine A, Nussenblatt RB, Parver LM, et al. Progressive subretinal fibrosis and uveitis. *Br J Ophthalmol.* 1984;(68):667–673.
112. Gandorfer A, Ulbig MW, Kampik A. Diffuse subretinal fibrosis syndrome. *Retina.* 2000;20:561–563.
113. Kaiser PK, Gragoudas ES. The subretinal fibrosis and uveitis syndrome. *Int Ophthalmol Clin.* 1996;36:145–152.
114. Wang RC, Zamir E, Dugel PU, et al. Progressive subretinal fibrosis and blindness associated with multifocal granulomatous chorioretinitis. A variant of sympathetic ophthalmia. *Ophthalmology.* 2002;109:1527–1531.
115. Amaro MH, Muccioli C, Motta MM. Progressive subretinal fibrosis and multifocal granulomatous chorioretinitis. *Arq Bras Oftalmol.* 2006;69(3):413–415.
116. Fuentes-Paez G, Martínez-Osorio H, Herreras JM, et al. Subretinal fibrosis and uveitis syndrome associated with ulcerative colitis. *Int J Colorectal Dis.* 2007;22(3):333–334.
117. Fuchs A. *Diseases of the Fundus Oculi with Atlas.* Philadelphia: The Blakiston Co; 1949.
118. Palestine A, Nussenblatt RB, Chan CC, et al. Histopathology of the subretinal fibrosis and uveitis syndrome. *Ophthalmology.* 1985;(92):838–844.
119. Kim M, Chan CC, Belfort R Jr, et al. Histopathologic and immunohistopathologic features of subretinal fibrosis and uveitis syndrome. *Am J Ophthalmol.* 1987;104:15–23.
120. Cantrill H, Folk J. Multifocal choroiditis associated with progressive subretinal fibrosis. *Am J Ophthalmol.* 1986;101:170–180.
121. Turbeville SD, Cowan LD, Gass JD. Acute macular neuroretinopathy: A review of the literature. *Surv Ophthalmol.* 2003;48:1–11.
122. Cornish KS, Kuffova L, Forrester JV. Treatment of diffuse subretinal fibrosis uveitis with rituximab. *Br J Ophthalmol.* 2015;99(2):153–154.
123. Adan A, Sanmartí R, Burés A, et al. Successful treatment with infliximab in a patient with diffuse subretinal fibrosis syndrome. *Am J Ophthalmol.* 2007;143(3):533–534.
124. Gass J. Acute zonal occult outer retinopathy. Donders lecture: The Netherlands Ophthalmological Society. Maastricht Holland. *J Clin Neuro-ophthalmol.* 1993;13(2):79–97.
125. Jacobson SG, Morales DS, Sun XK, et al. Pattern of retinal dysfunction in acute zonal occult outer retinopathy. *Ophthalmology.* 1995;102:1187–1198.
126. Francis PJ, Marinescu A, Fitzke FW, et al. Acute zonal occult outer retinopathy: towards a set of diagnostic criteria. *Br J Ophthalmol.* 2005;89(1):70–73.
127. Zibrandtsen N, Munch IC, Klemp K, et al. Photoreceptor atrophy in acute zonal occult outer retinopathy. *Acta Ophthalmol.* 2008;86(8):913–916.
128. Takai Y, Ishiko S, Kagokawa H, et al. Morphological study of acute zonal occult outer retinopathy (AZOOR) by multiplanar optical coherence tomography. *Acta Ophthalmol.* 2009;87(4):408–418.
129. Li D, Kishi S. Loss of photoreceptor outer segment in acute zonal occult outer retinopathy. *Arch Ophthalmol.* 2007;125(9):1194–1200.
130. Spaide RF. Collateral damage in acute zonal occult outer retinopathy. *Am J Ophthalmol.* 2004;138(5):887–889.
131. Gass JD, Agarwal A, Scott IU. Acute zonal occult outer retinopathy: A long-term follow-up study. *Am J Ophthalmol.* 2002;134:329–339.
132. Jacobson DM. Acute zonal occult outer retinopathy and central nervous system inflammation. *J Neuro-ophthalmol.* 1996;16:172–177.
133. Jampol LM, Becker KG. Perspective: White spot syndromes of the retina: a hypothesis based on the common genetic hypothesis of autoimmune/inflammatory disease. *Am J Ophthalmol.* 2003;135:376–379.
134. Song ZM, Sheng YJ, Chen QS, et al. Clinical characteristics of acute zonal occult outer retinopathy in Chinese patients. *Ophthalmologica.* 2008;222(3):149–156.
135. Sharma SM, Watzke RC, Weleber RG, et al. Acute zonal occult outer retinopathy (AZOOR) and pars planitis: a new association? *Br J Ophthalmol.* 2008;92(4):583–584.
136. Jones BE, Jampol LM, Yannuzzi LA, et al. Relentless placoid chorioretinitis: a new entity or an unusual variant of serpiginous chorioretinitis? *Arch Ophthalmol.* 2000;118(7):931–938.
137. Golchet PR, Jampol LM, Wilson D, Yannuzzi LA, Ober M, Stroh E. Persistent placoid maculopathy: a new clinical entity. *Ophthalmology.* 2007;114(8):1530–1540.
138. Jampol LM, Wiredu A. MEWDS, MFC, PIC, AMN, AIBSE, AZOOR: one disease or many? *Retina.* 1995;15(5):373–378.
139. Teyssot N, Bodaghi B, Cassoux N, et al. Acute posterior multifocal placoid pigment epitheliopathy, serpiginous and multifocal choroiditis: etiological and therapeutic management. *J Fr Ophthalmol.* 2006;29(5):510–518.
140. Matsumoto Y, Haen SP, Spaide RF. The white dot syndromes. *Compr Ophthalmol Update.* 2007;8(4):179–200. Discussion 203–204.
141. Machida S, Fujiwara T, Murai K, et al. Idiopathic choroidal neovascularization as an early manifestation of inflammatory chorioretinal diseases. *Retina.* 2008;28(5):703–710.
142. Sadaba LM, Moreno J, Sáinz C, et al. AZOOR. After whiplash injury. *Rev Med Univ Navarra.* 2001;45(4):35–38.

31

Masquerade Syndromes

Scott M. Whitcup

KEY CONCEPTS

- The masquerade syndromes comprise a group of disorders that mimic an ocular inflammatory disease but require specific treatment other than, or in addition to, anti-inflammatory therapy.
- Because many of the masquerade syndromes are malignancies or infectious processes, early diagnosis and prompt treatment are critical.
- Intraocular lymphomas, sometimes called *vitreoretinal lymphomas*, are frequently primary central nervous system (CNS) lymphomas (non-Hodgkin lymphoma [NHL] involving the CNS).
- Intraocular disease with concomitant brain involvement is a poor prognostic factor for primary CNS lymphoma.
- Diagnosis can be made by identifying malignant cells in the vitreous or cerebrospinal fluid; however, prompt and correct handling of specimens and review by an experienced cytopathologist are critical to making the correct diagnosis.
- Nonmalignant masquerade syndromes are often treated with unnecessary anti-inflammatory therapy.
- Response to anti-inflammatory therapy does not rule out a masquerade syndrome; however, lack of a response to therapy should suggest the possibility of a masquerade syndrome.
- The diagnosis of masquerade syndrome should be considered in all cases of idiopathic uveitis.

The masquerade syndromes comprise a group of disorders that mimic an ocular inflammatory disease requiring anti-inflammatory therapy. These disorders are often misdiagnosed as chronic idiopathic uveitis. The term *masquerade syndrome* was first used in the ophthalmic literature in 1967 to describe conjunctival carcinoma manifesting as a case of chronic conjunctivitis[1]; today, however, it is used most commonly to describe disorders simulating chronic uveitis. Because many of the masquerade syndromes are malignant processes, early diagnosis and prompt treatment are critical (Box 31.1). Other disorders, such as retinal degenerations and intraocular foreign body, can also masquerade as uveitis, and, again, misdiagnosis frequently leads to inappropriate therapy. There is a semantic debate on whether certain infectious conditions, such as *Propionibacterium acnes* endophthalmitis or herpes simplex virus–associated uveitis, should be considered a masquerade syndrome. Some experts exclude any ocular infections from the masquerade syndromes, but I prefer to include them when they are not easily recognized as infectious diseases, especially because these ocular infections can mimic idiopathic uveitis and cause adverse sequelae when treated with anti-inflammatory therapy alone. I prefer to limit the diagnosis of masquerade syndromes to malignancies and conditions where an underlying inflammatory disease or infection is not the main cause of the pathology and where anti-inflammatory therapy alone may be inappropriate to optimize patient outcomes. Examples include infections, where antimicrobial therapy is warranted; malignancy, where cancer treatment is required; adverse reactions to medications, where the offending therapy should be stopped; or trauma, where an intraocular foreign body should be removed. There are also conditions that mimic intraocular inflammation where no therapy is needed, such as asteroid hyalosis. The focus of this chapter is on the malignant conditions that can masquerade as uveitis, but nonmalignant disorders often misdiagnosed as chronic idiopathic ocular inflammatory disease are also discussed.

INTRAOCULAR LYMPHOMA

Although intraocular lymphoma can be a lethal disease, early diagnosis and treatment can improve the prognosis. This disease was previously misnamed "reticulum cell sarcoma" because the large malignant cells were thought to resemble sarcoma cells. However, these tumors are more appropriately classified as intraocular large-cell lymphomas. The term *primary vitreoretinal lymphoma* (PVRL) is being used to describe primary central nervous system lymphoma (PCNSL) involving the eye.

Several types of lymphoma can involve the eye and mimic uveitis. Hodgkin disease, which is characterized by painless lymphadenopathy, fever, night sweats, weight loss, and the presence of Reed-Sternberg cells on histologic examination, can involve the eye. Ocular involvement in Hodgkin lymphoma is relatively rare and usually occurs late in the course of the disease.[2] In one case reported in the ophthalmic literature, the patient with Hodgkin disease had retinal periphlebitis as the initial clinical finding.[3] Other ocular manifestations include iritis or chorioretinitis with associated vitritis. In addition, paraneoplastic retinopathy associated with Hodgkin lymphoma has been reported.[4]

Two clinically distinct forms of non-Hodgkin lymphoma (NHL) more frequently involve the eye: NHL of the central nervous system (CNS), more commonly called *PCNSL*; and systemic NHL, which metastasizes to the eye. Patients with systemic NHL metastatic to the eye are usually quite ill, with fever, lymphadenopathy, and weight loss. Diagnosis in these patients is rarely puzzling. In contrast, the patient with PCNSL with initial manifestation of ocular findings often poses a diagnostic dilemma.

Primary Central Nervous System Lymphoma

PCNSL arises from the brain, spinal cord, leptomeninges, or eyes and may then spread throughout the CNS.[5-7] Systemic spread outside the

BOX 31.1 Ophthalmic Conditions Masquerading as Idiopathic Uveitis

Malignant Disorders

Intraocular lymphomas
- Non-Hodgkin lymphoma of central nervous system
- Systemic non-Hodgkin lymphoma metastatic to eye
- Hodgkin lymphoma

Leukemia

Carcinoma metastatic to eye
- Lung
- Renal
- Breast

Uveal melanoma

Childhood malignancies
- Retinoblastoma
- Leukemia
- Medulloepithelioma
- Juvenile xanthogranuloma

Paraneoplastic syndromes
- Cancer-associated retinopathy
- Melanoma-associated retinopathy
- Bilateral diffuse uveal melanocytic proliferation

Nonmalignant Disorders

Intraocular foreign body

Retinal detachment

Myopic degeneration

Pigment dispersion syndrome

Retinal degenerations

Postoperative infections
- Fungal
- *Propionibacterium acnes*

Postvaccination disorders and drug reactions

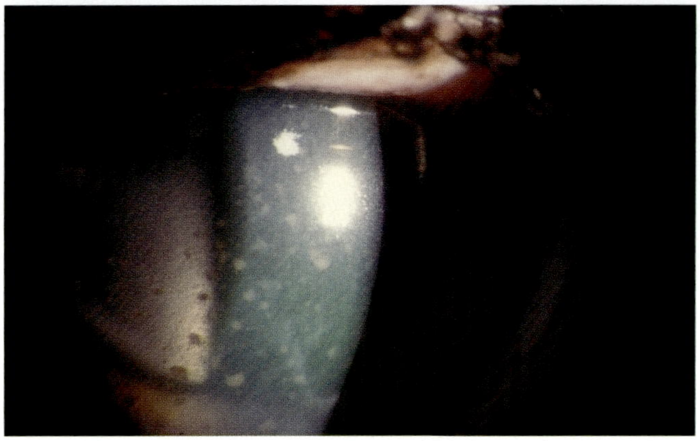

Fig. 31.1 Anterior segment of the eye of a patient with biopsy-proven intraocular large-cell lymphoma demonstrating corneal keratic precipitates.

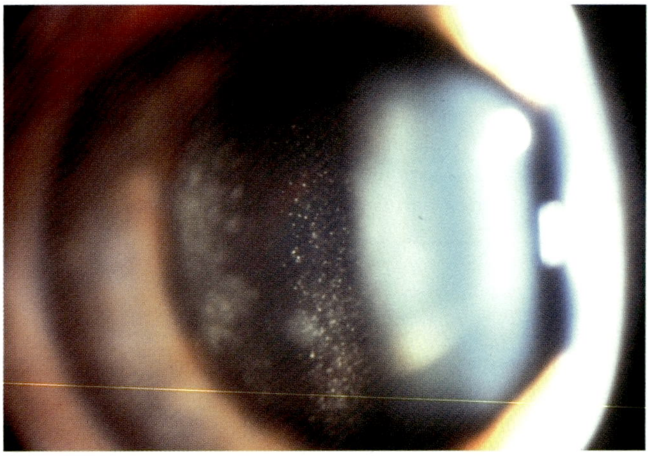

Fig. 31.2 Slit-lamp biomicroscopy examination revealing sheets of vitreous cells characteristic of intraocular lymphoma in two patients with primary central nervous system lymphoma (PCNSL).

CNS occurs more rarely and has been reported in fewer than 10% of autopsies.[8,9] Although PCNSL is a rare tumor, some data suggest that its incidence is increasing,—an increase that cannot be fully explained by the prevalence of acquired immunodeficiency syndrome (AIDS) or other causes of immunosuppression.[10] The incidence of PCNSL reported in the U.S. Central Brain Tumor Registry was 0.46 per 100,000 person-years in the period 2004 to 2007.[11] Ocular involvement has been reported in 15% to 25% of patients with PCNSL.[12]

The median age for patients with PCNSL is 50 to 60 years; there is a slight male preponderance.[5,10] Cases of PCNSL in children have been reported,[13,14] and intraocular lymphomas have been reported in patients 15 and 27 years of age.[15,16] Ocular lymphoma has now been associated with AIDS.[17] In addition, ocular lymphoma has been reported in a number of patients undergoing immunosuppression after organ transplantation.[18]

In a large case series by Hochberg and Miller,[10] four distinct clinical profiles were observed in patients with PCNSL: (1) solitary or multiple discrete intracranial nodules, (2) diffuse meningeal or periventricular lesions, (3) subretinal infiltrates or vitritis, and (4) localized intradural spinal masses. Ocular involvement may precede detectable disease in other parts of the CNS, although the percentage of patients in whom this occurs may be overestimated in the reports in the ophthalmic literature because of selection bias with regard to patients with ocular disease. In a study performed at the National Eye Institute (NEI), two-thirds of the patients with ocular disease had undiagnosed CNS disease at the time of their diagnosis.[19] The mean time between the onset of ocular symptoms and the onset of CNS symptoms in one study was 29 months (range, 7–108 months).[20] In this study, systemic spread outside the CNS was noted in 6% of patients, and disease was limited to the eye in 22%.

The most common ocular symptoms associated with intraocular lymphoma are blurred vision and floaters; redness and pain are rare. Patients have reduced visual acuity, although vision is usually better than one would expect from the clinical examination. Slit-lamp biomicroscopic examination often reveals mild anterior segment inflammation, with aqueous cells and flare and keratic precipitates (KPs) on the corneal endothelium (Fig. 31.1).[7,15,19-21] Anterior synechiae are not associated with the disease. Vitreous cells, occurring in sheets, are typical of the disease (Fig. 31.2), and examination of the fundus usually shows subretinal yellow infiltrates through a hazy vitreous (Fig. 31.3). Atypical presentations have been reported, including a hemorrhagic retinal vasculitis resembling viral retinitis (Fig. 31.4).[22] In some patients, the fundus may appear normal, and subretinal lesions may be noted only on fluorescein angiography (Fig. 31.5). Fundus autofluorescence (FAF) may demonstrate hyperfluorescent or hypofluorescent spots, depending on the location of tumor cells above or below the retinal pigment epithelium (RPE) and the presence of RPE atrophy.[23] Optical coherence tomography (OCT) may also be useful in identifying patients with lymphoma with vitreoretinal involvement. In a study

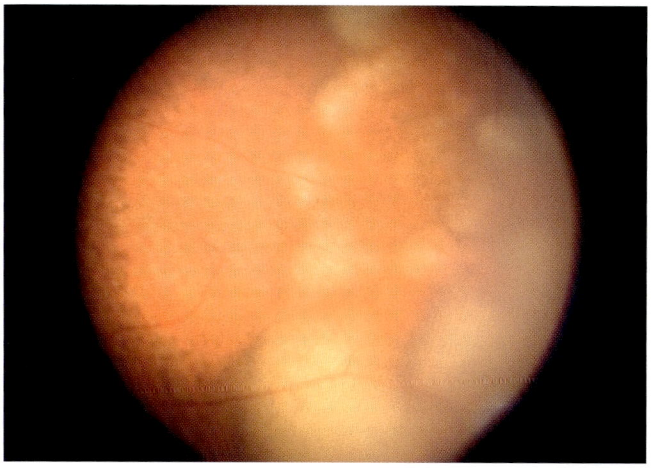

Fig. 31.3 Retinal photograph of a patient with biopsy-proven intraocular lymphoma demonstrating multiple yellow lesions deep to the retina.

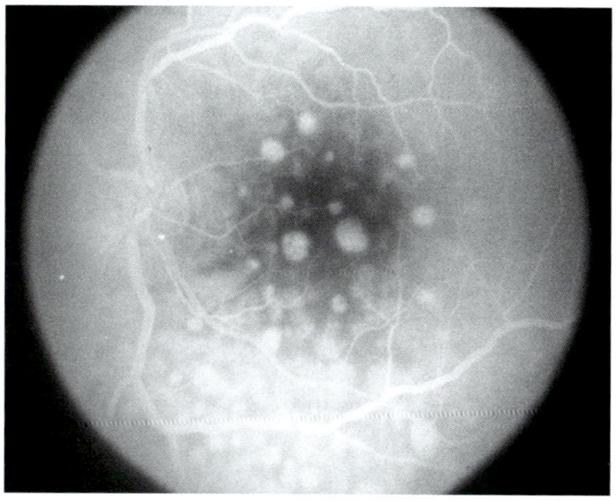

Fig. 31.5 Fluorescein angiogram from a patient with intraocular lymphoma showing multiple circular areas of hyperfluorescence corresponding to tumor infiltration.

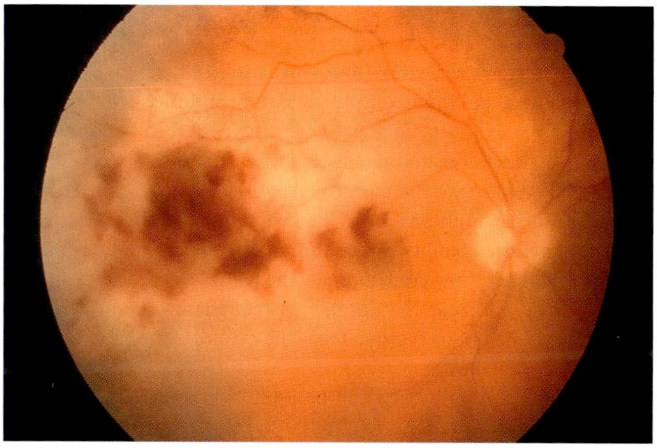

Fig. 31.4 Fundus photograph of patient with intraocular lymphoma showing retinal infiltrates and hemorrhage mimicking cytomegalovirus retinitis. Findings resolved with therapy for lymphoma.

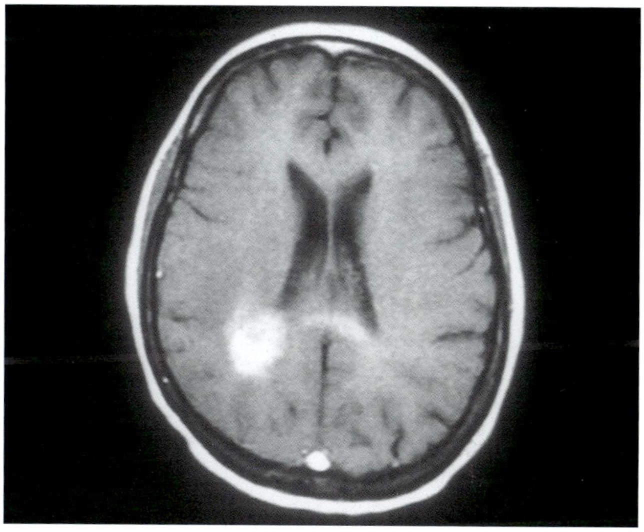

Fig. 31.6 Magnetic resonance imaging (MRI) scan showing a mass lesion in the temporal lobe of a patient with intraocular lymphoma.

of 61 eyes with biopsy-proven intraocular lymphoma with vitreoretinal involvement, nodular hyperreflective lesions were seen at the level of the RPE.[24] Although the disease may start in one eye, bilateral disease is common after several months.[15,19]

Diagnosis

Many patients with intraocular lymphoma have CNS disease at the time of presentation, and a thorough history and neurologic examination are warranted. CNS findings, such as headaches, focal weakness, sensory deficits, confusion, and difficulty with gait, are common. A history of recent seizure is also a strong indication of CNS involvement. Magnetic resonance imaging (MRI) and lumbar puncture should be performed on all patients suspected of having intraocular lymphoma, even if neurologic symptoms are absent (Fig. 31.6). Because lymphoma cells can be fragile, samples should be immediately hand-carried to the cytology laboratory for processing, and at least 5 to 10 mL of cerebrospinal fluid (CSF) should also be sent for cytologic examination. Repeat lumbar puncture may be necessary for the diagnosis.

If CSF shows no malignant cells, we perform pars plana vitrectomy in an attempt to diagnose lymphoma. Tissue culture medium added to the collection chamber of the vitrectomy machine may improve cell viability. An initial sample of core vitreous is also obtained at the start of vitrectomy and taken immediately to the cytology laboratory for processing. We prefer complete surgical vitrectomy to obtain as much vitreous as possible for analysis, but some investigators have used vitreous aspiration needle tap in patients with possible intraocular lymphoma.[25]

The methods used to process vitreous specimens have been delineated previously.[26,27] Typical lymphoma cells are large and pleomorphic with scanty cytoplasm, and hypersegmented nuclei with prominent nucleoli are often diagnostic (Fig. 31.7). Mitoses may be present or absent. Furthermore, only a few of these characteristic cells are present in any single specimen, and most vitreous samples contain mainly reactive lymphocytes, histiocytes, necrotic debris, and fibrinous material. Monoclonality is associated with the disease, and B-cell populations with a kappa or lambda restriction or T-cell populations can be identified with immunohistochemical staining or flow cytometry.[28] Because B cells are rarely associated with nonmalignant autoimmune uveitis, identification of CD20+ cells is useful in differentiating intraocular lymphoma from idiopathic uveitis.[28]

Gross examination of the eyes with PCNSL reveals large gray patches of subretinal and retinal infiltration above a thickened choroid (Fig. 31.8). Collections of lymphoma cells are characteristically found

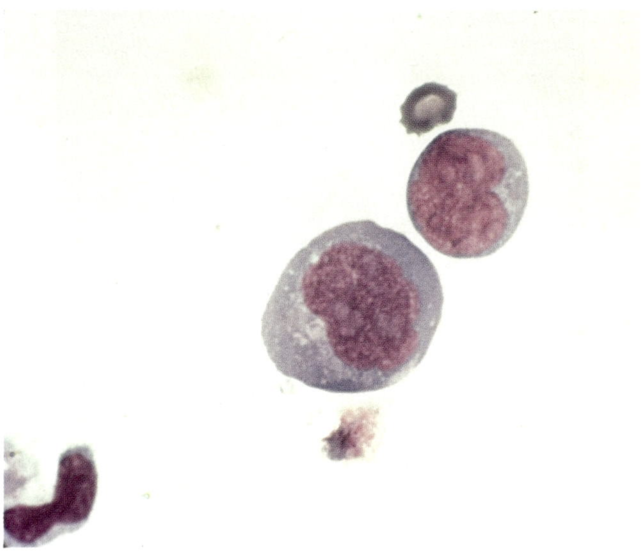

Fig. 31.7 Cells obtained from vitrectomy specimen from a patient with large-cell lymphoma demonstrating large cells with hyperchromatic, pleomorphic nuclei. (Diff Quick stain; original magnification ×1000). (Reproduced with permission from Whitcup SM, de Smet MD, Rubin BI, et al. Intraocular lymphoma: clinical and histopathologic diagnosis. *Ophthalmology.* 1993;100:1399–1406.)

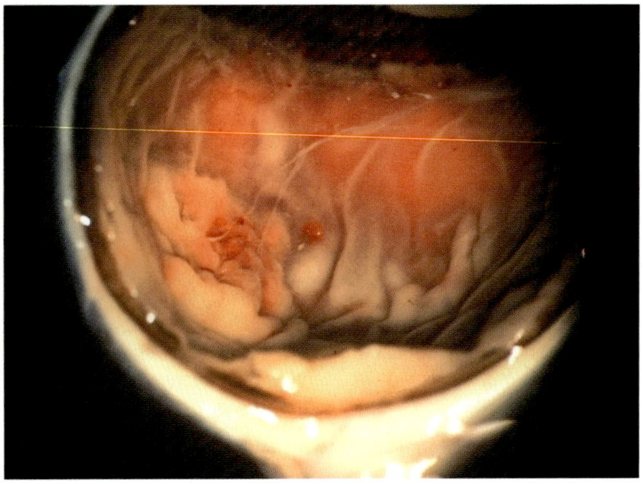

Fig. 31.8 Enucleation specimen from a patient with intraocular lymphoma shows multiple white areas of retinal and subretinal tumor infiltration with adjacent areas of retinal hemorrhage.

between the Bruch membrane and the RPE (Fig. 31.9). Reactive T lymphocytes can be seen in the retina and the choroid in areas surrounding the tumor cells.

Even when vitreous specimens are properly processed, diagnosis of intraocular lymphoma can be difficult. Multiple vitreous specimens may be needed to make the diagnosis. Char et al.[29] reported that in three of the 14 patients in whom ocular lymphoma was later diagnosed, more than one vitreous specimen was required, and we found that multiple samples were needed to make the correct diagnosis in three of 10 patients.[19] In another series of 84 vitrectomy specimens, 14% were diagnosed as definite "malignant lymphoma," 6% as "suspicious of neoplastic disease," 74% as "reactive cellular infiltrate," and 5% "insufficient for diagnosis."[30] Although mishandling of vitreous samples partially accounts for some of the difficulty in making the correct diagnosis, treatment with corticosteroids may obscure the

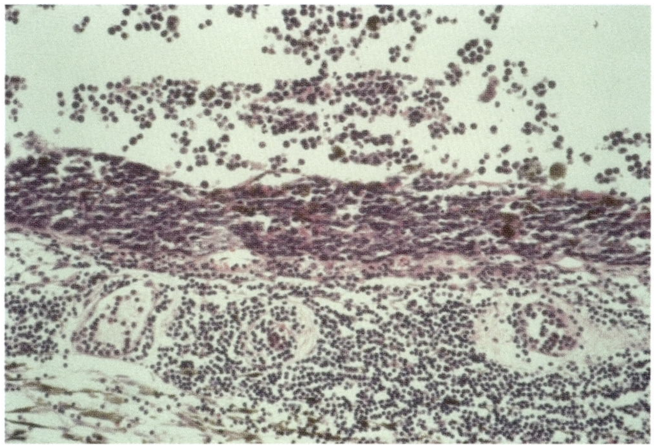

Fig. 31.9 Photomicrograph of enucleated globe shown in Fig. 31.8 reveals tumor infiltration between the Bruch membrane and the retinal pigment epithelium. Reactive lymphocytes and some tumor cells are seen in the overlying vitreous. (Hematoxylin & eosin stain; original magnification ×200.)

diagnosis of intraocular lymphoma. Corticosteroids can be cytolytic in CNS lymphoma, and this exquisite sensitivity of tumor cells appears to be unique to PCNSL. In some patients, corticosteroid therapy caused CNS lymphoma lesions to be reduced in size or to disappear, hindering the ability to make the correct diagnosis. Because many patients with intraocular lymphoma are treated with corticosteroids at the time of vitrectomy, the viability of the tumor cells in the samples may be diminished, which may contribute to the difficulty in diagnosing this disease. Finally, because the number of malignant cells in a vitreous specimen may be few, it is critical that the cytologist be experienced in the diagnosis of lymphoma.

Intravitreal cytokine levels can be useful in the diagnosis of intraocular lymphoma. Interleukin (IL)-10 can be produced by lymphoma cells, and levels of IL-10 are elevated in both the serum and vitreous of patients with intraocular lymphoma. In contrast, levels of IL-6 are elevated in the vitreous of patients with intraocular inflammation unrelated to a malignant neoplasm. We reported that levels of IL-10 exceeded those of IL-6 in all five patients with intraocular lymphoma examined but in none of the 13 patients with uveitis.[31] This test, however, is neither 100% sensitive nor 100% specific. We have seen patients with intraocular lymphoma with levels of IL-6 higher than those of IL-10.[32] However, when IL-10 is elevated in vitreous specimens, the clinician should remain suspicious about an underlying malignancy, and these patients should be closely followed up. A study of 51 patients with proven intraocular lymphoma and 108 patients with uveitis of other causes showed that measurement of IL-10 in the aqueous humor can be a good screening test for NHL-CNS.[33] A cutoff of 50 pg/mL in the aqueous humor was associated with sensitivity of 0.89 and specificity of 0.93, and the area under the respective receiver operating characteristic (ROC) curves was only slightly higher for vitreous levels (0.989) than for aqueous levels (0.962).

The differential diagnosis for patients suspected of having intraocular lymphoma often includes sarcoidosis. Therefore evaluation of these patients should include chest x-ray, angiotensin-converting enzyme (ACE) measurement, serum and urine calcium levels, and pulmonary function testing to rule out this diagnosis. Limited gallium scanning of the chest and lacrimal glands may also be useful. If patients have diminished diffusing capacity on pulmonary function testing, we often obtain a pulmonary consultation and consider computed tomography (CT) of the chest and bronchoscopic examination to make the diagnosis of sarcoidosis. Other diseases to consider include syphilis, tuberculosis, acute retinal necrosis, and cytomegalovirus retinitis.

Treatment

The treatment of PCNSL is controversial, and the ideal therapy is as yet unproven. Surgery, other than for diagnosis, was thought to provide little benefit; however, one randomized controlled trial (RCT) suggested that aggressive resection of PCNSL in select patients can improve progression-free survival.[34] Radiation therapy was first proposed for the treatment of chronic uveitis in 1911,[35] and, historically, radiotherapy has been recommended as the initial therapy for PCNSL.[36] However, the usefulness of whole-brain radiotherapy alone is limited by incomplete control of the lymphoma, dissemination of the lymphoma outside of the field of radiation, and the toxicity of radiation to the brain.[37]

The limitations of radiotherapy led oncologists to study induction chemotherapy as a therapeutic strategy for PCNSL. Early studies demonstrated the efficacy of therapy with the use of high-dose systemic methotrexate with leucovorin rescue.[38,39] Nevertheless, the optimal dose or number of cycles of methotrexate have not been definitively defined. One center suggested using eight cycles of high-dose methotrexate, based on the assumption that a complete remission is obtained by cycle 6.[40]

Combination chemotherapy for PCNSL has also been studied, including high-dose methotrexate with a number of agents with success. The National Cancer Institute and the NEI investigated a treatment protocol using systemic and intrathecal chemotherapy for the treatment of NHL-CNS.[41] In this trial, 14 nonimmunocompromised patients received a chemotherapy regimen that incorporated 24-hour infusion of high-dose methotrexate with leucovorin rescue, thiotepa, vincristine, dexamethasone, and intrathecal Ara-C with methotrexate. The chemotherapy was administered in 21-day cycles, and the response rate was 100%. Eleven patients (79%) had a complete response, and three (21%) had a partial response. At follow-up of more than 4.5 years, the cumulative survival rate was 68.8%, and the progression-free survival rate was 34.3%. Median survival had not been determined at the time of publication, and progression-free survival was 16.5 months. Improvement was also noted in the retinal lesions in patients with ocular involvement. Toxicity of the treatment regimen included severe drug-related leukoencephalopathy in two patients, grade 3 or 4 neutropenia in 50% of the cycles, ileus in one patient, and seizures in two. Nguyen et al.[42] looked at a subset of patients with PCNSL involving the eye in a larger trial comparing high-dose methotrexate regimens on the disease.[43] Their analysis confirmed the effect of systemic high-dose methotrexate–based polychemotherapy on the ocular disease in PCNSL but noted frequent ocular relapses.

Because many studies have indicated that CSF levels of systemically administered chemotherapeutic agents may be variable and short lived,[44] some experts recommend placement of an Ommaya reservoir for delivery of intrathecal methotrexate or the use of osmotic blood–brain barrier disruption to ensure adequate drug levels in CSF. Chemotherapy combined with stem cell transplantation is also being studied.[45,46]

DeAngelis et al.[5] showed that the addition of chemotherapy to cranial radiotherapy significantly improved disease-free survival and contributed to overall survival in patients with PCNSL. However, combined radiotherapy and chemotherapy can cause significant toxicity. Cranial radiotherapy produces significant CNS toxicity in long-term survivors. Furthermore, Bleyer[47] and DeAngelis et al.[5] emphasized that chemotherapy can exacerbate the toxicity produced by radiotherapy, especially with methotrexate. In contrast to the usual sequence of therapy for intraocular lymphoma, in which radiotherapy is administered before chemotherapy, the use of chemotherapy before radiotherapy may reduce the risk of leukoencephalopathy and protect against late toxicity.[47,48] Furthermore, combined chemotherapy and radiation therapy may improve progression-free survival but may not improve overall survival and does lead to increased risk of neurotoxicity in long-term survivors. In an RCT of 551 patients with PCNSL, the subjects were randomly assigned to chemotherapy with whole brain radiotherapy versus chemotherapy alone.[49] In this trial, 318 patients were treated per protocol (the primary analysis), and median overall survival was 32.4 months in patients receiving whole brain radiotherapy (n = 154) and 37.1 months in those not receiving radiotherapy. Median progression-free survival was 6.4 months longer in patients receiving radiotherapy, but the difference was not statistically significant.

PCNSL occurs in patients with human immunodeficiency virus (HIV) infection, and these patients tend to die as a result of advanced opportunistic infections regardless of therapy.[50] Although the prognosis in these patients remains poor, use of antiretroviral therapy combined with therapy for PCNSL and antimicrobial therapy may improve survival.

In patients with detectable lymphoma limited to the eyes, there is ongoing controversy that is focused on whether to limit therapy to the eye or to treat the CNS prophylactically. When the eye is involved, along with other areas of the CNS, therapy needs to be more aggressive, given the poorer overall prognosis. In analyzing the data from the G-PCNSL-SG1 trial—a large multicenter study of over 526 patients—of the 297 patients who had ophthalmologic examination at baseline, median progression-free survival was 3.5 months in those with intraocular involvement compared with 8.3 months in those without intraocular involvement.

As expected, treatment of intraocular lymphoma has followed from the advances made in the treatment of PCNSL. Initial small case series suggested that patients could be managed with ocular radiation alone, but subsequent larger, longer-term studies showed frequent CNS recurrences in patients receiving treatment limited to the eye. Char et al.[29] reported on two patients who had isolated ocular involvement treated with only ocular radiation and who had no recurrent disease 24 and 109 months after treatment. PCNSL tends to be quite radiosensitive and responds well to 15 to 45 Gy. However, many experts recommended cranial irradiation (45 Gy to the whole brain) in addition to orbital radiation in patients with isolated ocular involvement because many patients have subclinical CNS involvement by the time intraocular lymphoma manifests.[29,51] However, in the series by Peterson et al.,[16] in 10 of 11 patients with lymphoma limited to the eyes at initial presentation, CNS disease developed subsequently. In fact, Rouwen et al.[51] recommended using a combination of chemotherapy and radiotherapy for intraocular lymphoma even if CNS disease cannot be identified on MRI or lumbar puncture. Chemotherapy is now frequently recommended to treat possible CNS disease. In a retrospective review of 83 HIV-negative patients with primary intraocular lymphoma, the authors recommended local therapy with intravitreal methotrexate and rituximab alone or with local radiotherapy for select patients without CNS or systemic involvement.[28] If CNS disease with intraocular involvement is found, treatment with systemic chemotherapy, possibly combined with intravitreal chemotherapy, is often considered.

Similar chemotherapy regimens used for treating PCNSL have specifically been studied for the treatment of intraocular lymphoma, although few RCTs on this approach have been performed. Most experts use high-dose methotrexate for treating intraocular lymphoma, although the use of high-dose cytarabine (Ara-C) can lead to therapeutic drug levels in CSF, and there have been reports of successful treatment of intraocular lymphomas with this therapy alone.[52] A number of researchers have used intrathecal methotrexate for the treatment of intraocular lymphoma, but always in combination with radiotherapy.[29]

High-dose thiotepa, busulfan, and cyclophosphamide, followed by autologous bone marrow transplantation, appeared to be effective in some patients with refractory intraocular lymphoma.[53]

Local recurrence of NHL-CNS in the eye can be difficult to diagnose and treat. Definitive diagnosis requires obtaining a vitreous specimen for cytologic examination. One therapeutic option for ocular recurrence is radiation. However, we have seen a number of patients with ocular recurrence who had already received maximal radiation to the eyes. Intravitreal injections of multiple chemotherapeutic agents may be a useful therapeutic approach for these patients. Combinations of intravitreal methotrexate, fluorouracil, and dexamethasone have been studied.[54-57] The safety of intravitreal injections of rituximab is being assessed.[58]

The presence of intraocular lymphoma is usually associated with concomitant brain disease, and survival is similar to that in other presentations of PCNSL.[59] Some data suggested that patients whose ocular disease was identified and treated before CNS progression had a significantly improved survival,[60] thereby emphasizing the importance of early diagnosis and therapy. Although many patients with NHL-CNS have a good initial response to therapy, recurrence is common, and in some studies, the 5-year survival is less than 5%. Hochberg and Miller[10] reported an overall median survival time from diagnosis of 13.5 months in patients with PCNSL, and Freeman et al.[20] reported a mean survival time of 26 months for patients with intraocular lymphoma. However, some reports have suggested that intrathecal chemotherapy combined with radiotherapy of the orbits and whole brain may improve survival.[29] Hopefully, additional research into new therapeutic approaches will lead to improved survival for patients with this disease.

Finally, immunotherapy, including chimeric antigen receptor (CAR) T-cell therapy, have dramatically improved response rates and survival for patients with many forms of cancer, including lymphomas. In a study of the anti-CD19 CAR T-cell therapy with tisagenlecleucel, a best overall response rate of 52% and a complete response rate of 40% were achieved in 93 adult patients with relapsed or refractory diffuse large B-cell lymphoma.[61] Further studies are needed to confirm whether immunotherapy can favorably improve the outcome in patients with PCNSL.

Systemic Non-Hodgkin Lymphoma Metastatic to the Eye

Systemic NHL can metastasize to the eye and cause anterior or posterior uveitis. Unlike the location of PCNSL cells between the RPE and the Bruch membrane, lymphoma cells in patients with systemic NHL characteristically infiltrate the choroid and may be mistaken for ocular melanoma.[62] Metastatic lymphoma may also cause a hypopyon or hyphema in an otherwise uninflamed eye.[63] A case of a metastatic vitreoretinal lymphoma presenting as acute retinal necrosis has also been reported.[64] Although most patients with NHL have symptoms of lymphadenopathy, fever, and weight loss, ocular involvement may be the initial presentation of the disease.[62]

UVEAL LYMPHOMA

Uveal lymphoma is a usually indolent disorder characterized by infiltration of the uveal tract by well-differentiated small lymphocytes. The disease was initially referred to as *inflammatory pseudotumors of the uveal tract* or *intraocular pseudotumor*,[65,66] and, more recently, *reactive lymphoid hyperplasia*.[67] Although the disease is usually unilateral, bilateral cases have been reported. Clinical features include anterior uveitis, vitritis, choroidal infiltrates (Fig. 31.10), and iris heterochromia.[66,68] Open-angle glaucoma is common because of infiltration of the anterior chamber angle. Extraocular extension may occur, leading to conjunctival salmon-colored lesions and orbital masses that cause proptosis and diplopia.[66,69] Most patients present with decreased vision, and the disease is usually painless unless severe glaucoma develops.

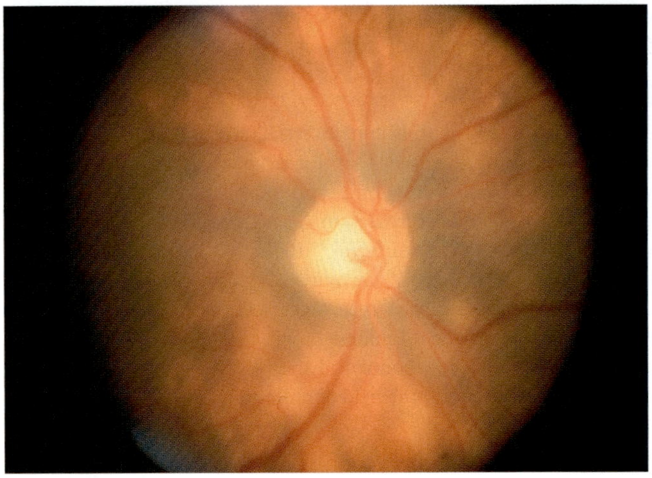

Fig. 31.10 Multiple yellow choroidal infiltrates in patient with lymphoid hyperplasia of uvea.

Diagnosis has often been based on histologic findings in enucleation specimens or biopsy specimens obtained from extraocular extensions of the tumor. In a study of 34 eyes, extranodal marginal zone lymphoma was the predominant (76.2%) histologic subtype.[70] We were able to make the diagnosis on the basis of chorioretinal biopsy in a 39-year-old man with painless choroidal thickening.[71] Many pathologists believe that uveal lymphoma is probably a low-grade lymphoid neoplasm. Ten cases of reactive lymphoid hyperplasia of the uvea were re-evaluated by using immunohistochemical and molecular analyses at the Armed Forces Institute of Pathology.[72] Eight of the 10 were low-grade lymphomas, as shown by histology and immunohistochemistry. The tumor can respond to therapy with corticosteroids, although some tumors warrant the use of moderate doses of radiotherapy; unlike in patients with NHL-CNS, the long-term prognosis for these patients is quite favorable.[68,69] In the study by Aronow et al., external beam radiotherapy was the modality commonly chosen for primary treatment, and the disease was localized to the eye in over three-fourths of cases. In this study, systemic disease did not develop in any of these patients with localized disease at diagnosis after a median follow-up of 30.3 months.[70]

OTHER MALIGNANT PROCESSES MANIFESTING AS UVEITIS

Uveal melanoma can manifest as unilateral uveitis.[73] Melanoma involving the ciliary body can produce dilated episcleral vessels called *sentinel vessels,* which may be misdiagnosed as episcleritis. Melanoma of the iris can produce anterior chamber cells and flare,[74] and choroidal melanoma is often associated with cataract and a focal choroidal mass that may be mistaken for sarcoid or tuberculous granuloma or posterior scleritis.[75] Leukemia can masquerade as uveitis in adults. Chronic myeloid leukemia in blast crisis and relapsing acute myeloid leukemia have been reported as masquerade syndromes.[76,77] Severe anterior segment cellular infiltration with hypopyon often occurs in these patients. Diagnosis can be made on the basis of cytologic findings from anterior chamber paracentesis. Panuveitis has been described more rarely in patients with leukemia.[78]

Choroidal metastases can produce signs and symptoms of uveitis. In some case series, up to half the ocular metastases were recognized before the diagnosis of an underlying malignant process.[79] Renal and lung carcinomas are the malignant conditions most likely to metastasize to the eye. Although breast carcinomas frequently metastasize to the eye, in greater than 90% of patients, the primary lesion is known at the time the ocular lesion is noted. Patients with possible metastatic disease to the eye should undergo a thorough medical evaluation to determine the underlying primary cancer. In some patients, needle aspiration of the ocular tumor may be helpful in the diagnosis.[80]

In children, retinoblastoma may manifest with tumor cells floating in the anterior chamber and be mistaken for iritis.[81] Because retinoblastoma is the most common intraocular malignant process in childhood, the possibility of retinoblastoma should be excluded in any young child with leukokoria, strabismus, or undiagnosed uveitis. Acute myelogenous leukemia can also manifest as uveitis in children, and in some cases, findings on anterior chamber paracentesis can be diagnostic.[82,83] Other tumors, such as medulloepitheliomas, and benign lesions, such as juvenile xanthogranuloma, can masquerade as idiopathic uveitis.[84]

PARANEOPLASTIC SYNDROMES

Paraneoplastic syndromes may cause intraocular inflammation with autoimmune retinopathy and masquerade as uveitis. Cancer-associated retinopathy (CAR) is a paraneoplastic syndrome that was initially described in three patients with oat cell carcinoma of the lung[85] but has now been reported in patients with a number of malignant conditions. Patients usually experience loss of vision, and although the fundus can appear normal early in the course of the disease, vascular sheathing, disturbances of the RPE, and optic disk pallor may ensue. Histologic studies show destruction of the photoreceptors.[86] Thirkill et al.[87] identified retinal autoantibodies in patients with CAR, and some patients have improved with corticosteroid therapy. These findings suggest that the retinal destruction may be partly immune mediated.

We have seen a patient with a clinical picture similar to that of CAR but with no underlying malignancy (Fig. 31.11).[88] This patient had elevated levels of antibody against recoverin, and we termed this immunologically and clinically distinctive condition *recoverin-associated retinopathy* (RARe). These cases of nonparaneoplastic autoimmune retinopathy may also include disorders such as acute zonal occult outer retinopathy (AZOOR) (Fig. 31.12); however, more research is needed to determine the pathogenesis of these diseases.[89]

Another paraneoplastic disorder that can masquerade as idiopathic uveitis has been named *bilateral diffuse uveal melanocytic proliferation* (BDUMP). Machemer[90] first reported bilateral diffuse uveal melanocytic tumors in a patient with a large retroperitoneal mass thought to be pancreatic carcinoma, and Barr et al.[91] reported on four similar bilateral diffuse melanocytic uveal tumors in patients with an associated systemic malignant process diagnosed with biopsy or at autopsy. Although the condition occurs in patients with carcinomas, the underlying malignant processes are often occult.[92] Gass and Glatzer[93] characterized the ocular findings on the basis of the presence of multiple, subtle, round and oval subretinal red patches that demonstrate early

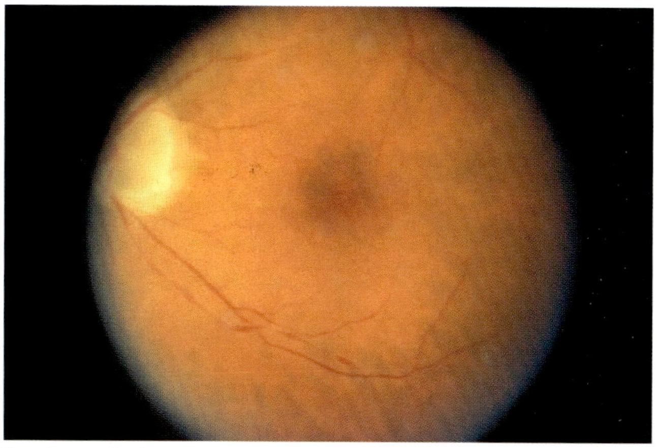

Fig. 31.11 Retina photograph of a patient with recoverin-associated retinopathy. Optic disk pallor, attenuated retinal vessels, and areas of retinal pigment epithelial atrophy are seen.

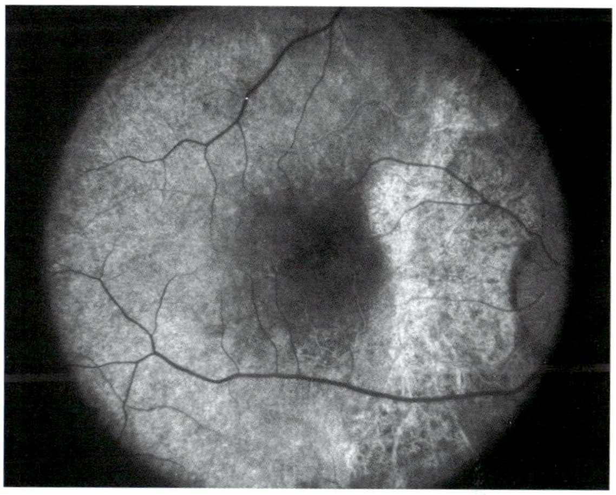

Fig. 31.12 Late-phase fluorescein angiogram from a patient with acute zonal occult outer retinopathy showing a large patch of hyperfluorescence extended from the optic disk to the macula. (Courtesy Muriel Kaiser-Kupfer, MD.)

hyperfluorescence on angiographic examination; multiple, slightly elevated, pigmented and nonpigmented uveal melanocytic tumors with evidence of diffuse thickening of the uveal tract; exudative retinal detachment; and the rapid development of cataracts. Episcleral injection, vitreous cells, and other signs of mild ocular inflammation can be seen.

Histopathologic findings in the ocular lesions are diffuse uveal tract infiltrates with apparently benign, spindle-shaped melanocytic cells. Some of these cells have vesiculated nuclei with prominent nucleoli, and many have foamy cytoplasm, but mitotic figures are not characteristic.[91] BDUMP should be suspected in patients with bilateral diffuse melanocytic uveal tumors, serous retinal detachments, and cataract. It is important to recognize this condition so that patients can be evaluated for underlying malignant conditions that may warrant immediate therapy to improve prognosis.

MULTIPLE SCLEROSIS

Ocular inflammatory disease classified as intermediate uveitis may occur in patients with multiple sclerosis. Although some authors

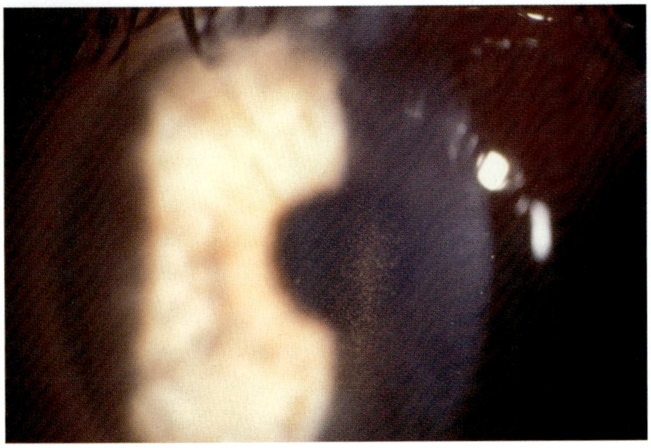

Fig. 31.13 Krukenberg spindle in a patient with pigment dispersion syndrome that masqueraded as anterior uveitis. (Courtesy Muriel Kaiser-Kupfer, MD.)

previously included multiple sclerosis in a list of masquerade syndromes, most consider multiple sclerosis as a cause of uveitis, such as other immune-based uveitic disorders with both CNS and ocular manifestations (e.g., Vogt-Koyanagi-Harada syndrome). Multiple sclerosis as a cause of uveitis is discussed in the chapter on intermediate uveitis (see Chapter 22).

OTHER NONMALIGNANT CONDITIONS

A number of nonmalignant conditions can masquerade as idiopathic uveitis. An intraocular foreign body may elicit anterior or posterior uveitis. Patients with uniocular uveitis should be questioned about possible antecedent trauma. Gonioscopic examination should be performed to rule out a foreign body in the angle, and patients at high risk for an intraocular foreign body, such as construction workers, may require ultrasonography or CT to make the diagnosis. Metastatic squamous epithelial downgrowth after cataract surgery has masqueraded as chronic inflammation.[94] Retinal detachment in atopic dermatitis can masquerade as panuveitis.[95]

A number of retinal diseases can masquerade as ocular inflammatory disease. Retinal detachment can sometimes produce enough intraocular inflammation to be misdiagnosed as uveitis, and myopic degeneration can produce cream-colored atrophic lesions that may be confused with focal choroiditis. We have also seen cases where advanced atrophic age-related macular degeneration was misdiagnosed as an idiopathic white-dot syndrome.

Ocular ischemia can lead not only to necrosis but also to infiltration of the eye by inflammatory cells. Ischemia may be associated with underlying vascular disease or cardiac disease or may be induced by drugs or environmental insults. For example, anterior segment ischemia with inflammatory signs mimicking uveitis has been reported after viper bites.[96]

Pigment dispersion syndrome is characterized by accumulation of pigment on the posterior surface of the central cornea in a vertical, spindle-shaped pattern (Krukenberg spindle) (Fig. 31.13). Pigment granules may also be deposited on the anterior surface of the lens and on the iris, leading to heterochromia. Pigment dispersion may be associated with glaucoma and, in some patients, may be mistaken for uveitis.[97] Mydriatic agents can cause pigmented cells in the aqueous humor and may lead to improper grading of anterior chamber inflammation.

Patients with retinal degenerations, such as retinitis pigmentosa (RP), may have a number of signs consistent with underlying inflammatory disease. Vitreous cells, posterior subcapsular cataract, and cystoid macular edema may occur,[98-100] and in patients in whom the characteristic bone spicule pigment is minimal, the underlying diagnosis of RP may be missed. With advances in genetic testing, additional retinal dystrophies have been associated with uveitis, especially in children.[101] Mutations in the *CRB1* gene have been associated with exudative maculopathy and cystoid macular edema.[102,103] It is of interest that some have suggested that the ocular inflammation in these patients may be caused by a secondary immunologic reaction against retinal antigens released into the vitreous as the retina degenerates. Thirkill et al.[104] showed that sera from 11 of 52 patients with RP (21%) exhibited a minimum of twice the clinically normal reactivity with retinal antigens on enzyme-linked immunosorbent assay (ELISA), and of these 11 patients, eight had antibodies to the retinal S-antigen. The authors concluded that patients with RP who have indications of immunologic hypersensitivity to known uveitopathogenic retinal antigens are at higher risk for autoimmune retinopathies. Williams et al.[105] demonstrated that activated RP peripheral lymphocytes adhered to and altered cultured human RPE cells, suggesting that immune-mediated cytopathologic effects may contribute to the retinal degeneration in RP. If this secondary immunologic response contributes to the deterioration of visual function in patients with RP, immunosuppressive therapy may have a role in the treatment of some patients with retinal degeneration, although this hypothesis needs to be tested in controlled studies.

Indolent ocular infections may mimic chronic idiopathic uveitis, and these infections are discussed in detail in Chapters 10 and 11. Fungal infections of the choroid, retina, and vitreous may occur in immunosuppressed patients, in patients with systemic fungal infections, or in patients who have recently had surgery. *P. acnes*, a pathogen that has been recognized as a cause of uveitis, may not appear clinically for months after cataract surgery. *P. acnes* endophthalmitis is discussed in detail in Chapter 19.

Uveitis has been associated with many medications, some which are listed in Table 31.1. Drug-induced uveitis can occur with both locally administered and systemic medications.[106] Even topical administration of corticosteroids has been associated with the development of an anterior uveitis.[107] Although some of the reported associations between uveitis and medications may not represent a direct causal effect of the drugs, patients with an anterior uveitis should still be asked whether they have recently started taking any new medications. Uveitis can also occur after vaccination or the purified protein derivative (PPD) skin test.[108] Interestingly, clusters of drug-induced uveitis may occur with increased clinical use of a particular medication. For example, cases of a triamcinolone-associated crystalline maculopathy were described after the increased use of intravitreal injections of the drug for treating retinal disease.[109]

With the development of new cancer immunotherapy, a number of ocular inflammatory conditions have been reported in patients receiving immune checkpoint inhibitor treatment for malignancy.[110-112] Immune checkpoint blockade increases immunity against cancer cells by blocking the intrinsic downregulators of immunity, including cytotoxic T-lymphocyte antigen 4 (CTLA-4) and programmed cell death 1 (PD-1) or its ligand programmed cell death ligand 1 (PD-L1). Although increasing overall immune system activity has led to dramatic survival in patients with a number of

TABLE 31.1 Uveitis Associated with Medications

	Predominant Uveitis
Topical Ophthalmic Medications	
Anticholinesterases and direct-acting agonists	Anterior uveitis
Corticosteroids	Anterior uveitis
Beta blockers	Anterior uveitis
Prostaglandin analogs	Anterior uveitis, cystoid macular edema
Alpha agonists	Anterior uveitis
Antibiotics	Anterior uveitis
Intraocular Medications	
Triamcinolone	Vitritis
Antibiotics	Posterior segment inflammation
Anti-VEGF antibodies	Posterior segment inflammation
Perfluorocarbons	Fibrinous anterior uveitis
Silicone oil	Anterior uveitis
Air	Anterior uveitis
Urokinase	Hypopyon uveitis
Plasmin	Anterior uveitis
Cidofovir	Anterior uveitis
Systemic Medications	
Hydralazine	Lupus-like syndrome with episcleritis and retinal vasculitis
Nitrogen mustard	Necrotizing uveitis with retinal vasculitis
Rifabutin	Hypopyon uveitis
Procainamide	Lupus-like syndrome with episcleritis
Diethylcarbamazine	Uveitis with punctate keratitis and retinal pigment epithelium atrophy
Quinidine	Anterior uveitis
Tumor necrosis factor (TNF)-α antagonists	Anterior uveitis
Bisphosphonates	Anterior uveitis, scleritis
Fluoroquinolones	Anterior uveitis
Sulfonamides	Anterior uveitis
Immune checkpoint inhibitors	Uveitis, anterior uveitis, panuveitis, peripheral ulcerative keratitis, choirdal neovascularization, scleritis, orbital inflammation
Hydroxychloroquine and chloroquine	"Bull's eye" maculopathy, macular edema, vitritis

malignancies, these medications have been associated with a number of immune-related, inflammatory side effects affecting multiple organ systems.[113] Reported ocular inflammatory side effects have included anterior uveitis, panuveitis, scleritis, choroidal neovascularization, and orbital inflammation. It is not clear whether the inflammation is secondary to an immune response to the therapy or an induced immune response to shared antigens between the tumor and the eye resulting in a paraneoplastic syndrome.

Uveitis is a rare presentation of hydroxychloroquine-induced retinal toxicity.[114] Because chloroquine and hydroxychloroquine are used to treat autoimmune diseases in which uveitis is common and because early recognition of chloroquine and hydroxychloroquine toxicity can prevent vision loss, it is important to carefully monitor patients on therapy and to consider this masquerade syndrome. Although "bull's eye" maculopathy is the common finding in chloroquine and hydroxychloroquine toxicity, the retinal lesions can masquerade as posterior uveitis with macular involvement. The American Academy of Ophthalmology (AAO) has revised recommendations on screening for chloroquine and hydroxychloroquine retinopathy.[115] In this statement, the AAO again highlights the fact that high dose and long duration of use are the most significant risk factors for toxicity. The AAO recommends a maximum daily dose of hydroxychloroquine of 5 mg/kg real weight or less. A fundus examination should be performed at baseline to rule out pre-existing maculopathy, and annual screening should begin after 5 years for patients on acceptable doses of the drug. The primary screening tests are automated visual fields plus spectral-domain optical coherence tomography (SD-OCT). The statement also notes that tests should examine the retina beyond the central macula in Asian patients because they often have extramacular damage. Multifocal electroretinography (ERG) findings can corroborate visual field changes, and FAF can identify areas of retinal damage. Because the retinopathy is not reversible and there is no current therapy for the toxicity, early recognition is needed so that therapy can be stopped, where indicated.

Most cases of drug-induced uveitis can be controlled with corticosteroids and the use of mydriatic and cycloplegic agents; however, if inflammation is severe and alternative medications are available, consideration should be given to stopping the presumed inciting drug.

Rarely, in addition to trauma, uveitis has been reported after electrical injury and laser procedures. Recurrent iritis and cataract was reported in 1946[116] and in two of 159 patients with high-voltage electrical burns.[117] Two cases of anterior uveitis were reported after laser-assisted epilation of eyebrow hair.[118] These cases of energy-induced uveitis can usually be controlled with topical corticosteroids and cycloplegia.

Finally, uveitis has been reported to occur after gene therapy for inherited retinal diseases. In a clinical trial of gene therapy for Leber hereditary optic neuropathy, uveitis was noted in two of 12 patients receiving adeno-associated virus 2 (AAV2) vector-based gene therapy delivered via subretinal injection.[119] These patients were asymptomatic, and the condition resolved without therapy; however, patients routinely receive systemic corticosteroids before and after the subretinal injections. This therapy has been approved by the U.S. Food and Drug Administration (FDA), and eye inflammation has been reported in 5% of treated eyes, and subretinal deposits, described as asymptomatic subretinal precipitates, inferior to the retinal injections site 1 to 6 days after injection were reported in 4% of treated eyes (FDA package insert). This inflammation may represent an immune response against the viral capsid or another component of the gene therapy. As clinical trials and use of gene therapies for this and other ocular diseases increase, inflammation associated with these therapies may become more common and require therapy with systemic or locally administered corticosteroids.

It is clear that a number of entities can masquerade as idiopathic uveitis, and in the absence of a correct diagnosis, inappropriate therapy may be prescribed. The diagnosis of a masquerade syndrome should therefore be considered in the evaluation of all patients with undiagnosed inflammatory eye disease.

CASE 31.1

A 32-year-old Caucasian man was diagnosed with chronic intermediate uveitis in both eyes characterized by vitreous cells and macular edema (Fig. 31.14A). Despite anti-inflammatory therapy, the patient reported decreasing vision and was referred for further evaluation. On detailed dilated retinal examination, characteristic bone spicules were noted in a quadrant of the retinal periphery (see Fig. 31.14B), and electroretinography findings were consistent with a diagnosis of sectoral retinitis pigmentosa.

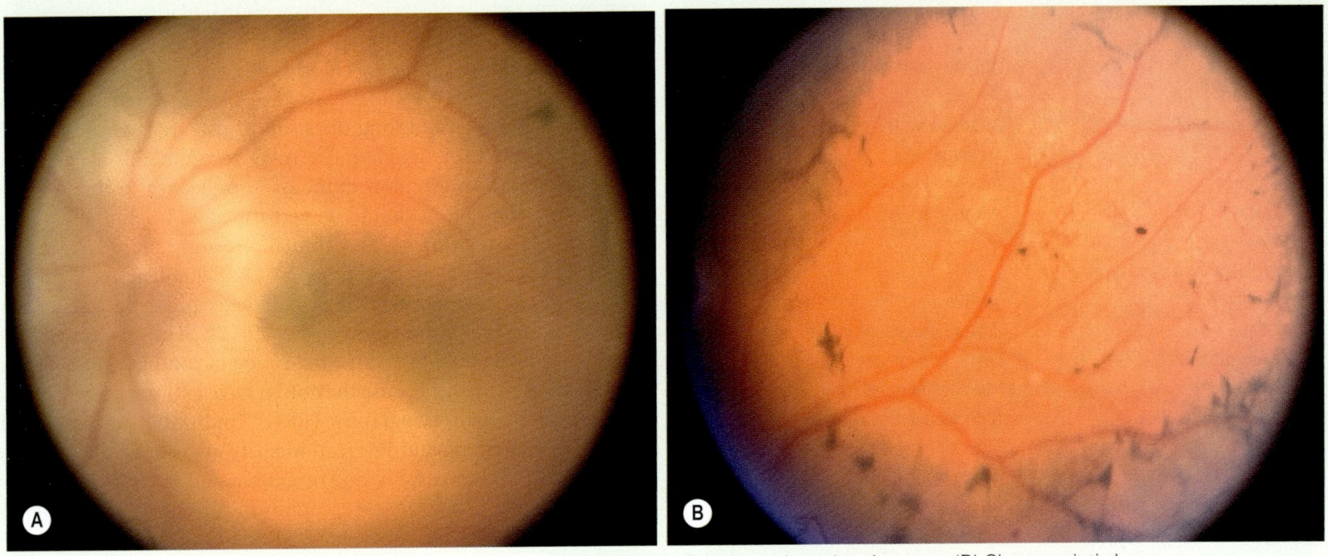

Fig. 31.14 (A) Photograph of the retina showing edema of the macula and optic nerve. (B) Characteristic bone spicules in a quadrant of the retinal periphery, consistent with a diagnosis of sectoral retinitis pigmentosa.

CASE 31.2

An African American woman with a long history of sarcoidosis was referred with progressive, severe vision loss in both eyes and retinal edema despite increased systemic therapy, and the patient was referred for further evaluation and treatment. On detailed medical history, the patient reported having received chloroquine therapy, and retinal examination revealed macular lesions in both eyes consistent with "bull's eye" maculopathy (Fig. 31.15). Findings on further evaluation, including visual fields, were consistent with a diagnosis of chloroquine retinopathy.

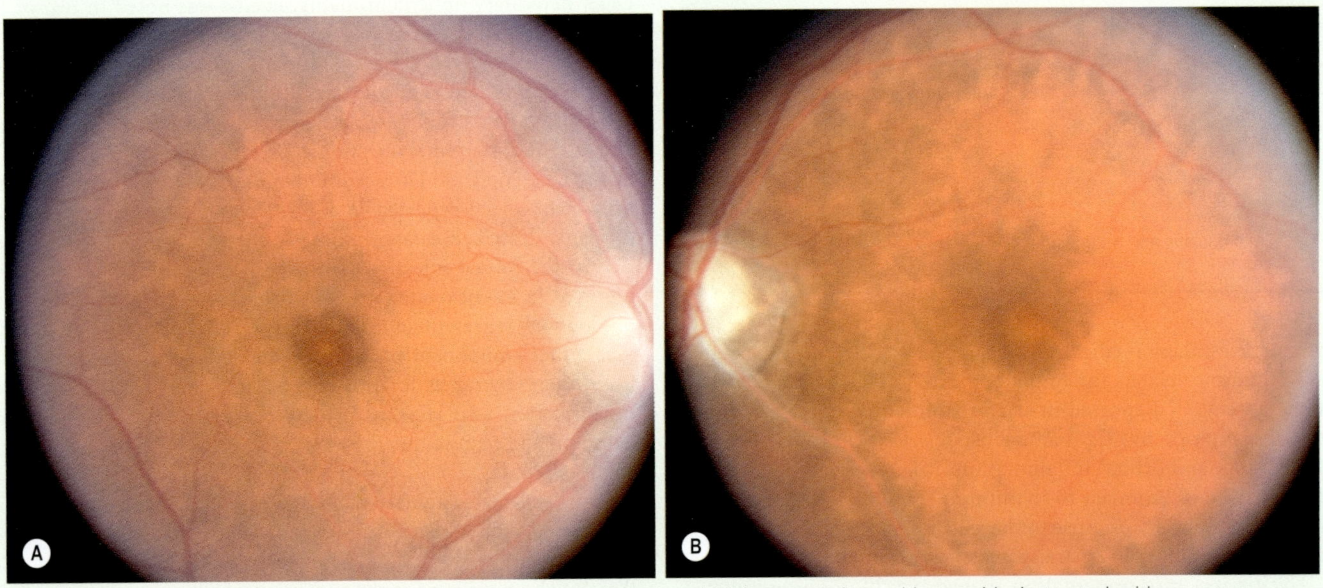

Fig. 31.15 "Bull's eye" maculopathy in both eyes (A and B) from a patient with sarcoidosis treated with chloroquine. Attenuated retinal vessels were also seen, especially in the left eye (B).

REFERENCES

1. Theodore FH. Conjunctival carcinoma masquerading as chronic conjunctivitis. *Eye Ear Nose Throat Mon*. 1967;46:1419–1420.
2. Kamellin S. Uveitis associated with Hodgkin's disease: report of a case. *Arch Ophthalmol*. 1944;31:517–519.
3. Barr CC, Joondeph HC. Retinal periphlebitis as the initial clinical finding in a patient with Hodgkin's disease. *Retina*. 1983;3:253–257.
4. To KW, Thirkill CE, Jakobiec FA, et al. Lymphoma-associated retinopathy. *Ophthalmology*. 2002;109:2149–2153.
5. DeAngelis LM, Yahalom J, Thaler H, et al. Combined modality therapy for primary CNS lymphoma. *J Clin Oncol*. 1992;10:635–643.
6. Appen RE. Posterior uveitis and primary cerebral reticulum cell sarcoma. *Arch Ophthalmol*. 1975;93:123–124.
7. Rockwood EJ, Zakov ZN, Bay JW. Combined malignant lymphoma of the eye and CNS (reticulum-cell sarcoma). *J Neurosurg*. 1984;61:369–374.
8. Henry JM, Heffner RR Jr, Dillard SH, et al. Primary malignant lymphomas of the central nervous system. *Cancer*. 1974;34:1293–1302.
9. Murray K, Kun L, Cox J. Primary malignant lymphoma of the central nervous system: results of treatment of 11 cases and review of the literature. *J Neurosurg*. 1986;65:600–607.
10. Hochberg FH, Miller DC. Primary central nervous system lymphoma. *J Neurosurg*. 1988;68:835–853.
11. Ostrom QT, Gittleman H, Liao P, et al. CBTRUS statistical report: primary brain and central nervous system tumors diagnosed in the United States in 2007-2011. *Neuro Oncol*. 2014;16 Suppl 4(Suppl 4):iv1-iv63.
12. Hong JT, Chae JB, Lee JY, et al. Ocular involvement in patients with primary CNS lymphoma. *J Neurooncol*. 2011;102:139–145.
13. Helle TL, Britt RH, Colby TV. Primary lymphoma of the central nervous system: clinicopathological study of experience at Stanford. *J Neurosurg*. 1984;60:94–103.
14. Cohen IJ, Vogel R, Matz S, et al. Successful non-neurotoxic therapy (without radiation) of a multifocal primary brain lymphoma with methotrexate, vincristine, and BCNY protocol (DEMOB). *Cancer*. 1986;57:6–11.
15. Qualman SJ, Mendelsohn G, Mann RB, et al. Intraocular lymphomas: natural history based on a clinicopathologic study of eight cases and review of the literature. *Cancer*. 1983;52:878–886.
16. Peterson K, Gordon KB, Heinemann M-H, et al. The clinical spectrum of ocular lymphoma. *Cancer*. 1993;72:843–849.
17. Schanzer CM, Font RL, O'Malley RE. Primary ocular malignant lymphoma associated with the acquired immune deficiency syndrome. *Ophthalmology*. 1991;98:88–91.
18. Johnson BL. Intraocular and central nervous system lymphoma in a cardiac transplant recipient. *Ophthalmology*. 1992;99:987–992.
19. Whitcup SM, de Smet MD, Rubin BI, et al. Intraocular lymphoma: clinical and histopathologic diagnosis. *Ophthalmology*. 1993;100:1399–1406.
20. Freeman LN, Schachat AP, Knox DL, et al. Clinical features, laboratory investigations, and survival in ocular reticulum cell sarcoma. *Ophthalmology*. 1987;94:1631–1639.
21. Barr CC, Green WR, Payne JW, et al. Intraocular reticulum-cell sarcoma: clinicopathologic study of four cases and review of the literature. *Surv Ophthalmol*. 1975;19:224–239.
22. de Smet MD, Nussenblatt RB, Davis JL, et al. Large cell lymphoma masquerading as a viral retinitis. *Int Ophthalmol*. 1990;14:413–417.
23. Ishida T, Hono-Matsui K, Kaneko Y, et al. Fundus autofluorescence patterns in eyes with primary intraocular lymphoma. *Retina*. 2010;30:23–32.
24. Fardeau C, Lee CP, Merle-Beral H, et al. Retinal fluorescein, indocyanine green angiography and optic coherence tomography in non-Hodgkin primary intraocular lymphoma. *Am J Ophthalmol*. 2009;147:886–894.
25. Lobo A, Lightman S. Vitreous aspiration needle tap in the diagnosis of intraocular inflammation. *Ophthalmology*. 2003;110:595–599.
26. Davis JL, Solomon D, Nussenblatt RB, et al. Immunocytochemical staining of vitreous cells: indications, techniques, and results. *Ophthalmology*. 1992;99:250–256.
27. Ljung BM, Char D, Miller TR, et al. Intraocular lymphoma: cytologic diagnosis and the role of immunologic markers. *Acta Cytol*. 1988;32:840–847.
28. Chan C-C, Rubenstein JL, Coupland SE, et al. Primary vitreoretinal lymphoma: a report from an international primary central nervous system lymphoma collaborative group symposium. *Oncologist*. 2011;16:1589–1599.
29. Char DH, Ljung B-M, Miller T, et al. Primary intraocular lymphoma (ocular reticulum cell sarcoma): diagnosis and management. *Ophthalmology*. 1988;95:625–630.
30. Coupland SE, Bechrakis NE, Anastassiou G, et al. Evaluation of vitrectomy specimens and chorioretinal biopsies in the diagnosis of primary intraocular lymphoma in patients with masquerade syndrome. *Graefes Arch Clin Exp Ophthalmol*. 2003;241:860–870.
31. Whitcup SM, Stark-Vancs V, Wittes RE, et al. Association of interleukin 10 in the vitreous and cerebrospinal fluid and primary central nervous system lymphoma. *Arch Ophthalmol*. 1997;115:1157–1160.
32. Buggage RR, Velez G, Myers-Powell B, et al. Primary intraocular lymphoma with a low interleukin 10 to interleukin 6 ratio and heterogeneous IgH gene rearrangement. *Arch Ophthalmol*. 2000;118:731–732.
33. Cassoux N, Giron A, Bodaghi B, et al. IL-10 measurement in aqueous humor for screening patients with suspicion of primary intraocular lymphoma. *Invest Ophthalmol Vis Sci*. 2007;48:3253–3259.
34. Weller M, Martus P, Roth P, et al. German PCNSL Study Group. Surgery for primary CNS lymphoma? Challenging a paradigm. *Neurooncol*. 2012;14:1481–1484.
35. Koster W. Über die Direkte Behandlung von Augenerkrankungen mit Radium und Metothorium. *Strahlentherapie*. 1913;3.
36. Margolis L, Fraser R, Lichter A, et al. The role of radiation therapy in the management of ocular reticulum cell sarcoma. *Cancer*. 1980;45:688–692.
37. Rubenstein JL, Gupta NK, Mannis GN, et al. How I treat CNS lymphomas. *Blood*. 2013;122:2318–2330.
38. Skarin AT, Zuckerman KS, Pitman SW, et al. High-dose methotrexate with folinic acid in the treatment of advanced non-Hodgkin lymphoma including CNS involvement. *Blood*. 1977;50:1039–1047.
39. Ervin T, Canellos GP. Successful treatment of recurrent primary central nervous system lymphoma with high-dose methotrexate. *Cancer*. 1980;45:1556–1557.
40. Fraser E, Gruenberg K, Rubenstein JL. New approaches in primary central nervous system lymphoma. *Chin Clin Oncol*. 2015;4:1.
41. Sandor V, Stark-Vancs V, Pearson D, et al. Phase II trial of chemotherapy alone for primary CNS and intraocular lymphoma. *J Clin Oncol*. 1998;16:3000–3006.
42. Nguyen D-T, Houillier C, Choquet S, et al. Primary oculocerebral lymphoma: MTX polychemotherapy alone on intraocular disease control. *Ophthalmology*. 2016;123:2047–2050.
43. Omuro A, Chinot O, Taillandier L, et al. Methotrexate and temozolamide versus methotrexate, procarbazine, vincristine, and cytarabine from primary NCS lymphoma in an elderly population: an intergroup ANOCEF-GOELAMS randomized phase 2 trial. *Lancet Haematol*. 2015;2:e251–e259.
44. Shapiro WR, Young DF, Tehta BM. Methotrexate: distribution in cerebrospinal fluid after intravenous, intraventricular and lumbar injections. *N Engl J Med*. 1975;293:161–166.
45. Soussain C, Suzan F, Hoang-Xuan K, et al. Intensive chemotherapy followed by hematopoietic stem-cell rescue in 22 patients with refractory or recurrent primary CNS lymphoma or intraocular lymphoma. *J Clin Oncol*. 2001;19:742–749.
46. Illerhaus G, Marks R, Ihorst G, et al. High-dose chemotherapy with autologous stem-cell transplantation and hyperfractionated radiotherapy as first-line treatment of primary CNS lymphoma. *J Clin Oncol*. 2006;24:3865–3870.
47. Bleyer WA. Neurologic sequelae of methotrexate and ionizing radiation: a new classification. *Cancer Treat Rep*. 1981;65(Suppl 1):89–98.
48. Geyer JR, Taylor EM, Milstein JM. Radiation, methotrexate, and white matter necrosis: laboratory evidence for neural radioprotection with pre-irradiation methotrexate. *Int J Radiat Oncol Biol Phys*. 1988;15:373–375.
49. Thiel E, Korfel A, Martus P, et al. High-dose methotrexate with or without whole brain radiotherapy for primary CNS lymphoma (G-PCNSL-SG-1): a phase 3, randomised, non-inferiority trial. *Lancet Oncol*. 2010;11:1036–1047.
50. Levine AM. Acquired immunodeficiency syndrome-related lymphoma. *Blood*. 1992;80:8–20.

51. Rouwen AJP, Wijermans PW, Boen-Tan TN, et al. Intraocular non-Hodgkin's lymphoma treated with systemic and intrathecal chemotherapy and radiotherapy: a case report and review of the literature. *Graefes Arch Clin Exp Ophthalmol.* 1989;227:355–359.
52. Baumann MA, Ritch PS, Hande KR, et al. Treatment of intraocular lymphoma with high-dose Ara-C. *Cancer.* 1986;57:1273–1275.
53. Soussain C, Merle-Beral H, Reux I, et al. A single-center study of 11 patients with intraocular lymphoma treated with conventional chemotherapy followed by high-dose chemotherapy and autologous bone marrow transplantation in 5 cases. *Leuk Lymphoma.* 1996;23:339–345.
54. Fishburne BC, Wilson DJ, Rosenbaum JT, et al. Intravitreal methotrexate as an adjunctive treatment of intraocular lymphoma. *Arch Ophthalmol.* 1997;115:1152–1156.
55. de Smet MD. Management of non-Hodgkin's intraocular lymphoma with intravitreal methotrexate. *Bull Soc Belge Ophthalmol.* 2001;279:91–95.
56. Velez G, Yuan P, Sung C, et al. Pharmacokinetics and toxicity of intravitreal chemotherapy for primary intraocular lymphoma. *Arch Ophthalmol.* 2001;119:1518–1524.
57. Sou R, Ohguro N, Maeda T, et al. Treatment of primary intraocular lymphoma with intravitreal methotrexate. *Jpn J Ophthalmol.* 2008;52:167–174.
58. Kitzmann AS, Pulido JS, Mohney BG, et al. Intraocular use of rituximab. *Eye.* 2007;21:1524–1527.
59. Ferreri AJ, Blay JY, Reni M, et al. International Extranodal Lymphoma Study Group (IELSG). Relevance of intraocular involvement in the management of primary central nervous system lymphomas. *Ann Oncol.* 2002;13:531–538.
60. Hormigo A, Abrey L, Heinemann MH, et al. Ocular presentation of primary central nervous system lymphoma: diagnosis and treatment. *Br J Haematol.* 2004;126:202–208.
61. Schuster SJ, Bishop MR, Tam CS, et al. Tisagenlecleucel in adult relapsed or refractory diffuse large B-cell lymphoma. *N Engl J Med.* 2019;380:45–56.
62. Fredrick DR, Char DH, Ljung BM, et al. Solitary intraocular lymphoma as an initial presentation of widespread disease. *Arch Ophthalmol.* 1989;107:395–397.
63. Guzak SV. Lymphoma as a cause of hyphema. *Arch Ophthalmol.* 1970;84:229–231.
64. Ryan ME, Shantha JG, Grossinklaus HE, et al. Secondary vitreoretinal lymphoma masquerading as acute retinal necrosis. *Ophthalmic Surg Lasers Imaging Retina.* 2015;46:1048–1050.
65. Ryan SJ, Frank RN, Green WR. Bilateral inflammatory pseudotumors of the ciliary body. *Am J Ophthalmol.* 1971;72:586–591.
66. Ryan SJ, Zimmerman LE, King FM. Reactive lymphoid hyperplasia: an unusual form of intraocular pseudotumor. *Trans Am Acad Ophthalmol Otolaryngol.* 1972;76:652–671.
67. Chute DJ, Biscotti CV, Singh AD. Uveal lymphoma. In: Biscotti CV, Singh AD, eds. *FNA Cytology of Ophthalmic Tumors. Monographs in Clinical Cytology.* Vol. 21. Basel: Karger; 2012:31–43.
68. Jakobiec FA, Sacks E, Kronish JW, et al. Multifocal static creamy choroidal infiltrates: an early sign of lymphoid neoplasia. *Ophthalmology.* 1987;94:397–406.
69. Desroches G, Abrams GW, Gass JDM. Reactive lymphoid hyperplasia of the uvea: a case with ultrasonographic and computed tomographic studies. *Arch Ophthalmol.* 1983;101:725–728.
70. Aronow ME, Portell CA, Sweetenham JW, Singh AD. Uveal lymphoma: clinical features, diagnostic studies, treatment selection, and outcomes. *Ophthalmology.* 2014;121:334–341.
71. Cheung MK, Martin DF, Chan CC, et al. Diagnosis of reactive lymphoid hyperplasia by chorioretinal biopsy. *Am J Ophthalmol.* 1994;118:457–462.
72. Cockerham GC, Hidayat AA, Bijwaard KE, et al. Re-evaluation of "reactive lymphoid hyperplasia of the uvea": an immunohistochemical and molecular analysis of 10 cases. *Ophthalmology.* 2000;107:151–158.
73. Read RW, Zamir E, Rao NA. Neoplastic masquerade syndromes. *Surv Ophthalmol.* 2002;47:81–124.
74. Litricin O. Diffuse malignant ring melanoma of the iris and ciliary body. *Ophthalmologica.* 1979;178:235–238.
75. Char DH, Schwartz A, Miller TR, et al. Ocular metastases from systemic malignant melanoma. *Am J Ophthalmol.* 1980;90:702–707.
76. Lipton JH, McGowan HD, Payne DG. Ocular masquerade syndrome in lymphoid blast crisis of chronic myeloid leukemia. *Leuk Lymphoma.* 1995;20:161–163.
77. Ayliffe W, Foster CS, Marcoux P, et al. Relapsing acute myeloid leukemia manifesting as hypopyon uveitis. *Am J Ophthalmol.* 1995;119:361–364.
78. Dhar-Munshi S, Alton P, Ayliffe WH. Masquerade syndrome: T-cell prolymphocytic leukemia presenting as panuveitis. *Am J Ophthalmol.* 2001;132:275–277.
79. Ferry AP, Font RL. Carcinoma metastatic to the eye and orbit. I. A clinicopathologic study of 227 cases. *Arch Ophthalmol.* 1974;92:276–286.
80. Shields JA, Shields CL, Ehya H, et al. Fine-needle aspiration biopsy of suspected intraocular tumors (the 1992 Urwick lecture). *Ophthalmology.* 1993;100:1677–1684.
81. Croxatto JO, Fernandez MR, Malbran ES. Retinoblastoma masquerading as ocular inflammation. *Ophthalmologica.* 1983;186:48–53.
82. Kincaid MC, Green WR. Ocular and orbital involvement in leukemia. *Surv Ophthalmol.* 1983;27:211–232.
83. Rosenthal AR. Ocular manifestations of leukemia: a review. *Ophthalmology.* 1983;90:899–905.
84. DeBarge LR, Chan CC, Greenberg S, et al. Chorioretinal, iris, and ciliary body infiltration by juvenile xanthogranuloma masquerading as uveitis. *Am J Ophthalmol.* 1994;39:65–71.
85. Sawyer RA, Selhorst JB, Zimmerman LE, et al. Blindness caused by photoreceptor degeneration as a remote effect of cancer. *Am J Ophthalmol.* 1976;81:606–613.
86. Buchanan TAS, Gardiner TA, Archer DB. An ultrastructural study of retinal photoreceptor degeneration associated with bronchial carcinoma. *Am J Ophthalmol.* 1984;97:277–287.
87. Thirkill CE, Roth AM, Keltner JL. Cancer-associated retinopathy. *Arch Ophthalmol.* 1987;105:372–375.
88. Whitcup SM, Vistica BA, Milam AH, et al. Recoverin-associated retinopathy: a clinically and immunologically distinctive disease. *Am J Ophthalmol.* 1998;126:230–237.
89. Heckenlively JR, Ferreyra HA. Autoimmune retinopathy: a review and summary. *Semin Immunopathol.* 2008;30:127–134.
90. Machemer R. Zur Pathogenese des flachenhaften malignen Melanoms. *Klin Monatsbl Augenheilkd.* 1966;148:641–652.
91. Barr CC, Zimmerman LE, Curtin VT, et al. Bilateral diffuse melanocytic uveal tumors associated with systemic malignant neoplasms: a recently recognized syndrome. *Arch Ophthalmol.* 1982;100:249–255.
92. Ryll DL, Campbell RJ, Robertson DM, et al. Pseudometastatic lesions of the choroid. *Ophthalmology.* 1980;87:1181–1186.
93. Gass JDM, Glatzer RJ. Acquired pigmentation simulating Peutz-Jeghers syndrome: initial manifestation of diffuse uveal melanocytic proliferation. *Br J Ophthalmol.* 1991;75:693–695.
94. Stone DU, Char DH, Crawford JB, et al. Metaplastic squamous epithelial downgrowth after clear corneal cataract surgery. *Am J Ophthalmol.* 2006;142:695–697.
95. Lim WK, Chee SP. Retinal detachment in atopic dermatitis can masquerade as acute panuveitis with rapidly progressive cataract. *Retina.* 2004;24:953–956.
96. Sivakumar RR, Rao NA. Anterior segment ischemia in viper bite. *Ocul Immunol Inflamm.* 2016;24:49–54.
97. Char DH. Intraocular masquerade syndromes. In: Tasman W, Jaeger EA, eds. *Duane's Clinical Ophthalmology.* Philadelphia: Lippincott; 1989.
98. Heckenlively JR. The frequency of posterior subcapsular cataract in the hereditary retinal degenerations. *Am J Ophthalmol.* 1982;93:733–738.
99. Fetkenhour CL, Choromokos E, Weinstein J, et al. Cystoid macular edema in retinitis pigmentosa. *Trans Am Acad Ophthalmol Otolaryngol.* 1977;83:515–521.
100. Fishman GA, Maggiero JM, Fishman M. Foveal lesions seen in retinitis. *Arch Ophthalmol.* 1977;95:1993–1996.
101. Stunkel M, Bhattarai S, Kemerley A, et al. Vitritis in pediatric genetic retinal disorders. *Ophthalmology.* 2015;122:192–199.
102. Den Hollander AI, Heckenlively JR, van den Born LI, et al. Leber congenital amaurosis and retinitis pigmentosa with Coats-like exudative vasculopathy are associated with mutations in the crumbs homologue 1 (CRB1) gene. *Am J Hum Genet.* 2001;69:198–203.
103. Wolfson Y, Applegate CD, Strauss RW, et al. CRB1-related maculopathy with cystoid macular edema. *JAMA Ophthalmol.* 2015;133:1357–1360.

104. Thirkill CE, Roth AM, Takemoto DJ, et al. Antibody indications of secondary and superimposed retinal hypersensitivity in retinitis pigmentosa. *Am J Ophthalmol*. 1991;112:132–137.
105. Williams LL, Lew HM, Shannon BT, et al. Activated retinitis pigmentosa peripheral lymphocytes adhere to and alter cultured human retinal pigment epithelial cells. *Invest Ophthalmol Vis Sci*. 1992;33:2848–2860.
106. London NJS, Garg SJ, Cunningham ET Jr. Drug-induced uveitis. *J Ophthalmic Inflamm Infect*. 2013;3:43.
107. Krupin T, LeBlanc RP, Becker B, et al. Uveitis in association with topically administered corticosteroid. *Am J Ophthalmol*. 1970;70:883–885.
108. Moorthy RS, Valluri S, Jampol LM. Drug-induced uveitis. *Surv Ophthalmol*. 1998;425:57–70.
109. Sarraf D, Vyas N, Jain A, et al. Triamcinolone-associated crystalline maculopathy. *Arch Ophthalmol*. 2010;128:685–690.
110. Hanna KS. A rare case of pembrolizumab-induced uveitis in a patient with metastatic melanoma. *Pharmacotherapy*. 2016;36:e183–e188.
111. Conrady CD, Larochelle M, Pecan P, et al. Checkpoint inhibitor-induced uveitis: a case series. *Graefes Arch Clin Exp Ophthalmol*. 2018;256(1):187–191.
112. Antoun J, Titah C, Cochereau I. Ocular and orbital side-effects of check point inhibitors: a review article. *Curr Opin Oncol*. 2016;4:288–294.
113. Postow MA, Sidlow R, Hellman MD. Immune-related adverse events associated with immune checkpoint blockade. *N Engl J Med*. 2018;378:158–168.
114. Chang CY, Sheu SJ. Macular edema might be a rare presentation of hydroxychloroquine-induced retinal toxicity. *Taiwan J Ophthalmol*. 2017;1:56–58.
115. Marmor MF, Kelner U, Lai TYY, et al. *American Academy of Ophthalmology Statement. Recommendations on screening for chloroquine and hydroxychloroquine retinopathy (2016 Revision)*. San Francisco: AAO; 2016.
116. Brobeck VH, Fleishli CA. Cataract, recurrent iritis, and deafness secondary to injury by lightning. *Am J Ophthalmol*. 1946;29:1309.
117. Boozalis GT, Purdue GF, Hunt JL, McCulley JP. Ocular changes from electrical burn injuries. A literature review and report of cases. *J Burn Care Rehabil*. 1991;12:458–462.
118. Gunes A, Yasar C, Tok L, Tok O. Two cases of anterior uveitis after laser eyebrow epilation. *Cornea*. 2015;34:101–102.
119. Guy J, Feuer WJ, Davis JL, et al. Gene therapy for Leber hereditary optic neuropathy: low- and medium-dose visual results. *Ophthalmology*. 2017;124:1621–1634.

APPENDIX

Sample Uveitis Questionnaire

FAMILY HISTORY

These questions refer to your parents, grandparents, children, grandchildren, brothers, sisters, aunts, and uncles.

Has anyone in your family had:

Cancer.......... Yes No
Diabetes.......... Yes No
Allergies.......... Yes No
Arthritis or rheumatism.......... Yes No
Syphilis.......... Yes No
Tuberculosis.......... Yes No
Sickle cell disease or trait.......... Yes No
Lyme disease.......... Yes No

Has anyone in your family had medical problems of the:

Eyes.......... Yes No
Skin.......... Yes No
Kidneys.......... Yes No
Lungs.......... Yes No
Stomach or bowel.......... Yes No
Nervous system or brain.......... Yes No

SOCIAL HISTORY

Age (years) ____________________
Current job ____________________
Have you lived outside of the United States?.......... Yes No
If Yes, where?
Have you traveled outside of the United States in the past year?.......... Yes No
If Yes, where?
Have you ever owned a dog?.......... Yes No
Have you ever owned a cat?.......... Yes No
Have you ever eaten raw meat or uncooked sausage?.......... Yes No
Have you ever been exposed to sick animals?.......... Yes No
Do you drink untreated stream, well, or lake water?.......... Yes No
Do you smoke cigarettes?.......... Yes No
How many alcoholic drinks do you have each day?____________
Have you ever used intravenous drugs?.......... Yes No
Have you ever taken birth control pills?.......... Yes No
Have you ever had a bisexual or homosexual relationship?.......... Yes No

PERSONAL MEDICAL HISTORY

Are you allergic to any medications?.......... Yes No
If Yes, which medications?
Please list the medicines you are currently taking, including nonprescription drugs, such as aspirin, ibuprofen, acetaminophen, antihistamines, and heartburn medications.

____
____
____
____

MEDICAL HISTORY

Please list all eye operations you have had (including laser surgery) and the dates of the surgeries.

____
____
____
____
____
____

Please list all other operations you have had and the dates of the surgeries.

____
____
____
____
____
____

Have you ever had any of the following illnesses?

Cancer.......... Yes No
Diabetes.......... Yes No
Hepatitis.......... Yes No
High blood pressure.......... Yes No

Have you ever had any of the following illnesses?

Anemia (low blood cell counts).......... Yes No Maybe
Pneumonia or pleurisy.......... Yes No Maybe
Tuberculosis.......... Yes No Maybe
Herpes (cold sores).......... Yes No Maybe
Chicken pox.......... Yes No Maybe
Shingles (zoster).......... Yes No Maybe
German measles (rubella).......... Yes No Maybe
Measles (rubeola).......... Yes No Maybe
Mumps.......... Yes No Maybe
Chlamydia or trachoma.......... Yes No Maybe
Syphilis.......... Yes No Maybe
Any other sexually transmitted disease.......... Yes No Maybe
Leprosy.......... Yes No Maybe
Leptospirosis.......... Yes No Maybe
Lyme disease.......... Yes No Maybe
Zika virus infection.......... Yes No Maybe
Histoplasmosis.......... Yes No Maybe
Candidiasis or moniliasis.......... Yes No Maybe
Coccidioidomycosis.......... Yes No Maybe
Sporotrichosis.......... Yes No Maybe
Cryptococcal infection.......... Yes No Maybe
Toxoplasmosis.......... Yes No Maybe
Ameba infection.......... Yes No Maybe
Giardiasis.......... Yes No Maybe
Toxocariasis.......... Yes No Maybe
Cysticercosis.......... Yes No Maybe
Trichinosis.......... Yes No Maybe

Whipple disease.......... Yes No Maybe
Human immunodeficiency virus/acquired immunodeficiency syndrome (HIV/AIDS).......... Yes No Maybe
Hay fever.......... Yes No Maybe
Allergies.......... Yes No Maybe
Vasculitis.......... Yes No Maybe
Arthritis.......... Yes No Maybe
Rheumatoid arthritis.......... Yes No Maybe
Lupus (systemic lupus erythematosus [SLE]).......... Yes No Maybe
Scleroderma.......... Yes No Maybe
Reiter syndrome.......... Yes No Maybe
Colitis.......... Yes No Maybe
Crohn disease.......... Yes No Maybe
Ulcerative colitis.......... Yes No Maybe
Behçet disease.......... Yes No Maybe
Sarcoidosis.......... Yes No Maybe
Ankylosing spondylitis.......... Yes No Maybe
Erythema nodosum.......... Yes No Maybe
Temporal arteritis.......... Yes No Maybe
Multiple sclerosis.......... Yes No Maybe
Serpiginous choroidopathy.......... Yes No Maybe
Fuchs heterochromic iridocyclitis.......... Yes No Maybe
Vogt-Koyanagi-Harada syndrome.......... Yes No Maybe

General Health

Chills.......... Yes No
Fevers (persistent or recurrent).......... Yes No
Night sweats.......... Yes No
Fatigue (tire easily).......... Yes No
Poor appetite.......... Yes No
Unexplained weight loss.......... Yes No
Do you feel sick?.......... Yes No

Neurologic

Frequent or severe headaches.......... Yes No
Fainting.......... Yes No
Numbness or tingling in your body.......... Yes No
Paralysis or weakness in parts of your body.......... Yes No
Seizures or convulsions.......... Yes No
Psychiatric conditions.......... Yes No

Ears

Hard of hearing or deafness.......... Yes No
Ringing or noises in your ears.......... Yes No
Frequent or severe ear infections.......... Yes No
Painful or swollen ear lobes.......... Yes No

Nose and Throat

Sores in your nose or mouth.......... Yes No
Severe or recurrent nosebleeds.......... Yes No
Frequent sneezing.......... Yes No
Sinus trouble.......... Yes No
Persistent hoarseness.......... Yes No
Tooth or gum infections.......... Yes No

Skin

Rashes.......... Yes No
Skin sores.......... Yes No
Sunburn easily (photosensitivity).......... Yes No
White patches of skin or hair (vitiligo or poliosis).......... Yes No
Loss of hair.......... Yes No
Tick or severe insect bites.......... Yes No
Painfully cold fingers.......... Yes No
Severe itching.......... Yes No

Respiratory

Severe or frequent colds.......... Yes No
Constant coughing.......... Yes No
Coughing up blood.......... Yes No
Recent flu or viral infection.......... Yes No
Wheezing or asthma attacks.......... Yes No
Difficulty breathing.......... Yes No

Cardiovascular

Chest pain.......... Yes No
Shortness of breath.......... Yes No
Swelling of legs.......... Yes No

Blood

Frequent or easy bruising.......... Yes No
Frequent or easy bleeding.......... Yes No
Have you received blood transfusions?.......... Yes No

Gastrointestinal

Trouble swallowing.......... Yes No
Diarrhea.......... Yes No
Bloody stools.......... Yes No
Stomach ulcers.......... Yes No
Jaundice or yellow skin.......... Yes No

Bones and Joints

Stiff joints.......... Yes No
Painful or swollen joints.......... Yes No
Stiff lower back.......... Yes No
Back pain while sleeping or on awakening.......... Yes No
Muscle aches.......... Yes No

Genitourinary

Kidney problems.......... Yes No
Bladder trouble.......... Yes No
Blood in urine.......... Yes No
Urinary discharge.......... Yes No
Genital sores or ulcers.......... Yes No
Prostatitis.......... Yes No
Testicular pain.......... Yes No
Are you pregnant?.......... Yes No
Do you plan to become pregnant in the near future?.......... Yes No

INDEX

Page numbers followed by "f" figures; "t" indicate tables; and "b" indicate boxes.